Pulmonary Involvement in Patients with Hematological Malignancies

Élie Azoulay
(Editor)

Pulmonary Involvement in Patients with Hematological Malignancies

Springer

Editor
Élie Azoulay, M.D., Ph.D
Service de Réanimation Médicale
Hôpital Saint-Louis
1 avenue Claude Vellefaux, 75010, Paris
France and
Medical Intensive Care Units, Saint-Louis
Hospital, Paris 7 University, Paris
France
elie.azoulay@sls.aphp.fr

ISBN 978-3-642-15741-7 e-ISBN 978-3-642-15742-4
DOI 10.1007/978-3-642-15742-4
Springer Heidelberg Dordrecht London New York

Library of Congress Control Number: 2011921694

Cover design: eStudioCalamar, Figueres/Berlin

Printed on acid-free paper

Springer is part of Springer Science+Business Media (www.springer.com)

This book is dedicated to all patients: you are the force that drives our work and our most important teachers. Thank you.

I would like to dedicate this book to all those who are important to me.

Foreword I

In the United States, cancer is the second most common cause of death. Over 560,000 people die of cancer each year. One in four deaths in the United States is due to cancer. Since the 1970s, the 5-year survival from cancer has increased from 50% to 66%. This improvement in survival reflects earlier diagnosis and more effective therapies and management strategies. As medical technology improves, even more progress is anticipated, but such progress requires experience and analysis, which only highly experienced clinicians and scientists can amass.

Patients with hematologic malignancies are a special challenge to health care providers. In the United States, over 130,000 persons are diagnosed with a hematologic malignancy each year, and over 50,000 individuals die. Half of these hematologic malignancies are acute or chronic leukemias, and the remainder is primarily lymphomas or multiple myeloma. These hematologic malignancies represent 9.5% of the cancer burden in the United States. These patients undergo a wide variety of immunosuppressive therapies that can have impressive results in terms of disease-free survival. However, the toxicities of these regimens can be substantial. Both disease and therapy can cause complications. These complications are very different for different cancers and for different therapies.

Our ability to improve the outcome of hematologic malignancies is due to more precise methods to identify the specific malignant process and to an expanding array of treatments for the underlying malignancies. These treatments are often used in combination regimens over periods of many months to years. These treatments include ionizing radiation, cytotoxic drugs, immunosuppressive agents, and stem cell transplantation. There are now over 50 drugs approved in the United States to treat hematologic malignancies. These drugs have an expanding number of mechanisms of action, ranging from traditional cytotoxic agents to newer drugs that are enzyme inhibitors, monoclonal antibodies, or proteasome inhibitors. Each of these approaches offers promise for specific indications, but also produces enormous complexity in terms of the effects on host immune and inflammatory response, and in terms of the specific organ toxicities they produce.

In this book, *Pulmonary Involvement in Patients with Hematological Malignancies*, Élie Azoulay has assembled experienced clinicians from around the world to focus on the infectious and non-infectious pulmonary complications that occur in these patients as they are managed with these diverse therapeutic modalities. Dr. Azoulay is renowned for his experience in dealing with such complications and for his careful investigations, which have improved patient care around the world. He has assembled well-published authorities to provide a comprehensive body of information on epidemiology, natural history, diagnosis, and therapy of pulmonary complications.

What makes this book especially useful is the focus on very specific clinical scenarios. Clinicians who care for patients with hematologic malignancies, which includes most oncologists, infectious disease specialists, and pulmonary-critical care physicians, will immediately be drawn to chapters on long-standing clinical controversies such as the role for various types of lung biopsies, new molecular techniques to enhance diagnostic accuracy, and chapters on specific pathogens such as *Candida*, *Aspergillus*, and CMV.

Also of special note are chapters that focus on non-infectious challenges such as diffuse alveolar hemorrhage and transfusion-related lung injury. Dr. Azoulay has also included chapters on management problems, such as invasive and non-invasive ventilation, transfusion policies, and palliative care, which clinicians will benefit from reviewing in order to be certain they are providing state-of-the-art care.

This book represents the work of experienced, thoughtful, evidence-based clinicians who provide the authoritative information that only a highly specialized, focused book such as this can supply. Health care providers who deal with this patient population will find the information and insights in this volume to be extremely valuable and will refer to this book often!

H. Masur

Foreword II

The number of immunocompromised patients has increased over the last decade. Improvements in solid-organ and hematopoietic stem cell transplantation techniques, the expanded use of chemotherapy and steroid use, and the appearance of immunomodulatory therapies are some of the reasons that explain this increase. The success of the different transplant techniques has generated a great deal of interest in the management of immunocompromised patients among clinicians and basic scientists.

The recognition and management of pulmonary complications that result from immunosuppression are challenging tasks. The lungs may be injured directly through infectious or toxic insults. Conversely, lung disease may result as a secondary event. Pulmonary complications in these patients require a multidisciplinary approach that often involves different specialties. This includes an appreciation of the epidemiology of post-transplant pulmonary complications, the different diagnoses for these processes, the appropriate diagnostic explorations, and the specific treatments and potential interactions. Some of these patients with pulmonary complications may need intensive care treatment.

The first part of this book is dedicated to non-infectious complications. Dr. Bekele Afessa describes the epidemiology, diagnosis, and treatment of diffuse alveolar hemorrhage, which is a frequent entity in hematological patients. Dr. Afessa provides a very comprehensive review of non-infectious pulmonary involvement after hematopoietic stem cell or bone marrow transplantation. The non-infectious complications comprise a series of entities that may respond to steroid treatment, although in some cases, they will lead to fatal outcomes (graft-versus-host disease).

Pulmonary veno-occlusive disease following hematopoietic stem cell transplantation is a rare complication that is difficult to manage. This subject is reviewed in depth by Drs. Bunte and Burns.

Not infrequently, drugs used to treat cancer patients have cardiovascular complications. One chapter describes how frequently these complications occur, which drugs may be responsible, and how we can decrease the severity of cardiovascular toxicity caused by these drugs.

Diagnosis of pulmonary infiltrates in hematologic malignancies is a difficult problem that often requires bronchoscopic evaluation. Post-mortem studies have helped us to provide the operative values of the techniques that we use in vivo. Dr. Pastores and colleagues have written a comprehensive chapter on this subject.

Hematologic malignancies often require transfusions that may be followed by acute lung injury, especially in children. Respiratory infections in patients with hematologic malignancies, neutropenia, and bone marrow transplants continue to be a serious problem triggered by abnormalities in the function and number of neutrophils, T and B lymphocytes, anatomic considerations, or a combination of factors. They range from bacterial pneumonias to opportunistic infections. Dr. Soubani et al. provide an update on the etiology, epidemiology, diagnosis, and management of these infections.

In summary, this book edited by Dr. Élie Azoulay gathers a series of excellent chapters written by experts in different problems that cause acute lung injury in hematological patients. The book will be very useful for specialists dealing with these types of problems, and this obviously includes intensive care physicians.

Prof. Antoni Torres

Acknowledgments

I am grateful to all the authors and co-authors who contributed to this book, spending their valuable time to write thoughtful presentations of difficult topics based on their own clinical experience acquired over the years and on a thorough knowledge of the most recent literature. Many thanks to all of you.

I have the deepest respect and consideration for the team working at the medical ICU at the Saint-Louis Hospital. Along with Benoit Schlemmer, I know how lucky we are to work with this group of people who care deeply about their patients and about communicating their skills to their young colleagues. They gladly accept the challenges raised by the sickest patients, while making every effort to avoid non-beneficial care. I learn everyday from them.

I am indebted to the hematologists who work closely with our medical ICU at the Saint Louis Hospital. We learn a lot from each other as we combine our energies to devise the best means of caring for our patients. Our close collaboration has nourished important research projects, shedding new light on topics such as the mechanisms underlying specific organ dysfunctions, emerging infections, and unexpected drug-related toxicities. This new understanding has helped us to improve patient outcomes.

I am grateful to Dr Francois Vincent for his critical revision of contributions to this book and his willingness to check every single reference. The huge amount of work he put into this book was invaluable.

I owe a debt of gratitude to Meike Stoeck from Springer for her assistance and willingness to adjust to my own pace, as well as to Ute Heilmann for her trust and kindness.

I have a personal thought for Dr Arnaud de Lassence who would certainly have written a contribution for this book. He was among those who knew the most about pulmonary involvement in patients with hematological malignancies. The memory of his bright mind and sparkling enthusiasm continues to nourish my work.

Contents

Part I

Preamble and Introduction

Managing Patients with Hematological Malignancies for 25 Years

1

Benoit Schlemmer

Contents

In 1986, just 25 years ago, three reports were published by Laufe [1], Maunder [2] and Ognibene [3], focusing on the occurrence of Adult Respiratory Distress Syndrome in neutropenic patients. Hematological patients had just begun to be included in the field of diffuse alveolar damage and pulmonary critical care medicine.

For many years, hematological patients were known to experience severe life-threatening conditions because of the course of their underlying disease or complications of therapy. Most of the latter were considered from infectious origin, resulting in sepsis, multiple organ failure and death. Doctors in the field of hematology or cancer were reluctant to admit such patients to the ICU, which was presumed to be futile because of poor results. Most intensivists agreed that this kind of patient was beyond any supportive care. Misknowledge about pathophysiology, concepts, diagnosis and therapy was equally distributed on both sides, in hematology and critical care. The flaws and fears were similar among these physicians.

Progress in the field of critical care and respiratory medicine along with therapeutic advances in the field of cancer has progressively changed medical attitudes regarding patients' medical presentations and the management of hematological patients with pulmonary disease. Medical teams in specialized centers have moved from "just say no" [4] to "consider saying yes" or "let's perform a trial" [5].

Twenty-five years have been necessary to distinguish among multiple complex medical entities, to increase our knowledge regarding both hematological diseases and complications of therapy. The role of the malignant process and its specific impact on organs and functions, or complex side effects of therapy, such as endothelial damage related to antineoplastic drugs or immune consequences of transplantation, have been

B. Schlemmer
Department of Intensive Care Medicine,
Saint-Louis Hospital, Paris, France and
University Paris-Diderot, Paris, France
e-mail: benoit.schlemmer@sls.aphp.fr

É. Azoulay (ed.), *Pulmonary Involvement in Patients with Hematological Malignancies*,
DOI: 10.1007/978-3-642-15742-4_1, © Springer-Verlag Berlin Heidelberg 2011

recognized. In addition, great progress has been made in the field of therapy, resulting in new opportunities and hopes for many patients previously considered to have rapidly fatal diseases.

In addition, better knowledge about critical care conditions and the impact of their management by intensivists has also resulted in new concepts and strategies. Where critical care physicians cooperate with their colleagues in hematological wards, they have developed new strategies regarding diagnosis and therapy. The respective benefits of invasive versus noninvasive diagnostic procedures have been discussed, along with the opportunity to use new diagnostic tools in the field of infection or lung injury, from inflammation to healing and fibrosis. Improvement in respiratory therapy, with the development of noninvasive ventilatory support and low tidal volume mechanical ventilation, has resulted in the opportunity to develop the concept of early management for many hematological patients with pulmonary disease before the occurrence of critical conditions, out of the scope of any hope.

Medical benefit for patients has been the result of improvement in basic science, pathophysiology and nosology in pulmonary medicine and hematology. Accordingly, better knowledge, better diagnosis and therapeutic advances should result in better strategies and improved patient outcomes. Widening the field of diagnostic and therapeutic tools in pulmonary medicine for hematological patients has highlighted the need for accurate medical decision-making, both from technical and ethical points of view. When faced with a patient with a history of hematological disease and pulmonary signs, one should now distinguish between several etiologies, choose a diagnostic strategy or empiric therapy, and discuss whether an invasive diagnostic procedure or ventilatory support would be valuable, taking into account probabilities, hope of reversibility, patient willingness and risk-benefit analysis. Intensive care therapy of hematological patients now has to be considered as a way to support critical conditions in order to allow diagnostic procedures and/or therapy to reverse such medical situations. Emergency decisions sometimes have to be made, including in non-specialized medical facilities, because of the great developments in ambulatory medicine for some hematological disorders. However, sometimes, withholding or withdrawal of some therapeutic options has to be discussed, as for many other patients in ICUs. The medical decision has to be based both on evidence, whenever possible, and experience.

Better knowledge in the field of pulmonary involvement in hematological malignant diseases has pushed intensivists and physicians in hematology to share their experience and to provide new opportunities for their patients. This has also resulted in the need for additional research in this field, not only related to acute conditions and their management, but also to long-term outcomes and quality of life.

This book will offer any intensivist, even non-specialized, and any physician in the field of hematology and cancer the opportunity to review 25 years of medical progress. Increasing medical knowledge would not only result in answers for hematological patients with pulmonary disease, but would also result in more comprehensive understanding, in new questions for the future and in the opening of new fields for medical research in which both intensivists and cancer physicians should cooperate.

In this respect, this book is exemplary. I want to thank all the contributors who have accepted the task of summarizing their outstanding experience for young physicians who need to be educated in the field of such difficult medical conditions. I want to congratulate my young colleague and friend, Elie Azoulay, who is a masterpiece in clinical training and supervision at Saint-Louis Hospital, but also a leader in clinical research, for initiating this huge work and succeeding in the challenge of gathering the most influent specialists in this field of medical care.

References

1. Laufe MD, Simon RH, Flint A, Keller JB (1986) Adult respiratory distress syndrome in neutropenic patients. Am J Med 80:1022–1026
2. Maunder RJ, Hackman RC, Riff E et al (1986) Occurrence of the adult respiratory distress syndrome in neutropenic patients. Am Rev Respir Dis 133:313–316
3. Ognibene FP, Martin SE, Parker MM et al (1986) Adult respiratory distress syndrome in patients with severe neutropenia. N Engl J Med 315:547–551
4. Carlon GC (1989) Just say no. Crit Care Med 17(1):106–107
5. Lecuyer L, Chevret S, Thiery G, Darmon M, Schlemmer B, Azoulay E (2007) The ICU trial: a new admission policy for cancer patients requiring mechanical ventilation. Crit Care Med 35(3):808–814

2 Pulmonary Involvement in Patients with Hematological Malignancies

Élie Azoulay

Acute pulmonary events are among the most common complications in patients with hematological malignancies. These events often raise difficult diagnostic and therapeutic challenges. In this book, readers faced with these challenges will find a vast array of clinically relevant information contributed by physicians in many specialties who have acquired considerable experience over the years. Pulmonary complications in patients with hematological malignancies may be related to many factors, including infection, tissue invasion by the malignant cells, toxicity and immune deficiency related to the disease or treatments. The multiplicity of the possible etiologies and frequent presence of more than one etiology in a given patient create diagnostic conundrums. Importantly, an early accurate diagnosis is crucial to improve patient outcomes. This book provides practical guidance on untangling complex diagnoses and selecting optimal treatments.

In addition to hematologists, intensivists, and pulmonologists, clinicians from many specialties may be called on to manage respiratory events in patients with hematological malignancies. This book was written to serve as an easily accessible source of information to primary-care physicians, emergency-room physicians, intensivists and physicians working in internal medicine, infectious diseases or pulmonary care departments. Furthermore, the problems encountered in patients with hematological malignancies are relevant to all specialties where patients require immunosuppressant treatments for systemic inflammatory diseases, including clinical immunology, rheumatology, hepatology, gastroenterology, nephrology, dermatology, neurology, and solid organ transplantation.

This book has six parts. After an introduction by Dr Soubani, who presents a comprehensive overview of infectious etiologies of respiratory events in patients with hematological malignancies, the first part focuses on epidemiology. International leaders draw attention to important points such as the specificities of bone marrow transplant recipients and the possibility of non-infectious pulmonary involvement, most notably heart failure with pulmonary edema whose diagnostic and therapeutic management differ fundamentally from those of other etiologies of respiratory events in hematological patients. The second part addresses ongoing controversies about the best diagnostic strategies, which are largely fueled by the fast pace at which new diagnostic tools are being introduced. Renowned researchers discuss the latest information on the benefit/risk ratio of diagnostic tools ranging from the least invasive (clinical examination) to the most invasive (surgical lung biopsy). This careful attention to diagnostic tools is warranted, as mortality is higher when no cause to the respiratory symptoms is identified. In patients who are not receiving mechanical ventilation, noninvasive diagnostic testing may provide comparable diagnostic yields to those obtained using bronchoscopy with bronchoalveolar lavage. Attention is drawn to the valuable information that can be derived by the optimal use and interpretation of lung computed tomography. In the third and the fourth parts of this book, leading researchers describe the spectrum of pulmonary infections in hematological patients because of pathogens ranging from common bacteria to opportunistic pathogens, and the spectrum of

É. Azoulay
Service de Réanimation Médicale, Hôpital Saint-Louis, 1 avenue Claude Vellefaux, 75010, Paris, France and Medical Intensive Care Units, Saint-Louis Hospital, Paris 7 University, Paris, France
e-mail: elie.azoulay@sls.aphp.fr

É. Azoulay (ed.), *Pulmonary Involvement in Patients with Hematological Malignancies*,
DOI: 10.1007/978-3-642-15742-4_2,

noninfectious causes, including drug-related toxicity, pulmonary embolism, diffuse alveolar hemorrhage, and alveolar proteinosis. The fifth part provides new insights into treatments and difficult decisions for patients with hematological malignancies. Contributions from physicians in various specialties were assembled to shed light on the many facets of this topic. Opinion leaders provide recommendations on the use (or withdrawal) of various therapeutic strategies. Last, the sixth part presents 15 carefully selected case reports about clinical situations that are rare but important. The goal is to improve the diagnosis of rare but treatable conditions. For each clinical situation, a literature review is reported. These case reports may constitute valuable teaching material for discussing patients with unusual problems. The abundance of tables, figures, radiographs, and computed tomography scans in the book considerably enriches the written material.

Three methods can be suggested for using this book. First, you can look up a clinical situation you are interested in (e.g., pneumonia in patients with chronic lymphocytic leukemia or pulmonary infiltrates at the earliest phase of acute leukemia). Second, you can look for the diagnostic strategy that is best for evaluating a clinical suspicion of infectious or noninfectious pulmonary involvement (e.g., induced sputum, transbronchial biopsy, or core needle biopsy). Third, you can find a description of the clinical picture related to a given form of pulmonary involvement or a given pathogen (e.g., *Pneumocystis* pneumonia, cytomegalovirus pneumonia, cardiogenic pulmonary edema, diffuse alveolar hemorrhage, or transfusion-related acute lung injury). These three methods can complement one another. Therapeutic alternatives are also available for all these situations.

I hope this book will spread ten important messages. First, in patients with hematological malignancies who experience respiratory complications, treating every possible etiology is not the best way to ensure a favorable outcome. Instead, identifying the exact cause improves survival. Second, within the first few hours the most likely causes of the respiratory symptoms should be determined based on the clinical findings (see the DIRECT strategy) and recorded in the medical chart. Treatments appropriate for these causes should be given immediately, while waiting for the results of further investigations. Third, computed tomography may help to support a clinical suspicion of an infectious or noninfectious cause and may also rule out a number of etiologies. However, computed tomography alone cannot establish a diagnosis. Furthermore, computed tomography should be performed only after a comprehensive clinical assessment, whose findings guide the choice of the imaging strategy.

Fourth, not all patients are at risk for all the possible etiologies. Knowledge of the specific risk factors for each cause is crucial. For instance, the type of immune deficiency indicates which pathogens are most likely to cause pulmonary involvement. A discerning risk factor assessment may show that some patients are at very low risk for some causes. Fifth, two diagnoses, cardiogenic pulmonary edema and bacterial infections, should be considered in all patients at all times during the course of the hematological malignancy. Sixth, positive tests (e.g., cytomegalovirus antigen test, PCR test for *Pneumocystis*, or virological studies of nasopharyngeal swabs) must be interpreted with great caution. A positive test does not always mean that the disease is present. Furthermore, several causes may be present in combination. For instance, even when the bronchoalveolar lavage fluid indicates alveolar hemorrhage, infections (e.g., aspergillosis, *Pseudomonas*, *Staphylococcus*, and other causes of necrotizing pneumonia), and noninfectious disorders (e.g., cardiogenic pulmonary edema, leukemic infiltrates, and drug-related toxicity) must be ruled out before accepting a diagnosis of diffuse alveolar hemorrhage and initiating the specific treatment for this condition. Another important point is that negative results do not always exclude diagnoses, such as cytomegalovirus pneumonia, *Pneumocystis* pneumonia, or invasive aspergillosis. The few diagnostic tests whose negative predictive value is close to 100% (e.g., PCR test for *Pneumocystis*) are extremely valuable. Seventh, thrombocytopenia does not protect against the occurrence of thromboembolic events. Eighth, core needle biopsy performed by an experienced operator can provide valuable diagnostic information. As with all invasive procedures, the ICU may be the safest place to monitor the patients before and after core needle biopsy. Ninth, each new diagnostic method must be carefully evaluated in a group of unselected patients with hematological malignancies. The diagnostic performance characteristics must be reported, together with the prevalence of the disease in the study group. Tenth, managing patients with pulmonary events and hematological malignancies requires considerable clinical skill, close collaboration among medical specialties and with the laboratories, and easy access to the ICU. Among patients with hematological malignancies, more than half experience critical illnesses, and early ICU admission may be the best means of providing them with optimal diagnostic and therapeutic care.

I owe an enormous debt of gratitude to the specialists who provided their valuable contributions to this book.

Élie Azoulay

Respiratory Infections in Patients with Hematological Malignancies

3

Ayman O. Soubani

Contents

A.O. Soubani
Associate Professor of Medicine, Division of Pulmonary, Allergy, Critical Care and Sleep Medicine Wayne State University School of Medicine, Harper University Hospital, 3990 John R-3 Hudson, Deotrit, MI 48201
e-mail: asoubani@med.wayne.edu

3.1 Introduction

Hematological malignancies are a variety of cancers that involve the hematopoietic cell lines. They include acute and chronic leukemias, Hodgkin's disease, non-Hodgkin's lymphomas, multiple myeloma and myelodysplastic syndrome. The age-adjusted incidences of leukemias and lymphomas in the United States are 12.2 and 22.3 per 100,000 population per year, respectively. While the age adjusted death rate for leukemias is 7.3 and for lymphomas is 7.5 per 100,000 population per year [1]. Bone marrow and hematopoietic stem cell transplantations (HSCT) are an important treatment for a variety of hematological malignancies as well as other diseases such as hematological disorders, solid tumors and autoimmune diseases. Annually, there are more than 30,000 cases of autologous HSCT and 15,000 cases of allogeneic HSCT performed worldwide [2]. Hematopoietic stem cells may be obtained from bone marrow, peripheral blood or umbilical cord blood. Depending on the source of these stem cells, HSCT is classified as autologous if the cells are taken from an individual patient and stored for reinfusion after high-dose chemotherapy, and it is classified as allogeneic if the stem cells are donated from another individual (who may or may not be related). In the case of allogeneic HSCT, the conditioning regimen before transplantation may be myeloablative, in which supralethal doses of chemotherapy and irradiation are given, leading to significant toxicity and immunosuppression. More recently, nonmyeloablative regimens have been used to minimize the toxicity related to the conditioning regimen and allow for more robust immunologically mediated killing of tumor cells (graft vs. tumor effect).

É. Azoulay (ed.), *Pulmonary Involvement in Patients with Hematological Malignancies*,
DOI: 10.1007/978-3-642-15742-4_3, © Springer-Verlag Berlin Heidelberg 2011

Pulmonary complications, both infectious and non-infectious, are important causes of morbidity and mortality in patients with hematological malignancies (Table 3.1). The incidence of these complications reaches 60% of patients [3, 4]. Mortality of pulmonary complications is 40% and approaches 90% in patients who require mechanical ventilation [5]. The pulmonary complications are generally related to the underlying malignancy or toxicity of the chemotherapeutic regimen. In the case of HSCT, there are additional complications related to graft-vs.-host disease (GVHD), which is a condition in which the donated cells recognize the recipient's cells as nonself and attack them. Efforts to prevent or treat GVHD include harvesting hematopoietic stem cells from an HLA-matched donor and use of immunosuppressive and immunomodulatroy therapy such as corticosteroids, cyclosporine or tacrolimus (FK506) or TNF-α blocking agents [6]. The use of these agents entails further hazards for infectious complications and the development of a new neoplastic disease.

Table 3.1 Spectrum of respiratory infectious and noninfectious complications in patients with hematological malignancies

Infectious
Bacteria
Mycobacteria
Nocardia
Aspergillus
Non-Aspergillus fungi
P. jiroveci
CMV
Community respiratory viruses
Non-infectious
Pulmonary edema (cardiogenic and noncardiogenic)
Transfusion-related lung injury
Engraftment syndrome
Diffuse alveolar hemorrhage
Idiopathic pneumonia syndrome
Organizing pneumonia
Drug induced pulmonary toxicity
Radiation pneumonitis
Pulmonary thromboembolic disease
Secondary alveolar proteinosis
Bronchiolitis obliterans
Progression of underlying malignancy

The etiology of pulmonary disease following hematological malignancies may be predicted based on variables such as the type of immunodeficiency, the presence of neutropenia, the prophylactic agents the patient is on and the temporal relation to the administration of chemotherapy. The pattern of pulmonary complications is best demonstrated following allogeneic HSCT (Fig. 3.1).

This chapter details the spectrum of respiratory infections in patients with hematological malignancy, focusing on HSCT as the prime example of immunosuppression that develops in these patients. The main respiratory infections in patients with hematological malignancies are described along the lines of incidence, risk factors, clinical presentation, and recent advances in the diagnosis and management. The designation of "patients with hematological malignancies" throughout the chapter is used to describe patients who have a malignancy such as leukemia, lymphoma, multiple myeloma or myelodysplastic syndrome; are on chemotherapy; are neutropenic; or underwent HSCT. Data that are unique to one subgroup are specifically mentioned.

3.2 The Immune System Changes in Patients with Hematological Malignancies

The risk of infection in patients with hematological malignancies primarily stems from defects in the number or function of neutrophils, T-cells and B-cells. Abnormalities in each of these cell lines increase the risk of specific infections (Table 3.2). However, the functions of these defense mechanisms are interdependent, so an abnormality in one cell line may compromise the function of other defense mechanisms. Neutropenia is the most frequent immunodeficiency in patients with hematological malignancies. It is seen in patients with acute leukemia and secondary to myelosuppression following chemotherapy. In addition to decreasing the production of neutrophils, cancer chemotherapy and radiation interfere with the chemotactic and phagocytic activity and the intracellular killing

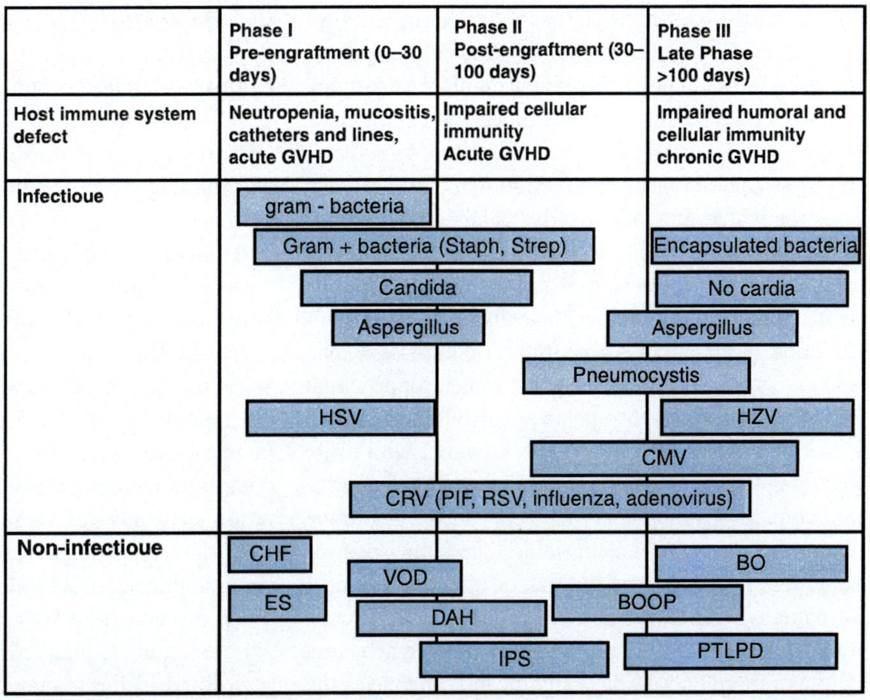

Fig. 3.1 The time line of pulmonary complications following HSCT. *HSV* herpes simplex virus, *HZV* herpes zoster virus, *CMV* cytomegalovirus, *RSV* respiratory syncytial virus, *CHF* congestive heart failure, *BO* bronchiolitis obliterans, *VOD* veno-occlusive disease, *ES* engraftment syndrome, *DAH* diffuse alveolar hemorrhage, *BOOP* bronchiolitis obliterans organizing pneumonia, *IPS* idiopathic pneumonia syndrome, *PTLPD* post transplant lymphoproliferative disorder

Table 3.2 Spectrum of immunosuppression in patients with hematological malignancies

Mechanism of immunosuppression	Causes of immunosuppression	Spectrum of respiratory infections
Neutropenia	Leukemia	Gram-negative bacilli
	Myelodysplastic syndrome	Gram-positive cocci
	Chemotherapy	Fungi (candida, Aspergillus)
	HSCT	
Neutrophil dysfunction	Lymphoma	Fungi (*P. jiroveci*, Aspergillus)
	Corticosteroids	
	Myelodysplastic Syndrome	
T-cell defects	Lymphoma	Bacteria (including nocardia, mycobacteria)
	Lymphoblastic leukemia	
	Chemotherapy	Viruses (CMV)
	Monoclonal antibodies	Fungi (Aspergillus, *P. jiroveci*)
	Corticosteroids	
	HSCT	Parasites
B-cell defects	Lymphoma	Encapsulated bacteria (*S. pneumoniae*, *H. influenza*)
	Leukemia	
	Multiple myeloma	
	Splenectomy	
	Monoclonal antibodies	
Anatomic	Tumor obstruction	Gram-positive cocci
	Mucositis	Gram-negative bacilli
	Indwelling catheters	Anaerobic bacteria
		Candida

of microorganisms by these cells. Furthermore, corticosteroids, used as part of chemotherapeutic regimens, decrease the accumulation of neutrophils at inflammation sites by reducing their adherence and chemotactic properties. The usual infections associated with abnormalities in the number or function of neutrophils are bacteria, including gram-negative bacilli, and opportunistic fungal infections, such as Aspergillus. The risk of infection increases significantly when the absolute neutrophil count falls below 500 cells/mm^3. The risk of infection is greatest with neutrophil counts less than 100 cells mm^3. The rate of decline in neutrophil count and the duration of neutropenia are also important factors in the risk of infection. Thus, a patient with acute leukemia is at higher risk of infection when the neutrophil count drops rapidly compared to one in whom the counts fall slowly or remain stable. The longer neutropenia lasts, the higher is the risk of infection. Almost all patients with neutrophil counts less than 100 cells mm^3 for more than 3 weeks develop fever. Neutropenia that lasts more than 10 days significantly increases the risk of invasive fungal infections. In one study, the risk of Aspergillus infection was increased by 1% each day of neutropenia for the first 3 weeks, then by 4% each day thereafter [7].

B cells differentiate and proliferate to antibody-producing plasma cells upon exposure to bacterial antigens. These cells are responsible for the humoral branch of the immune system. They produce different immunoglobulins, such as IgM and IgA, that protect the body against bacteria and viruses. The production of these immunoglobulins is decreased in lymphoproliferative disorders such as chronic lymphocytic leukemia and multiple myeloma, intensive chemotherapy and treatment with monoclonal antibodies such as rituximab. Abnormalities in the B cell number and function predispose to infection with encapsulated bacteria such as *Streptococcus pneumoniae*, *Haemophilus influenza* and *Staphylococcus aureus*.

T cells are responsible for cellular immunity and play a pivotal role in regulating monocyte-macrophage antigen handling and intracelullar microbial elimination by the release of various cytokines and chemokines. The function of T cells is compromised in patients with malignant lymphomas, especially Hodgkin's disease, lymphocytic leukemia and T-cell leukemia. Chemotherapeutic agents, such as cyclophosphamide, azathioprime, purine analogues including fludarabine and cladribine, and immunosuppressive agents including corticosteroids, cyclosporine, tacrolimus and sirolimus, suppress the T cell function. Also novel agents used in the management of lypmhoproliferative malignancies, such as monoclonal antibodies anti-CD52 (e.g., alemtuzumab), significantly affect the function of these cells. Abnormalities in T-cell function predispose patients to infections by fungi, including Aspergillus and *Pneumocystis jiroveci*, viruses, nocardia and mycobacteria.

Other factors that compromise the immune system in patients with hematological malignancies and increase the risk of infection include mucositis secondary to chemotherapy that may predispose to aspiration or translocation of microorganisms from the gastrointestinal tract. Vascular catheters inserted for chemotherapy, parenteral nutrition and transfusion of blood products may be a source of bacterial and fungal infections. Splenectomy, which is occasionally performed in the management of patients with malignant lymphoma, compromises the production of opsonizing antibodies and impairs the defense against encapsulated bacteria.

HSCT is the prototype of immunological abnormalities related to hematological malignancies. HSCT recipients develop profound changes in the immune system that affect all lines of defense against infection (Table 3.3). These patients develop neutropenia immediately following transplantation and may have both T- and B-cell problems related to chemotherapy, GVHD and immunosuppressive therapy. The patients typically follow a predictable pattern of immune system deficiency and recovery. During the first month after HSCT, the major host-defense deficits include neutropenia, damaged mucocutaneous barriers and indwelling intravenous catheters. The organisms that commonly cause infection during this period include gram-negative bacilli (e.g., Klebsiella, Escherichia and Pseudomonas), gram-positive cocci (e.g., coagulase-negative and coagulase-positive Staphylococci, Enterococcus), Candida species and herpes simplex virus. Aspergillus spp. may lead to infection if neutropenia persists. During preengraftment, the risks for infection are the same for autologous or allogeneic patients, and infection may present as febrile neutropenia. Although fever during this period is probably caused by a bacterial pathogen, an organism or site of infection is infrequently identified. Instead, such infections are usually treated

Table 3.3 Factors that increase the risk of respiratory infections following HSCT

Pre-transplantation	
	Older age
	Pre-transplant immune status
	Underlying pulmonary disease
	CMV status of the donor and recipient
	Residence in endemic areas
Transplantation	
	Allogeneic
	Type and intensity of conditioning regimen
	Total body irradiation
	Delayed engraftment
Post-transplantation	
	Mucositis
	Severity and duration of neutropenia
	GVHD
	T-cell depleting strategies
	Nosocomial factors (antibiotic-resistant organisms, indwelling catheters, construction, type of air filtration, transmission of infection by health-care providers)

preemptively or empirically until the neutropenia resolves. Growth factors can be administered to decrease neutropenia duration and complications. The risk of infection persists until the stem cells are engrafted, which is defined as sustained absolute neutrophil count of 500 cells/mm^3 and sustained platelet count of >20,000, lasting >3 consecutive days without transfusions. Among unrelated allogeneic recipients, engraftment occurs at a median of 22 days after HSCT (range 6–84 days) [8].

Following engraftment (30–100 days) and in the absence of corticosteroid therapy, neutrophil function is restored, which results in a decreased risk for bacterial and fungal infections. However, all HSCT recipients, and particularly allogeneic recipients, experience an immune system dysfunction for months after engraftment. They may have abnormal CD4/CD8 T-cell ratios, reflecting their decreased CD4 and increased CD8 T-cell counts [6]. They might also have IgG and IgA deficiencies for months after HSCT and have difficulty switching from IgM to IgG production after antigen exposure. Immune system recovery might be delayed further by CMV infection [9]. During this phase, allogeneic HSCT recipients usually develop acute GVHD that manifests as skin, gastrointestinal and liver injury. GVHD is associated with increased risk of infection due to delayed immunologic recovery. Furthermore, the immunosuppressive therapy used for GVHD prophylaxis and therapy puts HSCT recipients at an increased risk for opportunistic viral and fungal infections. The usual infectious agents during this phase include CMV, Aspergillus and *P. jiroveci*.

After 100 days following HSCT, some patients with allogeneic transplantation continue to have manifestations of chronic GVHD. This phase may be associated with cellular and humoral immunodeficiencies, including macrophage deficiency, impaired neutrophil chemotaxis and poor response to vaccination. Also patients may experience long-lasting IgA and IgG deficiencies, poor opsonization and impaired reticuloendothelial function [10, 11]. After chronic GVHD resolves, which might take years, cell-mediated and humoral immunity function are gradually restored. Patients in this phase are at an increased risk for infections caused by encapsulated organisms, such as *S. pneumoniae*, *H. influenzae* or *Neisseria meningitidis*. They may also develop infections as a result of cytomegalovirus (CMV), herpes zoster virus, community respiratory viral infections and Aspergillus.

3.3 Bacterial Pneumonia

Bacterial pneumonia caused by gram-positive or gram-negative organisms is a significant problem in patients with hematological malignancies. These bacteria may lead to community- or hospital-acquired pneumonia. They account for 15% of all respiratory infections [12]. Based on surgical lung biopsy, bacterial pneumonia is estimated to be 2%, but increases to more than 25% when documented by autopsy [13]. The mortality associated with bacterial pneumonia in these patients reaches 22% [14]. One of the main challenges in the diagnosis of bacterial pneumonia in patients with hematological malignancies is the inability to identify the organism in the majority of patients, which may underestimate the incidence of these infections. This is related to the contamination of respiratory samples by upper airway organisms, the fact that most of these patients are on prophylactic antibiotics and the limitations in performing invasive procedures such as bronchoscopy to confirm the cause of infection. There is ongoing controversy on the value of these invasive procedures in the diagnosis of bacterial pneumonia in these patients [8].

Factors that generally increase the risk of bacterial pneumonia in patients with hematological malignancies include their immune status, chemotherapeutic regimen, and degree and duration of neutropenia [4, 15]. The presence of GVHD in patients with allogeneic HSCT significantly increases the risk of bacterial pneumonia because of slower reconstitution of the immune system, impairment of the reticuloendothelial system and opsonization. Furthermore, the immunosuppressive therapy to treat GVHD increases the risk of bacterial pneumonia in these patients [15]. Other factors that predispose to bacterial pneumonia include mucositis that increases the risk of aspiration, especially with the use of narcotic analgesics. Indwelling catheters that increase the risk of bacteremia and septic embolization to the lungs (Fig. 3.2) [16]. The presentation of bacterial pneumonia in patients with hematological malignancies may be subtle, and not infrequently patients present with neutropenic fever with no localizing symptoms and signs due to blunted inflammatory response [17]. Radiological signs may also be scarce. The chest radiograph usually shows focal consolidation, however may be normal. The infiltrates may progress quickly to multifocal or diffuse changes that are compatible with acute respiratory distress syndrome. High-resolution computerized tomography of the chest is recommended in febrile neutropenic patients, which may show pulmonary infiltrates in up to 50% of patients with negative chest radiographs [18, 19]. A chapter from Heussel in this book details the different CT patterns in hematological patients with pulmonary infiltrates. The main organisms identified as causes of bacterial pneumonia in neutropenic patients and during the pre-engraftment phase of HSCT are usually gram-negative bacteria such as pseudomonas, klebseilla and enterobacter. In a recent report of the utility of bronchoscopy following HSCT, the most commonly isolated bacteria following HSCT was pseudomonas that was resistant to the current antibiotics [8]. There is also increasing incidence of gram-positive bacteria, such as *S. aureus*, *Enterococcus faecium* and α-hemolytic streptococcus, which may be associated with septic shock and acute respiratory distress syndrome. Anaerobic organisms may be causative agents in the case of aspiration [16, 20, 21].

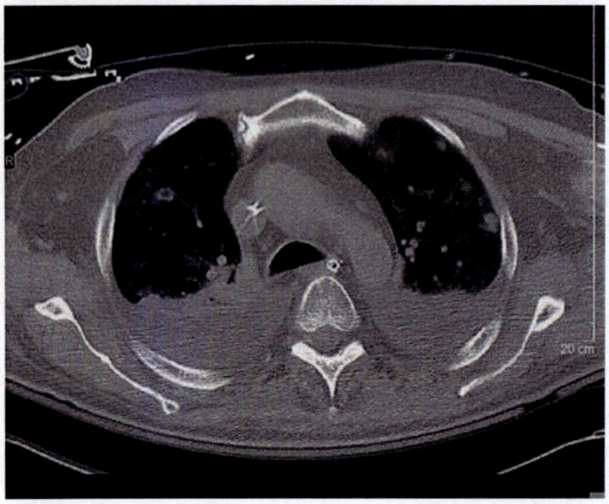

Fig. 3.2 CT scan of the chest showing multiple peripheral nodules, some with cavitation, consistent with septic pulmonary emboli in a HSCT recipient with methacillin resistant S aureus bactermia secondary to indwelling central venous catheter

Following HSCT, patients continue to be at risk for bacterial pneumonia post engraftment of the stem cells, albeit less frequently. The risk factors for bacterial pneumonias during this period are the presence of acute or chronic GVHD and the immunosuppressive therapy used to treat these patients. These patients are at risk of infection with encapsulated organisms such as *S. pneumoniae* and *H. influenza*. However, gram-negative organisms may be the etiology in up to 25% of patients [12, 14, 15, 22]. In a report of 1,359 HSCT recipients, 25% of the patients developed at least one episode of pneumonia. Bacterial pneumonia was documented in 9% of all patients and was the most common etiology in those in whom an organism was identified. The most frequent isolate was *S. pneumoniae*, and gram-negative organisms were isolated in 23% of those patients. The 1-year survival of patients after bacterial pneumonia was 71% [22]. In another report, *S. pneumoniae* pneumonia was documented in 0.7% of HSCT recipients. The majority of these patients underwent allogeneic HSCT and had chronic GVHD. Infection was more common in patients with a history of lymphoma and those on high-dose corticosteroid therapy. Pneumococcal vaccine breakthrough developed in 11% of the cases. The infection occurred a mean of 433 ± 669 days post transplantation, and 76% of the patients had bacteremia. Mortality due to pneumococcal infection was 13%. Admission to the critical care unit and higher APACHE II score were associated with worse outcome [23].

A retrospective report on invasive pseudomonas infection following HSCT revealed the incidence to be 1.65% a median of 63 days post HSCT. Attributable mortality was 36%. The risk factors for poor outcome were the presence of copathogens and high-dose corticosteroid therapy. Sixteen percent had recurrence of pseudomonas infection [24]. The clinical and radiological picture is usually classical for bacterial pneumonia. Antibiotic therapy during this period should be based on the organisms suspected or identified.

Patients with hematological malignancies are infrequently reported to develop Legionella pneumonia. A recent study of 49 patients found that lymphopenia, the use of systemic corticosteroids and chemotherapy were the most common underlying conditions. Positive DFA was the diagnostic method in 84% of patients. The case fatality rate was 31% [25]. A prolonged course of therapy with macrolide or fluroquinolone may be necessary in the majority of patients. Legionella pneumonia has also been reported following HSCT. Allogeneic HSCT recipients with GVHD seem to be at highest risk for this infection [17, 26].

Empiric broad-spectrum antibiotics should be started immediately when bacterial pneumonia is suspected in patients with hematological malignancies. The American Thoracic Society guidelines for the treatment of health-care associated pneumonia in patients with risk factors such as HSCT or neutropenia recommend a regimen that includes antipseudomonal cephalosporin or carbepenem, or B lactam, plus antipseudomonal fluroquinolone or aminoglycoside, plus linezolid or vancomycin if methicillin-resistant *S. aureus* is suspected. In patients who develop bacterial pneumonia late following HSCT, coverage of encapsulated organisms with a fluoroquinolone is recommended. The antibiotic regimen should be narrowed if the etiologic agent is identified [27, 28]. The institutional resistance pattern needs to be considered when determining the choice of antibiotics [19]. Further recommendations on the use of anti-bacterial agents in patients with hematological malignancies are provided in the chapter from Legrand et al.

Prophylactic measures against bacterial pneumonia include intravenous immunoglobulins in allogeneic HSCT recipients with low IgG level (Table 3.4) [29]. Antibiotics with activity against encapsulated organisms are recommended during the treatment of chronic GVHD. However, it should be noted that the routine use of prophylactic fluoroquinolones in the early post-transplant phase may be associated with an increased incidence of infections due to coagulase-negative staphylococci and gram-negative bacilli resistant to fluorquinolones [30].

Nocardia infection has been rarely reported in patients with hematological malignancies with an incidence ranging between 0.3 and 1.7% [31, 32]. In a study of 6,759 HSCT recipients, 22 cases of proven or probable nocardia infection were reported [32]. The infection was diagnosed a median of 210 days following transplantation. The main predisposing factors for developing nocardiosis were neutropenia, active acute or chronic GVHD, and lack of prophylaxis with trimethoprim-sulfamethoxezole (TMP-SMZ). In all except one patient, *Nocardia asteroides* was the causative agent. Pulmonary involvement occurs in 56% of patients, and the most common radiological findings are nodules with or without infiltrates. Cavitary lung lesions and empyema are other common features of nocardia infection (Fig. 3.3). The diagnosis of nocardia pneumonia is usually made by bronchoalveolar lavage (BAL), although occasionally the organism is detected by culture of sputum or tracheal secretions. If these methods are nondiagnostic, then the diagnosis could be confirmed by CT-guided aspirate of a pulmonary nodule or surgical lung biopsy. In 36% of patients there is co-infection with other organisms such as CMV and Aspergillus [32].

Treatment of nocardia infection is by prolonged administration of TMP-SMZ. Second-line agents are available if there are allergy or side effects associated with sulfa preparations. These second-line agents include amikacin, minocycline, cephalosporin or imipenem. Response to treatment is generally good, and long-term survival in patients with nocardiosis is not significantly different from controls [32]. Prophylaxis against *P. jiroveci* using low-dose TMP-SMZ has an added benefit of reducing the incidence of nocardia infection in high-risk patients.

An entire chapter on pulmonary tuberculosis and other mycobacterial infections in patients with

Table 3.4 Suggested prophylactic options against respiratory infections in patients with hematological malignancies

Infection	First choice	Alternate choice	Comments
Bacteria	Fluoroquinolone Intravenous immunoglobulins Pneumococcal vaccine *H. influenza* B vaccine	Macrolides	Intravenous immunoglobulins only if IgG level <400 mg/dL
Mycobacteria	Isoniazid 300 mg/day	Rifampin	9-month therapy Add pyridoxine 25–50 mg daily
Aspergillus	Posaconazole 200 mg three times daily	Voriconazole Itraconazole Echinocandins	
Candida	Fluconazole 400 mg/day orally or IV	Echinocandins Voriconazole	During neutropenia
P. jiroveci	TMP/SMZ double-strength one tablet/day or three times/week	Dapsone Aerosolized pentamidine	Prolonged corticosteroids treatment Allogeneic HSCT: from engraftment for 6 months and during immunosuppressive therapy for GVHD
CMV	Gancyclovir 5 mg/kg/dose twice daily for 7–14 days, followed by 5 mg/kg/day for 5 days/week	Foscarnet Valgancyclovir	Allogeneic HSCT: until day 100 or for a minimum of 3 weeks. Monitor CMV antigen for duration of treatment
RSV	RSV immunoglobulins 750 mg/kg/month	Aerosolized ribavirin	Based on pediatric HSCT during the high season months
Influenza	Lifelong annual seasonal Influenza vaccine	Rimantadine Amantadine Oseltamivir	
Herpes	Acyclovir 200 mg orally 3 times/day or 250 mg/m^2/dose twice daily intravenously	Valacyclovir	HSCT: Until engraftment or day 30
Herpes zoster virus	Herpes zoster immunoglobulin 625 U IM	Acycolvir Valacycolvir	

hematological malignancies is presented in this book by Dr. Al Anazi and colleagues. Briefly, *Mycobacterium tuberculosis* is rare in patients with hematological malignancies. The incidence of *M. tuberculosis* in patients with hematological malignancies varies significantly depending on whether the patients lived in an endemic area. In a large cancer center in the United States, the overall rate of active *M. tuberculosis* infection was 0.2 in 1,000 new cancer diagnoses. Five out of the 18 patients described had hematological malignancies, and 4 were neutropenic [33]. In a report from India of 130 patients with acute leukemia, 9 cases (6.9%) had active tuberculosis [34]. In HSCT recipients the reported incidence of M tuberculosis ranges from 0.4% to 5.5% [35–40] The prevalence of *M. tuberculosis* in autologous HSCT is similar to that in the general population, whereas in allogeneic HSCT recipients, *M. tuberculosis* infection increased by threefold [36].

A recent review of the literature reported the overall frequency of *M. tuberculosis* infection in HSCT recipients to be 0.4%, with only 2% of infections

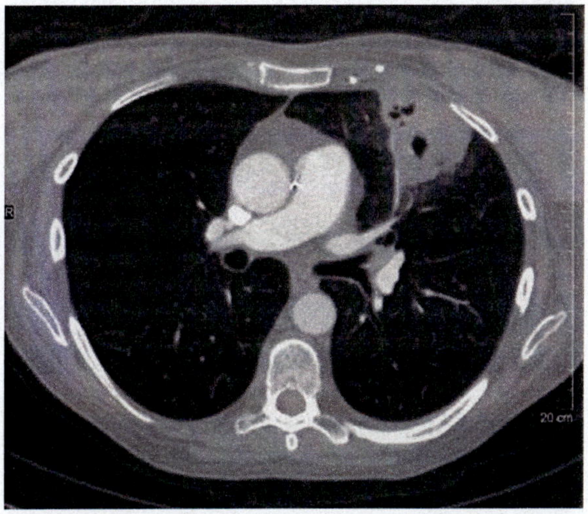

Fig. 3.3 CT scan of the chest showing a wedge shaped infiltrate in the left upper lobe with cavitation in a patient with GVHD on immunosuppressive therapy following HSCT who developed nocardia pneumonia

developing during neutropenia; 23% were during the first 100 days post-transplantation, and 75% were after the first 100 days [40]. In another review of 2,241 patients who underwent HSCT, only 11 patients (0.49%) had mycobacterial infection; 2 patients had *M. tuberculosis*, 2 *M. avium intracellulare* and the rest had rapidly growing mycobacteria organisms. All patients responded well to antimycobacterial treatment [35].

The main risk factors for *M. tuberculosis* in patients with hematological malignancies are allogeneic transplantation, total body irradiation, chronic GVHD, corticosteroid therapy and residence in endemic areas [36–40]. In HSCT recipients the median time for *M. tuberculosis* infection was 324 days in one study [36]. The clinical and radiological picture of *M. tuberculosis* infection in these patients is generally similar to non-immunocompromised patients. However, atypical presentations, including rapidly progressive disease, lack of cavitation and extrapulmonary manifestations, have been described in patients with hematological malignancies [33, 41]. The diagnosis of *M. tuberculosis* infection is usually made by smear and culture from sputum, BAL or pleural fluid samples. Rapid diagnosis of *M. tuberculosis* may be established by PCR test on the above samples. It is important to check the positive samples for drug susceptibility.

Treatment of *M. tuberculosis* infection in patients with hematological malignancies is similar to other patient populations. However, rifampin should be used with caution because of potential interaction with commonly used medications in this patient population, such as fluconazole and calcineurin inhibitors [19, 42]. Some studies suggested a full 1 year of treatment [40].

Diagnosis of latent *M. tuberculosis* may be difficult in patients with hematological malignancies given the degree of immunosuppression. The tuberculin skin test with 5 mm or more induration as well as a history of significant exposure to patients with active *M. tuberculosis* infection may be indications for treatment [19]. Diagnostic yield of T-cell interferon gamma release blood assays is important [43].

Nontuberculous mycobacterial infections (such as *M. avium* complex, *M. kansasii*, *M. chelonae*) are rare in patients with hematological malignancies. In HSCT recipients the incidence has been generally reported to be less than 1% of all patients [44]. However, in one report from Memorial Sloan Kettering Hospital, the incidence of nontuberculous mycobacterial infection was 2.8% of HSCT recipients [45]. This higher incidence was considered to be related to environmental and historical factors. In a review of 93 cases of nontuberculous mycobacterial infection in HSCT recipients reported in the literature, the median time to diagnosis was 4 months following transplantation, and 46% of patients had GVHD. The infection resolved with medical therapy in 62% of patients. The attributed mortality to nontuberculous mycobacteria was 7.5% [44]. Nontuberculous mycobacteria may colonize the airways of the patients having chronic lung disease, such as bronchiectasis, which may create a challenge in determining the significance of isolating these bacteria from lower respiratory tract samples. In the case of *M. avium intracellulare*, first-line therapeutic agents include clarithromycin, azithormycin, ethambutol, rifampin and rifabutin for 18 months (12 months after negative cultures) [46, 47].

3.4 Fungal Infections

3.4.1 *Aspergillus*

Aspergillus is a filamentous fungus that is ubiquitous in the environment. The Aspergillus species are present in the environment as small conidia that are regularly inhaled into the lungs. In the lungs, they change into hyphae that are short and septate, with acute angle branching. Alveolar macrophages and peripheral blood neutrophils are the primary defense mechanism against this fungus. T helper cells and their cytokines (such as TNF-α, interferon-γ, IL-12 and IL-15) augment the activity of macrophages and neutrophils against Aspergillus. Neutropenia and defects in T-helper cell function in patients with hematological malignancies make these patients especially vulnerable to invasive disease by Aspergillus. A chapter from Bougnoux and colleagues in this book reports an up-to-date and comprehensive review on invasive pulmonary aspergillosis in patients with hematological malignancies. Invasive pulmonary aspergillosis (IPA) is the most common invasive fungal infection in patients with hematological malignancies, with a steady rise in the documented cases. Following HSCT, the risk for IPA is much higher following allogeneic HSCT when compared to autologous transplantation (incidence is 0.5–4% in autologous HSCT compared to 2.3–15% in allogeneic HSCT [48–52]). After autologous HSCT, IPA is mainly seen during the neutropenic phase. In allogeneic HSCT, the highest risk is in patients with severe GVHD (grade III-IV). In a study by Marr et al., the probability of IPA following allogeneic HSCT reached approximately 5% at 2 months, 9% at 6 months and 10% at 1 year following allogeneic HSCT. By the third year after transplantation, the probability of IPA increased minimally to 11.1% [50]. In these patients, the timeline for IPA infection follows a bimodal distribution, with a peak in the first month following HSCT, which is associated with neutropenia. The second peak is during the treatment for GVHD (median 78–112 days post transplantation) [49, 51, 53]. The first peak is currently less significant due to the routine use of stem cell instead of bone marrow for transplantation, non-myeloablative regimens, the use of colony-stimulating factors during neutropenia and the widespread use of antifungal agents have significantly decreased the incidence of IPA during this period [49, 54]. On the other hand, the incidence of IPA during the treatment of GVHD has become more significant, especially with higher incidence of GVHD associated with unrelated allogeneic transplantation and nonmyeloablative HSCT. Cord blood HSCT is also associated with increased risk of IPA. In one study of patients who received low intensity cord blood transplantation, the 3-year accumulative incidence of IPA was 10% with mortality of 86%. All of these patients developed IPA in the first 100 days post transplantation (median 20 days) [55]. Also the risk of IPA increases with the use of Alemtuzumab, which is an anti-DC52 monoclonal antibody used to deplete peripheral B and T lymphocytes [49, 50, 52]. Treatment of GVHD with intensive immunosuppressive therapy, including corticosteroids, cyclosporine A and anti-TNF- α agents, further increases the risk of IPA [49, 50, 56–58]. There is also evidence that CMV infection in these patients increases the risk of IPA [50, 59]. The hazards ratio for IPA in the setting of CMV disease increases by 13.3 folds (95% CI 4.7–37.7) [51]. A recent retrospective review of 385 cases of suspected or documented IPA in patients with hematological malignancies over a 9-year period revealed that the overall and disease-specific survival rates were 52% and 60%, respectively. Factors that predicted mortality were allogeneic HSCT, neutropenia, progression of the underlying malignancy, prior respiratory disease, corticosteroids therapy, renal impairment, low monocyte counts, disseminated aspergillosis and pleural effusion [60].

Aspergillus is most often introduced to the lower respiratory tract by inhalation of the infectious spores. Less commonly, IPA may start in locations other than the lungs, like sinuses, the gastrointestinal tract, or the skin (intravenous catheters or prolonged skin contact with adhesive tapes) [61–64]. Patients present with symptoms that are usually non-specific and consistent with bronchopneumonia, with fever unresponsive to antibiotics, cough, sputum production and dyspnea. Patients may also present with pleuritic chest pain (due to vascular invasion leading to small pulmonary infarcts) and hemoptysis, which is usually mild, but could be massive. IPA is one of the most common causes of hemoptysis in neutropenic patients and has been reported to be associated with cavitation that occurs with neutrophil recovery [65]. Aspergillus infection may also disseminate hematogenously to other organs, most commonly the brain (leading to seizures, ring-enhancing lesions, cerebral infarctions, intracranial hemorrhage, meningitis and epidural abscess), and less frequently other organs such as skin, kidneys, pleura, heart, esophagus and liver may be involved [66].

The diagnosis of IPA is challenging. Early diagnosis of IPA in patients with hematological malignancies remains difficult, and a high index of suspicion is necessary in patients with risk factors for invasive disease. Histopathological diagnosis by examining lung tissue obtained by surgical lung biopsy remains the "gold standard" for the diagnosis of IPA [67]. The presence of septate, acute, branching hyphae invading the lung tissue samples along with a culture that is positive for Aspergillus species from the same site is diagnostic of IPA. Histopathological examination also allows for the exclusion of other diagnoses, such as malignancy or nonfungal infectious diseases. The histopathological findings associated with IPA have been recently shown to differ according to the underlying host. In patients with allogeneic HSCT and GVHD, there is intense inflammation with neutrophilic infiltration, minimal coagulation necrosis and low fungal burden. On the other hand, IPA in neutropenic patients is characterized by scant inflammation, extensive coagulation necrosis associated with hyphal angioinvasion and high fungal burden. Dissemination to other organs is equally high in both groups [68].

The chest radiograph has a small role in early stages of the disease because the incidence of non-specific changes is high. Usual findings include rounded densities, pleural-based infiltrates that are suggestive of pulmonary infarctions and cavitations. Pleural effusions are uncommon [69, 70]. Chest CT scan, especially when combined with high-resolution images, is a much more helpful tool in the diagnosis of IPA. The routine use of high-resolution CT of the chest early in the course of IPA has been shown to lead to earlier diagnosis and improved outcome of these patients [71, 72]. It also aids further diagnostic studies such as bronchoscopy and surgical lung biopsy [73]. The typical chest CT scan findings in patients suspected to have IPA include: multiple nodules and the halo sign, which is mainly seen in neutropenic patients early in the course of infection (usually in the first week), and appears as a zone of low attenuation due to hemorrhage surrounding the pulmonary nodule (Fig. 3.4). Another late radiological sign is the air crescent sign, which represents crescent-shaped lucency in the region of the original nodule secondary to necrosis [70, 74]. Neither the halo nor the air crescent signs are sensitive to or pathognomic of IPA. The halo sign may be found as a result of metastasis, organizing pneumonia or other fungal infection [75]. Greene et al. found that 94% of 235 patients with a confirmed diagnosis of IPA had at least one nodular region [76]. In another recent report of 27 patients with IPA following allogeneic HSCT, the most common radiological findings were ill-defined consolidation (48%), nodules with halo sign (44%), centrilobular nodules (44%), ground-glass-attenuation (22%) and pleural effusion (26%) [77]. In a large study of 236 patients with IPA, 86% of whom had hematological malignancies, the halo sign was detected in 61% of the cases. In the study population as a whole, and specifically in patients with hematological malignancies, the presence of the halo sign predicted better response to antifungal therapy [78]. On the other hand, in a retrospective study done on 45 patients, Horger et al. found that none of the early high-resolution CT scan signs (nodule, consolidation, peribronchial infiltrates) seems to predict patient outcome or the development of pulmonary hemorrhage [79]. However, pulmonary hemorrhage is expected to occur

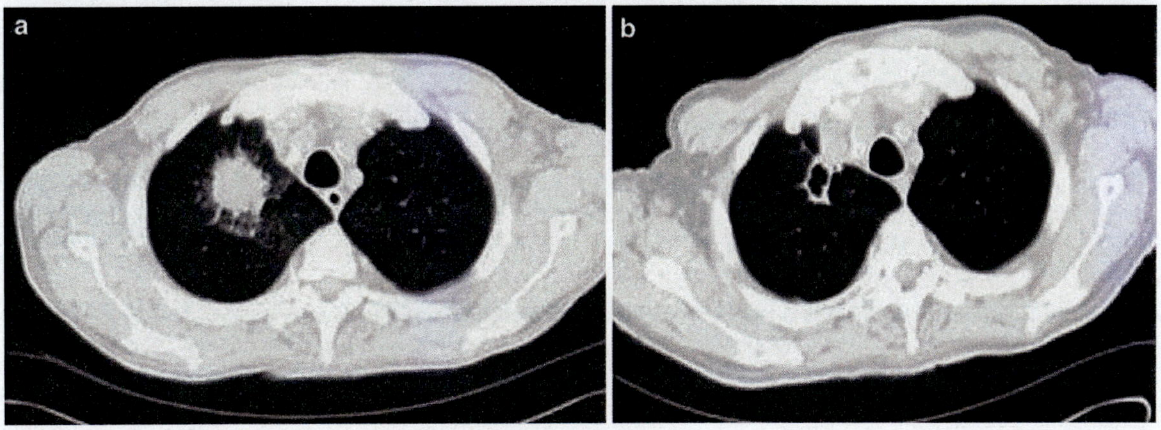

Fig. 3.4 (**a**) High resolution CT scan of the chest showing right upper lobe nodule with the Halo sign in a patient with non-Hodgkin's lymphoma and neutropenia who developed IPA. (**b**) Shows residual cavity formation after 2 months of treatment with antifungal agent

in the presence of large cavitating nodules or consolidations located close to larger pulmonary vessels.

The significance of isolating Aspergillus species in sputum samples depends on the immune status of the host. In patients with hematological malignancies, isolation of Aspergillus species from sputum is highly predictive of invasive disease. Studies have shown that sputum samples that are positive for Aspergillus in these patients have a positive predictive value of 80–90% [80–82]. However, sputum samples that are negative could not rule out IPA, since negative sputum studies have been noted in 70% of patients with confirmed IPA [82, 83]. Blood cultures are rarely positive in patients with confirmed IPA [84].

Bronchoscopy with BAL is generally helpful in the diagnosis of IPA, especially in patients with diffuse lung involvement. Visualization of the bronchial tree may also provide arguments for IPA in patients with airway-invasive IPA. The sensitivity and specificity of a positive result of BAL fluid are around 50% and 97%, respectively. The yield of BAL in the diagnosis of IPA is not consistent, and there are reports of much lower diagnostic yield [80, 81, 85–89]. BAL is generally a safe and useful tool in non-hypoxemic patients with hematological malignancies suspected to have IPA. In addition to obtaining samples for fungal stain and culture, it may be useful in detecting Aspergillus antigens in the BAL fluid and excluding other infections. Transbronchial biopsies usually do not add much to the diagnosis of IPA and are associated with increased risk of bleeding, so they are usually not performed [80].

In the setting of diagnostic workup for IPA, it is important to send samples such as sputum, BAL fluid or lung tissue for culture as well as for histological examination. This is because other fungal species, such as scedosporium, pseudallescheria and fusarium, may have a similar histological appearance as Aspergillus [90]. Furthermore, there are different species of Aspergillus that may lead to IPA. While *Aspergillus fumigatus* is the most common cause of IPA, there are increasing reports of IPA in patients with hematological malignancies due to other species such as *A. niger*, *A. terreus* and *A. flavus* [91–95]. Some of these species (such as *A. terreus* and *A. nidulans*) are resistant to amphotericin B [92, 95]. In a review of 300 patients with hematological malignancies (40% were HSCT recipients) with proven IPA, *A. terreus* was the second most common species isolated with a frequency of 23%. The risk factors and outcome for *A. terreus* infection were similar to those for *A. fumigatus* infection; however the former was significantly more likely to be nosocomial in origin and more likely to be resistant to amphotericin B [94]. The new triazole antifungal agents such as voriconazole and posaconazole have significantly better efficacy against *A. terreus* [92, 93, 96].

The most recent advances in the diagnosis of IPA are related to detecting Aspergillus antigens in body fluids. Galactomannan (GM) is a polysaccharide cell-wall component that is released by Aspergillus during growth. A double-sandwich ELISA for the detection of GM in serum was approved by the Food and Drug Administration for the diagnosis of IPA, with a threshold of 0.5 ng/mL. It is reported that serum GM can be detected several days before the presence of clinical signs, an abnormal chest radiograph or positive culture. Thus, GM detection may allow earlier confirmation of the diagnosis, and serial determination of serum GM values may be useful in assessing the evolution of infection during treatment [97, 98].

A meta-analysis study was undertaken by Pfeiffer et al. to assess the accuracy of a GM assay in diagnosing IPA. Twenty-seven studies from 1996 to 2005 were included, and cases were diagnosed to have IPA according to the European Organization for Research on Treatment of Cancer/Mycoses Study Group (EORTC/MSG) criteria. Overall, the GM assay had a sensitivity of 71% and specificity of 89% for proven cases of invasive aspergillosis. The negative predictive value was 92–98%, and the positive predictive value was between 25% and 62% [99]. Pfeiffer and colleagues concluded that GM assay is more useful in patients who have hematological malignancies or who have undergone allogeneic HSCT than in solid-organ transplant recipients or nonneutropenic patients.

GM is found in food and may be absorbed by the digestive tract, especially in patients with postchemotherapy mucositis, resulting in a false-positive reaction. Also medications such as β-lactam antibiotics (e.g., piperacillin/tazobactam) may be associated with false-positive GM assay, while antifungal agents with activity against Aspergillus may lead to a false-negative test [100–103]. It is noteworthy that GM assay is species specific, and it is not possible to exclude the involvement of other molds such as Fusarium, Zygomycetes and dematiaceous fungi by measuring serum GM [104].

There is evidence that GM is detected in other body fluids such as BAL, urine and cerebrospinal fluid, and that these tests may become positive prior to clinical and radiological findings suggestive of IPA [104–107].

A recent prospective study of 200 patients with hematological malignancies and profound neutropenia found that GM assay from BAL had a sensitivity of 100% for IPA compared to 71% by serum GM assay [108]. Another study done by Musher et al. showed that incorporating GM assay and quantitative PCR assay into standard BAL fluid analysis may enhance bronchoscopic identification of Aspergillus species as the cause pulmonary disease in patients with hematological malignancies [105]. Serial serum GM assay has also been shown to help in the early detection of IPA and as a surrogate to response to therapy. In a study of 70 neutropenic patients with IPA, serum GM assay was performed three times weekly after the start of antifungal therapy until GM index negativity or death. The patients who had normalization of the serum GM index did significantly better than those who continued to have positive serum GM [109].

Polymerase chain reaction (PCR) is another way to diagnose IPA by the detection of Aspergillus DNA in BAL fluid and serum. A positive Aspergillus PCR in BAL fluid has an estimated sensitivity of 67–100% and specificity between 55% and 95% [110]. PCR sensitivity and specificity have also been reported as 100% and 65–92%, respectively, in serum samples [110–113]. However, this test is often associated with false-positive results because it doesn't discriminate between colonization and infection. PCR for Aspergillus nucleic acid detection remains restricted to highly specialized laboratories and cannot be considered as a routine exam.

Detection of serum (1→3)-β-D-glucan, a fungal cell wall constituent, has recently received Food and Drug Administration approval. Determination of plasma (1→3)-β-D-glucan has been reported to be a highly sensitive and specific test for invasive deep mycosis, including candidiasis, fusariosis, Pneumocystosis and aspergillosis, and could be useful in the immunocompromised patients [114]. A prospective study of 95 patients with hematological malignancies and neutropenia evaluated the value of monitoring the serum level of (1→3)-β-D-glucan twice weekly in the absence of fever and daily in the presence of fever in the early diagnosis of IPA. Thirteen patients developed IPA, 15 patients had candidiasis, and 2 patients had mixed invasive fungal infections. The sensitivity, specificity, positive predictive value and negative predictive value of two consecutive positive (1→3)-β-D-glucan values were 0.63, 0.96, 0.79 and 0.91, respectively [115]. The utility of routine monitoring of this assay in patients with hematological malignancies at high risk for IPA is not yet defined.

The role of GM and other serological studies in the diagnosis of IPA is evolving. Furthermore, their role in different hosts, as surveillance tools, and their impact on the outcome of patients are not clear. There are ongoing prospective studies to address these issues. Until solid data are available, these tests should be considered as adjunct diagnostic studies, and should not replace appropriate clinical and radiological evaluation, and in selected cases, invasive procedures to confirm the diagnosis of IPA.

The EORTC/MSG has revised its criteria for the diagnosis of invasive fungal infections [116, 117]. These criteria consist of host factors, microbiologic, minor and major clinical criteria (Table 3.5). Positive serum GM, with the appropriate host and clinical

Table 3.5 The diagnostic criteria for IPA

Diagnosis	Criteria
Proven IPA	Histopathologic or cytopathologic examination of lung tissue showing hyphae from needle aspiration or biopsy specimen with evidence of associated tissue damage; *OR* Positive culture result for Aspergillus from a sample obtained by sterile procedure from the lung and clinically or radiologically abnormal site consistent with infection
Probable IPA	Host risk factor[a]; *AND* Microbiological criteria (positive Aspergillus microscopy or culture from the sputum or BAL, or positive GM assay); *AND* Clinical criteria consistent with the infection (1 major or 2 minor)[b]
Possible IPA	Host risk factor; *AND* Microbiological criteria (positive Aspergillus microscopy or culture from the sputum or BAL, or positive GM assay from one BAL or at least two serum samples); *OR* Clinical criteria consistent with the infection (1 major or 2 minor)[a]

[a]At least one of the following host factors include neutropenia (<500 cells/mm^3 for >10 days), allogeneic HSCT, prolonged corticosteroid therapy (>0.3 mg/kg/day of prednisone or equivalent for >3 weeks); T cell suppressant therapy

[b]Major clinical criteria are: new characteristic infiltrates on CT imaging (halo sign, air-crescent sign, or cavity within area of consolidation). Minor clinical criteria are: Symptoms of LRTI (cough, chest pain, hemoptysis, or dyspnea); physical finding of pleural rub; any new infiltrate not fulfilling major criterion; pleural effusion

factors, can be considered as "probable" IPA. The EORTC/MSG criteria are not evidence-based and are not prospectively validated. Instead, they are meant to serve as a guide for clinical and epidemiological research and need not be present in every patient to treat for IPA.

The treatment of IPA is difficult, and the mortality rate is still high despite the introduction of several new antifungal agents. Herbrecht and colleagues report in this book a very comprehensive and up-to-date contribution on antifungal agents. Therapy should be considered as soon as there is a clinical suspicion of IPA and while a workup is underway. For many years, amphotericin B has been the first line of therapy for IPA. The recommended dose is 1–1.5 mg/kg/day. Amphotericin B is known, however, to cause serious side effects, including nephrotoxicity, electrolyte disturbances and hypersensitivity. For these reasons, this agent nowadays has little role to play in the treatment of IPA, and newer lipid-based preparations of amphotericin B (e.g., liposomal amphotericin B and lipid complex amphotericin B) have been introduced to minimize these side effects. Higher doses of the lipid formulations are needed for equivalent antifungal efficacy to amphotericin B. Voriconazole is a new broad-spectrum triazole that is approved as the initial treatment of invasive aspergillosis and is currently considered the treatment of choice in many patients with IPA [118–120]. In a large prospective, randomized, multicenter trial, voriconazole was compared to amphotericin B as the primary therapy for IPA [121]. Patients receiving voriconazole had a higher favorable response rate at week 12 (53% compared with 32% in patients receiving amphotericin B) and a higher 12-week survival (71% compared with 58%). Voriconazole is available in both intravenous and oral formulations. The recommended dose is 6 mg/kg twice daily intravenously on day 1 followed by 4 mg/kg/day. After 7 days, switching to 200 mg orally twice daily may be considered. Voriconazole has a milder side effect profile and is much better tolerated than amphotericin B. The most frequent adverse effect is visual disturbances described as blurred vision, photophobia and altered color perception. Liver function test abnormalities and skin reactions are less common side effects associated with voriconazole treatment. It is important to note that voriconazole is associated with a significant number of drug-drug interactions such as cyclosporine, warfarin, terfenadine, carbamazepine, quinidine, rifampin, statins and sulfonylureas [118].

Posaconazole is another broad-spectrum triazole that has been shown to be effective and safe as salvage therapy in patients with invasive aspergillosis refractory to standard antifungal therapy [96, 122, 123].

Echinocandin derivatives such as caspofungin, micafungin and anidulafungin are effective agents in the treatment of IPA refractory to standard treatment or if the patient could not tolerate first line agents [124, 125]. In its recent guidelines, The Infectious Disease Society of America recommends voriconazole as the primary treatment for IPA in most patients and liposomal amphotericin B as an alternative treatment for some patients. For salvage therapy, agents include lipid-based preparations of amphotericin A, posaconazole, itraconazole, caspofungin or micafungin [126].

Some studies have suggested that combination antifungal therapy could be a strategy to treat refractory IPA [127, 128]. There are no prospective randomized studies that show superior efficacy of combination therapy over a single agent in the primary management of IPA. There are in vitro and limited clinical studies in the form of case reports and retrospective case series that show a benefit from combining antifungal agents as salvage therapy in refractory IPA [128–131]. The combination of caspofungin and liposomal amphotericin B as a salvage therapy showed an overall response rate of 42%; however, in patients with progressive documented IPA, the response rate was only 18% [128]. A survival advantage of voriconazole plus caspofungin compared with voriconazole alone was reported by Marr et al. in a retrospective analysis of salvage therapy for IPA [130]. On the other hand, the report by Denning et al. showed no difference in the response rate between patients who received micafungin alone or in combination with other antifungal agents as primary or salvage therapy for IPA [132]. Combination therapy of an echinocandin with either a lipid formulation of amphotericin B or triazole agent appears to be promising, however cannot be recommended for the routine treatment of primary IPA. Controlled randomized prospective studies are needed to document the value of this approach.

Surgical resection has a limited role in the management of patients with IPA; however, it should be considered in cases of massive hemoptysis or pulmonary lesions close to the great blood vessels or pericardium, or the resection of residual localized pulmonary lesions in patients with continuing immunosuppression. Several reports have shown the relative efficacy and safety of surgical intervention – in addition to antifungal therapy – in these situations [72, 133–138].

Immunomodulatory therapy, such as using colony-stimulating factors (i.e., granulocyte-colony stimulating factors, granulocyte macrophage-colony stimulating therapy) or interferon-γ, could be used to decrease the degree of immunosuppression and as an adjunct to antifungal therapy for the treatment of IPA. Colony-stimulating factors stimulate the bone marrow to produce more neutrophils and have been shown to augment the phagocytic activity of neutrophils against fungi, including Aspergillus species [139–141]. There is a theoretical advantage to adding these agents to the treatment of neutropenic patients suspected to have IPA. In one randomized study in patients receiving chemotherapy for acute myelogenous leukemia, prophylaxis with GM-CSF led to a lower frequency of fatal fungal infections compared with placebo (1.9% vs. 19%, respectively) and reduced overall mortality [142]. It is recommended to consider colony-stimulating factors in neutropenic patients with serious infections; however, there are no definitive studies that show benefit in patients with IPA [143]. Interferon-γ is another cytokine that has been shown in vitro and in animal models to augment immunity by increasing neutrophil and monocyte activity against Aspergillus [140, 144, 145]. The value of adding interferon-γ as an adjunct treatment of IPA is limited to case reports and small reports, and there are no guidelines on its role in the treatment of IPA [146]. There was a concern about the use of interferon-γ in allogeneic HSCT recipients, since it may worsen GVHD; however, a recent trial showed that GVHD may actually improve during this therapy [147]. Granulocyte transfusion is another potential supportive therapy for patients with prolonged neutropenia and life-threatening infections refractory to conventional therapy. It has been shown that it is safe for potential donors to donate neutrophils by granulocytophoresis; however, there are no randomized studies that prove the benefit of adjuvant granulocyte transfusion in the treatment of IPA [148]. A review of 66 observational studies of patients who received ganulocyte transfusions, either prophylactic or therapeutic, in the management of gram-negative bacterial or fungal infections suggested survival in 70% [149]. It is also important in patients with IPA, whenever possible, to decrease the dose of systemic corticosteroids and immunosuppressive agents.

The management of IPA is difficult and an important approach to this problem is prophylaxis for those patients who are at increased risk for this infection. Avoiding the hospitalization of patients in areas where there are construction and the use of high-efficiency particulate air (HEPA) filtration with or without laminar air flow ventilation have proven to be efficient [150]. A meta-analysis suggested that itraconazole was effective in preventing fungal infections in neutropenic patients [151]. Recent data also suggest the efficacy of posaconazole in the prophylaxis against IPA in patients with severe GVHD and other hematological malignancies [152, 153]. There are also preliminary data that suggest aerosolized treatment with antifungal agents such as liposomal amphotericin B and voriconzaole may be effective in the prevention of IPA in high risk population [154, 155].

3.4.2 Other Fungi

Other fungal infections may invade the lungs in hematological patients. An entire chapter on emerging fungal infections from Drs. Garnica and Nucci is provided in this book. These invasive fungal infections primarily involve the lungs, but may disseminate to other organs. They are mainly seen in patients with neutropenia, allogeneic HSCT, and GVHD [52, 156–159]. The main invasive fungal infections that are reported in these patients include hyaline hyphomycetes (such as fusarium and Scedosporium), zygomycetes and endemic fungi. In a Centers for Disease Control-sponsored surveillance program for invasive fungal infections, there were 886 patients with invasive fungal infections out of 20,000 HSCT and solid organ transplant recipients [160]. Non-apsergillus molds were responsible for 14% of infections, cryptococcus in 4%, endemic fungi in 3% and pneumoystis in 2%.

Hyaline hyphomycetes, such as fusarium and scedosporium, are the main non-aspergillus molds that are reported in patients with hematological malignancies. These organisms resemble Aspergillus histologically with septate hyphae that invade blood vessels [52, 161, 162]. Culture is the only means to distinguish these organisms from Aspergillus. The lungs are the primary site of infection; however, these organisms have the tendency to disseminate. In one study, fusarium infection involved the lungs in 81% of the cases, and was disseminated in 74% of the patients [52]. Fungemia due to fusarium is reported in 20–70% of patients [163]. These infections usually occur early (in the first 2 months) following allogeneic HSCT. The mortality in patients with pulmonary fusariosis is 65% within 1 month of diagnosis [164]. Factors that decrease survival are persistent neutropenia and corticosteroid therapy. Scedosporium has been isolated from the air in hospitals [162]. In the lungs, these organisms usually present with thin wall cavities or nodules with or without air-crescent sign that are refractory to antibiotics and antifungal therapy [165]. The diagnosis is usually confirmed by isolating the organisms by culture of BAL fluid or lung tissue obtained by surgical lung biopsy. Occasionally the diagnosis is obtained by fungal blood cultures. Mortality associated with these fungal infections remains very high, in the range of 70–100% [163, 166–168].

Zygomycetes such as Rhizopus and mucor are characterized by sparsely septate, broad hyphae with irregular branching. They have the tendency to invade blood vessels with thrombosis and tissue necrosis. They usually involve the sinopulmonary tree; however dissemination to other organs is rare. The incidence of zygomycetes infections in patients with hematological malignancies is rare (0.5–1.9%) [52, 158, 159]. It is important to note that these organisms may be resistant to voriconazole [169]. Recent reports suggest good response to posaconazole [170]. Mortality associated with zygomycetes infection in patients with hematological malignancies reaches 80% [52, 158, 159].

Cryptococcus infection in patients with hematological malignancies has been rarely reported. The widespread prophylaxis with fluconazole may account for the relatively low incidence in these patients. Patients with profound T cell depression (such as Hodgkin's disease, chronic leukemia and treatment with purine analogues) are at highest risk [171]. The diagnosis of pulmonary cryptococcal infection is usually made by detection of the fungus in BAL or lung tissue samples. Serum cryptococcal antigen has more than 95% sensitivity and specificity in the diagnosis of invasive cryptococcosis, however could be negative in patients with localized pulmonary infection [172]. The treatment of pulmonary cryptococcosis in hematological malignancies includes Amphotericin B for severe cases, and fluconazole or itraconazole for milder cases and for maintenance therapy [173].

As reported in the chapter from Carvajal et al., invasive Candida infection develops in 11–16% of patients with hematological malignancies, and pulmonary involvement is usually secondary to disseminated candidiasis or candidemia. Autopsy studies suggest that 50% of infected patients have pulmonary involvement [174]. In a study of 529 patients who died from leukemia or myelodysplastic syndrome and were affected by candidiasis, 45% had lung involvement. It is believed that Candida may have disseminated to all organs, including the lungs, prior to their death [175]. Primary Candida pneumonia is extremely rare. Histopathological confirmation is necessary in most of the cases. The universal prophylaxis with fluconazole has significantly decreased the incidence of Candida infections. However, there is a shift in the Candida species from *Candida albicans* to more resistant species such as *C. glabrata* or *C. krusei*.

As reported in the dedicated chapter, *Pneumocystis pneumonia* is caused by *P. jiroveci*, which is a fungal agent [176]. Infection is caused by inhalation of aerosolized organisms. The incidence of *P. pneumonia* was historically up to 20% of patients with hematological malignancies and 5–15% of HSCT recipients [4, 177]. However, the routine prophylaxis with TMX/SMZ during high-risk periods has significantly decreased the incidence of this infection to negligible values. Breakthrough infection in patients on TMP/SMZ prophylaxis is extremely rare, however is possible in patients on other prophylactic agents such as low-dose atovaquone or aerosolized pentamidine [178–180]. Patients with lymphoproliferative disorders appear to be at the highest risk for *P. jiroveci* infection. Also the prolonged administration of high-

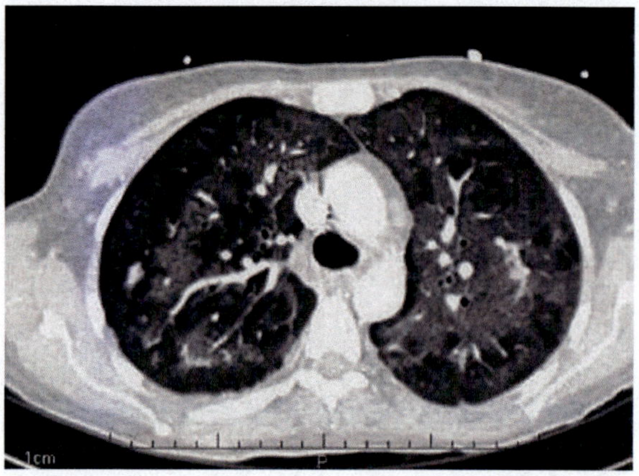

Fig. 3.5 High resolution CT scan of the chest showing diffuse ground glass infiltrates in a patient with non-Hodgkin's lymphoma on chemotherapy who developed P jiroveci pneumonia

dose corticosteroid therapy and purine analogues such as fludarabine–especially when combined with corticosteroids–significantly increase the risk of this infection [181–184]. In a recent report of 519 allogeneic HSCT recipients, *P. jiroveci* pneumonia was documented in 13 patients (2.5%). The majority of cases occurred late in the course following HSCT (median 14.5 months) after discontinuation of prophylactic agents [185]. The CD4+ T cell count was low, and 70% of patients were on immunosuppressive therapy for chronic GVHD.

The onset of *P. jiroveci* pneumonia is acute and rapidly progressive in the majority of cases, with dyspnea, nonproductive cough and fever. Hypoxemia is usually dramatic in these patients [183]. Radiologically, there are perihilar interstitial or alveolar infiltrates. Ground-glass opacities may be the prominent finding on high-resolution CT scan of the chest (Fig. 3.5). LDH may be elevated. The diagnosis is usually made by bronchoscopy with BAL; however, the sensitivity of this procedure is lower than that reported in patients with AIDS due to the lower burden of the organism [4]. Monoclonal antibodies for detecting *P. jiroveci* have higher sensitivity and specificity in induced sputum samples than conventional staining, but the difference between the two methods is insignificant in BAL fluid [186, 187].

Mortality has been recently reported to be 20% of patients with cancer, and the only predictor of poor outcome based on multivariate analysis was the need for mechanical ventilation [188, 189]. Prophylaxis against *P. jiroveci* pneumonia using TMP/SMZ is recommended for patients who are on chronic corticosteroid therapy and following engraftment in allogeneic HSCT recipients for 120 days. However, if the patient has chronic GVHD, prophylactic treatment is recommended as long as they are on immunosuppressive therapy for this condition.

Endemic mycoses, such as histoplasmosis, blastomycosis and coccidiomycosis, are rare in patients with hematological malignancies [190]. These infections tend to have geographical distribution and are usually caused by endogenous reactivation of a latent infection. The infection usually presents with progressive pulmonary disease that disseminates to other organs. Treatment is with a high-dose amphotericin B preparation [161]. After controlling the infection, an azole such as itraconazole (or fluconazole in the case of coccidiomycosis) can be used as a maintenance treatment [160].

3.5 Cytomegalovirus

It is important at the outset to define the different manifestations of CMV infection. CMV infection is defined as isolation of the CMV virus or its proteins or nucleic acid from body fluids or tissue specimens. CMV viremia is isolation of CMV from blood by culture. CMV antigenemia is detection of CMV pp65 in circulating leukocytes or CMV DNA by PCR techniques. CMV disease is the presence of signs and symptoms related to CMV infection, and may manifest as hepatitis, gastroenteritis, encephalitis or a systemic syndrome. CMV pneumonia is one of the most frequent and severe manifestations of CMV disease in patients with hematological malignancies, especially HSCT recipients. It is defined as pulmonary signs and symptoms combined with detection of CMV in pulmonary samples (BAL or lung tissue). It is important to note that some patients may shed CMV in BAL fluid in the absence of invasive disease. It is also significant to note that CMV affects the immune system and promotes other infections. Co-infection with other organisms, such as bacteria, *P. jiroveci*, Aspergillus or other viruses, is reported in up to one third of cases [191].

An entire very nice contribution from Dr. Vigil and Chemaly in this book provides a comprehensive overview on CMV pneumonia. Traditionally, CMV pneumonia was a relatively frequent infection in patients with hematological malignancies. It was diagnosed in 20–35% of allogeneic HSCT recipients and 60–80% of patients with diffuse pneumonitis following HSCT [29, 192, 193]. CMV pneumonia usually presented in the first 2 months post-transplantation (median 44 days), and was associated with high mortality ranging between 80% and 100% [192]. However, antiviral prophylaxis for high-risk patients and preemptive therapy has changed the epidemiology of CMV pneumonia in HSCT recipients. Currently in allogeneic HSCT recipients, the incidence of CMV pneumonia is about 10%, while in autologous recipients, CMV pneumonia is extremely rare (1–9%) [194–197]. An autopsy-based case control study evaluated the incidence and risk factors of fatal CMV pneumonia in patients with hematological malignancies. The incidence of fatal CMV pneumonia was 3.5% before 1997 compared to 0.8% after that date. Complete remission of the underlying malignancy and sustained lymphopenia were independent predictors of CMV pneumonia [198]. Prophylactic and preemptive antiviral therapy has also shifted the onset of CMV pneumonia in allogeneic HSCT to after the first 100 days (median 169 days), especially in patients with non-myeloablative HSCT and during the treatment of chronic GVHD [199, 200]. The risk of CMV pneumonia in patients with hematological malignancies is mainly seen in patients with leukemia or lymphoma who are on T-cell-depleting chemotherapeutic regimen (such as cytarabine, fludarabine, high-dose cyclophosphamide, corticosteroids or alemtuzumab). In HSCT recipients, CMV pneumonia is mainly seen after allogeneic transplantation and the highest risk is in seropositive recipients. CMV disease is reported in 14% of seropostive recipients who received a seropositive graft and in 12% of seropositive recipients and seronegative grafts. On the other hand, the risk of CMV disease is lower in seronegative recipients who had HSCT from seropositive donors (incidence is less than 5%) [201]. Additional risk factors for CMV pneumonia include older age, total body irradiation, myeloablative chemotherapy, the presence and acuity of acute GVHD, and the use of T-cell depletion strategies [192, 202, 203]. In autologous HSCT, the main risk factors for CMV pneumonia are the presence of CMV infection prior to transplantation, CD-34-enriched stem cells, probably due to lower number of T cells and delayed immunologic reconstitution [204].

CMV pneumonia presents clinically with rapid onset of fever, nonproductive cough, dyspnea and hypoxemia. Pleurisy may be present. The respiratory symptoms usually progress to acute respiratory failure within 2 weeks. Radiologically, the most common findings are an interstitial pattern with tiny pulmonary nodules and patchy areas of consolidation. Rarely CMV pneumonia may present with focal diseases [205, 206]. High-resolution CT scan of the chest is more sensitive in detecting the findings related to CMV pneumonia including diffuse or patchy ground-glass opacification, thickened interlobular septa and tree in bud nodular changes. Pleural effusion may be present in around quarter of patients [206]. The differential diagnosis of these clinical and radiological findings includes *P. jiroveci*, other viral infections, pulmonary hemorrhage, drug-induced lung injury, pulmonary edema or tumor recurrence. Some of these conditions may co-exist with CMV pneumonia. The hallmark of the histopathological findings of CMV pneumonia is demonstrating the intracytoplasmic inclusion bodies within areas of inflammation on lung biopsy. These eosinophilic bodies may be absent early in the process. There are also areas of mononuclear interstitial pneumonitis with or without alveolar epithelial desquamation and hyaline membrane formation. These findings can be rarely demonstrated by bronchoscopic biopsy; however, usually surgical lung biopsy by video-assisted thoracoscopy is necessary. Cytological examination of the BAL fluid to detect the inclusion bodies within the lower respiratory tract epithelial cells is highly specific (98%) for CMV pneumonia, but has low sensitivity, with a positive-predicted value of 73% and a negative predictive value of 99.5% [207]. On the other hand, rapid culture of the BAL fluid using the shell viral technique is highly sensitive (99%) in detecting the virus, but lacks the specificity (67–83%), since it cannot differentiate between viral shedding and invasive disease [207, 208]. The value of detecting CMV antigens in the diagnosis of CMV pneumonia is controversial. CMV pp65 antigen assay is based on staining blood neutrophils for the pp65 antigen. The test requires an adequate number of neutrophils (>1,000 cells mm^3), so it is not useful in the presence of neutropenia [209]. Another way to quantitatively measure CMV viral load is by detecting the viral DNA by PCR, which could be done on whole blood, plasma, leukocytes, BAL, urine and CSF. Detection of CMV viral DNA in the BAL fluid is suggestive of CMV pneumonia; however, false-positive results are frequent [210]. Detecting blood CMV antigens–by either method–correlates well with CMV pneumonia [211, 212]. However, it is possible for CMV pneumonia to develop without antigenemia [213]. CMV antigens in blood samples may precede clinical features of CMV pneumonia by up to 3 weeks [214]. These tests are also useful in monitoring the response to antiviral therapy. Persistence of CMV antigenemia after 2 weeks of therapy should raise suspicion of antiviral resistance. Gancyclovir as a single agent or in combination with CMV immunoglobulins has been shown to be effective in uncontrolled trials in the treatment of CMV pneumonia and is currently the standard of care in the management of this condition [194, 197]. This is reported in the reviews from Dr. Vigil and from Dr. Sandherr. With this approach, mortality has decreased to 0–47% provided treatment is started prior to the onset of acute respiratory failure. Survival of patients with respiratory failure at the time of initiation of therapy remains infrequent. Prevention of CMV infection is the best approach to avoid disease. Use of CMV negative stem cells for HSCT and seronegative or leukocyte-filtered blood products for CMV seronegative recipients decreases the risk of infection to 2–4% [215–217]. Antiviral prophylaxis and viral monitoring with pre-emptive therapy are at present the two main antiviral strategies used in the prevention of CMV infection and disease. Gancyclovir prophylaxis administered in seropositive patients or in seronegative subjects receiving graft from a seropositive donor from 5 days before engraftment to 100 days after HSCT reduces the risk of CMV infection and invasive disease, as well as mortality [218]. However, this approach did not change the overall survival owing to increased sepsis associated with gancyclovir-induced neutropenia and shift in the onset of the CMV disease later in the course following HSCT when the prophylactic treatment is discontinued [219]. Valgancyclovir showed promise as an alternative antiviral agent for preemptive treatment of CMV reactivation following allogeneic HSCT [220]. The use of a cutoff of the number of CMV DNA copies in whole blood samples (10,000 DNA copies/ml) may be useful in avoiding unnecessary antiviral treatment [221]. Other interventions that are under evaluation include infusion of donor-derived CMV-specific cytotoxic T lymphocyte infusion and CMV vaccine [222].

3.6 Community Respiratory Viruses

There are four community respiratory viral agents that commonly lead to serious infection in patients with hematological malignancies. These are respiratory syncytial virus (RSV), parainfluenza, influenza and adenovirus. In this book, Schnell and coworkers provide a comprehensive overview on pneumonia related to common viruses in hematological patients. The data on the significance of community respiratory viral infections in this patient population are limited for several reasons, including reports based on small case series, the seasonal nature of the infection that may change the frequency of these infections depending on the time and location of the study, and the fact that many of the patients with community respiratory viral infections are asymptomatic. Nevertheless, there have been recent large studies that improved our understanding of the role of community respiratory viral infections in patients with hematological malignancies, especially those who underwent HSCT. Overall, it appears that the incidence of these viral infections in patients with hematological malignancies ranges between 11 and 65% [223–226]. In one study of community respiratory viral infections following HSCT, the main viruses were RSV (35%), parainfluenza (30%), rhinovirus (25%) and influenza virus (11%). Of these, pneumonia occurred in 49% of patients with RSV infection, 22% of those with parainfluenza virus and 3% of rhinovirus infection [227]. In another recent review of 343 cases of community respiratory viral infections in 306 adult patients with hematological malignancies, parainfluenza (mainly type 3) accounted for 27% of infections, influenza (mainly type A) in 33% of infections and RSV in 31% of infections. Community respiratory viral infections progressed to pneumonia in 35% of patients with equal frequency among the three viruses. The patients at high risk for community respiratory viral infections included allogeneic HSCT, leukemia, age older than 65 years, and presence of severe neutropenia or lymphopenia. The overall mortality for community respiratory viral pneumonia was 15%. The only independent predictor of fatal outcome was absolute lymphopenia in patients with influenza pneumonia [226].

The diagnosis of lower respiratory tract community respiratory viral infection is usually suspected in patients with preceding upper respiratory tract infection. The high-resolution CT scan of the chest usually shows patchy or extensive ground-glass opacities, or a mixture of patterns including ground-glass attenuation, thickening of the bronchial walls, and multiple small nodules that may have centrilobular or random distribution. Consolidation and pleural effusions are less common [228]. The diagnosis is usually made using the combination of direct fluorescent antibody (DFA) and indirect fluorescent antibody (IFA) testing, and viral cultures of clinical specimens. The results of the former tests are usually available within 24 h, whereas cultures usually take 7–14 days. The clinical specimens are best obtained by nasopharyngeal wash or swabs. The sensitivity of direct DFA and IFA in detecting infection in patients with hematological malignancies ranges between 20% and 52% [229–231]. BAL fluid may also be helpful when lower respiratory tract infection is suspected with a sensitivity of around 70% [225]. It is important to note in this context that community respiratory viruses are often co-pathogens with other organisms, including bacteria, fungi (such as

Aspergillus and *P. jiroveci*) or other viruses (such as CMV) [232]. In one study of community respiratory viral pneumonia, 119 patients had BAL specimens, and 14% had other pathogens cultured [226]. This may create a challenge to clinicians, and every effort should be made to exclude such infections in which community respiratory viruses are isolated.

Community respiratory viruses associated with upper respiratory tract infections in patients with hematological malignancies are usually self-limiting and are not associated with increased mortality. However, not uncommonly these patients develop lower respiratory tract infection that is associated with higher mortality [226]. Another potential risk associated with community respiratory viral infections is the development of bronchiolitis obliterans following allogeneic HSCT. In a large series of new-onset airflow obstruction following allogeneic HSCT, one of the main risk factors was respiratory viral infections within the first 100 days following transplantation [233]. Lower respiratory tract parainfluenza [OR 17.9 (95% CI, 2.0–160) and RSV (OR 3.6, 95% CI, 1.0–13)] infections were independent risk factors for development of airflow decline 1 year after allogeneic HSCT [234].

Given the high mortality associated with community respiratory viral lower respiratory tract infections in hematological malignancies, preventive measures play an important role in avoiding infection in these patients. Simple measures such as hand washing are very effective against infection (except for influenza, which is transmitted by aerosolized droplets). In addition, isolating patients suspected to have community respiratory viral infection, even before the infection is confirmed, has been shown to be effective [19]. Symptomatic health-care providers should be restricted from contact with patients with hematological malignancies who are severely immunocompromised [235]. It is also advisable to limit visitors to these patients during the winter months [19].

3.6.1 Respiratory Syncytial Virus (RSV)

RSV is one of the most common community respiratory virus infection in patients with hematological malignancies [236–238]. The reported incidence of RSV infection in HSCT recipients ranges between 3.5% and 6.3% and 0.4–1.5% following allogeneic and autologous transplantation, respectively [239, 240]. RSV infection usually starts with upper respiratory tract symptoms including cough, rhinorrhea and sinus congestion. Wheezing may develop in 30%; however, fever may not be present even with lower respiratory tract infection [241]. The most serious complication of RSV infection in this patient population is the development of lower respiratory tract infection that happens in up to one third of patients and is associated with high mortality (19%) [226, 242]. Lack of RSV-directed antiviral therapy and older age are associated with increased risk of progression to pneumonia [226]. Other risk factors for RSV pneumonia include male gender, high APACHE II score, protracted lymphopenia and recent corticosteroid therapy [243]. Lower respiratory tract infection is characterized by progressive dyspnea and hypoxemia. The radiological findings of RSV pneumonia include multiple small nodules, bud on tree pattern, diffuse ground-glass infiltrates and bronchial thickening [244]. The diagnosis of RSV lower respiratory tract infection could be made by DFA, IFA or PCR of nasopharyngeal or BAL specimens [245].

The role of pharmacological therapy in RSV infection in patients with hematological malignancies remains controversial. Several studies have suggested benefit from ribavirin (intravenously, orally or aerosolized) with or without RSV-specific intravenous immunoglobulins [246, 247]. The efficacy of this treatment once the patient develops acute respiratory failure requiring mechanical ventilation is significantly lower [246]. Delivery of aerosolized ribavirin requires a special machine that is not widely available. Care should be taken during aerosolization of this medication since those who are exposed to it may develop headaches, skin rash and conjunctivitis. Furthermore, ribavirin has teratogenic effects, and pregnant women should not enter the patient's room during treatment [247]. Other therapeutic modalities, such as high titer monoclonal antibody against RSV, are under investigation [239, 248]. In a recent trial on HSCT, recipients with upper respiratory tract RSV infection were randomized to preemptive aerosolized ribavirin or supportive therapy to prevent progression to lower respiratory tract infection. The intervention was safe and associated with reduced viral load; however, the study could not prove the efficacy of aerosolized ribavirin in preventing progression to lower respiratory tract RSV infection [249].

3.6.2 Parainfluenza Virus

Parainfluenza is another important cause of community respiratory viral infections in patients with hematological malignancies [227, 250, 251]. Parainfluenza has four serotypes, and serotypes 1 and 3 are reportedly the most common causes of infection in these patients. Parainfluenza infection is variable throughout the year, with outbreaks reported in winter, and sometimes in spring and summer.

Parainfluenza infection usually presents with cough; however, rhinorrhea and fever are uncommon. Lower respiratory tract infection is the most serious complication of parainfluenza infection and is reported in 18–100% (mean 33%) of patients, with mortality ranging between 15% and 73% (mean 50%) [242]. It is estimated that up to 50% of patients with parainfluenza lower respiratory tract infection have co-infection with bacteria or fungi [251]. The diagnosis of parainfluenza infection is usually made by IFA or DFA and culture of respiratory samples. Real-time PCR is under development and is not available for clinical practice. Treatment of parainfluenza infection is supportive. Ribavirin has activity against parainfluenza and has been shown to be helpful in small studies; [247, 252] however, large studies failed to demonstrate benefit from this therapy [251]. It is recommended to consider aerosolized ribavirin in the treatment of parainfluenza lower respiratory tract infection, although experience to date provides little evidence of efficacy [247].

3.6.3 Influenza

Influenza infection has been described in patients with hematological malignancies as a community or nosocomial infection. It develops in the winter months, and the clinical picture is similar to normal hosts with fever, rhinorrhea, coryza, mayalgia and headache. Following HSCT, the frequency of influenza infection is similar with autologous and allogeneic transplantation. In one study of children with cancer, 40% of patients were on chemotherapy, and 63% were lymphopenic. Only one third of the patients were neutropenic [253]. Prognosis is worse in patients with lymphopenia and in those who develop infection early post HSCT [226, 254].

The treatment of influenza infection is supportive. Antiviral agents, such as amantadine, rimantadine, oseltamivir and zanamivir, may be considered in patients with severe infection [255]. In one report, early treatment with oseltamivir was associated with a trend to less progression to lower respiratory tract infection and decreased viral shedding [254]. Vaccination against influenza is effective; however, live attenuated preparations should be avoided in these patients, and that HSCT recipients may respond poorly to vaccination in the first 2 years following transplantation must be taken into consideration [247].

The pandemic of novel H1N1 influenza is another risk to patients with hematological malignancies. Patients with suspected or confirmed infection should be treated with either oseltamivir or zanamivir. Patients with immunocompromising conditions are advised to receive the inactivated novel H1N1 influenza vaccine [256].

3.6.4 Adenovirus

Adenovirus infection accounts for 0–21% of community respiratory viral infections in patients with hematological malignancies and is more common in children [242, 257]. Patients with allogeneic HSCT may have delayed adenovirus-specific T-cell immune recovery, which correlates with increased risk of adenovirus associated morbidity and mortality [258]. Approximately 20% of patients with adenovirus infection develop pneumonia [259]. Histologically, the diagnosis is suggested by the presence of the characteristic smudge cells [259]. There are limited antiviral agents with activity against adenovirus. Ribavirin and gancyclovir have no significant activity against this virus [260, 261].

3.6.5 Other Viruses

As reported in the paper from Shah and Chemaly, *Herpes simplex virus-1* reactivates in the majority of these patients and occasionally may be associated with pneumonia. HHV6 has been suggested to have a role in the pathogenesis of idiopathic pneumonia syndrome following HSCT [262]. It may act as a co-pathogen with CMV or as an isolated cause of pneumonia [262]. In a recent report, HHV-6 was isolated from 56.6% of peripheral blood or other specimen tested following HSCT; however, it was associated with interstitial/alveolar pneumonia in only 2% of patients. HHV-6 reactivation was significantly associated with GVHD, Epstein-Barr viral co-infection, and unrelated donor transplantation [263].

In the chapter from Dr. Schildgen, emerging viral infections are reviewed. *Human metapneumovirus* is another RNA respiratory virus that has been detected in 3.2% of patients with hematological malignancies. Around half of the patients have pulmonary radiological abnormalities. The prognosis of this infection is good, and the majority of patients do not require antiviral therapy [264].

3.7 Conclusion

Patients with hematological malignancies have defects in their immune system that involve one or more of the defense cell lines. These patients are at high risk for a variety of respiratory infectious and noninfectious complications that are related to their underlying malignancies or due to the aggressive therapy of these conditions. There have been significant advances in the diagnosis and management of respiratory infections in patients with hematological malignancies. *P. jiroveci* and CMV infections are very rare. The treatment of bacterial pneumonias has improved with the availability of broad-spectrum antibiotics. The management of fungal infections, including IPA, is enhanced by the introduction of noninvasive diagnostic methods such as galactomannan assay and better tolerated antifungal agents.

Future directions in the management of respiratory infections in patients with hematological malignancies need to focus on more robust and validated noninvasive diagnostic assays that allow for earlier detection and preemptive therapy of fungal and viral infections. Also more emphasis is needed on prevention of respiratory infections. More effective and safer antiviral agents should be another area of research and development as well as the role of combination antimicrobial agents in the management of severe viral and fungal infections. Respiratory infections in patients with hematological malignancies can also be minimized by improved treatment regimens including enhanced HSCT techniques that lead to better engraftment and less GVHD. More targeted chemotherapeutic regimens may also decrease the risk of opportunistic infections.

References

1. www.cancer.gov. In: wwwcancergov. Accessed Oct 2009
2. www.ibmtr.org. Accessed Oct 2009
3. Maschmeyer G, Link H, Hiddemann W et al (1994) Pulmonary infiltrations in febrile patients with neutropenia. Risk factors and outcome under empirical antimicrobial therapy in a randomized multicenter study. Cancer 73(9):2296–2304
4. Soubani AO, Miller KB, Hassoun PM (1996) Pulmonary complications of bone marrow transplantation. Chest 109(4):1066–1077
5. Ewig S, Torres A, Riquelme R et al (1998) Pulmonary complications in patients with haematological malignancies treated at a respiratory ICU. Eur Respir J 12(1): 116–122
6. Lazarus HM, Vogelsang GB, Rowe JM (1997) Prevention and treatment of acute graft-versus-host disease: the old and the new. A report from the Eastern Cooperative Oncology Group (ECOG). Bone Marrow Transplant 19(6): 577–600
7. Gerson SL, Talbot GH, Hurwitz S, Strom BL, Lusk EJ, Cassileth PA (1984) Prolonged granulocytopenia: the major risk factor for invasive pulmonary aspergillosis in patients with acute leukemia. Ann Intern Med 100(3):345–351
8. Hofmeister CC, Czerlanis C, Forsythe S, Stiff PJ (2006) Retrospective utility of bronchoscopy after hematopoietic stem cell transplant. Bone Marrow Transplant 38(10): 693–698
9. Paulin T, Ringden O, Lonnqvist B (1985) Faster immunological recovery after bone marrow transplantation in patients without cytomegalovirus infection. Transplantation 39(4):377–384
10. Witherspoon RP, Storb R, Ochs HD et al (1981) Recovery of antibody production in human allogeneic marrow graft recipients: influence of time posttransplantation, the presence or absence of chronic graft-versus-host disease, and antithymocyte globulin treatment. Blood 58(2):360–368
11. Aucouturier P, Barra A, Intrator L et al (1987) Long lasting IgG subclass and antibacterial polysaccharide antibody deficiency after allogeneic bone marrow transplantation. Blood 70(3):779–785
12. Kotloff RM, Ahya VN, Crawford SW (2004) Pulmonary complications of solid organ and hematopoietic stem cell transplantation. Am J Respir Crit Care Med 170(1): 22–48
13. Sloane JP, Depledge MH, Powles RL, Morgenstern GR, Trickey BS, Dady PJ (1983) Histopathology of the lung after bone marrow transplantation. J Clin Pathol 36(5):546–554

14. Lossos IS, Breuer R, Or R et al (1995) Bacterial pneumonia in recipients of bone marrow transplantation. A five-year prospective study. Transplantation 60(7):672–678
15. Wingard JR (1999) Opportunistic infections after blood and marrow transplantation. Transpl Infect Dis 1(1):3–20
16. Poutsiaka DD, Price LL, Ucuzian A, Chan GW, Miller KB, Snydman DR (2007) Blood stream infection after hematopoietic stem cell transplantation is associated with increased mortality. Bone Marrow Transplant 40(1):63–70
17. Rolston KV (2001) The spectrum of pulmonary infections in cancer patients. Curr Opin Oncol 13(4):218–223
18. Heussel CP, Kauczor HU, Heussel G, Fischer B, Mildenberger P, Thelen M (1997) Early detection of pneumonia in febrile neutropenic patients: use of thin-section CT. AJR Am J Roentgenol 169(5):1347–1353
19. Guidelines for preventing opportunistic infections among hematopoietic stem cell transplant recipients. MMWR Recomm Rep 2000;49(RR-10):1–125, CE1-7
20. Laws HJ, Kobbe G, Dilloo D et al (2006) Surveillance of nosocomial infections in paediatric recipients of bone marrow or peripheral blood stem cell transplantation during neutropenia, compared with adult recipients. J Hosp Infect 62(1):80–88
21. Narreddy S, Mellon-Reppen S, Abidi MH et al (2007) Non-bacterial infections in allogeneic non-myeloablative stem cell transplant recipients. Transpl Infect Dis 9(1):3–10
22. Chen CS, Boeckh M, Seidel K et al (2003) Incidence, risk factors, and mortality from pneumonia developing late after hematopoietic stem cell transplantation. Bone Marrow Transplant 32(5):515–522
23. Youssef S, Rodriguez G, Rolston KV, Champlin RE, Raad II, Safdar A (2007) Streptococcus pneumoniae infections in 47 hematopoietic stem cell transplantation recipients: clinical characteristics of infections and vaccine-breakthrough infections, 1989-2005. Medicine (Baltimore) 86(2):69–77
24. Hakki M, Limaye AP, Kim HW, Kirby KA, Corey L, Boeckh M (2007) Invasive Pseudomonas aeruginosa infections: high rate of recurrence and mortality after hematopoietic cell transplantation. Bone Marrow Transplant 39(11): 687–693
25. Jacobson KL, Miceli MH, Tarrand JJ, Kontoyiannis DP (2008) Legionella pneumonia in cancer patients. Medicine (Baltimore) 87(3):152–159
26. Oren I, Zuckerman T, Avivi I, Finkelstein R, Yigla M, Rowe JM (2002) Nosocomial outbreak of Legionella pneumophila serogroup 3 pneumonia in a new bone marrow transplant unit: evaluation, treatment and control. Bone Marrow Transplant 30(3):175–179
27. Niederman MS, Mandell LA, Anzueto A et al (2001) Guidelines for the management of adults with community-acquired pneumonia. Diagnosis, assessment of severity, antimicrobial therapy, and prevention. Am J Respir Crit Care Med 163(7):1730–1754
28. Niederman MS, Craven DE, Bonten MJ et al (2005) Guidelines for the management of adults with hospital-acquired, ventilator-associated, and healthcare-associated pneumonia. Am J Respir Crit Care Med 171(4): 388–416
29. Sullivan KM, Dykewicz CA, Longworth DL, et al (2001) Preventing opportunistic infections after hematopoietic stem cell transplantation: the Centers for Disease Control and Prevention, Infectious Diseases Society of America, and American Society for Blood and Marrow Transplantation Practice Guidelines and beyond. Hematol Am Soc Hematol Educ Program 1:392–421
30. Bonadio M, Morelli G, Mori S, Riccioni R, Papineschi F, Petrini M (2005) Fluoroquinolone resistance in hematopoietic stem cell transplant recipients with infectious complications. Biomed Pharmacother 59(9):511–516
31. Daly AS, McGeer A, Lipton JH (2003) Systemic nocardiosis following allogeneic bone marrow transplantation. Transpl Infect Dis 5(1):16–20
32. van Burik JA, Hackman RC, Nadeem SQ et al (1997) Nocardiosis after bone marrow transplantation: a retrospective study. Clin Infect Dis 24(6):1154–1160
33. Aisenberg GM, Jacobson K, Chemaly RF, Rolston KV, Raad II, Safdar A (2005) Extrapulmonary tuberculosis active infection misdiagnosed as cancer: mycobacterium tuberculosis disease in patients at a Comprehensive Cancer Center (2001–2005). Cancer 104(12):2882–2887
34. Mishra P, Kumar R, Mahapatra M et al (2006) Tuberculosis in acute leukemia: a clinico-hematological profile. Hematology 11(5):335–340
35. Roy V, Weisdorf D (1997) Mycobacterial infections following bone marrow transplantation: a 20 year retrospective review. Bone Marrow Transplant 19(5):467–470
36. de la Camara R, Martino R, Granados E et al (2000) Tuberculosis after hematopoietic stem cell transplantation: incidence, clinical characteristics and outcome. Spanish Group on infectious complications in hematopoietic transplantation. Bone Marrow Transplant 26(3):291–298
37. Cordonnier C, Martino R, Trabasso P et al (2004) Mycobacterial infection: a difficult and late diagnosis in stem cell transplant recipients. Clin Infect Dis 38(9): 1229–1236
38. Ip MS, Yuen KY, Woo PC et al (1998) Risk factors for pulmonary tuberculosis in bone marrow transplant recipients. Am J Respir Crit Care Med 158(4):1173–1177
39. Ku SC, Tang JL, Hsueh PR, Luh KT, Yu CJ, Yang PC (2001) Pulmonary tuberculosis in allogeneic hematopoietic stem cell transplantation. Bone Marrow Transplant 27(12): 1293–1297
40. Yuen KY, Woo PC (2002) Tuberculosis in blood and marrow transplant recipients. Hematol Oncol 20(2):51–62
41. Keung YK, Nugent K, Jumper C, Cobos E (1999) Mycobacterium tuberculosis infection masquerading as diffuse alveolar hemorrhage after autologous stem cell transplant. Bone Marrow Transplant 23(7):737–738
42. Mycobacterium tuberculosis. Am J Transplant 2004;4 (Suppl 10):37–41
43. Richeldi L, Losi M, D'Amico R et al (2009) Performance of tests for latent tuberculosis in different groups of immunocompromised patients. Chest 136(1):198–204
44. Doucette K, Fishman JA (2004) Nontuberculous mycobacterial infection in hematopoietic stem cell and solid organ transplant recipients. Clin Infect Dis 38(10):1428–1439
45. Weinstock DM, Feinstein MB, Sepkowitz KA, Jakubowski A (2003) High rates of infection and colonization by nontuberculous mycobacteria after allogeneic hematopoietic stem cell transplantation. Bone Marrow Transplant 31(11): 1015–1021

46. Nontuberculous mycobacteria. Am J Transplant 2004;4 (Suppl 10):42–46
47. Griffith DE, Aksamit T, Brown-Elliott BA et al (2007) An official ATS/IDSA statement: diagnosis, treatment, and prevention of nontuberculous mycobacterial diseases. Am J Respir Crit Care Med 175(4):367–416
48. Morgan J, Wannemuehler KA, Marr KA et al (2005) Incidence of invasive aspergillosis following hematopoietic stem cell and solid organ transplantation: interim results of a prospective multicenter surveillance program. Med Mycol 43(Suppl 1):S49–S58
49. Wald A, Leisenring W, van Burik JA, Bowden RA (1997) Epidemiology of Aspergillus infections in a large cohort of patients undergoing bone marrow transplantation. J Infect Dis 175(6):1459–1466
50. Marr KA, Carter RA, Boeckh M, Martin P, Corey L (2002) Invasive aspergillosis in allogeneic stem cell transplant recipients: changes in epidemiology and risk factors. Blood 100(13):4358–4366
51. Fukuda T, Boeckh M, Carter RA et al (2003) Risks and outcomes of invasive fungal infections in recipients of allogeneic hematopoietic stem cell transplants after nonmyeloablative conditioning. Blood 102(3):827–833
52. Marr KA, Carter RA, Crippa F, Wald A, Corey L (2002) Epidemiology and outcome of mould infections in hematopoietic stem cell transplant recipients. Clin Infect Dis 34(7):909–917
53. Baddley JW, Stroud TP, Salzman D, Pappas PG (2001) Invasive mold infections in allogeneic bone marrow transplant recipients. Clin Infect Dis 32(9):1319–1324
54. Junghanss C, Marr KA, Carter RA et al (2002) Incidence and outcome of bacterial and fungal infections following nonmyeloablative compared with myeloablative allogeneic hematopoietic stem cell transplantation: a matched control study. Biol Blood Marrow Transplant 8(9): 512–520
55. Miyakoshi S, Kusumi E, Matsumura T et al (2007) Invasive fungal infection following reduced-intensity cord blood transplantation for adult patients with hematologic diseases. Biol Blood Marrow Transplant 13(7):771–777
56. Warris A, Bjorneklett A, Gaustad P (2001) Invasive pulmonary aspergillosis associated with infliximab therapy. N Engl J Med 344(14):1099–1100
57. Cordonnier C, Ribaud P, Herbrecht R et al (2006) Prognostic factors for death due to invasive aspergillosis after hematopoietic stem cell transplantation: a 1-year retrospective study of consecutive patients at French transplantation centers. Clin Infect Dis 42(7):955–963
58. Ribaud P, Chastang C, Latge JP et al (1999) Survival and prognostic factors of invasive aspergillosis after allogeneic bone marrow transplantation. Clin Infect Dis 28(2): 322–330
59. Nichols WG, Corey L, Gooley T, Davis C, Boeckh M (2002) High risk of death due to bacterial and fungal infection among cytomegalovirus (CMV)-seronegative recipients of stem cell transplants from seropositive donors: evidence for indirect effects of primary CMV infection. J Infect Dis 185(3):273–282
60. Nivoix Y, Velten M, Letscher-Bru V et al (2008) Factors associated with overall and attributable mortality in invasive aspergillosis. Clin Infect Dis 47(9):1176–1184
61. Iwen PC, Rupp ME, Langnas AN, Reed EC, Hinrichs SH (1998) Invasive pulmonary aspergillosis due to Aspergillus terreus: 12-year experience and review of the literature. Clin Infect Dis 26(5):1092–1097
62. Young RC, Bennett JE, Vogel CL, Carbone PP, DeVita VT (1970) Aspergillosis. The spectrum of the disease in 98 patients. Medicine (Baltimore) 49(2):147–173
63. Prystowsky SD, Vogelstein B, Ettinger DS et al (1976) Invasive aspergillosis. N Engl J Med 295(12):655–658
64. Allo MD, Miller J, Townsend T, Tan C (1987) Primary cutaneous aspergillosis associated with Hickman intravenous catheters. N Engl J Med 317(18):1105–1108
65. Albelda SM, Talbot GH, Gerson SL, Miller WT, Cassileth PA (1985) Pulmonary cavitation and massive hemoptysis in invasive pulmonary aspergillosis. Influence of bone marrow recovery in patients with acute leukemia. Am Rev Respir Dis 131(1):115–120
66. Denning DW (1998) Invasive aspergillosis. Clin Infect Dis 26(4):781–803, quiz 4-5
67. Ruhnke M, Bohme A, Buchheidt D et al (2003) Diagnosis of invasive fungal infections in hematology and oncology – guidelines of the Infectious Diseases Working Party (AGIHO) of the German Society of Hematology and Oncology (DGHO). Ann Hematol 82(Suppl 2):S141–S148
68. Chamilos G, Luna M, Lewis RE et al (2006) Invasive fungal infections in patients with hematologic malignancies in a tertiary care cancer center: an autopsy study over a 15-year period (1989–2003). Haematologica 91(7): 986–989
69. Libshitz HI, Pagani JJ (1981) Aspergillosis and mucormycosis: two types of opportunistic fungal pneumonia. Radiology 140(2):301–306
70. Kuhlman JE, Fishman EK, Siegelman SS (1985) Invasive pulmonary aspergillosis in acute leukemia: characteristic findings on CT, the CT halo sign, and the role of CT in early diagnosis. Radiology 157(3):611–614
71. Caillot D, Casasnovas O, Bernard A et al (1997) Improved management of invasive pulmonary aspergillosis in neutropenic patients using early thoracic computed tomographic scan and surgery. J Clin Oncol 15(1):139–147
72. Caillot D, Mannone L, Cuisenier B, Couaillier JF (2001) Role of early diagnosis and aggressive surgery in the management of invasive pulmonary aspergillosis in neutropenic patients. Clin Microbiol Infect 7(Suppl 2):54–61
73. Kuhlman JE, Fishman EK, Burch PA, Karp JE, Zerhouni EA, Siegelman SS (1987) Invasive pulmonary aspergillosis in acute leukemia. The contribution of CT to early diagnosis and aggressive management. Chest 92(1):95–99
74. Curtis AM, Smith GJ, Ravin CE (1979) Air crescent sign of invasive aspergillosis. Radiology 133(1):17–21
75. Gaeta M, Blandino A, Scribano E, Minutoli F, Volta S, Pandolfo I (1999) Computed tomography halo sign in pulmonary nodules: frequency and diagnostic value. J Thorac Imaging 14(2):109–113
76. Greene R (2005) The radiological spectrum of pulmonary aspergillosis. Med Mycol 43(Suppl 1):S147–S154
77. Kojima R, Tateishi U, Kami M et al (2005) Chest computed tomography of late invasive aspergillosis after allogeneic hematopoietic stem cell transplantation. Biol Blood Marrow Transplant 11(7):506–511
78. Greene RE, Schlamm HT, Oestmann JW et al (2007) Imaging findings in acute invasive pulmonary aspergillosis:

clinical significance of the halo sign. Clin Infect Dis 44(3):373–379

79. Horger M, Hebart H, Einsele H et al (2005) Initial CT manifestations of invasive pulmonary aspergillosis in 45 non-HIV immunocompromised patients: association with patient outcome? Eur J Radiol 55(3):437–444
80. Soubani AO, Qureshi MA (2002) Invasive pulmonary aspergillosis following bone marrow transplantation: risk factors and diagnostic aspect. Haematologia (Budap) 32(4):427–437
81. Horvath JA, Dummer S (1996) The use of respiratory-tract cultures in the diagnosis of invasive pulmonary aspergillosis. Am J Med 100(2):171–178
82. Yu VL, Muder RR, Poorsattar A (1986) Significance of isolation of Aspergillus from the respiratory tract in diagnosis of invasive pulmonary aspergillosis.Results from a three-year prospective study. Am J Med 81(2):249–254
83. Tang CM, Cohen J (1992) Diagnosing fungal infections in immunocompromised hosts. J Clin Pathol 45(1):1–5
84. Duthie R, Denning DW (1995) Aspergillus fungemia: report of two cases and review. Clin Infect Dis 20(3): 598–605
85. Albelda SM, Talbot GH, Gerson SL, Miller WT, Cassileth PA (1984) Role of fiberoptic bronchoscopy in the diagnosis of invasive pulmonary aspergillosis in patients with acute leukemia. Am J Med 76(6):1027–1034
86. Kahn FW, Jones JM, England DM (1986) The role of bronchoalveolar lavage in the diagnosis of invasive pulmonary aspergillosis. Am J Clin Pathol 86(4):518–523
87. Levy H, Horak DA, Tegtmeier BR, Yokota SB, Forman SJ (1992) The value of bronchoalveolar lavage and bronchial washings in the diagnosis of invasive pulmonary aspergillosis. Respir Med 86(3):243–248
88. Reichenberger F, Habicht J, Matt P et al (1999) Diagnostic yield of bronchoscopy in histologically proven invasive pulmonary aspergillosis. Bone Marrow Transplant 24(11):1195–1199
89. Maschmeyer G, Beinert T, Buchheidt D et al (2003) Diagnosis and antimicrobial therapy of pulmonary infiltrates in febrile neutropenic patients – guidelines of the Infectious Diseases Working Party (AGIHO) of the German Society of Hematology and Oncology (DGHO). Ann Hematol 82(Suppl 2):S118–S126
90. Panackal AA, Marr KA (2004) Scedosporium/pseudallescheria infections. Semin Respir Crit Care Med 25(2):171–181
91. Walsh TJ, Groll AH (2001) Overview: non-fumigatus species of Aspergillus: perspectives on emerging pathogens in immunocompromised hosts. Curr Opin Investig Drugs 2(10):1366–1367
92. Lass-Florl C, Griff K, Mayr A et al (2005) Epidemiology and outcome of infections due to Aspergillus terreus: 10-year single centre experience. Br J Haematol 131(2): 201–207
93. Steinbach WJ, Benjamin DK Jr, Kontoyiannis DP et al (2004) Infections due to Aspergillus terreus: a multicenter retrospective analysis of 83 cases. Clin Infect Dis 39(2):192–198
94. Hachem RY, Kontoyiannis DP, Boktour MR et al (2004) Aspergillus terreus: an emerging amphotericin B-resistant opportunistic mold in patients with hematologic malignancies. Cancer 101(7):1594–1600
95. Kontoyiannis DP, Lewis RE, May GS, Osherov N, Rinaldi MG (2002) Aspergillus nidulans is frequently resistant to amphotericin B. Mycoses 45(9–10):406–407
96. Walsh TJ, Raad I, Patterson TF et al (2007) Treatment of invasive aspergillosis with posaconazole in patients who are refractory to or intolerant of conventional therapy: an externally controlled trial. Clin Infect Dis 44(1):2–12
97. Boutboul F, Alberti C, Leblanc T et al (2002) Invasive aspergillosis in allogeneic stem cell transplant recipients: increasing antigenemia is associated with progressive disease. Clin Infect Dis 34(7):939–943
98. Marr KA, Balajee SA, McLaughlin L, Tabouret M, Bentsen C, Walsh TJ (2004) Detection of galactomannan antigenemia by enzyme immunoassay for the diagnosis of invasive aspergillosis: variables that affect performance. J Infect Dis 190(3):641–649
99. Pfeiffer CD, Fine JP, Safdar N (2006) Diagnosis of invasive aspergillosis using a galactomannan assay: a meta-analysis. Clin Infect Dis 42(10):1417–1727
100. Herbrecht R, Letscher-Bru V, Oprea C et al (2002) Aspergillus galactomannan detection in the diagnosis of invasive aspergillosis in cancer patients. J Clin Oncol 20(7):1898–1906
101. Singh N, Obman A, Husain S, Aspinall S, Mietzner S, Stout JE (2004) Reactivity of platelia Aspergillus galactomannan antigen with piperacillin-tazobactam: clinical implications based on achievable concentrations in serum. Antimicrob Agents Chemother 48(6):1989–1992
102. Marr KA, Laverdiere M, Gugel A, Leisenring W (2005) Antifungal therapy decreases sensitivity of the Aspergillus galactomannan enzyme immunoassay. Clin Infect Dis 40(12):1762–1769
103. Ansorg R, van den Boom R, Rath PM (1997) Detection of Aspergillus galactomannan antigen in foods and antibiotics. Mycoses 40(9–10):353–357
104. Busca A, Locatelli F, Barbui A et al (2006) Usefulness of sequential Aspergillus galactomannan antigen detection combined with early radiologic evaluation for diagnosis of invasive pulmonary aspergillosis in patients undergoing allogeneic stem cell transplantation. Transplant Proc 38(5):1610–1613
105. Musher B, Fredricks D, Leisenring W, Balajee SA, Smith C, Marr KA (2004) Aspergillus galactomannan enzyme immunoassay and quantitative PCR for diagnosis of invasive aspergillosis with bronchoalveolar lavage fluid. J Clin Microbiol 42(12):5517–5522
106. Klont RR, Mennink-Kersten MA, Verweij PE (2004) Utility of Aspergillus antigen detection in specimens other than serum specimens. Clin Infect Dis 39(10): 1467–1474
107. Salonen J, Lehtonen OP, Terasjarvi MR, Nikoskelainen J (2000) Aspergillus antigen in serum, urine and bronchoalveolar lavage specimens of neutropenic patients in relation to clinical outcome. Scand J Infect Dis 32(5):485–490
108. Penack O, Rempf P, Graf B, Blau IW, Thiel E (2008) Aspergillus galactomannan testing in patients with long-term neutropenia: implications for clinical management. Ann Oncol 19(5):984–989
109. Maertens J, Buve K, Theunissen K et al (2009) Galactomannan serves as a surrogate endpoint for outcome of pulmonary invasive aspergillosis in neutropenic hematology patients. Cancer 115(2):355–362

110. Hizel K, Kokturk N, Kalkanci A, Ozturk C, Kustimur S, Tufan M (2004) Polymerase chain reaction in the diagnosis of invasive aspergillosis. Mycoses 47(7):338–342
111. Buchheidt D, Baust C, Skladny H et al (2001) Detection of Aspergillus species in blood and bronchoalveolar lavage samples from immunocompromised patients by means of 2-step polymerase chain reaction: clinical results. Clin Infect Dis 33(4):428–435
112. Loeffler J, Kloepfer K, Hebart H et al (2002) Polymerase chain reaction detection of aspergillus DNA in experimental models of invasive aspergillosis. J Infect Dis 185(8): 1203–1206
113. Halliday C, Hoile R, Sorrell T et al (2006) Role of prospective screening of blood for invasive aspergillosis by polymerase chain reaction in febrile neutropenic recipients of haematopoietic stem cell transplants and patients with acute leukaemia. Br J Haematol 132(4):478–486
114. Obayashi T, Yoshida M, Mori T et al (1995) Plasma (1 –>3)-beta-D-glucan measurement in diagnosis of invasive deep mycosis and fungal febrile episodes. Lancet 345(8941):17–20
115. Senn L, Robinson JO, Schmidt S et al (2008) 1, 3-Beta-D-glucan antigenemia for early diagnosis of invasive fungal infections in neutropenic patients with acute leukemia. Clin Infect Dis 46(6):878–885
116. Ascioglu S, Rex JH, de Pauw B et al (2002) Defining opportunistic invasive fungal infections in immunocompromised patients with cancer and hematopoietic stem cell transplants: an international consensus. Clin Infect Dis 34(1):7–14
117. De Pauw B, Walsh TJ, Donnelly JP et al (2008) Revised definitions of invasive fungal disease from the European Organization for Research and Treatment of Cancer/Invasive Fungal Infections Cooperative Group and the National Institute of Allergy and Infectious Diseases Mycoses Study Group (EORTC/MSG) Consensus Group. Clin Infect Dis 46(12):1813–1821
118. Johnson LB, Kauffman CA (2003) Voriconazole: a new triazole antifungal agent. Clin Infect Dis 36(5):630–637
119. Sambatakou H, Dupont B, Lode H, Denning DW (2006) Voriconazole treatment for subacute invasive and chronic pulmonary aspergillosis. Am J Med 119(6):527, e17-24
120. Ghannoum MA, Kuhn DM (2002) Voriconazole – better chances for patients with invasive mycoses. Eur J Med Res 7(5):242–256
121. Herbrecht R, Denning DW, Patterson TF et al (2002) Voriconazole versus amphotericin B for primary therapy of invasive aspergillosis. N Engl J Med 347(6):408–415
122. Segal BH, Barnhart LA, Anderson VL, Walsh TJ, Malech HL, Holland SM (2005) Posaconazole as salvage therapy in patients with chronic granulomatous disease and invasive filamentous fungal infection. Clin Infect Dis 40(11): 1684–1688
123. Pitisuttithum P, Negroni R, Graybill JR et al (2005) Activity of posaconazole in the treatment of central nervous system fungal infections. J Antimicrob Chemother 56(4):745–755
124. Spanakis EK, Aperis G, Mylonakis E (2006) New agents for the treatment of fungal infections: clinical efficacy and gaps in coverage. Clin Infect Dis 43(8):1060–1068
125. Cohen-Wolkowiez M, Benjamin DK Jr, Steinbach WJ, Smith PB (2006) Anidulafungin: a new echinocandin for the treatment of fungal infections. Drugs Today (Barc) 42(8):533–544
126. Walsh TJ, Anaissie EJ, Denning DW et al (2008) Treatment of aspergillosis: clinical practice guidelines of the Infectious Diseases Society of America. Clin Infect Dis 46(3): 327–360
127. Aliff TB, Maslak PG, Jurcic JG et al (2003) Refractory Aspergillus pneumonia in patients with acute leukemia: successful therapy with combination caspofungin and liposomal amphotericin. Cancer 97(4):1025–1032
128. Kontoyiannis DP, Hachem R, Lewis RE et al (2003) Efficacy and toxicity of caspofungin in combination with liposomal amphotericin B as primary or salvage treatment of invasive aspergillosis in patients with hematologic malignancies. Cancer 98(2):292–299
129. Graybill JR, Bocanegra R, Gonzalez GM, Najvar LK (2003) Combination antifungal therapy of murine aspergillosis: liposomal amphotericin B and micafungin. J Antimicrob Chemother 52(4):656–662
130. Marr KA, Boeckh M, Carter RA, Kim HW, Corey L (2004) Combination antifungal therapy for invasive aspergillosis. Clin Infect Dis 39(6):797–802
131. Perea S, Gonzalez G, Fothergill AW, Kirkpatrick WR, Rinaldi MG, Patterson TF (2002) In vitro interaction of caspofungin acetate with voriconazole against clinical isolates of Aspergillus spp. Antimicrob Agents Chemother 46(9):3039–3041
132. Denning DW, Marr KA, Lau WM et al (2006) Micafungin (FK463), alone or in combination with other systemic antifungal agents, for the treatment of acute invasive aspergillosis. J Infect 53(5):337–349
133. Moreau P, Zahar JR, Milpied N et al (1993) Localized invasive pulmonary aspergillosis in patients with neutropenia. Effectiveness of surgical resection. Cancer 72(11): 3223–3226
134. Reichenberger F, Habicht J, Kaim A et al (1998) Lung resection for invasive pulmonary aspergillosis in neutropenic patients with hematologic diseases. Am J Respir Crit Care Med 158(3):885–890
135. Habicht JM, Reichenberger F, Gratwohl A, Zerkowski HR, Tamm M (1999) Surgical aspects of resection for suspected invasive pulmonary fungal infection in neutropenic patients. Ann Thorac Surg 68(2):321–325
136. Pidhorecky I, Urschel J, Anderson T (2000) Resection of invasive pulmonary aspergillosis in immunocompromised patients. Ann Surg Oncol 7(4):312–317
137. Matt P, Bernet F, Habicht J et al (2004) Predicting outcome after lung resection for invasive pulmonary aspergillosis in patients with neutropenia. Chest 126(6): 1783–1788
138. Baron O, Guillaume B, Moreau P et al (1998) Aggressive surgical management in localized pulmonary mycotic and nonmycotic infections for neutropenic patients with acute leukemia: report of eighteen cases. J Thorac Cardiovasc Surg 115(1):63–68, discussion 8-9
139. Giles FJ (1998) Monocyte-macrophages, granulocyte-macrophage colony-stimulating factor, and prolonged survival among patients with acute myeloid leukemia and stem cell transplants. Clin Infect Dis 26(6):1282–1289
140. Roilides E, Holmes A, Blake C, Venzon D, Pizzo PA, Walsh TJ (1994) Antifungal activity of elutriated human monocytes against Aspergillus fumigatus hyphae: enhancement

by granulocyte-macrophage colony-stimulating factor and interferon-gamma. J Infect Dis 170(4):894–899
141. Roilides E, Sein T, Holmes A et al (1995) Effects of macrophage colony-stimulating factor on antifungal activity of mononuclear phagocytes against Aspergillus fumigatus. J Infect Dis 172(4):1028–1034
142. Rowe JM, Andersen JW, Mazza JJ et al (1995) A randomized placebo-controlled phase III study of granulocyte-macrophage colony-stimulating factor in adult patients (>55 to 70 years of age) with acute myelogenous leukemia: a study of the Eastern Cooperative Oncology Group (E1490). Blood 86(2):457–462
143. Ozer H, Armitage JO, Bennett CL et al (2000) 2000 Update of recommendations for the use of hematopoietic colony-stimulating factors: evidence-based, clinical practice guidelines. American Society of Clinical Oncology Growth Factors Expert Panel. J Clin Oncol 18(20): 3558–3585
144. Roilides E, Uhlig K, Venzon D, Pizzo PA, Walsh TJ (1993) Prevention of corticosteroid-induced suppression of human polymorphonuclear leukocyte-induced damage of Aspergillus fumigatus hyphae by granulocyte colony-stimulating factor and gamma interferon. Infect Immun 61(11): 4870–4877
145. Nagai H, Guo J, Choi H, Kurup V (1995) Interferon-gamma and tumor necrosis factor-alpha protect mice from invasive aspergillosis. J Infect Dis 172(6):1554–1560
146. Safdar A (2006) Strategies to enhance immune function in hematopoietic transplantation recipients who have fungal infections. Bone Marrow Transplant 38(5):327–337
147. Safdar A, Rodriguez G, Ohmagari N et al (2005) The safety of interferon-gamma-1b therapy for invasive fungal infections after hematopoietic stem cell transplantation. Cancer 103(4):731–739
148. Price TH, Bowden RA, Boeckh M et al (2000) Phase I/II trial of neutrophil transfusions from donors stimulated with G-CSF and dexamethasone for treatment of patients with infections in hematopoietic stem cell transplantation. Blood 95(11):3302–3309
149. van de Wetering MD, Weggelaar N, Offringa M, Caron HN, Kuijpers TW (2007) Granulocyte transfusions in neutropaenic children: a systematic review of the literature. Eur J Cancer 43(14):2082–2092
150. Sherertz RJ, Belani A, Kramer BS et al (1987) Impact of air filtration on nosocomial Aspergillus infections. Unique risk of bone marrow transplant recipients. Am J Med 83(4): 709–718
151. Mattiuzzi GN, Kantarjian H, O'Brien S et al (2004) Intravenous itraconazole for prophylaxis of systemic fungal infections in patients with acute myelogenous leukemia and high-risk myelodysplastic syndrome undergoing induction chemotherapy. Cancer 100(3):568–573
152. Ullmann AJ, Cornely OA (2006) Antifungal prophylaxis for invasive mycoses in high risk patients. Curr Opin Infect Dis 19(6):571–576
153. Ullmann AJ, Lipton JH, Vesole DH et al (2007) Posaconazole or fluconazole for prophylaxis in severe graft-versus-host disease. N Engl J Med 356(4): 335–347
154. Rijnders BJ, Cornelissen JJ, Slobbe L et al (2008) Aerosolized liposomal amphotericin B for the prevention of invasive pulmonary aspergillosis during prolonged neutropenia: a randomized, placebo-controlled trial. Clin Infect Dis 46(9):1401–1408
155. Tolman JA, Nelson NA, Son YJ, et al (2009) Characterization and pharmacokinetic analysis of aerosolized aqueous voriconazole solution. Eur J Pharm Biopharm 72(1):199–205
156. Nucci M, Marr KA, Queiroz-Telles F et al (2004) Fusarium infection in hematopoietic stem cell transplant recipients. Clin Infect Dis 38(9):1237–1242
157. Boutati EI, Anaissie EJ (1997) Fusarium, a significant emerging pathogen in patients with hematologic malignancy: ten years' experience at a cancer center and implications for management. Blood 90(3): 999–1008
158. Gaziev D, Baronciani D, Galimberti M et al (1996) Mucormycosis after bone marrow transplantation: report of four cases in thalassemia and review of the literature. Bone Marrow Transplant 17(3):409–414
159. Maertens J, Demuynck H, Verbeken EK et al (1999) Mucormycosis in allogeneic bone marrow transplant recipients: report of five cases and review of the role of iron overload in the pathogenesis. Bone Marrow Transplant 24(3):307–312
160. Costa SF, Alexander BD (2005) Non-aspergillus fungal pneumonia in transplant recipients. Clin Chest Med 26(4):675–690, vii
161. Groll AH, Walsh TJ (2001) Uncommon opportunistic fungi: new nosocomial threats. Clin Microbiol Infect 7(Suppl 2): 8–24
162. Jahagirdar BN, Morrison VA (2002) Emerging fungal pathogens in patients with hematologic malignancies and marrow/stem-cell transplant recipients. Semin Respir Infect 17(2):113–120
163. Sampathkumar P, Paya CV (2001) Fusarium infection after solid-organ transplantation. Clin Infect Dis 32(8): 1237–1240
164. Marom EM, Holmes AM, Bruzzi JF, Truong MT, O'Sullivan PJ, Kontoyiannis DP (2008) Imaging of pulmonary fusariosis in patients with hematologic malignancies. AJR Am J Roentgenol 190(6):1605–1609
165. Castiglioni B, Sutton DA, Rinaldi MG, Fung J, Kusne S (2002) Pseudallescheria boydii (Anamorph Scedosporium apiospermum). Infection in solid organ transplant recipients in a tertiary medical center and review of the literature. Medicine (Baltimore) 81(5):333–348
166. Berenguer J, Rodriguez-Tudela JL, Richard C et al (1997) Deep infections caused by Scedosporium prolificans. A report on 16 cases in Spain and a review of the literature. Scedosporium Prolificans Spanish Study Group. Medicine (Baltimore) 76(4):256–265
167. Espinel-Ingroff A (2001) In vitro fungicidal activities of voriconazole, itraconazole, and amphotericin B against opportunistic moniliaceous and dematiaceous fungi. J Clin Microbiol 39(3):954–958
168. Husain S, Munoz P, Forrest G et al (2005) Infections due to Scedosporium apiospermum and Scedosporium prolificans in transplant recipients: clinical characteristics and impact of antifungal agent therapy on outcome. Clin Infect Dis 40(1):89–99
169. Trifilio S, Singhal S, Williams S, et al (2007) Breakthrough fungal infections after allogeneic hematopoietic stem cell transplantation in patients on prophylactic voriconazole. Bone Marrow Transplant 40(5):451–456
170. Page RL 2nd, Schwiesow J, Hilts A (2007) Posaconazole as salvage therapy in a patient with disseminated zygomy-

cosis: case report and review of the literature. Pharmacotherapy 27(2):290–298
171. Anaissie EJ, Kontoyiannis DP, O'Brien S et al (1998) Infections in patients with chronic lymphocytic leukemia treated with fludarabine. Ann Intern Med 129(7): 559–566
172. Tanner DC, Weinstein MP, Fedorciw B, Joho KL, Thorpe JJ, Reller L (1994) Comparison of commercial kits for detection of cryptococcal antigen. J Clin Microbiol 32(7):1680–1684
173. Saag MS, Graybill RJ, Larsen RA et al (2000) Practice guidelines for the management of cryptococcal disease. Infectious Diseases Society of America. Clin Infect Dis 30(4):710–718
174. Goodrich JM, Reed EC, Mori M et al (1991) Clinical features and analysis of risk factors for invasive candidal infection after marrow transplantation. J Infect Dis 164(4):731–740
175. Kume H, Yamazaki T, Abe M, Tanuma H, Okudaira M, Okayasu I (2003) Increase in aspergillosis and severe mycotic infection in patients with leukemia and MDS: comparison of the data from the Annual of the Pathological Autopsy Cases in Japan in 1989, 1993 and 1997. Pathol Int 53(11):744–750
176. Stringer JR, Beard CB, Miller RF, Wakefield AE (2002) A new name (Pneumocystis jiroveci) for Pneumocystis from humans. Emerg Infect Dis 8(9):891–896
177. Hughes WT, Feldman S, Aur RJ, Verzosa MS, Hustu HO, Simone JV (1975) Intensity of immunosuppressive therapy and the incidence of Pneumocystis carinii pneumonitis. Cancer 36(6):2004–2009
178. Rodriguez M, Sifri CD, Fishman JA (2004) Failure of low-dose atovaquone prophylaxis against Pneumocystis jiroveci infection in transplant recipients. Clin Infect Dis 38(8): e76–e78
179. Torre-Cisneros J, De la Mata M, Pozo JC et al (1999) Randomized trial of weekly sulfadoxine/pyrimethamine vs. daily low-dose trimethoprim-sulfamethoxazole for the prophylaxis of Pneumocystis carinii pneumonia after liver transplantation. Clin Infect Dis 29(4): 771–774
180. Marras TK, Sanders K, Lipton JH, Messner HA, Conly J, Chan CK (2002) Aerosolized pentamidine prophylaxis for Pneumocystis carinii pneumonia after allogeneic marrow transplantation. Transpl Infect Dis 4(2):66–74
181. Varthalitis I, Aoun M, Daneau D, Meunier F (1993) Pneumocystis carinii pneumonia in patients with cancer. An increasing incidence. Cancer 71(2):481–485
182. Arend SM, Kroon FP, Van't Wout JW (1995) Pneumocystis carinii pneumonia in patients without AIDS, 1980 through 1993. An analysis of 78 cases. Arch Intern Med 155(22): 2436–2441
183. Pagano L, Fianchi L, Mele L et al (2002) Pneumocystis carinii pneumonia in patients with malignant haematological diseases: 10 years' experience of infection in GIMEMA centres. Br J Haematol 117(2):379–386
184. Wijermans PW, Gerrits WB, Haak HL (1993) Severe immunodeficiency in patients treated with fludarabine monophosphate. Eur J Haematol 50(5):292–296
185. De Castro N, Neuville S, Sarfati C et al (2005) Occurrence of Pneumocystis jiroveci pneumonia after allogeneic stem cell transplantation: a 6-year retrospective study. Bone Marrow Transplant 36(10):879–883
186. Naimey GL, Wuerker RB (1995) Comparison of histologic stains in the diagnosis of Pneumocystis carinii. Acta Cytol 39(6):1124–1127
187. Kovacs JA, Ng VL, Masur H et al (1988) Diagnosis of Pneumocystis carinii pneumonia: improved detection in sputum with use of monoclonal antibodies. N Engl J Med 318(10):589–593
188. Torres HA, Chemaly RF, Storey R et al (2006) Influence of type of cancer and hematopoietic stem cell transplantation on clinical presentation of Pneumocystis jiroveci pneumonia in cancer patients. Eur J Clin Microbiol Infect Dis 25(6):382–388
189. Bollee G, Sarfati C, Thiery G et al (2007) Clinical picture of Pneumocystis jiroveci pneumonia in cancer patients. Chest 132(4):1305–1310
190. Glenn TJ, Blair JE, Adams RH (2005) Coccidioidomycosis in hematopoietic stem cell transplant recipients. Med Mycol 43(8):705–710
191. Ison MG, Fishman JA (2005) Cytomegalovirus pneumonia in transplant recipients. Clin Chest Med 26(4):691–705, viii
192. Meyers JD, Flournoy N, Thomas ED (1982) Nonbacterial pneumonia after allogeneic marrow transplantation: a review of ten years' experience. Rev Infect Dis 4(6): 1119–1132
193. Crawford SW, Bowden RA, Hackman RC, Gleaves CA, Meyers JD, Clark JG (1988) Rapid detection of cytomegalovirus pulmonary infection by bronchoalveolar lavage and centrifugation culture. Ann Intern Med 108(2):180–185
194. Blacklock HA, Griffiths P, Stirk P, Prentice HG (1985) Specific hyperimmune globulin for cytomegalovirus pneumonitis. Lancet 2(8447):152–153
195. Taplitz RA, Jordan MC (2002) Pneumonia caused by herpesviruses in recipients of hematopoietic cell transplants. Semin Respir Infect 17(2):121–129
196. Konoplev S, Champlin RE, Giralt S et al (2001) Cytomegalovirus pneumonia in adult autologous blood and marrow transplant recipients. Bone Marrow Transplant 27(8):877–881
197. Shepp DH, Dandliker PS, de Miranda P et al (1985) Activity of 9-[2-hydroxy-1-(hydroxymethyl)ethoxymethyl]guanine in the treatment of cytomegalovirus pneumonia. Ann Intern Med 103(3):368–373
198. Torres HA, Aguilera E, Safdar A et al (2008) Fatal cytomegalovirus pneumonia in patients with haematological malignancies: an autopsy-based case-control study. Clin Microbiol Infect 14(12):1160–1166
199. Boeckh M, Leisenring W, Riddell SR et al (2003) Late cytomegalovirus disease and mortality in recipients of allogeneic hematopoietic stem cell transplants: importance of viral load and T-cell immunity. Blood 101(2):407–414
200. Junghanss C, Boeckh M, Carter RA et al (2002) Incidence and outcome of cytomegalovirus infections following nonmyeloablative compared with myeloablative allogeneic stem cell transplantation, a matched control study. Blood 99(6):1978–1985
201. Ljungman P, Aschan J, Lewensohn-Fuchs I et al (1998) Results of different strategies for reducing cytomegalovirus-associated mortality in allogeneic stem cell transplant recipients. Transplantation 66(10):1330–1334
202. Reusser P (1991) Cytomegalovirus infection and disease after bone marrow transplantation: epidemiology, prevention, and treatment. Bone Marrow Transplant 7(Suppl 3):52–56

203. Enright H, Haake R, Weisdorf D et al (1993) Cytomegalovirus pneumonia after bone marrow transplantation. Risk factors and response to therapy. Transplantation 55(6): 1339–1346
204. Holmberg LA, Boeckh M, Hooper H et al (1999) Increased incidence of cytomegalovirus disease after autologous CD34-selected peripheral blood stem cell transplantation. Blood 94(12):4029–4035
205. Leung AN, Gosselin MV, Napper CH et al (1999) Pulmonary infections after bone marrow transplantation: clinical and radiographic findings. Radiology 210(3): 699–710
206. Franquet T, Lee KS, Muller NL (2003) Thin-section CT findings in 32 immunocompromised patients with cytomegalovirus pneumonia who do not have AIDS. AJR Am J Roentgenol 181(4):1059–1063
207. Tamm M, Traenkle P, Grilli B et al (2001) Pulmonary cytomegalovirus infection in immunocompromised patients. Chest 119(3):838–843
208. Sakamaki H, Yuasa K, Goto H et al (1997) Comparison of cytomegalovirus (CMV) antigenemia and CMV in bronchoalveolar lavage fluid for diagnosis of CMV pulmonary infection after bone marrow transplantation. Bone Marrow Transplant 20(2):143–147
209. Michaelides A, Liolios L, Glare EM et al (2001) Increased human cytomegalovirus (HCMV) DNA load in peripheral blood leukocytes after lung transplantation correlates with HCMV pneumonitis. Transplantation 72(1):141–147
210. Westall GP, Michaelides A, Williams TJ, Snell GI, Kotsimbos TC (2004) Human cytomegalovirus load in plasma and bronchoalveolar lavage fluid: a longitudinal study of lung transplant recipients. J Infect Dis 190(6): 1076–1083
211. Humar A, Lipton J, Welsh S, Moussa G, Messner H, Mazzulli T (2001) A randomised trial comparing cytomegalovirus antigenemia assay vs screening bronchoscopy for the early detection and prevention of disease in allogeneic bone marrow and peripheral blood stem cell transplant recipients. Bone Marrow Transplant 28(5):485–490
212. Leruez-Ville M, Ouachee M, Delarue R et al (2003) Monitoring cytomegalovirus infection in adult and pediatric bone marrow transplant recipients by a real-time PCR assay performed with blood plasma. J Clin Microbiol 41(5):2040–2046
213. Reinke P, Prosch S, Kern F, Volk HD (1999) Mechanisms of human cytomegalovirus (HCMV) (re)activation and its impact on organ transplant patients. Transpl Infect Dis 1(3):157–164
214. Bordon V, Bravo S, Van Renterghem L, et al (2008) Surveillance of cytomegalovirus (CMV) DNAemia in pediatric allogeneic stem cell transplantation: incidence and outcome of CMV infection and disease. Transpl Infect Dis 10(1):19–23
215. Bacigalupo A, Bregante S, Tedone E et al (1996) Combined foscarnet -ganciclovir treatment for cytomegalovirus infections after allogeneic hemopoietic stem cell transplantation (Hsct). Bone Marrow Transplant 18(Suppl 2):110–114
216. Bowden RA, Slichter SJ, Sayers M et al (1995) A comparison of filtered leukocyte-reduced and cytomegalovirus (CMV) seronegative blood products for the prevention of transfusion-associated CMV infection after marrow transplant. Blood 86(9):3598–3603
217. Nichols WG, Price TH, Gooley T, Corey L, Boeckh M (2003) Transfusion-transmitted cytomegalovirus infection after receipt of leukoreduced blood products. Blood 101(10):4195–4200
218. Zaia JA (1993) Prevention and treatment of cytomegalovirus pneumonia in transplant recipients. Clin Infect Dis 17(Suppl 2):S392–S399
219. Goodrich JM, Bowden RA, Fisher L, Keller C, Schoch G, Meyers JD (1993) Ganciclovir prophylaxis to prevent cytomegalovirus disease after allogeneic marrow transplant. Ann Intern Med 118(3):173–178
220. Busca A, de Fabritiis P, Ghisetti V et al (2007) Oral valganciclovir as preemptive therapy for cytomegalovirus infection post allogeneic stem cell transplantation. Transpl Infect Dis 9(2):102–107
221. Lilleri D, Gerna G, Furione M, et al (2007) Use of a DNAemia cut-off for monitoring human cytomegalovirus infection reduces the number of pre-emptively treated children and young adults receiving haematopoietic stem cell transplantation as compared to qualitative pp65-antigenemia. Blood
222. Walter EA, Greenberg PD, Gilbert MJ et al (1995) Reconstitution of cellular immunity against cytomegalovirus in recipients of allogeneic bone marrow by transfer of T-cell clones from the donor. N Engl J Med 333(16): 1038–1044
223. Lujan-Zilbermann J, Benaim E, Tong X, Srivastava DK, Patrick CC, DeVincenzo JP (2001) Respiratory virus infections in pediatric hematopoietic stem cell transplantation. Clin Infect Dis 33(7):962–968
224. Roghmann M, Ball K, Erdman D, Lovchik J, Anderson LJ, Edelman R (2003) Active surveillance for respiratory virus infections in adults who have undergone bone marrow and peripheral blood stem cell transplantation. Bone Marrow Transplant 32(11):1085–1088
225. van Kraaij MG, van Elden LJ, van Loon AM et al (2005) Frequent detection of respiratory viruses in adult recipients of stem cell transplants with the use of real-time polymerase chain reaction, compared with viral culture. Clin Infect Dis 40(5):662–669
226. Chemaly RF, Ghosh S, Bodey GP et al (2006) Respiratory viral infections in adults with hematologic malignancies and human stem cell transplantation recipients: a retrospective study at a major cancer center. Medicine (Baltimore) 85(5):278–287
227. Bowden RA (1997) Respiratory virus infections after marrow transplant: the Fred Hutchinson Cancer Research Center experience. Am J Med 102(3A):27–30, discussion 42-3
228. Franquet T, Rodriguez S, Martino R, Gimenez A, Salinas T, Hidalgo A (2006) Thin-section CT findings in hematopoietic stem cell transplantation recipients with respiratory virus pneumonia. AJR Am J Roentgenol 187(4): 1085–1090
229. Whimbey E, Englund JA, Couch RB (1997) Community respiratory virus infections in immunocompromised patients with cancer. Am J Med 102(3A):10–18, discussion 25-6
230. Raboni SM, Nogueira MB, Tsuchiya LR et al (2003) Respiratory tract viral infections in bone marrow transplant patients. Transplantation 76(1):142–146
231. Bredius RG, Templeton KE, Scheltinga SA, Claas EC, Kroes AC, Vossen JM (2004) Prospective study of respira-

tory viral infections in pediatric hemopoietic stem cell transplantation patients. Pediatr Infect Dis J 23(6): 518–522

232. Nichols WG, Corey L, Gooley T, Davis C, Boeckh M (2001) Parainfluenza virus infections after hematopoietic stem cell transplantation: risk factors, response to antiviral therapy, and effect on transplant outcome. Blood 98(3):573–578
233. Soubani AO, Uberti JP (2007) Bronchiolitis obliterans following haematopoietic stem cell transplantation. Eur Respir J 29(5):1007–1019
234. Erard V, Chien JW, Kim HW et al (2006) Airflow decline after myeloablative allogeneic hematopoietic cell transplantation: the role of community respiratory viruses. J Infect Dis 193(12):1619–1625
235. Garcia R, Raad I, Abi-Said D et al (1997) Nosocomial respiratory syncytial virus infections: prevention and control in bone marrow transplant patients. Infect Control Hosp Epidemiol 18(6):412–416
236. Hall CB (2000) Nosocomial respiratory syncytial virus infections: the "Cold War" has not ended. Clin Infect Dis 31(2):590–596
237. Ghosh S, Champlin RE, Ueno NT et al (2001) Respiratory syncytial virus infections in autologous blood and marrow transplant recipients with breast cancer: combination therapy with aerosolized ribavirin and parenteral immunoglobulins. Bone Marrow Transplant 28(3): 271–275
238. Abdallah A, Rowland KE, Schepetiuk SK, To LB, Bardy P (2003) An outbreak of respiratory syncytial virus infection in a bone marrow transplant unit: effect on engraftment and outcome of pneumonia without specific antiviral treatment. Bone Marrow Transplant 32(2):195–203
239. Small TN, Casson A, Malak SF et al (2002) Respiratory syncytial virus infection following hematopoietic stem cell transplantation. Bone Marrow Transplant 29(4): 321–327
240. Ljungman P (1997) Respiratory virus infections in bone marrow transplant recipients: the European perspective. Am J Med 102(3A):44–47
241. Falsey AR, Walsh EE (2000) Respiratory syncytial virus infection in adults. Clin Microbiol Rev 13(3):371–384
242. Barton TD, Blumberg EA (2005) Viral pneumonias other than cytomegalovirus in transplant recipients. Clin Chest Med 26(4):707–720, viii
243. Khanna N, Widmer AF, Decker M et al (2008) Respiratory syncytial virus infection in patients with hematological diseases: single-center study and review of the literature. Clin Infect Dis 46(3):402–412
244. Escuissato DL, Gasparetto EL, Marchiori E et al (2005) Pulmonary infections after bone marrow transplantation: high-resolution CT findings in 111 patients. AJR Am J Roentgenol 185(3):608–615
245. Englund JA, Piedra PA, Jewell A, Patel K, Baxter BB, Whimbey E (1996) Rapid diagnosis of respiratory syncytial virus infections in immunocompromised adults. J Clin Microbiol 34(7):1649–1653
246. Englund JA, Piedra PA, Whimbey E (1997) Prevention and treatment of respiratory syncytial virus and parainfluenza viruses in immunocompromised patients. Am J Med 102(3A):61–70, discussion 5-6
247. Taylor-Robinson D (2004) Community-acquired respiratory viruses. Am J Transplant 4(4 Suppl):105–109
248. Ottolini MG, Curtis SR, Mathews A, Ottolini SR, Prince GA (2002) Palivizumab is highly effective in suppressing respiratory syncytial virus in an immunosuppressed animal model. Bone Marrow Transplant 29(2):117–120
249. Boeckh M, Englund J, Li Y et al (2007) Randomized controlled multicenter trial of aerosolized ribavirin for respiratory syncytial virus upper respiratory tract infection in hematopoietic cell transplant recipients. Clin Infect Dis 44(2):245–249
250. Whimbey E, Vartivarian SE, Champlin RE, Elting LS, Luna M, Bodey GP (1993) Parainfluenza virus infection in adult bone marrow transplant recipients. Eur J Clin Microbiol Infect Dis 12(9):699–701
251. Elizaga J, Olavarria E, Apperley J, Goldman J, Ward K (2001) Parainfluenza virus 3 infection after stem cell transplant: relevance to outcome of rapid diagnosis and ribavirin treatment. Clin Infect Dis 32(3):413–418
252. McCurdy LH, Milstone A, Dummer S (2003) Clinical features and outcomes of paramyxoviral infection in lung transplant recipients treated with ribavirin. J Heart Lung Transplant 22(7):745–753
253. Tasian SK, Park JR, Martin ET, Englund JA (2008) Influenza-associated morbidity in children with cancer. Pediatr Blood Cancer 50(5):983–987
254. Nichols WG, Guthrie KA, Corey L, Boeckh M (2004) Influenza infections after hematopoietic stem cell transplantation: risk factors, mortality, and the effect of antiviral therapy. Clin Infect Dis 39(9):1300–1306
255. Vu D, Peck AJ, Nichols WG et al (2007) Safety and tolerability of oseltamivir prophylaxis in hematopoietic stem cell transplant recipients: a retrospective case-control study. Clin Infect Dis 45(2):187–193
256. www.cdc.gov. Accessed Oct 2009
257. Symeonidis N, Jakubowski A, Pierre-Louis S et al (2007) Invasive adenoviral infections in T-cell-depleted allogeneic hematopoietic stem cell transplantation: high mortality in the era of cidofovir. Transpl Infect Dis 9(2):108–113
258. Myers GD, Bollard CM, Wu MF et al (2007) Reconstitution of adenovirus-specific cell-mediated immunity in pediatric patients after hematopoietic stem cell transplantation. Bone Marrow Transplant 39(11):677–686
259. Shields AF, Hackman RC, Fife KH, Corey L, Meyers JD (1985) Adenovirus infections in patients undergoing bone-marrow transplantation. N Engl J Med 312(9):529–533
260. Adenovirus. Am J Transplant 2004;4 (Suppl 10):101–104
261. Hassan IA, Chopra R, Swindell R, Mutton KJ (2003) Respiratory viral infections after bone marrow/peripheral stem-cell transplantation: the Christie hospital experience. Bone Marrow Transplant 32(1):73–77
262. Buchbinder S, Elmaagacli AH, Schaefer UW, Roggendorf M (2000) Human herpesvirus 6 is an important pathogen in infectious lung disease after allogeneic bone marrow transplantation. Bone Marrow Transplant 26(6):639–644
263. Hentrich M, Oruzio D, Jager G et al (2005) Impact of human herpesvirus-6 after haematopoietic stem cell transplantation. Br J Haematol 128(1):66–72
264. Kamboj M, Gerbin M, Huang CK et al (2008) Clinical characterization of human metapneumovirus infection among patients with cancer. J Infect 57(6):464–471

Part II

Epidemiology

Epidemiology of Respiratory Events in Patients with HM (Not Including ICU)

4

Georg Maschmeyer

Contents

G. Maschmeyer
Department of Hematology, Oncology and Palliative Care, Center for Hematology, Oncology and Radiotherapy, Klinikum Ernst von Bergmann, Charlottenstr. 72, D-14467 Potsdam, Germany
e-mail: gmaschmeyer@klinikumevb.de

4.1 Respiratory Events in Patients with Hematological Malignancies

Respiratory events, defined as episodes of respiratory symptoms or signs, such as dyspnea, cough, sputum, chest pain, rales, hemoptysis, oxygenation impairment or pulmonary infiltrates on chest radiograph or computed tomography scan, are frequent among patients with hematological malignancies (HM). Almost 50% of patients with acute leukemia undergoing chemotherapy may be affected [10], preferably those with preexisting pulmonary disease and smokers. Also among patients with chronic lymphocytic leukemia, respiratory events are frequent and are likely to take a complicated course caused by the complex immunodeficiency in these patients. Pulmonary events have been reported for up to 58% of patients with malignant lymphoma undergoing high-dose chemotherapy and autologous hematopoietic stem cell transplantation [18], but in general, less than 10% of all autologous stem cell transplant patients will develop pneumonia [27, 30].

The epidemiology of respiratory events has only rarely been investigated using invasive procedures, so that reliable data on specific causes in different subgroups of patients with HM are sparse. Chaoui et al. investigated consecutive patients with newly diagnosed acute leukemia over 1 year to evaluate the incidence and prognostic value of these events and found that the cause of respiratory events was infectious in 34% of cases, an established cause other than infection in 42% and an undetermined cause in 24%. Among patients with undetermined etiology, around 20% were cured by antibiotics and could be considered as probable bacterial pneumonia, increasing the proportion of infectious causes to 55%. Aspergillosis was proven in approximately 10% of cases. The majority of

É. Azoulay (ed.), *Pulmonary Involvement in Patients with Hematological Malignancies*,
DOI: 10.1007/978-3-642-15742-4_4, © Springer-Verlag Berlin Heidelberg 2011

respiratory events occurred after starting induction chemotherapy; however, almost all respiratory events of undetermined etiology were present at diagnosis of HM already, and respiratory events of non-infectious origin typically occurred within 10 days of leukemia diagnosis.

Among patients with chronic lymphocytic leukemia, pulmonary complications analyzed over a 9-year period were associated with a poor prognosis and a fatality rate of 40% [1]. Notably, 25% of these complications were not caused by pneumonia, but by pleural effusion or lung infiltration by the underlying malignancy (9%), pulmonary leukostasis (4%), secondary malignancies or Richter's syndrome (3%), or bronchial obstruction (2%). With respect to prognosis, granulocytopenia and renal failure had an unfavorable impact on clinical outcome.

4.2 Lung Infiltrates in Patients with HM

In febrile neutropenic patients, lung infiltrates emerge in up to 30% [31]. Clinical outcome deteriorates with increasing patient age, and is particularly dismal in patients with bacteremia and shock as well as in case of delayed appropriate antimicrobial treatment [7, 21]. Infiltrates become apparent in approximately two thirds of cases within 5 days after the onset of fever. As compared with other types of infections, lung infiltrates in neutropenic patients are associated with a higher risk of mortality [3, 15, 26], and their treatment is more difficult and costly [19]. Histopathological findings show that these infiltrates may have numerous different causes, including multi-resistant bacteria [32] and pathogens not susceptible to beta-lactam antibiotics [20], alveolar bleeding, infiltration by the underlying malignancy, cryptogenic organizing pneumonia, immune reconstitution syndrome, and lesions caused by chemotherapy or radiation [2, 4, 8, 13, 14, 35, 36], In particular, the differential diagnosis of drug-induced lung infiltrates should be kept in mind (Table 4.1).

Successful clinical response to broad-spectrum antibacterial treatment is observed in less than 30% of patients with pulmonary infiltrates in the course of febrile neutropenia [26, 29], whereas prompt addition of mold-active systemic antifungals increases the response rate to up to 78% [34]. The dramatic reduction of lung infiltrates in acute leukemia patients under voriconazole prophylaxis [38], along with histopathological and molecular [20] as well as autopsy studies [4, 9, 17], indicate that the majority of those infiltrates are caused by filamentous fungi, particularly by *Aspergillus* spp. Clinical outcome of microbiologically or histologically documented invasive aspergillosis in neutropenic patients is poor [12, 22, 28], so that early pre-emptive antifungal treatment is recommended in febrile patients with severe neutropenia and pulmonary infiltrates whose radiological morphology is not typical for non-fungal origin [24, 39]. This recommendation also takes into account that Aspergillus pneumonia will have an unfavorable impact on long-term prognosis and that early institution of systemic

Table 4.1 Drugs potentially associated with pulmonary toxicity in patients with hematological malignancies

Alkylating agents
Busulfan
Chlorambucil
Cyclophosphamide
Antimetabolites
Azathioprine
Cytosine arabinoside
Fludarabine
Gemcitabine
Methotrexate
Cytotoxic antibiotics
Bleomycin
Dactinomycin
Doxorubicin
Mitomycin
Nitrosoureas
BCNU (carmustine)
CCNU (lomustine)
Assorted agents
Procarbazine
Sirolimus
Taxanes
Vinca alkaloids

Modified after Shorr et al. [36]

antifungal treatment against *Aspergillus* spp. improves survival [5, 34].

In patients treated with nucleoside analog, microorganisms typically observed under prolonged cellular immunosuppression, such as cytomegalovirus, mycobacteria or yeasts, must be considered [33], as well as *Staphylococcus aureus*, *Pseudomonas aeruginosa*, *Aspergillus* spp. and pneumococci [1]. Respiratory viruses such as Influenza A or Respiratory Syncytial Virus have occasionally been identified as causes of pulmonary infiltrates in hospitalized, febrile neutropenic patients [23, 37], predominantly during wintertime, but they do not occur more frequently in immunocompromised than in non-immunocompromised patients [16]. Among patients affected, those who are older than 65 years of age or have severe lymphocytopenia may show a mortality rate of 5–15% [11].

4.3 Acute Respiratory Failure in Cancer Patients

[3] performed a prospective 5-year observational study in a medical intensive care unit treating 203 cancer patients with acute respiratory failure and reported that repiratory failure was mainly due to infectious pneumonia (58%), but also due to lung inflammation due to non-infectious causes in 9% and to congestive heart failure in 12% of patients, whereas no cause was identifiable in 21%.

Mortality of HM patients with respiratory events requiring referral to an intensive care unit is high, though decreases over time [10]. Half the patients do not survive their respiratory events (Fig. 4.1). Multivariate analysis shows the type and state of the underlying malignancy [3], proven pulmonary aspergillosis, the

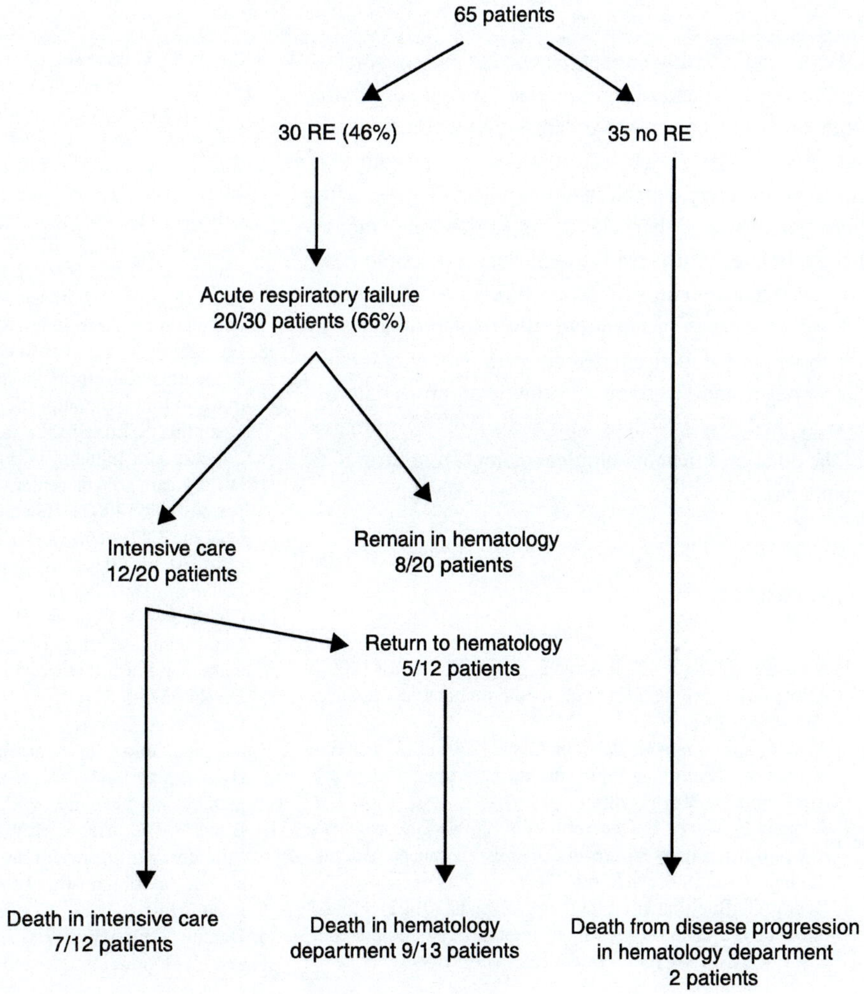

Fig. 4.1 Outcome of acute leukemia patients with respiratory events (RE) (end point: death within 45 days of the start of induction chemotherapy) (From [10])

Table 4.2 Multivariable analysis: independent predictors of hospital death in cancer patients with acute respiratory failure[a]

	Odds ratio	95% Confidence interval	*p* Value
Cause of ARF			
Congestive heart failure	0.16	0.03–0.72	0.01
Invasive aspergillosis	3.78	1.05–14.24	0.049
No definite diagnosis	3.85	1.26–11.70	0.01
Need for vasopressors	3.19	1.28–7.95	0.01
Need for respiratory support			
NIMV only	1.58	0.37–6.70	0.52
NIMV followed by conventional MV	17.46	5.04–60.52	<0.0001
First-line conventional MV	8.75	2.35–32.54	0.001
Late NIMV failure[b]	10.64	1.05–107.83	0.04

[a]Hosmer–Lemeshow chi-square p value = 0.78

[b]Late NIMV failure: need for conventional MV after 2 full days of NIMV

From Azoulay et al. [3]

lack of a definite diagnosis, the need for pressor support and the requirement of invasive mechanical ventilation after failure of non-invasive ventilation as independent poor-risk factors (Table 4.2); however, the prognosis is not unequivocally dismal. In a long-term analysis, it has been demonstrated that at least three unfavorable factors had to be present to clearly predict fatal outcome [25], so that intensive care should be offered to all patients who do not have an unequivocally fatal prognosis. In this book, two papers are dedicated to patient outcome. Dr. Groeger and Dr. Azoulay provide an up-to-date literature analysis, as well as an appraisal of determinants of the outcomes in hematological patients requiring ICU management.

References

1. Ahmed S, Siddiqui AK, Rossoff L, Sison CP, Rai KR (2003) Pulmonary complications in chronic lymphocytic leukemia. Cancer 98:1912–1917
2. Azoulay E, Darmon M, Delclaux C et al (2002) Deterioration of previous acute lung injury during neutropenia recovery. Crit Care Med 30:781–786
3. Azoulay E, Thiery G, Chevret S et al (2004) The prognosis of acute respiratory failure in critically ill cancer patients. Medicine (Baltimore) 83:360–370
4. Bodey G, Bueltmann B, Duguid W et al (1992) Fungal infections in cancer patients: an international autopsy survey. Eur J Clin Microbiol Infect Dis 11:99–109
5. Caillot D, Casasnovas O, Bernard A et al (1997) Improved management of invasive pulmonary aspergillosis in neutropenic patients using early thoracic computed tomographic scan and surgery. J Clin Oncol 15:139–147
6. Camus P, Costabel U (2005) Drug-induced respiratory disease in patients with hematological diseases. Semin Respir Crit Care Med 26:458–81
7. Carratalà J, Rosón B, Fernández-Sevilla A, Alcaide F, Gudiol F (1998) Bacteremic pneumonia in neutropenic patients with cancer: causes, empirical antibiotic therapy, and outcome. Arch Intern Med 158:868–872
8. Cazzadori A, di Perri G, Todeschini G et al (1995) Transbronchial biopsy in the diagnosis of pulmonary infiltrates in immunocompromised patients. Chest 107:101–106
9. Chamilos G, Luna M, Lewis RE et al (2006) Invasive fungal infections in patients with hematologic malignancies in a tertiary care cancer center: an autopsy study over a 15-year period (1989-2003). Haematologica 91:986–989
10. Chaoui D, Legrand O, Roche N et al (2004) Incidence and prognostic value of respiratory events in acute leukemia. Leukemia 18:670–675
11. Chemaly RF, Torres HA, Aguilera EA et al (2007) Neuraminidase inhibitors improve outcome of patients with leukemia and influenza: an observational study. Clin Infect Dis 44:964–967
12. Cornillet A, Camus C, Nimubona S et al (2006) Comparison of epidemiological, clinical, and biological features of invasive aspergillosis in neutropenic and nonneutropenic patients: a 6-year survey. Clin Infect Dis 43:577–584
13. Danés C, Gonzalez-Martin J, Pumarola T et al (2002) Pulmonary infiltrates in immunosuppressed patients: analysis of a diagnostic protocol. J Clin Microbiol 40: 2134–2140
14. Daniels CE, Myers JL, Utz JP, Markovic SN, Ryu JH (2007) Organizing pneumonia in patients with hematologic

malignancies: a steroid-responsive lesion. Respir Med 101: 162–168
15. Ewig S, Glasmacher A, Ulrich B et al (1998) Pulmonary infiltrates in neutropenic patients with acute leukemia during chemotherapy. Chest 114:444–451
16. Falsey AR, Hennessey PA, Formica MA, Cox C, Walsh EE (2005) Respiratory syncytial virus infection in elderly and high-risk adults. N Engl J Med 352:1749–1759
17. Groll AH, Shah PM, Mentzel C, Schneider M, Just-Nuebling G, Huebner K (1996) Trends in the postmortem epidemiology of invasive fungal infections at a university hospital. J Infect 33:23–32
18. Jules-Elysee K, Stover DE, Yahalom J, White DA, Gulati SC (1992) Pulmonary complications in lymphoma patients treated with high-dose therapy autologous bone marrow transplantation. Am Rev Respir Dis 146:485–491
19. Kuderer NM, Dale DC, Crawford J, Cosler LE, Lyman GH (2006) Mortality, morbidity, and cost associated with febrile neutropenia in adult cancer patients. Cancer 106: 2258–2266
20. Lass-Flörl C, Resch G, Nachbaur D (2007) The value of computed tomography-guided percutaneous lung biopsy for diagnosis of invasive fungal infection in immunocompromised patients. Clin Infect Dis 45:e101–e104
21. Lin MY, Weinstein RA, Hota B (2008) Delay of active antimicrobial therapy and mortality among patients with bacteremia: impact of severe neutropenia. Antimicrob Agents Chemother 52:3188–3194
22. Lin SJ, Schranz J, Teutsch SM (2001) Aspergillosis case-fatality rate: systematic review of the literature. Clin Infect Dis 32:358–366
23. Martino R, Ramila E, Rabella N et al (2003) Respiratory virus infections in adults with hematologic malignancies: a prospective study. Clin Infect Dis 36:1–8
24. Maschmeyer G, Beinert T, Buchheidt D et al (2009) Diagnosis and antimicrobial therapy of pulmonary infiltrates in febrile neutropenic patients. 2008 updated guidelines of the Infectious Diseases Working Party of the German Society of Hematology and Oncology. Eur J Cancer 45:2462–2472
25. Maschmeyer G, Bertschat FL, Häusler E et al (2003) Outcome analysis of 189 consecutive cancer patients referred to the intensive care unit as emergencies during a 2-year period. Eur J Cancer 39:783–792
26. Maschmeyer G, Link H, Hiddemann W et al (1994) Pulmonary infiltrations in febrile neutropenic patients. Risk factors and outcome under empirical antimicrobial therapy in a randomized multicenter trial. Cancer 73:2296–2304
27. Mossad SB, Longworth DL, Goormastic M, Serkey JM, Keys TF, Bolwell BJ (1996) Early infectious complications in autologous bone marrow transplantation: a review of 219 patients. Bone Marrow Transplant 18:265–271
28. Pagano L, Caira M, Candoni A et al (2006) The epidemiology of fungal infections in patients with hematologic malignancies: the SEIFEM-2004 study. Haematologica 91: 1068–1075
29. Raad II, Whimbey EE, Rolston KVI et al (1996) A comparison of aztreonam plus vancomycin and imipenem plus vancomycin as initial therapy for febrile neutropenic cancer patients. Cancer 77:1386–1394
30. Reich G, Mapara MY, Reichardt P, Dörken B, Maschmeyer G (2001) Infectious complications after high-dose chemotherapy and autologous stem cell transplantation: comparison between patients with lymphoma or multiple myeloma and patients with solid tumors. Bone Marrow Transplant 27:525–529
31. Rossini F, Verga M, Pioltelli P et al (2000) Incidence and outcome of pneumonia in patients with acute leukemia receiving first induction therapy with anthracycline-containing regimens. Haematologica 85:1255–1260
32. Safdar A, Rolston KV (2007) Stenotrophomonas maltophilia: changing spectrum of a serious bacterial pathogen in patients with cancer. Clin Infect Dis 45:1602–1609
33. Samonis G, Kontoyiannis DP (2001) Infectious complications of purine analog therapy. Curr Opin Infect Dis 14: 409–413
34. Schiel X, Link H, Maschmeyer G (2006) A prospective, randomized multicenter trial of the empirical addition of antifungal therapy for febrile neutropenic cancer patients. Infection 34:118–126
35. Shorr AF, Susla GM, O'Grady NP (2004) Pulmonary infiltrates in the non-HIV-infected immunocompromised patient: etiologies, diagnostic strategies, and outcomes. Chest 125:260–271
36. Suzuki HI, Asai T, Tamaki Z, Hangaishi A, Chiba S, Kurokawa M (2008) Drug-induced hypersensitivity syndrome with rapid hematopoietic reconstitution during treatment for acute myeloid leukemia. Haematologica 93: 469–470
37. Torres HA, Aguilera EA, Mattiuzzi GN et al (2007) Characteristics and outcome of Respiratory Syncytial Virus infection in patients with leukemia. Haematologica 92:1216–1223
38. Vehreschild JJ, Böhme A, Buchheidt D et al (2007) A double-blind trial on prophylactic voriconazole or placebo during induction chemotherapy for acute myelogenous leukaemia. J Infect 55:445–449
39. Walsh TJ, Anaissie EJ, Denning DW et al (2008) Treatment of aspergillosis: clinical practice guidelines of the Infectious Diseases Society of America. Clin Infect Dis 46: 327–360

Epidemiology of Acute Respiratory Failure in Patients with HM (ICU Only)

5

Carlos Agustí, Carmen Lucena, and Antoni Torres

Contents

C. Agustí (✉)
Pneumology Department, Clinic Institute of Thorax (ICT), Hospital Clinic of Barcelona – Insitut d'Investigacions Biomèdiques August Pi i Sunyer (IDIBAPS), Ciber de Enfermedades Respiratorias, University of Barcelona (UB), Villarroel 170, 08036 Barcelona, Spain
e-mail: cagusti@clinic.ub.es

C. Lucena and A. Torres
Pneumology Department, Clinic Institute of Thorax (ICT), Hospital Clinic of Barcelona – Insitut d'Investigacions Biomèdiques August Pi i Sunyer (IDIBAPS), University of Barcelona (UB), Villarroel 170, 08036 Barcelona, Spain and
Beca Josep Font. Hospital Clínic de Barcelona, Barcelona, Spain
e-mail: atorres@clinic.ub.es

5.1 Introduction

Great progress has been made in stem cell transplantation over the last years. Most of the progress can be ascribed to an understanding of the human leukocyte antigen (HLA) system for donor selection, immunosuppression for prevention and treatment of graft-versus host disease (GVHD), and significant advances in infectious disease prevention, therapy and supportive care. As a result of this progress, the number of potential candidates to receive a transplant has greatly increased, and the survival figures have been progressively encouraging. In fact, the term "hematopoietic stem cell transplantation" (HSCT) has supplanted the previously employed term "bone marrow transplantation" to reflect the broader range of donor stem cell sources available: bone marrow, fetal cord blood, and growth factor-stimulated peripheral blood [1]. Unfortunately, the use of aggressive chemotherapeutic regimens frequently results in life-threatening complications, requiring transfer to the intensive care unit (ICU). Pulmonary complications, both infectious and noninfectious, occur in up to 60% of HSCT recipients, and a significant percentage of them will require ICU admission [1–3]. Infectious complications are more common in allograft recipients because of the requirement of immunosuppressive agents to prevent and treat GVHD. In addition, GVHD itself causes an immunodeficient state. In contrast, noninfectious acute lung injury syndromes (e.g., idiopathic pneumonia syndrome, diffuse alveolar hemorrhage) occur after

Supported by: 2009 SGR 911, Ciber de Enfermedades Respiratorias (Ciberes CB06/06/0028), el Ciberes es una iniciativa del ISCIII.

É. Azoulay (ed.), *Pulmonary Involvement in Patients with Hematological Malignancies*,
DOI: 10.1007/978-3-642-15742-4_5,

both allogeneic and autologous transplantation with similar frequency [1]. The recognition as well as management of pulmonary complications that result from immunosuppression is a challenging task for clinicians. Although the above-described improvements in patient care have improved the overall survival, once a patient with a hematologic malignancy requires advanced intensive care support, the prognosis worsens significantly with high associated mortality rates, particularly in patients with acute respiratory failure (ARF). Although the survival rate of HSCT recipients admitted to the ICU has been steadily improving, it remains under 50%, with a long-term survival rate under 20% [4].

5.2 Main Indications for ICU Admission

It is estimated that 15–30% of the HSCT recipients are admitted to the medical ICU for the management of different complications, with 20% of them requiring mechanical ventilation (MV). In our experience from data collected within a 10-year period [5], 89 patients with hematological malignancies with pulmonary complications were admitted to a respiratory ICU. Fifty-two of 89 (58%) of these patients were HSCT recipients. Patients were admitted to the ICU because of ARF in 61 instances (68%; including 23 patients with acute respiratory distress syndrome, ARDS), sepsis syndrome (12%), pulmonary hemorrhage (9%), heart failure (8%), and miscellaneous conditions (2%). The most common cause of ARF was a pulmonary infection, which was diagnosed in 60% of the patients for whom a specific diagnosis was obtained. Other authors have also found that infection is the most frequent cause of admission to the ICU, particularly in those with neutropenia where up to 80% have a clinically documented infection [6–8]. Also, among organ failures at ICU admission, acute respiratory failure and severe sepsis or septic shock are present in up to 80% of critically ill cancer patients [2, 9] (Table 5.1).

Clinical management of infections in critically ill immunocompromised patients is complex since virtually any microorganism may be involved at any time in the evolution, mainly depending on the net state of immunosuppression. The high associated mortality requires a rapid and sometimes invasive diagnostic approach to trying to obtain an etiological diagnosis allowing the early introduction of specific treatment.

Table 5.1 Indications by organ system for ICU admission

Respiratory	48%
Sepsis	23%
Cardiac	19%
Neurologic	6%
Bleeding	2%
Others	2%

Modified from ref. [10]

5.3 Etiology of Pulmonary Infections

5.3.1 Bacterial Infections

Bacteria are the most frequent cause of pulmonary infections in patients with hematological malignances, accounting for 15–20% of all respiratory infections in HSCT recipients [1] with an associated mortality of 22% [10] (Table 5.2). Different series have shown that bacterial pneumonia is also the most common cause of admission to the ICU in HSCT recipients [11]. One of the problems in diagnosing bacterial pneumonia in hematological patients is the inability to identify the organism in the majority of these patients, which may underestimate the incidence of these infections. Factors that generally increase the risk of bacterial pneumonia following HSCT include pre-transplantation immune status, type of conditioning regimen, and degree and duration of neutropenia [12]. In transplant recipients, bacterial infections may occur at any time in the post-

Table 5.2 Etiologic diagnosis in HSCT recipients and in haematological patients

	HSCT recipients (%)	Hematologic patients (%)
Bacterial	11	23
Fungal	13	19
Polymicrobial	20	8
Other infections	2	4
Pulmonary edema	5	4
DAH	8	4
NOC	3	4
Other non-infections etiologies	7	6
Undetermined	23	28

Modified from ref. [7]

transplantation period; however, they seem to be more common in the pre-engraftment phase due to the presence of mucositis and neutropenia. Potential pathogens are myriad. Encapsulated organisms, such as *Streptococcus pneumoniae* and *Haemophilus influenzae*, are particularly prevalent; however, many other bacteria must also be considered, particularly *Staphyloccocus aureus* (including methicillin-resistant, MRSA) and multi-resistant gram-negative bacilli, such as *P. aeruginosa* [13]. Some epidemiological studies have shown that *Legionella* sp. pneumonia is more prevalent in the immunocompromised host [14]. It is important to consider that 15–30% of cases diagnosed as bacterial pneumonia are mixed bacterial/opportunistic infections [11–13]. This fact has to be considered, particularly in patients that do not respond to appropriate specific antibiotic treatment.

5.3.2 Invasive Fungal Infections

Since neutrophils are the key cells in the defense against a*spergillus* sp. and other molds, the neutropenic patient and particularly HSCT recipients are at highest risk for dissemination. A steady rise in the documented cases of invasive pulmonary aspergillosis (IPA) post-transplantation has been documented. The risk for IPA is much higher following allogeneic HSCT when compared to autologous transplantation (incidence is 2.3–15% and 0.5–4%, respectively) [15]. Mortality rates for HSCT recipients with IPA have historically been as high as 80%; however, during the past 2 decades, the outcome of this infection seems to be changing. Recently, the Prospective Antifungal Therapy Alliance Registry performed a multicenter study to assess the epidemiology and outcomes of invasive fungal infections in HSCT recipients [16]. In this study, a total of 250 proven or probable invasive fungal infections were included. Almost 70% of the patients had received an allogeneic HSCT, and 31% had received an autologous HSCT. In this series, mortality rates of 21% and 35% at 6 and 12 weeks of diagnosing proven or probable IPA were reported, numbers that are consistent with those reported by other authors, confirming the survival gain evidenced after the inclusion of azoles in the therapeutic armamentarium of invasive fungal infections. Interestingly, the absence of MV or/and hemodialysis was significantly associated with improved survival.

With regard to Candida infections, with the expanded use of the new antifungal therapies, a higher incidence of infections caused by *Candida kruseii* and *Candida glabrata* has been reported [17, 18]. Also infections due to fusarium, *Penicillium purpurogenum* [19], and *Scedosporium prolificans* [20, 21] are increasingly being reported. In contrast, a marked decrease in the incidence of *P. jiroveci* pneumonia has been observed over the last years, mainly because of prescription of specific prophylaxis in patients at risk [22]. In a recent report, *P. jiroveci* infection was documented in 2.5% of patients undergoing allogeneic HSCT (2.5%). The majority of cases occurred late in the course following HSCT (median 14.5 months) [23] and with a CD4+ count less than 200 cells/mm^3.

5.3.3 Cytomegalovirus (CMV)

Traditionally, CMV pneumonia has affected 20–35% of HSCT recipients [24], being a common cause of ICU admission. However, the application of antiviral prophylaxis and the systematic use of preemptive therapy have changed the epidemiology of CMV pneumonia in HSCT recipients. Currently, in allogeneic HSCT recipients, the incidence of CMV pneumonia is 10–30% [25]. Also mortality is revised downwards between 30% and 50%. In the pre-prophylaxis era, onset of CMV pneumonia almost invariably occurred between engraftment and day 100. The use of prophylaxis has also shifted the onset of CMV pneumonia in allogeneic HSCT to after the first 100 days, especially in patients with non-myeloablative HSCT and during the treatment of chronic GVHD [26].

Despite improvements in specific treatment, survival of patients with established respiratory failure requiring mechanical ventilation is very poor.

5.3.4 Respiratory Viruses

Recent developments in molecular-based diagnostic tools have shown that conventional respiratory viruses [influenza, parainfluenza, respiratory syncitial viruses (RSV), adenoviruses, enteroviruses, and rhinoviruses] may commonly cause respiratory illnesses with significant morbidity and mortality among HSCT recipients. The incidence of these viral infections following HSCT ranges between 11–65% [27]. Upper respiratory tract infections in HSCT recipients are usually self-limiting. However, the progression to pneumonia carries a significant associated mortality. In one study of community respiratory viral infections following HSCT, the main viruses were RSV (35%), parainfluenza (30%), rhinovirus (25%), and influenza virus (11%). Of these, pneumonia occurred in 49% of patients with RSV infection, 22% of those with parainfluenza virus, and 3% of rhinovirus infection [28]. In another recent review of 343 cases of community respiratory viral infections in 306 adults with hematological malignancies (mostly HSCT recipients), parainfluenza (mainly type 3) accounted for 27% of infections, influenza (mainly type A) for 33% of infections, and RSV for 31% of infections. Community respiratory viral infections progressed to pneumonia in 35% of patients with equal frequency among the three viruses [27]. Interestingly, community respiratory viruses are often co-pathogens with other organisms, including bacteria, fungi (aspergillus), or other viruses (CMV). Herpes simplex virus 1 reactivates in 80% of HSCT recipients and occasionally may be associated with pneumonia. However, universal prophylaxis with acyclovir and gancyclovir has significantly reduced the incidence [27, 29]. Human herpes virus (HHV-6) may act as a co-pathogen with CMV or act as an isolated cause of pneumonia [30].

5.4 Survival in the ICU

In this book, Groeger and colleagues report updated data on outcomes in patients with hematological malignancies admitted to the ICU. Suffering from hematologic malignances is one of the most powerful predictors of mortality due to ARF in the ICU, and this is particularly true when patients with HSCT are considered and when MV is required. For many years, survival was considered dismal, with physicians supporting either denial of ICU admission or considering early treatment limitation decisions. Shuster and Marion [31] found a mortality of 80% in 77 patients treated in the ICU. Our study, evaluating prognostic factors of non-HIV-positive immunocompromised patients with pulmonary complications, showed that the mortality rate among HSCT recipients was almost twofold higher than that of patients with hematological malignances or of those who had received solid organ transplants. The requirement of mechanical ventilation was a critical predictor of poor outcome with mortality rates approaching 95% [7]. Long-term survival rates after MV are also dismal in recipients of allogeneic HSCT with active GVHD, with approximately 5% of patients surviving 6 months. Consequently, some clinicians have questioned the utilization of mechanical ventilatory support for these patients.

Over the last years, the pessimistic vision of the dismal outcome of hematological patients admitted to the ICU seems to be changing. First, the number of hematological patients requiring further ICU admission or MV has been decreasing [9]. Second, recent series support the notion that the prognosis for hematological patients admitted to the ICU has improved compared to that reported in the 1980s and early 1990s [32, 33]. Benoit et al. [32], evaluating a cohort of 124 patients with a hematologic malignancy admitted to the ICU for a life-threatening complication, observed an ICU and in-hospital mortality of 42% and 54%, respectively. Soubani et al. [2] evaluated 85 patients admitted to the medical ICU, representing 11.4% of patients who had undergone HSCT during the study period. Fifty-two patients (61%) survived their ICU stay, and 35 patients (41%) were discharged alive from the hospital. The long-term survival rate (>6 months) in this cohort was 28%. Moreover, 19 patients receiving MV (37%) survived their ICU stay, and 33 (97%) patients who did not require MV survived. The study showed short-term and long-term survival rates among adult HSCT recipients who had been admitted to the ICU that were higher than those previously reported. Azoulay et al. [34], in a study evaluating a large group of cancer patients with ARF due to a variety of causes, reported a mortality rate of less than 50%, reaffirming the survival gains achieved in critically ill cancer patients in recent years.

Although the above-mentioned results are promising, some factors should lead us to temper this optimistic picture. A recent meta-analysis by Van Gestel et al. [35] in a population of children did not show survival improvement over time when the variable MV was considered. When the specific studies included in this meta-analysis were individually evaluated, it was shown that some of them showed improved survival in ventilated, post-HSCT patients, while others did not show such improvement. Even in those studies that reported improved survival, the need for MV was a strong indicator of worse prognosis. These controversial results may be due to many different variables accounting for survival in hematological patients requiring ICU admission.

In the following, we report some of the most determining variables that have been related to survival in HSCT recipients.

5.4.1 Selection of Patients

The number of HSCT recipients requiring ICU admission is decreasing [2]. This lower ratio of admissions is unlikely to be due to the underutilization of ICU resources. Rather, it is probably related to a shorter neutropenic phase, better antimicrobial prophylaxis and treatment, and improved experience in the management of these patients before their condition deteriorates. Also, the improved survival may partially be explained by the implantation of restrictive policies for selecting patients to ICU admission. Although the selection of the best candidates for ICU care is difficult and there are no objective data to support the decision [36], it is possible that selection of patients who are most likely to benefit from ICU admission might explain part of the survival gains. Also, it is possible that the decrease in mortality was, in fact, accompanied by a decrease in the number of patients requiring MV, a known risk factor for poor outcome. Reasons for a decrease in the number of HSCT patients who require MV may be related to a decrease in pulmonary complications in these patients or because hematologists and intensivists are better at the early management of pulmonary complications, thereby minimizing the number of patients who ultimately require MV [3, 37].

5.4.2 Transplant Specific Factors

HSCT recipients have "per se" an adverse prognostic factor in many studies. However the prognosis of both autologous and allogeneic HCT seems to be different. In allogeneic HSCT recipients, infectious complications are more common because they require the administration of immunosuppressive agents after transplantation to prevent or treat GVHD. In addition, GVHD itself causes an immunodeficient state by involving mucosal surfaces, the reticuloendothelial system, and bone marrow. Because of all this, the mortality of recipients of allogeneic HSCT, requiring life-sustaining measures, is extremely high [3, 9]. In contrast, autologous HSCT recipients, who receive a less intense conditioning regimen, have a similar prognosis to other critically ill cancer patients in that their short-term risk of death depends only on the number and type of organ dysfunctions. Few studies have emphasized the radically different outcomes between allogeneic and autologous HSCT recipients in the ICU. Shorr et al. [38] collected data focusing only on autologous HSCT, with the aim of determining the frequency of and risk factors for the use of MV in this population. These authors concluded that MV is infrequently needed following autotransplants. Of 159 patients included, only 17 required MV (10.7%), with 3 of them surviving the episode (17.6%). It is possible that the large proportion of autologous transplantation recipients included in the recently published cohorts might be a confounding factor and led to an underestimation of the mortality rate of allogeneic graft recipients. In particular, the recent series by Soubani et al. [2], which showed a significant improvement in survival in HSCT recipients, included a cohort with almost half of the patients (47%) having received an autologous HSC transplant.

Finally, other reasons related to the transplantation technique that can indicate an improved survival are the reduced toxicity of conditioning regimens, the use of alternative hematopoietic precursor sources, such as mobilized peripheral blood stem cells, and cytokines, such as hematopoietic cell colony-stimulating factors, which significantly shorten the time to engraftment, thus decreasing the incidence of infectious pulmonary complications.

5.4.3 Ventilatory Support

The outcome of alo-HSCT recipients requiring MV has not improved for 2 decades, with consistent survival rates of less than 20% [37, 39, 40] Patients requiring MV have a worse prognosis than similar patients matched for general severity-of-illness scoring systems such as APACHE II, because MV may be directly injurious through increasing the risk for nosocomial pneumonia [41, 42]. Moreover, the association of ARF requiring MV with other organ failures has been reported to be almost uniformly fatal (Fig. 5.1). The avoidance of intubation using ventilatory strategies aimed at minimizing further lung injury may change the dismal prognosis associated with MV in HSCT recipients. Different studies have shown that early implementation of noninvasive ventilation (NIV) is indicated in an early stage of hypoxemic ARF in immunocompromised patients, since it decreases both the requirement of intubation and the incidence of nosocomial pneumonia, and consequently this ventilatory support might improve survival [43–45]. However, caution should be used concerning the unselective use of NIV in immunocompromised patients. Azulay et al. [34] conducted a prospective study to identify factors associated with death in critically ill cancer patients admitted for ARF. These authors observed that mortality in patients treated with NIV who subsequently did not require conventional MV was only 15%, confirming the critical goal that this technique can add to the management of critically ill cancer patients. However, mortality in patients that required conventional MV after 72 h of NIV was very high. The absence of benefit from NIV in patients with severe lung involvement is in agreement with previous reports, suggesting that in selected cases NIV might have a deleterious impact by delaying conventional MV in patients who have ARDS and are managed with nonoptimal diagnostic and treatment strategies. Depuydt et al. [46], in a retrospective revision of 26 patients with hematologic malignancies treated with NIV for ARF, could not demonstrate a survival benefit for the use of NIV in comparison with control patients receiving MV and matched for SAPS II. In this study, NIV was mainly used for the treatment of patients with acute severe hypoxic failure, and 60% of them required immediate endotracheal intubation as well as vasopressor therapy because of circulatory shock [45]. They hypothesized that the protective effect of NIV might be exerted only if applied immediately in an early, more compensated phase of their critical illness.

In summary, based on the extremely poor prognosis of patients requiring MV and the promising results obtained with NIV, it seems logical to recommend the application of this type of ventilatory support to HSCT recipients with pulmonary infiltrates once significant respiratory failure has ensued. Further studies are needed to confirm these results and to determine the optimal duration of NIV in hematological patients.

5.4.4 Importance of Establishing a Specific Diagnosis

HSCT recipients with pulmonary infiltrates need to be managed aggressively, and the underlying etiology must be identified as early as possible. The possibility

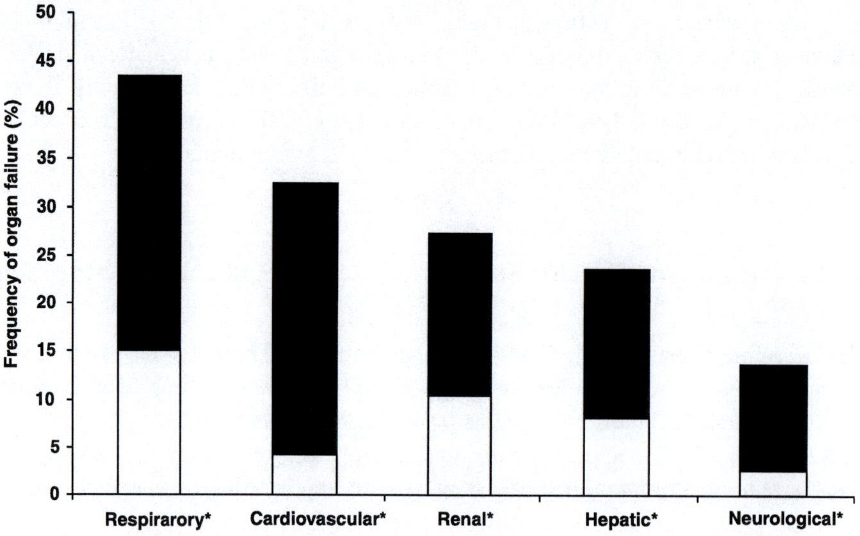

Fig. 5.1 Differences in the incidence of organ failure between survivors (*white segments*) and nonsurvivors (*black segments*) (From [10])

of non-infectious complications and the difficulty of making an antibiotic selection in light of growing resistance and the wide spectrum of potential etiologic factors emphasize the importance of designing strategies aimed at obtaining an early diagnosis. This is particularly true if we consider that inadequacy of the empirical treatment in the ICU setting increases the risk of death significantly [47]. In this sense, it has been shown that early diagnosis of both viral and fungal infections decreases mortality [48]. The use of both non-invasive and bronchoscopic techniques may facilitate the diagnosis in the majority of cases [49]. Some authors advocate the use of non-invasive diagnostic techniques as the cornerstone of the diagnostic workup of these patients, leaving bronchoscopic techniques for those selected patients with no evident risk of deterioration [50]. However, various studies in non-hypoxemic patients outside the ICU have shown that fiberoptic bronchoscopy is a low-risk procedure that can be performed in most patients and may add to the prompt identification of the specific etiologic agent, facilitating an etiology-guided treatment and avoiding unnecessary and potentially harmful additional treatment [51].

More controversial is whether or not the achievement of an early and specific diagnosis improves survival in HSCT recipients admitted to the ICU. Some investigators have reported that obtaining a specific diagnosis does not alter mortality in these patients [52–54]. Other researchers have reached different conclusions [51, 52]. The impact of diagnostic delay on mortality is an important emerging general theme in the care of seriously ill patients, particularly as it affects the adequacy of initial therapy [55]. Recommendations should focus on which is the best diagnostic strategy. In this sense, non-invasive techniques are increasingly used with success in these patients [52]. Bronchoscopy has, no doubt, an important role in the diagnosis, but a diligent analysis of its risk must be performed in each particular patient [52].

5.4.5 Other Factors Influencing Survival

Interestingly, in patients who are selected for ICU admission, the characteristics of the underlying malignancy are not associated with survival. Thus, the response to chemotherapy, stage of the malignancy, and other characteristics of the cancer have little or no impact on short-term survival [9]. The importance of leucopenia as a risk factor for mortality in critically ill patients with a hematologic malignancy is controversial. Different studies have reported a higher mortality in patients with prolonged neutropenia; however, this has not been confirmed by other authors [33]. The infectious etiology of the pulmonary complication has been classically considered as the most important cause of mortality in patients with a hematologic malignancy admitted to the ICU [7, 56], however, a recent study by Benoit et al. [8] reported a better prognosis in patients with documented bacterial infection than in those with non-bacterial pulmonary infections. Even in the absence of an identifiable bacterial microorganism, severely ill hematological patients admitted to the ICU with a clinical suspicion of bacterial infection had a better prognosis.

Other factors that have been considered as early predictors of poor outcome are the use of vasopressors, high urea levels [33], the number and severity of organ failures [9], liver failure, use of glucocorticoids for treating GVHD, and interval time between transplantation and ICU admission.

Although various retrospective analyses in immunocompromised patients indicate that higher APACHE II scores predict mortality [7], extrapolating a specific mortality rate to a particular patient is fraught with difficulty [55]. The information provided by general severity scores should only be considered in light of other clinical and more relevant variables.

Finally, some specific complications have been identified as predictors of favorable outcome, such as the engraftment syndrome, congestive heart failure, and diffuse pulmonary hemorrhage [57].

5.5 Conclusions

Over the last years, important advances in the management of hematological patients requiring ICU admission have taken place. As a result, survival in these patients has improved over the last decade. Thus, the general reluctance to admit patients with a hematologic malignancy to the ICU, even those with severe critical illness, is currently no longer justified. Not all transplanted patients with ARF can be expected to succumb. In the select, low-risk population of patients with autologous SCT with ARF, survival rates fall within a range that we see for many other diseases that are routinely managed in ICU, such as sepsis-related ARDS [42]. In these patients, dedicated and aggressive support in the early phases of respiratory failure to attempt to establish an etiology seems warranted, allowing the early introduction of specific treatment. Early diagnosis is advantageous, and bronchoscopy, when carefully indicated, substantially increases the diagnostic yield, causing changes in the empirical treatment in the majority of patients [7]. The appropriate timing for withholding or withdrawal of support is probably the most contentious issue surrounding the care of these patients [42]. In patients in whom potential benefits of ICU admission are in doubt, a trial of full intensive ICU management should be given for a limited time period, during which daily evaluation of organ dysfunction may provide a more accurate prediction of survival than at admission [9].

References

1. Kotloff RM, Ahya VN, Crawford SW (2004) Pulmonary complications of solid organ and hematopoietic stem cell transplantation. Am J Respir Crit Care Med 170:22–48
2. Soubani AO, Kseibi E, Bander JJ et al (2004) Outcome and prognostic factors of hematopoietic stem cell transplantation recipients admitted to a medical ICU. Chest 126:1604–1611
3. Pène F, Aubron C, Azoulay E et al (2006) Outcome of critically ill allogeneic hematopoietic stem cell transplantation recipients: a reappraisal of indications for organ failure supports. J Clin Oncol 24:643–649
4. Khassawneh BY, White P Jr, Anaissie EJ et al (2002) Outcome from mechanical ventilation after autologous peripheral blood stem cell transplantation. Chest 121: 185–188
5. Ewig S, Torres A, Riquelme R et al (1998) Pulmonary complications in patients with haematological malignancies treated at a respiratory ICU. Eur Respir J 12:116–122
6. Darmon M, Azoulay E, Alberti C et al (2002) Impact of neutropenia duration on short-term mortality in neutropenic critically ill cancer patients. Intensive Care Med 28: 1775–1780
7. Rañó A, Agustí C, Benito N et al (2002) Prognostic factors of non-HIV immunocompromised patients with pulmonary infiltrates. Chest 122:253–261
8. Benoit DD, Depydt PO, Peleman RA et al (2005) Documented and clinically suspected bacterial infection precipitating intensive care unit admission in patients with hematological malignancies: impact on outcome. Int Care Med 31:934–942
9. Darmon M, Azoulay E (2009) Critical care management of cancer patients: cause for optimism and need for objectivity. Curr Opin Oncol 21:318–326
10. Lossos IS, Breuer R, Or R et al (1995) Bacterial pneumonia in recipients of bone marrow transplantation. A five-year prospective study. Transplantation 60(7):672–678
11. Dunagan DP, Am B, Hurd DD, Haponik EF (1997) Bronchoscopic evaluation of pulmonary infiltrates following bone marrow transplantation. Chest 111:135–141
12. Wingard JR (1999) Opportunistic infections after blood and marrow transplantation. Transpl Infect Dis 1(1):3–20
13. BitMansour A, Burns SM, Traver D (2002) Myeloid progenitors protect against invasive aspergillosis and Pseudomonas aeruginosa infection following hematopoietic stem cell transplantation. Blood 100:4660–4667
14. Haley CE, Cohen ML, Halter J et al (1979) Nosocomial Legionnaire´s disease: a continuing common source epidemic at Wadsworth Medical Center. Ann Intern Med 90: 583–586
15. Marr KA, Carter RA, Boeckh M, Martin P, Corey L (2002) Invasive aspergillosis in allogeneic stem cell transplant recipients: changes in epidemiology and risk factors. Blood 100(13):4358–66
16. Neofytos D, Horn D, Annaisie E et al (2009) Epidemiology and outcome of invasive fungal infection in adult hematopoietic stem cell transplant recipients: analysis of Multicenter Prospective Antifungal Therapy (PATH) Alliance registry. Clin Infect Dis 48:265–273
17. Wingard J, Merz W, Rinaldi M et al (1991) Increase in candida krusei infection among patients with bone marrow transplantation and neutropenia treated prophylactically with fluconazole. N Engl J Med 325:1274–1277
18. Horn DL, Neofytos D, Anaissie EJ et al (2009) Epidemiology and outcomes of candidemia in 2019 patients: data from the prospective antifungal therapy alliance registry. Clin Infect Dis 48:1695–1703
19. Lyratzopoulos G, Ellis M, Nerringer R et al (2002) Invasive infection due to penicillium species other than *P. marneffei*. J Infect 45:184–195
20. Marr KA, Carter RA, Crippa F et al (2002) Epidemiology and outcome of mould infections in hematopoietic stem cell transplant recipients. Clin Infect Dis 34:909–917
21. De Hoog GS, Marvin-Sikkema FD, Lahpoor GA et al (1994) Ecology and physiology of the emerging opportunistic fungi *Pseudallescheria boydii* and *Scedosporium prolificans*. Mycoses 37:71
22. Kovacs JA, Masur H (2009) Evolving health effects of Pneumocystis: one hundred years of progress in diagnosis and treatment. JAMA 301:2578–2585
23. De Castro N, Neuville S, Sarfati C et al (2005) Occurrence of Pneumocystis jiroveci pneumonia after allogeneic stem cell transplantation: a 6-year retrospective study. Bone Marrow Transplant 36(10):879–883
24. Sullivan KM, Dykewicz CA, Longworth DL et al (2001) Preventing opportunistic infections after hematopoietic stem cell transplantation: the Centers for Disease Control and Prevention, Infectious Diseases Society of America, and American Society for Blood and Marrow Transplantation Practice Guidelines and beyond. Hematology Am Soc Hematol Educ Program 2001:392–421
25. Taplitz RA, Jordan MC (2002) Pneumonia caused by herpes viruses in recipients of hematopoietic cell transplants. Semin Respir Infect 17:121–129
26. Boeckh M, Leisenring W, Riddell SR et al (2003) Late cytomegalovirus disease and mortality in recipients of allogeneic

hematopoietic stem cell transplants: importance of viral load and T-cell immunity. Blood 101:407–414
27. Chemaly RF, Ghosh S, Bodey GP et al (2006) Respiratory viral infections in adults with hematologic malignancies and human stem cell transplantation recipients: a retrospective study at a major cancer center. Medicine (Baltimore) 85: 278–287
28. Bowden RA (1997) Respiratory virus infections after marrow transplant: the Fred Hutchinson Cancer Research Center experience. Am J Med 102:27–30, discussion 42-3
29. Fischer SA (2008) Emerging viruses in transplantation: there is more to infection after transplant than CMV and EBV. Transplantation 86:1327–1339
30. Buchbinder S, Elmaagacli AH, Schaefer UW, Roggendorf M (2000) Human herpesvirus 6 is an important pathogen in infectious lung disease after allogeneic bone marrow transplantation. Bone Marrow Transplant 26:639–44
31. Schuster DP, Marion JM (1983) Precedents for meaningful recovery during treatment in a medical intensive care unit. Am J Med 75:402–408
32. Benoit DD, Vandewoude KH, Decruyenaere JM, Hoste EA, Colardyn FA (2003) Outcome and early prognostic indicators in patients with a hematologic malignancy admitted to the intensive care unit for a life-threatening complication. Crit Care Med 31:104–112
33. Dane N, Maziarz RT, Haupt MT (1999) Mechanical ventilation in hematopoietic stem cell transplant patients: is there need for re-evaluation? Chest 116:857–859
34. Azoulay E, Thièry G, Chevret S et al (2004) The prognosis of acute respiratory failure in critically ill cancer patients. Medicine 83:360–370
35. Van Gestel J, Bollen C, Van der Tweel I et al (2008) Intensive care unit mortality trends in children after hematopoietic stem cell transplantation: a meta-regression analysis. Crit Care Med 36:2898–2904
36. Thiery G, Azoulay E, Darmon M et al (2005) Outcome of cancer patients considered for intensive care unit admission: a hospital-wide prospective study. J Clin Oncol 23: 4406–4413
37. Parker RI (2008) Paediatric intensive care unit outcome following paediatric hematopoietic stem cell transplantation: Quo Vadis? Crit Care Med 36:2954–2955
38. Shorr AF, Moores LK, Edenfield WJ et al (1999) Mechanical ventilation in hematopoietic stem cell transplantation. Can we effectively predict outcomes? Chest 116:1012–1018
39. Bach PB, Schrag D, Nierman DM et al (2001) Identification of poor prognostic features among patients requiring mechanical ventilation after hematopoietic stem cell transplantation. Blood 93:3234–3240
40. Price KJ, Thall PF, Kish SK et al (1998) Prognostic indicators for blood and marrow transplant patients admitted to an intensive care unit. Am J Respir Crit Care Med 158: 876–884
41. Nichols DJ, Maziarz RT, Haupt MT (1999) Mechanical ventilation in hematopoietic stem cell transplant recipients: is there need for reevaluation? Chest 116:857–859
42. Esteban A, Anzueto A, Frutos F et al (2002) Characteristics and outcomes in adult patients receiving mechanical ventilation. A 28-day international study. JAMA 287:345–355
43. Antonelli M, Conti C, Rocco M et al (1998) A comparison of noninvasive positive-pressure ventilation and conventional mechanical ventilation in patients with acute respiratory failure. N Engl J Med 339:429–435
44. Hilbert G, Gruson D, Vargas F et al (2001) Noninvasive ventilation in immunocompromised patients with pulmonary infiltrates, fever, and acute respiratory failure. N Engl J Med 95:358–364
45. Azoulay E, Alberti C, Bornstain C et al (2001) Improved survival in cancer patients requiring mechanical ventilatory support: impact of noninvasive mechanical ventilatory support. Crit Care Med 29:519–525
46. Depuydt PO, Benoit DD, Vandewoude KH et al (2004) Outcome in noninvasively and invasively ventilated hematologic patients with acute respiratory failure. Chest 126: 1299–1306
47. Ibrahim EH, Sherman G, Ward S et al (2000) The influence of inadequate antimicrobial treatment of blood stream infections on patient outcomes in the ICU setting. Chest 118: 146–155
48. Elizaga J, Olavarria E, Apperley JF et al (2001) Parainfluenzae virus 3 infection after stem cell transplant: relevance to outcome of rapid diagnosis and ribavirin treatment. Clin Infect Dis 32:413–418
49. Rañó A, Agustí C, Jiménez P et al (2001) Pulmonary infiltrates in non-HIV immunocompromised patients: a diagnostic approach using non-invasive and bronchoscopic procedures. Thorax 56:379–387
50. Azoulay E, Mokart D, Rabbat A et al (2008) Diagnostic bronchoscopy in hematology and oncology patients with acute respiratory failure: prospective multicenter data. Crit Care Med 36:100–107
51. Shorr AF, Susla GM, O'Grady NP (2004) Pulmonary infiltrates in the non-HIV-infected immunocompromised patient: etiologies, diagnostic strategies and outcomes. Chest 125: 260–271
52. White D, Bonacum JT, Miller CB (1997) Utility of fiberoptic bonchoscopy in bone marrow transplant patients. Bone Marrow Transplant 20:681–687
53. Murray PV, O'Brien ME, Padhani AR et al (2001) Use of first line bronchoalveolar lavage in the immunosuppressed oncology patient. Bone Marrow Transplant 27:967–71
54. Poe RH, Wahl GW, Qazi R et al (1986) Predictors of mortality in immunocompromised patients with pulmonary infiltrates. Arch Intern Med 146:1304–1308
55. Shorr AF, Kollef MH (2002) The quick and the dead: the importance of rapid evaluation of infiltrates in the immunocompromised patient. Chest 122:9–12
56. Groeger JS, White P, Nierman DM et al (1999) Outcome for cancer patients requiring mechanical ventilation. J Clin Oncol 17:991–997
57. Lee CK, Gingrich RD, Hohl RJ et al (1995) Engraftment syndrome in autologous bone marrow and peripheral stem cell transplantation. Bone Marrow Transplant 16:175–182

Noninfectious Lung Involvement in Patients with Hematological Malignancies (Excluding BMT)

6

Bernard Maitre

Contents

B. Maitre
Service de Pneumologie, Hôpitaux Henri Mondor et intercommunal, Créteil,
Université Paris XII, PRES EST France
e-mail: antenne.pneumo@hmn.aphp.fr

6.1 Epidemiology

Patients with hematological malignancies frequently experience pulmonary diseases, and these complications represent a difficult challenge for physicians. The aim of this chapter is not to give an exhaustive review of noninfectious causes of lung involvement in these patients, but to highlight the frequency of some of well-known lung diseases. We have made the choice to examine three different aspects of noninfectious lung involvement in hematological patients that are also covered in three different chapters in this book, namely, thromboembolism, secondary cancers and treatment-related pulmonary toxicity. Our major goal is to illustrate the wide spectrum of lung diseases in hematological patients.

6.2 Venous Thromboembolism in the Hematologic Malignancies

Patients with hematological malignancies are well known to be at high risk of hemorrhagic complications, but are also at high risk of venous thromboembolism (VTE) [11]. Dr. Khorana has contributed a specific chapter on this topic in this book. Compared with the estimated annual incidence of VTE in the general population, the incidence of 0.1–0.5% in the cancer population appears in the ranges of VTE in patients with high-risk solid tumors [18]. Immobility, age, previous thrombotic history, venous stasis and infection are all disease-host risk factors for VTE. Treatment-related risk factors, such as chemotherapy, hormone therapy, erythropoiesis-stimulating factor or central venous devices, can participate to the general risk [15].

É. Azoulay (ed.), *Pulmonary Involvement in Patients with Hematological Malignancies*,
DOI: 10.1007/978-3-642-15742-4_6, © Springer-Verlag Berlin Heidelberg 2011

Current published data allow estimation of VTE rates in patients with lymphoma, acute leukemia (AL) and multiple myeloma (MM).

6.2.1 Lymphoma

In a large cohort study from Khorana et al., lymphoma was associated with the third risk level of thrombosis after upper gastrointestinal cancers and lung cancers [15]. The retrospective analysis from [24] found a global VTE incidence of 7.7%, with a significantly higher rate in patients with high-grade lymphoma (10.6%). The thrombosis incidence is even higher in CNS lymphoma patients mostly receiving methotrexate (59.5%) [12]. Two studies have prospectively evaluated the incidence of VTE in lymphoma. The VTE rate was estimated between 6.6% and 8.6% depending on the type of lymphoma (Hodgkin's disease versus non-Hodgkin's lymphoma) and chemotherapy regimens [15, 26]. A platelet count higher than 350,000 mm^3 and vessel compression by the tumor were risk factors for VTE.

6.2.2 Acute Leukemia

Thrombotic events have been described to be less frequent than hemorrhages in AL patients, particularly in acute promyelocytic leukemia. However, recent studies suggest a significant rate of thrombosis, which can vary from 1.4% to 12% depending on the timing: at diagnosis or during remission induction therapy. A large population-based cohort study of patients with AL, AML or ALL was used to determine the incidence and risk factors associated with development of VTE. The 2-year cumulative incidence of VTE was 5.2% in AML and 4.5% in ALL [17]. In AML patients, female sex, older age, number of chronic comorbidities, and presence of a catheter were significant predictors of development of VTE within 1 year. A diagnosis of VTE was not associated with reduced survival in AML patients. Risk factors for VTE in ALL patients were presence of a central venous catheter, older age and number of chronic comorbidities. In the patients with ALL, development of VTE was associated with a 40% increase in the risk of dying within 1 year. In acute lymphoid leukemia, two meta-analyses found an incidence of 5.2% (children) to 5.9% (adults) of thrombotic events [5, 6].

6.2.3 Multiple Myeloma

Ten percent of patients with MM will develop a VTE. Thalidomide and its derivative increase the response of treatment, but when these drugs are associated with doxorubicin or dexamethasone, the risk of VTE is two or three times more likely [3, 10]. Few data are available for lenalidomide, but it seems associated with an increase of thrombotic events, particularly in combination with dexamethasone (6% vs. 2%) [22]. A recent study combining results and follow-up of two randomized protocols, including 353 patients with MM, showed a thromboembolic event in 17% of patients. However, contrary to patients with solid cancer, it is not associated with shorter survival [32].

6.3 Drug-Induced Lung Toxicity

Infiltrative lung diseases related to the use of antineoplastic agents are being increasingly described in patients with hematological malignancies. A chapter from Camus and coworkers covers this topic very well in this book. Although the pulmonary toxicity of old agents is well known, they contribute little to significant pulmonary disease. However, newer drugs or old drugs with new indications (such as thalidomide in MM) increase the incidence of such complications substantially.

Regarding epidemiological data, conversely to VTE, no specific diagnostic criteria are set up to report on precise the incidence of drug-induced lung diseases. Drugs can produce all histological patterns of interstitial pneumonia, and there are no specific histological criteria for drug-induced lung disease. The diagnosis rests on a temporal association between exposure and the development of respiratory symptoms. Since patients with hematological malignancies are often being treated at the same time by different antineoplastic drugs or exposed to a wide variety of others medications, with potential lung toxicity, increased difficulties exist when trying to affirm the relation between one drug and lung toxicity.

The incidence of drug-induced lung toxicities varies considerably from 0.1% to 15% of patients with hematological malignancies. It has to be noted that concomitant use of steroids does not necessarily prevent the development of lung toxicities (Table 6.1).

Table 6.1 Antineoplastic agents associated with lung disease

Agent	Class	Incidence	Frequency
Anthracyclines	Cytotoxic antibiotics	<0.1	
Azacytidine	Demethylating agent	<5	a
Bleomycin	Antineoplastic antibiotic		c
Bortezomib	Proteasome inhibitor	15	a
Busulfan	Alkylating agent		c
Carmustine	Nitrosourea		c
Cladribine	Purine analog	<0.1	a
Cyclophosphamide	Alkylating agent		c
Cytosine Arabinoside	Antimetabolite analog		b
Dasatinib	Tyrosine kinase inhibitor	<0.1	b
Etoposide	Topoisomerase inhibitor		c
Fludarabine	Purine analog	<9	b
Gemcitabine	Antimetabolite		b
Hydroxyurea	Antimetabolite		b
Imatinib	Tyrosine kinase inhibitor	<1.3	a
Interferon-alpha	Interferon	1.5	b
Lenalidomine	Thalidomide derivative	6	a
Lomustine	Nitrosourea		b
Melphalan	Alkylating agent		b
Methotrexate	Antimetabolite agent		c
Procarbazine	Alkylating agent	<0.1	b
Rituximab	Monoclonal antibody	<0.1	b
Thalidomide	Thalidomide	<0.1	a
Trofosfamide	Alkykating agent	<0.1	a
Vinblastine	Vinca alkaloid		c

Pneumotox® website [4]

[a]Isolated cases

[b]10 cases reported

[c]20–100 cases reported

Adapted from http://pneumotox.com

6.4 Lung Diseases Induced by Radiation of the Chest

Radiation lung toxicity can develop during or following radiation therapy for Hodgkin's or non-Hodgkin's lymphoma, or total body irradiation (TBI). Gallego and Rello have covered this topic very nicely in this book. Variation in study population, treatment regimen and criteria for radiation pneumonia diagnosis hampers the comparison of patient cohorts across different studies. In contrast to allogeneic BMT studies, the incidence of pneumonitis is low (between 0% and 16%). In a study of 94 patients who underwent BMT using an escalated TBI-containing conditioning regimen, Chen and coworkers looked at pretransplant variables that predict radiation-induced pneumonitis [7]. They failed to find predictable variables other than pretransplant hemoglobin less than 100 g/L. This suggests that TBI itself is the main factor, and this has been confirmed by comparison with others cohorts of patients with lymphoma who have been treated by the same conditioning regimen with or without TBI [7]. This has been confirmed in patients with MM. Unacceptable risk of pulmonary fibrosis has been described in regimens combining radiation and drugs, such as gemcitabin, vinblastin, bleomycin and methotrexate. However, in one study of 60 early stage Hodgkin's lymphoma (HL) patients receiving an ABVD regimen, adding mediastinal radiotherapy was associated with a significant decrease in FVC and DLCO. This worsening respiratory function was observed in 37% of patients, but with no translation into clinical symptoms [14].

Mediastinal emphysema and pneumothorax have also been described in case series, and a frequency of 2.2% has been proposed for Hodgkin's patient without previous lung disease and treated by mantle radiation therapy [27, 28]. This suggests a pathophysiologic link between apical fibrosis and onset of pneumothorax. Strikingly, most patients were asymptomatic.

Radiation can also cause vasculopathy with intimal damage in both arterioles and veinules. Different case reports have emphasized the risk of veno-occlusive disease of the liver but also the lung following TBI and a conditioned regimen before bone marrow transplantation, but case reports described this complication in patients following radiation in a mantle distribution [16, 19].

6.5 Secondary Lung Cancers

Although the possibility of a malignant involvement in different organs is possible and frequent in hematological malignancies, secondary malignancy as a result of long-term complications of treatment is one of the most concerning problems for physicians.

6.5.1 Hodgkin's Lymphoma

Solid tumors account for more than one-half of second malignancies developing after 15 or more years of follow-up in patients treated for HL. Although no prospective study has reported the occurrence of a new second cancer, 20 retrospective studies with long-term outcomes have been published [20]. In this study, relative risk and absolute excess risk of second malignant disease in 32,591 patients treated for HL were as follows: for all solid tumors, RR 2.0 (1.9–2.4) and absolute excess risks of 33.1; for esophagus, 2.8 (1.8–4.0) and 0.7, for stomach, 1.5 (0.3–3.5) and 0.1; for small intestine 1.9 (1.5–2.4) and 1.5; for colon, 2.9 (2.6–3.2) and 9.7; for the lung 1.6 (1.4–1.9) and 2.0; for female breast, 9.9 (8.7–11.2) and 8.8 [20].

Lung cancer frequencies varied across studies: 1/3 of solid tumors in the British National Lymphoma Organization and less than 10% in the American study [29, 30].

Risk of lung cancer is significantly increased in patients who have been treated for HL[21, 25]. The median relative risk of a second lung cancer ranges from 2.6 to 7. Several risk factors have been described: (1) age at treatment older than 45 years; (2) time since treatment, but above 20–30 years after treatment the risk falls to that of the untreated population; (3) the treatment modality is an important risk factor: an increased number of cycles >9 or a MOPP regimen; radiotherapy is a more important factor than chemotherapy itself, increasing the radiation dose up to 40 Gy; (4) the smoking habit, smoking at the time of treatment or current smokers can increase the risk for lung cancer [30], but not the amount smoked before diagnosis [31].

There appears to be a more than multiplicative relation between smoking-related and radiation-related or alkylating agent risk (Table 6.2). Contrarily, gender, splenic involvement or splenectomy and combined modality do not appear to be associated with a high risk.

6.5.2 Second Cancers Following Bone Marrow Transplantation

In the largest study conducted to date among 19,229 recipients of allogeneic and syngeneic HCT, the cumulative incidence of second cancers at 5, 10 and 15 years after transplantation was 0.7%, 2.2% and 6.7%, respectively. In the general population, these rates are of 0.3%, 0.6% and 0.8% [23].

Table 6.2 Risk of developing lung cancer in Hodgkin's lymphoma patients depending on treatment regimens and smoking habits

Radiation > 5 Gy	Alkylating agents	Smoking habits in the 5 years before diagnosis of lung cancer	Relative risk [95% CI]
–	–	–	1.0[a]
–	+	–	4.3 [2–12]
–	–	+	6.0 [2–20]
+	–	–	7.2 [3–21]
+	+	–	7.2 [3–22]
–	+	+	16.8 [6–53]
+	–	+	20.2 [7–68]
+	+	+	49.1 [15–187]

Data from Travis et al. [30]

[a]The reference group consisted of 21 patients with lung cancer and 98 control patients who received a radiation dose of less than 5 Gy to the specific location in the lung where the cancer was diagnosed

6.6 Other Lung Diseases

6.6.1 Pulmonary Extramedullary Hematopoiesis

Acute respiratory failure and pulmonary fibrosis have been described in patients with agnogenic myeloid metaplasia, but parenchymal nodules and pleural effusion have been described as well [1, 2].

6.6.2 Pulmonary Hypertension and Myelofibrosis

An association between pulmonary hypertension and myeloproliferative diseases has been suggested in small series [9]. For these reasons, it is difficult to estimate the incidence of this complication, but it is probably a rare disease. It has been suggested that there are two distinct forms of pulmonary hypertension [13]. Chronic thromboembolism disease is a common complication of myeloproliferative disease and can induce pulmonary hypertension. This form of pulmonary hypertension occurred more frequently in the first 2 years. Arterial pulmonary hypertension seems less frequent and occurred in a late course of the disease, suggesting that myeloid infiltration participates in the physiopathology.

6.6.3 Alveolar Proteinosis

In a retrospective study, Fleury Feith and colleagues estimated the incidence of this rare complication at 5.3% among all the hematologic population and 10% in patients with myeloid disorders [8]. The study is based on a BAL retrospective study, but may represent in most cases a more surfactant dysfunction than a lung disease. Alveolar proteinosis is covered by the contribution to this book by Vincent and Tandjaoui.

6.7 Summary

Noninfectious lung involvement in patients with hematological malignancies is a frequent condition. If infectious disease and cardiogenic pulmonary edema are the most frequent complications, VTE and drug-induced lung toxicity could potentially be detected early during the hematological disease. Risk of lung cancers is significantly increased in patients with CLL, those treated for lymphoma or those who underwent bone marrow transplantation. This emphasized the need to encourage patients to stop smoking, and a screening program for lung cancer in high-risk patients (age >45 years, chest irradiation and smokers) should be discussed.

References

1. Asakura S, Colby TV (1994) Agnogenic myeloid metaplasia with extramedullary hematopoiesis and fibrosis in the lung. Report of two cases. Chest 105:1866–1868
2. Bartlett RP, Greipp PR, Tefferi A et al (1995) Extramedullary hematopoiesis manifesting as a symptomatic pleural effusion. Mayo Clin Proc 70:1161–1164
3. Baz R, Li L, Kottke-Marchant K et al (2005) The role of aspirin in the prevention of thrombotic complications of thalidomide and anthracycline-based chemotherapy for multiple myeloma. Mayo Clin Proc 80:1568–1574
4. Camus P, Foucher P Pneumotox® website (1997) Last update 2009 http//pneumotox.com.
5. Caruso V, Iacoviello L, Di Castelnuovo A et al (2007) Venous thrombotic complications in adults undergoing induction treatment for acute lymphoblastic leukemia: results from a meta-analysis. J Thromb Haemost 5:621–623
6. Caruso V, Iacoviello L, Castelnuovo D et al (2006) Thrombotic complications in childhood acute lymphoblastic leukemia: a meta-analysis of 17 prospective studies comprising 1, 752 pediatric patients. Blood 108:2216–2222
7. Chen CI, Abraham R, Tsang et al (2001) Radiation-associated pneumonitis following autologous stem cell transplantation: predictive factors, disease characteristics and treatment outcomes. Bone Marrow Transplant 27: 177–182
8. Cordonnier C, Fleury-Feith J, Escudier E et al (1994) Secondary alveolar proteinosis is a reversible cause of respiratory failure in leukemic patients. Am J Respir Crit Care Med 149:788–794
9. Dingli D, Utz JP, Krowka MJ et al (2001) Unexplained pulmonary hypertension in chronic myeloproliferative disorders. Chest 120:801–808
10. El Accaoui RN, Shamseddeen WA, Taher AT (2007) Thalidomide and thrombosis. A meta-analysis. Thromb Haemost 97:1031–1036
11. Falanga A, Marchetti M (2009) Venous thromboembolism in the hematologic malignancies. J Clin Oncol 27: 4848–4857
12. Goldschmidt N, Linetsky E, Shalom E, Varon D, Siegal T (2003) High incidence of thromboembolism in patients with central nervous system lymphoma. Cancer 98: 1239–1242
13. Guilpain P, Montani D, Damaj G et al (2008) Pulmonary hypertension associated with myeloproliferative disorders: a retrospective study of ten cases. Respiration 76:295–302
14. Hirsch A, Vander Els N, Straus DJ et al (1996) Effect of ABVD chemotherapy with and without mantle or mediastinal irradiation on pulmonary function and symptoms in early-stage Hodgkin's disease. J Clin Oncol 14: 1297–1305
15. Khorana AA, Francis CW, Culakova E et al (2005) Risk factors for chemotherapy-associated venous thromboembolism in a prospective observational study. Cancer 104: 2822–2829
16. Kramer MR, Estenne M, Berkman N et al (1993) Radiation-induced pulmonary veno-occlusive disease. Chest 104: 1282–1284
17. Ku GH, White RH, Chew HK et al (2009) Venous thromboembolism in patients with acute leukemia: incidence, risk factors, and effect on survival. Blood 113:3911–3917
18. Lee AY, Levine MN (2003) Venous thromboembolism and cancer: risks and outcomes. Circulation 107:I17–21
19. Lombard CM, Churg A, Winokur S (1987) Pulmonary veno-occlusive disease following therapy for malignant neoplasms. Chest 92:871–876
20. Lorigan P, Radford J, Howell A et al (2005) Lung cancer after treatment for Hodgkin's lymphoma: a systematic review. Lancet Oncol 6:773–779
21. Mauch PM, Kalish LA, Marcus KC et al (1996) Second malignancies after treatment for laparotomy staged IA-IIIB Hodgkin's disease: long-term analysis of risk factors and outcome. Blood 87:3625–3632
22. Menon SP, Rajkumar SV, Lacy M et al (2008) Thromboembolic events with lenalidomide-based therapy for multiple myeloma. Cancer 112:1522–1528
23. Metayer C, Curtis RE, Vose J et al (2003) Myelodysplastic syndrome and acute myeloid leukemia after autotransplantation for lymphoma: a multicenter case-control study. Blood 101:2015–2023
24. Mohren M, Markmann I, Jentsch-Ullrich et al (2006) Increased risk of venous thromboembolism in patients with acute leukaemia. Br J Cancer 94:200–202
25. Ng AK, Bernardo P, Weller E et al (2002) Second malignancy after Hodgkin disease treated with radiation therapy with or without chemotherapy: long-term risks and risk factors. Blood 100:1989–1996
26. Ottinger H, Belka C, Kozol et al (1995) Deep venous thrombosis and pulmonary artery embolism in high-grade non Hodgkin's lymphoma: incidence, causes and prognostic relevance. Eur J Haematol 54:186–194
27. Pezner RD, Horak DA, Sayegh HO et al (1990) Spontaneous pneumothorax in patients irradiated for Hodgkin's disease and other malignant lymphomas. Int J Radiat Oncol Biol Phys 18:193–198
28. Shapiro SJ, Shapiro SD, Mill WB et al (1990) Prospective study of long-term pulmonary manifestations of mantle irradiation. Int J Radiat Oncol Biol Phys 19:707–714
29. Swerdlow AJ, Douglas AJ, Hudson GV et al (1992) Risk of second primary cancers after Hodgkin's disease by type of treatment: analysis of 2846 patients in the British National Lymphoma Investigation. BMJ 304:1137–1143
30. Travis LB, Gospodarowicz M, Curtis RE et al (2002) Lung cancer following chemotherapy and radiotherapy for Hodgkin's disease. J Natl Cancer Inst 94:182–192
31. van Leeuwen FE, Klokman WJ, Stovall M et al (1995) Roles of radiotherapy and smoking in lung cancer following Hodgkin's disease. J Natl Cancer Inst 87:1530–1537
32. Zangari M, Tricot G, Polavaram L et al (2010) Survival effect of venous thromboembolism in patients with multiple myeloma treated with lenalidomide and high-dose dexamethasone. J Clin Oncol 28:132–135

Noninfectious Pulmonary Involvement in Hematopoietic Stem Cell or Bone Marrow Transplant Recipients

7

Bekele Afessa

Contents

7.1 Introduction

Worldwide, tens of thousands of patients undergo blood and marrow transplants (BMT) each year, mainly for hematologic disorders [1]. BMT recipients are often treated with a conditioning regimen before the transplant. Conditioning regimens with total body irradiation ≥500 cGY, single fractionated dose ≥800 cGY, busulfan doses of >9 mg/kg, or malphalan doses of >150 mg/m² given as single agents or in combination with other agents are considered *myeloablative*. Conditioning regimens with lower doses of total body irradiation, fractionated doses, busulfan, and malphalan than those used in myeloablative regimens are considered *non-myeloablative* or *lower intensity* conditioning regimens. The majority of BMT performed worldwide is autologous. Mobilized peripheral blood stem cells are the main graft source for autologous BMT, accounting for >90% [1]. Bone marrow is the primary graft source in children undergoing allogeneic BMT. However, the use of peripheral blood and umbilical blood grafts in children is increasing. During the period

B. Afessa
Division of Pulmonary and Critical Care Medicine, Mayo Clinic College of Medicine, 200 First St SW, Rochester, MN 55905, USA
e-mail: afessa.bekele@mayo.edu

É. Azoulay (ed.), *Pulmonary Involvement in Patients with Hematological Malignancies*,
DOI: 10.1007/978-3-642-15742-4_7, © Springer-Verlag Berlin Heidelberg 2011

from 2003 to 2007, peripheral blood and umbilical cord blood grafts accounted for 28% and 20%, respectively, of allogeneic BMT in children [1]. Peripheral blood is the source of allogeneic graft in approximately 80% of BMT recipients older than 20 years. The most common indications for BMT are multiple myeloma and lymphoma, accounting for 63% in North America [1]. Multiple myeloma is the most common indication for autologous transplantation and acute myelogeneic leukemia for allogeneic transplantation.

The post-transplant period is divided into three phases: pre-engraftment (0–30 days), early post-engraftment (30–100 days), and late post-transplant (>100 days). BMT recipients' underlying diseases, the chemotherapy and radiation therapy they receive to treat the underlying diseases, and the conditioning regimen result in damage to multiple organ systems. Pulmonary complications develop in 30–60% of BMT recipients [2–4]. The pulmonary complications follow characteristic time patterns [5]. With the widespread use of prophylaxis for certain infections, the spectrum of pulmonary complications following BMT has shifted from more infectious to non-infectious complications [6]. Among the non-infectious pulmonary complications, pulmonary edema, diffuse alveolar hemorrhage (DAH), and peri-engraftment respiratory distress syndrome (PERDS) usually occur during the first 30 days following transplant (Fig. 7.1). Idiopathic pneumonia syndrome (IPS) can occur at any time following transplant. We will review the main non-infectious pulmonary complications in this chapter (Tables 7.1 and 7.2).

Table 7.1 Noninfectious pulmonary complications in blood and marrow transplant recipients

Isolated abnormality in pulmonary function
Asthma
Acute pulmonary edema
Bronchiolitis obliterans
Bronchiolitis obliterans organizing pneumonia
Idiopathic pneumonia syndrome
Diffuse alveolar hemorrhage
Peri-engraftment respiratory distress syndrome
Delayed pulmonary toxicity syndrome
Pulmonary cytolytic thrombi
Pulmonary veno-occlusive disease
Progressive pulmonary fibrosis
Pulmonary hypertension
Hepatopulmonary syndrome
Pulmonary alveolar proteinosis
Eosinophilic pneumonia

7.2 Pulmonary Function Abnormalities

Pulmonary function test (PFT) in BMT recipients has shown that restrictive and obstructive ventilatory defects and gas transfer abnormalities are frequent

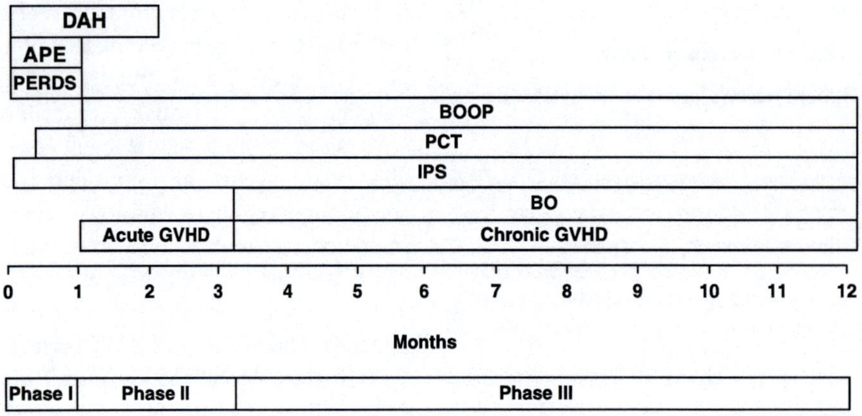

Fig. 7.1 Timing of the major non-infectious complications following blood and marrow transplantation. *BO* Bronchiolitis obliterans, *DAH* diffuse alveolar hemorrhage, *GVHD* graft-versus-host-disease, *IPS* idiopathic pneumonia syndrome, *P edema* pulmonary edema, *PERDS* peri-engraftment respiratory distress syndrome, *Phase I* pre-engraftment period, *Phase II* early post-engraftment period, *phase III* late post-engraftment period

Table 7.2 Characteristics of selected pulmonary complications in BMT recipients

Characteristics	BO	BOOP	DAH	PERDS	IPS
Incidence	3.8% in allogeneic, rare in autologous	Low	5%	5%	10%
Clinical features	Dyspnea Cough Wheezing	Dyspnea Cough Fever	Dyspnea Cough Fever	Dyspnea Fever	Cough Dyspnea
PFT	Airway obstruction	↓ TLC ↓ DLCO			↓ TLC ↓ DLCO
Radiographic features	Air trapping Hyperinflation Normal	Consolidation Ground-glass opacity Nodular opacity	Infiltrates Ground-glass opacities	Infiltrates	Diffuse infiltrates
Definite diagnosis	Surgical biopsy	Surgical biopsy Transbronchial biopsy	Bronchoscopy	Clinical Bronchoscopy	Bronchoscopy Surgical biopsy
Treatment	Immuno-suppressant	Steroids	Steroids	Steroids	None
Case fatality	High (59%)	Low (19%)	High (80%)	26%	74%

BMT Hematopoietic peripheral blood and bone marrow stem cell transplant, *BO* bronchiolitis obliterans, *BOOP* bronchiolitis obliterans organizing pneumonia, *DAH* diffuse alveolar hemorrhage, *DLCO* diffusion of carbon monooxide, *IPS* idiopathic pneumonia syndrome, *PERDS* peri-engraftment respiratory distress syndrome, *PFT* pulmonary function test, *TLC* total lung capacity

long-term sequelae, particularly following allogeneic transplantation [6, 7]. A systematic review of 20 publications published between 1996 and 2001 found decreased carbon monoxide diffusion (DLCO) in 83%, restriction in 35%, and obstruction in 23% of allogeneic BMT recipients [8]. A retrospective cohort study of over 500 BMT recipients from the University of Toronto covering a more contemporary period of 1980–1997 documented somewhat lower frequencies: impaired diffusion in 35%, restriction in 12%, and obstruction in only 6% of long-term survivors [9]. While the frequency of restriction and impaired diffusion appeared constant over time, this study suggested a declining frequency of airflow obstruction: 15% in patients transplanted before 1987 compared to 5% for those receiving transplantation after 1987. The extremely low incidence of airflow obstruction documented in this study likely reflects the very stringent diagnostic criteria utilized by the authors. Utilizing a more sensitive definition, Chien and colleagues identified airflow obstruction in 26% of long-term survivors of allogeneic BMT in a contemporary series from the Fred Hutchinson Cancer Center [10]. Notably, the development of airflow obstruction serves as a marker for increased risk of mortality following transplantation [9–11].

Risk factors for the development of PFT abnormalities following BMT include smoking history, pre-transplant pulmonary infection and viral infection in the early post-transplant period, older age, underlying disease, pre-transplant chemotherapy and conditioning regimen, graft-versus-host-disease (GVHD), and HLA-mismatch [9, 10, 12–26]. Respiratory muscle weakness due to GVHD-associated myositis has been described following allogeneic BMT and may rarely be a contributing factor to restrictive pulmonary function abnormalities [27–29].

Several studies have suggested that abnormal pulmonary function may be a risk factor for the subsequent development of pulmonary complications in BMT recipients [14, 30–34]. However, some investigators have reported conflicting data showing no significant association between baseline pulmonary function values and subsequent pulmonary complications or mortality [15, 26]. Moreover, there is considerable variability among published studies in the particular pulmonary parameters deemed to be predictive, the post-transplant complications that they predict, and the strength of the association [35].

7.3 Asthma

There are case reports of asthma developing after allogeneic BMT [36–40]. Limited data suggest that the serum IgE level, of donor origin, is elevated following transplantation [41]. Allergen-specific IgE-mediated hypersensitivity can be transferred from donor to recipient by B cells with allergen-specific memory leading to atopic dermatitis, allergic rhinitis, and asthma [36, 37, 41, 42]. The management of asthma in BMT recipients is similar to that of the other population.

7.4 Acute Pulmonary Edema

Acute pulmonary edema in BMT recipients commonly occurs during the neutropenic phase and results from a combination of both hydrostatic and non-hydrostatic (capillary leak) factors [43]. Hydrostatic pulmonary edema may result from high volumes of fluid for medications, total parenteral nutrition, and multiple transfusions. The heart may also be compromised by a number of chemotherapeutic drugs, such as adriamycin and high-dose cyclophosphamide. Clinical features include weight gain, dyspnea, and bibasilar crackles. The radiographic findings may include vascular redistribution, increased interstitial markings, Kerley B lines, and ground-glass opacities. Cardiomegaly is generally absent unless there is associated cardiac dysfunction. Acute pulmonary edema can be prevented and treated with fluid restriction and diuretics.

7.5 Bronchiolitis Obliterans

Graft-versus-host disease (GVHD) is a major complication of allogeneic BMT, with an overall incidence between 30% and 60% [44]. Infectious and non-infectious pulmonary complications are common in BMT recipients with GVHD. The pulmonary histology of BMT recipients with GVHD may show diffuse alveolar damage, lymphocytic bronchitis/ bronchiolitis with interstitial pneumonitis, bronchiolitis obliterans organizing pneumonia (BOOP), and bronchiolitis obliterans (BO) [45]. BO is a nonspecific inflammatory injury affecting primarily the small airways, often sparing the interstitium [46]. The term bronchiolitis obliterans has been used to describe a heterogeneous group of conditions [47]. This has been well depicted by Dr. Bergeron and colleagues in this book (see the Pearls section). In the clinical literature, it has been used to describe various conditions that result in airflow limitation. Philit et al. have recommended the term "post-transplant obstructive lung disease" instead of "bronchiolitis obliterans" because it takes into account both the functional definition and the clinical context of the syndrome [48]. Although BO can be idiopathic, it is often associated with connective tissue disease, inhaled toxins, infections, drugs, and chronic GVHD [46]. In the BMT recipient, BO is in most cases considered to be a severe manifestation of chronic GVHD, though infection and drug toxicity may be contributing factors [49].

7.5.1 Incidence and Risk Factors

Airway disease as a complication of BMT was first recognized in the early 1980s [50]. BO almost exclusively affects allogeneic recipients with GVHD. There are only rare case reports of BO in autologous recipients [51]. In a study of 1,789 allogeneic BMT recipients, 47 (2.6%) developed BO compared to none of the 1,070 autologous recipients [52]. The reported incidence of BO varies among studies, related in part to patient population, and to variable definitions and diagnostic criteria. Although some studies have included pathologic findings, most of the reported cases of BO were defined by the presence of airflow limitation in the appropriate clinical setting. The frequency of BO was 3.9% among 4,180 allogeneic BMT recipients reported in 13 studies [53]. A recent study employing a highly sensitive definition of airflow obstruction documented an incidence of 26% [10]. The incidence varies between 6% and 35% in long-term survivors with GVHD [13, 49, 52, 54, 55].

GVHD, older donor and recipient age, methotrexate use, antecedent respiratory infection, and serum immunoglobulin deficiency are risk factors for BO [10, 13, 17, 49, 52, 56]. Patients who receive allogeneic T-cell depleted stem cells or are treated with a non-myeloablative conditioning regimen have a lower incidence of pulmonary complications, including BO [57, 58]. Although pulmonary infections are identified in many patients with BO, it is not clear whether they are directly related to airway disease or whether they result from immune suppression.

7.5.2 Pathogenesis

The pathogenesis of BO in BMT recipients is not well understood. The association between BO and chronic GVHD suggests that host bronchiolar epithelial cells serve as a target for donor cytotoxic T-lymphocytes [59]. Recurrent aspiration of oral material due to esophagitis associated with GVHD, abnormal local immunoglobulin secretory function in the lungs, and unrecognized infections may also play roles [49, 59]. The variations in histopathology, bronchoalveolar lavage cellular composition, and clinical course; the frequency of associated pulmonary infection; the increased risk associated with methotrexate and the rare occurrence after autologous BMT suggest multi-factorial pathogenesis [51, 52, 59, 60].

7.5.3 Clinical Findings and Diagnostic Evaluation

BO can occur 2 months to 9 years after transplantation [17, 52, 55, 56, 61]. The majority of patients with BO present insidiously with dry cough and dyspnea, 40% develop wheezing, and 20% report antecedent "cold" symptoms; fever is notably absent [55, 56]. Twenty percent of the patients with BO had no respiratory symptoms at the time of the abnormal pulmonary function testing. Since the presenting respiratory symptoms are non-specific, a complete history, including prior medications and infections, and thorough physical examination focusing on signs of chronic GVHD should be obtained. Appropriate microbiology studies and laboratory evaluations, including complete blood count with differential, blood urea nitrogen, creatinine, total bilirubin, hepatic transaminases, gammaglobulin levels and subclasses, and urinalysis, are recommended to exclude infection and complications of GVHD [59]. Since there is a high prevalence of sinusitis in allogeneic BMT recipients with GVHD, radiographic assessment of the paranasal sinuses is also recommended [59, 62–65]. If gastrointestinal GVHD or aspiration is a consideration, esophageal studies should be performed [59, 66].

PFT is the mainstay of diagnosis of BO [67]. Although normal airflow has been reported in BMT recipients with histologically proven BO [51], irreversible airflow obstruction is the hallmark of clinically significant disease. In lung transplant recipients, BO is classified based on spirometry into stage1 (FEV1 66–80% of peak post-transplant baseline), stage 2 (FEV1 51–65% of baseline) and stage 3 (FEV1 < 51% of baseline) [68]. The utility of this classification scheme in defining the severity or prognosis in BMT recipients has not been established.

The chest radiograph is usually normal or may show hyperinflation. High-resolution computed tomography (HRCT) of the chest may show decreased lung attenuation, segmental or subsegmental bronchial dilatation, diminution of peripheral vascularity, centrilobular nodules, and expiratory air trapping (Fig. 7.2) [16, 48, 69, 70]. The most common finding on HRCT of the chest is decreased lung attenuation. The decreased lung attenuation and bronchial dilatations are more frequent and extensive in the lower lobes [69].

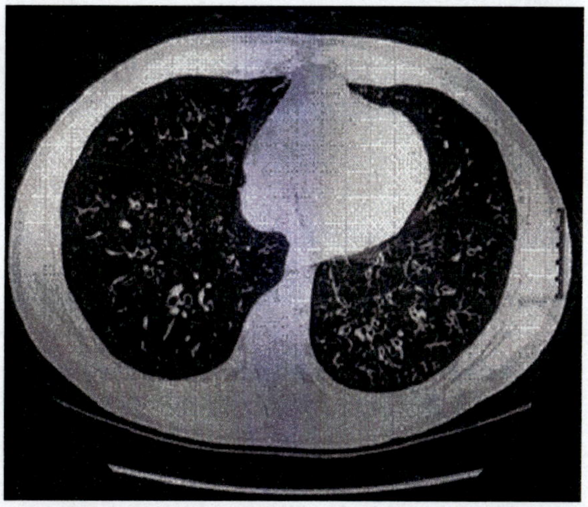

Fig. 7.2 Computed tomography of the chest in a patient with bronchiolitis obliterans showing diffuse areas of parenchymal hypoattenuation, proximal bronchiectasis, and subsegemental bronchial dilatation (Reprinted by permission from Afessa et al. [53], Copyright 2001 Macmillan Publishers Ltd.)

Fiberoptic bronchoscopy with bronchoalveolar lavage (BAL) is used in BMT recipients with suspected BO mainly to exclude infection as the cause of airflow obstruction. Because BO involves the respiratory and membranous bronchioles and is patchy in distribution, transbronchial lung biopsy rarely demonstrates the characteristic histological changes and is consequently of limited utility. Furthermore, transbronchial lung biopsy is contraindicated in the presence of severe airways obstruction or thrombocytopenia. BAL shows neutrophilic and/or lymphocytic inflammation, but this is a non-specific finding [60, 71].

Video-assisted thoracoscopic lung biopsy is required to make a definitive histologic diagnosis. Lung biopsies show small airway involvement with fibrinous obliteration of the lumen with or without associated interstitial pneumonia, fibrosis, or diffuse alveolar damage (Fig. 7.3) [48, 55, 72–74]. Necrotizing bronchitis and bronchiolitis have been reported [72]. The inflammatory cellular infiltrates are usually peribronchiolar and consist of neutrophils and lymphocytes in varying proportions [75]. Surgical biopsies are rarely indicated since the diagnosis usually can be made on clinical grounds. The diagnostic criteria for BO in BMT recipients have not been clearly defined. Obstructive airways disease and BO may exist as distinct clinical entities in BMT recipients. Bronchiolitis may occur without airway obstruction [59], and, conversely, airflow obstruction can occur for a number of reasons other than BO (e.g., asthma, pre-existent chronic obstructive pulmonary disease, viral bronchiolitis). BO is usually established by the presence of irreversible airflow obstruction and the exclusion of other causes of this functional abnormality. BO should be suspected in allogeneic BMT recipients, particularly those with chronic GVHD, who present with chronic cough, wheezing, dyspnea, or hypoxemia with a normal chest radiograph and no evidence of respiratory infection [53, 59]. Similarly, the diagnosis should be considered in asymptomatic patients with new onset of airflow obstruction on screening spirometry. Other chronic diseases such as pulmonary veno-occlusive disease and early diffuse interstitial disease can present with similar signs and symptoms. However, pulmonary veno-occlusive disease is rare and unlikely to show airflow obstruction. Interstitial lung disease is typically associated with a restrictive defect on pulmonary function testing and parenchymal abnormalities on HRCT of the chest.

7.5.4 Treatment

The treatment of BO in the BMT recipient is empiric, and typically consists of corticosteroids and augmented immunosuppression, targeting chronic GVHD. However, only a minority of the patients shows clinical

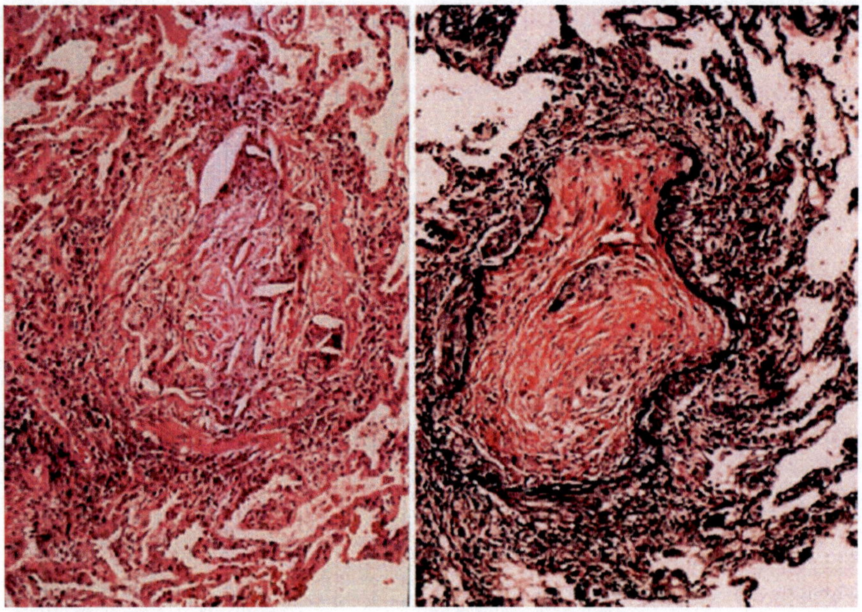

Fig. 7.3 Lung pathology in bronchiolitis obliterans showing bronchiolar inflammation and luminal obliteration associated with excess fibrous connective tissue. Alveoli and their ducts are spared. (Hematoxylin and eosin and Verhoeff-Van Gieson elastic tissue stain.) (Reprinted by permission from Afessa et al. [53], Copyright 2001 Macmillan Publishers Ltd.)

improvement in response to treatment [52, 53]. Prednisone in a range of 1–1.5 mg kg^{-1} day^{-1} is typically given for 4–6 weeks [59]. If the respiratory status remains stable, corticosteroid therapy is tapered and discontinued over 6–12 months. If no improvement is noted within 1 month, or if deterioration continues, cyclosporin or azathioprine can be added [59]. Antithymocyte globulin and high-dose intravenous methylprednisolone have also been used with mixed results [52]. There is a case report of an allogeneic BMT recipient with BO whose pulmonary status improved following treatment with Imatinib mesylate, a specific tyrosine kinase inhibitor with antifibrinogenic properties [76].

Macrolide antibiotics are known to have anti-inflammatory properties, and have been shown to improve symptoms, lung function, and mortality in patients with panbronchiolitis [77–83]. Additionally, there are recent reports of improved lung function in lung transplant recipients with bronchiolitis obliterans syndrome who received macrolide therapy [84, 85]. Currently, there is only one published study examining the effects of macrolides in BMT recipients with BO. Khalid and colleagues reported on eight BMT recipients with BO who were given azithromycin at an initial dose of 500 mg daily for 3 days followed by 250 mg three times weekly [86]. All patients demonstrated improvement in spirometric parameters, with a mean improvement in FEV1 of 20.6% (range 7.3–42.9%). This preliminary evidence, coupled with the lack of significant adverse effects, makes macrolide therapy an attractive therapeutic option, but validation with a prospective, randomized trial is necessary before this approach can be strongly endorsed.

Although there are case reports suggesting beneficial response to thalidomide in BMT recipients with BO, a recent study showed no benefit [52, 87, 88]. While hypogammaglobulinemia has been described as a risk factor for chronic GVHD, prophylaxis with intravenous immunoglobulin has not been shown to prevent BO [89]. Cyclosporin may play a protective role against BO, but its role in established BO is unproven [90]. A randomized clinical trial showed inhaled corticosteroids to be ineffective in lung transplant recipients with bronchiolitis obliterans syndrome, and there is no reason to suspect that this intervention would be any more efficacious when applied to post-BMT BO [91].

In addition to immunosuppression and anti-inflammatory therapy, adjunctive treatments are important in the management of BMT recipients with BO. Prophylaxis for *Pneumocystis jiroveccii* pneumonia and *Streptococcus pneumoniae* should be maintained. Since bacterial infections, especially sinusitis, are common in patients with BO, they should be treated aggressively. Bronchodilator therapy is recommended, although only a minority of patients responds [56, 63, 72].

In selected BMT recipients with respiratory failure secondary to BO who were deemed to be cured of the underlying malignancy for which BMT was performed, lung transplantation is an option [45, 92–95].

7.5.5 Clinical Course

Serial pulmonary function tests in allogeneic BMT recipients with BO have shown that the rate of decline in FEV1 is widely variable [56]. Deterioration in FEV1 correlates with increased mortality rate [56]. The FEV1 improves in only 8–20% [55, 59, 67, 70]. The reported case fatality rates vary widely, ranging from 14% to 100%, with an average case fatality rate of 59% [96]. In one study published 2 decades ago, the 3-year mortality rate of 35 allogeneic BMT recipients with GVHD and obstructive airway disease was 65% compared to 44% for those with GVHD without obstructive airway disease [56]. In a more recent study, the 5-year survival rate of 47 BMT recipients with BO was 10% compared to 40% for those without BO, highlighting the lack of progress in the management of BO over the last 2 decades [52].

7.6 Bronchiolitis Obliterans Organizing Pneumonia (BOOP)

7.6.1 Incidence and Pathogenesis

BOOP is an uncommon lung disease characterized by the presence of granulation tissue within the terminal and respiratory bronchioles, the alveolar ducts, and alveoli. It was first described as a distinct clinical entity in 1985 [97]. BOOP can be either idiopathic or associated with other conditions such as infections, drugs, radiation, or connective tissue diseases [98]. The first cases of BOOP in BMT recipients were reported in the early 1990s [99, 100].

BOOP is not as common as BO in BMT recipients. In a report of 296 patients with BOOP from 63 publications, BMT recipients accounted for four (1.4%) [101]. At Vancouver General Hospital, 5 of the 25 (20%) patients identified as having BOOP over an 8-year period were allogeneic BMT recipients [101]. At the author's institution, the incidence of BOOP was 1.7% among 179 allogeneic BMT recipients who survived for 3 months or longer [70]. The published medical literature on BOOP in BMT recipients is limited to case reports, with a maximum number of five patients [45, 70, 99–107].

Idiopathic BOOP is an inflammatory lung disease of unknown etiology [98]. Its occurrence almost exclusively in allogeneic recipients with GVHD suggests that it may represent a form of alloimmune injury to the lung by the transplanted stem cell [101]. BOOP is uncommon in BMT recipients treated with T-cell lymphocyte-depleted stem cells, highlighting the role T-cell lymphocytes may play in its pathogenesis [57, 108]. The higher frequency of human leukocyte antigen (HLA) B35 in BMT recipients with BOOP, compared to those without BOOP, suggests HLA B35 may play a role in its pathogenesis [109]. The exhaled nitric oxide level is increased in allogeneic BMT recipients with BOOP [104]. The rare occurrence of BOOP in autologous recipients suggests that other mechanisms may be involved as well [102]. A case report of BOOP associated with human herpes virus-6 in a BMT recipient suggests unrecognized infections may play role [110].

7.6.2 Clinical Presentation and Diagnostic Evaluation

The onset of BOOP is usually 1 month to 2 years after transplant [70, 99–101, 103–107, 111]. The presenting symptoms of BOOP include dry cough, dyspnea, and fever. Rarely, the disease may be asymptomatic [70]. Physical examination may reveal inspiratory crackles.

BOOP should be included in the differential diagnosis of airspace disease in BMT recipients not responding to antibiotics. Although the airspace disease is usually bilateral, it can be unilateral [102]. Pulmonary function tests usually show a restrictive defect, decreased DLCO, and normal flow rates [99, 101, 104, 112]. Arterial blood gas analysis may reveal mild hypoxemia [101]. Chest radiographs and computed tomography show patchy air space consolidation, ground-glass attenuation, and nodular opacities [99–101, 104, 113, 114]. The radiographic abnormalities usually have a peripheral distribution [115]. One recent study demonstrated increased exhaled nitric oxide concentration in BMT recipients with BOOP that decreases with response to treatment [104].

Although pulmonary function test and CT scan findings in conjunction with the clinical features may suggest the diagnosis, confirmation requires either surgical or transbronchial lung biopsy. Although the diagnosis of BOOP in the BMT recipient occasionally can be made with transbronchial lung biopsy in the appropriate clinical setting, about 85% of the patients require surgical lung biopsy [101]. Histologic confirmation of the diagnosis is particularly warranted before the patient is subjected to long-term corticosteroid therapy. Surgical lung biopsy, usually via video-assisted thoracoscopy, is considered the gold standard for the diagnosis of BOOP. The histologic hallmark of BOOP is the presence of patchy intraluminal fibrosis, consisting of polypoid plugs of immature fibroblast tissue resembling granulation tissue obliterating the distal airways, alveolar ducts, and peribronchial alveolar space (Fig. 7.4) [47].

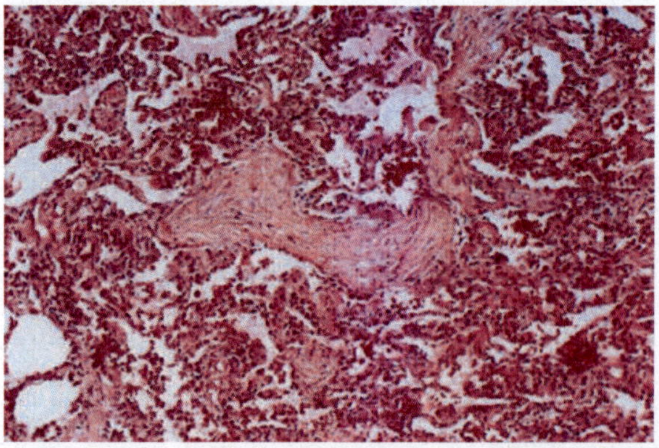

Fig. 7.4 Lung pathology in bronchiolitis obliterans organizing pneumonia showing the presence of intraluminal granulation tissue in bronchioli, alveolar ducts, and alveoli. There is also interstitial infiltration with mononuclear cells and foamy macrophages. (Hematoxylin and eosin stain.) (Reprinted by permission from Afessa et al. [53], Copyright 2001 Macmillan Publishers Ltd.)

7.6.3 Treatment and Prognosis

Corticosteroid therapy is the treatment of choice for symptomatic patients with BOOP [70, 98–101, 104]. About 80% of BMT recipients with BOOP respond favorably to treatment [70, 99–101, 103–106, 111]. The duration and dosage of corticosteroid therapy in the BMT recipient with BOOP have not been clearly defined. Based on the experience from other patients, the initial dose of prednisone is in the range of 0.75–1.5 mg kg^{-1} day^{-1} to a maximum daily dose of 100 mg, administered for 1–3 months, then 40 mg/day for 3 months, and then 10–20 mg/day or every other day for a total of 1 year [98, 116]. Radiographic abnormalities usually clear within 1–3 months of initiating corticosteroid therapy [100, 101, 104, 105]. Erythromycin 10 mg kg^{-1} day^{-1} for 14 months has been used in conjunction with corticosteroid to treat BOOP in one allogeneic BMT recipient [103].

The case fatality rate of treated BOOP is 7.9% in the general population, but appears to be higher in BMT recipients [101]. Among 27 BMT recipients with BOOP documented in the literature, the overall case fatality rate was 19% [45, 70, 99–107, 111].

7.7 Idiopathic Pneumonia Syndrome (IPS)

7.7.1 Epidemiology

IPS is characterized by clinical features of pneumonia and diffuse lung injury in the absence of an identified infection. The overall frequency of IPS is 10%, with a reported range of 2–17% [53, 117, 118]. Its median time of onset is between 21 and 87 days after transplant. Risk factors for IPS include old age, transplant for malignancy other than leukemia, pre-transplant chemotherapy, total body irradiation, GVHD, and positive donor cytomegalovirus serology [53].

7.7.2 Clinical Findings and Diagnostic Evaluation

IPS is defined by the presence of widespread alveolar injury in the absence of lower respiratory tract infection characterized by the presence of acute, bilateral pulmonary infiltrates, associated symptoms of cough and dyspnea, hypoxemia, and restrictive physiology, in the absence of infection or heart failure [119]. The pathogenesis is not well defined [120–122]. Lung tissue injury, inflammation, and cytokine release are implicated. The clinical spectrum of IPS is broad, ranging from acute respiratory failure to incidental radiographic abnormalities [119]. The usual presentations include dyspnea, dry cough, hypoxemia, and non-lobar infiltrates [119]. Because IPS mimics infectious pneumonia, the majority of the patients are on antibiotics at the time of diagnosis [123]. Infection is excluded by the absence of a pathogen in BAL fluid and by the lack of clinical response to antimicrobial therapy. Diffuse alveolar hemorrhage (DAH) and peri-engraftment respiratory syndrome (PERDS) also fulfill the diagnostic criteria of IPS [124, 125]. Despite overlap in the clinical features of IPS, DAH, and PERDS, their responses to treatment and clinical courses are different [124]. In my diagnostic approach to patients with suspected IPS, I perform BAL and, if there are no contraindications, transbronchial lung biopsy. We proceed to video-assisted thoracoscopic lung biopsy if transbronchial lung biopsy is contraindicated or if the transbronchial specimen is inadequate. Lung biopsies of patients with IPS may show diffuse alveolar damage, organizing or acute pneumonia, and interstitial lymphocytic inflammation [6, 123].

7.7.3 Treatment

There have been no randomized clinical trials addressing the treatment of IPS. Despite case reports of patients with IPS responding to treatment with corticosteroids, studies with larger sample sizes have not shown any outcome benefit [6, 123, 126]. Currently, management consists of supportive care and prevention and treatment of infection. There is a report of three cases of BMT recipients with IPS whose lung function improved following the administration of etanercept [122]. This observation awaits further confirmation by an ongoing clinical trial.

7.7.4 Clinical Course and Prognosis

The clinical course of BMT recipients with IPS is usually complicated by viral and fungal infections as well as pneumothorax, pneumomediastinum, subcutaneous emphysema, pulmonary fibrosis, and auto-immune polyserositis [53]. The overall mortality of IPS is 74%, with a reported range between 60% and 86% [53]. The 1-year survival rate is less than 15% [123, 126]. For those who require mechanical ventilation, the hospital mortality exceeds 95% [123].

7.8 Diffuse Alveolar Hemorrhage (DAH)

DAH is discussed in Chap. 3.

7.9 Periengraftment Respiratory Distress Syndrome (PERDS)

7.9.1 Epidemiology

PERDS occurs in approximately 5% of autologous BMT recipients [125]. About one-third of DAH occurs during the peri-engraftment period, and about one-third of patients with PERDS have DAH [125, 127].

7.9.2 Clinical Findings and Diagnostic Evaluation

PERDS is a subset of IPS characterized by acute lung injury during the neutrophil peri-engraftment period. It represents the pulmonary component of the engraftment syndrome, which may also present with diarrhea and skin rash [125, 128, 129]. The diagnostic criteria of PERDS include the presence of fever and evidence of pulmonary injury in the form of hypoxia (arterial oxygen saturation <90%) and/or pulmonary infiltrates on chest radiograph, in the absence of cardiac dysfunction or infection, within 5 days of neutrophil engraftment [125]. The median time to onset of PERDS is 11 days (range, 4–25 days) after transplant [125].

BAL in patients with PERDS may show neutrophilic alveolitis [125]. Transbronchial lung biopsy is usually contraindicated because of thrombocytopenia. Surgical lung biopsy is rarely necessary, but may show diffuse alveolar damage [125].

7.9.3 Treatment and Prognosis

High-dose corticosteroid therapy often leads to rapid clinical improvement [125]. Unlike DAH and IPS, only about one-third of BMT recipients with PERDS require ICU admission and mechanical ventilation [125]. The reported mortality rate of PERDS is about 26% [125].

7.10 Delayed Pulmonary Toxicity Syndrome (DPTS)

Chemotherapeutic agents and radiation therapy have been associated with pulmonary toxicities that manifest weeks to years later [130, 131]. In the 1990s, many patients with breast cancer were treated with a high-dose chemotherapy regimen consisting of cyclophosphamide, cisplatin, and bischloroethylinitrosurea (BCNU), followed by autologous BMT [132]. Following transplant, a significant number of these patients developed pulmonary complications, one of the more common referred to as the delayed pulmonary toxicity syndrome (DPTS) [118, 133–139]. DPTS develops in up to 72% of autologous BMT recipients who have received high-dose chemotherapy for breast cancer [134, 135, 140]. The relatively high frequency, low mortality, and good response to corticosteroid treatment distinguish DPTS from IPS [134, 138, 139, 141]. Because recent studies have not shown a survival benefit, the use of autologous BMT following high-dose chemotherapy for breast cancer has declined [142, 143].

The pathogenesis of DPTS is not known. The depletion of reduced glutathione and impaired antioxidant defenses caused by cyclophosphamide and BCNU have been implicated [138]. One study showed no significant correlation between patient age, stage of breast cancer, chemotherapy regimen, chest wall radiotherapy, tobacco use, prior lung disease, or baseline pulmonary function and the development of DPTS [140].

7.10.1 Clinical Findings and Diagnostic Evaluation

Patients with DPTS present with cough, dyspnea, and fever [135, 139, 140]. The onset of symptoms ranges from 2 weeks to 4 months following transplantation [139, 140]. In the context of prior breast cancer treated with high-dose chemotherapy and autologous BMT, DPTS is diagnosed by demonstration of a decline in DLCO and exclusion of infectious causes [139, 140]. The DLCO declines in over 70% of patients with breast cancer treated with high-dose chemotherapy and autologous BMT [136]. In patients with DPTS, the median absolute DLCO decrement is 26% (range, 10–73%), and a nadir is reached in 15–18 weeks following transplant [139, 140]. The most common findings on CT of the chest are ground-glass opacities [139]. Other abnormalities include linear or nodular opacities and consolidation. Many patients may have a normal chest CT at the onset of DPTS [139]. Because of the typical clinical presentation and response to therapy, invasive procedures such as bronchoscopy are rarely required [134, 135, 139, 140].

7.10.2 Treatment and Prognosis

Corticosteroid therapy for DPTS usually results in resolution of symptoms and improvement in DLCO without long-term pulmonary sequelae [135, 139, 140]. Treatment usually consists of prednisone initiated at a dose of 60 mg/day for 14 days and subsequently tapered over 5–7 weeks [134]. While patients are being treated with steroids, they should also receive oral trimethoprim-sulfamethoxazole or aerosolized pentamidine prophylaxis against *Pneumocystis jiroveccii* pneumonia [134, 140]. One case of DPTS refractory to steroid was treated successfully with interferon-gamma [144]. A study using prophylactic inhaled fluticasone propionate 880 μg every 12 h for 12 weeks starting from the day of high-dose chemotherapy demonstrated a reduction in the frequency of DPTS to 35% compared to 73% in historical controls [145].

No deaths attributable to DPTS have been reported [134, 135, 139, 140]. The 3-year survival of stage II and III breast cancer patients who developed DPTS is 84%, which is not significantly different from those of patients who did not develop DPTS [140].

7.11 Pulmonary Cytolytic Thrombi (PCT)

Pulmonary cytolytic thrombi (PCT) is a non-infectious pulmonary complication of unknown etiology. Among BMT recipients, PCT occurs exclusively after allogeneic procedures, typically in the setting of GVHD. PCT has also been described at autopsy in a non-transplant patient who died following hip replacement surgery [146]. All except 1 of the 16 BMT recipients with PCT reported in the medical literature are from a single institution [147, 148]. Fifteen of the 16 patients were under age 18 years at the time of diagnosis [147, 148]. Despite the seemingly rare and previously unrecognized nature of PCT, it was found in 15 of 33 (45%) BMT recipients who underwent surgical lung biopsy for diagnosis of pulmonary nodules at the University of Minnesota [147].

7.11.1 Pathogenesis

The pathogenesis of PCT is not known. Although the hemorrhagic infarcts in PCT are similar to those seen in angioinvasive fungal infections, none of the lung biopsies in the reported PCT cases had evidence of infection [147, 148]. The development of PCT exclusively in allogeneic BMT, and chiefly in those with GVHD, suggests that it may be a manifestation of GVHD targeting the endothelium of the lungs [147]. Demonstration of clinical and radiological improvement following increased immunosuppression also favors GVHD as the underlying pathogenic mechanism [147, 148].

7.11.2 Clinical Findings and Diagnostic Evaluation

Most BMT recipients with PCT have active GVHD at the time of presentation [148–150]. The onset of PCT is between 8 and 343 days (median 72) after transplantation [148–150]. All patients are febrile, and some have cough at presentation [148–150]. Dyspnea has not been reported at presentation.

Chest radiographs, usually performed as part of the evaluation of persistent fever, may be normal in 25% of the patients with PCT [150]. Abnormal chest radiographic findings include nodules, interstitial prominence, and atelectasis [150]. Chest CT shows multiple peripheral pulmonary nodules, ranging from a few millimeters to 4 cm in size. In one study, pleural effusion was reported in 1 of 13 patients who had undergone chest CT examination [150].

Bronchoscopy with bronchoalveolar lavage is used to exclude infection. Because of the peripheral and intravascular location of the nodules in PCT, transbronchial lung biopsy is unlikely to yield a diagnosis. Histological demonstration of PCT requires surgical lung biopsy or necropsy [148, 150]. The histologic features of PCT include occlusive vascular lesions and hemorrhagic infarcts due to thrombi that consist of intensely basophilic, amorphous material that may extend into the adjacent tissue through the vascular wall [147]. The amorphous material suggests cellular breakdown products [149]. Immunohistochemical studies show a discontinuous endothelial cell layer.

7.11.3 Treatment and Prognosis

Because of the unclear etiology of PCT and concerns about an infectious cause of lung nodules, patients have been treated with broad-spectrum antibiotics, antifungals, and systemic corticosteroids [150]. In one recent case report, treatment with intravenous methylprednisolone 2 mg kg^{-1} day^{-1} and cyclosporin 3 mg/kg three times daily for 1 week followed by oral prednisone 30 mg/day and 125 mg cyclosporin twice daily resulted in improvement [148]. Although it is unclear which of these various interventions is actually beneficial, most of the patients with PCT described in the literature improved clinically within 1–2 weeks and radiographically over weeks to months [150]. There has been no reported death attributed to PCT [147, 148]. Of the 15 BMT recipients with PCT reported from the University of Minnesota, 10 were still alive at an average of 13 months after diagnosis and 5 died, 1 from GVHD and 4 from infectious complications [147]. The one patient reported from Mayo Clinic died of progressive pulmonary hypertension 4 months after the diagnosis of PCT, with no evidence of PCT at autopsy [148].

7.12 Pulmonary Veno-Occlusive Disease (PVOD)

PVOD is a rare cause of pulmonary hypertension that has been associated with various conditions including BMT. Pulmonary hypertension in PVOD results from intimal fibrosis obstructing the pulmonary veins and venules.

The incidence of PVOD in BMT recipients is not known. Wingard et al. reported PVOD in 19 of 154 autopsies of allogeneic BMT recipients (12%) [151]. However, in a recent autopsy review of 71 adult BMT recipients from the Mayo Clinic (39 allogeneic), we did not identify any case of PVOD [152]. PVOD affects both genders. There are about 28 cases of BMT recipients with PVOD in the published literature [148, 151, 153–159]. The predominant underlying disease in BMT recipients with PVOD is hematologic malignancy. However, PVOD has been found following BMT for neuroblastoma and aplastic anemia [148, 157]. Only 2 of the 28 BMT recipients with PVOD had autologous grafts [155, 157]. The frequency of PVOD is particularly high in allogeneic BMT recipients who have concurrent interstitial pneumonia and hepatic veno-occlusive disease [151]. PVOD has been reported at autopsy following resolution of PCT [148].

7.12.1 Pathogenesis

Since the reported cases of BMT recipients with PVOD are limited in scope and number, its etiology is not well defined. Infection, radiation, and chemotherapy are hypothesized to be contributing factors for the development of PVOD [153–155, 157, 160–162]. BCNU, mitomycin C, and bleomycin are among the chemotherapeutic agents implicated as potential causes of vascular injury [160, 162–165].

7.12.2 Clinical Findings and Diagnostic Evaluation

Presenting symptoms are non-specific and include dyspnea, lethargy, and chronic cough [162]. As the pulmonary hypertension worsens, orthopnea, cyanosis, chest pain, abdominal pain due to hepatic congestion, and exertional syncope may be noted. Physical examination is also nonspecific and may reveal bibasilar crackles and inspiratory squeaks on auscultation of the lungs and findings indicative of pulmonary hypertension including right ventricular heave, loud pulmonic heart sound, lower extremity edema, and elevated jugular venous pressure [159].

Radiographic findings include Kerley B lines, prominent central pulmonary arteries, and scattered patchy opacities [159, 162]. Unlike other forms of primary pulmonary hypertension, pleural effusions are common in PVOD [162]. Echocardiogram and right heart catheterization show elevated pulmonary artery pressure. Pulmonary arteriogram may show delayed runoff and venous filling without arterial filling defects [159]. PFT demonstrates a decreased DLCO and restrictive ventilatory defect [159, 162, 166].

The triad of pulmonary arterial hypertension, radiographic evidence of pulmonary edema, and normal pulmonary artery occlusion pressure suggests PVOD. However, many patients with PVOD do not have this triad, and it is often difficult to get an accurate pulmonary artery occlusion pressure tracing in these patients [162].

The diagnosis cannot be made by bronchoscopy, although the findings of hemosiderosis and sclerosed venules in transbronchial lung biopsies suggest PVOD [158]. The definitive diagnosis of PVOD requires surgical lung biopsy. In the absence of this, most cases are diagnosed at postmortem examination [151, 157]. The pathologic hallmark of PVOD is the extensive and diffuse occlusion of pulmonary veins and venules by fibrous tissue [151, 162, 167].

7.12.3 Treatment and Prognosis

There is no proven therapy for PVOD. Because observational trials involving patients with primary pulmonary hypertension have suggested improved survival in those treated with anticoagulation, some advocate treating PVOD with long-term warfarin [162]. There are case reports suggesting that steroids may be beneficial in BMT recipients with PVOD [153, 159]. However, the data supporting the use of steroid therapy and anticoagulation are limited to case reports [153, 159]. In one report of two BMT recipients with PVOD, methylprednisolone 2 mg/kg daily resulted in improvement of arterial oxygenation and dyspnea within 1–2 weeks [153]. In one of these two patients, discontinuation of steroid therapy led to recurrent disease that responded to additional treatment [153]. On the other hand, there are reports of BMT recipients with PVOD who deteriorated and died despite treatment with steroid therapy [155]. The role of vasodilators in PVOD is unclear. Despite case reports of successful therapy with oral vasodilators or intravenous administration of prostacyclin in PVOD, these agents can dilate the arterial vessels without concomitant venodilation, leading to increased transcapillary hydrostatic pressures, acute pulmonary edema, and death [162, 168].

Lung transplantation is a consideration in patients free of other comorbidities, including the underlying condition for which BMT was performed, but there is currently no published experience on outcomes of lung transplantation in this unique setting [161, 162]. In light of the limited treatment options and the generally progressive nature of the disease, it is not surprising that most patients with PVOD die within 2 years of diagnosis [162].

7.13 Other Pulmonary Complications

7.13.1 Pulmonary Arterial Hypertension

Several cases of pulmonary arterial hypertension have been reported in BMT recipients [156, 169–171]. The pathogenesis is not clearly defined. Normal pulmonary endothelium releases vasodilators, such as prostacyclin and endothelial-derived relaxing factors. Radiation- and chemotherapy-associated endothelial damage may be the mechanism for the development of the pulmonary hypertension [156, 169–171]. Prostacyclin infusion and calcium channel antagonists have been used for the treatment of pulmonary arterial hypertension in BMT recipients [169–171].

7.13.2 Pulmonary Alveolar Proteinosis

Pulmonary alveolar proteinosis is characterized by excessive accumulation of surfactant lipoprotein in the alveoli leading to abnormal gas exchange [172]. The diagnosis of pulmonary alveolar proteinosis is made by the presence of periodic acid Schiff proteineceaous material in bronchoalveolar fluid [173]. Cordonnier et al. described three BMT recipients with pulmonary alveolar proteinosis [173]. All three had received allogeneic transplant for leukemia between 12 and 90 days before the onset of pulmonary symptoms. Chest radiographs showed diffuse infiltrates. The clinicians had suspected infection in two and alveolar hemorrhage in one. Only one of the three survived. A very didactical case of pulmonary alveolar proteinosis is depicted in this book by Drs. Vincent and Tandjaoui (see Pearl's section).

7.13.3 Chronic Eosinophilic Pneumonia

Three cases of chronic eosinophilic pneumonia have been reported in BMT recipients, one autologous and two allogeneic [174–176]. Despite initial response to steroid therapy, one patient had a fatal course [174].

References

1. Pasquini MC, Wang Z (2009) Current use and outcome of hematopoietic stem cell transplantation: Part I. *CIBMTR Newsletter* [serial on line], 2009;1:7–11. www.cibmtr.org/PUBLICATIONS/Newsletter. Accessed Oct 2009
2. Breuer R, Lossos IS, Berkman N et al (1993) Pulmonary complications of bone marrow transplantation. Respir Med 87:571–579
3. Jules-Elysee K, Stover DE, Yahalom J et al (1992) Pulmonary complications in lymphoma patients treated with high-dose therapy autologous bone marrow transplantation. Am Rev Respir Dis 146:485–491
4. Cordonnier C, Bernaudin JF, Bierling P et al (1986) Pulmonary complications occurring after allogeneic bone marrow transplantation. A study of 130 consecutive transplanted patients. Cancer 58:1047–1054
5. Afessa B, Peters SG (2006) Major complications following hematopoietic stem cell transplantation. Semin Respir Crit Care Med 27:297–309
6. Griese M, Rampf U, Hofmann D et al (2000) Pulmonary complications after bone marrow transplantation in children: twenty-four years of experience in a single pediatric center. Pediatr Pulmonol 30:393–401
7. Cerveri I, Zoia MC, Fulgoni P et al (1999) Late pulmonary sequelae after childhood bone marrow transplantation. Thorax 54:131–135
8. Marras TK, Szalai JP, Chan CK et al (2002) Pulmonary function abnormalities after allogeneic marrow transplantation: a systematic review and assessment of an existing predictive instrument. Bone Marrow Transplant 30: 599–607
9. Marras TK, Chan CK, Lipton JH et al (2004) Long-term pulmonary function abnormalities and survival after allogeneic marrow transplantation. Bone Marrow Transplant 33:509–517
10. Chien JW, Martin PJ, Gooley TA et al (2003) Airflow obstruction after myeloablative allogeneic hematopoietic stem cell transplantation. Am J Respir Crit Care Med 168: 208–214
11. Chien JW, Martin PJ, Flowers ME et al (2004) Implications of early airflow decline after myeloablative allogeneic stem cell transplantation. Bone Marrow Transplant 33: 759–764
12. Schwarer AP, Hughes JM, Trotman-Dickenson B et al (1992) A chronic pulmonary syndrome associated with graft-versus-host disease after allogeneic marrow transplantation. Transplantation 54:1002–1008
13. Clark JG, Schwartz DA, Flournoy N et al (1987) Risk factors for airflow obstruction in recipients of bone marrow transplants. Ann Intern Med 107:648–656
14. Badier M, Guillot C, Delpierre S et al (1993) Pulmonary function changes 100 days and 1 year after bone marrow transplantation. Bone Marrow Transplant 12:457–461
15. Lund MB, Kongerud J, Brinch L et al (1995) Decreased lung function in 1 year survivors of allogeneic bone marrow transplantation conditioned with high-dose busulphan and cyclophosphamide. Eur Respir J 8:1269–1274
16. Schultz KR, Green GJ, Wensley D et al (1994) Obstructive lung disease in children after allogeneic bone marrow transplantation. Blood 84:3212–3220
17. Curtis DJ, Smale A, Thien F et al (1995) Chronic airflow obstruction in long-term survivors of allogeneic bone marrow transplantation. Bone Marrow Transplant 16:169–173
18. Burgart LJ, Heller MJ, Reznicek MJ et al (1991) Cytomegalovirus detection in bone marrow transplant patients with idiopathic pneumonitis. A clinicopathologic study of the clinical utility of the polymerase chain reaction on open lung biopsy specimen tissue. Am J Clin Pathol 96:572–576
19. Lund MB, Brinch L, Kongerud J et al (2004) Lung function 5 yrs after allogeneic bone marrow transplantation conditioned with busulphan and cyclophosphamide. Eur Respir J 23:901–905
20. Chiou TJ, Tung SL, Wang WS et al (2002) Pulmonary function changes in long-term survivors of chronic myelogenous leukemia after allogeneic bone marrow transplantation: a Taiwan experience. Cancer Invest 20:880–888
21. Frisk P, Arvidson J, Bratteby LE et al (2004) Pulmonary function after autologous bone marrow transplantation in children: a long-term prospective study. Bone Marrow Transplant 33:645–650
22. Tait RC, Burnett AK, Robertson AG et al (1991) Subclinical pulmonary function defects following autologous and allogeneic bone marrow transplantation: relationship to total body irradiation and graft-versus-host disease. Int J Radiat Oncol Biol Phys 20:1219–1227
23. Gore EM, Lawton CA, Ash RC et al (1996) Pulmonary function changes in long-term survivors of bone marrow transplantation. Int J Radiat Oncol Biol Phys 36:67–75
24. Leneveu H, Bremont F, Rubie H et al (1999) Respiratory function in children undergoing bone marrow transplantation. Pediatr Pulmonol 28:31–38
25. Fanfulla F, Locatelli F, Zoia MC et al (1997) Pulmonary complications and respiratory function changes after bone marrow transplantation in children. Eur Respir J 10:2301–2306
26. Mancuzo EV, da Silva WE, de Rezende NA (2007) Preoperative and post-operative spirometry in bone marrow transplant patients. J Bras Pneumol 33:36–42
27. Oshima Y, Takahashi S, Nagayama H et al (1997) Fatal GVHD demonstrating an involvement of respiratory muscle following donor leukocyte transfusion (DLT). Bone Marrow Transplant 19:737–740
28. Oya Y, Kobayashi S, Nakamura K et al (2001) Skeletal muscle pathology of chronic graft versus host disease accompanied with myositis, affecting predominantly respiratory and distal muscles, and hemosiderosis. Rinsho Shinkeigaku 41:612–616

29. Stephenson AL, Mackenzie IR, Levy RD et al (2001) Myositis associated graft-versus-host-disease presenting as respiratory muscle weakness [In Process Citation]. Thorax 56:82–84
30. Baddley JW, Stroud TP, Salzman D et al (2001) Invasive mold infections in allogeneic bone marrow transplant recipients. Clin Infect Dis 32:1319–1324
31. Crawford SW, Fisher L (1992) Predictive value of pulmonary function tests before marrow transplantation [see comments]. Chest 101:1257–1264
32. Horak DA, Schmidt GM, Zaia JA et al (1992) Pretransplant pulmonary function predicts cytomegalovirus-associated interstitial pneumonia following bone marrow transplantation. Chest 102:1484–1490
33. Kaya Z, Weiner DJ, Yilmaz D et al (2009) Lung function, pulmonary complications, and mortality after allogeneic blood and marrow transplantation in children. Biol Blood Marrow Transplant 15:817–826
34. Milburn HJ, Prentice HG, du Bois RM (1992) Can lung function measurements be used to predict which patients will be at risk of developing interstitial pneumonitis after bone marrow transplantation? Thorax 47:421–425
35. Afessa B (2005) Pretransplant pulmonary evaluation of the blood and marrow transplant recipient. Chest 128:8–10
36. Agosti JM, Sprenger JD, Lum LG et al (1988) Transfer of allergen-specific IgE-mediated hypersensitivity with allogeneic bone marrow transplantation. N Engl J Med 319:1623–1628
37. Hallstrand TS, Sprenger JD, Agosti JM et al (2004) Long-term acquisition of allergen-specific IgE and asthma following allogeneic bone marrow transplantation from allergic donors. Blood 104:3086–3090
38. Hirayama M, Azuma E, Kumamoto T et al (1998) Late-onset unilateral renal dysfunction combined with non-insulin-dependent diabetes mellitus and bronchial asthma following allogeneic bone marrow transplantation for acute lymphoblastic leukemia in a child. Bone Marrow Transplant 22:923–926
39. Rietz H, Plummer AL, Gal AA (2002) Asthma as a consequence of bone marrow transplantation. Chest 122:369–370
40. Tabbara KF, Nassar A, Ahmed SO et al (2008) Acquisition of vernal and atopic keratoconjunctivitis after bone marrow transplantation. Am J Ophthalmol 146:462–465
41. Schuurman HJ, Verdonck LF, Geertzema JG et al (1986) Monotypic immunoglobulin E plasma cells in an allogeneic bone marrow transplant recipient. Histopathology 10:963–969
42. Bellou A, Kanny G, Fremont S et al (1997) Transfer of atopy following bone marrow transplantation. Ann Allergy Asthma Immunol 78:513–516
43. Gosselin MV, Adams RH (2002) Pulmonary complications in bone marrow transplantation. J Thorac Imaging 17:132–144
44. Barton-Burke M, Dwinell DM, Kafkas L et al (2008) Graft-versus-host disease: a complex long-term side effect of hematopoietic stem cell transplant. Oncology (Williston Park) 22:31–45
45. Yousem SA (1995) The histological spectrum of pulmonary graft-versus-host disease in bone marrow transplant recipients. Hum Pathol 26:668–675
46. King TE Jr (1993) Overview of bronchiolitis. Clin Chest Med 14:607–610
47. Myers JL, Colby TV (1993) Pathologic manifestations of bronchiolitis, constrictive bronchiolitis, cryptogenic organizing pneumonia, and diffuse panbronchiolitis. Clin Chest Med 14:611–622
48. Philit F, Wiesendanger T, Archimbaud E et al (1995) Post-transplant obstructive lung disease ("bronchiolitis obliterans"): a clinical comparative study of bone marrow and lung transplant patients. Eur Respir J 8:551–558
49. Holland HK, Wingard JR, Beschorner WE et al (1988) Bronchiolitis obliterans in bone marrow transplantation and its relationship to chronic graft-v-host disease and low serum IgG. Blood 72:621–627
50. Roca J, Granena A, Rodriguez-Roisin R et al (1982) Fatal airway disease in an adult with chronic graft-versus-host disease. Thorax 37:77–78
51. Paz HL, Crilley P, Patchefsky A et al (1992) Bronchiolitis obliterans after autologous bone marrow transplantation. Chest 101:775–778
52. Dudek AZ, Mahaseth H, DeFor TE et al (2003) Bronchiolitis obliterans in chronic graft-versus-host disease: analysis of risk factors and treatment outcomes. Biol Blood Marrow Transplant 9:657–666
53. Afessa B, Litzow MR, Tefferi A (2001) Bronchiolitis obliterans and other late onset non-infectious pulmonary complications in hematopoietic stem cell transplantation. Bone Marrow Transplant 28:425–434
54. Alonso RR, Villa A Jr, Sequeiros GA et al (2004) Obstructive lung disease after allogenic stem cell transplantation in children. An Pediatr (Barc) 61:124–130
55. Chan CK, Hyland RH, Hutcheon MA et al (1987) Small-airways disease in recipients of allogeneic bone marrow transplants. An analysis of 11 cases and a review of the literature. Medicine (Baltimore) 66:327–340
56. Clark JG, Crawford SW, Madtes DK et al (1989) Obstructive lung disease after allogeneic marrow transplantation. Clinical presentation and course. Ann Intern Med 111: 368–376
57. Ditschkowski M, Elmaagacli AH, Trenschel R et al (2007) T-cell depletion prevents from bronchiolitis obliterans and bronchiolitis obliterans with organizing pneumonia after allogeneic hematopoietic stem cell transplantation with related donors. Haematologica 92:558–561
58. Nusair S, Breuer R, Shapira MY et al (2004) Low incidence of pulmonary complications following nonmyeloablative stem cell transplantation. Eur Respir J 23: 440–445
59. Crawford SW, Clark JG (1993) Bronchiolitis associated with bone marrow transplantation. Clin Chest Med 14: 741–749
60. St.John RC, Gadek JE, Tutschka PJ et al (1990) Analysis of airflow obstruction by bronchoalveolar lavage following bone marrow transplantation. Implications for pathogenesis and treatment. Chest 98:600–607
61. Krowka MJ, Rosenow EC III, Hoagland HC (1985) Pulmonary complications of bone marrow transplantation. Chest 87:237–246
62. Billings KR, Lowe LH, Aquino VM et al (2000) Screening sinus CT scans in pediatric bone marrow transplant patients. Int J Pediatr Otorhinolaryngol 52:253–260

63. Ralph DD, Springmeyer SC, Sullivan KM et al (1984) Rapidly progressive air-flow obstruction in marrow transplant recipients. Possible association between obliterative bronchiolitis and chronic graft-versus-host disease. Am Rev Respir Dis 129:641–644
64. Savage DG, Taylor P, Blackwell J et al (1997) Paranasal sinusitis following allogeneic bone marrow transplant. Bone Marrow Transplant 19:55–59
65. Thompson AM, Couch M, Zahurak ML et al (2002) Risk factors for post-stem cell transplant sinusitis. Bone Marrow Transplant 29:257–261
66. McDonald GB, Sullivan KM, Plumley TF (1984) Radiographic features of esophageal involvement in chronic graft-vs.- host disease. AJR Am J Roentgenol 142: 501–506
67. Hyland RH, Chan CK, Hutcheon MA, Fyles G, Virdee M, Jaidka RK et al (1988) Early diagnosis of obstructive airways disease after allogeneic bone marrow transplantation may improve outcome. Am Rev Respir Dis 137(Supplement):111
68. Estenne M, Maurer JR, Boehler A et al (2002) Bronchiolitis obliterans syndrome 2001: an update of the diagnostic criteria. J Heart Lung Transplant 21:297–310
69. Jung JI, Jung WS, Hahn ST et al (2004) Bronchiolitis obliterans after allogenic bone marrow transplantation: HRCT findings. Korean J Radiol 5:107–113
70. Palmas A, Tefferi A, Myers JL et al (1998) Late-onset noninfectious pulmonary complications after allogeneic bone marrow transplantation. Br J Haematol 100:680–687
71. Trisolini R, Stanzani M, Agli LL et al (2001) Delayed noninfectious lung disease in allogeneic bone marrow transplant recipients. Sarcoidosis Vasc Diffuse Lung Dis 18: 75–84
72. Johnson FL, Stokes DC, Ruggiero M et al (1984) Chronic obstructive airways disease after bone marrow transplantation. J Pediatr 105:370–376
73. Ostrow D, Buskard N, Hill RS et al (1985) Bronchiolitis obliterans complicating bone marrow transplantation. Chest 87:828–830
74. Wyatt SE, Nunn P, Hows JM et al (1984) Airways obstruction associated with graft versus host disease after bone marrow transplantation. Thorax 39:887–894
75. Urbanski SJ, Kossakowska AE, Curtis J et al (1987) Idiopathic small airways pathology in patients with graft-versus-host disease following allogeneic bone marrow transplantation. Am J Surg Pathol 11:965–971
76. Majhail NS, Schiffer CA, Weisdorf DJ (2006) Improvement of pulmonary function with imatinib mesylate in bronchiolitis obliterans following allogeneic hematopoietic cell transplantation. Biol Blood Marrow Transplant 12: 789–791
77. Culic O, Erakovic V, Parnham MJ (2001) Anti-inflammatory effects of macrolide antibiotics. Eur J Pharmacol 429: 209–229
78. Ichikawa Y, Ninomiya H, Koga H et al (1992) Erythromycin reduces neutrophils and neutrophil-derived elastolytic- like activity in the lower respiratory tract of bronchiolitis patients [see comments]. Am Rev Respir Dis 146: 196–203
79. Kanazawa S, Nomura S, Muramatsu M et al (2004) Azithromycin and bronchiolitis obliterans. Am J Respir Crit Care Med 169:654–655
80. Kudoh S, Azuma A, Yamamoto M et al (1998) Improvement of survival in patients with diffuse panbronchiolitis treated with low-dose erythromycin. Am J Respir Crit Care Med 157:1829–1832
81. Kudoh S (1998) Erythromycin treatment in diffuse panbronchiolitis. Curr Opin Pulm Med 4:116–121
82. Nagai H, Shishido H, Yoneda R et al (1991) Long-term low-dose administration of erythromycin to patients with diffuse panbronchiolitis. Respiration 58:145–149
83. Oda H, Kadota J, Kohno S et al (1994) Erythromycin inhibits neutrophil chemotaxis in bronchoalveoli of diffuse panbronchiolitis. Chest 106:1116–1123
84. Gerhardt SG, McDyer JF, Girgis RE et al (2003) Maintenance azithromycin therapy for bronchiolitis obliterans syndrome: results of a pilot study. Am J Respir Crit Care Med 168:121–125
85. Verleden GM, Dupont LJ (2004) Azithromycin therapy for patients with bronchiolitis obliterans syndrome after lung transplantation. Transplantation 77:1465–1467
86. Khalid M, Al Saghir A, Saleemi S et al (2005) Azithromycin in bronchiolitis obliterans complicating bone marrow transplantation: a preliminary study. Eur Respir J 25: 490–493
87. Browne PV, Weisdorf DJ, DeFor T et al (2000) Response to thalidomide therapy in refractory chronic graft-versus-host disease. Bone Marrow Transplant 26:865–869
88. Forsyth CJ, Cremer PD, Torzillo P et al (1996) Thalidomide responsive chronic pulmonary GVHD. Bone Marrow Transplant 17:291–293
89. Sullivan KM, Storek J, Kopecky KJ et al (1996) A controlled trial of long-term administration of intravenous immunoglobulin to prevent late infection and chronic graft-vs.-host disease after marrow transplantation: clinical outcome and effect on subsequent immune recovery. Biol Blood Marrow Transplant 2:44–53
90. Payne L, Chan CK, Fyles G et al (1993) Cyclosporine as possible prophylaxis for obstructive airways disease after allogeneic bone marrow transplantation. Chest 104: 114–118
91. Whitford H, Walters EH, Levvey B et al (2002) Addition of inhaled corticosteroids to systemic immunosuppression after lung transplantation: a double-blind, placebo-controlled trial. Transplantation 73:1793–1799
92. Boas SR, Noyes BE, Kurland G et al (1994) Pediatric lung transplantation for graft-versus-host disease following bone marrow transplantation. Chest 105:1584–1586
93. Favaloro R, Bertolotti A, Gomez C et al (2004) Lung transplant at the Favaloro Foundation: a 13-year experience. Transplant Proc 36:1689–1691
94. Pechet TV, de le MM, Mendeloff EN et al (2003) Lung transplantation in children following treatment for malignancy. J Heart Lung Transplant 22:154–160
95. Rabitsch W, Deviatko E, Keil F et al (2001) Successful lung transplantation for bronchiolitis obliterans after allogeneic marrow transplantation. Transplantation 71:1341–1343
96. Afessa B, Peters SG (2005) Chronic lung disease after hematopoietic stem cell transplantation. Clin Chest Med 26:571–586
97. Epler GR, Colby TV, McLoud TC et al (1985) Bronchiolitis obliterans organizing pneumonia. N Engl J Med 312: 152–158

98. Epler GR (2001) Bronchiolitis obliterans organizing pneumonia. Arch Intern Med 161:158–164
99. Thirman MJ, Devine SM, O'Toole K et al (1992) Bronchiolitis obliterans organizing pneumonia as a complication of allogeneic bone marrow transplantation. Bone Marrow Transplant 10:307–311
100. Mathew P, Bozeman P, Krance RA et al (1994) Bronchiolitis obliterans organizing pneumonia (BOOP) in children after allogeneic bone marrow transplantation. Bone Marrow Transplant 13:221–223
101. Alasaly K, Muller N, Ostrow DN et al (1995) Cryptogenic organizing pneumonia. A report of 25 cases and a review of the literature. Medicine (Baltimore) 74:201–211
102. Hayes-Jordan A, Benaim E, Richardson S et al (2002) Open lung biopsy in pediatric bone marrow transplant patients. J Pediatr Surg 37:446–452
103. Ishii T, Manabe A, Ebihara Y et al (2000) Improvement in bronchiolitis obliterans organizing pneumonia in a child after allogeneic bone marrow transplantation by a combination of oral prednisolone and low dose erythromycin [In Process Citation]. Bone Marrow Transplant 26:907–910
104. Kanamori H, Fujisawa S, Tsuburai T et al (2002) Increased exhaled nitric oxide in bronchiolitis obliterans organizing pneumonia after allogeneic bone marrow transplantation. Transplantation 74:1356–1358
105. Kanda Y, Takahashi T, Imai Y et al (1997) Bronchiolitis obliterans organizing pneumonia after syngeneic bone marrow transplantation for acute lymphoblastic leukemia. Bone Marrow Transplant 19:1251–1253
106. Kleinau I, Perez-Canto A, Schmid HJ et al (1997) Bronchiolitis obliterans organizing pneumonia and chronic graft-versus-host disease in a child after allogeneic bone marrow transplantation. Bone Marrow Transplant 19: 841–844
107. Przepiorka D, Abu-Elmagd K, Huaringa A et al (1993) Bronchiolitis obliterans organizing pneumonia in a BMT patient receiving FK506 [letter; comment]. Bone Marrow Transplant 11:502
108. Huisman C, van der Straaten HM, Canninga-van Dijk MR et al (2006) Pulmonary complications after T-cell-depleted allogeneic stem cell transplantation: low incidence and strong association with acute graft-versus-host disease. Bone Marrow Transplant 38:561–566
109. Yotsumoto S, Okada F, Yotsumoto S et al (2007) Bronchiolitis obliterans organizing pneumonia after bone marrow transplantation: association with human leukocyte antigens. J Comput Assist Tomogr 31:132–137
110. Yata K, Nakajima M, Takemoto Y et al (2002) Pneumonitis with a bronchiolitis obliterans organizing pneumonia-like shadow in a patient with human herpes virus-6 viremia after allogeneic bone marrow transplantation. Kansenshogaku Zasshi 76:385–390
111. Baron FA, Hermanne JP, Dowlati A et al (1998) Bronchiolitis obliterans organizing pneumonia and ulcerative colitis after allogeneic bone marrow transplantation. Bone Marrow Transplant 21:951–954
112. Epler GR (1995) Bronchiolitis obliterans organizing pneumonia. Semin Respir Infect 10:65–77
113. Muller NL, Staples CA, Miller RR (1990) Bronchiolitis obliterans organizing pneumonia: CT features in 14 patients. AJR Am J Roentgenol 154:983–987
114. Worthy SA, Flint JD, Muller NL (1997) Pulmonary complications after bone marrow transplantation: high-resolution CT and pathologic findings. Radiographics 17:1359–1371
115. Graham NJ, Muller NL, Miller RR et al (1991) Intrathoracic complications following allogeneic bone marrow transplantation: CT findings. Radiology 181:153–156
116. Cordier JF (2000) Organising pneumonia. Thorax 55:318–328
117. Chen CS, Boeckh M, Seidel K et al (2003) Incidence, risk factors, and mortality from pneumonia developing late after hematopoietic stem cell transplantation. Bone Marrow Transplant 32:515–522
118. Wong R, Rondon G, Saliba RM et al (2003) Idiopathic pneumonia syndrome after high-dose chemotherapy and autologous hematopoietic stem cell transplantation for high-risk breast cancer. Bone Marrow Transplant 31: 1157–1163
119. Clark JG, Hansen JA, Hertz MI et al (1993) NHLBI workshop summary. Idiopathic pneumonia syndrome after bone marrow transplantation. Am Rev Respir Dis 147: 1601–1606
120. Hauber HP, Mikkila A, Erich JM et al (2002) TNFalpha, interleukin-10 and interleukin-18 expression in cells of the bronchoalveolar lavage in patients with pulmonary complications following bone marrow or peripheral stem cell transplantation: a preliminary study. Bone Marrow Transplant 30:485–490
121. Schots R, Kaufman L, Van RI et al (2003) Proinflammatory cytokines and their role in the development of major transplant-related complications in the early phase after allogeneic bone marrow transplantation. Leukemia 17: 1150–1156
122. Yanik G, Hellerstedt B, Custer J et al (2002) Etanercept (Enbrel) administration for idiopathic pneumonia syndrome after allogeneic hematopoietic stem cell transplantation. Biol Blood Marrow Transplant 8:395–400
123. Kantrow SP, Hackman RC, Boeckh M et al (1997) Idiopathic pneumonia syndrome: changing spectrum of lung injury after marrow transplantation. Transplantation 63:1079–1086
124. Afessa B, Tefferi A, Litzow MR et al (2002) Diffuse alveolar hemorrhage in hematopoietic stem cell transplant recipients. Am J Respir Crit Care Med 166:641–645
125. Capizzi SA, Kumar S, Huneke NE et al (2001) Peri-engraftment respiratory distress syndrome during autologous hematopoietic stem cell transplantation. Bone Marrow Transplant 27:1299–1303
126. Crawford SW, Hackman RC (1993) Clinical course of idiopathic pneumonia after bone marrow transplantation. Am Rev Respir Dis 147:1393–1400
127. Afessa B, Tefferi A, Litzow MR et al (2002) Outcome of diffuse alveolar hemorrhage in hematopoietic stem cell transplant recipients. Am J Respir Crit Care Med 166: 1364–1368
128. Akasheh M, Eastwood D, Vesole DH (2003) Engraftment syndrome after autologous hematopoietic stem cell transplant supported by granulocyte-colony-stimulating factor (G-CSF) versus granulocyte-macrophage colony-stimulating factor (GM-CSF). Bone Marrow Transplant 31: 113–116

129. Maiolino A, Biasoli I, Lima J et al (2003) Engraftment syndrome following autologous hematopoietic stem cell transplantation: definition of diagnostic criteria. Bone Marrow Transplant 31:393–397
130. Abratt RP, Morgan GW, Silvestri G et al (2004) Pulmonary complications of radiation therapy. Clin Chest Med 25: 167–177
131. Limper AH (2004) Chemotherapy-induced lung disease. Clin Chest Med 25:53–64
132. Pedrazzoli P, Ferrante P, Kulekci A et al (2003) Autologous hematopoietic stem cell transplantation for breast cancer in Europe: critical evaluation of data from the European Group for Blood and Marrow Transplantation (EBMT) Registry 1990–1999. Bone Marrow Transplant 32: 489–494
133. Bearman SI, Overmoyer BA, Bolwell BJ et al (1997) High-dose chemotherapy with autologous peripheral blood progenitor cell support for primary breast cancer in patients with 4–9 involved axillary lymph nodes. Bone Marrow Transplant 20:931–937
134. Bhalla KS, Wilczynski SW, Abushamaa AM et al (2000) Pulmonary toxicity of induction chemotherapy prior to standard or high- dose chemotherapy with autologous hematopoietic support. Am J Respir Crit Care Med 161:17–25
135. Chap L, Shpiner R, Levine M et al (1997) Pulmonary toxicity of high-dose chemotherapy for breast cancer: a non-invasive approach to diagnosis and treatment. Bone Marrow Transplant 20:1063–1067
136. Fanfulla F, Pedrazzoli P, Da Prada GA et al (2000) Pulmonary function and complications following chemotherapy and stem cell support in breast cancer. Eur Respir J 15:56–61
137. Jones RB, Matthes S, Shpall EJ et al (1993) Acute lung injury following treatment with high-dose cyclophosphamide, cisplatin, and carmustine: pharmacodynamic evaluation of carmustine. J Natl Cancer Inst 85:640–647
138. Todd NW, Peters WP, Ost AH et al (1993) Pulmonary drug toxicity in patients with primary breast cancer treated with high-dose combination chemotherapy and autologous bone marrow transplantation. Am Rev Respir Dis 147: 1264–1270
139. Wilczynski SW, Erasmus JJ, Petros WP et al (1998) Delayed pulmonary toxicity syndrome following high-dose chemotherapy and bone marrow transplantation for breast cancer. Am J Respir Crit Care Med 157:565–573
140. Cao TM, Negrin RS, Stockerl-Goldstein KE et al (2000) Pulmonary toxicity syndrome in breast cancer patients undergoing BCNU-containing high-dose chemotherapy and autologous hematopoietic cell transplantation. Biol Blood Marrow Transplant 6:387–394
141. Peters WP, Ross M, Vredenburgh JJ et al (1993) High-dose chemotherapy and autologous bone marrow support as consolidation after standard-dose adjuvant therapy for high-risk primary breast cancer. J Clin Oncol 11: 1132–1143
142. Report on state of the art in blood and marrow transplantation. *IBMTR/ABMTR Newsletter* 2003; 10:7–10
143. Stadtmauer EA, O'Neill A, Goldstein LJ et al (2000) Conventional-dose chemotherapy compared with high-dose chemotherapy plus autologous hematopoietic stem-cell transplantation for metastatic breast cancer. Philadelphia Bone Marrow Transplant Group. N Engl J Med 342: 1069–1076
144. Suratt BT, Lynch DA, Cool CD et al (2003) Interferon-gamma for delayed pulmonary toxicity syndrome resistant to steroids. Bone Marrow Transplant 31:939–941
145. McGaughey DS, Nikcevich DA, Long GD et al (2001) Inhaled steroids as prophylaxis for delayed pulmonary toxicity syndrome in breast cancer patients undergoing high-dose chemotherapy and autologous stem cell transplantation. Biol Blood Marrow Transplant 7:274–278
146. Castellano-Sanchez AA, Poppiti RJ (2001) Pulmonary cytolytic thrombi (PCT). A previously unrecognized complication of bone marrow transplantation (BMT). Am J Surg Pathol 25:829–831
147. Gulbahce HE, Pambuccian SE, Jessurun J et al (2004) Pulmonary nodular lesions in bone marrow transplant recipients: impact of histologic diagnosis on patient management and prognosis. Am J Clin Pathol 121:205–210
148. Morales IJ, Anderson PM, Tazelaar HD et al (2003) Pulmonary cytolytic thrombi: unusual complication of hematopoietic stem cell transplantation. J Pediatr Hematol Oncol 25:89–92
149. Gulbahce HE, Manivel JC, Jessurun J (2000) Pulmonary cytolytic thrombi: a previously unrecognized complication of bone marrow transplantation. Am J Surg Pathol 24: 1147–1152
150. Woodard JP, Gulbahce E, Shreve M et al (2000) Pulmonary cytolytic thrombi: a newly recognized complication of stem cell transplantation. Bone Marrow Transplant 25:293–300
151. Wingard JR, Mellits ED, Jones RJ et al (1989) Association of hepatic veno-occlusive disease with interstitial pneumonitis in bone marrow transplant recipients. Bone Marrow Transplant 4:685–689
152. Sharma S, Nadrous HF, Peters SG et al (2005) Pulmonary complications in adult blood and marrow transplant recipients: autopsy findings. Chest 128:1385–1392
153. Hackman RC, Madtes DK, Petersen FB et al (1989) Pulmonary venoocclusive disease following bone marrow transplantation. Transplantation 47:989–992
154. Kuga T, Kohda K, Hirayama Y et al (1996) Pulmonary veno-occlusive disease accompanied by microangiopathic hemolytic anemia 1 year after a second bone marrow transplantation for acute lymphoblastic leukemia. Int J Hematol 64:143–150
155. Salzman D, Adkins DR, Craig F et al (1996) Malignancy-associated pulmonary veno-occlusive disease: report of a case following autologous bone marrow transplantation and review. Bone Marrow Transplant 18:755–760
156. Seguchi M, Hirabayashi N, Fujii Y et al (2000) Pulmonary hypertension associated with pulmonary occlusive vasculopathy after allogeneic bone marrow transplantation. Transplantation 69:177–179
157. Trobaugh-Lotrario AD, Greffe B, Deterding R et al (2003) Pulmonary veno-occlusive disease after autologous bone marrow transplant in a child with stage IV neuroblastoma: case report and literature review. J Pediatr Hematol Oncol 25:405–409
158. Troussard X, Bernaudin JF, Cordonnier C et al (1984) Pulmonary veno-occlusive disease after bone marrow transplantation. Thorax 39:956–957
159. Williams LM, Fussell S, Veith RW et al (1996) Pulmonary veno-occlusive disease in an adult following bone marrow

transplantation. Case report and review of the literature. Chest 109:1388–1391

160. Kotloff RM, Ahya VN, Crawford SW (2004) Pulmonary complications of solid organ and hematopoietic stem cell transplantation. Am J Respir Crit Care Med 170:22–48
161. Kramer MR, Estenne M, Berkman N et al (1993) Radiation-induced pulmonary veno-occlusive disease. Chest 104: 1282–1284
162. Mandel J, Mark EJ, Hales CA (2000) Pulmonary veno-occlusive disease. Am J Respir Crit Care Med 162: 1964–1973
163. Doll DC, Yarbro JW (1992) Vascular toxicity associated with antineoplastic agents. Semin Oncol 19:580–596
164. Doll DC, Yarbro JW (1994) Vascular toxicity associated with chemotherapy and hormonotherapy. Curr Opin Oncol 6:345–350
165. Gagnadoux F, Capron F, Lebeau B (2002) Pulmonary veno-occlusive disease after neoadjuvant mitomycin chemotherapy and surgery for lung carcinoma. Lung Cancer 36: 213–215
166. Elliott CG, Colby TV, Hill T et al (1988) Pulmonary veno-occlusive disease associated with severe reduction of single-breath carbon monoxide diffusing capacity. Respiration 53:262–266
167. Wagenvoort CA, Wagenvoort N, Takahashi T (1985) Pulmonary veno-occlusive disease: involvement of pulmonary arteries and review of the literature. Hum Pathol 16:1033–1041
168. Palmer SM, Robinson LJ, Wang A et al (1998) Massive pulmonary edema and death after prostacyclin infusion in a patient with pulmonary veno-occlusive disease. Chest 113:237–240
169. Shankar S, Choi JK, Dermody TS et al (2004) Pulmonary hypertension complicating bone marrow transplantation for idiopathic myelofibrosis. J Pediatr Hematol Oncol 26:393–397
170. Vaksmann G, Nelken B, Deshildre A et al (2002) Pulmonary arterial occlusive disease following chemotherapy and bone marrow transplantation for leukaemia. Eur J Pediatr 161:247–249
171. Bruckmann C, Lindner W, Roos R et al (1991) Severe pulmonary vascular occlusive disease following bone marrow transplantation in Omenn syndrome. Eur J Pediatr 150: 242–245
172. Presneill JJ, Nakata K, Inoue Y et al (2004) Pulmonary alveolar proteinosis. Clin Chest Med 25:593–613, viii
173. Cordonnier C, Fleury-Feith J, Escudier E et al (1994) Secondary alveolar proteinosis is a reversible cause of respiratory failure in leukemic patients. Am J Respir Crit Care Med 149:788–794
174. Gross TG, Hoge FJ, Jackson JD et al (1994) Fatal eosinophilic disease following autologous bone marrow transplantation. Bone Marrow Transplant 14:333–337
175. Brunet S, Muniz-Diaz E, Baiget M (1994) Chronic eosinophilic pneumonia in a patient treated with allogeneic bone marrow transplantation. Med Clin (Barc) 103:677
176. Richard C, Calavia J, Loyola I et al (1994) Chronic eosinophilic pneumonia in a patient treated with allogenic bone marrow transplantation. Med Clin (Barc) 102: 462–464

Are There Any Pulmonary Issues Specifically Related to Cord Blood Transplants?

8

Jonathan Gutman

Contents

J. Gutman
Fred Hutchinson Cancer Research Center, Seattle, Washington, USA
e-mail: jgutman@fhcrc.org

8.1 Introduction

A growing body of evidence supports the efficacy of umbilical cord blood as a donor source for hematopoietic stem cell transplantation, and the number of cord blood transplants (CBTs) is increasing [1]. Among pediatric patients, data suggest that outcomes following CBT are comparable to outcomes following unrelated donor transplants and that outcomes following well-matched CBT may be superior to outcomes following matched unrelated donor transplants. For adult patients, data continue to accumulate demonstrating outcomes similar to unrelated donor transplants, but early transplant-related mortality (TRM) due to delayed engraftment, increased graft failures, and infectious complications remains an important challenge. Broadly speaking, CBT patients can be expected to have similar pulmonary complications as non-CBT patients, and there is no significant literature describing distinct patterns of pulmonary complications following CBT. Given the unique immunologic characteristics of cord blood, however, larger studies may demonstrate unique pulmonary complications following CBT, and several pulmonary issues specifically related to CBT are worthy of consideration. In this brief report, we highlight complications that have been reported or that are based on our experience in recipients of CBT.

8.2 Infusional Toxicities

Unlike matched sibling and unrelated donor transplants, where stem cell products are typically infused fresh, cord blood units are processed, frozen, and

É. Azoulay (ed.), *Pulmonary Involvement in Patients with Hematological Malignancies*,
DOI: 10.1007/978-3-642-15742-4_8,

stored for subsequent use. Cord blood banks use a variety of strategies to process units for storage, ranging from plasma depletion only to intensive red cell depletion. Transplant centers use a variety of techniques to process frozen units prior to infusion, ranging from bedside thaw and infusion to albumin dilution and infusion to wash and infusion. In the United States, the National Marrow Donor Program (NMDP) has recently issued a warning describing four cases of serious adverse events involving heart failure and acute pulmonary edema following the use of plasma-depleted, red blood cell-replete units that were not washed prior to infusion. Based on these findings, the NMDP recommends washing of cord blood units, particularly red blood cell-replete units, prior to infusion. Physicians should be aware of this potential pulmonary/cardiovascular complication [2]. Larger studies will better characterize the incidence and pathophysiology underlying this phenomenon.

8.3 Preengraftment Syndrome

Following CBT, "preengraftment" syndrome has been reported to occur at an increased frequency as compared to related or unrelated donor transplant. The syndrome is being increasingly well characterized. It develops before or at the time of engraftment, and its clinical manifestations include high fever in the absence of infection as well as diffuse erythematous skin rash resembling acute graft-versus-host disease (aGVHD) and may include fluid retention. Those patients who experience fluid retention may develop pulmonary infilitrates. The syndrome frequently responds to a brief burst of steroids (common dosing 3 days of 1 mg/kg methylpredinsolone) and appears to be distinct from early onset acute GVHD. Some data suggest, however, the preengraftment syndrome may be predictive of the subsequent development of GVHD [3].

8.4 Infections

Infectious complications, including pulmonary infections, are a significant concern following CBT [4, 5]. Delayed neutrophil engraftment exposes patients to prolonged vulnerability to bacterial and fungal infections [5]. Several series have reported high rates of early TRM following CBT, and pulmonary infections account for a portion of these early events. Delayed T-cell reconstitution following CBT raises concerns about prolonged and increased risk for viral infections [6], including respiratory infections [7, 8]. No large studies, however, have quantified the incidence of respiratory viral infections following CBT. Pulmonary physicians should have a high suspicion for infectious etiologies of pulmonary symptoms following CBT.

8.5 Pulmonary Immune Reactions

In numerous studies, cord blood is associated with a lower incidence of chronic GVHD than transplant with unrelated donors. It is reasonable to speculate, therefore, that CBT may be associated with lower incidences of pulmonary transplant complications attributed to immune reactions between the donor and host [9]. The incidences of bronchiolitis obliterans (BO) and bronchiolitis obliterans organizing pneumonia (BOOP) may be lower following CBT [10, 11], but no studies to date have examined this outcome.

In conclusion, although there is no sound evidence of increased incidence of respiratory events in recipients of CBTs, clinicians must be aware of some infectious or noninfectious conditions that may occur in CBT patients. Given the unique immunologic characteristics of cord blood, several pulmonary issues specifically related to CBT (infusional toxicity, preengraftment syndrome, pulmonary infections, and pulmonary immune reactions) are worthy of consideration.

References

1. Rocha V, Labopin M, Sanz G, Arcese W, Schwerdtfeger R, Bosi A, Jacobsen N, Ruutu T, De Lima M, Finke J, Frassoni F, Gluckman E, Acute Leukemia Working Party of European Blood and Marrow Transplant Group, Eurocord-Netcord Registry (2004) Transplants of umbilical-cord blood or bone marrow from unrelated donors in adults with acute leukemia. N Engl J Med 351(22):2276–2285, 25 Nov 2004

2. Konuma T, Ooi J, Takahashi S, Tomonari A, Tsukada N, Kobayashi T, Sato A, Kato S, Kasahara S, Ebihara Y, Nagamura-Inoue T, Tsuji K, Tojo A, Asano S (2008) Cardiovascular toxicity of cryopreserved cord blood cell infusion. Bone Marrow Transplant 41(10):861–865
3. Patel KJ, Rice RD, Hawke R, Abboud M, Heller G, Scaradavou A, Young JW, Barker JN (2010) Pre-engraftment syndrome after double-unit cord blood transplantation: a distinct syndrome not associated with acute graft-versus-host disease. Biol Blood Marrow Transplant 16(3):435–440
4. Cahu X, Rialland F, Touzeau C, Chevallier P, Guillaume T, Delaunay J, Ayari S, Dubruille V, Le Gouill S, Mahe B, Gastinne T, Blin N, Saulquin B, Harousseau JL, Moreau P, Mohty M (2009) Infectious complications after unrelated umbilical cord blood transplantation in adult patients with hematologic malignancies. Biol Blood Marrow Transplant 15(12):1531–1537
5. Szabolcs P, Cairo MS (2010) Unrelated umbilical cord blood transplantation and immune reconstitution. Semin Hematol 47(1):22–36
6. Montesinos P, Sanz J, Cantero S, Lorenzo I, Martín G, Saavedra S, Palau J, Romero M, Montava A, Senent L, Martínez J, Jarque I, Salavert M, Córdoba J, Gómez L, Weiss S, Moscardó F, De la Rubia J, Larrea L, Sanz MA, Sanz GF (2009) Incidence, risk factors, and outcome of cytomegalovirus infection and disease in patients receiving prophylaxis with oral valganciclovir or intravenous ganciclovir after umbilical cord blood transplantation. Biol Blood Marrow Transplant 15(6):730–740, Epub 2009, Apr 11
7. Almyroudis NG, Fabian J, Hahn T, Segal BH, Wetzler M, McCarthy PL Jr (2009) Late infectious complications after cord blood stem cell transplantation. Eur J Clin Microbiol Infect Dis 28(11):1405–1408
8. Yazaki M, Atsuta Y, Kato K, Kato S, Taniguchi S, Takahashi S, Ogawa H, Kouzai Y, Kobayashi T, Inoue M, Kobayashi R, Nagamura-Inoue T, Azuma H, Takanashi M, Kai S, Nakabayashi M, Saito H, Japan Cord Blood Bank Network (2009) Incidence and risk factors of early bacterial infections after unrelated cord blood transplantation. Biol Blood Marrow Transplant 15(4):439–446
9. Shima T, Yoshimoto G, Miyamoto T, Yoshida S, Kamezaki K, Takenaka K, Iwasaki H, Harada N, Nagafuji K, Teshima T, Shimono N, Akashi K (2009) Disseminated tuberculosis following second unrelated cord blood transplantation for acute myelogenous leukemia. Transpl Infect Dis 11(1): 75–77
10. Gutman JA, Leisenring W, Appelbaum FR, Woolfrey AE, Delaney C (2009) Low relapse without excessive transplant-related mortality following myeloablative cord blood transplantation for acute leukemia in complete remission: a matched cohort analysis. Biol Blood Marrow Transplant 15(9):1122–1129
11. Majhail NS, Parks K, Defor TE, Weisdorf DJ (2006) Diffuse alveolar hemorrhage and infection-associated alveolar hemorrhage following hematopoietic stem cell transplantation: related and high-risk clinical syndromes. Biol Blood Marrow Transplant 12(10):1038–1046

Cardiovascular Complications of Cancer Therapeutics

9

Aarif Y. Khakoo and Callie S. Kwartler

Contents

A.Y. Khakoo (✉)
Department of Cardiology,
University of Texas MD Anderson Cancer Center,
Houston, TX, 77030
e-mail: aykhakoo@mdanderson.org

C.S. Kwartler
Department of Internal Medicine,
University of Texas Health Science Center at Houston,
Houston, TX, 77030

9.1 Introduction

As treatment for cancer has modernized and the number of anticancer drugs has multiplied, survival of cancer patients beyond their initial disease has improved dramatically. Perversely, the same agents that bring about a "cure" for cancer can also lead to devastating cardiovascular side effects, including cardiomyopathy, myocardial infarction, thromboembolism, hypertension, arrhythmias, and QT prolongation. In fact, cancer survivors are in many cases more likely to develop cardiovascular disease than experience a recurrence of their malignancy.

Cardiovascular toxicities not only increase morbidity and mortality for these patients, but also impair the ability of clinicians to manage a patient's anticancer regimen with maximal efficiency. This chapter provides

É. Azoulay (ed.), *Pulmonary Involvement in Patients with Hematological Malignancies*,
DOI: 10.1007/978-3-642-15742-4_9, © Springer-Verlag Berlin Heidelberg 2011

Table 9.1 Cardiotoxic drugs by disease presentation

Drug	Incidence	Notes
Cardiomyopathy		
Anthracyclines (chronic)	4–26% [3, 6]	Symptomatic dilated cardiomyopathy or heart failure; irreversible
Mitoxantrone (chronic)	2.6% [54, 55]	Symptomatic heart failure; irreversible
Trastuzumab	1–10% [26, 63–65]	LV dysfunction in up to 10%, heart failure in 1–4%; reversible
Lapatinib	0.2–2% [66, 72]	LV dysfunction in 2%, symptomatic heart failure in 0.2%; reversible
Imatinib	1.7–4% [191, 192]	Symptomatic heart failure
Sunitinib	11–19% [86, 87]	LV dysfunction in 19%, grade 3 dysfunction or clinical heart failure in 7%
Cyclophosphamide	10–28% [110, 193]	Typically acute onset within 1–10 days of first dose
Mitomycin	Rare [54, 194]	
Interferon α	Unknown [88]	Dilated cardiomyopathy; incidence suspected to be underreported due to similar symptoms with other complications
Gemcitabine	1.8% [136]	Cardiac dysfunction with decline in LVEF
Bortezomib	Up to 10% [163, 195]	Mostly based on case reports and one study that found a 10% incidence of heart failure serious enough to cause hospitalization
All-trans retinoic acid	17% [194]	Described as "substantial decline" in LVEF, symptomatic of "retinoic acid syndrome"
Thromboembolism		
Alemtuzumab	Rare [101, 196]	Controversial; events observed in some studies but not others
Cisplatin	Up to 12.9% [119, 120]	Includes DVT, PE, arterial thromboses, CVA, and angina pectoris; high risk of grade 4 or 5 events
Irinotecan	Up to 20% [131]	Both venous and arterial thromboembolic events
Oxaliplatin	1–2% [5]	Increased incidence (8%) when combined with capecitabine
Estramustine	Up to 10% [54]	Includes coronary ischemia, cerebrovascular ischemia, PE, and venous thromboembolism
Tamoxifen	1.2% [156, 197]	Includes DVT and PE
Thalidomide	12–20% [95, 167]	Includes lower extremity DVT and PE most commonly, but rarely stroke, unstable angina, and cerebral venous sinus thrombosis reported
Denileukin diftitox	11% [194]	Results from vascular leak syndrome
Bevacizumab	2–11% [5, 96, 97]	mostly arterial thromboembolism; includes CVA, angina, sudden death, and other manifestations
Hypertension		
Sunitinib	17–47% [86, 198]	Any grade 47%, grade 3 or higher 17%
Sorafenib	"Common" [91]	Mechanistically similar to sunitinib, so incidence is likely similar
Bevacizumab	8–18% [96]	Grade 3 or higher hypertension 8–18%

Table 9.1 (continued)

Hypertension		
Drug	Incidence	Notes
Vinorelbine	Rare [145]	Based on case reports
Docetaxel	Unknown [5]	Can cause either hypo- or hypertension
QT prolongation		
Dasatinib	1% [78, 199]	Grade 3–4 QT prolongation
Nilotinib	3% [77–79]	Grade 3–4 QT prolongation
Arsenic trioxide	Up to 63% [169–172]	Can lead to tachyarrhythmias, torsades de pointes, or sudden death
Vorinostat	3.5–6% [194]	
Myocardial infarction		
Gefitinib	Rare [200]	Case reports only
Sorafenib	2.9% [92, 93]	Acute coronary symptoms including MI
Cisplatin	12.9% [116–118]	Ischemic disease; more common in elderly; possibly related to thromboembolic disease (see above)
Bleomycin	<3% [130]	Severe chest pain; rare ischemia or MI in young patients
Etoposide	Rare [194, 201]	Case reports only; rechallenge worsens cardiac function
Gemcitabine	Rare [137, 138]	Case reports only
Vinca alkaloids	1% [54, 144, 145]	
5-Fluorouracil	4% [106]	Myocardial ischemia or infarction, likely due to coronary vasospasm
Capecitabine	<4% [108]	Similar to 5-fluorouracil
Aromatase inhibitors	1–2% [155, 202, 203]	Increased incidence relative to tamoxifen, but controversial as to whether incidence is increased relative to controls
IL2	More than 1.5% [176]	1.5% treatment-related deaths; MI and ischemia are more common
Pentostatin	Rare [194]	Case reports only; incidence increases when co-treated with cyclophosphamide
Methotrexate	Rare [54]	Case reports only
Arrhythmias		
Anthracyclines (acute)	Rare [1, 5]	Transient ventricular arrhythmias
Mitoxantrone (acute)	Rare [54, 55]	Transient ventricular arrhythmias
Nilotinib	2% [79]	
Alemtuzumab	Rare [101, 196]	Controversial; events observed in some studies but not in others
Rituximab	1–7% [204]	Various types of arrhythmias
Gemcitabine	2–3% [136, 139, 140]	Case reports of atrial fibrillation; grade 1–4 ventricular tachyarrhythmias in 2.3%
5-fluorouracil	>2.2% [105]	2.2% suffer cardiac death due to arrhythmias

(continued)

Table 9.1 (continued)

Arrhythmias		
Drug	Incidence	Notes
Paclitaxel	5% [146, 151]	Sinus bradycardia in up to 30%, more serious arrhythmias in 5%; typically transient
Docetaxel	Up to 5% [5]	Dysrhythmias or tachycardia
Bortezomib	Rare [163, 195]	Mostly case reports
Interferon α	Up to 20% [54, 168]	Supraventricular arrhythmias most common; can be lethal
IL-2	6% [54]	
Homoharringtonine	Rare [194]	Most common presentation is hypotension; arrhythmias are rare
Pentostatin	Rare [194]	Case reports only; incidence increases when co-treated with cyclophosphamide
Methotrexate	Rare [54, 205]	Case reports only, no typical clinical presentation of arrhythmia

LV left ventricular, *LVEF* left ventricular ejection fraction, *DVT* deep venous thrombosis, *PE* pulmonary embolism, *CVA* cerebrovascular accident, *MI* myocardial infarction

an overview of the cardiovascular complications associated with specific anticancer drugs (see Table 9.1 for a list of effects categorized by disease presentation). We specifically focus on the drugs most strongly associated with cardiotoxicities, and present information on the risk factors, incidence, and specific mechanisms of the effect on the cardiovascular system.

9.2 Anthracyclines

Anthracyclines are a class of drugs originally isolated from microorganisms that are used to treat a wide spectrum of cancers. Doxorubicin (also called adriamycin) and daunorubicin were the original anthracyclines, and are still the most potent antitumor drugs in the class [1]. Epirubicin, idarubicin, and others have since been developed in attempts to create a better anthracycline with more potent antitumor effects and less cardiotoxicity. Daunorubicin and idarubicin are typically used to treat acute lymphoblastic and myeloblastic leukemias, while doxorubicin and epirubicin are used to treat a broader spectrum of solid and hematological cancers [2].

The antitumor effects of anthracyclines are mediated by their DNA intercalating effects and inhibition of topoisomerase II [3]. The potency of the antitumor effect, however, is counterbalanced by a severe dose-dependent toxic effect causing irreversible cardiomyopathy. However, cardiotoxicity may not be mediated through the same mechanisms as antineoplastic effects, and appears to be independent of tumor type [4]. There are four general categories of cardiotoxicity related to anthracyclines: acute (during or immediately after treatment), subchronic (within 1–3 days after treatment), early chronic (develops late in the treatment course or up to months after completion of treatment), and delayed or late-onset (manifests years to decades after therapy). Acute cardiotoxicity, which is not dose-dependent, most frequently manifests as transient arrhythmias [5]. In rare cases, however, acute doxorubicin toxicity has been shown to cause acute heart failure with a decrease in left ventricular ejection fraction down to 10%. By contrast, subchronic cardiotoxicity is most frequently seen as a pericarditis-myocarditis syndrome, and the chronic and late-onset cardiotoxicities are usually characterized by dilated cardiomyopathy, which results in a decline in systolic or diastolic cardiac function and eventually congestive heart failure [6]. Delayed cardiotoxicity most frequently manifests in survivors of childhood cancer and can be particularly brought to the surface by stressors such as pregnancy.

Risk factors contributing to the incidence of anthracycline cardiotoxicity include the extremes of age, preexisting cardiac disease, female gender, African-American race, and trisomy 21. Use of certain other chemotherapeutic agents or mediastinal radiation along with anthracyclines also increases risk [7]. These risk factors apply to both acute and all chronic types of cardiotoxicity [8]. However, the most significant (and in some studies the only independent) predictor of developing anthracycline-induced cardiomyopathy is cumulative dose. Dosing limits have been set for each drug above which the incidence of cardiotoxicity becomes unacceptably high: for doxorubicin dose is limited to 400–450 mg/m^2, whereas for the modified anthracycline epirubicin the limiting dose is 750 mg/m^2[5]. Even at these confined doses, reports cite incidences of chronic cardiotoxicity ranging from <4% to 26%.

Studies have suggested that children respond differently to anthracyclines than adults, with possibly less risk of developing acute or chronic cardiomyopathy but significantly increasing risk with time from treatment of developing delayed cardiomyopathy. Indeed, one clinical trial that looked at 607 children found a cumulative incidence of anthracycline-induced heart failure of 2.8% 6.3 years after treatment, but that risk increased significantly up to 5% after 15 years of follow-up [9]. Longer follow-up times would likely yield even higher incidences of cardiac dysfunction in childhood cancer survivors treated with anthracyclines [4]. The cumulative dose above which incidence was significantly increased was also lower in children: only 300 mg/m^2 of doxorubicin [8].

9.2.1 Genetic Risk

Some recent work has shown that genetic factors influence the development of anthracycline cardiotoxicity. Strong support for a genetic role in determining risk originally came from knockout and transgenic animal studies that showed increased sensitivity or resistance to anthracyclines. For example, overexpression of the multi-drug resistance gene MDR1 is protective, while overexpression of the carbonyl reductase gene is sensitizing. In humans [10], higher incidences of anthracycline cardiotoxicity have been found associated not only with SNPs in NADPH oxidase, but also with polymorphisms in GSTP, a phase II detox enzyme, and CBR3, a paralog of the carbonyl reductase CBR1 [11]. One group sequenced candidate genes in patients who did or did not develop cardiotoxic responses to anthracycline therapy. They found significantly associated SNPs in multiple NADPH oxidase subunits, suggesting the importance of this protein complex in modulating risk of anthracycline cardiotoxicity. They also found that SNPs in three transmembrane efflux receptors responsible for transport of anthracyclines correlated strongly with acute cardiotoxic responses. Polymorphisms in adrenergic receptors and angiotensin-converting enzymes were not associated with increased cardiotoxicity [10].

With the sequencing of the human genome and the development of more advanced methods for genome-wide association studies, continued research into this area could be crucial both to understanding the mechanisms and to predicting risk of individual patients. In the future, patients with alleles increasing their risk could be put on lower doses of anthracyclines or be treated with alternative drugs to decrease the overall incidence of cardiotoxicity substantially.

9.2.2 Mechanistic Insights

Recent focus has been on determining mechanisms of cardiotoxicity in the hope of identifying possible cardioprotective mechanisms or deriving a new anthracycline that is less cardiotoxic but no less potent against tumors. Endomyocardial biopsies of affected hearts reveal characteristic ultrastructural features of anthracycline-induced cardiac damage. Cytoplasmic vacuolization, swelling of mitochondria, increased numbers of lysosomes, loss of myofibrils, and dilation of the sarcoplasmic reticulum are all frequently observed changes [12]. Treatment of cultured cardiomyocytes with anthracyclines induces an apoptosis-like cell death phenotype similar to that observed in the tissue [13].

Interference with multiple aspects of cardiomyocyte cellular function have been observed after exposure to anthracyclines, including effects on myocardial calcium handling [14], adrenergic receptor signaling [14], myocardial protein synthesis [15], and mitochondrial function [16]. In addition, multiple studies have demonstrated that anthracyclines induce cardiomyocyte myofibrillar disarray [17] and apoptosis [12]. While it is difficult to completely unify these diverse cytotoxic effects to one mechanism of cellular injury, many studies have suggested a central role of oxidative stress, leading to increased reactive oxygen species, lipid peroxidation, and iron-regulated oxidative damage. Such studies have provided the mechanistic basis for cardioprotective strategies (discussed below), which have had mixed results in the clinical setting. Over the past 2 decades data have emerged to suggest that alternative mechanisms independent of ROS-mediated damage are important in anthracycline-induced cardiotoxicity [1]. Such alternative mechanisms may be better targets for more effective cardioprotective strategies.

One such alternative theory proposes that oxidative stress (mediated by the formation of ROS by redox cycling of anthracyclines) plays a primary role only in the development of *acute* anthracycline cardiotoxicity, while secondary alcohol metabolites of anthracyclines accumulate in cardiac tissue over time and lead to chronic cardiotoxicity [2]. Anthracycline molecules bear a quinone moiety that can be reduced by two electrons to form secondary alcohol metabolites such as doxorubicinol [18]. Such metabolites potently impair cardiomyocyte calcium handling to a much greater degree than their parent compounds through effects on calcium handling proteins [19] and on sarcoplasmic reticulum Ca^{2+}-induced Ca^{2+} release [20] in a free-radical independent manner.

9.2.3 Synergistic Interactions

Anticancer agents that are commonly co-administered with anthracyclines or commonly administered in patients previously treated with anthracyclines may enhance cardiac toxicity of anthracyclines, despite the fact that such agents alone exhibit minimal cardiac toxicity. One such class of drugs is the taxanes, which are microtubule-stabilizing drugs that inhibit tumor growth by causing cell-cycle arrest. Paclitaxel and docetaxel, both widely used taxanes, have both been shown to increase formation of doxorubicinol, the secondary alcohol metabolite of doxorubicin. Kinetic studies showed that at low doses (such as those given to patients), taxanes bind with high affinity to a regulatory or allosteric site of the aldehyde reductase enzymes that convert anthracyclines to their metabolites. However, at high doses taxanes begin to compete with anthracyclines to bind to the active sites of these enzymes and thus prevent alcohol formation [21]. Clinically, initial studies demonstrated an enhancement of anthracycline-induced cardiac toxicity occurring when co-administered with paclitaxel; [22] however, subsequent adjusted dosing regimens have minimized this effect [23]. The use of docetaxel simultaneously with doxorubicin does not appear to enhance the rates of clinically significant cardiac toxicity compared with anthracyclines administered as a single agent [23].

Co-administration of anthracyclines and the anti-ErbB2 antibody trastuzumab results in a high rate of heart failure. Up to 28% of patients treated with this regimen experienced a cardiac event [24, 25] with 15% experiencing a grade 3 or 4 complication [26]. One hypothesis to explain this synergistic relationship is that trastuzumab alters ErbB2 signaling to interfere with the regulation of cytoskeletal proteins, while anthracyclines directly affect biosynthesis of sarcomeric proteins. These two independent mechanisms both leading to an effective contractile dysfunction could be causing the additive effect of cardiotoxicity [27]. More frequently cited, however, is the "multiple hit" hypothesis: that anthracyclines induce oxidative stress, and myocytes typically signal through survival pathways like ErbB2 in response to that stress. In fact, data in anthracycline-treated patients suggest that ErbB2-dependent signaling in the myocardium may be particularly important in the setting of anthracycline treatment. Myocardial uptake of indium-labeled trastuzumab was seen in 50% of patients within 3 weeks after anthracycline treatment, while only 9% of patients exhibit myocardial uptake of labeled trastuzumab 11 months after anthracyline administration, and no uptake is detected in the hearts of patients with heart failure not due to anthracyclines [28].

It is essential to be wary of combining new drugs with anthracyclines, as these examples show. Another study on pharmacokinetics of doxorubicin showed that even drugs that do not react with the quinone moiety to increase ROS formation or with the reductase enzymes to speed secondary alcohol metabolite formation can still cause increased cardiotoxicity by competing sterically for anthracycline-degrading factors like $Mb_{IV\text{-}O}$. Even drugs with no cardiotoxic effects themselves could interfere with doxorubicin metabolism in this way [29].

9.2.4 Cardioprotective Strategies

Since anthracycline-induced cardiotoxicity is irreversible and usually unresponsive to traditional heart failure treatments like digitalis, ACE inhibitors, and beta-blockers, several strategies have been developed to reduce the risk of heart failure due to anthracyclines. Table 9.2 summarizes the results of several strategies to reduce the risk of cardiotoxicity resulting from anthracyclines. Continuous infusion of anthracycline as opposed to standard, bolus therapy showed initial promise as a cardioprotective strategy [30]. Enthusiasm for this approach was tempered by other reports that were unable to reproduce this cardioprotective effect [31]. Thus, there remains a wide spectrum of administration protocols for anthracycline infusion at different centers, with continuous infusion reserved for patients at high risk for cardiotoxicity.

Table 9.2 Cardioprotective strategies for anthracyclines

Strategy	Doxil (Pegylated Lipoxomal Doxorubicin) [34, 35, 206, 207]	Slow infusion (>6 hours) [30, 31, 208]	Dexrazoxane[40]	ACE inhibitors [46, 209]	Beta blockers [45, 209]
Net decrease of Cardiotoxicity	RR= 0.38 for heart failure combined	RR = 0.27 for clinical heart failure, also protective against subclinical disease	RR = 0.29 for heart failure combined	Significant increase in average LVEF after treatment	Significant increase in avg LVEF after treatment
Effect on Cancer therapy efficacy	RR = 1.01 for tumor response, 1.01 for progression free survival	RR = 1.2 for tumor response, 1.42 for overall survival (difference not statistically significant)	RR = 0.89 for tumor response, 1.01 for progression-free survival	None reported	None reported
Adverse effects	increased skin toxicity (PPE), bone marrow toxicity, and infusion reactionsp; decreased alopecia, myelosuppression, mucositis	Decreased gastrointestinal effects, no effect on myelosuppression or alopecia	No change in thrombocytopenia, neutropenia, slight increase in abnormal white blood cell count and anemia (RR=1.19); increased pain on injection; increased phlebitis and fever; decreased stomatitis, nausea/vomiting; one studied suggested high risk of secondary malignant disease	Incraesed incidence of dizziness, hypotension, and fatigue Fetal kidney damage if taken during pregnancy	None specifically reported Beta-blockers can increase risk of hypoglycemic shock in diabetic patients, and can reduce circulation to extremitie, dizziness and clinical depression are also common
Other notes	Doxil formulation has greatly increased half-life and higher uptake in tumor cells	This strategy is used routinely at MD Anderson Cancer Center; some evidence suggests it is not effective in children	Dexrazoxane is the only co-drug that has been proven to be cardioprotective by several rigorous clinical trials	ACE is are also used to slow progression of cardiomyopathy once it occurs	Beta-blockers are also used to slow progression of cardiomyopathy once it occurs

RR risk ratio (<0.5 is significantly beneficial, >2 is significantly harmful)

Changes in the chemical structure or method of formulation of anthracyclines have also been devised in an effort to reduce cardiotoxicity without reducing tumor efficacy. Epirubicin is a structurally modified analog of doxorubicin, which has less toxicity on an equimolar basis [32], but comparative studies have not detected a significant difference in cardiotoxicity between these two drugs when used at dosages that are efficacious in cancer therapy [33]. Pre-clinical studies strongly suggest that epirubicin is converted to its secondary alcohol metabolite epirubicnol at a much lower efficiency than conversion of doxorubicin to doxorubicinol [2]. Thus, one would predict that epirubicin would have significantly lower incidence of chronic cardiac toxicity compared with doxorubicin when used at dosages with equivalent anticancer efficacy, but this has not yet been clearly demonstrated in head-to-head clinical trials. Furthermore, a meta-analysis of five randomized, controlled trials found no significant difference between rates of cardiotoxicity associated with epirubicin compared with that of doxorubicin [34].

More favorable findings have been demonstrated with the use of liposomal anthracycline formulations, particularly with pegylated liposomal doxorubicin (PLD, Doxil) [35, 36]. In a large phase III trial of patients with metastatic breast cancer that compared conventional doxorubicin and PLD, the latter was associated with a highly significant ($P<0.0001$), threefold decreased risk in cardiotoxicity, with no difference in antitumor efficacy [35, 36].

The EDTA-like iron chelator dexrazoxane has also shown promise in preventing anthracycline-induced cardiotoxicity. Dexrazoxane was originally itself an anticancer drug whose cardioprotective effects were discovered accidentally [3]. Treatment of cultured cardiomyocytes with doxorubicin causes loss of mitochondrial DNA and cell death, pre- or co-treatment with dexrazoxane significantly reduces these effects [37]. Dexrazoxane has two mechanisms of action: in tumor cells it, like anthracyclines, is a strong inhibitor of topoisomerase II. In cardiomyocytes, meanwhile, it is metabolized to an EDTA-type form that chelates iron and prevents oxidative damage to the cells [38].

In one of the first randomized trials of this agent, patients treated with dexrazoxane had significant decreases in the incidence of cardiotoxicity caused by doxorubicin as determined by the development of congestive heart failure (CHF) left ventricular dysfunction (LVD) and changes on endomyocardial biopsy consistent with anthracycline cardiotoxicity [39]. A meta-analysis of six randomized, controlled trials concluded that dexrazoxane significantly reduces the incidence of anthracycline-induced heart failure [relative risk (RR) = 0.28, CI 0.18–0.42, $P<0.000001$] [40]. This same meta-analysis identified a trend towards decreased tumor response in patients receiving dexrazoxane (RR = 0.88, CI 0.77–1.01, P = 0.06), although a significant worsening in tumor response rate in patients treated with dexrzoxane has only been observed in one study [41].

Notably, although dexrazoxane can worsen both thrombocytopenia and granulocytopenia during cancer therapy, no significant difference in the incidence of these adverse effects was identified in the meta-analysis. Furthermore, an overall survival benefit has not been observed in patients receiving dexrazoxane for cardioprotection in either a large randomized trial [41] or in the meta-analysis of six randomized studies [40]. For all of these reasons, the usage of dexrazoxane is limited to subsets of pediatric patients and patients at high-risk of cardiotoxicity due to anthracyclines, such as those with pre-existing cardiac disease.

The nonspecific beta-blocker carvedilol, a mainstay of therapy for patients with heart failure, has potent antioxidant and antiapoptotic properties, which suggest that it may be effective as a protective agent for anthracycline-induced cardiotoxicity [42]. Preclinical studies have demonstrated that carvedilol protects cardiomyocytes from anthracycline-induced damage in vitro [43] and in animal model studies [44]. A recent small, placebo-controlled study demonstrated a similar cardioprotective effect of once-daily carvedilol in patients receiving anthracycline-based chemotherapy [45]. Larger, randomized clinical studies are needed to confirm the utility of carvedilol as a cardioprotective agent for patients receiving anthracycline-based chemotherapy.

A recent report integrating the use of cardiac biomarkers with the use of the angiotensin-converting enzyme (ACE) inhibitors as a chemoprotective strategy demonstrated a promising approach [46]. In a randomized study of patients who received high-dose chemotherapy with elevated serum troponin I levels, none of the 56 patients randomized to receive enalapril developed heart failure, while 14 of 58 (24%) control patients developed heart failure. This finding was consistent with pre-clinical observations demonstrating that ACE-inhibitors provide a powerful cardioprotective effect in animals receiving anthracyclines [47, 48]. While we await further large trials of these chemoprotection strategies, it is reasonable to use ACE-inhibitors prophylactically in patients receiving anthracyclines who have a high-risk of developing cardiotoxicity or in whom antihypertensive therapy is indicated. This approach is in accordance with the recently updated American Heart Association/American College of Cardiology guidelines for the treatment of heart failure [49].

Many other molecules and drugs have been tested as potential cardioprotective agents, with several showing promise in cell culture or animal studies. For example, probucol is an antioxidant with lipid-lowering effects, and has been shown to effect doxorubicin pharmacokinetics without affecting antitumor efficacy. Pretreatment with probucol significantly decreases doxorubicin concentrations in plasma and also reduces markers of cardiac damage in pre-clinical studies [12, 50]. Two hypotheses about its mechanism have been proposed: either probucol could inhibit conversion of doxorubicin into its toxic secondary alcohol metabolite doxorubicinol or its effect may be to accelerate excretion of the drug through the kidney through an antioxidant effect, thus reducing dosage to the heart.

Modulation of diet and exercise has also been shown to be potentially cardioprotective. In mice, increased exercise training has been shown to be protective particularly against acute anthracycline cardiotoxicity and may also protect against chronic effects [51]. Meanwhile, rats fed with a high-fat diet show an increased sensitivity to doxorubicin that may be due to preexisting cardiac stress [52], suggesting that restricting diet or increasing exercise to improve overall cardiac health may reduce cardiotoxicity caused by anthracyclines.

9.2.5 Conclusions

Although recent studies have significantly advanced our understanding of anthracycline-induced cardiotoxicity, many questions still remain. The search for human genetic variants, the use of cell culture and animal models to probe specific mechanisms, and the preclinical and clinical studies of treatments that may be cardioprotective or sensitizing have so far yielded strong results that are just beginning to make sense together. Since the cardiac damage caused by anthracyclines is irreversible, clinically relevant, and potentially fatal, the urgency of this research is not diminishing. Reducing the incidence of anthracycline cardiotoxicity through better drug development, cardioprotective strategies, and modulation of treatment based on genetic risk will improve outlook for many cancer survivors.

9.3 Mitoxantrone

Mitoxantrone is a broad-spectrum anticancer drug with a similar structure to anthracyclines called an anthraquinone. It is a DNA intercalating agent and a topoisomerase II inhibitor with similar antitumor mechanisms to anthracyclines [53]. Phase I and II trials for mitoxantrone revealed incidents of cardiac failure and arrhythmias, including a 13% rate of LVEF decline and a 2.6% rate of heart failure. These reactions appeared to be dose dependent [54]. Mitoxantrone-induced cardiotoxicity, like anthracycline cardiotoxicity, can manifest as either an acute or chronic type [55].

An early randomized clinical trial comparing mitoxantrone to doxorubicin showed that although cardiac function declined on both drugs, treatment with doxorubicin caused a more accelerated drop. Risk of leaving the study due to cardiac events and risk of developing full-blown congestive heart failure were both also higher in doxorubicin-treated than mitoxantrone-treated patients [56]. A more recent trial again comparing mitoxantrone to anthracyclines in Hodgkin's disease patients had the reverse result, demonstrating a significantly increased incidence of clinically relevant cardiac events and cardiac mortality on mitoxantrone compared with doxorubicin or epirubicin [57].

9.3.1 Mechanistic Insights

Mitoxantrone causes similar ultrastructural pathology in the heart to that seen with anthracyclines: features of myofibrillar loss, sarcotubular dilation, and mitochondrial swelling [58]. These similarities suggest similar mechanisms to induce cardiac damage. Indeed, as discussed above, doxorubicin induces mitochondrial-mediated apoptosis pathways in cardiomyocytes. Similar apoptotic induction was observed with mitoxantrone [53].

Mitoxantrone has been shown to be a potent blocker of certain potassium channels, which causes a prolongation of the action potential in cardiomyocytes and may predispose to arrhythmias [58]. A comparison of cellular effects of doxorubicin vs. mitoxantrone showed that both drugs also delay calcium uptake by the sarcoplasmic reticulum (SR), but while doxorubicin also inhibits SR calcium release, mitoxantrone enhances SR calcium release [59]. Further studies need to be done to continue to clarify in what ways mitoxantrone cardiotoxicity is similar to and different from anthracycline cardiotoxicity, and to determine whether similar cardioprotective methods could be applied to mitoxantrone.

9.4 Tyrosine Kinase Inhibitors

Tyrosine kinase inhibitors (TKIs) are targeted therapies in the form of either monoclonal antibodies or small molecule inhibitors that restrict cell signaling through kinases known to be important in cancer, for example, the ErbB2 receptor in breast cancer. Conceptually, by specifically inhibiting tyrosine kinases overexpressed in tumor cells, these therapies will be more effective against cancer cells and cause less damage to normal organs [60]. While these therapies are very effective for the treatment of cancer, some of them turned out to cause cardiotoxic effects. For multitargeted kinase inhibitors especially it is important to determine which pathways are causing the cardiac effects so better TKIs can be developed without those "off-target" effects [61].

9.4.1 Trastuzumab

Trastuzumab is a monoclonal antibody against the ErbB2 receptor (also known as HER-2) approved for the treatment of ErbB2 positive breast cancer in 1998. ErbB2 is a member of the epidermal growth factor receptor family which includes EGFR and ErbB2-4. Approximately 1/3 of all breast cancers show a 10- to 100-fold increase in ErbB2 expression, and this phenotype is associated with poor prognosis [30]. Treatment with trastuzumab has significantly improved overall survival and disease-free survival rates in women with breast cancer [62]. Several studies have reported left ventricular dysfunction in up to 10% of patients and development of congestive heart failure in 1–4% of patients treated with trastuzumab alone [63–65]. Cumulative dose of the drug does not appear to be related to cardiac complications, and the effects are mostly reversible upon discontinuation of treatment [66]. No ultrastructural changes are observed in the myocardium of these patients, including no vacuolization or myocyte loss [64].

Risk factors for trastuzumab-induced cardiac dysfunction include older age, preexisting cardiovascular disease including coronary artery disease, diabetes, and valvular disease, and possibly prior radiation therapy to the left breast. Trastuzumab also causes synergistically increased toxicity when combined with anthracyclines (see anthracyclines section) or paclitaxel: up to 28% of women treated with anthracyclines and trastuzumab and 13% of women treated with paclitaxel and trastuzumab developed significant cardiac dysfunction [25, 67]. Paclitaxel, a taxane drug, causes a decrease in ERK1/2 phosphorylation, which leads to an increase in myofilament degradation; similar effects are seen with ErbB2 inhibitors. The combination of these two drugs increases diastolic calcium, shortens relaxation time, and reduces fractional shortening in heart tissue, suggesting an additive effect of cardiac dysfunction [68].

The question remains why cardiac tissue is sensitive to trastuzumab in spite of a relatively low level of ErbB2 receptor expression. ErbB2 was known to be required for formation of the heart, as knockout mice cause embryonic lethality due to defects in cardiac development. However, the role of ErbB2 signaling in the adult heart was unknown, until clinical cardiotoxicity associated with trastuzumab prompted a closer look. Conditional, cardiac-specific ErbB2 knockout mice have a dilated cardiomyopathy phenotype and exhibit excess mortality in response to pressure overload stress [69].

Trastuzumab has been shown to effectively phosphorylate ErbB2 in the human heart, and treatment over the course of weeks has been shown to induce breakdown of myocardial fibers and loss of the beating contractions [27]. Two hypotheses have been suggested. First, ErbB2 may be nonrandomly localized on the cell surface in such a way that it is easily targeted by trastuzumab. There is evidence that ErbB2 heterodimerizes with ErbB4 to signal in the heart and that both proteins localize specifically to the T-tubule. Alternatively, minor perturbations in ErbB2 signaling may be particularly devastating to cardiomyocytes. In chimeras where a subset of cells was ErbB2 negative, the entire heart was still unable to contract properly [27].

Another question is why only a small subset of patients develops cardiac dysfunction on trastuzumab if the ErbB2 pathway is so critical for cardiomyocyte function and survival. One hypothesis is that multiple "hits" are required: a heart with preexisting or concurrent stress, caused by prior heart disease or anthracycline treatment, would need to signal through ErbB2 more in order to maintain function [63]. Patients with these risk factors do show increased sensitivity to trastuzumab, supporting this theory. Another theory is that natural variability in expression of neuregulin genes NRG1 and NRG2 in the heart leaves some patients more vulnerable to trastuzumab-induced cardiac damage. One study showed that only a subset of patients absorbs the drug into the myocardium, and all of these patients developed cardiotoxicity [27, 70]. It is unknown what makes these patients more susceptible, but higher levels of ErbB2 expression or lower levels of ErbB4 expression (effectively mimicking higher levels of ErbB2) could also contribute to sensitivity.

Despite a significant incidence of CHF as a result of trastuzumab treatment, cardiotoxicity caused by trastuzumab results in substantially lower morbidity and mortality compared with CHF due to anthracyclines [71]. The reversibility of cardiac dysfunction caused by trastuzumab was suggested by a study of 38 anthracycline-treated breast cancer patients who subsequently developed cardiac dysfunction (mean pre-treatment ejection fraction 61%; mean post-trastuzumab ejection fraction 45%) [64]. After discontinuation of trastuzumab and aggressive treatment with ACE inhibitors and beta blockers (BB), cardiac function returned to near-baseline levels in nearly all of these patients. Moreover, 25 of these patients were maintained on standard heart-failure therapy and were successfully rechallenged with trastuzumab without a subsequent decline in cardiac function.

9.4.2 Lapatinib

Lapatinib is also an ErbB2 inhibitor, but is a small molecule rather than a monoclonal antibody targeting the EGF-receptor [61]. In a study of 3,700 patients, 60 (2%) experienced cardiac events. No risk factors were identified, and cumulative dose was not related to incidence of cardiotoxicity. Cardiac events, including cardiac failure and palpitations, were generally reversible [72]. An analysis of multiple trials of patients treated with lapatinib for a variety of solid tumors showed that 1.6% of patients had a decline in the left ventricular ejection fraction, while 0.2% developed symptomatic congestive heart failure.

The difference in cardiotoxicity between trastuzumab and lapatinib has not yet been explained. One possibility is that since trastuzumab is a monoclonal antibody, it may have immune-mediated effects on cardiomyocytes that are not replicated by the small molecule inhibitor lapatinib. Another explanation could be that these two drugs, despite targeting the same receptor, may trigger different intracellular signaling responses in cardiomyocytes, but not in cancer cells. A detailed molecular understanding of the differences between trastuzumab and lapatinib on cardiac function may provide key insights into the role of ErbB2 in cardiac function and may also provide insights into novel strategies for cardioprotection. A third possibility is that there is not a great inherent difference in cardiotoxicity, but that because of the findings with trastuzumab, patients were more carefully selected for lapatinib trials. For example, after the discovery of a severe increase in toxicity when trastuzumab and anthracyclines are used concurrently, patients receiving anthracycline treatment were screened more heavily for lapatinib trials [66].

9.4.3 Imatinib

Imatinib was designed to inhibit Abl kinase, but also targets PDGF-receptors, c-Kit, and other pathways. It is used in the treatment of hematological malignancies and gastrointestinal stromal tumor (GIST). More than 80% of chronic myelogenous leukemia patients achieve full remission with imatinib treatment. Initial clinical trials, which likely excluded patients at high risk for cardiovascular disease, found no evidence of cardiotoxicity caused by imatinib. In 2006, however, a study was published on ten individuals who developed severe congestive heart failure during imatinib therapy. The pathology of these patients' myocardiums revealed membrane whorls, pleomorphic mitochondria, and glycogen accumulation [73]. The same study reported that mice treated with imatinib developed cardiac dysfunction associated with activation of the ER stress response and resulting in histological findings similar to those observed in patients. The toxic effects of imatinib on cardiomyocytes were linked to inhibition of Abl kinase. Consistent with these findings, a modified form of imatinib, which has a specific reduction in activity against Abl kinase, produces substantially less cardiac toxicity in a murine model [74].

Despite these compelling findings, the incidence of clinically significant cardiomyopathy and heart failure attributable to imatinib appears to be low. A retrospective study of patients with CML treated with imatinib found that 1.7% of patients develop heart failure [75]. Risk factors included older age, prior treatment with anthracyclines or interferon, and prior history of cardiac disease or risk factors, but did not include increased dose of imatinib. Similarly, a retrospective study of gastrointestinal stromal tumor patients reported an incidence of heart failure and cardiomyopathy attributable to imatinib of less than 1% [76]. It is important to note that retrospective studies can underestimate the incidence of cardiotoxicity, particularly overlooking subclinical decreases in cardiac function. Nevertheless, based upon the existing data, the clinical significance of cardiotoxicity due to imatinib seems to be small. However, in light of preclinical findings suggesting that imatinib impairs aspects of the cardiac stress response, the long-term consequences of imatinib therapy warrant further, prospective study, particularly in patients with preexisting cardiovascular disease and when combined in anticancer regimens containing other established cardiotoxins.

9.4.4 Dasatinib and Nilotinib

Dasatinib and nilotinib are both Abl kinase inhibitors developed for use in imatinib-resistant or -intolerant patients with leukemias [77, 78]. Dasatinib also inhibits Src family kinases, c-Kit, PDGF-receptors, and ephrin-A. *In vitro* studies suggested both drugs could potentially cause prolonged QT interval. Only 1% of patients treated with dasatinib, however, developed significant QT prolongation [78], whereas 3% of nilotinib treated patients develop significant QT prolongation [79]. QT prolongation should be managed by discontinuation of the drug or dose reduction.

A clinically significant incidence of cardiomyopathy or heart failure associated with nilotinib or dasatinib has not been reported. Up to 35% of CML patients treated with dasatinib develop pleural effusions [80], with a significant number of such patients also developing pericardial effusions. However, these adverse effects do not appear to be the result of cardiac dysfunction. The etiology of such effusions appears to be multifactorial, due in part to generalized fluid retention, and possibly also attributable to immune-mediated effects [81]. Nilotinib is also associated with both pleural and pericardial effusions, albeit at a much lower frequency [77].

9.4.5 Sunitinib

Sunitinib is an extremely promiscuous multiple tyrosine kinase inhibitor. In one study, sunitinib reacted with 18% of all kinases tested, a percentage that suggests the possibility of an extremely high number of kinases inhibited in vivo [82]. Sunitinib activity against both VEGFR and PDGFR make it a highly antiangiogenic agent, which is the dominant mechanism of its antitumor effect. Sunitinib is approved for treatment of metastatic renal cell carcinoma and imatinib-resistant gastrointestinal stromal tumors. Questions about the cardiac safety of sunitinib emerged from early clinical trials of the drug. In one study of patients with GIST, 10% of patients experienced left ventricular dysfunction compared with 3% treated with placebo [83]. Similarly, in one study, patients with metastatic renal cell carcinoma treated with sunitinib developed LVD 15% of the time [84]. In a study of 75 sunitinib-treated patients with no prior history of cardiac dysfunction, 19% of patients experienced a 15% or greater decline in ejection fraction, whereas 8% of patients developed cardiac dysfunction along with advanced heart failure symptoms [85]. Forty-seven percent of these patients experienced hypertension, including 17% with grade 3 or greater hypertension. In another study of metastatic renal cell carcinoma patients, 19% had substantial declines in left ventricular function with 7% experiencing left ventricular dysfunction and advanced heart failure. All of the heart failure patients also had grade

3 hypertension [86]. In a referral-based study, six sunitinib-treated patients (3%) with no history of heart disease developed severe left ventricular dysfunction and heart failure associated with marked cardiac morbidity or mortality [87]. In each of these studies, the onset of cardiac toxicity from initiation of therapy was less than 6 months and was associated with the development of profound hypertension.

Risk factors for development of sunitinib cardiotoxicity included history of hypertension and history of coronary artery disease. Studies reporting a higher incidence of hypertension also reported a higher percentage of patients developing heart failure [86]. Cardiotoxicity does not appear to be dose-dependent, and cardiac damage appears to be incompletely reversible after discontinuation of treatment [88].

Endomyocardial biopsies from patients with sunitinib cardiotoxicity showed hypertrophy and swollen mitochondria with membrane whorls. No inflammation or fibrosis was seen [85]. In the patients examined, there were no signs of ischemia or valvular damage, but histology showed loss of cellular mass with fragmented myocardial muscle bundles [89]. Few mechanistic studies have been done, but it appears hypertension may precede or contribute to sunitinib toxicity. Inhibition of PDGF-receptor signaling has been suggested as a possible mechanism for sunitinib cardiotoxicity. PDGF-receptor signaling stimulates myocyte growth in response to hypertensive stress [87]. However, endogenous PDGF signaling has not been shown to be cardioprotective, though overexpression of PDGF has [61]. A combination of hypertension and inhibition of key tyrosine kinases may be the cause of cardiotoxicity.

9.4.6 Sorafenib

Sorafenib is also a multi-kinase inhibitor used in the treatment of renal cell and hepatocellular carcinoma, and is in trials for treatment of metastatic melanoma and non-small-cell lung cancer. Its targets include Raf-1, b-Raf, PDGF-receptor, VEGF-receptor, c-Kit, and Flt3 [90]. As Raf kinases and VEGF-receptor signaling are important in angiogenesis, sorafenib can be considered an antiangiogenic drug. A common side effect of all antiangiogenic drugs, including sorafenib, is hypertension [91]. Treatment with sorafenib reduces proliferation of vascular smooth muscle cells and increases apoptosis of these cells [90]. Its hypertensive effect is likely mediated through effects on vascular rarefaction and nitric oxide production associated with vascular endothelial dysfunction.

Sorafenib also induces acute coronary symptoms, including myocardial infarction, in 2.9% of patients [92]. Some patients developed severe cardiac effects without prior history of heart disease or hypertension [93]. It may also cause a higher incidence of less dramatic cardiac events. Reinitiation of therapy after treatment of cardiovascular complications did not cause further problems [94]. In patients with poorly controlled hypertension, pressure load on the heart increases, and the normal response is to increase angiogenesis in the heart. Inhibition of angiogenesis by sorafenib may lead to heart failure in these patients [61, 95]. Sorafenib is significantly more toxic to cells relying entirely on mitochondria for energy generation. The drug has been shown to inhibit all complexes (I–V) in the mitochondrial electron transport chain. These experiments suggest that damages to mitochondrial energy metabolism processes might be a key cardiotoxic effect of sorafenib [92].

9.4.7 Bevacizumab

Bevacizumab is a monoclonal anti-VEGF antibody approved to treat metastatic colon cancer, renal cell cancer, breast cancer, kidney cancer, and non-small-cell lung cancer. It is an angiogenesis inhibitor that also affects tumor vasculature in a way that improves delivery of other chemotherapeutic drugs and decreases pressure inside tumors. Like other angiogenesis inhibitors, it causes a significant percentage of patients to develop hypertension [96, 97]. Grade 3 or 4 hypertension is seen in 8–18% of patients, and the incidence appears to be dose-dependent. Risk of hypertension also increases with age over 75, African-American race, and specifically renal cell cancers [96].

This drug also causes an increase in severe cardiovascular complications. One study reported 2.1% of patients had myocardial infarctions, 2.5% had cerebrovascular accidents, 1.8% had hemorrhagic bleed in the gastrointestinal tract, 2.0% developed congestive heart failure, 3.0% developed angina, and 1.8% died suddenly over a 1 1/2-year period of bevacizumab treatment. Prior history of cardiovascular disease was a significant risk factor, and anthracycline treatment or radiation to the heart may also increase risk [98]. Many of these cardiovascular events were probably related to an increase in risk of arterial thromboembolism with bevacizumab treatment [5]. Age over 65 and prior history of thromboembolism are risk factors, but cumulative dose is not. Therapy with bevacizumab should be permanently discontinued in case of this type of complication.

Thromboembolic effects may be mediated by a persistent inflammatory state that results from VEGF inhibition [96]. Mice with an endothelial-specific deletion of VEGF experience progressive endothelial degeneration leading to thrombosis [95]. The complication of hypertension is most likely due to inhibition of nitrous oxide synthase, causing vasoconstriction and a decrease in sodium ion excretion. These effects both raise blood pressure. Decreased capillary density, increased vascular resistance, disrupted balance of endothelin, and vascular rarefaction may also contribute to the hypertensive phenotype. Although most adult blood vessels were previously thought not to require VEGF signaling for maintenance, many recent studies refute that claim. Capillaries with endothelial fenestrations are most dependent on VEGF signaling and regress with VEGF inhibition [99]. This finding may help identify tumors most likely to respond to this therapy. Treatment with anticoagulants, ACE inhibitors, and calcium channel blockers may help to prevent the vascular side effects of bevacizumab.

9.4.8 Conclusions

Contrary to the initial goals of targeted molecular therapeutics, it appears that tyrosine kinase inhibitors are frequently associated with a small but clinically important risk of severe cardiovascular complications. Prospective studies of cardiac function are needed for all of these drugs to determine the true incidence of hypertension, arrhythmias, cardiac ischemia, and congestive heart failure. Retrospective studies based on adverse event reports are likely to underestimate risks.

As more targeted therapies are designed, researchers and clinicians should be aware of potential cardiotoxic effects. Many kinases have a known role in the heart, and as drugs are designed against them we should be especially careful. For example, loss of Jak1, Jak2, or Stat3 in the heart increases sensitivity to cardiac damage including that caused by anthracyclines. The drug lestaurtinib inhibits Jak2, and patients should be monitored for cardiac function during clinical tests of this drug. Another example is the drug perifosine, an inhibitor of Akt kinase, which has recently been identified as important for normal cardiac growth and response to stress. Vigilant monitoring for cardiotoxicity in patients treated with this agent may also be warranted.

9.5 Monoclonal Antibody Therapies

9.5.1 Alemtuzumab

Alemtuzumab is a monoclonal antibody against CD52 and is used to treat chronic myelogenous leukemia. Initial infusion-related toxicity symptoms can include dyspnea and hypotension, but with a gradual increase of dose this reaction can be avoided [100]. Mycosis fungoides and Sezary syndrome are also sometimes treated with alemtuzumab, and one small study of this patient population reported an unacceptably high incidence of cardiac effects, including congestive heart failure, arrhythmias, deep venous thrombosis, severe hypotension, and vascular leak syndrome [101]. However, a subsequent retrospective analysis by another group identified no clinically significant cardiotoxicity in mycosis fungoides/Sezary syndrome patients treated with alemtuzumab [102]. CD52 is not expressed in cardiomyocytes or endothelial cells, so direct cardiovascular toxicity is unlikely, but rare incidences of cardiac effects may be mediated by inflammatory cytokine release leading to coronary spasm.

9.5.2 Rituximab

Rituximab is a chimeric monoclonal antibody against CD20 used to treat multiple malignant and benign hematological conditions. Rituximab can cause severe infusion reactions that include hypotension and angioedema, with very severe reactions occurring in 1% of patients [103]. Rituximab is generally well tolerated with minimal cardiovascular toxicities, such as angina, which has been reported in less than 1% of infusions.

9.5.3 Cetuximab

Cetuximab is a monoclonal anti-EGF-receptor antibody used to treat metastatic colon cancer either as a single agent or with irinotecan. It can cause a severe infusion reaction with hypotension in up to 3% of patients. This reaction can sometimes be fatal [103].

9.6 5-Fluorouracil and Capecitabine

5-Fluorouracil (5-FU) is an antimetabolite used to treat solid tumors of the breast, head, neck, and GI tract [95]. It inhibits thymidylate synthase in cancer cells and ultimately causes cell death [104], 5-FU is well known to cause myocardial ischemia and rarely myocardial infarction. The incidence of 5-FU cardiotoxicity has been reported in the range of 1.2–18%, depending on the treatment regimen and co-drugs. In a prospective analysis of patients receiving high-dose 5-fluoruracil by continuous infusion (600–1,000 mg/m2/day), 7.6% experienced cardiac events during infusion [105]. Although the symptoms were transient in most of these patients, 2.2% of patients experienced cardiac death due to arrhythmias or circulatory collapse. More recently, a series of 427 patients receiving high-dose, continuous infusion 5-fluorouracil identified symptomatic cardiac toxicity with ischemic EKG changes in 17 treated patients (4%) during drug infusion [106]. Clinical improvement was noted in most patients with termination of infusion and administration of nitrates, but one patient died of an arrhythmia. Patients with established coronary artery disease may be at higher risk of developing myocardial ischemia during infusion of 5-FU [107]. Chest pain and EKG changes suggestive of myocardial ischemia have also been described in patients treated with capecitabine, an orally administered prodrug of 5-fluorouracil [108]. The nature and extent of capecitabine-induced myocardial ischemia may be similar to that of infusional 5-fluorouracil, although larger studies are needed to evaluate the risk of myocardial ischemia and infarction attributable to these two agents.

Coronary vasospasm is an important mechanism leading to myocardial ischemia and/or infarction associated with 5-FU. *In vitro* experiments show that therapeutic levels of 5-FU cause a vasoconstriction effect in smooth muscle, possibly mediated by effects on protein kinase C and reversible by nitrate therapy [109]. Clinical research confirms that patients have a significantly decreased brachial artery diameter upon treatment with 5-FU. In addition, some reports suggest 5-FU can also cause non-ischemic cardiomyopathy and myocarditis [104], although this does not appear to occur commonly in clinical practice at usual dosage regimens.

9.7 Cyclophosphamide

Cyclophosphamide is used in combination chemotherapy for several solid tumors and lymphomas, and is used at high dosages as a conditioning regimen prior to bone marrow transplantation. Although cyclophosphamide is well tolerated at lower dosages, LV dysfunction and CHF have been reported with high-dose regimens [110]. The myocardial injury due to high-dose cyclophosphamide may be largely reversible [111], but significant morbidity and mortality have been seen in patients with cyclophosphamide-induced cardiac dysfunction [111]. Similarly, Quezado et al. [112] have also reported a significant, dose-related incidence of CHF and arrhythmias in patients given ifosfamide. As with cyclophsphamide, ifosfamide-induced cardiac dysfunction appears to be transient and reversible.

Pericarditis is another established cardiovascular toxicity associated with cyclophosphamide therapy [113]. The risk of cardiovascular toxicity due to cyclophosphamide increases with greater one-time doses of cyclophosphamide, but does not increase with cumulative dose [114]. Prior anthracycline treatment, prior irradiation to the heart, and a history of cardiovascular disease appear to increase the risk of cyclophosphamide cardiotoxicity [113–115].

9.8 Cisplatin and Cisplatin-Based Combination Therapies

Cisplatin is an alkylating chemotherapy agent that produces interstrand DNA cross-links. Early case reports suggested that vascular ischemic events could be associated with cisplatin-based therapy: myocardial infarction, cerebrovascular accident, and hypertensive events were reported in young patients with no risk factors for cardiovascular disease [116–118]. A retrospective analysis of urothelial transitional cell carcinoma patients revealed vascular events in 12.9% of patients receiving cisplatin, including deep venous thrombosis (DVT), pulmonary embolisms, arterial thromboses, cerebrovascular accidents, and angina pectoris. Risk factors for these events included history of peripheral vascular disease or coronary artery disease and a large tumor size in the pelvis [119]. While older studies report a low rate of thrombosis, more recent studies show a significantly heightened risk on cisplatin-based therapies, including a particularly dangerous risk of grade 4 or 5 thrombotic events [120]. Treatment with prophylactic anticoagulation or calcium channel blockers may allow patients to continue use of cisplatin [116, 119], which is a very effective drug for the treatment of solid tumors.

Although the exact mechanism of cisplatin-induced vascular toxicity is unknown, some indications and theories have been reported. Alterations to the clotting cascade affecting coagulability have been suggested as a possible mechanism particularly for thrombotic-type events [120]. Hypomagnesemia is reported to occur in 77–87% of patients after cisplatin-based chemotherapy, likely because cisplatin induces a tubular injury in the kidney that decreases the rate of reabsorption of magnesium. Lower Mg^{2+} concentration increases Ca^{2+} influx and results in constriction of the blood vessels. Elevation of plasma levels of von Willebrand factor (vWF) may also contribute to development of vascular disease. Cisplatin is known to stimulate endothelial cells to secrete increased levels of vWF [118]. This mechanism may be more frequently responsible for cerebrovascular accident or thrombosis, particularly in elderly patients, as these events typically occur earlier in the treatment course, while hypomagnesemia may contribute more to development of later events, which are predominantly myocardial infarctions without endovascular disease.

9.8.1 *Toxicity with Combination Therapies*

There are two commonly used cisplatin-based chemotherapy regimens for the treatment of cancers, in particular testicular seminoma and germ cell tumors: PVB (cisplatin, vinblastine, and bleomycin) and BEP (bleomycin, etoposide, cisplatin). Cisplatin-based combination chemotherapies have shown a "cure rate" for testicular cancer of over 80%. Both treatment courses have been associated with vascular toxicities, including development of Reynaud's phenomenon in 37% of patients on either regimen [121]. Risk factors for Reynaud's phenomenon include a cumulative dose of bleomycin, PVB treatment rather than BEP treatment, and hypertension [122]. Age, tumor histology, and other toxicities were not predictive factors [123].

Several other vascular events were seen more rarely: myocardial infarction [122, 124], angina pectoris [125, 126], cerebrovascular events [121], heart failure [126], major thromboembolic events (DVT, pulmonary embolisms (PE)) [127], and transient ischemia of the toes [125]. Digital ischemia occurred in 21% of patients treated without cisplatin compared with 41% treated with cisplatin [123]. Bleomycin is thought to be the most important drug in the pathogenesis of Reynaud's phenomenon, while cisplatin is the most likely cause of the other vascular toxicities.

9.9 Other Chemotherapeutic Agents

9.9.1 *Bleomycin*

Bleomycin is a glycoprotein used in the treatment of lymphomas, germ cell testicular cancer, and squamous cell cancers. In addition to peripheral vascular toxicities that have been reported with combination cisplatin/blemyocin treatment (described above), bleomycin has been associated with a 2.8% incidence of severe chest pain of unclear etiology [128]. It also has been associated with the development of acute pericarditis in a small subset of patients [128, 129]. In rare cases with young patients there have been reports of myocardial infarction or myocardial ischemia associated with bleomycin treatment [130].

9.9.2 Irinotecan

Used in the treatment of gastric and colorectal cancer, irinotecan may be associated with increased incidence of venous and arterial thromboembolic events. Eleven of 50 patients over two clinical trials developed drug-related thromboembolism when treated with irinotecan or irinotecan plus bevacizumab (no difference in incidence between the two treatment groups) [131]. These findings have not been reported subsequently by other groups.

9.9.3 Cytarabine

Cytarabine, also known as cytosine arabinoside, is a pyrimidine agonist used to treat acute myeloid leukemia [54]. Pericarditis is a rare side effect of this drug, mostly published in case reports [132, 133]. Cardiac tamponade has been reported to occur in conjunction with pericarditis in some patients [134], and capillary leak syndrome with pulmonary edema and pericardial effusion has also been reported [135]. Most published cases of pericarditis also report simultaneous pulmonary failure [135]. In all cases of pericardial disease appear to be directly related to the toxicity of cytarabine. Corticosteroid treatment may be an appropriate therapy for pericardial damage in these patients [132, 133].

9.9.4 Gemcitabine

Gemcitabine is an antimetabolic drug, related to cytarabine, used in the treatment of solid tumors (most frequently breast and GI cancers). Original phase I trials of the drug used as a daily infusion caused severe hypertension, but the currently approved treatment regimen eliminates that side effect [136]. There have been case reports of gemcitabine-caused myocardial infarction [137, 138] and atrial fibrillation [136, 139]. The time frame to development of arrhythmic complications is within 12-24 h after infusion [140]. Gemcitabine has been reported to cause ventricular tachyarrhythmias of grade 1–4 in 2.3% of patients, cardiac dysfunction (with decline in LVEF) in 1.8% of patients, and mild pericarditis in 0.2% of patients [136]. It has also been reportedly associated with cases of thromboembolism [140]. The pathophysiology of these toxicities is unknown.

9.10 Microtubule-Altering Therapies

9.10.1 Vinca Alkaloids

The vinca alkaloids are a class of microtubule-targeting drugs used to treat a wide array of solid and hematological cancers. Their mechanism of action is to disrupt microtubule assembly and arrest cells at metaphase [141]. There have been reports of hypertension, myocardial ischemia, myocardial infarction, and other vaso-occlusive disease with these compounds [54]. Vinorelbine is used to treat non-small-cell lung cancer, ovarian cancer, and breast cancer [142–144], and has been reported to cause an acute ischemic event or infarction during or very shortly after treatment [144]. A meta-analysis suggested an incidence of cardiotoxicity of 1% with vinorelbine [145]. Vinblastine, vincristine, and vindesine are three other vinca alkaloids shown to cause repolarization disorders, precordial pain, acute ischemia, or infarction [144].

Risk factors for vinca alkaloid toxicity include female gender [145], prior cardiac history [145], prior irradiation [144], and prior anthracycline therapy [144]. Several mechanisms have been proposed, including direct toxicity to myofibrils [143], coronary vasospasm [142], progressive dissolution of the sarcoplasm and formation of membranous bodies [146], an affect on coagulation leading to arterial occlusion [144], and disorganization of cellular microtubules leading to impairment of metabolism and impairment of contractility [144].

Interestingly, several reports of vincristine interactions with doxorubicin have been published, some suggesting a higher incidence of ischemic toxicity [147], and others suggesting vincristine is cardioprotective against doxorubicin effects [141, 148]. Cell culture studies show vincristine increases myocyte survival signaling [141] and decreases oxidative stress and apoptosis [148]. More studies are needed to confirm and further probe these effects.

9.10.2 Taxanes

Taxanes work by stabilizing microtubules and preventing depolymerization [149], and are used to treat breast, ovarian, and non-small-cell lung cancers [5]. As described above, pre-clinical studies have suggested that combination taxane/anthracycline therapy may enhance formation of cardiotoxic anthracycline metabolites, potentially offering an explanation of excess cardiac toxicity observed when doxorubicin and paclitaxel were co-administered in bolus-dosing regimens to patients with metastatic breast cancer [22]. Importantly, a similar enhancement of clinical cardiotoxicity has not been observed when docetaxel is co-administered with doxorubicin [150].

However, taxanes can cause cardiotoxicity as single agents as well. Paclitaxel may cause sinus bradycardia in up to 30% of patients, although this rarely results in significant symptoms, while more serious arrhythmias such as conduction blocks or ventricular tachycardia can develop in up to 5% of treated patients [146, 151]. Complete heart block [152] and myocardial infarction [153] are rare but serious complications associated with taxane treatment. However, cardiac abnormalities caused by taxanes are typically asymptomatic and transient [153]. For these reasons, routine cardiac monitoring is not necessary for patients without preexisting cardiac risk factors, but monitoring is recommended for those with preexisting heart disease [152].

9.11 Hormone Therapies

Breast cancer patients are often treated with some form of hormonal therapy in the adjuvant setting, depending upon the level of expression of hormonal receptors identified in tumor biopsy specimens. Such regimens usually consist of tamoxifen (an estrogen receptor antagonist) or aromatase inhibitors (which block the synthesis of estrogen). Several large trials have demonstrated an LDL cholesterol lowering effect of tamoxifen in breast cancer patients compared with placebo-treated or aromatase inhibitor-treated patients, suggesting a potential protective effect of tamoxifen [154]. Consistent with such an effect, women treated with tamoxifen had 50% fewer serious (grades 3–5) ischemic cardiac events compared with those treated the aromatase inhibitor letrozole [155]. However, in the same study, tamoxifen treatment was associated with a two-fold increase in thromboembolic events ($p<0.001$) compared with letrozole-treated patients. As further evidence of a pro-thrombotic effect of tamoxifen, 1.2% of women with breast cancer treated with tamoxifen developed VTE compared with 0.5% of placebo treated controls [156]. The risk of thromboembolism due to tamoxifen is highest in older women and in the first 2 years of therapy, while the addition of chemotherapies to treatment regimens does not affect risk [156].

Hormonal therapy also has an important role in the treatment of patients with metastatic prostate cancer. Diethylstilbestrol (DES), a synthetic estrogen showed promise in the treatment of metastatic prostate cancer, but at higher dosages (5 mg/day), was found to result in an excess number of cardiovascular deaths compared to placebo, defined as death from myocardial infarction, stroke, heart failure, or pulmonary embolism [157]. Importantly, at lower dosages of DES (1 mg/day), a significant anticancer benefit is observed without an increase in cardiovascular deaths [158]. When used at this dosage, VTE remains the principal toxicity of DES and appears to occur in spite of prophylactic anticoagulation regimens that include low dose warfarin and aspirin [159]. The optimal prophylactic antithrombotic regimen in patients treated with DES has not yet been established.

Another form of hormone therapy is androgen deprivation therapy for prostate cancer patients. This is achieved using several strategies, including orchiectomy, treatment with GnRH agonists, or treatment with antiandrogens. Patients treated with GnRh agonists had significantly more cases of diabetes, coronary artery disease, myocardial infarction, and sudden cardiac death than untreated patients [160, 161]. GnRh agonists increase fat mass and fasting insulin levels, and decrease insulin sensitivity [161], providing a mechanistic basis for this increased risk.

9.12 Other Miscellaneous Drugs

9.12.1 Bortezomib

Bortezomib is a reversible proteasome inhibitor, resulting in cells accumulating poly-ubiquitylated proteins and eventually triggering apoptosis. It is used to treat multiple myeloma and non-small-cell lung cancer [162]. A 2007 study revealed an unexpected increase of cardiac complications in patients with multiple myeloma or non-Hodgkin's lymphoma on bortezomib alone or in combination. Eight of 69 patients in the study developed serious cardiac effects, including heart failure and arrhythmias, requiring hospitalization or pacemaker implantation [163]. In contrast, the incidence of cardiac events in a large, phase III trial comparing bortezomib with dexamethasone for the treatment of multiple myeloma did not identify an excess of cardiac toxicity in the bortezomib-treated group and reported an incidence of heart failure of 2% in both treatment arms [164]. Since routine cardiac monitoring (e.g., echocardiography, electrocardiography, or clinical assessment by a cardiologist) was not mandated in this trial, the incidence of cardiac toxicity due to bortezomib may be underestimated. Importantly, the incidence of fatigue (a nonspecific symptom of cardiac failure) was significantly greater in the bortezomib-treated group despite a superior objective anticancer response compared with dexamethasone. Thus, the clinical significance of cardiac toxicity due to bortezomib remains unclear and will only be resolved with a prospective study with close cardiac monitoring.

Cardiac toxicity due to bortezomib and other proteosome inhibitors is mechanistically plausible. The ubiquitin-proteasome system is crucial for the proper regulation of protein degradation within cardiomyocytes, and abnormalities in the proteasomal pathways and accumulation of damaged proteins are well recognized in several forms of cardiac failure [164]. In addition, a number of pre-clinical studies have linked proteosome inhibition with impaired protein quality control in the vascular endothelium, leading to accelerated atherosclerotic lesion formation [165, 166]. While the clinical significance of these findings is being explored, patients being treated with bortezomib who have preexisting heart disease or significant atherosclerotic risk factors should be closely monitored and receive therapies designed to reduce their cardiovascular risk.

9.12.2 Thalidomide

Thalidomide, though most well known for its teratogenic effects, is currently in use for treatment of many solid organ and hematological cancers, particularly multiple myeloma. Thalidomide is an antiangiogeneic therapy that inhibits TNFα and modulates the immune system [167]. It has been linked with high incidences of deep venous thrombosis – up to 58% of patients experience an event in some drug combinations. More commonly reported incidences range from 12% to 20% [95]. Lower extremity thrombosis and pulmonary embolism are the most common manifestations, but cerebral venous sinus thrombosis, unstable angina, myocardial infarction, and stroke have also been reported [167]. Possible mechanisms of this adverse effect include inhibition of Cox2, overstimulation of immune response, and modulation of adhesion molecules [95]. Thalidomide acts directly on vascular endothelial cells, particularly those that have been previously damaged [167]. A structural analog of thalidomide, lenalidomide, is associated with similar toxicity. Both drugs are recommended to be used with prophylactic anticoagulant therapies [95].

9.12.3 Interferon-α

High-dose interferon is used to treat cutaneous melanoma and other malignancies [168]. Two studies (one of Kaposi's sarcoma patients and one of chronic myelogenous leukemia) both revealed increased rates of cardiomyopathy associated with interferon therapy [88]. The most common adverse effects reported are transient hypotension, atrial extrasystoles, and supraventricular arrhythmias, but lethal arrhythmias, myocardial infarction, and dilated cardiomyopathy have also been described [168]. Reported incidence of arrhythmias is up to 20% [54], but incidence of other cardiac effects may be underreported due to similarity of symptoms with more common interferon side effects [88].

Pathology of interferon-treated myocardium shows no myocyte necrosis or anticardiac antibodies, with ultrastructural findings of endothelial tubuloreticular structures (this is an interferon signature) [88]. Interferon may damage endothelial cells, thicken capillary walls, and induce deposition of immune complexes. An inflammatory mechanism has been proposed to play a role in interferon cardiomyopathy [88, 168]. The most effective treatment of cardiac complications is discontinuation of interferon therapy [88].

9.12.4 Arsenic Trioxide

Arsenic trioxide is an effective treatment for relapsed or refractory acute promyelocytic leukemia, but it can cause cardiotoxicity usually manifesting as QT prolongation [169]. Arsenic prolongs action potential duration in the heart, which can also lead to tachyarrhythmias or sudden death [170]. Patients can also develop torsades de pointes or vascular leak syndrome [171]. The toxicity profile in children is similar to that in adults [171], with up to 63% of patients experiencing QT prolongation [54]. Risk factors for development of conduction abnormalities include hypomagnesaemia, hypokalemia, and hypocalcaemia [171]. Prior chemotherapy-induced cardiac damage may also contribute to increased incidence of cardiotoxicity [170]. Patients treated with arsenic who develop QT prolongation should be monitored for arrhythmias, and any electrolyte imbalances in these patients should be corrected before proceeding with therapy [172].

Possible mechanisms of arsenic cardiotoxicity include alterations in DNA methylation and repair, generation of reactive oxygen species, changes in cardiac ion channels, and apoptosis [169]. Apoptosis has been observed in a cell culture model of arsenic cardiotoxicity with caspase-3 activation, intracellular calcium overload, and increased reactive oxygen species [173]. Inhibition of caspase-3, or treatment with vitamin E or verapamil (both antioxidants) alleviated the apoptotic phenotype in this model, suggesting a possible cardioprotective mechanism [173]. Resveratrol, an antioxidant with antiapoptotic and antiarrhythmic effects, was also cardioprotective: concurrent treatment prevented QT prolongation, decreased myocardial injury, inhibited production of reactive oxygen species, and reduced the number of apoptotic cells [169].

9.12.5 IL-2

Interleukin-2 is used at high doses to treat metastatic melanoma and renal cell carcinoma [174]. Hemodynamic alterations including severe hypotension and tachyarrhythmias are frequently observed adverse effects of IL-2 [175]. Treatment-related deaths occur in only 1.5% of patients, but serious complications including myocardial ischemia and myocarditis have been reported [176]. Histopathologic analysis suggests a diffuse lymphocytic and eosinophilic form of myocarditis with myocyte necrosis [177]. Capillary leak syndrome, which causes vascular permeability and hypotension, is observed in the majority of IL-2 patients, with vasopressor treatment required in 30–50% [178].

Case reports of more rare cardiotoxicities include global myocardial dysfunction [179], regional aneurysmal and dyskinetic cardiomyopathies [175], and acute myocardial infarction [176]. In addition to an inflammatory cardiomyopathy, direct myocardial toxicity may be due to myocardial stunning accompanied by excessive production of nitric oxide [175]. In an animal model, IL-2 treatment caused myocyte vaculization, myofibrillar loss, swelling of endothelial cells, migration of lymphocytes into the interstitium, and interstitial hemorrhage and edema [180]. These results suggest that IL-2 activates lymphocytes that first attack endothelial cells, then cardiac myocytes, causing lesions in both cardiac vessels and the myocardium itself [180].

9.13 Cardiotoxicity as a Discovery Platform

The value of studying cardiotoxic drugs is not limited to identifying the mechanisms of cardiotoxicity itself. Cardiotoxic effects of molecularly targeted anticancer therapies can shed light on the function of signaling pathways whose role in regulating cardiovascular function was previously unknown. Following such a discovery paradigm, researchers can discover new pathways that are important to the maintenance of adult human cardiac structure and function. Eventually this information may lead not just to better therapeutic strategies for cancer patients with cardiotoxicity, but also to therapies for diseases like cardiomyopathies and ischemic heart disease that are among the most common causes of death in our society.

For example, as described above, the monoclonal anti-ErbB2 antibody trastuzumab was found to cause cardiotoxic effects, particularly when combined with anthracyclines. This result was surprising when it first appeared in the clinical trial data because previously ErbB2 was known to be required for embryonic heart development, but expression was thought to be too low to be relevant in the adult heart [210]. Recognition of trastuzumab's cardiotoxicity led to the development of a conditional cardiac-specific knockout mouse model of ErbB2, which has a progressive dilated cardiomyopathy phenotype, and these mice also are more sensitive to anthracycline treatment than wild-type mice [181]. Pressure overload in the rat heart leads to decreased levels of ErbB2 signaling as hypertrophic responses develop into cardiomyopathy, suggesting a protective role of this signaling pathway [27].

Further work on these mice and their cells revealed an important role for ErbB2 signaling in cardiomyocyte survival and mitochondrial function [182]. More recent functional studies have concluded that impaired ErbB2-neuregulin signaling does not consistently lead to apoptosis in vivo, but suggests an interaction instead with neurohormonal regulatory systems. Neuregulin synthesis by endothelial cells appears to be regulated by epinephrine, angiotensin, endothelin, and mechanical stress [183]. Treatment with neuregulin (the ErbB ligand) prolongs survival in several animal models of cardiomyopathies [184]. Clinical trials testing the efficacy of neuregulin as a therapeutic for patients with cardiomyopathy are currently ongoing.

The initial evidence of neuregulin-ErbB2 signaling as a cardioprotective pathway emerged as a result of the surprising finding of cardiotoxicity from the anti-ErbB2 antibody in trastuzumab. The result is a better understanding of the heart itself and a new potential therapeutic target for cardiomyopathy in humans. This same paradigm can be applied to cardiotoxicity caused by other targeted therapies to build a more complete picture of cardioprotective signaling pathways and further our understanding of human heart disease.

9.14 Conclusion

Treatment of cardiovascular complications of cancer or cancer therapies first relies on identifying the underlying problem. Excluding nontreatment-related causes of cardiovascular damage suggests that cardiotoxicity of one or more agents in the patient's treatment regimen is at fault. For many of these drugs, cardiac effects are reversible upon discontinuation of treatment, so this should be the first step undertaken. After resolving or stabilizing the cardiovascular disease, rechallenge with the same drug or a change in the treatment regimen can be considered depending on the circumstances.

Treatment of cardiomyopathy caused by cardiotoxicity should begin with preventative treatments in those patients at greatest risk. In patients undergoing treatment with potentially cardiotoxic anticancer therapy, we propose that such patients can be classified as stage A patients (at risk for heart failure) per the recently established guidelines for the prevention and treatment of heart failure from the American Heart Association/American College of Cardiology [60] (see Fig. 9.1). Such guidelines recommend patients receive aggressive treatment for risk factors for cardiovascular disease including diabetes, smoking, hypertension, and hyperlipidemia [49]. Patients who develop asymptomatic cardiac dysfunction (the stage B patient) should be treated with angiotensin-converting enzyme inhibitors, angiotensin receptor blockers, or beta-blockers [185, 186]. More aggressive drug and/or device treatments are reserved for patients with symptomatic cardiac dysfunction [1].

For patients with myocardial ischemia, treatment with calcium channel blockers or nitrates can be helpful. Prophylactic vasodilators are sometimes used when rechallenging with a drug that produced ischemia, but may not always be effective [187]. It can be especially challenging to treat acute myocardial infarctions in cancer patients, since many cancer therapies cause a high rate of adverse effects like thrombocytopenia that significantly complicate or prevent use of typical therapies [142]. Aspirin therapy does provide a substantial survival benefit, even in patients with thrombocytopenia, so its use is recommended in most patients with acute myocardial infarction [188], and statin therapy is also usually safe and effective in these patients [189].

For most other cardiac effects, including arrhythmias, QT prolongation, hypertension, and thromboembolism, there are limited specific guidelines for treatment in patients with cancer [190]. Caution and monitoring in patients with higher than average risk are the best ways to detect cardiovascular complications. Treatment should be undertaken as with any other patient, but with an awareness of the patient's other disease and treatment-based toxicities in mind.

Cardiovascular diseases are a considerable worry for cancer survivors. As reviewed here, many cancer

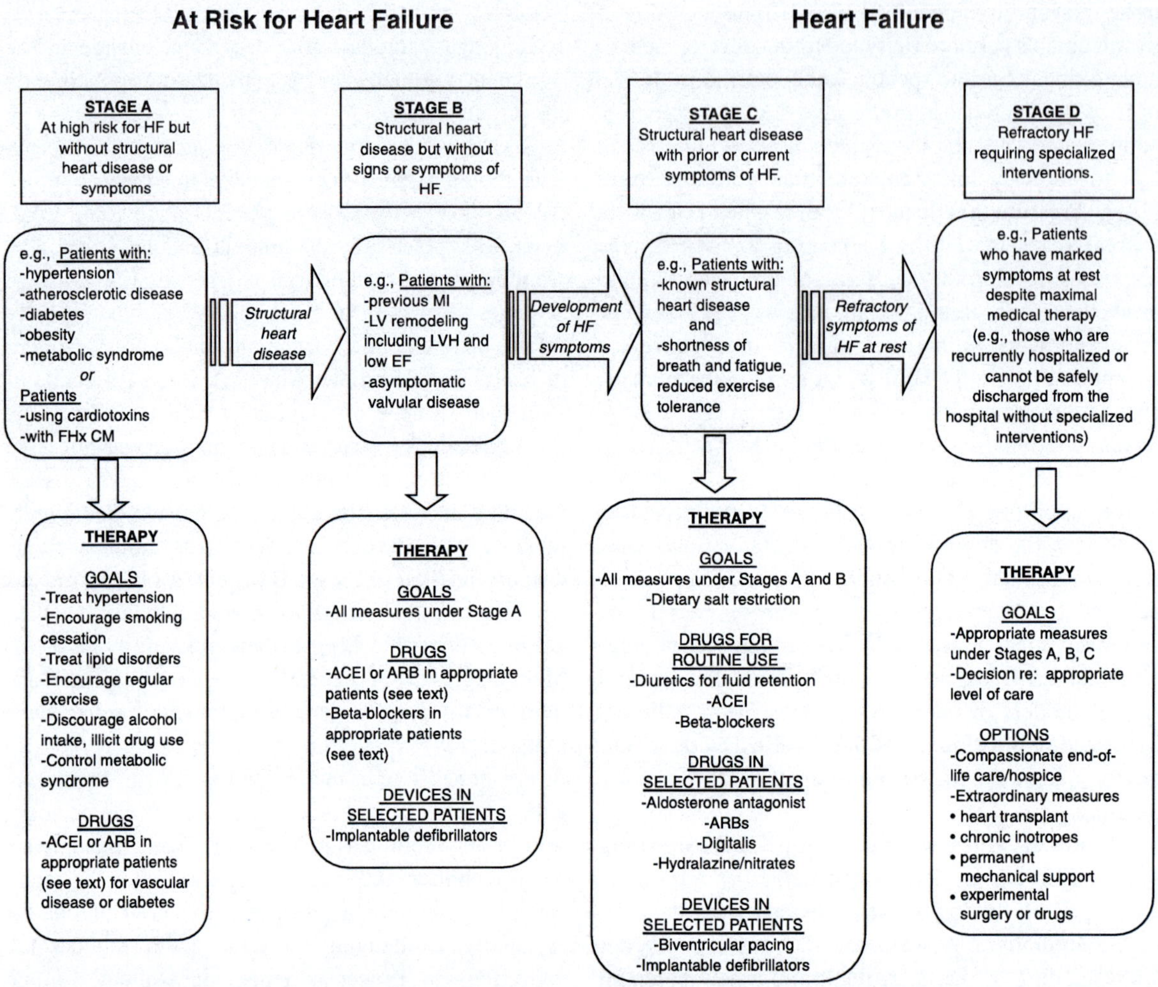

Fig. 9.1 AHA Guidelines for the Classification and Treatment of Congestive Heart Failure. Stages in the development of heart failure/recommended therapy by stage. Cancer patients treated with potentially cardiotoxic chemotherapy (reviewed within) are at risk for the development of heart failure and should be treated according to the treatment recommendations for stage A patients. Reprinted with permission from the American Heart Association. *HF* heart failure, *FHx CM* family history of cardiomyopathy, *ACEI* angiotensin-converting enzyme inhibitor, *ARB* angiotensin receptor blocker, *MI* myocardial infarction, *LVH* left ventricular hypertrophy, *EF* ejection fraction

therapies cause significant cardiotoxicity, and in some cases those effects may be underestimated due to the nature of clinical trials. Clinicians should be watchful for early signs or symptoms of cardiotoxicity in their patients. Prevention and treatment of these adverse effects is crucial, and more work needs to be done to define methods of prevention and optimize treatment in the specific population of cancer survivors. Research into the mechanisms of cardiotoxicity will help better identify prevention strategies, as well as enhancing our scientific knowledge of how these drugs work.

References

1. Simůnek T, Stérba M, Popelová O, Adamcová M, Hrdina R, Gersl V (2009) Anthracycline-induced cardiotoxicity: overview of studies examining the roles of oxidative stress and free cellular iron. Pharmacol Rep 61:154–171
2. Menna P, Minotti G, Salvatorelli E (2007) In vitro modeling of the structure-activity determinants of anthracycline cardiotoxicity. Cell Biol Toxicol 23:49–62
3. Minotti G, Menna P, Salvatorelli E, Cairo G, Gianni L (2004) Anthracyclines: molecular advances and pharmacologic developments in antitumor activity and cardiotoxicity. Pharmacol Rev 56:185–229

4. Carver JR, Shapiro CL, Ng A et al (2007) American Society of Clinical Oncology clinical evidence review on the ongoing care of adult cancer survivors: cardiac and pulmonary late effects. J Clin Oncol 25:3991–4008
5. Sereno M, Brunello A, Chiappori A et al (2008) Cardiac toxicity: old and new issues in anti-cancer drugs. Clin Transl Oncol 10:35–46
6. Jannazzo A, Hoffman J, Lutz M (2008) Monitoring of anthracycline-induced cardiotoxicity. Ann Pharmacother 42:99–104
7. Miller KD, Triano LR (2008) Medical issues in cancer survivors – a review. Cancer J 14:375–387
8. Kremer LC, van Dalen EC, Offringa M, Ottenkamp J, Voûte PA (2001) Anthracycline-induced clinical heart failure in a cohort of 607 children: long-term follow-up study. J Clin Oncol 19:191–196
9. Kremer LC, Caron HN (2004) Anthracycline cardiotoxicity in children. N Engl J Med 351:120–121
10. Wojnowski L, Kulle B, Schirmer M et al (2005) NAD(P)H oxidase and multidrug resistance protein genetic polymorphisms are associated with doxorubicin-induced cardiotoxicity. Circulation 112:3754–3762
11. Deng S, Wojnowski L (2007) Genotyping the risk of anthracycline-induced cardiotoxicity. Cardiovasc Toxicol 7: 129–134
12. Singal P, Li T, Kumar D, Danelisen I, Iliskovic N (2000) Adriamycin-induced heart failure: mechanisms and modulation. Mol Cell Biochem 207:77–86
13. Delpy E, Hatem SN, Andrieu N et al (1999) Doxorubicin induces slow ceramide accumulation and late apoptosis in cultured adult rat ventricular myocytes. Cardiovasc Res 43:398–407
14. Singal PK, Panagia V (1984) Direct effects of adriamycin on the rat heart sarcolemma. Res Commun Chem Pathol Pharmacol 43:67–77
15. Shan YX, Liu TJ, Su HF, Samsamshariat A, Mestril R, Wang PH (2003) Hsp10 and Hsp60 modulate Bcl-2 family and mitochondria apoptosis signaling induced by doxorubicin in cardiac muscle cells. J Mol Cell Cardiol 35:1135–1143
16. Green PS, Leeuwenburgh C (2002) Mitochondrial dysfunction is an early indicator of doxorubicin-induced apoptosis. Biochim Biophys Acta 1588:94–101
17. Lim CC, Zuppinger C, Guo X et al (2004) Anthracyclines induce calpain-dependent titin proteolysis and necrosis in cardiomyocytes. J Biol Chem 279:8290–8299
18. Olson RD, Mushlin PS, Brenner DE et al (1988) Doxorubicin cardiotoxicity may be caused by its metabolite, doxorubicinol. Proc Natl Acad Sci USA 85:3585–3589
19. Charlier HA Jr, Olson RD, Thornock CM et al (2005) Investigations of calsequestrin as a target for anthracyclines: comparison of functional effects of daunorubicin, daunorubicinol, and trifluoperazine. Mol Pharmacol 67:1505–1512
20. Olson RD, Li X, Palade P et al (2000) Sarcoplasmic reticulum calcium release is stimulated and inhibited by daunorubicin and daunorubicinol. Toxicol Appl Pharmacol 169: 168–176
21. Salvatorelli E, Guarnieri S, Menna P et al (2006) Defective one- or two-electron reduction of the anticancer anthracycline epirubicin in human heart. Relative importance of vesicular sequestration and impaired efficiency of electron addition. J Biol Chem 281:10990–11001
22. Giordano SH, Booser DJ, Murray JL et al (2002) A detailed evaluation of cardiac toxicity: a phase II study of doxorubicin and one- or three-hour-infusion paclitaxel in patients with metastatic breast cancer. Clin Cancer Res 8: 3360–3368
23. Valero V, Perez E, Dieras V (2001) Doxorubicin and taxane combination regimens for metastatic breast cancer: focus on cardiac effects. Semin Oncol 28:15–23
24. Ewer MS, Gibbs HR, Swafford J, Benjamin RS (1999) Cardiotoxicity in patients receiving transtuzumab (Herceptin): primary toxicity, synergistic or sequential stress, or surveillance artifact? Semin Oncol 26:96–101
25. Levine MN (2005) Trastuzumab cardiac side effects: only time will tell. J Clin Oncol 23:7775
26. Tan-Chiu E, Yothers G, Romond E et al (2005) Assessment of cardiac dysfunction in a randomized trial comparing doxorubicin and cyclophosphamide followed by paclitaxel, with or without trastuzumab as adjuvant therapy in node-positive, human epidermal growth factor receptor 2-overexpressing breast cancer: NSABP B-31. J Clin Oncol 23:7811–7819
27. Schneider JW, Chang AY, Rocco TP (2001) Cardiotoxicity in signal transduction therapeutics: erbB2 antibodies and the heart. Semin Oncol 28:18–26
28. de Korte MA, de Vries EG, Lub-de Hooge MN et al (2007) 111Indium-trastuzumab visualises myocardial human epidermal growth factor receptor 2 expression shortly after anthracycline treatment but not during heart failure: a clue to uncover the mechanisms of trastuzumab-related cardiotoxicity. Eur J Cancer 43:2046–2051
29. Menna P, Salvatorelli E, Minotti G (2007) Doxorubicin degradation in cardiomyocytes. J Pharmacol Exp Ther 322: 408–419
30. Legha SS, Benjamin RS, Mackay B et al (1982) Reduction of doxorubicin cardiotoxicity by prolonged continuous intravenous infusion. Ann Intern Med 96:133–139
31. Lipshultz SE, Giantris AL, Lipsitz SR et al (2002) Doxorubicin administration by continuous infusion is not cardioprotective: the Dana-Farber 91-01 Acute Lymphoblastic Leukemia protocol. J Clin Oncol 20: 1677–1682
32. Coukell AJ, Epirubicin FD (1997) An updated review of its pharmacodynamic and pharmacokinetic properties and therapeutic efficacy in the management of breast cancer. Drugs 53:453–482
33. Nair R, Ramakrishnan G, Nair NN et al (1998) A randomized comparison of the efficacy and toxicity of epirubicin and doxorubicin in the treatment of patients with non-Hodgkin's lymphoma. Cancer 82:2282–2288
34. van Dalen EC, Michiels EMC, Caron HN, Kremer LCM (2006) Different anthracycline derivates for reducing cardiotoxicity in cancer patients. Cochrane Database Syst Rev CD005006
35. O'Brien ME, Wigler N, Inbar M et al (2004) Reduced cardiotoxicity and comparable efficacy in a phase III trial of pegylated liposomal doxorubicin HCl (CAELYX/Doxil) versus conventional doxorubicin for first-line treatment of metastatic breast cancer. Ann Oncol 15:440–449
36. Safra T (2003) Cardiac safety of liposomal anthracyclines. Oncologist 8(Suppl 2):17–24
37. Lebrecht D, Geist A, Ketelsen U-P, Haberstroh J, Setzer B, Walker UA (2007) Dexrazoxane prevents doxorubicin-

induced long-term cardiotoxicity and protects myocardial mitochondria from genetic and functional lesions in rats. Br J Pharmacol 151:771–778
38. Hasinoff BB, Herman EH (2007) Dexrazoxane: how it works in cardiac and tumor cells. Is it a prodrug or is it a drug? Cardiovasc Toxicol 7:140–144
39. Speyer JL, Green MD, Zeleniuch-Jacquotte A et al (1992) ICRF-187 permits longer treatment with doxorubicin in women with breast cancer. J Clin Oncol 10:117–127
40. van Dalen EC, Caron HN, Dickinson HO, Kremer LC (2005) Cardioprotective interventions for cancer patients receiving anthracyclines. Cochrane Database Syst Rev. CD003917
41. Swain SM, Whaley FS, Gerber MC et al (1997) Cardioprotection with dexrazoxane for doxorubicin-containing therapy in advanced breast cancer. J Clin Oncol 15:1318–1332
42. Cheng J, Kamiya K, Kodama I (2001) Carvedilol: molecular and cellular basis for its multifaceted therapeutic potential. Cardiovasc Drug Rev 19:152–171
43. Spallarossa P, Garibaldi S, Altieri P et al (2004) Carvedilol prevents doxorubicin-induced free radical release and apoptosis in cardiomyocytes in vitro. J Mol Cell Cardiol 37: 837–846
44. Matsui H, Morishima I, Numaguchi Y, Toki Y, Okumura K, Hayakawa T (1999) Protective effects of carvedilol against doxorubicin-induced cardiomyopathy in rats. Life Sci 65:1265–1274
45. Kalay N, Basar E, Ozdogru I et al (2006) Protective effects of carvedilol against anthracycline-induced cardiomyopathy. J Am Coll Cardiol 48:2258–2262
46. Cardinale D, Colombo A, Sandri MT et al (2006) Prevention of high-dose chemotherapy-induced cardiotoxicity in high-risk patients by angiotensin-converting enzyme inhibition. Circulation 114:2474–2481
47. Vaynblat M, Shah HR, Bhaskaran D et al (2002) Simultaneous angiotensin converting enzyme inhibition moderates ventricular dysfunction caused by doxorubicin. Eur J Heart Fail 4:583–586
48. Sacco G, Bigioni M, Evangelista S, Goso C, Manzini S, Maggi CA (2001) Cardioprotective effects of zofenopril, a new angiotensin-converting enzyme inhibitor, on doxorubicin-induced cardiotoxicity in the rat. Eur J Pharmacol 414:71–78
49. Hunt SA, Abraham WT, Chin MH et al (2005) ACC/AHA 2005 Guideline Update for the Diagnosis and Management of Chronic Heart Failure in the Adult: a report of the American College of Cardiology/American Heart Association Task Force on Practice Guidelines (Writing Committee to Update the 2001 Guidelines for the Evaluation and Management of Heart Failure): developed in collaboration with the American College of Chest Physicians and the International Society for Heart and Lung Transplantation: endorsed by the Heart Rhythm Society. Circulation 112:e154–e235
50. El-Demerdash E, Ali AA, Sayed-Ahmed MM, Osman A-MM (2003) New aspects in probucol cardioprotection against doxorubicin-induced cardiotoxicity. Cancer Chemother Pharmacol 52:411–416
51. Hydock DS, Lien C-Y, Schneider CM, Hayward R (2008) Exercise preconditioning protects against doxorubicin-induced cardiac dysfunction. Med Sci Sports Exerc 40:808–817
52. Mitra MS, Donthamsetty S, White B, Mehendale HM (2008) High fat diet-fed obese rats are highly sensitive to doxorubicin-induced cardiotoxicity. Toxicol Appl Pharmacol 231:413–422
53. Kluza J, Marchetti P, Gallego M-A et al (2004) Mitochondrial proliferation during apoptosis induced by anticancer agents: effects of doxorubicin and mitoxantrone on cancer and cardiac cells. Oncogene 23:7018–7030
54. Floyd JD, Nguyen DT, Lobins RL, Bashir Q, Doll DC, Perry MC (2005) Cardiotoxicity of cancer therapy. J Clin Oncol 23:7685–7696
55. van Dalen EC, van der Pal HJH, Bakker PJM, Caron HN, Kremer LCM (2004) Cumulative incidence and risk factors of mitoxantrone-induced cardiotoxicity in children: a systematic review. Eur J Cancer 40:643–652
56. Henderson IC, Allegra JC, Woodcock T et al (1989) Randomized clinical trial comparing mitoxantrone with doxorubicin in previously treated patients with metastatic breast cancer. J Clin Oncol 7:560
57. Avilés A, Neri N, Nambo JM, Huerta-Guzman J, Talavera A, Cleto S (2005) Late cardiac toxicity secondary to treatment in Hodgkin's disease. A study comparing doxorubicin, epirubicin and mitoxantrone in combined therapy. Leuk Lymphoma 46:1023–1028
58. Wang GX, Zhou XB, Eschenhagen T, Korth M (1999) Effects of mitoxantrone on action potential and membrane currents in isolated cardiac myocytes. Br J Pharmacol 127:321–330
59. Chugun A, Uchide T, Tsurimaki C et al (2008) Mechanisms responsible for reduced cardiotoxicity of mitoxantrone compared to doxorubicin examined in isolated guinea-pig heart preparations. J Vet Med Sci 70:255–264
60. Chintalgattu V, Patel SS, Khakoo AY (2009) Cardiovascular effects of tyrosine kinase inhibitors used for gastrointestinal stromal tumors. Hematol Oncol Clin North Am 23:97–107, viii-ix
61. Force T, Krause DS, Van Etten RA (2007) Molecular mechanisms of cardiotoxicity of tyrosine kinase inhibition. Nat Rev Cancer 7:332–344
62. Hudis CA (2007) Trastuzumab–mechanism of action and use in clinical practice. N Engl J Med 357:39–51
63. Chien KR (2006) Herceptin and the heart – a molecular modifier of cardiac failure. N Engl J Med 354:789–790
64. Ewer MS, Vooletich MT, Durand J-B et al (2005) Reversibility of trastuzumab-related cardiotoxicity: new insights based on clinical course and response to medical treatment. J Clin Oncol 23:7820–7826
65. Hayes DF, Picard MH (2006) Heart of darkness: the downside of trastuzumab. J Clin Oncol 24(25):4056–4059
66. Perez EA (2008) Cardiac toxicity of ErbB2-targeted therapies: what do we know? Clin Breast Cancer 8(Suppl 3):S114–S120
67. Jerian S, Keegan P, Perez EA (1999) Cardiotoxicity associated with paclitaxel/trastuzumab combination therapy. J Clin Oncol 17:1644e
68. Pentassuglia L, Graf M, Lane H et al (2009) Inhibition of ErbB2 by receptor tyrosine kinase inhibitors causes myofibrillar structural damage without cell death in adult rat cardiomyocytes. Exp Cell Res 315:1302–1312
69. Ozcelik C, Erdmann B, Pilz B et al (2002) Conditional mutation of the ErbB2 (HER2) receptor in cardiomyocytes leads to dilated cardiomyopathy. Proc Natl Acad Sci USA 99:8880–8885

70. Schneider JW, Chang AY, Garratt A (2002) Trastuzumab cardiotoxicity: speculations regarding pathophysiology and targets for further study. Semin Oncol 29:22–28
71. Guarneri V, Lenihan DJ, Valero V et al (2006) Long-term cardiac tolerability of trastuzumab in metastatic breast cancer: the M.D. Anderson Cancer Center experience. J Clin Oncol 24:4107–4115
72. Perez EA, Koehler M, Byrne J, Preston AJ, Rappold E, Ewer MS (2008) Cardiac safety of lapatinib: pooled analysis of 3689 patients enrolled in clinical trials. Mayo Clin Proc 83:679–686
73. Kerkelä R, Grazette L, Yacobi R et al (2006) Cardiotoxicity of the cancer therapeutic agent imatinib mesylate. Nat Med 12:908–916
74. Fernandez A, Sanguino A, Peng Z et al (2007) An anticancer C-Kit kinase inhibitor is reengineered to make it more active and less cardiotoxic. J Clin Invest 117:4044–4054
75. Atallah E, Durand J-B, Kantarjian H, Cortes J (2007) Congestive heart failure is a rare event in patients receiving imatinib therapy. Blood 110:1233–1237
76. Trent JC, Patel SS, Zhang J et al (2009) Rare incidence of congestive heart failure in gastrointestinal stromal tumor and other sarcoma patients receiving imatinib mesylate. Cancer 116(184):192
77. Kantarjian HM, Giles F, Gattermann N et al (2007) Nilotinib (formerly AMN107), a highly selective BCR-ABL tyrosine kinase inhibitor, is effective in patients with Philadelphia chromosome-positive chronic myelogenous leukemia in chronic phase following imatinib resistance and intolerance. Blood 110:3540–3546
78. Wong S-F (2009) New dosing schedules of dasatinib for CML and adverse event management. J Haematol Oncol 2:10
79. Hazarika M, Jiang X, Liu Q et al (2008) Tasigna for chronic and accelerated phase Philadelphia chromosome–positive chronic myelogenous leukemia resistant to or intolerant of imatinib. Clin Cancer Res 14:5325–5331
80. Quintas-Cardama A, Kantarjian H, O'Brien S et al (2007) Pleural effusion in patients with chronic myelogenous leukemia treated with dasatinib after imatinib failure. J Clin Oncol 25:3908–3914
81. de Lavallade H, Punnialingam S, Milojkovic D et al (2008) Pleural effusions in patients with chronic myeloid leukaemia treated with dasatinib may have an immune-mediated pathogenesis. Br J Haematol 141:745–747
82. Hasinoff BB, Patel D, O'Hara KA (2008) Mechanisms of myocyte cytotoxicity induced by the multiple receptor tyrosine kinase inhibitor sunitinib. Mol Pharmacol 74:1722–1728
83. Rock EP, Goodman V, Jiang JX et al (2007) Food and Drug Administration drug approval summary: sunitinib malate for the treatment of gastrointestinal stromal tumor and advanced renal cell carcinoma. Oncologist 12:107–113
84. Abrams TJ, Murray LJ, Pesenti E et al (2003) Preclinical evaluation of the tyrosine kinase inhibitor SU11248 as a single agent and in combination with "standard of care" therapeutic agents for the treatment of breast cancer. Mol Cancer Ther 2:1011–1021
85. Chu TF, Rupnick MA, Kerkela R et al (2007) Cardiotoxicity associated with tyrosine kinase inhibitor sunitinib. Lancet 370:2011–2019
86. Di Lorenzo G, Autorino R, Bruni G, et al (2009) Cardiovascular toxicity following sunitinib therapy in metastatic renal cell carcinoma: a multicenter analysis. Ann Oncol. doi:10.1093/annonc/mdp025
87. Khakoo AY, Kassiotis CM, Tannir N et al (2008) Heart failure associated with sunitinib malate: a multitargeted receptor tyrosine kinase inhibitor. Cancer 112:2500–2508
88. Khakoo AY, Halushka MK, Rame JE, Rodriguez ER, Kasper EK, Judge DP (2005) Reversible cardiomyopathy caused by administration of interferon alpha. Nat Clin Pract Cardiovasc Med 2:53–57
89. Machiels JP, Bletard N, Pirenne P, Jacquet L, Bonbled F, Duck L (2008) Acute cardiac failure after sunitinib. Ann Oncol. doi:10.1093/annonc/mdn019
90. Klein M, Schermuly RT, Ellinghaus P et al (2008) Combined tyrosine and serine/threonine kinase inhibition by sorafenib prevents progression of experimental pulmonary hypertension and myocardial remodeling. Circulation 118: 2081–2090
91. Veronese ML, Mosenkis A, Flaherty KT et al (2006) Mechanisms of hypertension associated with BAY 43-9006. J Clin Oncol 24:1363–1369
92. Will Y, Dykens JA, Nadanaciva S et al (2008) Effect of the multitargeted tyrosine kinase inhibitors imatinib, dasatinib, sunitinib, and sorafenib on mitochondrial function in isolated rat heart mitochondria and H9c2 cells. Toxicol Sci 106:153–161
93. Mego M, Reckova M, Obertova J, Sycova-Mila Z, Brozmanova K, Mardiak J (2007) Increased cardiotoxicity of sorafenib in sunitinib-pretreated patients with metastatic renal cell carcinoma. Ann Oncol 18:1906
94. Schmidinger M, Zielinski CC, Vogl UM et al (2008) Cardiac toxicity of sunitinib and sorafenib in patients with metastatic renal cell carcinoma. J Clin Oncol 26:5204–5212
95. Daher IN, Yeh ETH (2008) Vascular complications of selected cancer therapies. Nat Clin Pract Cardiovasc Med 5:797–805
96. Gressett SM, Shah SR (2009) Intricacies of bevacizumab-induced toxicities and their management. Ann Pharmacother 43:490–501
97. Roth DB, King A, Weiss M, Klein D (2009) Systemic adverse events after bevacizumab. Ophthalmology 116:1226, e1
98. Hospitalaria F, Hosp F (2007) Insuficiencia cardiaca grave por bevacizumab en paciente tratado con antraciclinas. Farm Hosp 31:251–259
99. Kamba T, McDonald DM (2007) Mechanisms of adverse effects of anti-VEGF therapy for cancer. Br J Cancer 96:1788–1795
100. Alinari L, Lapalombella R, Andritsos L, Baiocchi RA, Lin TS, Byrd JC (2007) Alemtuzumab (Campath-1H) in the treatment of chronic lymphocytic leukemia. Oncogene 26:3644–3653
101. Lenihan DJ, Alencar AJ, Yang D, Kurzrock R, Keating MJ, Duvic M (2004) Cardiac toxicity of alemtuzumab in patients with mycosis fungoides/Sézary syndrome. Blood 104:655–658
102. Lundin J, Kennedy B, Dearden C, Dyer MJS, Osterborg A (2005) No cardiac toxicity associated with alemtuzumab therapy for mycosis fungoides/Sézary syndrome. Blood 105:4148–4149
103. Yeh ETH (2006) Cardiotoxicity induced by chemotherapy and antibody therapy. Annu Rev Med 57:485–498

104. Dalzell JR, Samuel LM (2009) The spectrum of 5-fluorouracil cardiotoxicity. Anticancer Drugs 20:79
105. de Forni M, Malet-Martino MC, Jaillais P et al (1992) Cardiotoxicity of high-dose continuous infusion fluorouracil: a prospective clinical study. J Clin Oncol 10:1795–1801
106. Tsavaris N, Kosmas C, Vadiaka M et al (2002) Cardiotoxicity following different doses and schedules of 5-fluorouracil administration for malignancy – a survey of 427 patients. Med Sci Monit 8:PI51–PI57
107. Labianca R, Beretta G, Clerici M, Fraschini P, Luporini G. Cardiac toxicity of 5-fluorouracil: a study on 1083 patients (1982) Tumori 68:505–510
108. Kosmas C, Kallistratos MS, Kopterides P et al (2007) Cardiotoxicity of fluoropyrimidines in different schedules of administration: a prospective study. J Cancer Res Clin Oncol 134(1):75–82
109. Mosseri M, Fingert HJ, Varticovski L, Chokshi S, Isner JM (1993) In vitro evidence that myocardial ischemia resulting from 5-fluorouracil chemotherapy is due to protein kinase C-mediated vasoconstriction of vascular smooth muscle. Cancer Res 53:3028–3033
110. Zver S, Zadnik V, Bunc M, Rogel P, Cernelc P, Kozelj M (2007) Cardiac toxicity of high-dose cyclophosphamide in patients with multiple myeloma undergoing autologous hematopoietic stem cell transplantation. Int J Hematol 85:408–414
111. Gottdiener JS, Appelbaum FR, Ferrans VJ, Deisseroth A, Ziegler J (1981) Cardiotoxicity associated with high-dose cyclophosphamide therapy. Arch Intern Med 141:758–763
112. Quezado ZM, Wilson WH, Cunnion RE et al (1993) High-dose ifosfamide is associated with severe, reversible cardiac dysfunction. Ann Intern Med 118:31–36
113. Tiersten A, Wo J, Jacobson C et al (2004) Cardiac toxicity observed in association with high-dose cyclophosphamide-based chemotherapy for metastatic breast cancer. Breast 13:341–346
114. Taniguchi I (2005) Clinical significance of cyclophosphamide-induced cardiotoxicity. Internal Med 44:89–90 (Tokyo 1992)
115. Kamezaki K, Fukuda T, Makino S, Harada M (2005) Cyclophosphamide-induced cardiomyopathy in a patient with seminoma and a history of mediastinal irradiation. Intern Med 44:120–123
116. Berliner S, Rahima M, Sidi Y et al (1990) Acute coronary events following cisplatin-based chemotherapy. Cancer Invest 8:583–586
117. Doll DC, List AF, Greco FA, Hainsworth JD, Hande KR, Johnson DH (1986) Acute vascular ischemic events after cisplatin-based combination chemotherapy for germ-cell tumors of the testis. Ann Intern Med 105:48–51
118. Içli F, Karao uz H, Dinçol D et al (1993) Severe vascular toxicity associated with cisplatin-based chemotherapy. Cancer 72:587–593
119. Czaykowski PM, Moore MJ, Tannock IF (1998) High risk of vascular events in patients with urothelial transitional cell carcinoma treated with cisplatin based chemotherapy. J Urol 160:2021–2024
120. Anders JC, Grigsby PW, Singh AK (2006) Cisplatin chemotherapy (without erythropoietin) and risk of life-threatening thromboembolic events in carcinoma of the uterine cervix: the tip of the iceberg? A review of the literature. Radiat Oncol 1:14
121. Chaudhary UB, Haldas JR (2003) Long-term complications of chemotherapy for germ cell tumours. Drugs 63:1565–1577
122. Berger CC, Bokemeyer C, Schneider M, Kuczyk MA, Schmoll HJ (1995) Secondary Raynaud's phenomenon and other late vascular complications following chemotherapy for testicular cancer. Eur J Cancer 31A:2229–2238
123. Vogelzang NJ, Bosl GJ, Johnson K, Kennedy BJ (1981) Raynaud's phenomenon: a common toxicity after combination chemotherapy for testicular cancer. Ann Intern Med 95:288–292
124. Bachmeyer C, Joly H, Jorest R (2000) Early myocardial infarction during chemotherapy for testicular cancer. Tumori 86:428–430
125. Stefenelli T, Kuzmits R, Ulrich W, Glogar D (1988) Acute vascular toxicity after combination chemotherapy with cisplatin, vinblastine, and bleomycin for testicular cancer. Eur Heart J 9:552–556
126. van den Belt-Dusebout AW, Nuver J, de Wit R et al (2006) Long-term risk of cardiovascular disease in 5-year survivors of testicular cancer. J Clin Oncol 24:467–475
127. Weijl NI, Rutten MFJ, Zwinderman AH et al (2000) Thromboembolic events during chemotherapy for germ cell cancer: a cohort study and review of the literature. J Clin Oncol 18:2169
128. White DA, Schwartzberg LS, Kris MG, Bosl GJ (1987) Acute chest pain syndrome during bleomycin infusions. Cancer 59:1582–1585
129. Ben Yosef R, Gez E, Catane R (1990) Acute pericarditis following bleomycin: a case report and literature analysis. J Chemother 2:70–71
130. Schwarzer S, Eber B, Greinix H, Lind P (1991) Non-Q-wave myocardial infarction associated with bleomycin and etoposide chemotherapy. Eur Heart J 12:748–750
131. Shah MA, Ilson D, Kelsen DP (2005) Thromboembolic events in gastric cancer: high incidence in patients receiving irinotecan- and bevacizumab-based therapy. J Clin Oncol 23:2574–2576
132. Gähler A, Hitz F, Hess U, Cerny T (2003) Acute pericarditis and pleural effusion complicating cytarabine chemotherapy. Onkologie 26:348–350
133. Hermans C, Straetmans N, Michaux JL, Ferrant A (1997) Pericarditis induced by high-dose cytosine arabinoside chemotherapy. Ann Hematol 75:55–57
134. Vaickus L, Letendre L (1984) Pericarditis induced by high-dose cytarabine therapy. Arch Intern Med 144:1868–1869
135. Reykdal S, Sham R, Kouides P (1995) Cytarabine-induced pericarditis: a case report and review of the literature of the cardio-pulmonary complications of cytarabine therapy. Leuk Res 19:141–144
136. Santini D, Tonini G, Abbate A et al (2000) Gemcitabine-induced atrial fibrillation: a hitherto unreported manifestation of drug toxicity. Ann Oncol 11:479–481
137. Bdair FM, Graham SP, Smith PF, Javle MM (2006) Gemcitabine and acute myocardial infarction – a case report. Angiology 57:367–371

138. Kalapura T, Krishnamurthy M, Reddy CV (1999) Acute myocardial infarction following gemcitabine therapy – a case report. Angiology 50:1021–1025
139. Tavil Y, Arslan U, Okyay K, Sen N, Boyaci B (2007) Atrial fibrillation induced by gemcitabine treatment in a 65-year-old man. Onkologie 30:253–255
140. Ferrari D, Carbone C, Codecà C et al (2006) Gemcitabine and atrial fibrillation: a rare manifestation of chemotherapy toxicity. Anticancer Drugs 17:359–361
141. Chatterjee K, Zhang J, Honbo N, Simonis U, Shaw R, Karliner JS (2007) Acute vincristine pretreatment protects adult mouse cardiac myocytes from oxidative stress. J Mol Cell Cardiol 43:327–336
142. Khakoo AY, Yeh ETH (2008) Therapy insight: management of cardiovascular disease in patients with cancer and cardiac complications of cancer therapy. Nat Clin Pract Oncol 5:655–667
143. Bergeron A, Raffy O, Vannetzel JM (1995) Myocardial ischemia and infarction associated with vinorelbine. J Clin Oncol 13:531–532
144. Karminsky N, Merimsky O, Kovner F, Inbar M (1999) Vinorelbine-related acute cardiopulmonary toxicity. Cancer Chemother Pharmacol 43:180–182
145. Lapeyre-Mestre M, Gregoire N, Bugat R, Montastruc JL (2004) Vinorelbine-related cardiac events: a meta-analysis of randomized clinical trials. Fundam Clin Pharmacol 18:97–105
146. Rowinsky EK, McGuire WP, Guarnieri T, Fisherman JS, Christian MC, Donehower RC (1991) Cardiac disturbances during the administration of taxol. J Clin Oncol 9:1704–1712
147. Calvo-Romero JM, Fernández-Soria-Pantoja R, Arrebola-Garcia JD, Gil-Cubero M (2001) Ischemic heart disease associated with vincristine and doxorubicin chemotherapy. Ann Pharmacother 35:1403–1405
148. Chatterjee K, Zhang J, Tao R, Honbo N, Karliner JS (2008) Vincristine attenuates doxorubicin cardiotoxicity. Biochem Biophys Res Commun 373:555–560
149. Shimoyama M, Murata Y, Sumi K-I, Hamazoe R, Komuro I (2001) Docetaxel induced cardiotoxicity. Heart 86:219
150. Nabholtz JM, North S, Smylie M et al (2000) Docetaxel (Taxotere) in combination with anthracyclines in the treatment of breast cancer. Semin Oncol 27:11–18
151. Bird BRJH, Swain SM (2008) Cardiac toxicity in breast cancer survivors: review of potential cardiac problems. Clin Cancer Res 14:14–24
152. Arbuck SG, Strauss H, Rowinsky E et al (1993) A reassessment of cardiac toxicity associated with taxol. J Natl Cancer Inst Monogr 15:117–130
153. Hekmat E (1996) Fatal myocardial infarction potentially induced by paclitaxel. Ann Pharmacother 30:1110–1112
154. Ewer MS, Glück S (2009) A woman's heart: the impact of adjuvant endocrine therapy on cardiovascular health. Cancer 115:1813–1826
155. Coates AS, Keshaviah A, Thurlimann B et al (2007) Five years of letrozole compared with tamoxifen as initial adjuvant therapy for postmenopausal women with endocrine-responsive early breast cancer: update of study BIG 1-98. J Clin Oncol 25:486–492
156. Hernandez RK, Sørensen HT, Pedersen L, Jacobsen J, Lash TL (2009) Tamoxifen treatment and risk of deep venous thrombosis and pulmonary embolism: a Danish population-based cohort study. Cancer 19:4442–4449
157. Byar DP (1973) Proceedings: The Veterans Administration Cooperative Urological Research Group's studies of cancer of the prostate. Cancer 32:1126–1130
158. Brawer MK (2006) Hormonal therapy for prostate cancer. Rev Urol 8(Suppl 2):S35–S47
159. Montgomery RB, Nelson PS, Lin D, Ryan CW, Garzotto M, Beer TM (2007) Diethylstilbestrol and docetaxel: a Phase II study of tubulin active agents in patients with metastatic, androgen-independent prostate cancer. Cancer 110:996–1002
160. Keating NL, O'Malley AJ, Smith MR (2006) Diabetes and cardiovascular disease during androgen deprivation therapy for prostate cancer. J Clin Oncol 24:4448–4456
161. Saylor PJ, Keating NL, Smith MR (2009) Prostate cancer survivorship: prevention and treatment of the adverse effects of androgen deprivation therapy. J Gen Intern Med 24(Suppl 2):S389–S394
162. Voortman J, Giaccone G (2006) Severe reversible cardiac failure after bortezomib treatment combined with chemotherapy in a non-small cell lung cancer patient: a case report. BMC Cancer 6:129
163. Enrico O, Gabriele B, Nadia C et al (2007) Unexpected cardiotoxicity in haematological bortezomib treated patients. Br J Haematol 138:396–397
164. Richardson PG, Sonneveld P, Schuster MW et al (2005) Bortezomib or high-dose dexamethasone for relapsed multiple myeloma. N Engl J Med 352:2487–2498
165. Herrmann J, Lerman LO, Lerman A (2010) On to the road to degradation: atherosclerosis and the proteasome. Cardiovasc Res 85:291–302
166. Herrmann J, Saguner AM, Versari D et al (2007) Chronic proteasome inhibition contributes to coronary atherosclerosis. Circ Res 101:865–874
167. Rajkumar SV (2005) Thalidomide therapy and deep venous thrombosis in multiple myeloma. Mayo Clin Proc 80:1549–1551
168. Benjamini O, Kimhi O, Lishner M (2007) Severe pleuropericarditis and cardiomyopathy induced by high dose interferon alpha-2b. Isr Med Assoc J 9:486–487
169. Zhao X-Y, Li G-Y, Liu Y et al (2008) Resveratrol protects against arsenic trioxide-induced cardiotoxicity in vitro and in vivo. Br J Pharmacol 154:105–113
170. Vizzardi E, Zanini G, Antonioli E, D'Aloia A, Raddino R, Cas LD (2008) QT prolongation: a case of arsenical pericardial and pleural effusion. Cardiovasc Toxicol 8:41–44
171. Fox E, Razzouk BI, Widemann BC et al (2008) Phase 1 trial and pharmacokinetic study of arsenic trioxide in children and adolescents with refractory or relapsed acute leukemia, including acute promyelocytic leukemia or lymphoma. Blood 111:566–573
172. Ohnishi K, Yoshida H, Shigeno K et al (2000) Prolongation of the QT interval and ventricular tachycardia in patients treated with arsenic trioxide for acute promyelocytic leukemia. Ann Intern Med 133:881–885
173. Zhao X, Feng T, Chen H et al (2008) Arsenic trioxide-induced apoptosis in H9c2 cardiomyocytes: implications in

cardiotoxicity. Basic Clin Pharmacol Toxicol 102: 419–425
174. Eisner RM, Husain A, Clark JI (2004) Case report and brief review: IL-2-induced myocarditis. Cancer Invest 22:401–404
175. Du Bois JS, Udelson JE, Atkins MB (1995) Severe reversible global and regional ventricular dysfunction associated with high-dose interleukin-2 immunotherapy. J Immunother Emphasis Tumor Immunol 18:119–123
176. Kragel AH, Travis WD, Steis RG, Rosenberg SA, Roberts WC (1990) Myocarditis or acute myocardial infarction associated with interleukin-2 therapy for cancer. Cancer 66:1513–1516
177. Samlowski WE, Ward JH, Craven CM, Freedman RA (1989) Severe myocarditis following high-dose interleukin-2 administration. Arch Pathol Lab Med 113:838–841
178. Acquavella N, Kluger H, Rhee J et al (2008) Toxicity and activity of a twice daily high-dose bolus interleukin 2 regimen in patients with metastatic melanoma and metastatic renal cell cancer. J Immunother 31:569–576
179. Goel M, Flaherty L, Lavine S, Redman BG (1992) Reversible cardiomyopathy after high-dose interleukin-2 therapy (1991). J Immunother 11:225–229
180. Zhang J, Yu ZX, Hilbert SL et al (1993) Cardiotoxicity of human recombinant interleukin-2 in rats. A morphological study. Circulation 87:1340–1353
181. Crone SA, Zhao Y-Y, Fan L et al (2002) ErbB2 is essential in the prevention of dilated cardiomyopathy. Nat Med 8:459–465
182. Grazette LP, Boecker W, Matsui T et al (2004) Inhibition of ErbB2 causes mitochondrial dysfunction in cardiomyocytes: implications for herceptin-induced cardiomyopathy. J Am Coll Cardiol 44:2231–2238
183. Lemmens K, Doggen K, De Keulenaer GW (2007) Role of neuregulin-1/ErbB signaling in cardiovascular physiology and disease: implications for therapy of heart failure. Circulation 116:954–960
184. Doggen K, Ray L, Mathieu M, Mc Entee K, Lemmens K, De Keulenaer GW (2009) Ventricular ErbB2/ErbB4 activation and downstream signaling in pacing-induced heart failure. J Mol Cell Cardiol 46:33–38
185. Demetri GD, von Mehren M, Blanke CD et al (2002) Efficacy and safety of imatinib mesylate in advanced gastrointestinal stromal tumors. N Engl J Med 347:472–480
186. Felker GM, Thompson RE, Hare JM et al (2000) Underlying causes and long-term survival in patients with initially unexplained cardiomyopathy. N Engl J Med 342: 1077–1084
187. Patel B, Kloner RA, Ensley J, Al-Sarraf M, Kish J, Wynne J (1987) 5-Fluorouracil cardiotoxicity: left ventricular dysfunction and effect of coronary vasodilators. Am J Med Sci 294:238–243
188. Sarkiss MG, Yusuf SW, Warneke CL et al (2007) Impact of aspirin therapy in cancer patients with thrombocytopenia and acute coronary syndromes. Cancer 109:621–627
189. Cannon CP, Braunwald E, McCabe CH et al (2004) Pravastatin or Atorvastatin Evaluation and Infection Therapy-Thrombolysis in Myocardial Infarction 22 Investigators. Intensive versus moderate lipid lowering with statins after acute coronary syndromes. N Engl J Med 350:1495–1504
190. Yeh ETH, Bickford CL (2009) Cardiovascular complications of cancer therapy: incidence, pathogenesis, diagnosis, and management. J Am Coll Cardiol 53:2231–2247
191. Perik PJ, Rikhof B, de Jong FA, Verweij J, Gietema JA, van der Graaf WTA (2008) Results of plasma N-terminal pro B-type natriuretic peptide and cardiac troponin monitoring in GIST patients do not support the existence of imatinib-induced cardiotoxicity. Ann Oncol 19:359–361
192. Turrisi G, Montagnani F, Grotti S, Marinozzi C, Bolognese L, Fiorentini G (2009) Congestive heart failure during imatinib mesylate treatment. Int J Cardiol
193. Todorova V, Vanderpool D, Blossom S et al (2009) Oral glutamine protects against cyclophosphamide-induced cardiotoxicity in experimental rats through increase of cardiac glutathione. Nutrition 25:812–817
194. Yeh ETH, Tong AT, Lenihan DJ et al (2004) Cardiovascular complications of cancer therapy: diagnosis, pathogenesis, and management. Circulation 109:3122–3131
195. Hacihanefioglu A, Tarkun P, Gonullu E (2008) Acute severe cardiac failure in a myeloma patient due to proteasome inhibitor bortezomib. Int J Hematol 88:219–222
196. Ferrajoli A, O'Brien SM, Cortes JE et al (2003) Phase II study of alemtuzumab in chronic lymphoproliferative disorders. Cancer 98:773–778
197. Fisher B, Costantino JP, Wickerham DL et al (1998) Tamoxifen for prevention of breast cancer: report of the National Surgical Adjuvant Breast and Bowel Project P-1 study. J Natl Cancer Inst 90:1371–1388
198. Chu TF, Rupnick MA, Kerkela R et al (2007) Cardiotoxicity associated with the tyrosine kinase inhibitor sunitinib. Lancet 370:2011–2019
199. Khoury HJ, Guilhot F, Hughes TP, Kim D-W, Cortes JE (2009) Dasatinib treatment for Philadelphia chromosome-positive leukemias: practical considerations. Cancer 115:1381–1394
200. Yamaguchi K, Kanazawa S, Kinoshita Y, Muramatsu M, Nomura S (2005) Acute myocardial infarction with lung cancer during treatment with gefitinib: the possibility of gefitinib-induced thrombosis. Pathophysiol Haemost Thromb 34:48–50
201. Law H (1996) Chemotherapy-induced myocardial infarction. Eur Heart J 17(6):966
202. Smith I (2005) A comparison of letrozole and tamoxifen in postmenopausal women with early breast cancer. New Engl J Med 353:2747–2757
203. Coombes RC, Hall E, Gibson LJ et al (2004) A randomized trial of exemestane after 2 to 3 years of tamoxifen therapy in postmenopausal women with primary breast cancer. N Engl J Med 350:1081–1092
204. Arai Y, Tadokoro J, Mitani K (2005) Ventricular tachycardia associated with infusion of rituximab in mantle cell lymphoma. Am J Hematol 78(4):317–318
205. Perez-Verdia A, Angulo F, Hardwicke FL, Nugent KM (2005) Acute cardiac toxicity associated with high-dose intravenous methotrexate therapy: case report and review of the literature. Pharmacotherapy 25:1271–1276
206. Judson I, Radford JA, Harris M et al (2001) Randomised phase II trial of pegylated liposomal doxorubicin (DOXIL/CAELYX) versus doxorubicin in the treatment of advanced or metastatic soft tissue sarcoma: a study by the EORTC

Soft Tissue and Bone Sarcoma Group. Eur J Cancer 37:870–877

207. Lyass O, Uziely B, Ben-Yosef R et al (2000) Correlation of toxicity with pharmacokinetics of pegylated liposomal doxorubicin (Doxil) in metastatic breast carcinoma. Cancer 89:1037–1047
208. van Dalen EC, van der Pal HJH, Caron HN, Kremer LC (2009) Different dosage schedules for reducing cardiotoxicity in cancer patients receiving anthracycline chemotherapy. Cochrane Database Syst Rev 4:CD005008
209. de Nigris F, Rienzo M, Schiano C, Fiorito C, Casamassimi A, Napoli C (2008) Prominent cardioprotective effects of third generation beta blocker nebivolol against anthracycline-induced cardiotoxicity using the model of isolated perfused rat heart. Eur J Cancer 44:334–340
210. de Azambuja E, Bedard PL, Suter T, Piccart-Gebhart M (2009) Cardiac toxicity with anti-HER-2 therapies-what have we learned so far? Target Oncol 4:77–88

Prophylaxis: Peace of Mind?

10

Benoit Guery and Karine Faure

Contents

In 2005, Bucaneve et al. reported the results of a randomized placebo-controlled double-blind trial showing that prophylactic levofloxacin given to cancer patients with chemotherapy-induced neutropenia significantly decreased the rate of febrile episodes [1]. However, mortality was not affected, and the long-term ecological impact of levofloxacin prophylaxis was not assessed [1]. Over the following years, many studies assessed the impact of antibiotic selection pressure on microbial ecology. In a prospective study done in a hematology unit, routine levofloxacin prophylaxis was associated with increases in the rates of enterococci, *Streptococcus viridans*, and *Pseudomonas aeruginosa* [2]. Another study also found an increase in *S. viridans* with levofloxacin prophylaxis [3]. These changes in bacterial ecology did not affect mortality rates. In several studies, the implementation of routine levofloxacin prophylaxis was followed by increases in the incidence of fluoroquinolone-resistant gram-negative bacterial strains [4, 5]. Interestingly, these changes had no impact on the incidence of gram-negative infections in the treated population. Other studies found no impact on bacterial ecology. In patients with febrile neutropenia compared to a retrospective cohort in the USA, levofloxacin prophylaxis decreased the rate of gram-negative bacteremia without affecting the rate of gram-positive bacteremia [6]. Neither mortality nor rates of resistance to antibiotics were significantly affected [6].

Studies of emerging resistant strains and antibiotic cycling have supplied useful information. In a prospective cohort of 388 patients in a surgical intensive care unit (ICU), cycling from cefpirome to piperacillin-tazobactam to finally levofloxacin, each molecule used for 4 months, failed to control the emergence of resistant gram-negative strains [7]. In 13 ICUs, selective gastrointestinal tract decontamination, including

B. Guery (✉) and K. Faure
Service de Gestion du Risque Infectieux et des Vigilances, CHRU Lille, Hôpital Calmette, Pavillon Christiaens, Lille Cedex 59037, France
e-mail: bguery@invivo.edu

É. Azoulay (ed.), *Pulmonary Involvement in Patients with Hematological Malignancies*,
DOI: 10.1007/978-3-642-15742-4_10, © Springer-Verlag Berlin Heidelberg 2011

cefotaxime, 4 g/day intravenously for 4 consecutive days, was associated with a significant increase in resistant strains recovered from the respiratory tract [8]. Adding metronidazole to ciprofloxacin-fluconazole for selective gastrointestinal decontamination in patients undergoing allogeneic bone marrow transplantation increased the rate of fungal gastrointestinal colonization but not the rate of invasive fungal infections [9]. We will not discuss the efficacy of selective gastrointestinal decontamination, which remains highly controversial in some patient populations. The reader is referred to the abundant literature on the topic.

Prophylactic antibiotic therapy affects bacterial ecology not only at the level of patient populations, but also at the level of hospital departments. Similar changes have been found in response to prophylactic antifungal treatment. Pooled data from two large studies of prophylactic posaconazole, itraconazole, or fluconazole in allogeneic BMT recipients or patients with acute myelogenous leukemia showed that the number of cultures positive for *Candida albicans* decreased with all three drugs [10]. In contrast, *C. glabrata*-positive cultures increased significantly with posaconazole and itraconazole therapy, and *C. krusei*-positive cultures increased significantly with fluconazole therapy. However, the rate of invasive fungal infection during prophylactic antifungal therapy was extremely low (about 1%). Other studies also found evidence of *C. glabrata* emergence during fluconazole therapy [11]. On the opposite, a study performed in Sweden to assess curative-dose fluconazole in patients with acute leukemia found a significant decrease in invasive fungal infections with no emergence of non-albicans *Candida* strains but with an increase in gram-positive bacterial infections [12]. No relation was found between fluconazole use over an 11-year period (1994–2004) and the ratio of albicans/non-albicans *Candida* strains in a university hospital, despite a high level of fluconazole consumption (defined daily doses, 5,013–6,807/100,000 patient-days [13]).

Conflicting data have also been obtained in ICUs. Over a 2-year period, fluconazole prophylaxis was associated with a significant decrease in invasive fungal infections but had no impact on mortality [14]. The flora was not extensively studied, and the potential impact of fluconazole use on fungal ecology was not assessed. A 2006 systematic review and meta-analysis of randomized controlled trials of fluconazole or ketoconazole prophylaxis in non-neutropenic ICU patients identified 12 trials [15,16]. Invasive infections decreased, and no significant increase in resistant strains was noted. However, the authors pointed out that the trials were not adequately powered to rule out an increase in resistant strains [15,16]. Another metaanalysis published 1 year earlier also found that antifungal prophylaxis was effective without increasing the proportion of resistant strains [17]. Thus, the potential impact of antifungal prophylaxis on fungal ecology remains unclear. The many studies published in recent years produced somewhat conflicting data [18–20].

In addition to the selection of resistant strains, infection prophylaxis may promote the occurrence of opportunistic infections by selecting rare pathogens resistant to the prophylactic agents used. For instance, posaconazole prophylaxis of fungal infections in high-risk patients has been associated with the emergence of zygomycosis [21–23] and *Scedosporium* infections [24].

The last few years have witnessed profound changes in our medical practice. Advances in the management of many diseases have led to the emergence of high-risk patient populations. Thus, intensive chemotherapy regimens and aggressive supportive care generate immune system impairments associated with a high risk of infection. Prophylactic interventions targeting bacterial and fungal infections seem reasonable in these patients. Several studies have highlighted a number of important points. First, long-term effects must be assessed in uniform patient populations. Second, although some studies found increased resistance rates after prophylactic therapy, with no impact on mortality, most studies were not designed to assess changes in resistance rates. Finally, the body of available evidence indicates that antibacterial or antifungal prophylactic therapy modifies the microbial ecology, thereby leading to the emergence of new risks. A crucial point is to weigh the benefits – often measured as decreases in infection rates or, preferably, in mortality rates – against the rate and severity of new infectious complications. In available studies, the amount of detail on the expected benefits contrasts with the uncertainty surrounding the risks, as designing studies to assess risks is challenging. Infection prophylaxis has considerably benefited the management of high-risk patients. However, we will be able to assess the risk/benefit ratio only when detailed information on the long-term impact of infection prophylaxis becomes available.

References

1. Bucaneve G, Micozzi A, Menichetti F et al (2005) N Engl J Med 353:977–987
2. Cattaneo C, Casari S, Bracchi F et al (2010) Scand J Infect Dis 42:324–332
3. Timmers GJ, Dijstelbloem Y, Simoons-Smit AM et al (2004) Bone Marrow Transplant 33:847–853
4. Kern WV, Klose K, Jellen-Ritter AS et al (2005) Eur J Clin Microbiol Infect Dis 24:111–118
5. Sahagún Pareja J, Castillo FJ, Andrés R et al (2005) Revista espanola de quimioterapia: publicacion oficial de la Sociedad Espanola de Quimioterapia, vol 18, pp 32–38
6. Craig M, Cumpston AD, Hobbs GR et al (2007) Bone Marrow Transplant 39:477–482
7. van Loon HJ, Vriens MR, Fluit AC et al (2005) Am J Respir Crit Care Med 171:480–487
8. Oostdijk E, De Smet A, Blok H et al (2010) Am J Respir Crit Care Med 181:452–457
9. Trenschel R, Peceny R, Runde V et al (2000) Bone Marrow Transplant 26:993–997
10. Mann P, McNicholas P, Chau A et al (2009) Antimicrob Agents Chemother 53:5026–5034
11. Tumbarello M, Sanguinetti M, Trecarichi E et al (2008) J Antimicrob Chemother 62:1379–1385
12. Nihtinen A, Anttila VJ, Elonen E et al (2008) Eur J Haematol 80:391–396
13. Blot S, Janssens R, Claeys G et al (2006) J Antimicrob Chemother 58:474–477
14. Faiz S, Neale B, Rios E et al (2009) Eur J Clin Microbiol Infect Dis 28:689–692
15. Playford EG, Webster AC, Sorrell TC et al (2006) J Antimicrob Chemother 57:628–638
16. Playford EG, Webster AC, Sorrell TC et al (2006) Cochrane Database of Systematic Reviews (Online) CD004920 http://onlinelibrary.wiley.com/o/cochrane/clsysrev/articles/CD004920/frame.html
17. Cruciani M, de Lalla F, Mengoli C (2005) Intensive Care Med 31:1479–1487
18. Bassetti M, Ansaldi F, Nicolini L et al (2009) J Antimicrob Chemother 64:625–629
19. Magill SS, Swoboda SM, Shields CE et al (2009) Ann Surg 249:657–665
20. Manzoni P, Leonessa M, Galletto P et al (2008) Pediatr Infect Dis J 27:731–737
21. Mousset S, Bug G, Heinz W et al (2009) Transpl Infect Dis 12:261–264
22. Kishel J, Sivik J (2008) J Oncol Pharm Pract 14:189–193
23. Schlemmer F, Lagrange-Xélot M, Lacroix C et al (2008) Breakthrough Rhizopus infection on posaconazole prophylaxis following allogeneic stem cell transplantation. Bone Marrow Transplant 42:551–552
24. Ananda-Rajah M, Grigg A, Slavin M (2008) Mycopathologia 166:83–86

Part III

Diagnostic Strategy in HM Patients

How Type of Malignancy and Treatment Assist in the Etiological Diagnosis

11

Alexandre Boyer and Didier Gruson

Contents

11.1 Introduction

Acute respiratory failure (ARF) in cancer patients is a major cause of morbidity and mortality. The number of cancer patients managed for ARF has increased with the prevalence of cancer and use of bone marrow transplantation (BMT) [1]. Identifying the cause of ARF improves patient outcomes [2, 3]. Many causes of ARF exist in cancer patients, and several causes may be present in the same patient, raising diagnostic challenges. The type of immune deficiency affects the risk of specific pulmonary complications and varies with the type of malignancy and cytotoxic drug exposure, which are therefore useful for guiding the diagnostic strategy [4]. This point is particularly important for diagnosing infections. Cancer chemotherapy severely affects the components of both humoral and cellular immunity, including monocytes/macrophages, neutrophils, the complement cascade, immunoglobulin production, and T lymphocytes. The risk of infection is particularly high when neutropenia develops as a result of cytotoxic chemotherapy or of bone marrow involvement by a hematological malignancy. B-lymphocyte dysfunction due to chemotherapy, bone marrow transplantation, or lymphoproliferative disorders is associated with bacterial infections, whereas T-lymphocyte dysfunction or steroid therapy is associated with viral and fungal infections and with infections due to intracellular bacteria.

This chapter reviews the diagnosis of infectious and noninfectious causes of ARF in cancer patients.

A. Boyer and D. Gruson (✉)
Medical Intensive Care Unit, Hôpital Pellegrin-Tripode, Place Amélie Raba Léon, 33076, Bordeaux cedex, France
e-mail: didier.gruson@chu-bordeaux.fr

É. Azoulay (ed.), *Pulmonary Involvement in Patients with Hematological Malignancies*,
DOI: 10.1007/978-3-642-15742-4_11, © Springer-Verlag Berlin Heidelberg 2011

11.2 Risk Factors for Acute Respiratory Failure

11.2.1 Neutropenia

Neutropenia related to myelosuppressive chemotherapy or the disease itself is a major risk factor for lung infections in immunocompromised patients. As the leukocyte count decreases, the risk of infection increases. Neutrophils are involved in the phagocytosis of microorganisms, and neutropenia is therefore chiefly associated with infections by extracellular pyogenic bacteria and fungi [5]. Common culprits in patients with ARF and fever during the phase of neutropenia include *Streptococcus pneumoniae, Streptococcus viridans, Staphylococcus aureus, Pseudomonas aeruginosa, Klebsiella* spp., and *Escherichia coli.* The risk of bacterial infection is highest early in the neutropenic phase. Fungal lung infections (*Aspergillus* sp., *Fusarium*, and *Candida* spp.) are more common after a prolonged period of neutropenia and in patients with complex immune deficiencies (e.g., allogeneic BMT or exposure to the new targeted chemotherapeutic agents such as anti-CD52 antibodies).

11.2.2 Deficiencies in Cellular and Humoral Immunity

The B-lymphocytes, which are antibody-secreting plasma cells, are the main immune cells affected in lymphoproliferative disorders and after immunosuppressive therapy or allogeneic BMT. B-lymphocyte impairments cause deficiencies in humoral immunity that may lead to lung infections because of *S. pneumoniae* or gram-negative organisms.

Cellular immunity is mediated by the T-lymphocytes. Cellular immunity is impaired in patients with lymphoproliferative disorders, those taking cancer chemotherapeutic agents or steroids, and after BMT. Patients with T-cell dysfunction are susceptible to unusual pathogens such as viruses, protozoa (*Toxoplasma gondii*), fungi (*Aspergillus* spp., *P. jirovecii, Candida* spp.), and bacteria (*Legionella pneumophila, Nocardia asteroides, Listeria monocytogenes* and mycobacteria).

11.2.3 Allogeneic Bone Marrow and Stem Cell Transplantation

After BMT, specific complications tend to occur within well-defined time periods, which facilitates the diagnosis. In general, three periods are defined after allogeneic BMT or stem cell transplantation: the preengraftment phase, the postengraftment phase, and the late posttransplantation phase. ARF is more common after allogeneic BMT than after autologous transplantation. Allogeneic BMT requires conditioning followed by chronic treatment with several immunosuppressive agents to prevent or treat graft-versus-host disease (GVHD). Furthermore, GVHD causes immune system impairments by affecting the mucosal surfaces and reticuloendothelial system. In addition, several noninfectious causes of ARF are related to GHVD, such as idiopathic pneumonia syndrome, chronic airway disease, bronchiolitis obliterans, and the engraftment syndrome. After both allogeneic and autologous BMT or stem-cell transplantation, rapid immune system reconstitution may promote the development of inflammatory pulmonary complications.

Severe immune dysfunction is present following BMT. The profound neutropenia related to high-dose cytotoxic chemotherapy and total body irradiation lasts 2–4 weeks, and the deficiency in humoral immunity lasts 6 months. During this period, 30% of patients require ICU admission for life-threatening ARF, which is often due to noninfectious diseases.

During the preengraftment phase after allogeneic BMT, i.e., for the first 2–4 weeks after the conditioning regimen, severe neutropenia may promote the development of lung infections due to extracellular bacteria and opportunistic fungi. *Aspergillus* spp. is the most common cause of fungal infections at this phase, whereas *Fusarium* spp., *Cryptococcus neoformans, Candida* spp., and *Mucormycosis* are less common. Other major pulmonary complications during these first 4 weeks include diffuse alveolar hemorrhage, pulmonary edema, and drug-related pulmonary toxicity.

The postengraftment phase covers the second and third months after allogeneic BMT. During this period, the neutrophil count begins to increase, but major deficiencies in cellular and humoral immunity persist. Initially, donor lymphocytes may convey passive T-cell immunity, which is partially effective for approximately 2 months. Host lymphocytes that survive radiation therapy and chemotherapy may also provide limited cellular immunity during this period. The immune system impairments are greatest after native immunity and passive donor immunity are lost and before immune function is restored by the transplanted marrow. GVHD further increases the immune deficiencies and delays the recovery of normal immune function. At this phase, cytomegalovirus (CMV) is the most common cause of infection, followed by other viruses and by protozoa.

The late phase after allogeneic BMT starts after the third month. Recovery of cellular and humoral immunity occurs gradually. During this period, chronic GVHD may delay the recovery of normal immune function. Chronic GVHD occurs in more than 30% of patients after allogeneic BMT and impairs intrinsic immunity. Both infectious and noninfectious diseases may occur. Encapsulated bacteria and *P. jiroveci* are the main causes of pulmonary infection, and bronchiolitis obliterans and organizing pneumonia may cause acute and chronic pulmonary dysfunction.

11.3 Bacterial Pneumonia

During the early stages of immune compromise, bacteria are the most common causes of lung infection in cancer patients. Predisposing factors include bacteremia, disruption of mucosal barriers, defective ciliary function in the tracheobronchial tree, aspiration, and endotracheal intubation. Routine early administration of empiric broad-spectrum antibiotics in febrile neutropenic patients has decreased the incidence of bacterial pneumonia. Bacterial pneumonia may occur at any time after transplantation, but is particularly prevalent during the preengraftment period characterized by profound neutropenia. Bacterial pneumonia develops in about 15% of patients after BMT. Nearly half the cases occur within the first 100 days after BMT and, overall, 22% of cases are fatal.

Patients with cancer are at increased risk for gram-negative pneumonia. In patients who are ill or hospitalized, the oropharynx becomes colonized with gram-negative bacilli that are more virulent than the normal flora. Gram-negative pathogens, especially *P. aeruginosa* and *K. pneumoniae*, predominate in the first 100 days, whereas gram-positive organisms such as *S. pneumoniae* cause most of the infections seen later on [6]. *Legionella* spp. has been reported to be an important cause of nosocomial pneumonia in some centers [7, 8].

Among gram-negative organisms, *Pseudomonas* spp. is a common cause of pneumonia in neutropenic patients. There are increasing reports of pneumonia due to gram-positive microorganisms in immunocompromised patients, a trend that is probably ascribable to the widespread use of indwelling central venous catheters. *S. pneumoniae* has become more common in neutropenic patients and as a late infection after allogeneic BMT with chronic GVHD. Of growing concern is the rise of antibiotic-resistant strains of *S. pneumoniae. S. viridans* is increasingly common in leukemia patients with severe oropharyngeal mucositis following high-dose cytarabine therapy.

Nocardia asteroides is an opportunistic bacterium that occurs in patients with impaired cellular immunity. Neutropenia is usually not present, but a history of steroid therapy is common. The nodules may be single or multiple, and cavitation may occur. The mass-like infiltrate may extend to the pleura, causing a pleural effusion. *N. asteroides* may also involve the skin, brain, and meninges.

Bacterial pneumonia is commonly heralded by a fever, although the usual respiratory symptoms and signs may be absent in neutropenic hosts. The chest X-ray abnormalities may be subtle or absent, probably because of the paucity of neutrophils. In one series, high-resolution computed tomography revealed evidence of pneumonia in more than 50% of febrile neutropenic patients with normal chest X-rays [9]. Broad-spectrum antibiotics (with antipseudomonal activity) should be initiated expeditiously in all patients with suspected bacterial pneumonia and in febrile neutropenic patients with no identified site of infection. There is currently no consensus on the routine use of prophylactic antibiotics in afebrile asymptomatic neutropenic patients during the preengraftment period [10]. Intravenous immunoglobulin therapy may reduce the risk of bacterial infections in the subset of allogeneic BMT recipients who experience severe hypogammaglobulinemia during the first 100 days [10].

In nonendemic areas, tuberculosis is rare after BMT, with a frequency of only 0.1–0.25% in two large surveys [11]. For this book, Dr. El Anazi has produced a comprehensive analysis of tuberculosis in patients with hematological malignancies. Risk factors for developing tuberculosis include allogeneic BMT, total body irradiation, and chronic GVHD [12]. Infection with nontuberculous mycobacteria has generally been uncommon among BMT recipients, except with the use of T cell-depleted marrow grafts [12].

11.4 Fungal Pneumonia

Pulmonary fungal infections are a major cause of death in immunocompromised patients. In this book, two chapters (by Dr. Bougnoux and Dr. Nucci) focus on invasive fungal pneumonia in patients with hematological malignancies. Neutropenic patients are at risk for opportunistic infections with *Aspergillus* spp., *Candida* spp, *C. neoformans*, and *Mucor* spp. Reactivation of indolent infection with organisms, such as *Histoplasma* and *Coccidioides*, may be seen in patients with impaired cellular immunity. Invasive aspergillosis is among the most devastating complications of allogeneic BMT and is the most common cause of fungal pneumonia in neutropenic patients. *Aspergillus* infection has been reported in up to 20% of patients after BMT. Risk factors for invasive aspergillosis include prolonged neutropenia, steroid therapy, broad-spectrum antibiotics, GVHD, and transplantation of T cell-depleted marrow.

Recipients of both allogeneic and autologous BMT are at increased risk for invasive aspergillosis during the preengraftment phase, when neutropenia is the main risk factor. During the postengraftment period, the risk of invasive aspergillosis remains high after allogeneic BMT. During this period, immunosuppressive agents must be given and GVHD may develop. There has been a notable decline in preengraftment infections, probably because the introduction of hematopoietic growth factors and peripheral blood-stem-cell donation has shortened the period of neutropenia. In contrast, there has been an increase in the frequency of postengraftment infections caused by *Aspergillus* spp. These risk factors are reported in detail in the chapter by Dr. Bougnoux et al.

Other causes of fungal pneumonia are far less common in cancer patients. Emerging fungal infections are covered in the chapter by Dr. Nucci. The zygomycetes, including *Mucor* and *Rhizopus*, rarely cause invasive fungal infections after BMT (prevalence of up to 2% of patients). *Mucor* occurs occasionally in patients with neutropenia, lymphoproliferative disorders, and prior antibiotic therapy. Risk factors include severe and prolonged neutropenia, steroid-treated acute or chronic GVHD, and severe transfusion-related iron overload. Other emerging fungal pathogens that occasionally cause pulmonary infections include *Fusarium* and *Scedosporium* spp.

Pneumocystis jiroveci, first identified as a protozoan nearly 100 years ago by C. Chagas and reclassified as a fungus in 1988, is a major cause of pneumonia and ARF in patients with impaired cellular immunity. A chapter of this book focuses on *P. jiroveci* infection. Most cases are associated with HIV infection rather than with lymphoproliferative disorders, immunosuppressive therapy, or stem-cell transplantation. *P. jiroveci* infection has rarely been reported in patients with myelodysplastic syndromes. *P. jiroveci* pneumonia is more common in patients with hematological malignancies compared to those with solid tumors. However, patients with brain tumors from carcinomatous lymphangitis receiving high-dose steroid therapy are at risk for *P. jiroveci* pneumonia.

11.5 Viral Pneumonia

Respiratory viruses can cause severe pneumonia in patients with hematological malignancies [13–17]. A chapter by Dr. Schnell et al. covers pulmonary involvement by common respiratory viruses. Respiratory syncytial virus, influenza A and B viruses, and parainfluenza viruses are well-documented causes of severe respiratory morbidity and mortality, especially after BMT or hematopoietic stem-cell transplantation. Although lymphopenia is the main risk factor for viral pneumonia, screening for respiratory viruses should be incorporated into the routine diagnostic workup of patients with hematological malignancies until more clinical data become available [18]. The new multiplex PCR tests need further evaluation. Adenovirus infection is an uncommon cause of pneumonia that almost invariably develops within the first 3 months after BMT.

CMV can still cause viral pneumonia after allogeneic BMT. For this book, Dr. Vigil and coworkers contributed a very comprehensive review of CMV pneumonia. Although CMV pneumonia usually starts

50–60 days after BMT, the onset may occur at any time during the postengraftment phase (50–100 days after transplantation). After BMT, 10–40% of patients experience CMV pneumonia, which is fatal in 85% of cases. Among BMT recipients who are seropositive for CMV, 70% experience CMV infection because of reactivation of latent endogenous virus; among patients who are seronegative for CMV, approximately 36% experience CMV infection. Risk factors for CMV pneumonia include seropositivity in the recipient, seropositive donor and seronegative recipient, older age, total body irradiation, severe acute GVHD, frequent blood transfusions, and use of anti-rejection drugs causing T-cell depletion. Patients with chronic GVHD appear particularly prone to late-onset CMV pneumonia.

Herpes simplex virus is a less common cause of viral pneumonia, affecting fewer than 5% of BMT patients. The infection generally occurs during the period of profound neutropenia within 3 weeks after BMT. Idiopathic interstitial pneumonia associated with other herpes viruses (HHV6) has been reported in BMT patients. This book has a chapter on herpes pneumonia, written by Dr. Shah and co-workers.

11.6 Noninfectious Causes of Acute Respiratory Failure

Noninfectious conditions have accounted for an increased proportion of ARF cases among cancer patients since the introduction of prophylactic measures against bacterial, fungal, and viral infections [19]. Noninfectious causes of ARF include cardiogenic pulmonary edema, drug-related pulmonary toxicity, and pulmonary alveolar proteinosis. Most of these complications emerge during the first 3 months after stem-cell transplantation. The main pathogenic mechanisms are activation of the inflammatory cascades and T-cell alloreactivity.

11.6.1 Pulmonary Edema

Hydrostatic pulmonary edema is a common early complication that is related to the large amounts of intravenous fluids needed to administer antibiotics, blood products, cytotoxic drugs (anthracyclin), and parenteral nutrition [20]. Noncardiogenic edema during the preengraftment phase after BMT is often ascribable to lung injury from chemotherapy or total body irradiation combined with episodes of sepsis. Cardiac dysfunction and pulmonary edema may be exacerbated by the development of acute renal failure due to the cancer, drug-related tubular toxicity, or malignant cell lysis.

11.6.2 Pulmonary Toxicity Syndrome

This nonspecific syndrome is a manifestation of chemotherapy-induced lung injury. Lung biopsy findings are consistent with drug-related pulmonary toxicity. Chemotherapy regimens well known to be associated with lung injury and ARF are those containing carmustine or high-dose cyclophosphamide or methotrexate.

11.6.3 Diffuse Alveolar Hemorrhage

Diffuse alveolar hemorrhage may develop in patients with newly diagnosed or treated myeloblastic leukemia, most notably after autologous or allogeneic BMT or stem-cell transplantation [21, 22]. Profound thrombocytopenia is common in these patients, but is not the cause of the bleeding, which is ascribable to inflammation caused by the influx of neutrophils in the lungs.

11.6.4 Idiopathic Pneumonia Syndrome

This idiopathic syndrome defined as diffuse lung injury in the absence of infection is a diagnosis of exclusion [23]. It may be a manifestation of pulmonary toxicity related to pretreatment regimens, especially conventional high-dose conditioning regimens including total body radiation. Other risk factors are malignancy other than leukemia, older age, and high-grade acute GHVD. It is difficult to eliminate an immune-mediated injury because of the frequent association with GHVD. This fact suggests alloreactive T-cell-mediated alveolar injury.

11.6.5 Graft-Versus-Host Disease

GVHD is an immune reaction resulting from minor incompatibilities between the donor and the recipient of an HLA-matched transplant. The donor T lymphocytes recognize the recipient's tissue as a foreign body. Within the first 100 days after allogeneic BMT or stem cell transplantation, acute GVHD develops in 25–75% of patients. Acute GVHD primarily affects the skin, liver, and gastrointestinal tract, whereas the lungs are rarely involved. Chronic GHVD is more likely to cause ARF than is acute GHVD. In addition, infections and lymphoid interstitial pneumonia may cause ARF in patients with GVHD. Histologically, pulmonary GVHD may manifest as diffuse alveolar damage, lymphocytic interstitial pneumonia, lymphocytic bronchitis, and/or bronchiolitis obliterans.

11.6.6 Bronchiolitis Obliterans

Bronchiolitis obliterans is an obstructive pulmonary disorder affecting the small airways. It is a late complication of allogeneic BMT or stem-cell transplantation (5–10%), and is rare in autologous transplant recipients. Bronchiolitis obliterans is associated with chronic GHVD. Although the cause of bronchiolitis obliterans remains unclear, an autoimmune process affecting the small airways in the setting of GHVD is suspected [24–27].

11.6.7 Pulmonary Alveolar Proteinosis

Alveolar proteinosis is characterized by the deposition in the alveoli of a granular, extracellular, PAS-positive material [28]. This material is a mixture of surfactants, proteins, and lipids. An entire chapter is dedicated to this complication in the Pearl's section, in the last part of this book.

11.7 Conclusion

Patients with cancer and those treated with BMT exhibit a variety of immunological impairments associated with overwhelming opportunistic lung infections, as well as community-acquired pneumonia. The morbidity and mortality from these infections can be high. The organisms most likely to cause pneumonia in immunocompromised patients vary with the nature of the immunological impairment and the period during the course of the immune deficiency.

References

1. Aronchick JM (2000) Pulmonary infections in cancer and bone marrow transplant patients. Semin Roentgenol 35:140–151
2. Benoit DD, Depuydt PO, Peleman RA et al (2005) Documented and clinically suspected bacterial infection precipitating intensive care unit admission in patients with hematological malignancies: impact on outcome. Intensive Care Med 31:934–942
3. Larché J, Azouley E, Fieux F et al (2003) Improved survival of critically ill cancer patients with septic shock. Intensive Care Med 29:1688–1695
4. Azoulay E, Schlemmer B (2006) Diagnostic strategy in cancer patients with acute respiratory failure. Intensive Care Med 32:808–822
5. Schimpff S (1977) Therapy of infection in patients with granulocytopenia. Med Clin North Am 61:1101–1118
6. Junghanss C, Marr KA, Carter RA et al (2002) Incidence and outcome of bacterial and fungal infections following nonmyeloablative compared with myeloablative allogeneic hematopoietic stem cell transplantation: a matched control study. Biol Blood Marrow Transplant 8:512–520
7. Clark JG, Crawford SW (1987) Diagnostic approaches to pulmonary complications of marrow transplantation. Chest 91:477–479
8. Harrington RD, Woolfrey AE, Bowden R et al (1996) Legionellosis in a bone marrow transplant center. Bone Marrow Transplant 18:361–368
9. Heussel CP, Kauczor HU, Heussel G et al (1997) Early detection of pneumonia in febrile neutropenic patients: use of thin-section CT. AJR Am J Roentgenol 169:1347–1353
10. Sullivan KM, Dykewicz CA, Longworth DL, et al. (2001) Preventing opportunistic infections after hematopoietic stem cell transplantation: the Centers for Disease Control and Prevention, Infectious Diseases Society of America, and American Society for Blood and Marrow Transplantation practice guidelines and beyond. Hematol Am Soc Hematol Educ Program 2001:392–421
11. de la Camara R, Martino R, Granados E et al (2000) Spanish group on infectious complications in hematopoietic transplantation. Tuberculosis after hematopoietic stem cell transplantation: incidence, clinical characteristics and outcome. Bone Marrow Transplant 26:291–298
12. Kotloff RM, Ahya VN, Crawford SW (2004) Pulmonary complications of solid organ and hematopoietic stem cell transplantation. Am J Respir Crit Care Med 170:22–48
13. Cordonnier C, Bernaudin JF, Bierling P et al (1986) Pulmonary complications occurring after allogeneic bone

marrow transplantation: a study of 130 consecutive transplanted patients. Cancer 58:1047–1054
14. Soubani AO, Miller KB, Hassoun PM (1996) Pulmonary complications of bone marrow transplantation. Chest 109:1066–1077
15. Wick MR, Moore SB, Gastineau DA et al (1983) Immunologic, clinical, and pathologic aspects of human graft-versus-host disease. Mayo Clin Proc 58:603–612
16. Kantrow SP, Hackman RC, Boeckh M et al (1997) Idiopathic pneumonia syndrome: changing spectrum of lung injury after marrow transplantation. Transplantation 63:1079–1086
17. Afessa B, Tefferi A, Litzow MR et al (2002) Diffuse alveolar hemorrhage in hematopoietic stem cell transplant recipients. Am J Respir Crit Care Med 166:641–645
18. Martino R, Ramila E, Rabella N et al (2003) Respiratory virus infections in adults with hematologic malignancies: A prospective study. Clin Infect Dis 36:1–8
19. Khurshid I, Anderson LC (2002) Non-infectious pulmonary complications after bone marrow transplantation. Postgrad Med J 78:257–262
20. Hamilton PJ, Pearson ADJ (1986) Bone marrow transplantation and the lung. Thorax 41:497–502
21. Raptis A, Mavroudis D, Suffredini AF et al (1999) High-dose corticosteroid therapy for diffuse alveolar hemorrhage in allogeneic bone marrow stem cell transplant recipients. Bone Marrow Transplant 24:879–883
22. Lewis ID, Defor T, Weisdorf DJ (2000) Increasing incidence of diffuse alveolar hemorrhage following allogeneic bone marrow transplantation: cryptic etiology and uncertain therapy. Bone Marrow Transplant 26:539–543
23. Clark JG, Hansen JA, Hertz MI et al (1993) Idiopathic pneumonia syndrome after bone marrow transplantation. Am Rev Respir Dis 147:1601–1606
24. Chan CK, Hyland RH, Hutcheon MA (1990) Pulmonary complications following bone marrow transplantation. Clin Chest Med 11:323–332
25. Jules-Elysee K, Stover DE, Yahalom J et al (1992) Pulmonary complications in lymphoma patients treated with high-dose therapy and autologous bone marrow transplantation. Am Rev Respir Dis 146:485–491
26. Holland KH, Wingard JR, Beschorner WE et al (1988) Bronchiolitis obliterans in bone marrow transplantation and its relationship to chronic graft-v-host disease and low serum IgG. Blood 72:621–627
27. Paz HL, Crilley P, Patchefsky A et al (1992) Bronchiolitis obliterans after autologous bone marrow transplantation. Chest 102:775–778
28. Cordonnier C, Fleury-Feith J, Escudier E et al (1994) Secondary alveolar proteinosis is a reversible cause of respiratory failure in leukemic patients. Am J Respir Crit Care Med 149:788–794

Contribution of Radiology in Patients with Hematological Malignancies and Pulmonary Involvement

12

Claus Peter Heussel

Contents

C.P. Heussel
Diagnostic and Interventional Radiology, Chest Clinic, Heidelberg University Hospital, Amalienstrasse 5, 69126, Heidelberg, Germany

12.1 Early Detection of Pneumonia

In patients with hematological malignancies, infections are associated with high mortality rates, and mortality increases sharply with increasing time to antimicrobial treatment, even within a range of only a few hours [1, 2]. Therefore, early detection of foci of infection is crucial. Furthermore, early detection and treatment of infections may decrease hospital stay length, thereby limiting the cost of treatment. Non-enhanced computed tomography (CT) is about 230€ in Germany (including the interpretation and comparison to previous CT scans).

Physical and laboratory findings should be used to determine which organ system or systems are most likely to be involved [3, 4]. The appropriate imaging technique should then be selected with the goal of achieving high sensitivity and a useful negative predictive value [5].

The exact frequencies of organ infections in neutropenic patients are difficult to determine and differ between evidence of microorganisms (colonization), clinically diagnosed infections (patients alive), and infections diagnosed by postmortem examination. Clinically, the lungs are affected in 30% of neutropenic patients with infection. The paranasal sinuses are involved in 3% of these patients overall and in 30% of allogeneic transplant recipients (concomitantly with pneumonia). The gastrointestinal tract, liver, spleen, central nervous system (especially after allogeneic transplantation), and kidneys are rarely affected [6].

É. Azoulay (ed.), *Pulmonary Involvement in Patients with Hematological Malignancies*,
DOI: 10.1007/978-3-642-15742-4_12, © Springer-Verlag Berlin Heidelberg 2011

12.2 Imaging Techniques

12.2.1 Chest X-Ray

Chest X-ray (CXR) is widely performed when pneumonia is suspected or must be excluded [7]. Advantages of CXR include rapidity, wide availability (even on the ward), low cost, and low radiation dose. CXR in the supine position can be performed on the ward in isolated neutropenic patients. A major disadvantage of CXR is the occurrence of superimpositions that considerably limit the sensitivity of this method for detecting pneumonia (Figs. 12.1 and 12.2) [8, 9]. In the supine position, lung inflation is limited, and no lateral projection can be obtained, which limits image quality, in addition to other technical issues. In 40 patients with fever of unknown origin after bone-marrow transplantation, digital CXR in the supine position had only 46% sensitivity for early pneumonia detection [10]. Thus, although CXR provides clinically relevant information on central venous catheters (CVC), pleural effusion, and pulmonary congestion [10], it often fails to detect early pneumonia and to rule out pneumonia, two key goals in immunocompromised patients. Therefore, supine CXR alone is not recommended for early pneumonia detection in immunocompromised hosts [11]. Also, when an infiltrate is seen, CXR provides only limited information on its characteristics. Thus, when pneumonia is suspected in an immunocompromised patient, thin-section CT should be preferred at any time, whenever possible [12].

12.2.2 CT

After studies documented the limitations of CXR in patients with hematological malignancies [9], a prospective study compared High resolution CT scan (HRCT) to CXR for early pneumonia detection in 188 neutropenic patients who were still febrile after 48 h on empirical antimicrobial therapy [20]. Patients with normal CXR findings at this time underwent HRCT on the same day, which showed infiltrates in about 60% of cases (Fig. 12.3). During the following days, the diagnosis of pneumonia was confirmed by the microbiological tests or CXR in approximately 50% of these patients (30% of the overall population). In the 40% of patients with normal CXR and HRCT findings at study

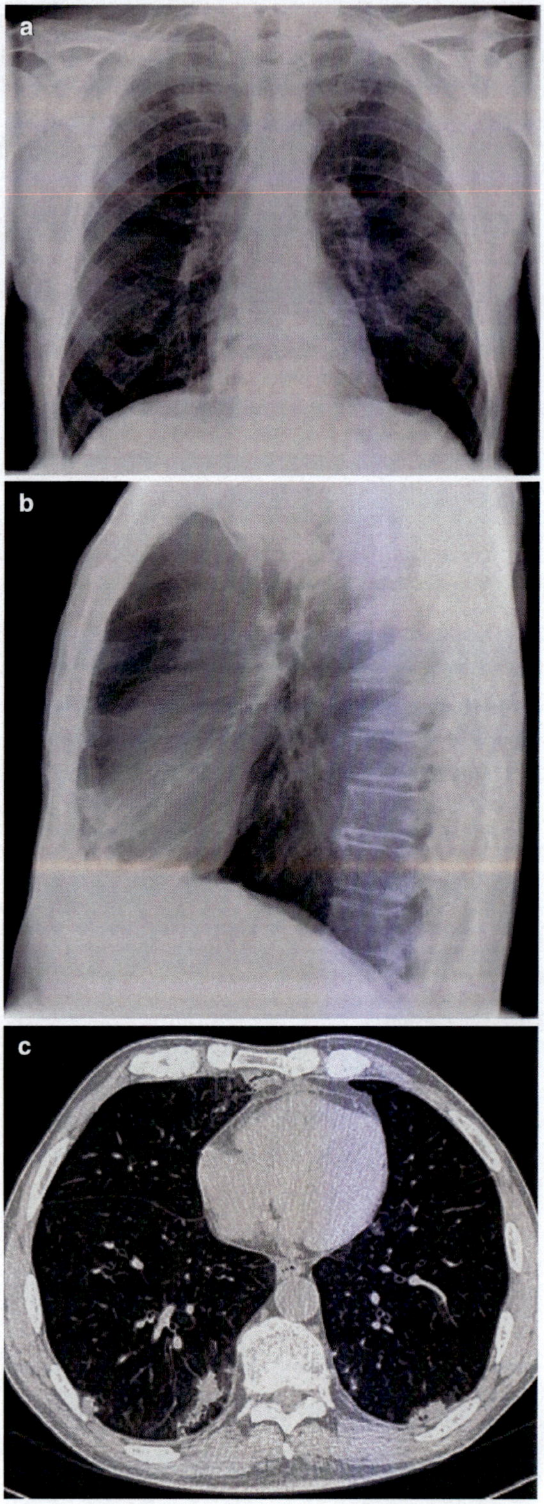

Fig. 12.1 Neutropenic febrile patient receiving broad-spectrum antibiotic therapy. CXR was normal on day 3 of fever (**a**, **b**). HRCT performed on the same day demonstrated bilateral infiltrates, which were hidden behind the heart on the posterior-anterior projection and obscured by the spine on the lateral projection (**c**)

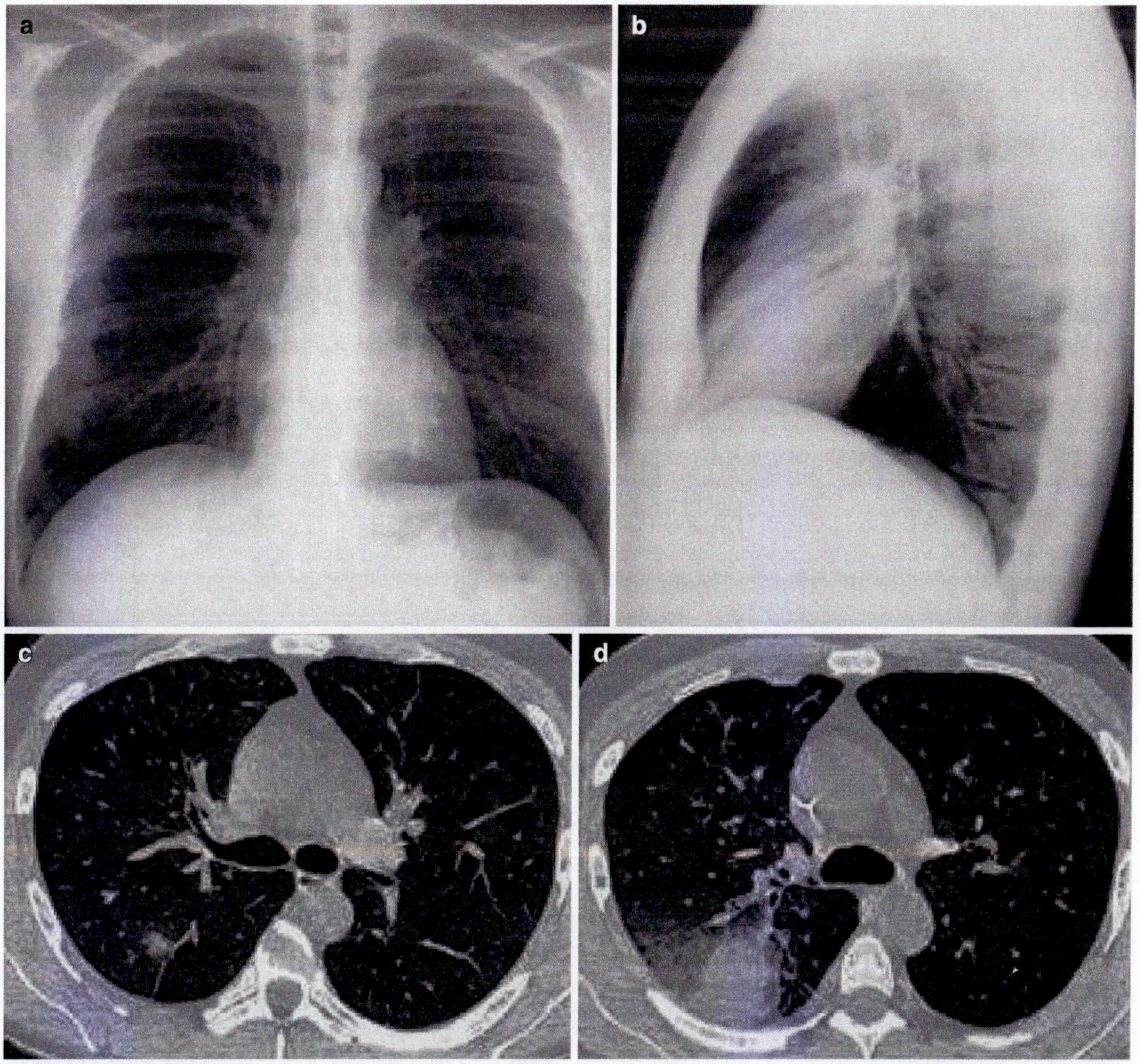

Fig. 12.2 The small ill-defined nodule in the right upper lobe (**c**) of this 34-year-old neutropenic patient with acute myelogenous leukemia was not visible on the chest X-ray, even upon retrospective evaluation (**a**, **b**). Amphotericin B treatment was started because fungal pneumonia was suspected. However, the nodule increased in size during neutropenia recovery 2 weeks later (**d**). To prepare for bone-marrow transplantation, the lesion was resected to prevent spreading. Examination of the specimen showed *Aspergillus*

inclusion, the rate of pneumonia during follow-up was only 10% [20]. The enrollment of both patients managed using conventional chemotherapy and transplant recipients is a weakness of this study. Another limitation is inherent in the imperfect performance of microbiological testing for diagnosing pneumonia [20].

In addition to detecting pneumonia, ruling out pneumonia is clinically useful. Therefore, the negative predictive value of HRCT has been assessed by determining the rate of, and time to, pneumonia documented by microbiological tests or CXR after a normal HRCT scan [20]. Pneumonia was rarely found in these patients and was never diagnosed within the first 5 days after a normal HRCT. The rare cases of pneumonia developed later on and were spread over the entire follow-up period (Fig. 12.4). In patients with infiltrates by HRCT, pneumonia was usually documented during the next 5–10 days (Fig. 12.4) [20].

Thus, CT holds considerable promise as a screening technique for pneumonia in neutropenic patients. Sensitivity was 87% and negative predictive value 88%. The discrepancies between HRCT and other

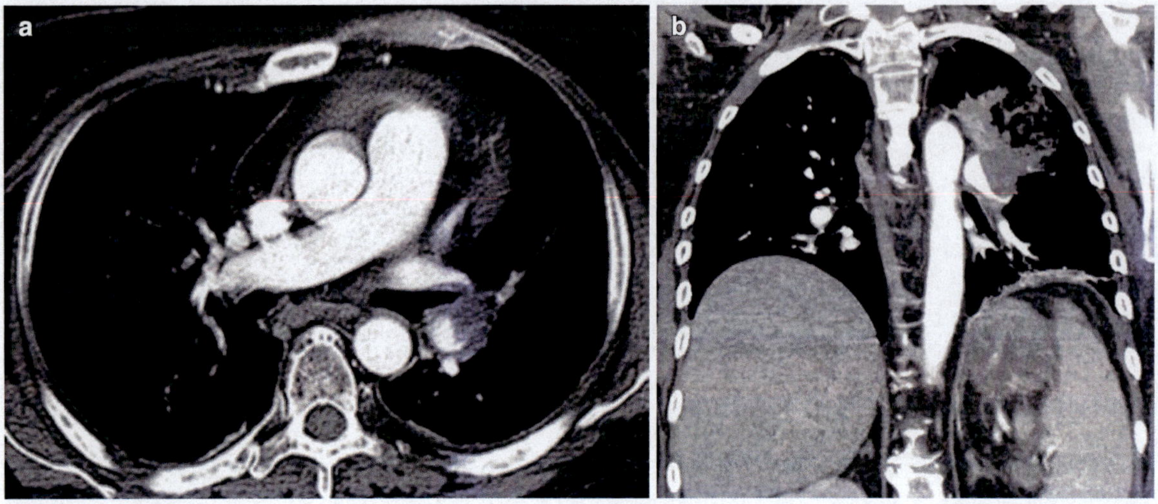

Fig. 12.3 A 45-year-old patient with acute myelogenous leukemia and a history of unrelated peripheral blood stem cell transplantation 6 months earlier. Contrast-enhanced CT demonstrating vessel erosion in a consolidating infiltrate in the left lung. An apposition thrombus is visible in the pulmonary artery of the left lower lobe. She died 2 days later from brain infarction

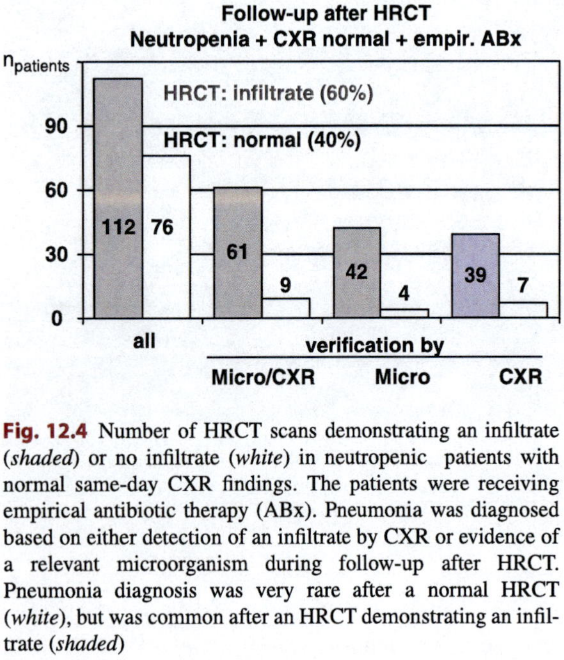

Fig. 12.4 Number of HRCT scans demonstrating an infiltrate (*shaded*) or no infiltrate (*white*) in neutropenic patients with normal same-day CXR findings. The patients were receiving empirical antibiotic therapy (ABx). Pneumonia was diagnosed based on either detection of an infiltrate by CXR or evidence of a relevant microorganism during follow-up after HRCT. Pneumonia diagnosis was very rare after a normal HRCT (*white*), but was common after an HRCT demonstrating an infiltrate (*shaded*)

investigations were mainly ascribable to delayed pneumonia after a negative HRCT (classified as false-negative HRCT results) and to minor infiltrates detected by HRCT and treated immediately so that the CXR remained normal (classified as false-positive results). The additional early use of HRCT achieved the diagnosis of pneumonia about 5 days earlier, and a normal HRCT virtually excluded pneumonia during the next 5 days [11]. Both the early diagnosis and the exclusion of pneumonia are valuable in immunocompromised patients [7].

12.2.2.1 CT Technique

The radiation dose is of limited concern in patients treated with total body irradiation (14,000 mGy) and cytotoxic agents. Current CT techniques deliver 1–10 mSv per lung scan (in this diagnostic scenario, 1 mSv = 1 mGy) [13, 14]. Thus, even when repeated CT scans are performed, the risk of radiation-induced malignancy is low compared to the high mortality associated with the primary malignancy and infections or to the risk of treatment-related secondary malignancies [1].

Terms such as "incremental CT," "high-resolution CT (HRCT)," "spiral CT," "thin-section CT," "multislice CT (MSCT)," and "low-dose CT" are widely used and may confuse non-radiologists. HRCT is an incremental scanning technique with several breath-holds. This early technique uses thin sections (e.g., 1 mm) separated by gaps (e.g., 10 mm), resulting in a representative but detailed image of the lungs. However, the non-contiguous scanning limits nodule detection, quantification, and monitoring. The volumetric techniques used in spiral CT and MSCT acquire slices with no gaps, but they are frequently reconstructed using greater slice thickness (e.g., 5 mm), which are associated with spatial volume effects. This characteristic limits the detection of inflammatory lung disease, especially ground-glass opacities [15]. Thin-section multislice CT (MSCT), in contrast, allows volumetric scanning and produces detailed images at the same time [16]. Thin-section MSCT is a good technique for monitoring lung disease, since the anatomical position can be accurately replicated from one scan to the next [16]. Given the fast pace of technological developments in the field of CT, the term "CT" is used in the rest of this chapter.

In general, contrast enhancement is not necessary for detecting and characterizing pneumonia [12, 17]. In specific situations, however, such as suspected pulmonary embolism or hemoptysis (e.g., due to vessel erosion), CT angiography is beneficial (Fig. 12.5). In allogeneic transplant recipients, bronchiolitis obliterans must be considered [18, 19]. To look for air trapping, a sign of bronchiolitis obliterans, an additional expiratory CT scan is helpful [18, 19].

12.2.3 MRI

Magnetic radiography imaging (MRI) has been evaluated for investigating pulmonary disease, since it is known to be effective in lesion characterization [21]. An intraindividual comparison showed that, compared to CT, MRI had 95% sensitivity, 88% specificity, 95% positive predictive value, and 88% negative predictive value [22]. Apart from the absence of radiation exposure (of nearly no benefit in this patient population, as mentioned above), MRI does not help in the early detection of pneumonia (Fig. 12.6). In patients with advanced pneumonia, CT and MRI perform similarly for visualizing the infiltrates [21]. However, CT is widely available, easier, and faster to perform, and less susceptible to breathing artifacts. MRI is superior over CT in detecting abscesses, as central necrosis is visualized clearly on T2-weighted images and rim enhancement after contrast injection on T1-weighted images [21]. Nevertheless, this fact has limited clinical impact. Furthermore, MRI takes longer and requires a higher degree of patient cooperation than does CT. MRI may fail to visualize small lesions, and cardiac motion may limit the detection of lesions adjacent to the left ventricle [22].

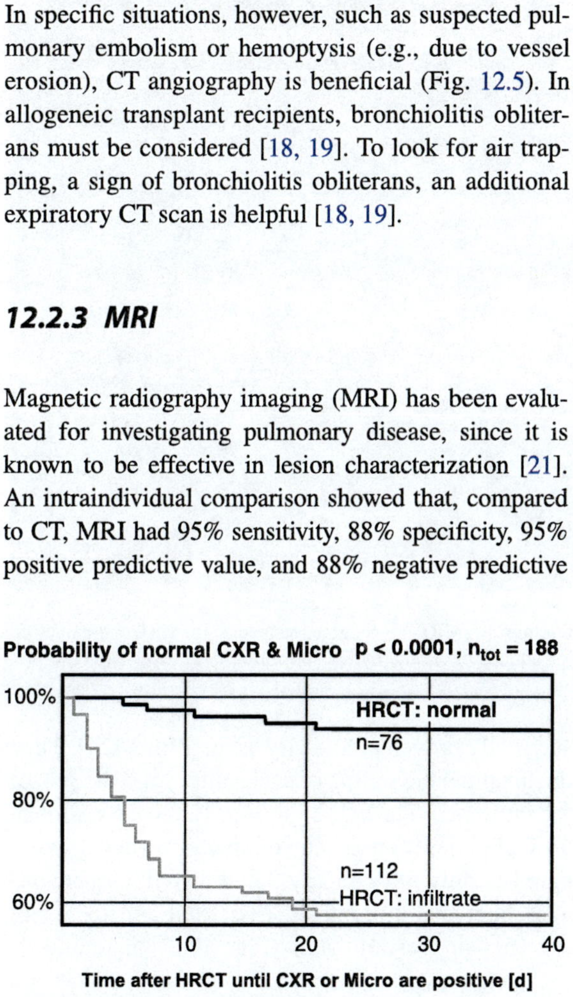

Fig. 12.5 Probability of pneumonia diagnosis based on a CXR infiltrate or evidence of a relevant microorganism during followup after HRCT. Kaplan-Meier analysis for patients with normal HRCT scans (*grey line*) and patients with evidence of pneumonia on HRCT scans (*black line*). The difference was highly significant ($P < 0.0001$). Very few cases of pneumonia were diagnosed after a normal HRCT, and the diagnoses were usually made late after HRCT. In patients with infiltrates by HRCT, most pneumonia diagnoses occurred within 5–10 days

12.2.4 Standard Recommendation

Identification of the causative organism is considerably more challenging in patients with pneumonia than in those with systemic infections. Attempts to increase the rate of organism recovery failed to significantly improve patient outcomes [23]. Therefore, a widely used strategy in febrile immunocompromised patients is empirical antimicrobial therapy guided by the imaging study results. However, noninvasive testing of sputum, blood, and nasopharyngeal aspirates is both safe and effective, and can be widely used.

CT is recommended for the early detection of pneumonia [23]. Importantly, CT findings help to determine whether invasive investigations are in order and which sites they should target. Thus, CT is valuable for guiding bronchoalveolar lavage (BAL) or lung biopsy [54]. Furthermore, CT excludes pneumonia with greater confidence than does CXR. The sequence shown in Fig. 12.7 can be modified if CT capabilities obviate the need for CXR.

12.3 Infectious Pneumonia

12.3.1 Identifying Pneumonia

Enlarging infiltrates may develop during hematological reconstitution [24]. Caillot et al. evaluated weekly HRCT findings in 25 neutropenic patients with

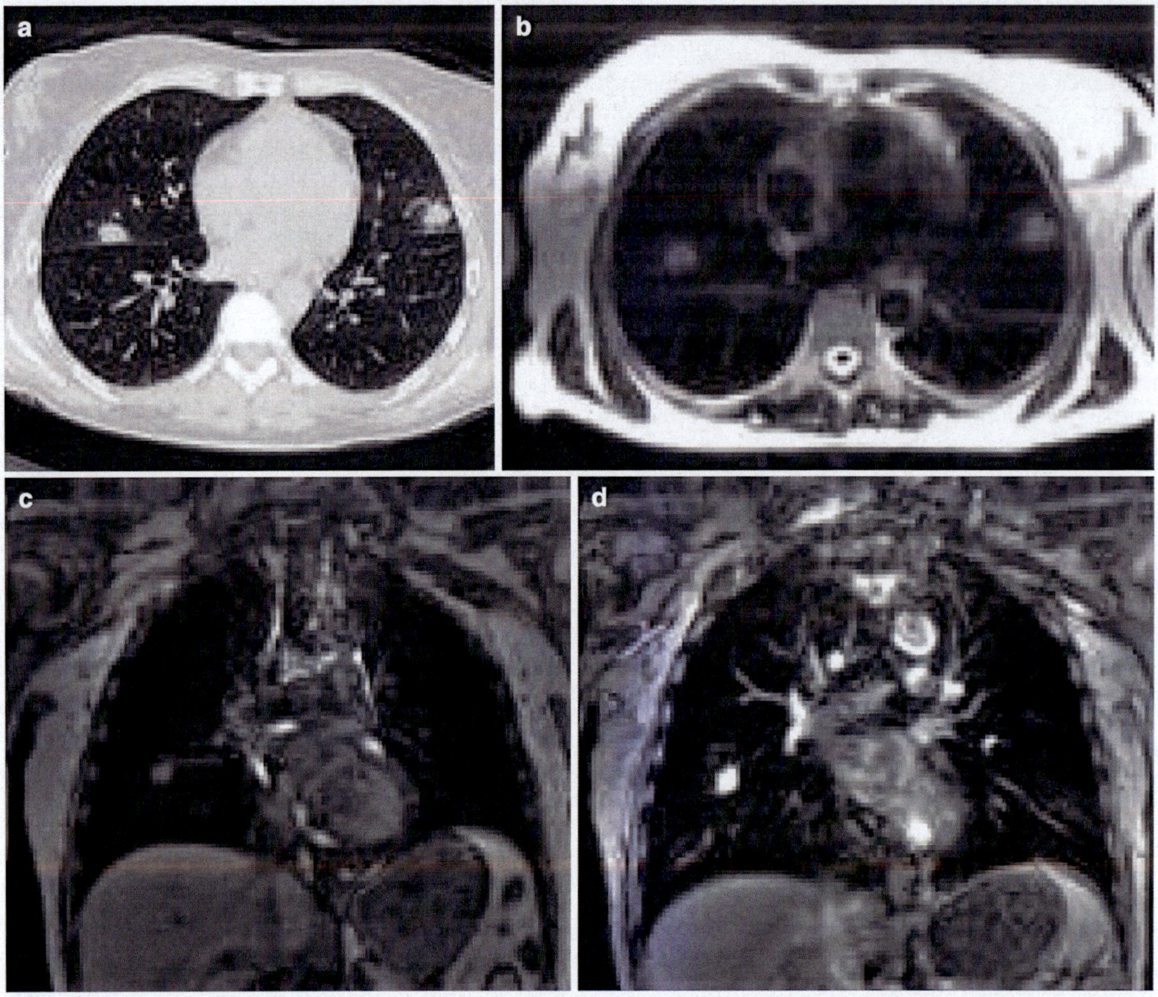

Fig. 12.6 Fungal pneumonia. Same-day HRCT and MRI. (**a**) HRCT findings. (**b**) MRI, T2-weighted sequence. (**c**) MRI, non-enhanced T1-weighted gradient-echo sequence. (**d**) Post-gadolinium MRI. Lesion contrast is similar by CT and contrast-enhanced MRI

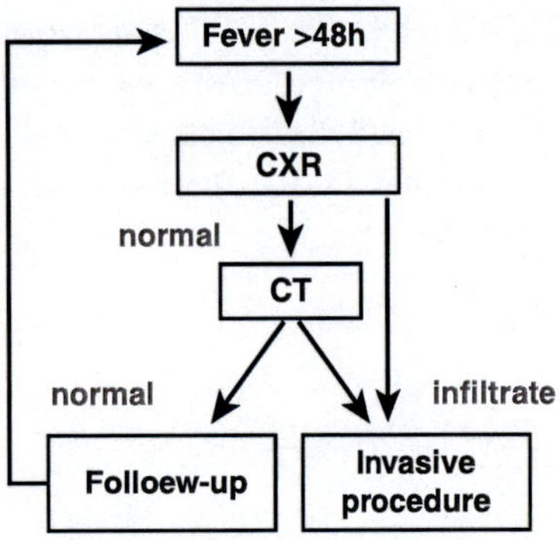

Fig. 12.7 Guidelines issued by the Infectious Diseases Working Party (AGIHO) of the German Society of Haematology and Oncology (DGHO) [23]. Since initial CXR is of limited usefulness, this diagnostic step is more and more often omitted and CT performed initially

surgically proven pulmonary aspergillosis [24]. They documented the timing of each pattern and the size of the infiltrates. The halo sign (Fig. 12.8) was visible in 96% of patients on the day of diagnosis (day 0) compared to only 68% on day 3 and dwindling percentages later on. In contrast, cavitation and the more specific air-crescent sign (Fig. 12.9) increased in prevalence over time (from 8% on day 3 to 63% on day 14). Lesion volume increased fourfold from day 0 to day 7 despite successful treatment and neutropenia recovery. The increase in lesion size is probably ascribable to the influx of neutrophils during neutropenia recovery. In critically ill patients, neutropenia recovery has been identified as a risk factor for acute respiratory distress syndrome [8]. In this study [24],

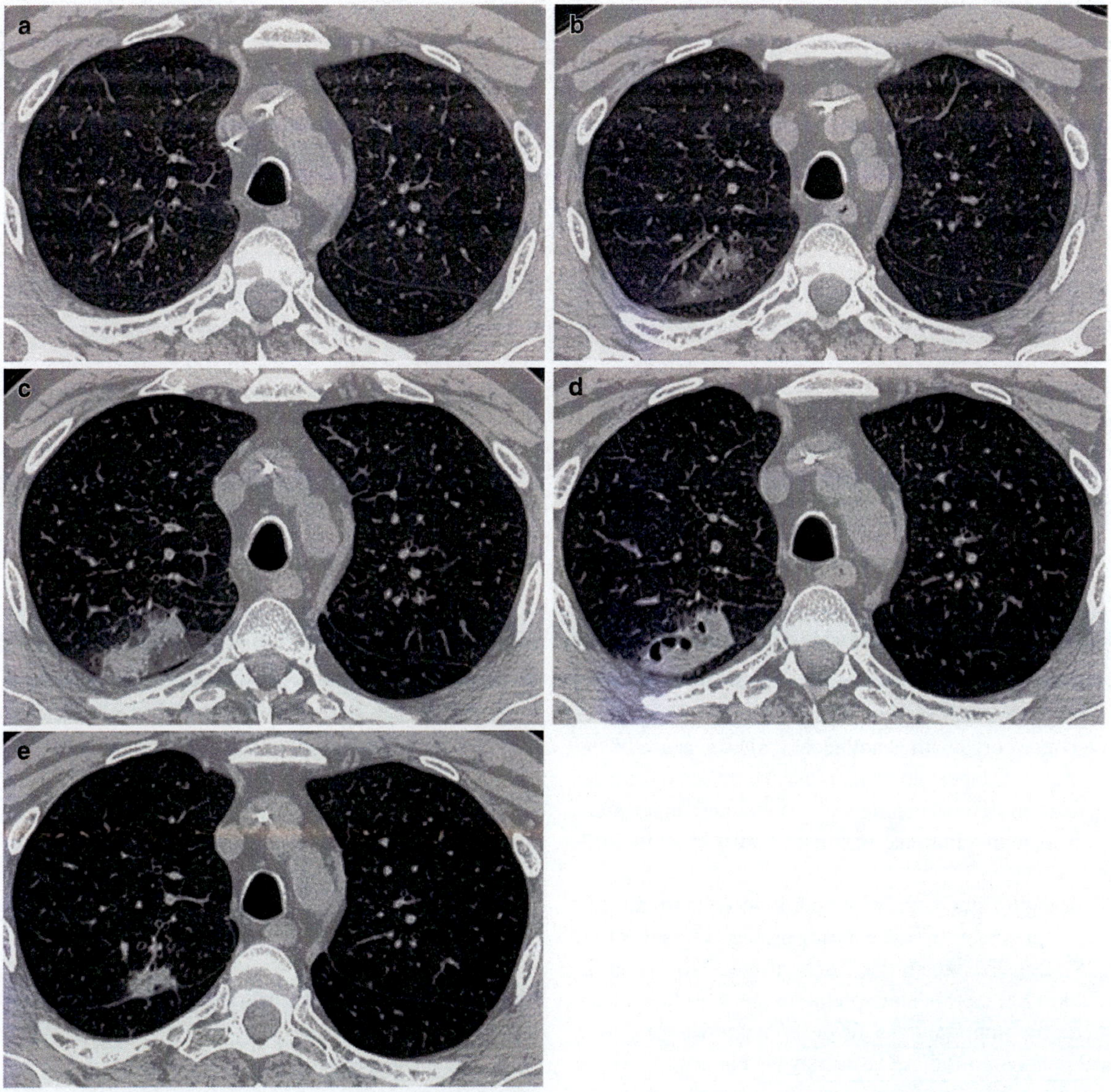

Fig. 12.8 Neutropenic febrile patient with non-Hodgkin lymphoma treated with autologous peripheral blood stem-cell transplantation. On day 2 after transplantation, neutropenia and fever occurred, prompting empirical antifungal treatment (**a**). Ill-defined pulmonary nodules were detected on day 7 (**b**). Neutropenia recovery occurred on day 13 when the infiltrate size was greatest (**c**). Under continuous antifungal treatment and with nearly normal leukocyte counts, the halo faded, and central cavitation developed (**d**), day 33. The lesions shrank considerably but did not disappear until day 108 (**e**)

the median time from neutropenia onset to the diagnosis of invasive pulmonary aspergillosis was 19 days. In our study of early HRCT for diagnosing pneumonia in febrile neutropenic patients, the duration of neutropenia was 11 days at pneumonia diagnosis [20].

12.3.2 Identifying the Cause of Pneumonia

Ideally, the microorganism causing pneumonia should be identified. However, several days are needed to obtain the results of microbiological and pathological investigations. Furthermore, these investigations fail to

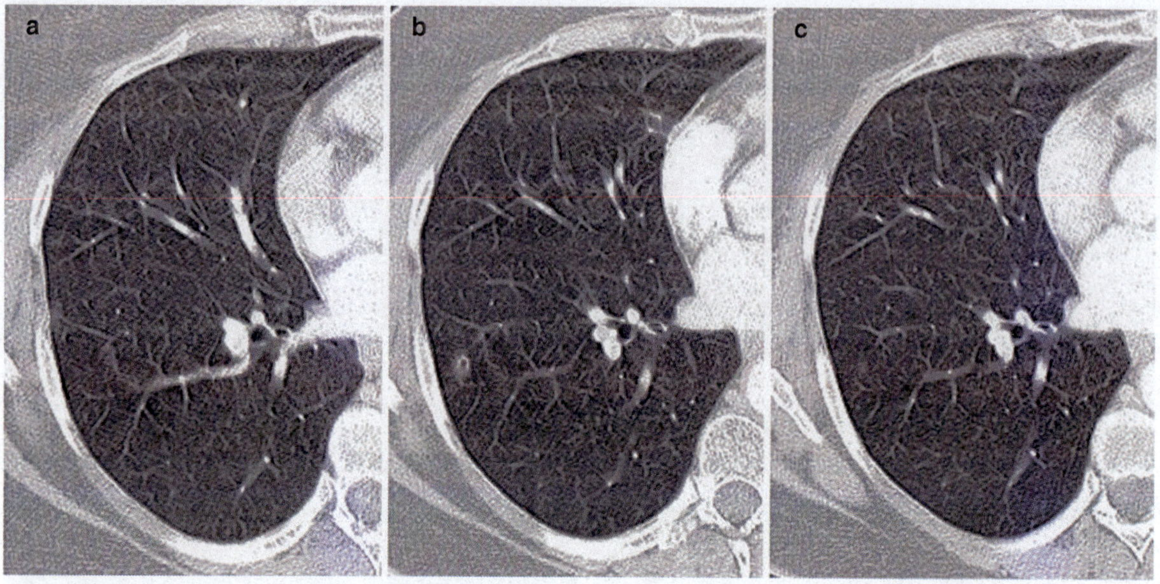

Fig. 12.9 The ill-defined nodules with cavitation were detected by CT done to evaluate repeated brief febrile episodes (**b**). They suggested fungal pneumonia and were not visible on the baseline CT (**a**). After port resection, both pulmonary lesions resolved, and no further febrile episodes occurred (**c**)

recover the organism in some patients [25]. Finally, the recovered organism is not necessarily the cause of the disease. Surface colonization may complicate the interpretation of microbiological results, and superinfection with an additional organism occurs in about 20% of cases [26, 27].

Imaging study findings cannot prove the nature of the pulmonary disease, but may provide valuable clues [28, 29], of which the most useful are listed in Table 12.1. Optimal interpretation of these clues is particularly important, as fever of unknown origin in immunocompromised hosts may be related to a variety of diseases, whose clinical presentations may be closely similar. Therefore, the imaging studies should be read by experienced radiologists, who should work in close collaboration with the clinicians. Radiologists should be informed about patient characteristics, such as neutropenia, allogeneic or autologous transplantation, positive tests for viral disease in the transplant and recipient, and exposure to cytotoxic agents or conditioning regimens (Table 12.1).

12.3.2.1 Bacterial Pneumonia

Since bacteria are responsible for approximately 90% of infections during the early phase of neutropenia [27], their empirical treatment has been optimized in recent years. Radiological features may include consolidation, especially in bronchopneumonia, and a positive bronchogram (Table 12.1) [29, 30]. Ground-glass opacities are more common than in immunocompetent patients, but are of course not specific of bacterial infection.

12.3.2.2 Fungal Pneumonia

Persistent fever in neutropenic patients may indicate invasive fungal infection [1]. In Europe, the main causative organism is *Aspergillus* spp. Rarely, *Candida* spp. is shown antemortem to be a cause of pneumonia (Fig. 12.10) [11]. *Candida* isolates may merely indicate surface colonization.

The typical findings of fungal and non-fungal pneumonia and of lung infiltrates caused by non-infectious diseases are detailed in a specific review [31]. Radiological studies may show pulmonary infiltrates, ill-defined nodules, and the halo sign at the earliest phase. Cavitation or even the air crescent sign may be visible later on.

For clinical and epidemiological research in neutropenic patients, the EORTC and BAMSO defined recommendations for interpreting radiological findings in

Table 12.1 Clinical and radiological appearance in various infectious and non-infectious lung diseases in neutropenic patients and bone marrow or stem cell transplant recipients

Diagnosis	Clinical setting	Radiological appearance
Infection bacterial	Early phase neutropenia	Consolidation, bronchopneumonia positive pneumobronchogram, GGO
Fungal	Prolonged neutropenia (>10 days)	Halo = ill-defined nodules (early phase)consolidations, negative pneumobronchogram Air crescent sign/cavitation (late phase)
Pneumocystis	Allogeneic transplantation	GGO, sparing of the subpleural space Intralobular septa (late phase)
Tuberculosis	Various	Small, ill-defined nodules/cavitations, tree-in-bud, homogeneous consolidation
Viral	Transplantation history in graft or host	GGO – mosaic pattern
Graft versus host	Allogeneic transplantation	GGO – mosaic pattern Intralobular septa become visible Tree-in-bud Air trapping (expiratory CT)
Radiation toxicity	Total body irradiation	GGO – paramediastinal distribution, also after TBI Intralobular septa become visible
Drug toxicity	Bleomycin, methotrexate, cytarabine, carmustine, etc.	GGO – mosaic pattern Intralobular septa become visible Peripheral consolidations of secondary lobule Traction bronchiectasis
Pulmonary congestion	Extensive hydration, renal impairment, hypoproteinosis	GGO Interlobular septa become visible
Leukemic infiltration	Chronic leukemic infiltration	Bronchovascular bundle thickening Interlobular septa become visible GGO
Pulmonary hemorrhage	Thrombocytopenia, intervention, hemoptysis	GGO Sedimentation phenomenon

GGO ground-glass opacity, *TBI* total body irradiation

invasive fungal infections in 2002 [32], then issued an update in 2008 [33]. The new occurrence of "typical" CT patterns (dense, well-circumscribed lesions with or without a halo sign, air crescent sign) constitutes a criterion for fungal pneumonia (Figs. 12.9 and 12.10). The halo sign was first described in 1984 [34, 35]. Although promising observations were made in 1986, the halo sign is non-specific [29] and is not required in the 2008 EORTC recommendations [33]. A non-specific infiltrate was considered a minor criterion in the 2002 recommendations [32], but was dropped in 2008 [33]. In a study of baseline CT findings in 235 patients with invasive pulmonary aspergillosis who were enrolled in a trial of antifungal treatment, presence of the halo sign (143 patients) was associated with a higher response rate (52% vs. 29%; $P<0.001$) and with a higher 3-month survival rate (71% vs. 53%; $P<0.01$), compared to the 79 patients without a halo sign [36].

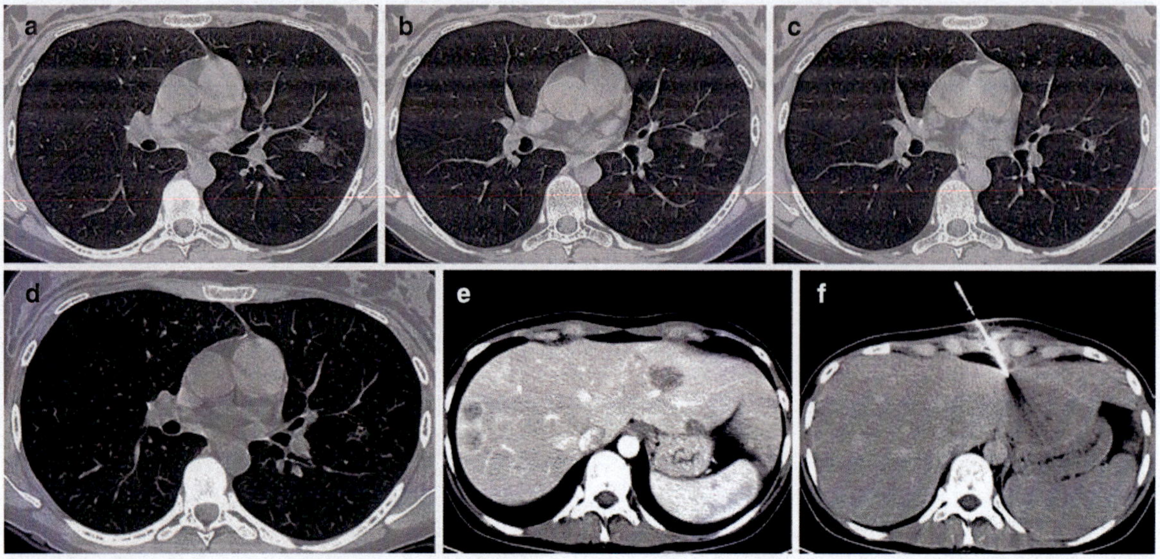

Fig. 12.10 Bilateral ill-defined nodules suggested a fungal infection (**a**, **b**), and antifungal treatment was given. Candida spp. Was identified in blood cultures and suspected as a cause of pneumonia. The small lesions developed into cavitations upon haematological reconstitution (**c**) then decreased in size (**d**). Liver enzyme levels increased, suggesting hepatosplenic candidiasis related to the candidemia. Contrast-enhanced CT showed liver lesions (**e**), which were biopsied. Candida spp. was found in the biopsy specimens (**f**)

Major limitations of this study include the use of thick-section CT instead of thin-section CT and the evaluation of hard copies instead of monitor reading [35]. In a study of 31 patients with hematological malignancies and suspected invasive pulmonary aspergillosis based on highly suggestive CT findings, open lung biopsy confirmed this diagnosis in only 17 (53%) patients [37]. The halo sign may be seen in patients with cryptogenic organizing pneumonia (COP, formerly known as bronchiolitis obliterans organizing pneumonia, BOOP), pulmonary hemorrhage, pulmonary involvement by the malignancy, and other infections (e.g., cytomegalovirus, tuberculosis, abscesses, and Candida) (Figs. 12.9 and 12.10) [37]. In sum, the halo sign suggests fungal pneumonia in neutropenic patients, but is not specific. Further diagnostic investigations are therefore in order, particularly when there is no response to antifungal treatment.

The air-crescent sign and cavitation develop concomitantly with hematological reconstitution during the late phase of fungal pneumonia [37]. Thus, both findings are associated with a good prognosis. However, they lack specificity, and differential diagnoses should be considered (Figs. 12.9 and 12.10) [38]. Another useful clue to fungal pneumonia is the feeding vessel sign characterized by lesion distribution along the bronchovascular bundle.

Advances in the field of antifungal drugs have affected the radiological appearance of fungal pneumonia. Mycetomas are rare with prophylactic or early antifungal treatment. In the near future radiologists will strive not only to determine whether the findings suggest fungal pneumonia, but also whether they suggest non-*Aspergillus* fungal pneumonia.

12.3.2.3 Pneumocystis Jiroveci Pneumonia (Pcp)

Pneumocystis jiroveci pneumonia (PcP) is not a typical event in patients with hematological malignancies other than lymphoproliferative disorders, except when high-dose or prolonged immunosuppressive therapy is used, most notably in allogeneic transplant recipients with chronic graft-versus-host disease [39–43, 54]. With standard trimethoprim/sulfamethoxazole prophylaxis, PcP may develop in about 8% of patients [43]. Prophylaxis is highly effective. In patients with hematological malignancies and PcP, mortality is 4–15% overall and up to 50% in the subset requiring ICU admission [43].

CT is valuable for differentiating PcP from pneumonia due to other organisms [12, 17, 28, 29]. A combination of ground-glass opacities and intralobular septa sparing the subpleural space (i.e., in a perihilar distribution) is very typical for PcP (Fig. 12.11) [29, 44].

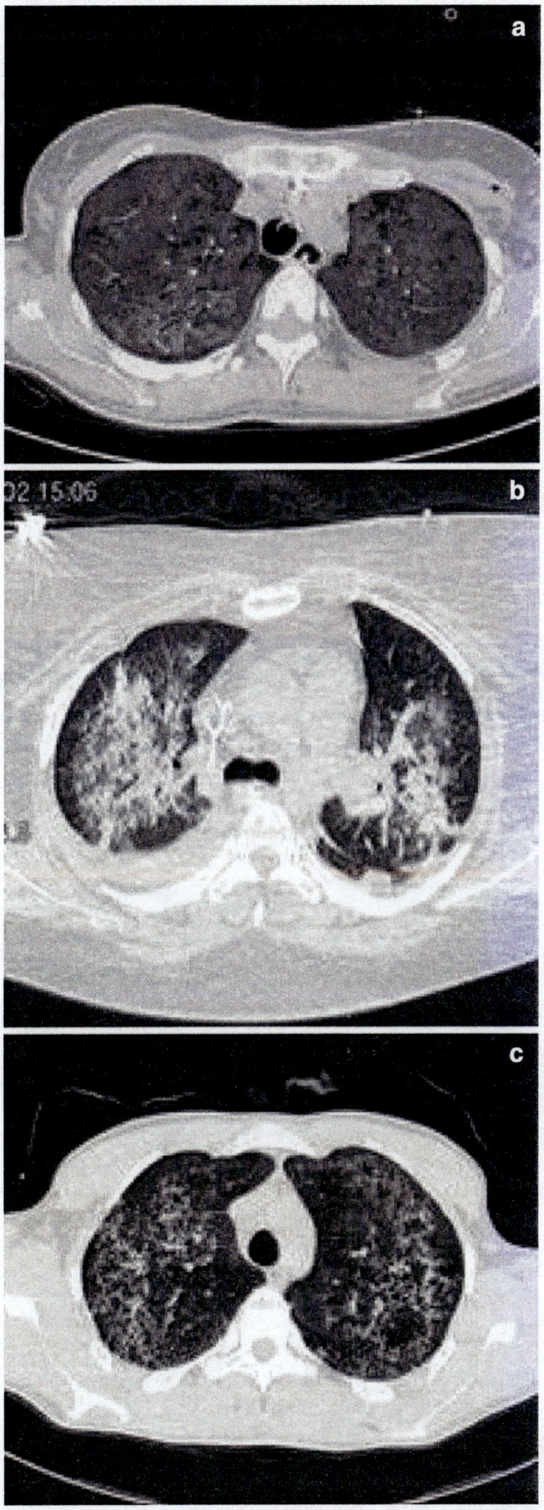

Fig. 12.11 Bilateral pneumonia caused by *Pneumocystis jiroveci* (PcP) at different stages of immunosuppression. The subpleural space is typically spared. Diffuse ground-glass opacities typically appear at the early phase of infection (**a**), while consolidations appear when the disease runs a fulminant course (**b**). Intralobular linear densities predominate in later stage or treated PcP (**c**)

12.3.2.4 Tuberculosis

Tuberculosis is a rare but relevant differential diagnosis in patients with hematological malignancies and suspected pneumonia [54]. The features of tuberculosis differ between immunocompromised patients and immunocompetent patients (e.g., primary gangliopulmonary disease) [45]. Immunocompromised patients tend to suffer greater lymphogenic and hematogenous dissemination, which may lead to a fulminant clinical course [45, 46]. Furthermore, tuberculosis may mimic or occur concomitantly with other infections such as pulmonary aspergillosis or systemic candidiasis [46].

In immunocompromised hosts, segmental bronchial spread (resulting in the "tree-in-bud" sign) of small, sometimes cavitated, ill-defined nodules may be seen, as well as military shadows [45, 46]. Primary gangliopulmonary involvement may be seen as heterogeneous consolidation and necrotic mediastinal and hilar lymphadenopathy [45].

12.3.2.5 Viral Pneumonia

Interstitial pneumonia in neutropenic patients and, most notably, after neutropenia recovery is frequently caused by a viral infection. Common culprits are cytomegalovirus, herpes viruses, influenza, parainfluenza, adenovirus, and respiratory syncytial viruses. There are no useful radiological patterns for differentiating the various forms of viral pneumonia. However, even a suspicion of viral pneumonia is very valuable information for the radiologist. Appropriate drug regimens are available for many of the causative viruses. The typical appearance of early-stage viral pneumonia is ground-glass opacification [29] and a mosaic pattern with affected and non-affected secondary lobules lying adjacent to one another (Fig. 12.12).

12.4 Non-infectious Pulmonary Disease

Several non-infectious diseases may affect the lungs in patients with hematological malignancies, such as graft-versus-host disease (GvHD), radiation toxicity, drug toxicity, pulmonary congestion, and bleeding. A fever may be related to the malignancy. For instance, in GvHD, the treatment of non-infectious infiltrates differs from that of infectious infiltrates. Thus, differentiating GvHD and infection is very helpful for

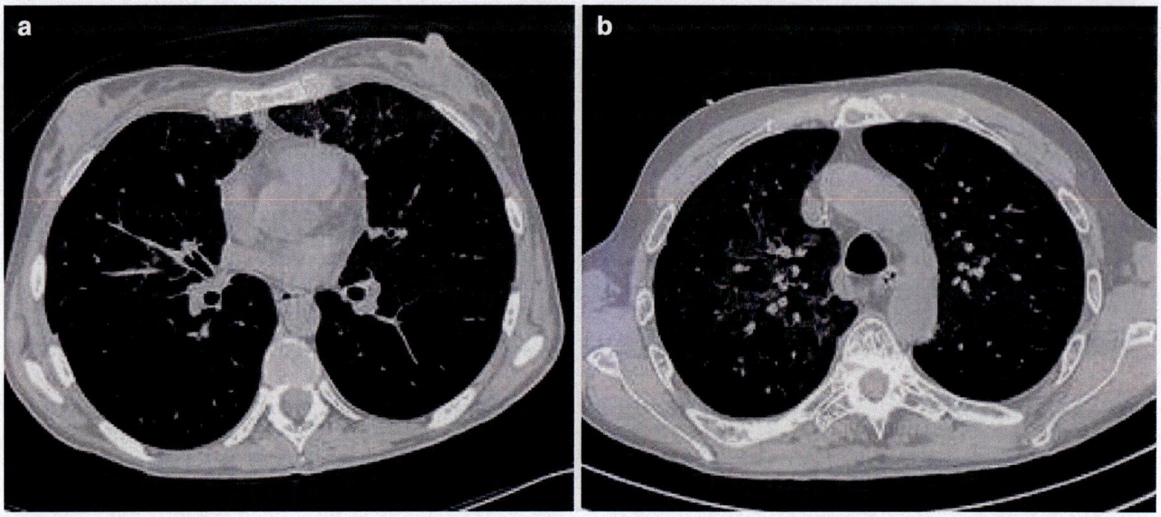

Fig. 12.12 Bilateral ground-glass opacities and mosaic pattern in two patients, A and B. However, the causative organism is cytomegalovirus in patient A (**a**) and respiratory syncytial virus in patient B (**b**). Note the mosaic pattern produced by affected and non-affected secondary lobules lying adjacent to one another

clinicians. CT can assist in detecting and characterizing non-infectious pulmonary diseases [12, 28].

12.4.1 Graft-Versus-Host Disease

Pulmonary manifestations of chronic GvHD occur in approximately 10% of allogeneic transplant recipients, usually about 9 months after the procedure (Fig. 12.13) [47] Bronchiolitis obliterans is among the pulmonary complications of GvHD [18, 54]. Unfortunately, the radiological appearance is similar to that of viral pneumonia, and the clinical signs are not specific. In early stage GvHD, pulmonary imaging may show ground-glass opacities and a mosaic pattern, as well as signs of bronchiolitis obliterans such as air trapping [18, 19] and bronchus wall thickening (Fig. 12.13), whereas intralobular septa and tree-in-bud images develop later on [47, 48].

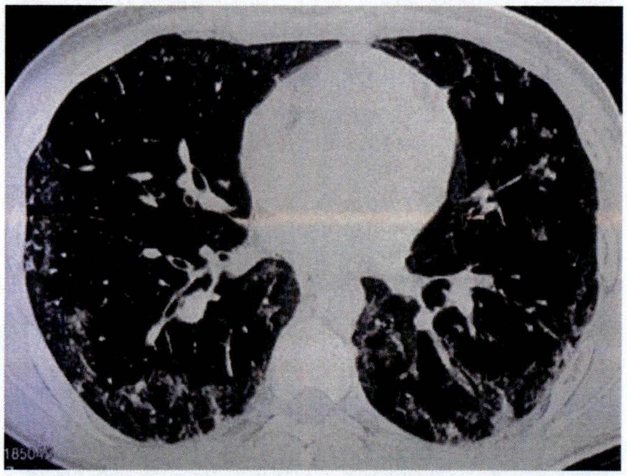

Fig. 12.13 A 28-year-old male after allogeneic re-transplantation for chronic myelogenous leukemia. HRCT was performed on post-transplantation day 91 to evaluate a fever with a cough and dyspnea. Peripheral intralobular septa (*arrow*) and ground-glass opacities were seen. The tree-in-bud pattern (*arrowhead*) suggests bronchiolitis obliterans. Acute GvHD was diagnosed by a transbronchial biopsy. The immunosuppressive treatment regimen was stepped up, after which the clinical symptoms and radiological signs disappeared. Note the similarity to Fig. 12.15

12.4.2 Radiation Toxicity

Radiation-induced pulmonary toxicity has been reported in 5–25% of patients, even after total body irradiation for conditioning before bone marrow or stem cell transplantation [49]. One problem in diagnosing radiation toxicity is that the manifestations are delayed, usually by about 3 weeks but occasionally by several months [48, 49].

CT shows ground-glass opacities with transition to consolidations (Fig. 12.14) [48, 49]. The key finding is

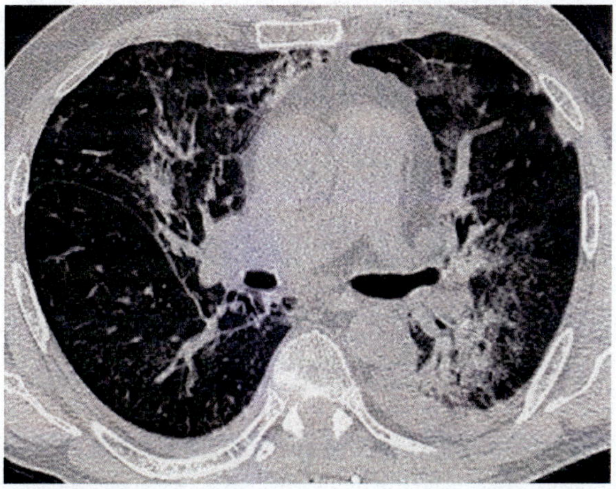

Fig. 12.14 Three weeks after local irradiation for an osteolytic vertebral tumor, this patient started experiencing a fever and dyspnea. Perihilar infiltrates appeared suddenly. HRCT showed intralobular septa, consolidation, and ground-glass opacities. The paramediastinal distribution of the infiltrates strongly suggested radiation pneumonitis. After failure of antibiotic escalation (given because of a concomitant abscess), corticosteroid therapy was added. The symptoms improved promptly and the infiltrates decreased

that these changes are confined to the radiation field. During total body irradiation, the lung parenchyma is protected, and toxicity chiefly involves the paramediastinal and apical regions. However, distortion of the lung parenchyma and the development of adhesions may blur the demarcation between exposed and non-exposed regions.

12.4.3 Drug Toxicity

Drug-induced pulmonary toxicity is particularly common with the high doses of cytotoxic agents used for conditioning. Widely used agents include bleomycin, methotrexate, cytarabine, and carmustine (Fig. 12.15) [50]. Radiologists must inform themselves about the cytotoxic agents used in their patients.

The term "drug-induced pneumonitis" encompasses several disorders, of which the most common are non-specific interstitial pneumonia and cryptogenic organizing pneumonia (COP, formerly known as bronchiolitis obliterans organizing pneumonia or BOOP) [50, 54]. The CT appearance of non-specific interstitial pneumonia consists of ground-glass opacities with transition to consolidations, intralobular septa, traction bronchiectasis, air trapping, and at a later stage the non-specific crazy-paving pattern [48, 50]. These findings are similar to those produced by radiation toxicity, but they are not limited to the radiation field. When lung toxicity is suspected but the agent is unclear, valuable information can be obtained from the French website www.pneumotox.com, which has versions in English and Spanish.

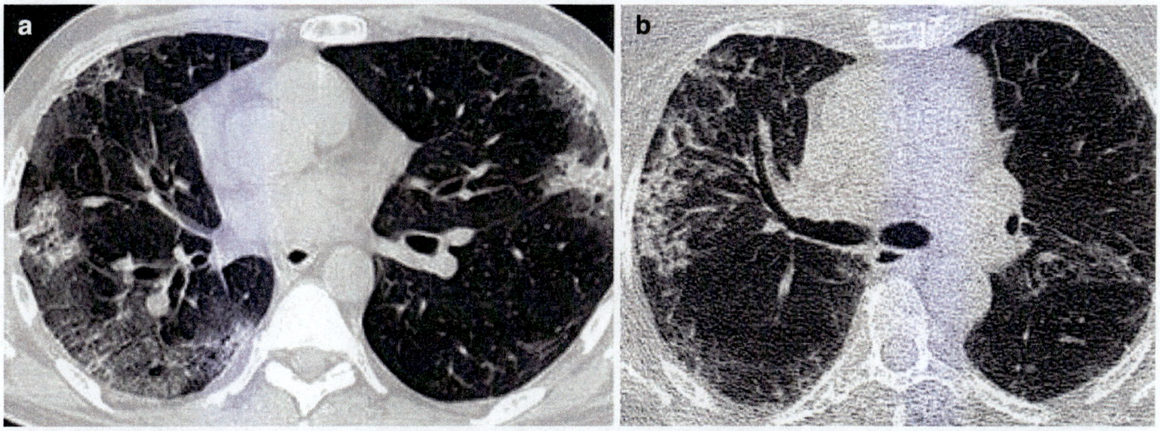

Fig. 12.15 (**a**) A 40-year-old male given chemotherapy including bleomycin (PEB protocol) for testicular cancer. CT was performed to evaluate a fever with a cough and dyspnea. Peripheral intralobular septa and ground-glass opacities were seen (**a**). The known pulmonary toxicity of the bleomycin suggested drug toxicity, which was confirmed by an open lung biopsy. Corticosteroid therapy was given. The symptoms resolved and the radiological abnormalities decreased. Note the similarity to Fig. 12.13. (**b**) In a similar clinical setting, non-specific interstitial pneumonia in a patient given cytarabine for acute myelogenous leukemia

12.4.4 Pulmonary Congestion

Pulmonary congestion is common even in younger patients, with contributing factors including central venous catheterization, extensive hydration for renal protection during chemotherapy, transient renal function impairment, and low serum protein levels. Pulmonary congestion is among the most common disorders in ICU patients with hematological malignancies. Dyspnea and lung infiltrates are common in patients with pulmonary congestion. CT shows thickening of the lymphatic vessels seen as Kerley lines (Fig. 12.16).

12.4.5 Leukemic Infiltration

Leukemic pulmonary infiltration is less common. The perilymphatic pulmonary interstitium is predominantly involved [51]. CT may show thickening of the bronchovascular bundles and interlobular septa. Nonlobular and non-segmental ground-glass opacities may be visible [28]. This pattern may mimic pulmonary congestion (Fig. 12.16).

12.4.6 Pulmonary Hemorrhage

In patients with pancytopenia, pulmonary bleeding may occur spontaneously after procedures such as bronchoalveolar lavage or during hematological reconstitution after fungal pneumonia [52]. The bleeding may be focal or diffuse. Sedimentation within the secondary lobules may be visible for a few days (Fig. 12.17).

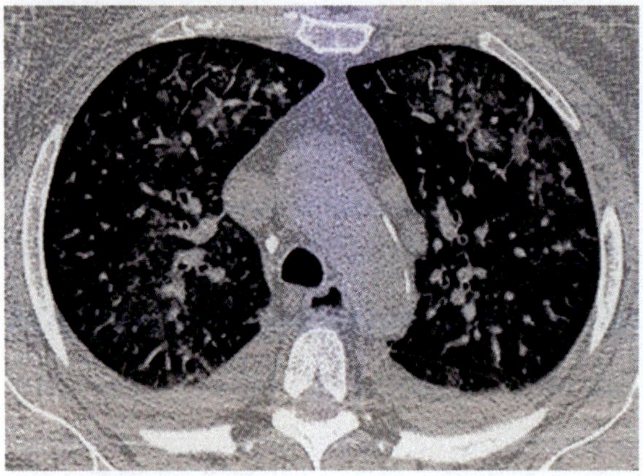

Fig. 12.16 Thickening of the intralobular septa related to fluid overload in the lymphatic vessels

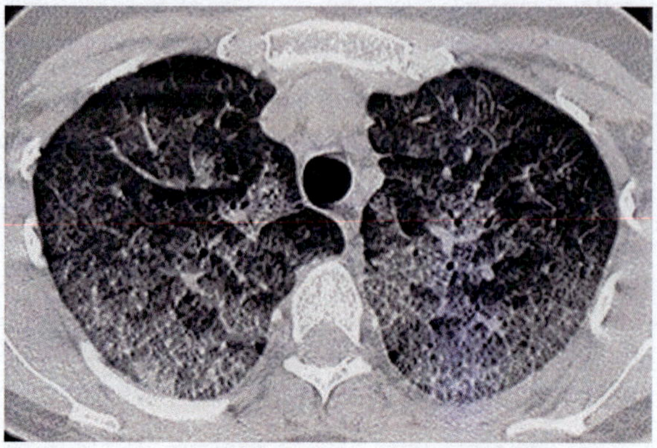

Fig. 12.17 Bilateral ground-glass opacities with an anterior-posterior gradient [1] over the entire lung and [2] within some of the secondary lobules. This gravity-dependent sedimentation phenomenon may occur temporarily and may be localized (e.g., after BAL) or a sign of diffuse pulmonary bleeding

12.5 Extrapulmonary Involvement

A global clinical approach is mandatory in these high-risk patients. Imaging can investigate liver and spleen for deep-seated infections (*Candida*, tuberculosis) or specific diseases (GvHD, VOD), gastrointestinal involvement such as infectious (CMV) or specific colitis (GvHD), infectious or non-infectious brain involvement. Interestingly since the sinuses are part of the respiratory tract, sinus infection correlates with pneumonia [53]. Sinus infections occur in up to 30% of allogeneic transplant recipients. Bone erosion and orbital or brain invasion are classified in the 2008 EORTC guideline as criteria for probable invasive fungal disease [33].

12.6 Conclusion

Many lung complications may develop in patients with neutropenia, most notably after bone marrow or stem cell transplantation. Supine CXR is not recommended for the early detection of infiltrates in these patients. When pneumonia is suspected, early thin-section CT is advisable, either to identify the cause of the fever (when lesions are seen) or to exclude the occurrence of pneumonia over the next few days (when findings are normal).

Imaging studies may show features that strongly suggest the nature of the lung disease. Close cooperation between clinicians and radiologists starting before CT scanning, together with careful image interpretation by experienced radiologists, may rapidly provide the etiological diagnosis.

References

1. Pizzo PA, Robichaud KJ, Gill FA, Witebsky FG (1982) Empiric antibiotic and antifungal therapy for cancer patients with prolonged fever and granulocytopenia. Am J Med 72:101–111
2. Hiddemann W, Maschmeyer G, Runde V, Einsele H (1996) Prevention, diagnosis and therapy of infections in patients with malignant diseases. Internist 37:1212–1224
3. Azoulay E, Thiery G, Chevret S, Moreau D, Darmon M, Bergeron A, Yang K, Meignin V, Ciroldi M, Le Gall JR, Tazi A, Schlemmer B (2004) The prognosis of acute respiratory failure in critically ill cancer patients. Medicine (Baltimore) 83(6):360–370
4. Azoulay E, Schlemmer B (2006) Diagnostic strategy in cancer patients with acute respiratory failure. Intensive Care Med 32(6):808–822
5. Maschmeyer G, Link H, Hiddemann W, Meyer P, Helmerking M, Eisenmann E, Schmitt J, Adam D (1994) Empirical antimicrobial therapy in neutropenic patients. Results of a multicenter study by the Infections in Hematology Study Group of the Paul Ehrlich Society. Med Klin 89:114–123
6. Maschmeyer G, Link H, Hiddemann W, Meyer P, Helmerking M, Eisenmann E, Schmitt J, Adam D (1994) Pulmonary infiltrations in febrile neutropenic patients. Risk factors and outcome under empirical antimicrobial therapy in a randomized multicenter trial. Cancer 73:2296–2304
7. Navigante AH, Cerchietti LC, Costantini P, Salgado H, Castro MA, Lutteral MA, Cabalar ME (2002) Conventional chest radiography in the initial assessment of adult cancer patients with fever and neutropenia. Cancer Control 9:346–351
8. Azoulay E, Darmon M, Delclaux C, Fieux F, Bornstain C, Moreau D, Attalah H, Le Gall JR, Schlemmer B (2002) Deterioration of previous acute lung injury during neutropenia recovery. Crit Care Med 30:781–786
9. Barloon TJ, Galvin JR, Mori M, Stanford W, Gingrich RD (1991) High-resolution ultrafast chest CT in the clinical management of febrile bone marrow transplant patients with normal or nonspecific chest roentgenograms. Chest 99: 928–933
10. Weber C, Maas R, Steiner P, Kramer J, Bumann D, Zander AR, Bucheler E (1999) Importance of digital thoracic radiography in the diagnosis of pulmonary infiltrates in patients with bone marrow transplantation during aplasia. Fortschr Röntgenstr 171:294–301
11. Maschmeyer G (2001) Pneumonia in febrile neutropenic patients: radiologic diagnosis. Curr Opin Oncol 13: 229–235
12. McLoud TC, Naidich DP (1992) Thoracic disease in the immunocompromised patient. Radiol Clin North Am 30:525–554
13. Cardillo I, Boal TJ, Einsiedel PF (1997) Patient doses from chest radiography in Victoria Australas. Phys Eng Sci Med 20:92–101
14. Schöpf UJ, Becker CXR, Obuchowski NA, Rust G-F, Ohnesorge BM, Kohl G, Schaller S, Modic MT, Reiser MF (2001) Multi-slice computed tomography as a screening tool for colon cancer, lung cancer and coronary artery disease. Eur Radiol 11:1975–1985
15. Remy-Jardin M, Giraud F, Remy J, Copin MC, Gosselin B, Duhamel A (1993) Computed tomography assessment of ground-glass opacity: Semiology and significance. J Thorac Imaging 8:249–264
16. Grenier PA, Beigelman-Aubry C, Fetita C, Preteux F, Brauner MW, Lenoir S (2002) New frontiers in CT imaging of airway disease. Eur Radiol 12:1022–1044
17. Schaefer-Prokop C, Prokop M, Fleischmann D, Herold C (2001) High-resolution CT of diffuse interstitial lung disease: key findings in common disorders. Eur Radiol 11: 373–392
18. Conces DJ (1999) Noninfectious lung disease in immunocompromised patients. J Thoracic Imaging 14:9–24
19. Grenier PA, Beigelman-Aubry C, Fetita C, Preteux F, Brauner MW, Lenoir S (2002) New frontiers in CT imaging of airway disease. Eur Radiol 12:1022–1044
20. Heussel CP, Kauczor H-U, Heussel G, Fischer B, Begrich M, Mildenberger P, Thelen M (1999) Pneumonia in Febrile Neutropenic Patients, Bone-Marrow and Blood Stem-Cell Recipients: use of High-Resolution CT. J Clin Oncol 17:796–805
21. Leutner CC, Gieseke J, Lutterbey G, Kuhl CK, Glasmacher A, Wardelmann E, Theisen A, Schild HH (2000) MR imaging of pneumonia in immunocompromised patients: comparison with helical CT. AJR 175:391–397
22. Eibel R, Herzog P, Dietrich O, Rieger CT, Ostermann H, Reiser MF, Schoenberg SO (2006) Pulmonary abnormalities in immunocompromised patients: comparative detection with parallel acquisition MR imaging and thin-section helical CT. Radiology 241:880–891
23. Maschmeyer G, Buchheidt D, Einsele H, Heußel CP, Holler E, Lorenz J, Schweigert M (1999) Diagnostik und Therapie von Lungeninfiltraten bei febrilen neutropenischen Patienten – Leitlinien der Arbeitsgemeinschaft Infektionen in der Hämatologie und Onkologie der Deutschen Gesellschaft für Hämatologie und Onkologie. Dtsch Med Wochenschr 9; 124(Suppl 1):S18–23
24. Caillot D, Couaillier JF, Bernard A, Casasnovas O, Denning DW, Mannone L, Lopez J, Couillault G, Piard F, Vagner O, Guy H (2001) Increasing volume and changing characteristics of invasive pulmonary aspergillosis on sequential thoracic computed tomography scans in patients with neutropenia. J Clin Oncol 19:253–259
25. Davies SF (1994) Fungal pneumonia. Med Clin North Am 78:1049–1065
26. Serra P, Santini C, Venditti M, Mandelli F, Martino P (1985) Superinfections during antimicrobial treatment with betalactam-aminoglycoside combinations in neutropenic patients with hematologic malignancies. Infection 13(Suppl 1):S115–S122
27. Azoulay E, Mokart D, Rabbat A, Pene F, Kouatchet A, Bruneel F, Vincent F, Hamidfar R, Moreau D, Mohammedi I, Epinette G, Beduneau G, Castelain V, de Lassence A, Gruson D, Lemiale V, Renard B, Chevret S, Schlemmer B (2008) Diagnostic bronchoscopy in hematology and oncology patients with acute respiratory failure: prospective multicenter data. Crit Care Med 36(1): 100–107

28. Tanaka N, Matsumoto T, Miura G, Emoto T, Matsunaga N (2002) HRCT findings of chest complications in patients with leukemia. Eur Radiol 12:1512–1522
29. Reittner P, Ward S, Heyneman L, Johkoh T, Müller NL (2003) Pneumonia: high-resolution CT findings in 114 patients. Eur Radiol 13:515–521
30. Conces DJ (1998) Bacterial pneumonia in immunocompromised patients. J Thoracic Imaging 13:261–270
31. Heußel CP, Ullmann AJ, Kauczor H-U (2000) Fungal pneumonia. Radiologe 40:518–529
32. Ascioglu S, Rex JH, de Pauw B, Bennett JE, Bille J, Crokaert F, Denning DW, Donnelly JP, Edwards JE, Erjavec Z, Fiere D, Lortholary O, Maertens J, Meis JF, Patterson TF, Ritter J, Selleslag D, Shah PM, Stevens DA, Walsh TJ (2002) Defining opportunistic invasive fungal infections in immunocompromised patients with cancer and hematopoietic stem cell transplants: An International Consensus. Clin Infect Dis 34:7–14
33. De Pauw B, Walsh TJ, Donnelly JP, Stevens DA, Edwards JE, Calandra T, Pappas PG, Maertens J, Lortholary O, Kauffman CA, Denning DW, Patterson TF, Maschmeyer G, Bille J, Dismukes WE, Herbrecht R, Hope WW, Kibbler CC, Kullberg BJ, Marr KA, Muñoz P, Odds FC, Perfect JR, Restrepo A, Ruhnke M, Segal BH, Sobel JD, Sorrell TC, Viscoli C, Wingard JR, Zaoutis T, Bennett JE (2008) European Organization for Research and Treatment of Cancer/Invasive Fungal Infections Cooperative Group; National Institute of Allergy and Infectious Diseases Mycoses Study Group (EORTC/MSG) Consensus Group: Revised definitions of invasive fungal disease from the European Organization for Research and Treatment of Cancer/Invasive Fungal Infections Cooperative Group and the National Institute of Allergy and Infectious Diseases Mycoses Study Group (EORTC/MSG) Consensus Group. Clin Infect Dis 46:1813–1821
34. Gefter WB, Albelda S, Talbot G, Gerson S, Cassileth P, Miller WT (1984) New observations on the significance of the air crescent in invasive pulmonary aspergillosis. Radiology 153:136
35. Kuhlman JE, Fishman EK, Siegelman SS (1985) Invasive pulmonary aspergillosis in acute leukemia: characteristic findings on CT, the CT halo sign, and the role of CT in early diagnosis. Radiology 157:611–614
36. Greene RE, Schlamm HT, Oestmann JW, Stark P, Durand C, Lortholary O, Wingard JR, Herbrecht R, Ribaud P, Patterson TF, Troke PF, Denning DW, Bennett JE, de Pauw BE, Rubin RH (2007) Imaging findings in acute invasive pulmonary aspergillosis: clinical significance of the halo sign. Clin Infect Dis 44:373–379
37. Kim K, Lee MH, Kim J, Lee KS, Kim SM, Jung MP, Han J, Sung KW, Kim WS, Jung CW, Yoon SS, Im YH, Kang WK, Park K, Park CH (2002) Importance of open lung biopsy in the diagnosis of invasive pulmonary aspergillosis in patients with hematologic malignancies. Am J Hematol 71:75–79
38. Kim MJ, Lee KS, Kim J, Jung KJ, Lee HG, Kim TS (2001) Crescent sign in invasive pulmonary aspergillosis: frequency and related CT and clinical factors. J Comput Assist Tomogr 25:305–310
39. Saito T, Seo S, Kanda Y, Shoji N, Ogasawara T, Murakami J, Tanosaki R, Tobinai K, Takaue Y, Mineishi S (2001) Early onset Pneumocystis carinii pneumonia after allogeneic peripheral blood stem cell transplantation. Am J Hematol 67(3):206–209
40. Kovacs JA, Hiemenz JW, Macher AM, Stover D, Murray HW, Shelhamer J, Lane HC, Urmacher C, Honig C, Longo DL et al (1984) Pneumocystis carinii pneumonia: a comparison between patients with the acquired immunodeficiency syndrome and patients with other immunodeficiencies. Ann Intern Med 100(5):663–671
41. Zahar JR, Robin M, Azoulay E, Fieux F, Nitenberg G, Schlemmer B (2002) Pneumocystis carinii pneumonia in critically ill patients with malignancy: a descriptive study. Clin Infect Dis 35(8):929–934
42. De Castro N, Neuville S, Sarfati C, Ribaud P, Derouin F, Gluckman E, Socié G, Molina JM (2005 Nov) Occurrence of Pneumocystis jiroveci pneumonia after allogeneic stem cell transplantation: a 6-year retrospective study. Bone Marrow Transplant 36(10):879–883
43. Bollée G, Sarfati C, Thiéry G, Bergeron A, de Miranda S, Menotti J, de Castro N, Tazi A, Schlemmer B, Azoulay E (2007 Oct) Clinical picture of Pneumocystis jiroveci pneumonia in cancer patients. Chest 132(4):1305–1310
44. McGuinness G, Gruden JF (1999) Viral and Pneumocystis carinii infections of the lung in the immunocompromized host. J Thorac Imaging 14:25–36
45. Van Dyck P, Vanhoenacker FM, Van den Brande P, De Schepper AM (2003 Aug) Imaging of pulmonary tuberculosis. Eur Radiol 13(8):1771–1785
46. Goo JM, Im JG (2002) CT of tuberculosis and nontuberculous mycobacterial infections. Radiol Clin North Am 40:73–87
47. Leblond V, Zouabi H, Sutton L, Guillon JM, Mayaud CM, Similowski T, Beigelman C, Autran B (1994) Late CD8+ lymphocytic alveolitis after allogeneic bone marrow transplantation and chronic graft-versus-host disease. Am J Respir Crit Care Med 150:1056–1061
48. Oikonomou A, Hansell DM (2002) Organizing pneumonia: the many morphological faces. Eur Radiol 12: 1486–1496
49. Monson JM, Stark P, Reilly JJ, Sugarbaker DJ, Strauss GM, Swanson SJ, Decamp MM, Mentzer SJ, Baldini EH (1998) Clinical radiation pneumonitis and radiographic changes after thoracic radiation therapy for lung carcinoma. Cancer 82:842–850
50. Erasmus JJ, McAdams HP, Rossi SE (2002) High-resolution CT of drug-induced lung disease. Radiol Clin North Am 40:61–72
51. Heyneman LE, Johkoh T, Ward S, Honda O, Yoshida S, Muller NL (2000) Pulmonary leukemic infiltrates: high-resolution CT findings in ten patients. AJR Am J Roentgenol 174:517–521
52. Heussel CP, Kauczor HU, Heussel G, Mildenberger P, Dueber C (1997) Aneurysms complicating inflammatory diseases in immunocompromised hosts: value of contrast-enhanced CT. Eur Radiol 7:316–319
53. Savage DG, Taylor P, Blackwell J et al (1997) Paranasal sinusitis following allogeneic bone marrow transplant. BMT 19:55–59
54. Lass-Florl C, Resch G, Nachbaur D, Mayr A, Gastl G, Auberger J, Bialek R, Freund MC (2007) The value of computed tomography guided percutaneous lung biopsy for diagnosis of invasive fungal infection in immunocompromised patients. Clin Infect Dis 45:e101–e104

Is There Still a Place for Transbronchial Lung Biopsy or Other Lung Biopsy Techniques?

13

Christophe Dooms and Vincent Ninane

Contents

C. Dooms
University Hospitals Leuven,
49, Herestraat, 3000,
Leuven, Belgium

V. Ninane (✉)
C.H.U. St Pierre – Clinique de Pneumologie,
Saint-Pierre University Hospital Brussels,
322, rue Haute, 1000,
Brussels, Belgium
e-mail: vincent_ninane@stpierre-bru.be,
ninanev@scarlet.be

13.1 Introduction

With the expanding use of immunosuppression (e.g., hematopoietic stem cell transplantation and high-dose chemotherapy for aggressive malignancies), respiratory and critical care physicians are increasingly providing care to immunocompromised patients. In patients with hematological malignancies, several conditions can cause immunodeficiency, including the malignancy itself (e.g., leukemia or lymphoma); chemotherapy within the last 3 months; long-term corticosteroid therapy (i.e., ≥20 mg/day prednisone for ≥2 months); high-dose corticosteroid therapy (≥60 mg/day prednisone for ≥2 weeks within the last 3 months); bone marrow or stem cell transplantation; and use of immunosuppressive drugs. The clinical presentation of immunocompromised patients with lung infiltrates seems nonspecific. Symptoms consist of shortness of breath, a cough, fever, and, in many cases, progressive hypoxemia. In patients with known immunosuppression, an opportunistic infection is immediately suspected, but many infectious and noninfectious causes should be considered also. Noninfectious processes are responsible for about 25–50% of pulmonary infiltrates in immunocompromised patients [1, 2]. The radiological changes caused by opportunistic infections may be difficult to distinguish from malignant lung infiltration, heart failure, or cancer chemotherapy toxicity. Moreover, radiation therapy, graft-versus-host disease, acute or chronic rejection, and idiopathic pulmonary disorders (i.e., alveolar proteinosis, diffuse alveolar damage, organizing pneumonia, and diffuse alveolar hemorrhage) may also contribute to the development of pulmonary complications in this setting. As an example, in a series of patients with hematological malignancies and lung infiltrates assessed by open

É. Azoulay (ed.), *Pulmonary Involvement in Patients with Hematological Malignancies*,
DOI: 10.1007/978-3-642-15742-4_13, © Springer-Verlag Berlin Heidelberg 2011

lung biopsy, infections accounted for only 36% of the specific diagnoses, and 67% of the cases were related to the malignancy or to inflammatory processes [3]. Another retrospective series including 213 patients with hematological malignancies and pulmonary lesions found that computed tomography (CT)-guided percutaneous biopsy provided a specific diagnosis in 60% of cases; the most common specific diagnoses were malignancy (63%) and infection (34%) [4]. In addition, two or more different processes may affect the lung simultaneously in immunocompromised patients. Malignancy is more often the cause of the pulmonary infiltrates in patients with lung lesions but no respiratory signs/symptoms or fever, whereas infection is more common in patients with acute leukemia, neutropenia, ongoing chemotherapy, or bone marrow transplantation.

Pulmonary infiltrates are a frequent cause of morbidity and mortality in immunocompromised patients and remain a diagnostic challenge. In a study of HIV-negative immunocompromised patients with pulmonary infiltrates, three factors predicted mortality: severity of illness as measured by the APACHE II score, need for mechanical ventilation, and longer time to a specific diagnosis [5]. A greater than 5day delay in identifying the cause of the pulmonary infiltrates independently increased the risk of death by more than threefold [5]. One hypothesis is that this effect of time-to-diagnosis reflects the fact that noninfectious causes are both more severe and more difficult to diagnose. However, the early diagnosis of both viral and fungal infections has also been shown to decrease mortality [6]. The early etiological diagnosis of focal or diffuse pulmonary infiltrates can be achieved by serological testing (including polymerase chain reaction technologies), sputum analysis, and bronchoscopic techniques, including bronchoalveolar lavage (BAL). Although BAL is the main invasive diagnostic procedure used in immunocompromised patients with pulmonary infiltrates, its diagnostic yield is only about 50% [7], and additional invasive procedures such as transbronchial biopsy (TBB), CT-guided percutaneous lung biopsy, or surgical lung biopsy (SLB) are often considered. These invasive techniques can supply tissue samples measuring about 1 mm to several centimeters in size, which may allow the identification of both infectious and noninfectious processes. No randomized trial comparing invasive and noninvasive tools has been performed in immunocompromised patients. In this population, only retrospective and prospective observational studies are available.

Pulmonary lesions in patients with hematological malignancies vary in their severity and etiology according to the type of underlying malignancy, clinical presentation, and time of lung lesion discovery during the course of the disease. The efficacy of TBB, CT-guided percutaneous lung biopsy, or SLB depends largely on the clinical setting and radiological pattern of the pulmonary infiltrate.

13.2 Is There Still a Place for Transbronchial Lung Biopsy?

As long as BAL remains the cornerstone of the diagnostic evaluation of immunocompromised patients with pulmonary involvement, the role for TBB will be a matter of interest because a forceps can be introduced through the operating channel of the bronchoscope to biopsy peripheral lesions or infiltrates. Several technical aspects and limitations of TBB should, however, be taken into account before discussing the potential of TBB for providing additional information in patients with hematological malignancies.

In patients with nodules or masses (but not diffuse involvement), fluoroscopy may be helpful and may increase the diagnostic yield of TBB provided the lesion is larger than 2 cm [8]. Similarly, lung CT may allow site-directed (but not real-time-guided) TBB, which is associated with an increased diagnostic yield (Fig. 13.1) [9]. The size of the forceps used for TBB has an impact, as larger forceps retrieve larger samples that have a higher diagnostic yield with no additional risk of bleeding [10]. One frequent contraindication in these patients is thrombocytopenia, and it is important to stress that TBB can be performed safely after a platelet transfusion [11, 12], although no specific recommendations have been published. As an example, White and colleagues suggested that the platelet count should exceed $30 \cdot 10^9$/L for TBB [13]. The main complications of TBB are pneumothorax and bleeding, but these are seldom encountered [14]. More often, bronchoscopy is associated with a (temporary) decrease in arterial oxygen tension. Therefore, bronchoscopy has been considered relatively contraindicated when, despite supplemental O_2 delivery, PaO_2 remains lower than 75 mmHg or oxygen saturation lower than 90% [15].

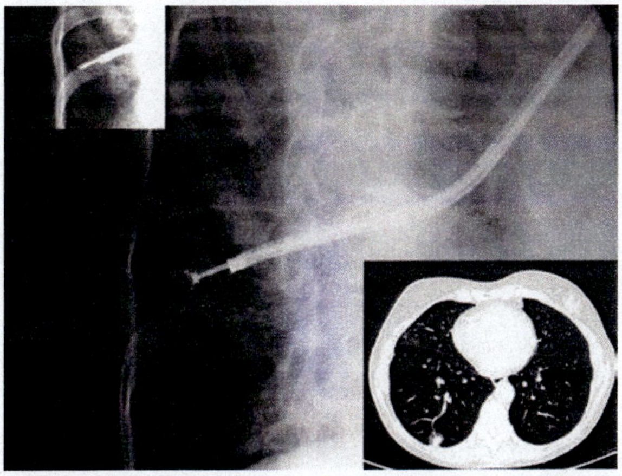

Fig. 13.1 A 47-year-old patient presented with fever and elevated liver enzymes 4 months after allogeneic BMT for relapsing AML. He was receiving steroids for acute GVHD (isolated skin involvement for 3 weeks). Liver biopsy was diagnostic of uncontrolled GVHD, and immunosuppressants were increased. CT was diagnostic of an isolated pulmonary nodule. Sputa examinations as well as BAL fluid analysis were negative. Invasive pulmonary aspergillosis was confirmed by trans-bronchial biopsy

Oxygenation strategies maintain sufficient oxygenation during bronchoscopy and increase the safety of bronchoscopy. In selected patients, bronchoscopy and BAL performed using Boussignac continuous positive airway pressure was safe, with no subsequent respiratory deterioration [16]. Safety is crucial since mechanical ventilation required by complications of BAL with TBB is associated with a high mortality rate that tends to override the expected benefit from the procedure [7, 11, 14].

13.2.1 TBB Increases the Diagnostic Yield of BAL in Non-neutropenic Patients

In non-neutropenic, non-HIV-infected immunocompromised patients, TBB has been shown to increase the diagnostic yield of BAL by 30% [17–20]. TBB may contribute to the diagnostic yield of BAL both in infectious processes (by allowing histopathological confirmation of cytomegalovirus pneumonitis or granulomatous lung diseases such as tuberculosis) and in noninfectious processes (by allowing histopathological confirmation of underlying malignant infiltration, lymphoma, organizing pneumonia, graft-versus-host disease, radiation-induced pneumonitis, or diffuse alveolar damage).

In a retrospective study [18], only 11 of 95 immunocompromised patients with hematological disorders had sufficient platelet counts to allow TBB, but the procedure was diagnostic in 7 (64%) of them. Similarly, a prospective study [1] of 200 immunocompromised patients showed that TBB was performed in only 11 patients but was diagnostic in 6 (55%) of them, most of whom had their treatment changed as a result of the findings. In another prospective study [19], TBB was possible in 45 of 104 immunocompromised patients (46% with hematological malignancies, 60% receiving chemotherapy, and >75% receiving long-term systemic corticosteroid therapy). Overall, BAL had a diagnostic yield of 38%. In the 45 patients who underwent TBB, the diagnostic yield was 44% for TBB and 70% for BAL plus TBB. TBB was the only investigation that provided the diagnosis in 28% of patients, of whom all but two had noninfectious infiltrates. Pneumothorax was the most frequent complication after TBB, with a rate of 4%. In a study evaluating the diagnostic usefulness of adding TBB to BAL in immunocompromised patients with hematological malignancies [20], BAL performed well for diagnosing infections (particularly fungal infections), whereas combined BAL and TBB was superior over BAL alone for diagnosing neoplastic infiltrates and toxic pneumonitis.

13.2.2 TBB Does Not Increase the Diagnostic Yield of BAL in Patients with Neutropenic Fever or in Patients on Mechanical Ventilation

In a retrospective study of a population with febrile neutropenia (neutrophils <1,000 $\times 10^9$/L), including 80% of patients with hematological malignancies [21], more than 75% of all pulmonary infiltrates were attributable to infections. The diagnostic yield of BAL was 49%, and sputum analysis increased the yield to 63%. TBB provided additional information in only 1% of patients. Thus, TBB should be considered of limited usefulness in neutropenic patients.

A retrospective study in mechanically ventilated immunocompromised patients showed that TBB was diagnostic in 35% of cases, but that the diagnoses (mainly *Pneumocystis* and CMV pneumonia) would also have been made by BAL [22]. In a small retrospective study, TBB performed during mechanical ventilation was diagnostic in only 31% of immunocompromised patients [23]. In mechanically ventilated patients, TBB is often contraindicated because of the patient's oxygen requirements or of the procedure's low sensitivity and high morbidity (40% pneumothorax rate) in severely hypoxemic patients. Recent data indicate that invasive aspergillosis may be underestimated in immunocompromised ICU patients with pneumonia [24]. Early galactomannan detection in BAL was 88% sensitive and 87% specific when a cutoff of 0.5 was used, which was significantly better than fungal culture and/or microscopic BAL examination or galactomannan detection in serum [25].

13.3 Is There Still a Place for CT-Guided Percutaneous Lung Biopsies or Surgical Lung Biopsies?

13.3.1 CT-Guided Percutaneous Lung Biopsy

CT-guided percutaneous lung biopsy requires transportation of the patient to the radiology department and may therefore not be the procedure of choice for patients with severe acute respiratory failure and/or mechanical ventilation with high FiO_2 values. As with TBB, CT-guided percutaneous lung biopsy can be performed after platelet transfusion to correct low platelet counts, as done in as many as 46 among 213 patients in a recent non-ICU study [4]. The diagnostic yield is up to 60%. However, pneumothorax occurred in 38.5% of cases and required chest tube drainage, usually on an ambulatory basis, a finding that deserves consideration as most of these patients initially had no respiratory signs or symptoms [4].

13.3.2 Open Lung Biopsy

Open lung biopsy is believed to be safe and reliable in patients with non-severe events and may be associated with a substantial diagnostic yield in those with diffuse lung disease [26]. Video-assisted thoracoscopy is being increasingly used as an alternative to open thoracotomy. In the only prospective randomized study available to date, thoracostomy was not associated with lower morbidity and mortality rates compared to thoracotomy [27]. An open procedure is often preferred in patients with severe hypoxemia. A bedside 10-cm lateral thoracotomy can be performed in patients with acute respiratory distress syndrome to obtain specimens 3–5 cm in size with no risk of death and with only a small decrease in the PaO_2/FiO_2 ratio [28].

13.3.3 CT-Guided Lung Biopsy Has a High Diagnostic Yield in Patients with Known Hematological Malignancies and Focal Pulmonary Lesions

In a retrospective study of 213 patients, CT-guided percutaneous biopsy provided a specific diagnosis in 60% of patients; the most common specific diagnoses were malignancy (63%) and infection (34%) [4]. Most of these patients had no respiratory signs/symptoms or positive cultures from BAL or TBB specimens, but chest CT disclosed nodules (59%), masses (12%), cavitary lesions (10%), or consolidation (19%). Importantly, biopsies of focal lesions (mainly cavitary lesions or lung masses) had a higher diagnostic yield than biopsies of diffuse lesions. CT-guided percutaneous biopsy yielded a specific diagnosis in 37 (53%) of the 70 patients with a previous non-diagnostic BAL, TBB, or both (but it is unknown whether these procedures were image-guided). In addition, in 14 patients with no specific diagnosis after CT-guided lung biopsy, BAL and TBB were performed and provided a specific diagnosis in only 4 patients, who had positive cultures of BAL or TBB specimens [4].

Other small retrospective studies have confirmed the usefulness of CT-guided transthoracic lung biopsy for the diagnosis of focal pulmonary lesions in patients with hematological malignancies. As an example, in a study of 24 patients with suspected pulmonary infection including 8 patients with hematological malignancies [29], CT-guided needle biopsy of parenchymal consolidation with or without cavitation identified one or more etiologic microorganisms in 19 (79.2%) patients.

Importantly, similar diagnostic yields have been reported using fluoroscopic-guided transthoracic biopsy, without CT [30, 31]. Thus, one possibility is that BAL combined with fluoroscopy-guided TBB [8] during the same procedure may be comparable with CT-guided lung biopsy for the diagnosis of focal lesions in patients with hematological malignancies, while, however, being associated with a lower risk of pneumothorax.

13.3.4 The Diagnostic Yield of Surgical Lung Biopsy (SLB) in Patients with Hematological Malignancies and Lung Infiltrates Varies with the Presentation

In general, SLB is considered the reference standard for diagnosing interstitial lung disease. Several recent retrospective studies reassessed the role for SLB in patients with hematological malignancies and lung infiltrates. In one of these studies, 63 patients with hematological malignancies underwent SLB for lung processes of unknown etiology [3]. A specific diagnosis was found in 62% of patients and led to a change in treatment in 57%. Survival rates after 1 and 3 months were also higher in patients with a specific diagnosis. Infections accounted for only 33% of the specific diagnoses and malignancy or inflammatory processes for the remaining 67%. The authors attributed this finding to widespread use of preemptive, prophylactic, and empiric strategies, as well as to the widespread use of invasive bronchoscopic (and other) diagnostic tests. Interestingly, they also studied the relationships between clinical factors and achieving a specific diagnosis. In the seven patients on mechanical ventilation or with neutropenia, SLB provided no specific diagnosis. In addition, a specific diagnosis was less frequently obtained in the group with prior bronchoscopy ($n = 35$, specific diagnosis in 48%) than in the group without previous bronchoscopy ($n = 32$, specific diagnosis in 75%). Finally, a focal radiographic pattern was associated with a higher specific diagnosis rate ($n = 39$; specific diagnosis in 79%) than a diffuse radiographic pattern ($n = 28$; specific diagnosis in 32%), as previously reported in similar patient populations [32, 33]. In another retrospective study [34], 39 immunocompromised patients (including 30 with hematological malignancies) were studied, and a clinical benefit defined as changes in treatment was observed in 46% of the patients; however, the overall mortality rate was high (39%).

In a retrospective study [35] in 62 patients with hematological malignancies or hematopoietic stem cell transplantation, SLB provided a specific diagnosis in 67% of patients and led to changes in treatment in 40%. The main specific diagnoses were infection (29%, mainly aspergillosis), malignancy (27%), and inflammatory conditions (11%). Mortality was lower in the patients who had a specific diagnosis. BAL was performed before SLB in 34 (54%) patients and was non-diagnostic in 28. Of the 13 patients on mechanical ventilation, only 4 (30%) had a specific diagnosis. A focal radiographic pattern was not associated with a significantly higher specific diagnosis rate ($n = 33$; specific diagnosis in 70%) than a diffuse pattern ($n = 29$; specific diagnosis in 58%). In contrast, in stem cell transplantation recipients with pulmonary infiltrates, SLB findings led to treatment changes in only a few cases, and eight of the nine patients who required mechanical ventilation died [36]. Finally, the impact of bedside open lung biopsies on the management of mechanically ventilated immunocompromised patients with acute respiratory distress syndrome was studied [37]. Among the 19 patients, 10 had hematological malignancies, and most of them had extensive investigations including chest CT and bronchoscopy. SLB provided a specific diagnosis in 13 (68%) patients and prompted major changes in management in 89%. However, 9 of the 13 specific diagnoses consisted in diffuse alveolar damage, which was classified among nonspecific diagnoses in previous studies, and 17 of the 19 patients died in the ICU [3, 35].

13.4 Conclusion

A prompt diagnosis seems crucial for improving the survival of immunocompromised patients with pulmonary infiltrates [5, 38]. Pulmonary involvement in patients with hematological malignancies can be due to a variety of causes, among which the most common are malignancy and infection. Early noninvasive tests should be performed, with or without invasive tests depending on the clinical presentation. Thoracic CT should be performed routinely before invasive procedures (TBB, CT-guided biopsy, or SLB), as it provides important diagnostic information and may increase the diagnostic yield of the invasive procedure by improving selection of the technique and sampling site.

In patients with hematological malignancies who are selected for bronchoscopy with BAL, TBB is a source of additional information in up to 30% of cases and is best performed under fluoroscopic guidance. The diagnostic yield of TBB ranged from 26% to 68% in published studies. Routine TBB is not recommended in immunocompromised patients, due to safety issues and to uncertainty about the clinical relevance of TBB in some situations. In non-neutropenic patients scheduled for diagnostic bronchoscopy, TBB (if not contraindicated) should be combined with BAL in the initial diagnostic workup only when non-infectious causes of lung infiltrates are suspected, to avoid sequential procedures. In neutropenic patients scheduled for bronchoscopy, TBB should not be performed, as it adds little to the diagnostic yield but increases the complication rate.

Both CT-guided biopsy and SLB seem relatively safe but are clearly more invasive than BAL plus TBB. Their diagnostic yield is good, most notably in patients who have focal lesions. Studies of SLB suggest that performing a bronchoscopy first may decrease the need for SLB [3]. Thus, the best initial procedure may be BAL with or without TBB under fluoroscopic guidance, in particular in patients with focal lesions.

In the ICU and in mechanically ventilated patients, BAL and TBB are not recommended, although they occasionally constitute useful alternatives to SLB. In this setting, TBB has a low diagnostic yield and can cause pneumothorax with potentially severe consequences. CT-guided biopsy should be reserved for selected patients, because it requires patient transportation to the radiology department. Last, SLB is rarely performed because studies clearly suggest a very low diagnostic yield in ICU and mechanically ventilated patients, with a questionable impact on the already elevated mortality rate.

References

1. Rano A, Agusti C, Jimenez P et al (2001) Pulmonary infiltrates in non-HIV immunocompromised patients: a diagnostic approach using non-invasive and bronchoscopic procedures. Thorax 56:379–387
2. Torres A, Ewig S, Insausti J et al (2000) Etiology and microbial patterns of pulmonary infiltrates in patients with orthotopic liver transplantation. Chest 117:494–502
3. White D, Wong P, Downey R (2000) The utility of open lung biopsy in patients with hematologic malignancies. Am J Respir Crit Care Med 161:723–729
4. Gupta S, Sultenfuss M, Romaguera J et al (2009) CT-guided percutaneous lung biopsies in patients with haematologic malignancies and undiagnosed pulmonary lesions. Hematol Oncol 28(2):75–81
5. Rano A, Agusti C, Benito N et al (2002) Prognostic factors of non-HIV immunocompromised patients with pulmonary infiltrates. Chest 122:253–261
6. Von Eiff M, Roos N, Schulten R (1995) Pulmonary aspergillosis: early diagnosis improves survival. Respiration 62: 341–347
7. Azoulay E, de Miranda S, Bèle N, Schlemmer B (2008) Stratégie diagnostique dans l'insuffisance respiratoire aiguë des patients d'oncohématologie. Rev Mal Respir 25: 433–448
8. Chechani V (1996) Bronchoscopic diagnosis of solitary pulmonary nodules and lung masses in the absence of endobronchial abnormality. Chest 109:620–625
9. Cadranel J, Gillet-Juvin K, Antoine M, Carnot F, Reynaud P, Parrot A, Carette MF, Mayaud C, Israël-Biet D (1995) Site-directed bronchoalveolar lavage and transbronchial biopsy in HIV-infected patients with pneumonia. Am J Respir Crit Care Med 52:1103–1106
10. Loube DI, Johnson JE, Wiener D, Anders GT, Blanton HM, Hayes JA (1993) The effect of forceps size on the adequacy of specimens obtained by transbronchial biopsy. Am Rev Respir Dis 148(5):1411–1413
11. Weiss SM, Hert RC, Gianola FJ, Clark JG, Crawford SW (1993) Complications of fiberoptic bronchoscopy in thrombocytopenic patients. Chest 104:1025–1028
12. Papin TA, Lynch JP, Weg JG (1985) Transbronchial biopsy in the thrombocytopenic patient. Chest 88:549–552
13. White P, Bonacum JT, Miller CG (1997) Utility of fiberoptic bronchoscopy in bone marrow transplant patients. Bone Marrow Transplant 20:681–687
14. Pue CA, Pacht ER (1995) Complications of fiberoptic bronchoscopy at a university hospital. Chest 107:430–432
15. American Thoracic Society (1990) Clinical role of bronchoalveolar lavage in adults with pulmonary disease. Am Rev Respir Dis 142:481–486
16. Maitre B, Jaber S, Maggiore SM, Bergot E, Richard JC, Bakthiari H, Housset B, Boussignac G, Brochard L (2000) Continuous positive airway pressure during fiberoptic bronchoscopy in hypoxemic patients. A randomized double-blind study using a new device. Am J Respir Crit Care Med 162:1063–1067
17. Cazzadori A, Di Perri G, Todeschini G et al (1995) Transbronchial biopsy in the diagnosis of pulmonary infiltrates in immunocompromised patients. Chest 107:101–106

18. Hohenadel I, Kiworr M, Genitsariotis R et al (2001) Role of bronchoalveolar lavage in immunocompromised patients with pneumonia treated with a broad spectrum antibiotic and antifungal regimen. Thorax 56:115–120
19. Jain P, Sandur S, Meli Y et al (2004) Role of bronchoscopy in immunocompromised patients with lung infiltrates. Chest 125:712–722
20. Mulabecirovic A, Gaulhofer P, Auner H et al (2004) Pulmonary infiltrates in patients with hematologic malignancies: transbronchial lung biopsy increases the diagnostic yield with respect to neoplastic infiltrates and toxic pneumonitis. Ann Hematol 83:420–422
21. Peikert T, Rana S, Edell E (2005) Safety, diagnostic yield, and therapeutic implications of flexible bronchoscopy in patients with febrile neutropenia and pulmonary infiltrates. Mayo Clin Proc 80:1414–1420
22. O'Brien J, Ettinger N, Shevlin D et al (1997) Safety and yield of transbronchial biopsy in mechanically ventilated patients. Crit Care Med 25:440–446
23. Bulpa P, Dive A, Mertens L et al (2003) Combined bronchoalveolar lavage and transbronchial lung biopsy: safety and yield in ventilated patients. Eur Respir J 21:489–494
24. Meersseman W, Vandecasteele S, Wilmer A et al (2004) Invasive aspergillosis in critically ill patients without malignancy. Am J Respir Crit Care Med 170:621–625
25. Meersseman W, Lagrou K, Maertens J et al (2008) Galactomannan in BAL fluid: a tool for diagnosing aspergillus in intensive care unit patients. Am J Respir Crit Care Med 177:27–34
26. Shah SS, Tsang V, Goldstraw P (1992) Open lung biopsy: a safe reliable and accurate method for diagnosis in diffuse lung disease. Respiration 59:243–246
27. Miller JD, Urschel JD, Cox G, Olak J, Young JE, Kay JM, McDonald E (2000) A randomized, controlled trial comparing thoracoscopy and limited thoracotomy for lung biopsy in interstitial lung disease. Ann Thorac Surg 70:1647–1650
28. Papazian L, Thomas P, Bregeon F, Garbe L, Zandotti C, Saux P, Gaillat F, Drancourt M, Auffray JP, Gouin F (1998) Open-lung biopsy in patients with acute respiratory distress syndrome. Anesthesiology 88(4):935–944
29. Hwang SS, Kim HH, Park SH, Jung JI, Jang HS (2000) The value of CT-guided percutaneous needle aspiration in immunocompromised patients with suspected pulmonary infection. Am J Roentgenol 175(1):235–238
30. Wong PW, Stefanec T, Brown K, White DA (2002) Role of fine-needle aspirates of focal lung lesions in patients with hematologic malignancies. Chest 121:527–532
31. Castellino RA, Blank N (1979) Etiologic diagnosis of focal pulmonary infection in immunocompromised patients by fluoroscopically guided percutaneous needle aspiration. Radiology 132:563–567
32. Catterall JR, McCabe RE, Brooks RG, Remington JS (1898) Open lung biopsy in patients with Hodgkin's disease and pulmonary infiltrates. Am Rev Respir Dis 139: 1274–1279
33. McCabe RE, Brooks RG, Catterall JR, Remington JS (1989) Open lung biopsy in patients with non-Hodgkin's lymphoma and pulmonary infiltrates. Chest 96:319–324
34. Kramer MR, Berkman N, Mintz B, Godfrey S, Saute M, Amir G (1998) The role of open lung biopsy in the management and outcome of patients with diffuse lung disease. Ann Thorac Surg 65:198–202
35. Zihlif M, Khanchandani G, Ahmed HP, Soubani AO (2005 Feb) Surgical lung biopsy in patients with hematological malignancy or hematopoietic stem cell transplantation and unexplained pulmonary infiltrates: improved outcome with specific diagnosis. Am J Hematol 78(2):94–99
36. Dunn JC, West KW, Rescorla FJ, Tres Scherer LR, Engum SA, Rouse TM, Smith JW, Grosfeld JL (2001) The utility of lung biopsy in recipients of stem cell transplantation. J Pediatr Surg 36:1302–1303
37. Charbonney E, Robert J, Pache JC, Chevrolet JC, Eggimann P (2009) Impact of bedside open lung biopsies on the management of mechanically ventilated immunocompromised patients with acute respiratory distress syndrome of unknown etiology. J Crit Care 24:122–128
38. Shorr A, Kollef M (2002) The quick and the dead: the importance of rapid evaluation of infiltrates in the immunocompromised patient. Chest 122:9–12

The Increasing Role for Core Needle Biopsy of Pulmonary Lesions in Immunocompromised Patients

14

Cédric de Bazelaire, Raphael Calmon, Marion Chapelier, Amélie Pluvinage, and Eric de Kerviler

Contents

C. de Bazelaire (✉), R. Calmon, M. Chapelier, A. Pluvinage, and E. de Kerviler
Service de radiologie, Hôpital Saint-Louis, Université Paris VII, 1 avenue Claude Vellefaux, 75475 Paris Cedex, France
e-mail: cedric.de-bazelaire@sls.aphp.fr

14.1 Introduction

Although immunocompromised patients now have a better prognosis than in the past, they remain exposed to a variety of complications including tumors, infections, and inflammatory or immunological disorders. Many of these complications affect the lungs. The numerous treatments used by immunocompromised patients affect the computed tomography appearance of the lung lesions, thus raising diagnostic challenges. Percutaneous transthoracic needle biopsy is a well-established method for achieving the cytological diagnosis of lung lesions that is being increasingly used to solve difficult diagnostic problems. In 1976, Haaga and Alfidi [1] reported that computed tomography (CT) was the most accurate method for guiding percutaneous needle biopsies, and, since then, many studies have shown that percutaneous transthoracic needle biopsy is effective and accurate [2–8]. Diagnostic accuracy was greater than 80% for benign disease and greater than 90% for malignant disease [2–8].

Lung biopsy indications and methods have changed over the years with the increased use of CT and introduction of new treatments for various diseases. Lung biopsy is being increasingly performed. As with all invasive procedures, lung biopsy is associated with morbidity and mortality and, therefore, requires a multidisciplinary discussion to determine whether a biopsy is appropriate and, if so, which method is best. At least a pulmonologist and a radiologist with special expertise in chest diseases should be involved. Factors that weigh heavily on the decision to perform a lung biopsy include the respiratory status and coagulation test results.

Fine-needle aspiration biopsy (FNAB) was the first technique used for lung biopsy. However, FNAB yields only cytological specimens. Core needle biopsy using

É. Azoulay (ed.), *Pulmonary Involvement in Patients with Hematological Malignancies*, DOI: 10.1007/978-3-642-15742-4_14, © Springer-Verlag Berlin Heidelberg 2011

cutting needles of similar diameter to those used for FNAB yields tissue cores that can be used for histological studies. In this chapter, the term percutaneous transthoracic needle biopsy refers to core needle biopsy.

The purpose of this chapter is to describe percutaneous transthoracic needle biopsy and to discuss the risks and diagnostic performance of this method.

14.2 Acronyms

Several acronyms are used in the field of percutaneous biopsies, as shown in Table 14.1. Biopsies in which needle positioning is guided by an imaging modality are called image-guided needle biopsies (IGNB). Over time, the techniques have evolved, and the names have changed. In the 1980s, the only needles available on the market were small needles (20G or less) intended for aspiration. Biopsies obtained using these needles were called fine-needle aspiration (FNA) or fine-needle aspiration cytology (FNAC), as the specimens consisted of cell suspensions that did not preserve tissue architecture. The diagnostic yield varied considerably across diseases, being fairly high for malignant epithelial tumors and much lower for lymphoproliferative disorders and infectious diseases. In the 1990s, cutting needles were developed. Cutting needles are larger in diameter than aspiration needles, between 20 and 14G, and are frequently used with a co-axial introducer to allow multiple passes and multiple sample harvesting through a single biopsy track. These needles are used with semi-automated or automated biopsy guns to harvest cores of tissue (core needle biopsy, CNB) that preserve tissue architecture and contain a far larger number of cells than do aspiration samples. At the chest, percutaneous biopsies performed using fine-needle aspiration are called transthoracic needle aspiration biopsies (TTNAB or TNAB), and those performed using cutting needles are known as transthoracic needle biopsies (TNB). When comparing results published in the literature, the reader must be aware of these subtle differences, which may account in part for the discrepancies in diagnostic yields and complication rates. Indeed, the needle diameter and the number of passes probably play an important role in both, as discussed later. As indicated above, the term percutaneous transthoracic needle biopsy refers to core needle biopsy in this chapter.

Table 14.1 Abbreviations

Acronyms	Legend
TNB	Thoracic needle biopsy
IGNB	Image-guided needle biopsy
FNAB	Fine-needle aspiration biopsy
FNAC	Fine-needle aspiration cytology
PNAB	Percutaneous needle aspiration biopsy
CNB	Core needle biopsy

14.3 Techniques

14.3.1 *Preoperative Investigations*

14.3.1.1 Coagulation Indices

Guidelines about routine clotting studies before performing percutaneous lung biopsy recommend that the platelet count, prothrombin time (PT), and activated partial thromboplastin time (APTT) be checked [9]. Opinion in the world literature suggests that a PT reported as the international normalized ratio (INR) or an APTT ratio greater than 1.4, or a platelet count below 100,000/mL may be relative contraindications to percutaneous lung biopsy (Fig. 14.1) [10]. Oral anticoagulation should be stopped before the procedure, and, depending on the risk of thrombosis associated with the condition warranting anticoagulant therapy, the INR can be measured and, if necessary, heparin instituted once the INR falls below the therapeutic range. There is no evidence to support withholding antiplatelet drugs before the procedure.

14.3.1.2 Pulmonary Function

The FEV1 cutoff below which percutaneous transthoracic needle biopsy lung biopsy is contraindicated has not been specified. Most practicing physicians and radiologists use a FEV1 cutoff of 1 L.

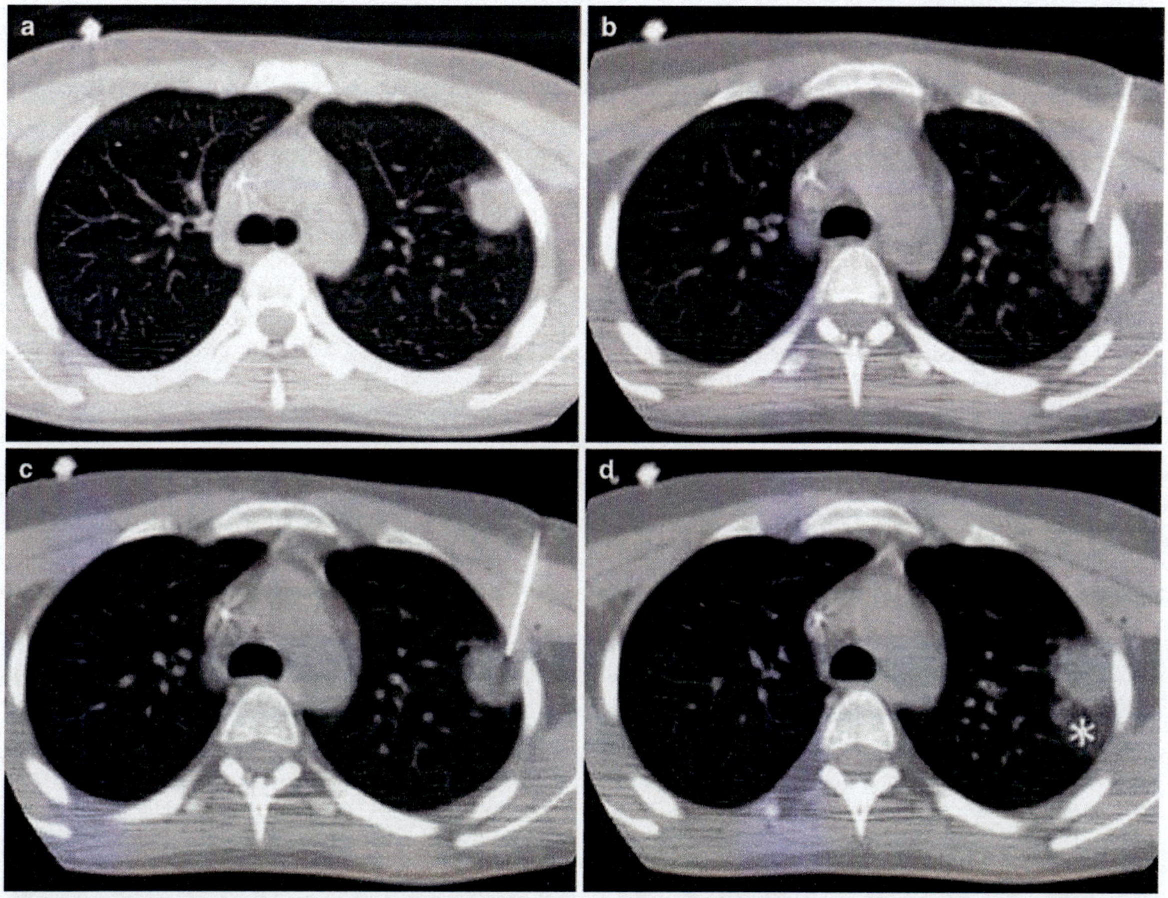

Fig. 14.1 CT-guided lung biopsy in a patient treated by allogeneic BMT for acute lymphoblastic leukemia and thought to have invasive lung aspergillosis. The platelet count remained below 30,000/mm^3 despite platelet transfusion. Mild alveolar hemorrhage (*asterisk*) occurred during the procedure but required no specific treatment. The biopsy confirmed the diagnosis of invasive pulmonary aspergillosis

14.3.1.3 Computed Tomography (CT)

Obtaining a CT scan before any further intervention in patients believed to have lung disease has several advantages. Performing CT before fiberoptic bronchoscopy (FOB) has been shown to increase the diagnostic yield of FOB by directing the bronchoscopist to the site most likely to give a diagnosis. CT can also show peripheral masses not visible by bronchoscopy and may suggest that histological specimens would be best obtained using other methods, such as percutaneous biopsy. On the contrary, diffuse consolidation or ground-glass opacities may be better investigated by noninvasive tests or bronchoalveolar lavage (BAL) than by percutaneous biopsy.

CT scans and all previous radiological investigations should be carefully reviewed to decide whether a biopsy is appropriate and must be available to the radiologist at the time of the biopsy. Repeat imaging should be performed if there has been a substantial change in the patient's clinical condition or a long time between the last imaging studies and the biopsy. Finally, the localizing CT scan done at the time of the biopsy may show major changes that may affect the decision to perform a biopsy, the target, or the expected needle trajectory.

14.3.2 Biopsy

Lung biopsies are usually performed under CT guidance. Ultrasound guidance may be used when the mass is in contact with the chest wall. When the lesion is deep, however, the ultrasound beam is scattered as it passes through the aerated lung. Conversely, ultrasound is particularly useful for large apical lesions, which can be better approached from the supraclavicular area (Fig. 14.2).

The method used for imaging guidance is selected by the interventional radiologist based on a careful review of the pre-biopsy CT scan. For CT-guided procedures, patients are positioned prone, supine, or in lateral decubitus to ensure easy and safe access to the target lesion. Then, a short spiral CT acquisition of the region of interest is obtained. Because anatomical landmarks change substantially with patient position, this new set of images obtained in the biopsy position is used to determine the entry site of the needle on the patient's skin and to plan the most direct and safest needle trajectory. The needle must avoid lung fissures, bullae, large airways, and large vessels (Fig. 14.3). To minimize the risk of pneumothorax, the needle tip must be kept at a distance from the pleuropulmonary interface (Figs. 14.3 and 14.4). Care should be taken to avoid the internal mammary vessels if the biopsy is performed via an anterior approach. For ultrasound-guided procedures, the patient is placed in the supine, lateral, or prone position. The trajectory to the pulmonary lesion is determined and the entry site marked on the skin.

Percutaneous transthoracic needle biopsy of the lung should be performed using standard universal precautions. Protective gloves should be worn. The entry site is cleaned and sterilely draped, and a 1% lidocaine solution is administered for local anesthesia. A co-axial technique should be used for both CT and ultrasound

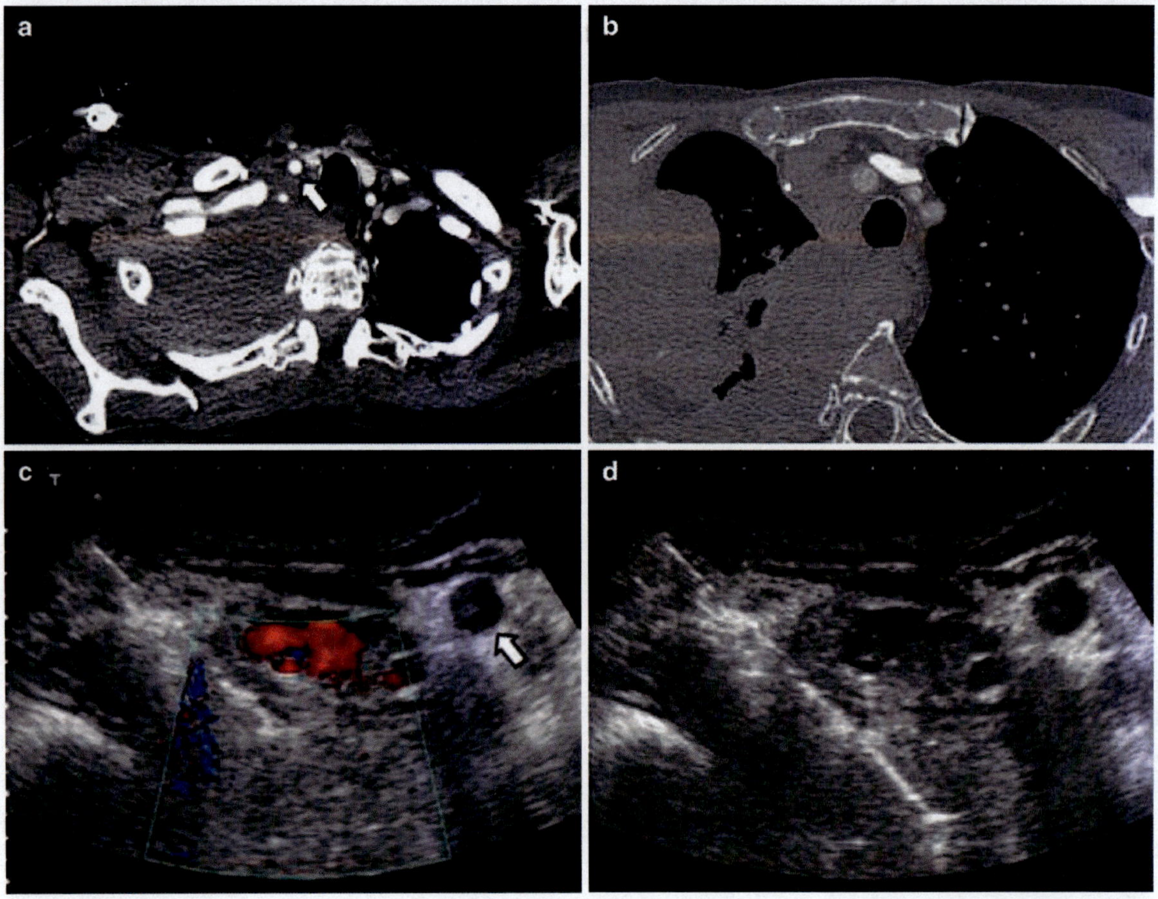

Fig. 14.2 Ultrasound-guided biopsy in a 65-year-old patient with lymphoma. Ultrasonography allowed real-time control of needle progression near the right subclavian vessel (in *red* with color Doppler, image **c**) and right carotid (*arrows*, images **a** and **c**). Image **b** shows pleural extension of the lymphoma

guidance to allow multiple passes and to minimize the number of pleural punctures [10, 11]. With ultrasound guidance, needle progression is monitored in real time. With CT, axial 3- to 6-mm-thick slices are acquired to monitor the needle progression toward the target. When appropriate positioning of the co-axial introducer is confirmed, a semi-automatic 18- to 20-G cutting needle is inserted. Collected samples are conditioned according to the clinical requirements (Fig. 14.5). This technique is supported by several recent studies indicating that the use of 18- or 20-G cutting needles, as well as co-axial techniques, improve the diagnostic yield and achieve diagnostic accuracies of 74–95% for malignancies [12–14]. False-negative results for malignancies may be due to a variety of factors including the patient's inability to cooperate, small lesion size, overlying bone partly or completely masking the lesion, and sampling of necrotic tissue or pneumonitis distal to an obstructing lesion [15, 16]. The false-negative rate has been shown to be significantly lower with cutting needles than with aspiration [17]. No data are available on the immediate assessment of core adequacy, and visual inspection to confirm that the sample is adequate seems reasonable. However, touch preparations (imprints) of core biopsy specimens used to allow a rapid cytological evaluation may be as accurate as conventional cytopathological methods [18].

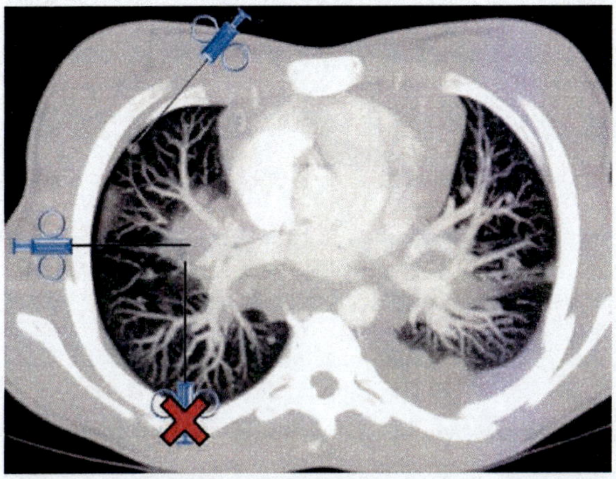

Fig. 14.3 Simulation of CT-guided lung biopsy. Keeping the needle in the peripheral lung parenchyma avoids injury of the large vessels. When proximal biopsies are needed (pulmonary hilum), the needle trajectory should be parallel to the vessels to avoid injury

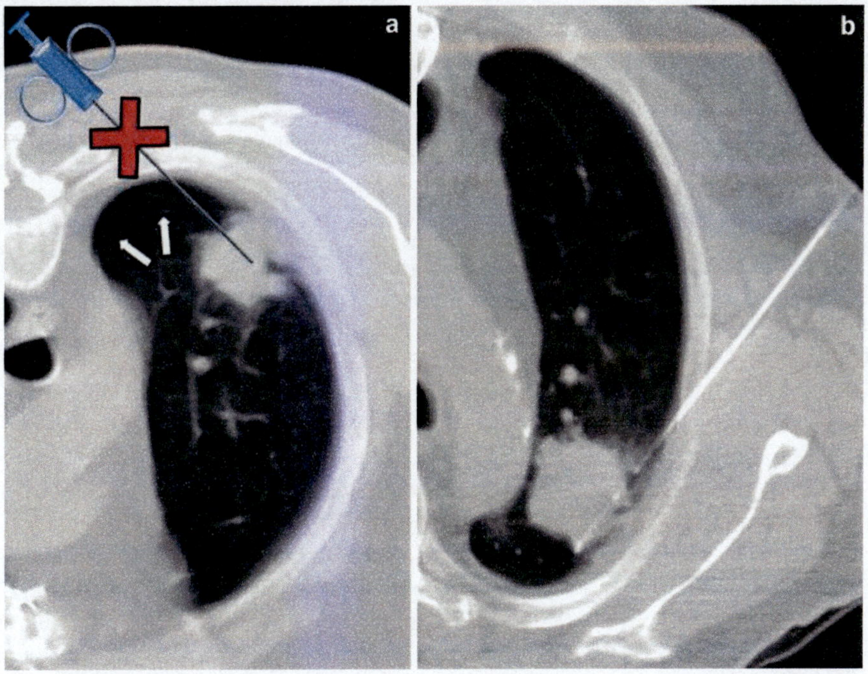

Fig. 14.4 CT-guided lung biopsy. The needle trajectory should avoid the lung fissures, and the needle tip should be kept as far as possible from the pleuropulmonary interface to minimize the risk of pneumothorax. Here, the patient was first placed in the prone position (**a**). However, the major fissure (*arrows*) was along the planned needle trajectory. The patient was placed in the supine position, which allowed safe performance of the biopsy (**b**)

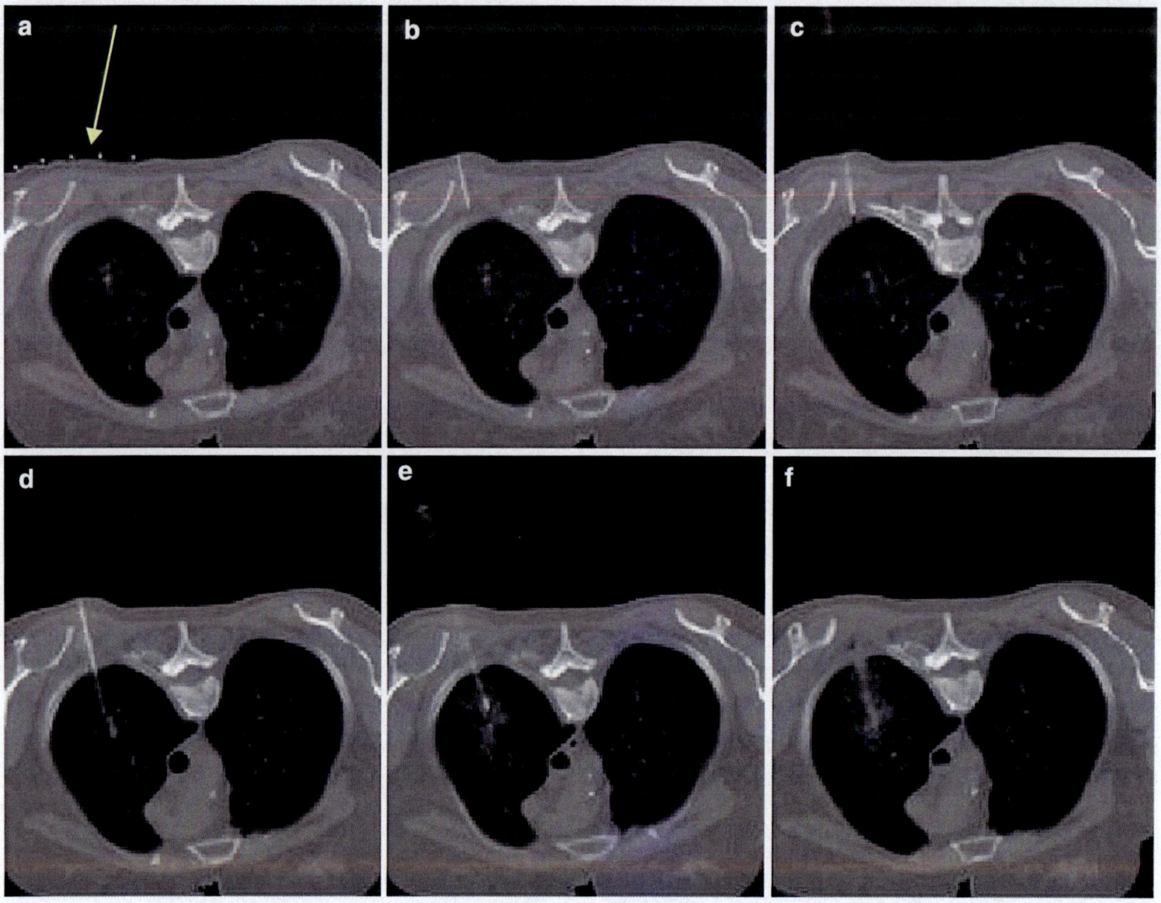

Fig. 14.5 CT-guided lung biopsy in a patient with chronic lymphoid leukemia who developed small lung nodules. The procedure started with a short CT acquisition used to localize the lesion and to plan the needle trajectory. Radioopaque markers were placed on the skin to indicate the entry site (*arrow* on (**a**)). Successive axial slices (**b**–**d**) were acquired to monitor needle progression toward the target. After the biopsy, alveolar hemorrhage developed (**e** and **f**). This unexpected minor complication plugs the needle track and prevents pneumothorax

After the lung biopsy, patients should be monitored for 4–6 h for delayed side effects such as pneumothorax. Simple clinical monitoring ensures the early detection of complications during the time needed for clotting of the needle track to occur.

14.3.3 Sample Conditioning

The referring clinician, pathologist, microbiologist, and interventional radiologist should work together. In particular, the referring clinician should discuss the suspected diagnoses with the interventional radiologist to assist in selecting the sample conditioning method and to determine the priorities should the amount of biopsy material be limited. Optimal conditioning is crucial to obtain a high diagnostic yield.

In all patients, at least one core biopsy should be fixed in a solution of acetic acid, formaldehyde, and alcohol (AFA solution). AFA solution fixation was selected based on its ability to allow high-quality structural analysis and its satisfactory performance in preliminary immunohistochemistry (IHC) studies. Although the AFA solution preserves the membrane and cytoplasmic epitopes and allows a number of molecular biology studies, nuclear antigens are not well preserved. Formaldehyde solutions allow the full range of immunohistochemical studies but

Table 14.2 Different staining available on lung specimens

Stain	Utility
Hematoxylin and eosin	Basic structural diagnosis
Reticulin	Fibers (sarcoma, fibrosis)
PAS (periodic acid Schiff)	Pathogens
MGG (May-Grünwald-Giemsa)	Basophilic cytoplasmic proteins
	Pathogens (*Pneumocystis*)
Ziehl	Acid-fast bacilli
GMS (Grocott methenamine silver)	Fungi

are not used as they produce inferior-quality structural data.

After fixation, the samples are embedded in paraffin, sliced, and stained according to the underlying disease and suspected diagnoses (Table 14.2). IHC uses monoclonal antibodies to target specific antigens. These antibodies are then targeted by a secondary antibody that is later marked with the staining agent. IHC provides additional structural information, thus benefiting the diagnosis, and may help to select targeted treatments (e.g., rituximab to target CD20+ cells).

Whenever possible, one of the cores should be frozen in liquid nitrogen as soon as possible after the biopsy. Frozen samples are highly versatile. They can be used for further structural analysis when the fixed specimens are not contributive, with good results. In addition, bacteria, fungi, and viruses can be reactivated. Last, preservation in frozen samples of intact proteins and nuclear material allows cytogenetic and molecular biology tests.

Samples from severely immunocompromised patients should be placed in a sterile tube with saline for ancillary studies to detect pathogens.

Structural studies can provide information on pathogens (fungi and acid-fast bacilli). When needed, this information can be acquired from fresh samples. Fresh samples require rapid conditioning and processing but allow extensive investigations for fungi, bacteria, and viruses by microscopic examination and culture. Viral infections can be detected using molecular biology tests on either fresh samples or cell culture extracts, and the results should be compared to serum viral load.

14.3.4 Safety, Major and Minor Complications

Operators should routinely audit their own practice and calculate their complication rates to inform their patients before asking them to consent to the procedure. They should strive to achieve rates at the lower end of the reported range. In an international survey, major complications included pneumothorax (20.5% of biopsies), pneumothorax requiring a chest drain (3.1%), hemoptysis (5.3%), and death (0.15%) [19].

14.3.4.1 Serious Complications

Serious complications requiring specific treatment are rare. They include pneumothorax requiring drainage, hemopericardium (Fig. 14.6), hemothorax, hemoptysis, and severe pain [2, 12, 20–24]. The rates of the main complications are reported in Table 14.3.

Pneumothorax

Chest tube placement is required for post-procedural pneumothorax in 3–15% of all lung biopsies [25]. Most patients with pneumothorax necessitating chest tube drainage have lesions located less than 2 cm from the pleural membrane [26]. The tube can usually be removed within 48 h. In patients with severe pulmonary destruction, due for instance to emphysema or graft-versus-host disease, the chest tube may need to be left in place for several days because of the decreased pulmonary compliance (Fig. 14.7).

Bleeding

Intrapulmonary hemorrhage occurs during lung biopsy in 5–30% of patients and hemoptysis in 1.25–5% [19, 27]. Lesion depth has been identified as the most important risk factor for hemorrhage, with an increased risk of bleeding in lesions deeper than 2 cm [28]. The hemothorax rate is about 1.5%. Clinically significant hemorrhage is rare. Hemothorax may result from injury to an intercostal or internal thoracic artery (Fig. 14.8) or vein [29].

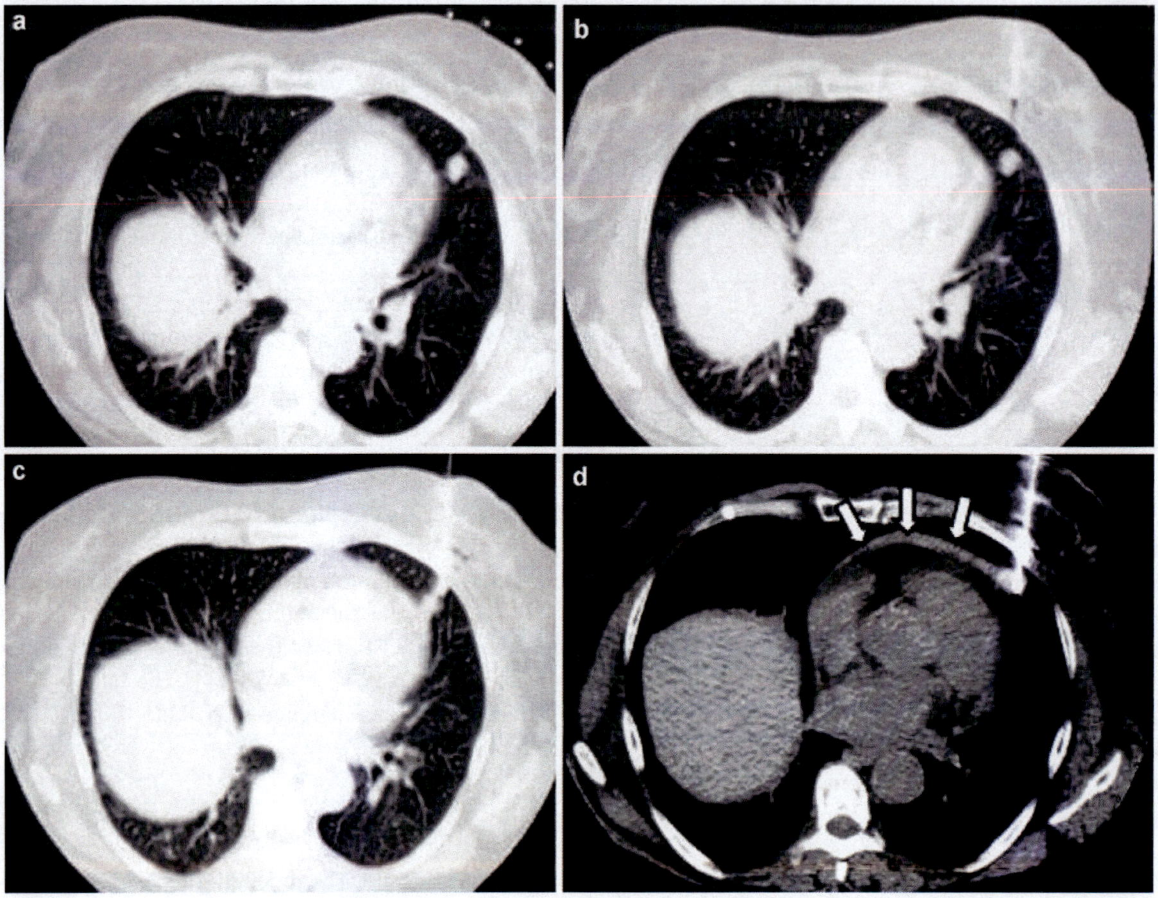

Fig. 14.6 CT-guided biopsy in an uncooperative 73-year-old patient. The patient moved during the procedure despite having previously received explanations on the risks of moving. A control image showed the needle in the pericardial sac, and a pericardial effusion developed rapidly (*arrows*, image **d**). Pericardial drainage was successful

Table 14.3 Major side effects reported after CT-controlled pulmonary biopsies in the literature

	Risk	No. of procedures	Needle	References
Pneumothorax (total/chest tube)	23/5%	660	19G CNB	[31]
	62/31%	61	18G PNAB	[39]
	28/2.5%	162	22G PNAB	[47]
	26/8%	846	19G PNAB	[30]
	21/2%	97	19G PNAB	[6]
	17/2%	135	17G CNB	[26]
	17/0.5%	605	19G CNB	[64]
Bleeding (total/hemoptysis)	30/4%	660	19G CNB	[31]
	–/2%	846	19G PNAB	[30]
	27/6%	135	17G CNB	[26]
	20/3.8%	604	19G CNB	[64]
Vasovagal response	0.3%	846	19G PNAB	[30]

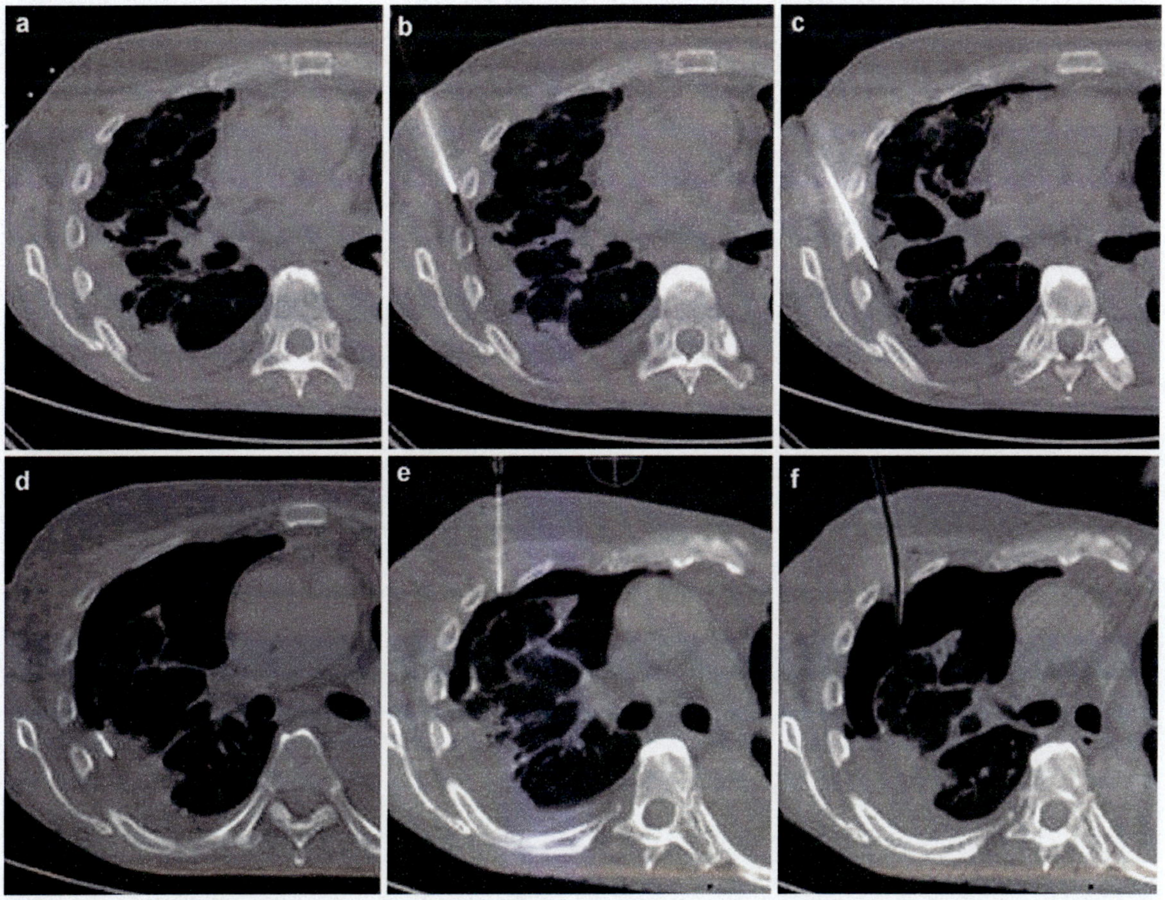

Fig. 14.7 CT-guided lung biopsy in a 55-year-old patient after allogeneic bone marrow transplantation for lymphoma. The target lesion is located less than 2 cm from the thoracic wall. Despite careful needle placement, a large pneumothorax occurred and failed to resolve with aspiration, necessitating chest tube placement. The biopsy demonstrated organizing pneumonia due to graft-versus-host disease

Pain

Pain is a rare complication (0.3% of the patients) that may occur in the absence of a specific injury, despite careful local anesthesia. Pain may be accompanied by vasovagal syncope, a drop in arterial oxygen saturation, or hypotension. These manifestations usually resolve spontaneously. However, acute pain during lung biopsy mandates close monitoring of the patient for evidence of a serious complication. After the procedure, patients are in general monitored in the emergency room for a few hours, after which they are discharged if no adverse events have occurred (Fig. 14.9).

14.3.4.2 Minor Complications

Minor complications occur in 30–60% of lung biopsies. Among these asymptomatic biopsy-related events, the most common are small pneumothorax (17–60%) and alveolar hemorrhage (5–30%) [26]. Usually, these asymptomatic complications resolve spontaneously and require no treatment after the biopsy (Fig. 14.10). The rate of pneumothorax/bleeding is highest with lesions smaller than 2 cm (tenfold higher risk of pneumothorax and sixfold higher risk of bleeding). The risk of pneumothorax is seven times higher when the lesion is less than 2 cm from the chest wall (Fig. 14.10). However,

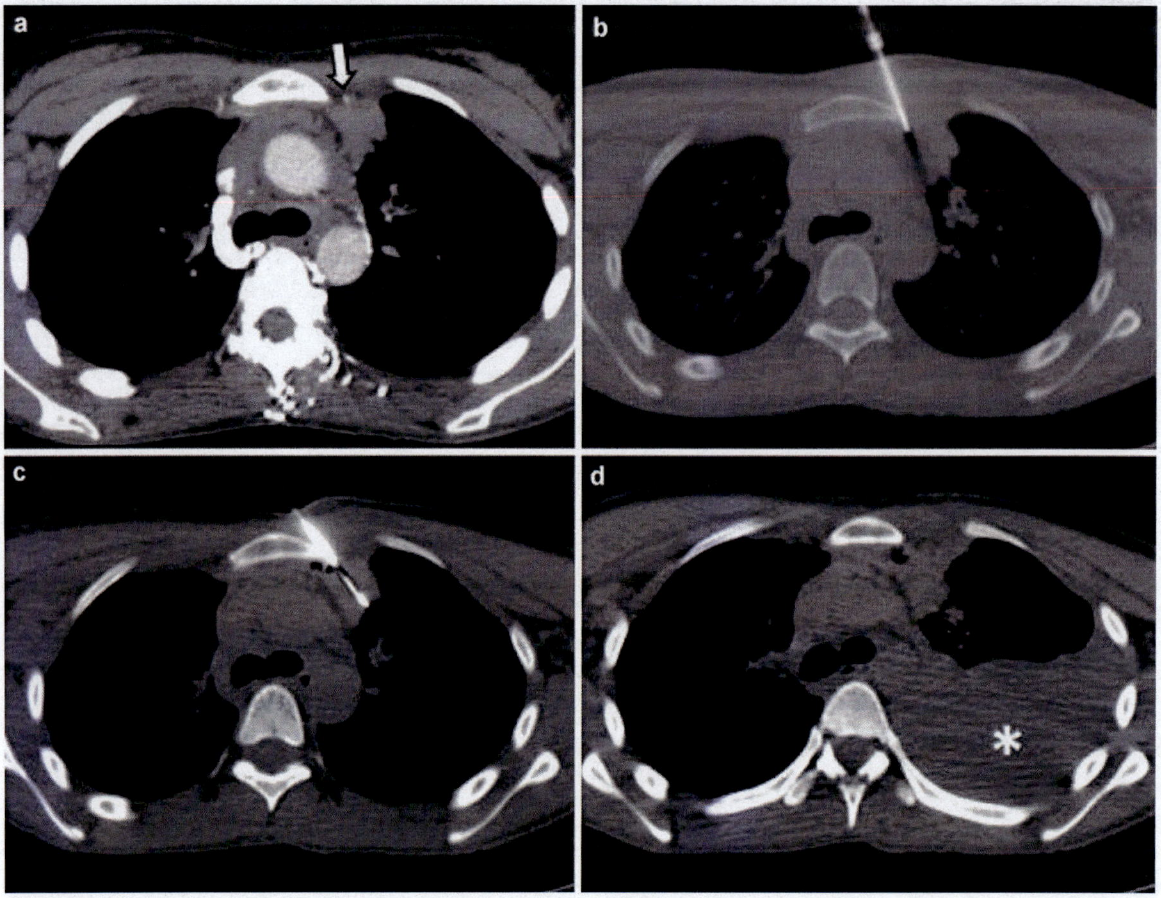

Fig. 14.8 CT-guided lung biopsy in an 18-year-old patient with suspected relapsing Hodgkin's disease. Care was taken to stay close to the manubrium (image **b**) to avoid the internal thoracic artery (*arrow*, image **a**). However, after three biopsies the artery was injured and severe hemothorax developed (*asterisk*, image **d**). Treatment was successful

CT-guided biopsy of lesions more than 2 cm from the chest wall is associated with a tenfold increase in the bleeding rate [31]. Longer length of the intrapulmonary needle track (>4 cm) is also associated with higher rates of bleeding around the track and of pneumothorax [26]. Bleeding and pneumothorax are more common when the pleural membrane is crossed twice by the needle. The risk of pneumothorax is also higher in patients with bullae and in those receiving mechanical ventilation. An oblique trajectory of the needle relative to the pleural membrane may increase the risk of pneumothorax [31]. Decreasing the duration of the procedure diminishes the pneumothorax rate [26].

The use of smaller co-axial introducers (19 G instead of 17 G) substantially decreases the risk of pneumothorax without affecting diagnostic accuracy, sensitivity, or specificity of the histopathologic diagnosis of pulmonary nodules [30]. Although pneumothorax rates are similar with FNAB and automated core biopsy, the automated devices are associated with a small and nonsignificant increase in the rate of bleeding with hemoptysis [12, 32]. However, no statistically significant relationship has been found between complication rates, number of passes through the co-axial system with the introducer needle or core gun (up to 4), and smoking history. The complication rate seems similar for masses, consolidations, and ground-glass opacities [33]. In our experience, the number of biopsy-related complications is not different between immunocompromised and immunocompetent patients.

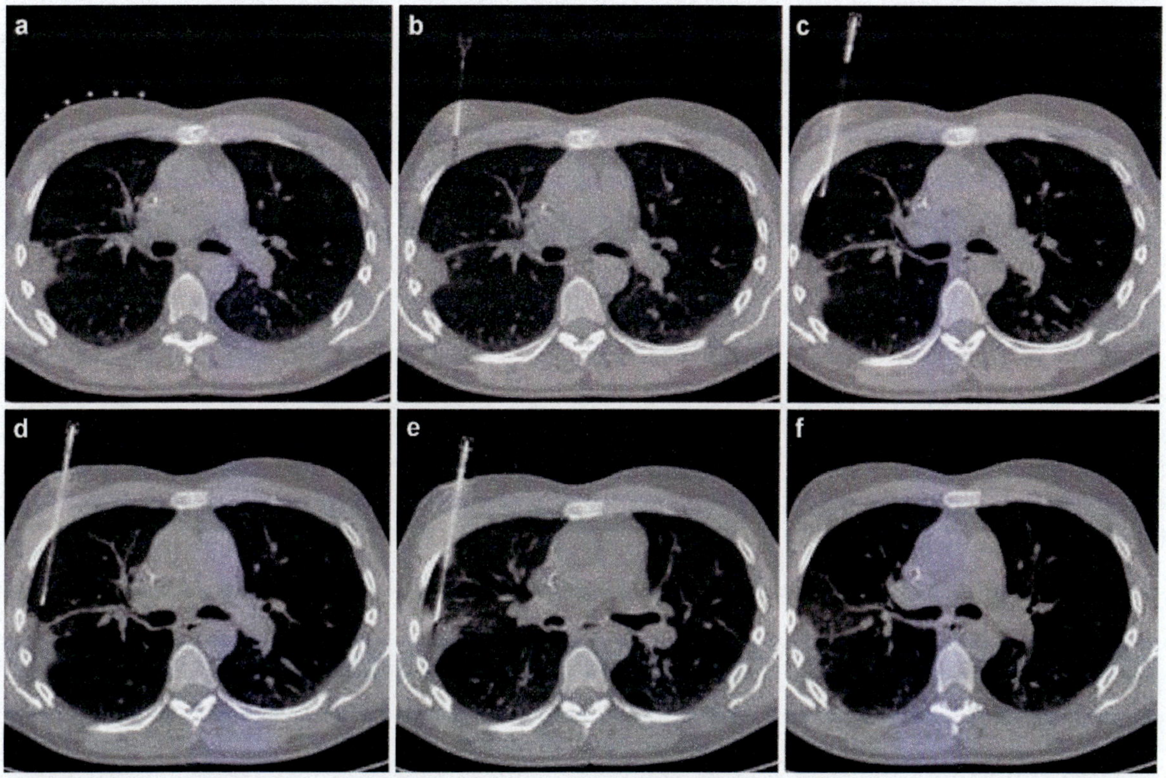

Fig. 14.9 CT-guided lung biopsy in a 65-year-old patient with organizing pneumonia. The patient experienced severe pain at the end of the procedure with a vasovagal syncope. The control image shows alveolar hemorrhage, but no hemoptysis occurred. The patient was monitored in the emergency room for 6 h then discharged

Monitoring

Most complications occur immediately or within the first hour of the transcutaneous lung biopsy. A limited number of CT slices are acquired at the end of the procedure to detect early complications. Pneumothorax is usually detectable by chest X-ray 1 h after the biopsy [22, 34–36], although recent reports describe delayed pneumothorax occurring 24 h after the biopsy despite normal chest X-rays 1 and 4 h post-biopsy [37]. No specific monitoring is required following an uncomplicated biopsy procedure, but patients should remain hospitalized for at least 1 h, or longer if further radiographs are required to monitor a pneumothorax. Patients should be in a supervised area so staff can be alerted if they develop shortness of breath, chest pain, or other symptoms. Last, they should be given complete information before they are discharged so that they can be alert to symptoms possibly indicating the development of a complication.

14.4 Efficiency

14.4.1 Sensitivity and Adequacy

The number of lung biopsies has increased considerably over the last decade. As fine-needle aspiration gained in popularity, its accuracy came under scrutiny. Audits showed that fine-needle biopsy was more likely to detect malignant disease than were any of the noninvasive tests or endoscopic bronchial sampling [38].

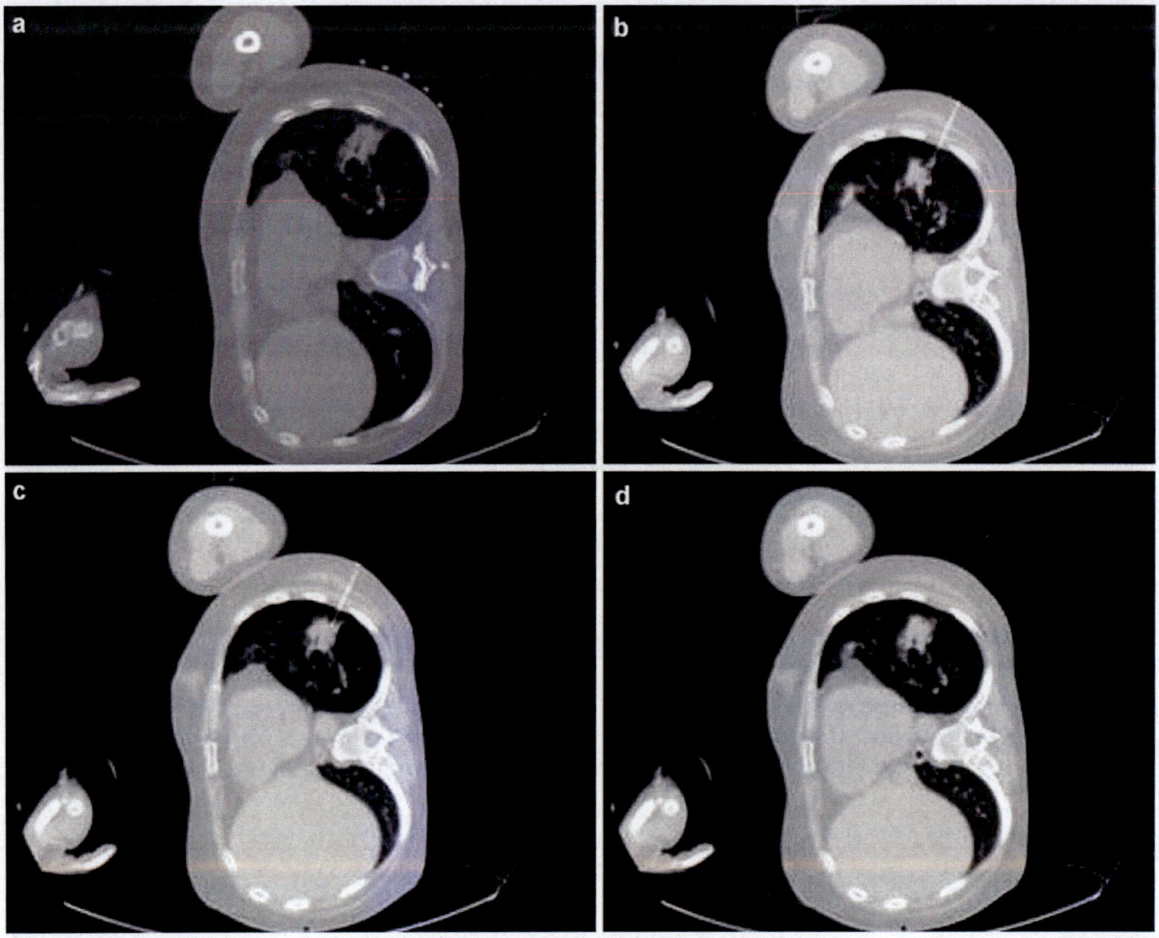

Fig. 14.10 CT-guided lung biopsy in a 32-year-old patient after stem cell transplantation for acute leukemia. The target lesion is located less than 10 mm from the chest wall. A small and stable pneumothorax developed during the procedure. No specific treatment was required. The small pneumothorax was not visible by chest X-ray. The biopsy showed organizing pneumonia

Several large studies of the efficiency of percutaneous transthoracic needle biopsy have been reported. Greater than 80% sensitivity and accuracy can be achieved (Table 14.4) [39]. The false-positive rate is usually less than 1% [40, 41] and the false-negative rate less than 5–10% [42–45]. Diagnostic accuracy depends on the size and location of the lesion, operator experience, needle type, needle path length, biopsy technique, and expertise of the cytopathologist [10, 46, 47]. Larger lesions are more likely to enable a positive diagnosis of malignancy [10, 48–52], although some operators have reported no significant difference between lesions smaller than 2 cm and lesions ≥2 cm in diameter [53, 54]. With CT-guided percutaneous transthoracic needle biopsy, accuracy is 91% and sensitivity 94% for large nodules (>15 mm) compared to 88% and 82%, respectively, for small nodules (<10 mm) (Fig. 14.11) [39]. Diagnostic accuracy for needle path lengths of 40 mm or less is significantly greater (>90%) than that for lengths greater than 40 mm (<56%). The overall diagnostic accuracy is 96% for procedures performed with 18-G needles and 92% for procedures performed with 19-G needles, with 95% and 89% sensitivity and 100% and 99% specificity, respectively [30]. Whether lung biopsy should be considered for persistent focal ground-glass opacities remains unclear. However, in a 2009 study of 28 patients with ground-glass opacities, 17 with malignant and 11 with benign lesions, percutaneous transthoracic needle biopsy had 71% overall sensitivity and 82% accuracy [33].

Table 14.4 Effectiveness of the biopsy according to the type of pulmonary lesions

	Sensitivity (%)	Accuracy (%)	No. of procedures	References
Overall	82	88	61	[39]
	87	77	162	[47]
	91	94	846	[30]
Malignancy	89	91	604	[64]
<10 mm	88	92	47	[39]
<10 mm	67	80	10	[33]
<15 mm	72	74	70	[6]
>15 mm	94	96	27	[6]
>20 mm	75	88	8	[33]
Infection fungal	70.6	76.4	17	[57]

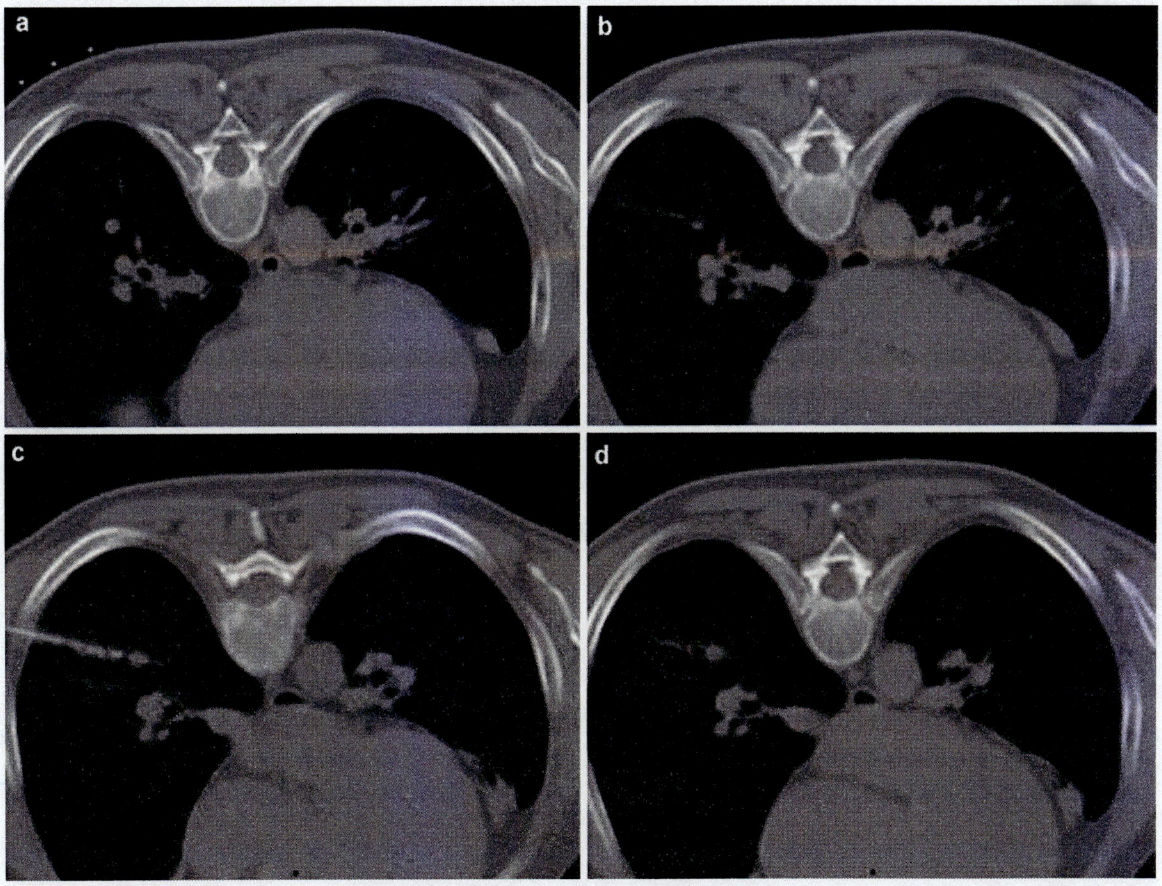

Fig. 14.11 CT-guided biopsy in a patient treated for MALT lymphoma. The biopsy of the 8-mm nodule located in the lower right lobe showed a metastasis from an unsuspected melanoma

In our experience, the diagnostic yield is higher for masses and nodules than for consolidations or diffuse infiltrates. Agreement between biopsy results and the final diagnosis is generally good (kappa, 0.80; $P<0.0001$). Eighty percent of percutaneous lung biopsies harvest a sufficient amount of tissue for the pathologic diagnosis [55].

14.4.2 Specific Diagnoses

In patients with lung infections, lung biopsy has been reported to have 70% sensitivity and 100% positive predictive value [56, 57]. Lung biopsy performs better for diagnosing bacterial infections (Fig. 14.12) (100% sensitivity) than fungal infections (Fig. 14.13) (30–70% sensitivity). The diagnosis of invasive fungal infection is rarely achieved by commonly used diagnostic procedures such as CT, sputum examination, BAL, fungal cultures, and antigen detection. BAL is usually performed in neutropenic patients if the imaging features suggest a fungal infection, but is only 50% sensitive for aspergillosis [58–60]. Bronchoscopy and BAL may fail to differentiate colonization from invasive infection. Transbronchial biopsy, performed only when the platelet count is $>50 \cdot 10^9$/L, improves diagnostic accuracy by only 6.5% [58]. Histology is more effective than culturing for the diagnosis of bacterial and fungal infections. Cultures are usually positive in fewer than 40% of patients with aspergillosis or mucormycosis [57]. Cultures are often negative in neutropenic patients and in patients given empirical antifungal or antibacterial agents before sampling [61]. Fungal and bacterial cultures may produce false-negative results. For instance, *Aspergillus* is a common saprophyte, and a positive

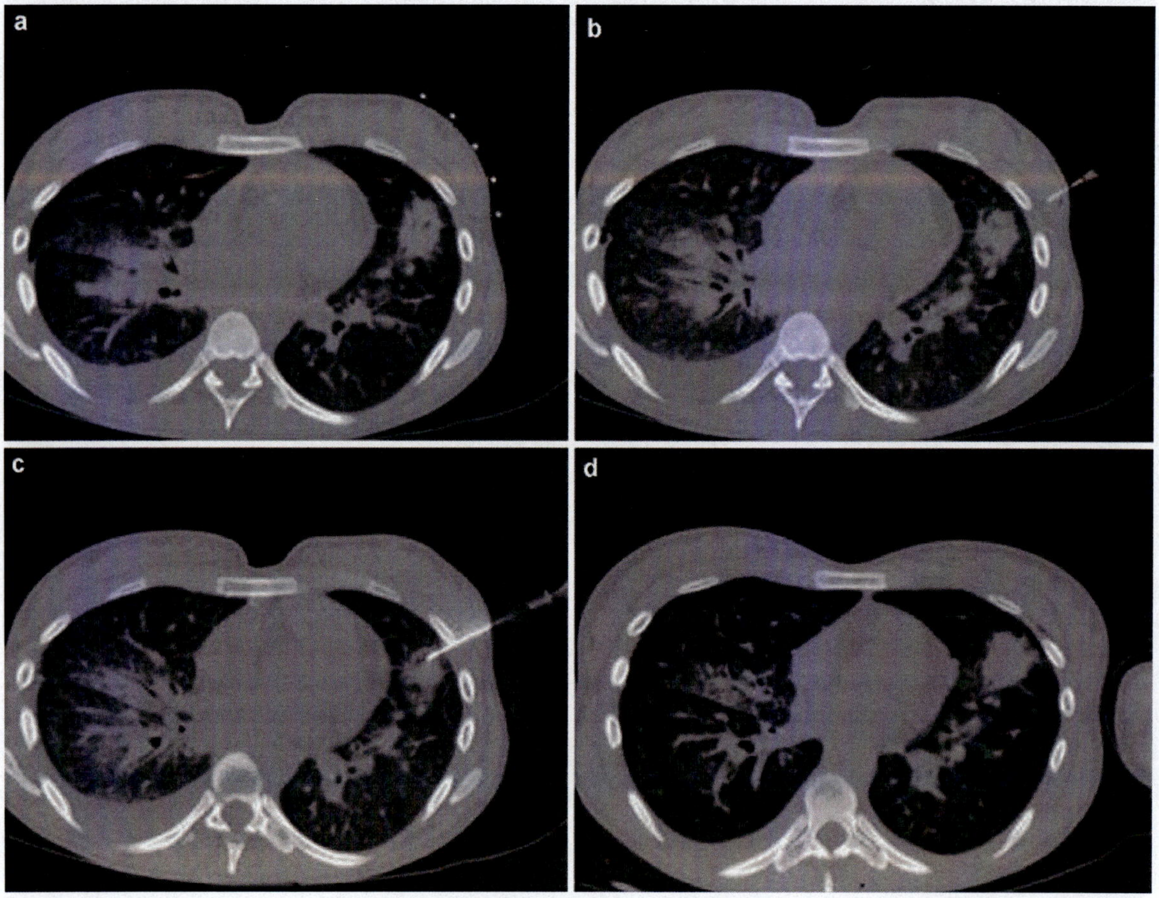

Fig. 14.12 CT-guided lung biopsy in a 64-year-old patient with a long history of chronic lymphoid leukemia and a new lung mass, suggesting aggressive lymphomatous transformation. The biopsy showed tuberculosis

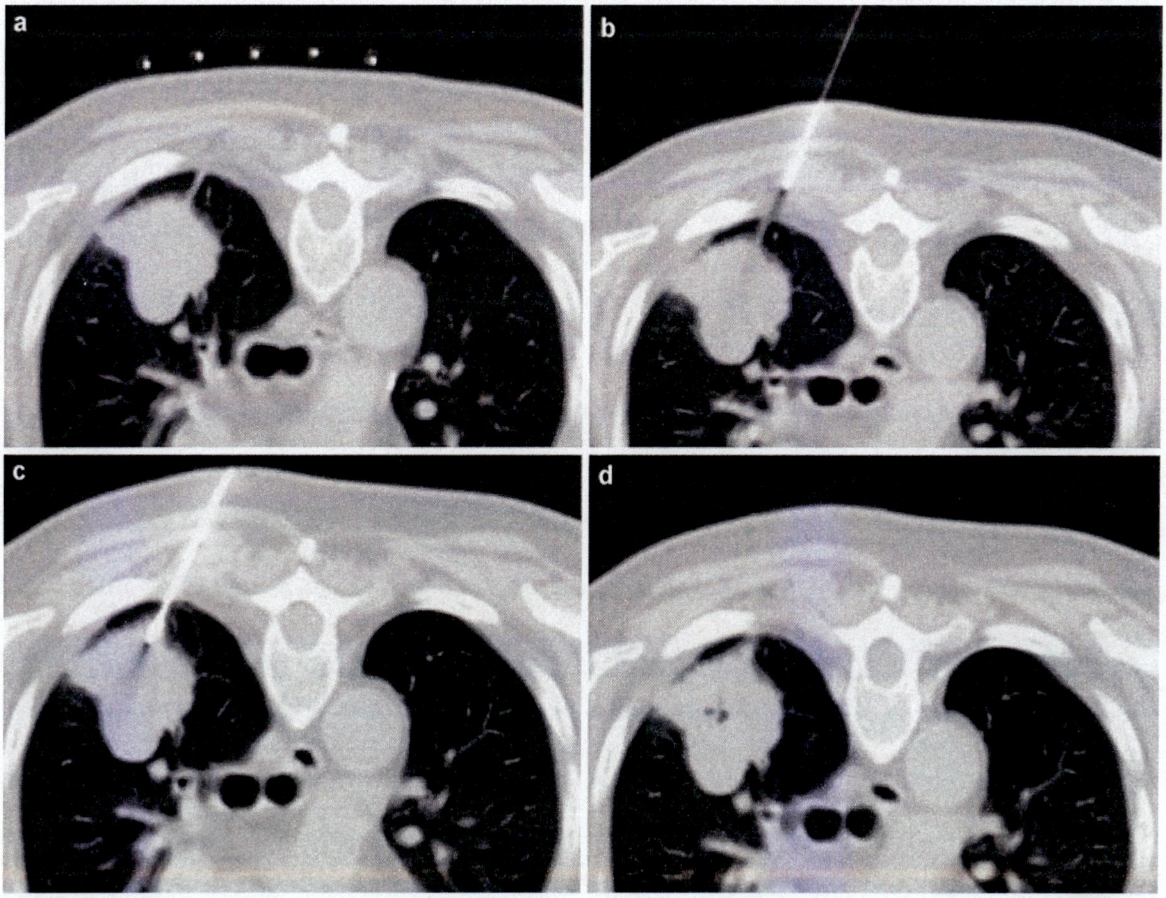

Fig. 14.13 CT-guided lung biopsy in a patient treated for B-cell lymphoma. The planned needle trajectory passed through a pleural tail to avoid the lung parenchyma. The biopsy demonstrated invasive pulmonary aspergillosis

culture is therefore not proof of infection. Hence, the gold standard is mycological and/or histological evidence of tissue invasion. Biopsy allows differentiation between aspergillosis and mucormycosis, which is important, as Mucorales are usually resistant to azoles and echinocandins and consequently require amphotericin B for curative treatment and secondary prophylaxis during bone marrow transplantation. Also, histology provides the diagnosis immediately. Histological studies show necrotic foci containing numerous filamentous fungi in patients with fungal infection and granulomas and infiltrates composed of histiocytes or neutrophils in those with bacterial infection.

Image-guided percutaneous transthoracic fine-needle aspiration biopsy (FNAB) has proved reliable for differentiating benign and malignant pulmonary lesions. Diagnostic accuracy exceeded 93% [49, 62] and sensitivity exceeded 95% [12, 54, 62]. For nodules <10 mm, overall sensitivity was 68% and accuracy was 78% [63], compared to 93% and 95%, respectively, for nodules <15 mm [53]. In a study of 605 biopsies, lesion size ≤10 mm was associated with a tenfold increase in the false-negative rate [64]. The positive and negative predictive values of 100% and 60–81%, respectively, have been reported [30, 63]. In patients with lymphoma, lung biopsy establishes the diagnosis in up to 90% of cases. In false-negative cases, histology may show inflammatory changes and necrosis. De novo non-hematological malignancies involving the lung are diagnosed by lung biopsy in 90% of cases [30]. Lung biopsy may assist in the diagnosis of organizing pneumonia, graft-versus-host disease with pulmonary complications, and benign tumors. Figures 14.14 and 14.15 show the diagnostic yield of lung biopsy in patients with non-infectious conditions. Figure 14.16 describes a case of pulmonary nocardiosis in a patient with chronic lymphocytic leukemia who was thought to have aggressive lymphoma.

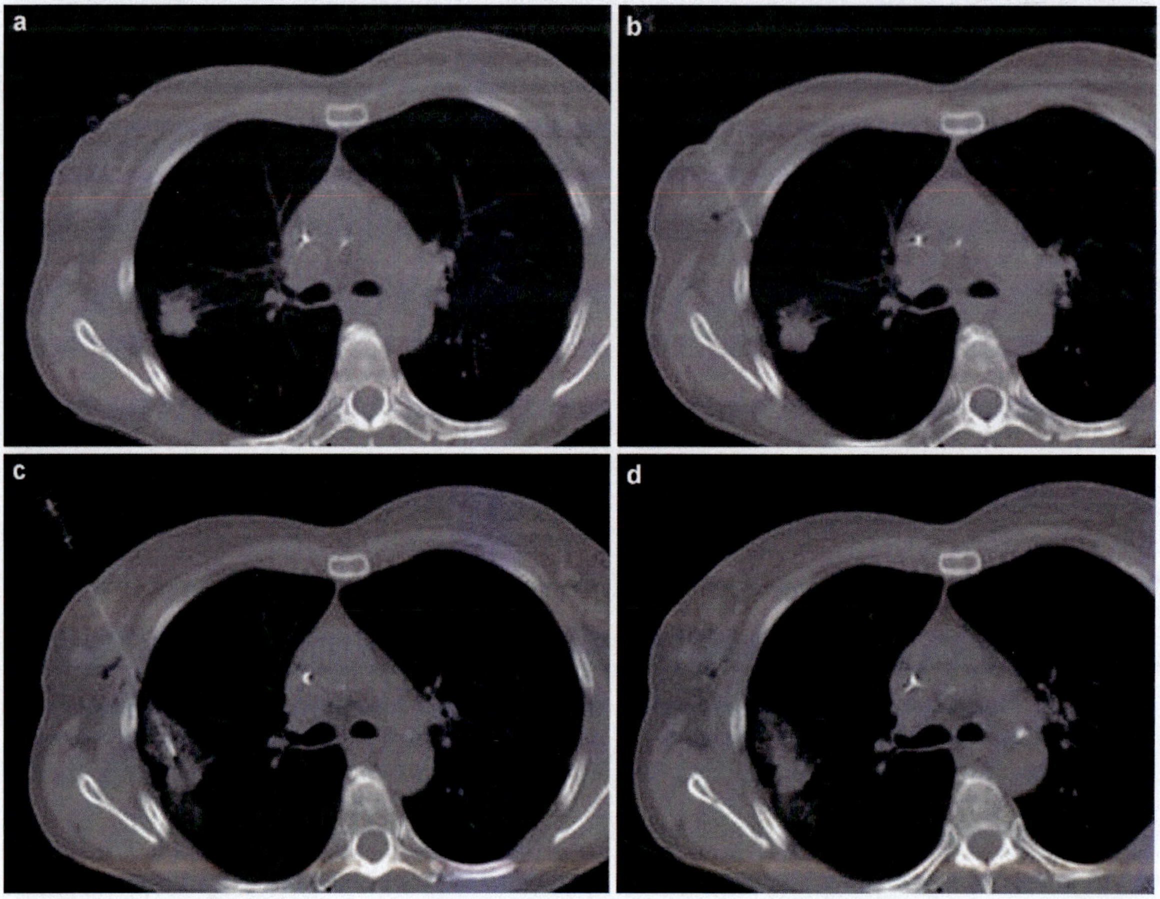

Fig. 14.14 CT-guided lung biopsy in a 63-year-old patient with a history of non-Hodgkin's lymphoma and a suspected pulmonary relapse. The biopsy unexpectedly showed an adenocarcinoma

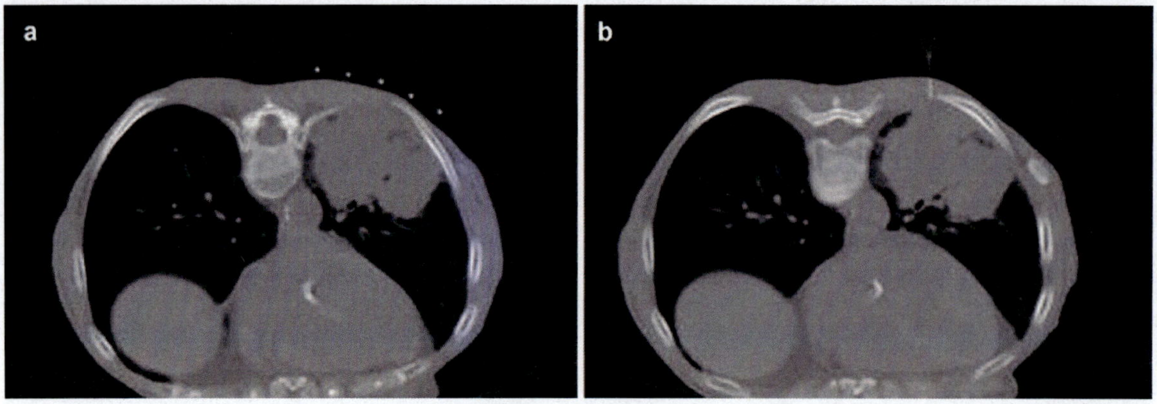

Fig. 14.15 CT-guided lung biopsy in an 83-year-old patient with a history of non-Hodgkin's lymphoma and a suspected pulmonary relapse. The biopsy confirmed the relapse

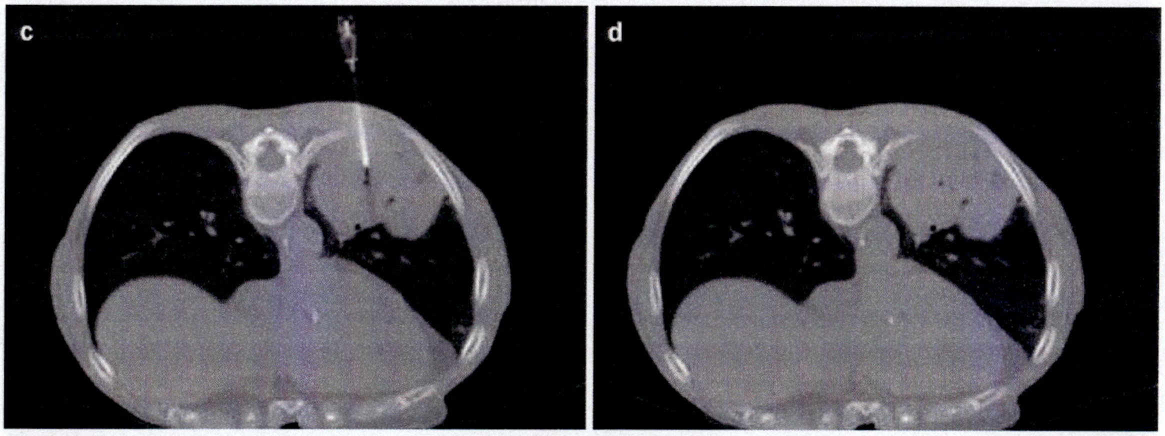

Fig. 14.15 (continued)

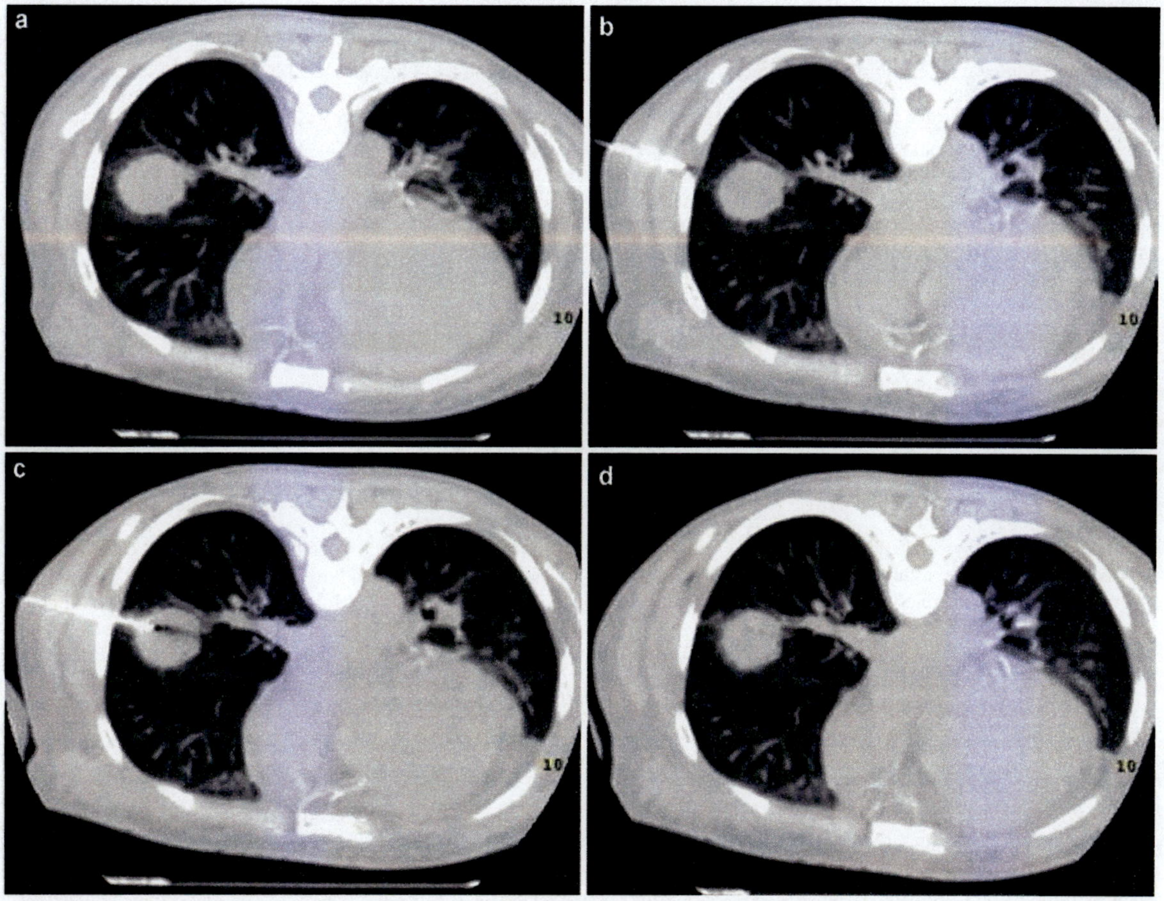

Fig. 14.16 CT-guided lung biopsy in a patient with chronic lymphocytic leukemia who was thought to have aggressive lymphoma. The biopsy diagnosis was pulmonary nocardiosis

14.5 Conclusion

CT-guided transthoracic lung biopsy is highly accurate for diagnosing malignancies and valuable for detecting infections in immunocompromised patients, provided the processing and routing of the biopsy samples are optimal. This technique is generally safe, the main complications being pneumothorax and hemorrhage. Both complications are associated with variables such as lesion size, lesion depth, number of pleural needle passes, and procedure duration. Most complications are minor and easily managed in the CT room. In-depth knowledge of predisposing factors allows clinicians and radiologists to anticipate complications and to ensure that the patient receives optimal monitoring after the procedure.

References

1. Haaga JR, Alfidi RJ (1976) Precise biopsy localization by computer tomography. Radiology 118:603–607
2. Westcott JL (1988) Percutaneous transthoracic needle biopsy. Radiology 169:593–601
3. van Sonnenberg E, Lin AS, Deutsch AL, Mattrey RF (1983) Percutaneous biopsy of difficult mediastinal, hilar, and pulmonary lesions by computed tomographic guidance and a modified coaxial technique. Radiology 148:300–302
4. Stanley JH, Fish GD, Andriole JG et al (1987) Lung lesions: cytologic diagnosis by fine-needle biopsy. Radiology 162: 389–391
5. Khouri NF, Stitik FP, Erozan YS et al (1985) Transthoracic needle aspiration biopsy of benign and malignant lung lesions. Am J Roentgenol 144:281–288
6. Li H, Boiselle PM, Shepard JO, Trotman-Dickenson B, McLoud TC (1996) Diagnostic accuracy and safety of CT-guided percutaneous needle aspiration biopsy of the lung: comparison of small and large pulmonary nodules. Am J Roentgenol 167:105–109
7. Larscheid RC, Thorpe PE, Scott WJ (1998) Percutaneous transthoracic needle aspiration biopsy: a comprehensive review of its current role in the diagnosis and treatment of lung tumors. Chest 114:704–709
8. Tsukada H, Satou T, Iwashima A, Souma T (2000) Diagnostic accuracy of CT-guided automated needle biopsy of lung nodules. Am J Roentgenol 175:239–243
9. British Thoracic Society guidelines on diagnostic flexible bronchoscopy. Thorax 2001 56(1):1–21
10. Moore EH (1998) Technical aspects of needle aspiration lung biopsy: a personal perspective. Radiology 208: 303–318
11. Yankelevitz DF, Vazquez M, Henschke CI (2000) Special techniques in transthoracic needle biopsy of pulmonary nodules. Radiol Clin North Am 38:267–279
12. Klein JS, Salomon G, Stewart EA (1996) Transthoracic needle biopsy with a coaxially placed 20-gauge automated cutting needle: results in 122 patients. Radiology 198:715–720
13. Boiselle PM, Shepard JA, Mark EJ et al (1997) Routine addition of an automated biopsy device to fine-needle aspiration of the lung: a prospective assessment. AJR Am J Roentgenol 169:661–666
14. Moulton JS, Moore PT (1993) Coaxial percutaneous biopsy technique with automated biopsy devices: value in improving accuracy and negative predictive value. Radiology 186:515–522
15. Poe RH, Kallay MC, Wicks CM, Odoroff CL (1984) Predicting risk of pneumothorax in needle biopsy of the lung. Chest 85:232–235
16. Miller JA, Pramanik BK, Lavenhar MA (1998) Predicting the rates of success and complications of computed tomography-guided percutaneous core-needle biopsies of the thorax from the findings of the preprocedure chest computed tomography scan. J Thorac Imaging 13:7–13
17. Laurent F, Latrabe V, Vergier B, Michel P (2000) Percutaneous CT-guided biopsy of the lung: comparison between aspiration and automated cutting needles using a coaxial technique. Cardiovasc Intervent Radiol 23: 266–272
18. Hahn PF, Eisenberg PJ, Pitman MB, Gazelle GS, Mueller PR (1995) Cytopathologic touch preparations (imprints) from core needle biopsies: accuracy compared with that of fine-needle aspirates. AJR Am J Roentgenol 165: 1277–1279
19. Richardson CM, Pointon KS, Manhire AR, Macfarlane JT (2002) Percutaneous lung biopsies: a survey of UK practice based on 5444 biopsies. Br J Radiol 75:731–735
20. Charig MJ, Phillips AJ (2000) CT-guided cutting needle biopsy of lung lesions–safety and efficacy of an out-patient service. Clin Radiol 55:964–969
21. Sakai T, Hayashi N, Kimoto T et al (1994) CT-guided biopsy of the chest: usefulness of fine-needle core biopsy combined with frozen-section pathologic diagnosis. Radiology 190: 243–246
22. Kazerooni EA, Lim FT, Mikhail A, Martinez FJ (1996) Risk of pneumothorax in CT-guided transthoracic needle aspiration biopsy of the lung. Radiology 198:371–375
23. Haramati LB, Austin JH (1991) Complications after CT-guided needle biopsy through aerated versus nonaerated lung. Radiology 181:778
24. Bungay HK, Berger J, Traill ZC, Gleeson FV (1999) Pneumothorax post CT-guided lung biopsy: a comparison between detection on chest radiographs and CT. Br J Radiol 72:1160–1163
25. Manhire A, Charig M, Clelland C et al (2003) Guidelines for radiologically guided lung biopsy. Thorax 58:920–936
26. Khan MF, Straub R, Moghaddam SR et al (2008) Variables affecting the risk of pneumothorax and intrapulmonal hemorrhage in CT-guided transthoracic biopsy. Eur Radiol 18: 1356–1363
27. Sinner WN (1976) Complications of percutaneous transthoracic needle aspiration biopsy. Acta Radiol Diagn (Stockh) 17:813–828
28. Yeow KM, See LC, Lui KW et al (2001) Risk factors for pneumothorax and bleeding after CT-guided percutaneous coaxial cutting needle biopsy of lung lesions. J Vasc Interv Radiol 12:1305–1312
29. Glassberg RM, Sussman SK (1990) Life-threatening hemorrhage due to percutaneous transthoracic intervention: importance of the internal mammary artery. AJR Am J Roentgenol 154:47–49

30. Geraghty PR, Kee ST, McFarlane G, Razavi MK, Sze DY, Dake MD (2003) CT-guided transthoracic needle aspiration biopsy of pulmonary nodules: needle size and pneumothorax rate. Radiology 229:475–481
31. Yeow KM, Su IH, Pan KT et al (2004) Risk factors of pneumothorax and bleeding: multivariate analysis of 660 CT-guided coaxial cutting needle lung biopsies. Chest 126:748–754
32. Lucidarme O, Howarth N, Finet JF, Grenier PA (1998) Intrapulmonary lesions: percutaneous automated biopsy with a detachable, 18-gauge, coaxial cutting needle. Radiology 207:759–765
33. Hur J, Lee HJ, Nam JE et al (2009) Diagnostic accuracy of CT fluoroscopy-guided needle aspiration biopsy of ground-glass opacity pulmonary lesions. AJR Am J Roentgenol 192:629–634
34. Poe RH, Kallay MC (1987) Transthoracic needle biopsy of lung in nonhospitalized patients. Chest 92:676–678
35. Stevens GM, Jackman RJ (1984) Outpatient needle biopsy of the lung: its safety and utility. Radiology 151:301–304
36. Perlmutt LM, Braun SD, Newman GE, Oke EJ, Dunnick NR (1986) Timing of chest film follow-up after transthoracic needle aspiration. AJR Am J Roentgenol 146: 1049–1050
37. Brown KT, Brody LA, Getrajdman GI, Napp TE (1997) Outpatient treatment of iatrogenic pneumothorax after needle biopsy. Radiology 205:249–252
38. Johnston WW (1988) Fine needle aspiration biopsy versus sputum and bronchial material in the diagnosis of lung cancer. A comparative study of 168 patients. Acta Cytol 32:641–646
39. Wallace MJ, Krishnamurthy S, Broemeling LD et al (2002) CT-guided percutaneous fine-needle aspiration biopsy of small (< or =1-cm) pulmonary lesions. Radiology 225: 823–828
40. Denley H, Singh N, Clelland CA (1997) Transthoracic fine needle aspiration cytology of lung for suspected malignancy: an audit of cytological findings with histopathological correlation. Cytopathology 8:223–229
41. Simpson RW, Johnson DA, Wold LE, Goellner JR (1988) Transthoracic needle aspiration biopsy. Review of 233 cases. Acta Cytol 32:101–104
42. Komiya T, Kusunoki Y, Kobayashi M et al (1997) Transcutaneous needle biopsy of the lung. Acta Radiol 38: 821–825
43. Greif J, Marmor S, Schwarz Y, Staroselsky AN (1999) Percutaneous core needle biopsy vs. fine needle aspiration in diagnosing benign lung lesions. Acta Cytol 43:756–760
44. Bocking A, Klose KC, Kyll HJ, Hauptmann S (1995) Cytologic versus histologic evaluation of needle biopsy of the lung, hilum and mediastinum. Sensitivity, specificity and typing accuracy. Acta Cytol 39:463–471
45. DiBonito L, Colautti I, Patriarca S, Falconieri G, Barbazza R, Vielh P (1991) Cytological typing of primary lung cancer: study of 100 cases with autopsy confirmation. Diagn Cytopathol 7:7–10
46. Murphy JM, Gleeson FV, Flower CD (2001) Percutaneous needle biopsy of the lung and its impact on patient management. World J Surg 25:373–379, discussion 379–380
47. Ohno Y, Hatabu H, Takenaka D et al (2003) CT-guided transthoracic needle aspiration biopsy of small (< or = 20 mm) solitary pulmonary nodules. AJR Am J Roentgenol 180: 1665–1669
48. Flower CD, Verney GI (1979) Percutaneous needle biopsy of thoracic lesions–an evaluation of 300 biopsies. Clin Radiol 30:215–218
49. Westcott JL (1980) Direct percutaneous needle aspiration of localized pulmonary lesions: result in 422 patients. Radiology 137:31–35
50. Protopapas Z, Westcott JL (2000) Transthoracic hilar and mediastinal biopsy. Radiol Clin North Am 38:281–291
51. Protopapas Z, Westcott JL (1997) Transthoracic hilar and mediastinal biopsy. J Thorac Imaging 12:250–258
52. van Sonnenberg E, Varney RR, Casola G (1988) Antibiotic commentary. Radiology 166:901–902
53. Westcott JL, Rao N, Colley DP (1997) Transthoracic needle biopsy of small pulmonary nodules. Radiology 202: 97–103
54. Laurent F, Latrabe V, Vergier B, Montaudon M, Vernejoux JM, Dubrez J (2000) CT-guided transthoracic needle biopsy of pulmonary nodules smaller than 20 mm: results with an automated 20-gauge coaxial cutting needle. Clin Radiol 55: 281–287
55. Hayes-Jordan A, Connolly B, Temple M et al (2003) Image-guided percutaneous approach is superior to the thoracoscopic approach in the diagnosis of pulmonary nodules in children. J Pediatr Surg 38:745–748
56. Shi JM, Cai Z, Huang H et al (2009) Role of CT-guided percutaneous lung biopsy in diagnosis of pulmonary fungal infection in patients with hematologic diseases. Int J Hematol 89:624–627
57. Nosari A, Anghilieri M, Carrafiello G et al (2003) Utility of percutaneous lung biopsy for diagnosing filamentous fungal infections in hematologic malignancies. Haematologica 88:1405–1409
58. Albelda SM, Talbot GH, Gerson SL, Miller WT, Cassileth PA (1984) Role of fiberoptic bronchoscopy in the diagnosis of invasive pulmonary aspergillosis in patients with acute leukemia. Am J Med 76:1027–1034
59. Nosari A, Oreste P, Cairoli R et al (2001) Invasive aspergillosis in haematological malignancies: clinical findings and management for intensive chemotherapy completion. Am J Hematol 68:231–236
60. Caillot D, Casasnovas O, Bernard A et al (1997) Improved management of invasive pulmonary aspergillosis in neutropenic patients using early thoracic computed tomographic scan and surgery. J Clin Oncol 15: 139–147
61. McCabe RE, Brooks RG, Mark JB, Remington JS (1985) Open lung biopsy in patients with acute leukemia. Am J Med 78:609–616
62. Swischuk JL, Castaneda F, Patel JC et al (1998) Percutaneous transthoracic needle biopsy of the lung: review of 612 lesions. J Vasc Interv Radiol 9:347–352
63. Ng YL, Patsios D, Roberts H et al (2008) CT-guided percutaneous fine-needle aspiration biopsy of pulmonary nodules measuring 10 mm or less. Clin Radiol 63: 272–277
64. Montaudon M, Latrabe V, Pariente A, Corneloup O, Begueret H, Laurent F (2004) Factors influencing accuracy of CT-guided percutaneous biopsies of pulmonary lesions. Eur Radiol 14:1234–1240

Minimally Invasive Diagnostic Strategy in Immunocompromised Patients with Pulmonary Infiltrates

15

Laurent Camous, Virginie Lemiale, Achille Kouatchet, David Schnell, Sandra de Miranda, and Élie Azoulay

Contents

15.1 Introduction

Physicians in most medical specialties are seeing a growing number of patients with solid tumours and haematological malignancies. The implementation of routine screening policies has improved the early diagnosis of cancer, and treatment advances have been achieved, with the result that prolonged survival or complete recovery can be obtained in many patients. Intensive and prolonged treatment regimens introduced over the last decade have increased the overall survival rates among patients with various types of malignancies [1]. For instance, intensified and shortened cyclical chemotherapy for acute lymphoblastic leukaemia in adults has improved survival [2], advances in the understanding of multiple myeloma have led to the development of new drugs [3], targeted therapies have proved useful in patients with lymphoma and chronic myeloid leukaemia [4, 5], and growth factors that hasten neutropenia recovery have allowed higher-dose chemotherapy regimens that increase the chances for a cure [6]. However, treatment-related toxic and infectious complications have increased in lockstep with the expanding use of aggressive cancer treatments.

Pulmonary events are the leading complications in patients treated for cancer. These events are frequently severe, with diffuse pulmonary infiltrates, hypoxaemia, and secondary dysfunction of other organs (i.e., shock and kidney injury) [7]. ARF is the most common reason for admission of cancer patients to the intensive care unit (ICU) [8–10]. In cancer patients admitted to the ICU for ARF, the mortality rate is about 50% overall, 60–70% when invasive mechanical ventilation is needed, and 80–90% in recipients of allogeneic bone marrow or

L. Camous, V. Lemiale, A. Kouatchet, D. Schnell, and S. de Miranda
Paris-7 Paris-Diderot University, UFR de Médecine, 1 avenue Claude Vellefaux, 75010 Paris, France

É. Azoulay (✉) and V. Lemiale
Service de Réanimation Médicale, Hôpital Saint-Louis, 1 avenue Claude Vellefaux, 75010, Paris, France and Medical Intensive Care Units, Saint-Louis Hospital, Paris 7 University, Paris, France
e-mail: elie.azoulay@sls.aphp.fr

É. Azoulay (ed.), *Pulmonary Involvement in Patients with Hematological Malignancies*,
DOI: 10.1007/978-3-642-15742-4_15, © Springer-Verlag Berlin Heidelberg 2011

Table 15.1 Causes of pulmonary infiltrates in patients with solid tumors or hematological malignancies (Adapted from [16])

Infections
Bacterial infections
Common pyogenic bacteria
Streptococcus pneumoniae
Staphylococcus aureus
Haemophilus influenzae
Pseudomonas aeruginosa and Enterobacteriaceae
Intracellular bacteria
Legionella pneumophila
Chlamydia and *Mycoplasma pneumoniae*
Other bacteria
Actinomyces israelii
Nocardia spp.
Pneumocystis jirovecii
Invasive fungal Infections
Molds
Aspergillosis
Emerging mycotic infection: trichosporosis, fusariosis, zygomycetes
Yeasts
Lung involvement during candidemia
Endemic fungal infections
Histoplasmosis, coccidioidomycosise, blastomycosis
Viral infections (primary infections or reactivations)
Seasonal respiratory viruses
Influenzae, parainfluenzae, rhinovirus
Respiratory syncytial virus
Herpes virus
Cytomegalovirus, herpes virus, zoster virus and HHV6
Other viruses: adenovirus
Mycobacterial infections
Tuberculosis and atypical mycobacteria
Noninfectious causes
Cardiogenic pulmonary edema
Capillary leak syndrome
Lung infiltration
Drug-induced toxicity
Alveolar hemorrhage
Transfusion-related acute lung injury
Radiation-induced lung damage
Alveolar proteinosis
Diffuse alveolar damage
Bronchiolitis
Cryptogenic organized pneumonia
Second malignancy

stem cell transplants who require mechanical ventilation [11]. Non-invasive mechanical ventilation has improved survival in cancer patients requiring ventilation by reducing the need for endotracheal intubation [12–15].

A vast array of conditions can manifest as pulmonary infiltrates in patients with cancer (Table 15.1). Although the need for early treatment, most notably with antimicrobials, is universally recognized, debate continues about the best diagnostic strategy in cancer patients with pulmonary infiltrates [16]. Suggested diagnostic strategies cover an extensive spectrum ranging from empirical treatment without diagnostic investigations to diagnostic lung biopsy. However, most groups recommend diagnostic investigations. The main difference across strategies consists in whether fiberoptic bronchoscopy with bronchoalveolar lavage (FO-BAL) is performed (Table 15.2) [16]. The debate about the appropriateness of FO-BAL is particularly relevant in patients with hypoxemic ARF, among whom 40% experience respiratory status deterioration when FO-BAL is performed [17–19]. This risk must be weighed against the increased risk of death that is independently associated with failure to identify the cause of pulmonary infiltrates in patients with cancer [11, 20–22].

This review focuses on the diagnostic strategy for cancer patients with pulmonary infiltrates. We will start by briefly reviewing our DIRECT approach designed to increase the likelihood of appropriate anti-infectious therapy being given within 2 h after ICU admission (Fig. 15.1). We do not recommend a strategy based solely on the DIRECT approach, because identifying the cause of the pulmonary infiltrates increases the chances of survival. We describe the two

Table 15.2 The diagnostic strategy without bronchoscopy in cancer patients with pulmonary infiltrates (Adapted from [16])

Radiography Chest radiography Thin-section high-resolution computed tomography Echocardiography or pleural ultrasonography
Sputum Bacteria Tubercle bacillus Fungi (aspergillus)
Tests for *Pneumocystis jirovecii* (MGG staining and immuno-fluorescence)
PCR for *Pneumocystis jirovecii*
Blood cultures
Serum tests Serology: Chlamydia, Mycoplasma, Legionella Herpes consensus PCR test Circulating aspergillus antigen Circulating cytomegalovirus antigen
Nasopharyngeal aspiration Tests for viruses (PCR and immunofluorescence)
Urine tests Cytology, bacteriology *Legionella* antigen
Biological markers Brain natriuretic peptide (BNP) or ProBNP Creactive protein Fibrin Procalcitonin

The DIRECT approach: a guide to select initial antimicrobial treatments and appropriate investigations
Delay since malignancy onset or BMT
Patterns of Immune deficiency
Radiographic appearance
Clinical Experience and Knowledge of the literature
Clinical picture
Findings by the high resolution computed Tomodensitometry (HRCT)

Fig. 15.1 The DIRECT approach for selecting the initial antimicrobial treatment (Adapted from [16]). This approach does not obviate the need for diagnostic investigations

main strategies for identifying the cause of pulmonary infiltrates, i.e., with and without FO-BAL. Because the diagnostic efficiency of FO-BAL was evaluated recently [16], we will focus on the strategy that does not include FO-BAL. In our ICU experience, although FO-BAL combined with other investigations fails to identify the cause of ARF in 10–15% of patients [11, 23], severe hypoxemia and associated organ dysfunctions limit the feasibility of lung biopsy in many cases. However, studies have found lung biopsy to be highly efficient, and we raise this point in the last section of this review, which identifies areas for future research that may help us to improve the management of these very vulnerable patients.

15.2 The DIRECT Approach: A Guide for Selecting the Initial Antimicrobial Treatment and Investigations

We recently proposed a clinical approach designed to help clinicians make hypotheses about the cause of pulmonary infiltrates in patients with haematological malignancies or solid tumours (Fig. 15.1) [16]. This empiric approach is being evaluated prospectively. In the next paragraphs, we describe this strategy and provide one or two examples for each situation. The main goal of the DIRECT approach is to target diagnostic and therapeutic efforts toward those conditions that are most likely to be present in the individual patient, instead of running through the entire list of causes of pulmonary infiltrates in cancer patients. By identifying the two or three diagnoses that are plausible in a given patient, the DIRECT approach may help to initiate appropriate treatment within a few hours after admission.

D stands for *D*elay and refers to three time intervals that should be taken into account: (1) time from the diagnosis of malignancy, (2) time from respiratory symptom onset and (3) where relevant, time from allogeneic bone marrow transplantation (BMT). For example, pulmonary leukaemic infiltration or leukostasis occurs in patients with high counts of circulating blast cells, i.e., at the earliest stage of acute leukaemia or during relapses [24]. Gradually worsening dyspnea over the last 4 weeks is more likely to indicate pulmonary infiltration by the malignancy or congestive heart failure and pulmonary oedema than bacterial infection or *Pneumocystis* pneumonia (PCP). In allogeneic BMT recipients, cytomegalovirus pneumonia may occur during graft-versus-host disease (GVHD) but is unlikely to explain pulmonary infiltrates during the first 30 days after transplantation [25].

I indicates the type of *I*mmune deficiency. This point is crucial when making hypotheses about the type of infection responsible for pulmonary infiltrates. Patients with lymphocyte abnormalities (e.g., acute or chronic lymphocytic leukaemia or lymphoma) are at risk for viral or fungal infections [e.g., herpes simplex virus (HSV), PCP, and emerging fungal infections], diseases affecting monocytes and macrophages (e.g., hairy cell leukaemia, chronic myelomonocytic leukaemia, and chronic myeloid leukaemia) are associated with intracellular bacterial infections (e.g., *Legionella*, *Mycoplasma*, and tuberculosis), and neutrophil abnormalities (e.g., absolute or relative neutropenia, myelodysplastic syndrome, and chronic myeloid leukaemia) increase the risk for bacterial and fungal infections. In addition, hypogammaglobulinaemia in patients with chronic lymphocytic leukaemia or myeloma is specifically associated with infection by encapsulated bacteria. However, all these patterns need to be re-evaluated using new technologies to assess the cellular defects. In addition, the increasing use of intensive and prolonged cancer chemotherapy regimens and of targeted therapies (e.g., rituximab and alemtuzumab) can be expected to change the patterns of immune deficiency seen in cancer patients and, therefore, qualitative studies are needed.

R indicates the chest *R*adiograph findings.

E refers to *E*xperience and knowledge of the literature. For example, although diffuse alveolar haemorrhage can theoretically cause pulmonary infiltrates in immunosuppressed patients, this complication seems virtually confined to BMT recipients [26, 27]. Similarly, pulmonary aspergillosis, although possible in every cancer patient, occurs chiefly in patients with prolonged neutropenia (e.g., acute leukaemia patients), long-term steroid therapy [28, 29], and BMT [30].

T refers to findings by high-resolution computed *T*omography (HRCT).

15.3 Bronchoscopy and Bronchoalveolar (FO-BAL) Lavage in Cancer Patients with Pulmonary Infiltrates

In the late 1980s, FO-BAL became the most widely used investigation for identifying the cause of pulmonary infiltrates in immunosuppressed patients [31–36]. FO-BAL superseded lung biopsy, as it was easier, simpler, and less invasive. These advantages were reported to be particularly helpful in patients at very high risk of death if treated with mechanical ventilation [37]. The results of 18 studies (in 1,537 patients) indicated that FO-BAL provided the diagnosis in about half the patients and led to treatment modifications in one-third (Table 15.3). These data were confirmed by a recent retrospective study [38], including 175 haematological patients admitted to the ICU for ARF and showing a 10% rate of life-threatening complications after FO-BAL. Moreover, the diagnostic yield was only 50%, and the therapeutic impact was significant in only 17% of the patients [38].

Data from 764 BMT recipients in 15 studies showed that FO-BAL supplied the diagnosis in 55% of cases, but caused the respiratory status to deteriorate in up to 40% (Table 15.4) [17–19].

The limited diagnostic efficiency of FO-BAL in immunocompromised patients may be related to several factors. First, most patients are already on antimicrobial therapy at the time of FO-BAL. Therefore, bacterial pneumonia is usually documented clinically but not bacteriologically, although FO-BAL may detect resistant pathogens that require adjustment of the antimicrobial regimen. Second, BAL fluid analysis is often confined to tests for infections, and most studies fail to report the appearance of the alveolar cells, which may suggest drug toxicity, or the presence of malignant cells, indicating pulmonary infiltration. Third, most studies were conducted in the 1990s, before the introduction of new tools for diagnosing infections with viruses, parasites, and fungi [39]. However, the diagnostic yield of FO-BAL was not better in recent studies [11, 40]. Last, FO-BAL may be less efficient in patients with cancer than in those with AIDS because of pathophysiological differences in the development of pulmonary invasion by *Aspergillus* or *Pneumocystis* [30, 41–45]. For instance, a study of PCP in cancer patients showed marked inflammation and scarce *Pneumocystis* bodies, indicating that negative BAL fluid findings did not rule out PCP [43].

15.4 Diagnostic Strategy Without Bronchoscopy

Table 15.2 lists the investigations used in the diagnostic strategy without FO-BAL. Routinely performing all these tests may be an alternative to FO-BAL in most

Table 15.3 Studies of fiberoptic bronchoscopy with bronchoalveolar lavage in patients with malignancies and pulmonary infiltrates (Adapted from [16])

Reference	*n*	Diagnosis	Diagnostic impact	Therapeutic impact
Stover et al. [96]	97	HM	66	–
Martin et al. [109]	100	HM	30	–
Xaubet et al. [110]	96	HM	49	31
Campbell et al. [111]	22	HM	55	–
Pisani et al. [112]	150	HM	39	–
Maschmeyer et al. [113]	46	Neutropenia	30	–
Cordonnier et al. [100]	56	Neutropenia	53	24
Cazzadori et al. [114]	142	HM	36	–
Von Eiff et al. [40]	90	HM	66	65
White et al. [3]	68	HM	31	24
Ewig et al. [28]	49	HM	31	16
Gruson et al. [18]	41	Neutropenia	63	28
Hilbert et al. [22]	24/46	HM	62	71
Murray et al. [2]	27	HM	33	28
Azoulay et al. [4]	203	HM	49.5	45.1
Pagano et al. [115]	127	HM	53	14
Jain et al. [82]	104	HM	56	–
Hohenadel et al. [81]	95	HM	30	–
Total	1537		46.2	34.6

cancer patients with pulmonary infiltrates (Fig. 15.2 and 15.3). We review available data on the use of each of these investigations in cancer patients. Imaging findings are discussed in another chapter 12. We will focus on laboratory methods to diagnose pulmonary infiltrates.

15.4.1 Laboratory Tests for Diagnosing Infectious

15.4.1.1 Bacterial Infections

Bacterial pneumonia in immunocompromised patients is usually due to gram-negative bacilli or *Staphylococcus aureus*. Selection pressure due to the use of broad-spectrum antibiotics explains the emergence of resistant gram-negative strains. As discussed above, FO-BAL often fails to establish the exact diagnosis. Moreover, identified organisms may indicate colonisation rather than infection. In a population of allogeneic BMT recipients, no pathogen was isolated in 70% of the patients, and some of the isolated microorganisms (such as *Candida* spp., coagulase-negative staphylococci, and enterococci) were probably mere contaminants [46].

As shown by studies of FO-BAL, conventional microbiological testing may fail to identify the cause of lower respiratory tract infection. In patients on broad-spectrum antibiotics at the time of sample collection, gram staining and culturing have low sensitivity, and cultures require time. Furthermore, these methods fail to distinguish colonisation from infection. Serological testing is slow and often lacks both sensitivity and specificity. In most cases, the causative pathogen is not found, despite optimal investigations. Methods that rapidly identify the causative pathogen would help physicians to select the best treatment strategy. Such methods are already available for

Table 15.4 Studies of fiberoptic bronchoscopy with bronchoalveolar lavage in bone marrow transplant recipients with pulmonary infiltrates (Adapted from [16])

Author	*n*	Type of patients	Diagnostic impact	Therapeutic impact	Complications
Springmeyer et al. [20]	22	Auto-allo	58	–	13
Corodonnier et al. [17]	52	Allo	50	–	0
Cordonnier et al. [9]	69	Allo	66	–	–
Milburn et al. [19]	40	Allo	80	76	0
Springmeyer [78]	15	Auto-allo	89	–	40
Heurlin et al. [116]	18	Auto-allo	61	–	–
Weiss et al. [80]	47	Auto-allo	47	–	12
Campbell et al. [79]	27	–	74	63	11
AbuFarsakh et al. [117]	77	Auto-allo	42	–	–
White et al. [93]	68	Auto-allo	31	24	15 (7% MV)
Dunagan et al. [1][a]	71	Auto-allo	38	42	27 (4% MV)
Glazer et al. [118]	79	Auto-allo	67	62	–
Gruson et al. [39]	38	Auto-allo	42	–	–
Gruson et al. [18]	52	Auto-allo	38	28	17
Huaringa et al. [108]	89	Auto-allo	42	–	–
Total	764	Auto-allo	55	49	0–40%

[a]32% Mechanical ventilation

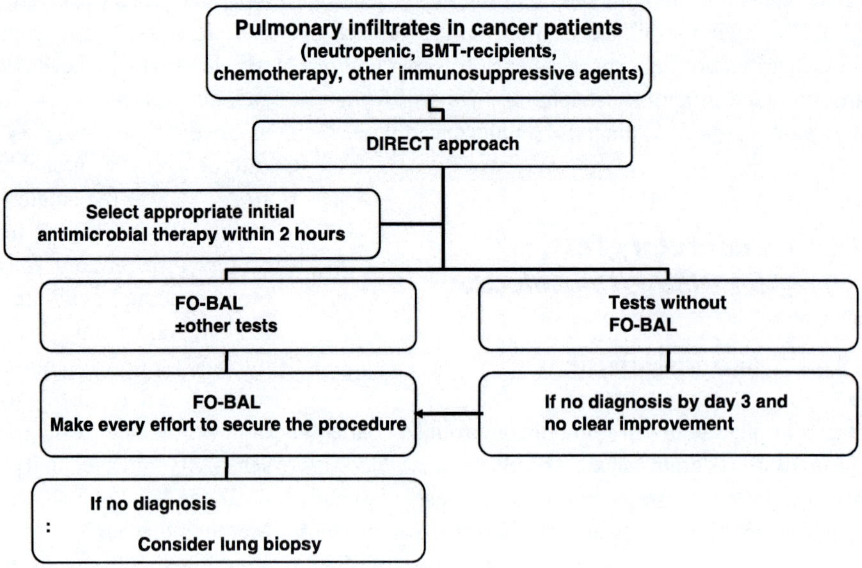

Fig. 15.2 Diagnostic strategy for cancer patients with pulmonary infiltrates

Legionella pneumophila and *Streptococcus pneumoniae* and are being developed for other bacteria. It seems, however, that the incidence of these pathogens may have been overestimated in haematological patients.

Legionella pneumophila

Antibodies to *Legionella pneumophila* were first detected using indirect immunofluorescence or microagglutination tests. Since then, numerous ELISAs based on different antigen-extraction methods have been developed. The reported sensitivities of these assays vary substantially, from 41% to 75% [47, 48]. Low titres of antibodies against *Legionella* spp. have been found in healthy volunteers, blood donors, outpatients, and hospitalised patients [49, 50]. These low titres seem to indicate previous exposure to *Legionella* spp. The urinary antigen test produced positive results 1–3 days after the clinical onset and remained positive for almost 1 year in a small proportion of patients [51, 52]. Importantly, the urinary antigen test showed greater than 99% specificity [53]. Sensitivity for *L. pneumophila* infections ranged from 56% to 99% [54]. Low sensitivity of urinary antigen assays for serogroups other than *L. pneumophila* serogroup 1 has been reported, the range being 14–69% [55, 56]. In the future, an easy-to-perform PCR test with high sensitivity and greater than 99% specificity will probably become available on a wider scale [57].

Streptococcus pneumoniae

The diagnosis of pneumococcal infection requires recovery of the microorganism from an uncontaminated specimen (e.g., blood or pleural fluid). Blood culture results are positive in only about one-fourth of cases, and prior antibiotic therapy significantly reduces the proportion of positive blood culture results. Bacteraemia may be absent in 70–80% of cases of *S. pneumoniae* pneumonia. Sputum cultures provide only a probable diagnosis, since *S. pneumoniae* carriage in the nasopharynx is common. PCR assays for *S. pneumoniae* have shown inadequate sensitivity when used on blood or urine and inadequate specificity for infection when used on respiratory samples. Several publications have described antigen detection assays. Good sensitivity and specificity have been reported with commercial kits for urinary C polysaccharide detection in adults. For example, the Binax NOW *S. pneumoniae* urinary antigen test was 82% sensitive and 97% specific when positive blood cultures were used as the reference standard. The test is simple to perform, detects the C polysaccharide cell wall antigen common to all *S. pneumoniae* strains, and provides results within 15 min. Urinary antigen was still detected in 83% of patients who were retested on treatment day 3 and persisted for at least 7 days in many patients [58]. Additional studies produced similar results (Table 15.5) [59–61]. A nested PCR assay targeting the pneumolysin gene was used to detect *S. pneumoniae* DNA in multiple sample types from 474 adults with community-acquired pneumonia and 183 control patients without pneumonia. The assay added little to information from existing diagnostic tests for *S. pneumoniae* and was unable to distinguish colonisation from infection when used on respiratory samples [59, 61]. Studies of *S. pneumoniae* antigen tests involving latex agglutination or counter-current immunoelectrophoresis showed detection rates ranging from 0% to 88%, and specificity was often poorly defined.

Table 15.5 Binax NOW *Streptococcus pneumoniae* urinary antigen test: sensitivity and specificity

Reference	Type of infection	Number of patients	Sensitivity (%)	Specificity (%)
Smith, J Clin Microbiol 2003 [58]	Pneumococcal bacteremia	107	82	97
Murdoch, J Clin Microbiol 2001 [61]	Community-acquired pneumonia	420	80	100
Dominguez, Chest 2001 [60]	Bacteremic and nonbacteremic pneumonia	51	82	97

Mycoplasma pneumoniae

The diagnosis of hard-to-culture pathogens such as *Mycoplasma pneumoniae* classically relies on testing paired sera to demonstrate a rise in the antibody titre. This method is of uncertain value in immunocompromised patients, most notably those with impaired cell-mediated immunity. Culturing is relatively insensitive and time-consuming, requiring up to 3 weeks for pathogen detection [62]. A number of PCR assays for *M. pneumoniae* have been evaluated in various respiratory specimens and patient populations, with promising results. PCR is more sensitive and considerably faster than culturing. In general, PCR results correlate well with serological results [63]. Both upper and lower respiratory tract samples are suitable for PCR testing. Upper respiratory tract samples (throat swabs and nasopharyngeal samples) may be the preferred sample types, as they are easy to obtain and ensure high sensitivity [59]. PCR on throat swabs may be the best existing diagnostic test for *M. pneumoniae.* However, standardised protocols will have to be developed before this test is recommended for widespread use [64].

Chlamydia pneumoniae

Cell cultures for *C. pneumoniae* detection are technically demanding and time-consuming, and their yield is generally low. Therefore, the diagnosis of *C. pneumoniae* infection relies largely on serological testing, whose value in immunocompromised patients is uncertain. Furthermore, both acute- and convalescent-phase sera must be tested, which can only provide a retrospective diagnosis. These major limitations have prompted many studies of PCR for diagnosing *C. pneumoniae* infection. Unfortunately, the results have been conflicting. Overall, PCR was at least as sensitive as culturing, but its specificity was difficult to assess given the absence of an appropriate reference standard [59]. *C. pneumoniae* DNA can be detected in both upper and lower respiratory tract samples, but it is unclear which sampling site is better. Highly sensitive PCR techniques may increase the ability to detect *C. pneumoniae* carriage, the clinical relevance of which is unclear.

15.4.1.2 Diagnosis of Viral Respiratory Infections Using Nasopharyngeal Aspirates

In the past, viral cultures were the reference standard for the laboratory diagnosis of respiratory viral infections. However, 2–10 days were usually needed to obtain the results. To overcome this major limitation, faster diagnostic techniques, such as viral antigen detection, were introduced. These faster techniques are generally considered less sensitive and less specific than cell cultures. Moreover, viral antigen detection is not feasible for all respiratory viruses. PCR has proven extremely specific and sensitive for detecting respiratory viruses: it is now the reference standard for diagnosing respiratory viral infections and the only method available for detecting some viruses [39]. PCR was not only more sensitive than viral culture or antigen or antibody tests for detecting respiratory viruses in patients with haematological malignancies, but also decreased the time to diagnosis [65, 66]. Parainfluenza viruses 1–3, respiratory syncytial virus, rhinovirus, influenza viruses A and B, enteroviruses, and coronaviruses were reliably detected by PCR [67–69]. Nose-throat swabs yielded the same results with PCR as did BAL samples [39]. In a recent study of patients with haematological malignancies and respiratory viral infections, PCR on nasopharyngeal aspirates usually provided the diagnosis [70]. In the near future, widespread use of multiplex PCRs in patients with haematological malignancies will raise additional concerns about the relevance of virus retrieval from nasopharyngeal aspirates in patients with lung infiltrates [69].

Cytomegalovirus frequently causes severe disease after stem cell transplantation. The cytomegalovirus antigen assay is a rapid quantitative tool for monitoring cytomegalovirus infection. However, this method is tedious, as it requires counting the cells in the samples. In addition, the results may be influenced by factors such as storage and fixation methods. PCR assays have been used to diagnose cytomegalovirus infection. Real-time PCR provides a qualitative assessment of viral load. However, although the antigenaemia cutoff has been determined, the viral load cutoff is unknown [39, 71].

BMT recipients and patients with haematological malignancies who have severe impairments of cell-mediated immunity are at risk for HSV pneumonia. Although HSV type 1 accounts for most cases, other herpes viruses such as cytomegalovirus, varicella zoster virus, Epstein-Barr virus, HHV-6, and HHV-8 are also common causes of pneumonia in this population. Advances in diagnostic techniques and the use of preventive or pre-emptive treatments have altered the epidemiology of some of the herpes virus infections. However, herpes viruses continue to cause significant morbidity and mortality in stem cell recipients [72]. A multiplex PCR assay designed to amplify herpes virus DNA in a diverse range of clinical specimens yielded higher detection rates for the viruses represented in the assay than did virus isolation and immunofluorescence-based antigen detection [73]. The turnaround time was far less than for the other techniques. Overall, the multiplex PCR detected substantially more herpes viruses, in some cases in specimens or at body sites where these viruses were found only rarely or never using conventional methods. Multiplex PCR has not yet been evaluated as a tool for diagnosing herpes virus pneumonia in patients with cancer. However, multiplex PCR may help to assess the pathogenic role for herpes viruses found in respiratory samples. An oligonucleotide microarray for herpes virus detection in clinical samples has been developed and needs to be evaluated in clinical practice.

15.4.1.3 Non-invasive Diagnostic Strategy for Diagnosing Pneumocystis Pneumonia (PCP)

The standard method for diagnosing PCP pneumonia is microscopic identification of the organism using stains (methenamine silver, Giemsa, or toluidine blue O) or antibodies in BAL or induced sputum samples [74]. Several studies confirmed that PCR was more sensitive than microscopy for detecting *P. jiroveci* [75]. PCR is useful to rule out *P. jiroveci* infection in HIV-negative immunocompromised patients, who often have lower parasite counts than AIDS patients [43]. Nested PCR methods tend to have low specificity with high false-positive rates, whereas real-time PCR seems more specific [39, 76–78]. Samples similar to those used for microscopy can serve for PCR [75]. BAL specimens have the best yield; induced sputum samples, which are commonly used for HIV-infected patients, may be diagnostic but have not been evaluated in patients with other causes of immunodeficiency. [77]. Oral washes may be used as alternative non-invasive samples, despite lower sensitivity of PCR compared to lower respiratory tract samples [42, 79]. In a recent study [80], 448 patients were screened for *P. jiroveci* pneumonia with PCR and Gromori-Grocott staining. BAL was performed in 351 patients and induced sputum was diagnostic in 39 patients. PCR sensitivity was 87% and specificity was 92%, Negative predictive value on BAL samples was 98.7%. Given this excellent negative predictive value, we recommend PCR as the leading method for excluding PCP in cancer patients with pulmonary infiltrates. Negative PCR results on BAL fluid or induced sputum indicate that PCP treatment can be safely discontinued [81].

15.4.1.4 Diagnosis of Fungal Infection

The diagnosis of invasive aspergillosis in haematological patients is often challenging. Until recently, only specimens from normally sterile sites were considered necessary for the definitive diagnosis of invasive fungal infections. Specimens from sites that may be colonised (e.g., sputum, BAL fluid, or sinus aspirate) were rarely diagnostic. BAL fluid cultures positive for *Aspergillus* spp. may indicate colonisation instead of invasive infection. Cultures may require days or weeks. The reference standard is histologically proven hyphal invasion in tissue specimens obtained by invasive procedures, but these may be deemed unsafe in patients with cytopenia [44, 82]. The first prospective, pathology-verified evaluation of a sandwich ELISA using a monoclonal antibody to galactomannan (GM) showed that serial monitoring was 92.6% sensitive and 95.4% specific [83]. The positive predictive value was 93%, and the negative predictive value was 95% [83]. In more than half the cases, antigenaemia was detected before invasive aspergillosis was suspected clinically [84, 85]. Based on this study and others, the European Organization for Research and Treatment of Cancer/ Invasive Fungal Infections Cooperative Group and the National Institute of Allergy and Infectious Diseases Mycoses Study Group convened a consensus panel to develop standard definitions for invasive fungal infections, introducing *Aspergillus* antigenaemia testing as an important diagnostic tool. The panel recommended that *Aspergillus* antigenaemia testing be used to support a probable diagnosis [44]. The value of this diagnostic strategy has been clinically validated [86, 87] and shown to be clinically relevant. Moreover, the diagnostic yield of *Aspergillus* antigenaemia may be higher in neutropenic patients [88]. Finally, PCR has been used to detect *Aspergillus* spp., but false-positive results were noted, and no standardised commercial method is available [89–91].

15.4.1.5 Microbial DNA Identification by Blood PCR

Numerous multivariate analyses have shown that inadequate antibiotic therapy in patients with severe sepsis is a strong and independent risk factor for death [92]. In clinical practice, diagnostic uncertainty regarding the causative microorganism leads to the use of broad-spectrum combinations of antibiotics. The high selection pressure created by these combinations may lead to the emergence of multi-drug resistant bacteria. Moreover, in patients with haematological malignancies, who are often neutropenic, the diagnostic yield of blood samples is low (25% in one study [93] and probably even less in patients on concomitant antibiotic therapy), and more than half the clinically diagnosed infections are treated empirically. These data may reflect the presumed low bacterial/fungal load necessary for clinical infection. Therefore, rapid diagnostic tests are needed [94]. In recent years, several diagnostic tools based on culture-independent molecular biology-based techniques, such as real-time polymerase chain reaction, were developed [95]. However, their usefulness in clinical practice needs to be demonstrated. Numerous studies are ongoing. In severe sepsis [96], the match between PCR and blood culture results seems disappointing, with only 70% of positive PCRs in patients with positive blood cultures. However, positive PCR results showed statistically significant associations with higher organ dysfunction scores, as well as a trend toward an association with higher mortality. In immunocompromised patients, the results of preliminary studies of PCR seem more promising, although the true accuracy of these methods needs to be determined [97, 98]. PCR seems more sensitive than blood cultures, with a 100% match between positive blood cultures and positive PCR, as well as a high negative predictive value (98.6%) of negative PCR. However, these results require confirmation in larger studies, and their clinical usefulness needs to be tested in terms of antibiotic use and treatment reduction.

15.4.1.6 Biomarkers

ARF in cancer patients can be related to many conditions, including infections (opportunistic or bacterial) and non-infectious events (infiltration by malignant cells, drug-related pulmonary toxicity, or cardiogenic pulmonary oedema) [11]. Identification of the exact cause of ARF is associated with a marked improvement in survival. Rapid evaluation of the contribution of left ventricular failure to ARF enables prompt adequate treatment, obviating the need for invasive diagnostic procedures. Echocardiography is the reference standard for diagnosing left ventricular dysfunction but requires the availability of an experienced sonographer. B-type natriuretic peptide (BNP) is a predominantly ventricular cardiac hormone whose levels increase in the event of cardiac overdistension [99]. BNP measurement has been found highly sensitive and specific for the diagnosis of heart failure [100]. However, in the initial cohort, no cancer patients were included.

The accuracy of BNP in cancer patients with ARF was evaluated in a recent study [101] of 100 patients. This study showed that BNP was useful only for ruling out a role for cardiac dysfunction in ARF, when NT-pro BNP was under 500 pg/mL (100% specificity and 100% negative predictive value). However, due to the direct cardiac toxicity of anti-cancer chemotherapy and high rate of renal failure among cancer patients, BNP elevation was not accurate for diagnosing cardiac dysfunction.

The morbidity of anti-infectious treatment can be high. Systemic inflammatory response syndrome (SIRS) can be related to various causes (i.e., toxicity of chemotherapy), and a highly specific marker for sepsis would therefore be valuable. In non-neutropenic patients, procalcitonin (PCT), produced by the reticulo-endothelial cells, is a specific and sensitive marker for bacterial infections [102]. For example, PCT can differentiate between bacterial and viral meningitis. Data from neutropenic patients are scarce except in the paediatric population, where small studies [103, 104] suggested that PCT might be a good marker for bacterial sepsis with more than 95% negative predictive value and more than 85% sensitivity. In adults, no convincing data are available. Some studies in neutropenic patients [105] indicated that PCT was unhelpful (although we have personal data that seems somewhat more promising). Therefore, we cannot recommend PCT as a diagnostic tool in patients with haematological malignancies or other forms of cancer.

15.5 Conclusion and Avenues for Future Research

The diagnostic and therapeutic impact of FO-BAL has been evaluated in several studies, and other diagnostic investigations have been evaluated individually. However, the routine use of all available investigations except FO-BAL has not been assessed, nor have the diagnostic strategy and outcomes been compared in cancer patients managed with versus without FO-BAL. The number of patients in whom non-invasive investigations obviates the need for FO-BAL may also deserve to be determined.

In the future, the development of new tools will contribute to improve the diagnosis of bacterial pneumonia (16S RNA) and viral pneumonia (oligonucleotide microarray). These new tools can be expected to improve the diagnostic yield of BAL analysis, and non-bronchoscopic lavage may cause less respiratory deterioration than FO-BAL [106]. Markers for heart failure (brain natriuretic peptide) or bacterial infection (procalcitonin) need to be evaluated in cancer patients.

We predict that advances in diagnostic tools will decrease the role for FO-BAL, just as in the past FO-BAL decreased the role for lung biopsy [107]. When the diagnosis remains uncertain despite extensive investigations including FO-BAL, the feasibility, safety, and diagnostic yield of lung biopsy should be evaluated, since identifying the cause of pulmonary infiltrates is known to reduce mortality [11, 16].

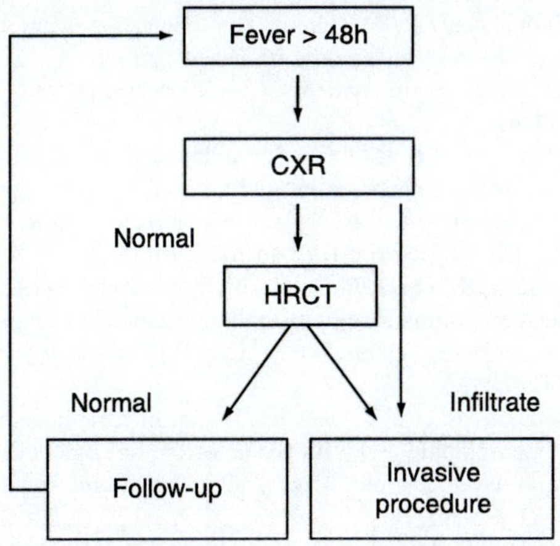

Fig. 15.3 Recommendations from the Infectious Diseases Working Party of the German Society of Haematology and Oncology (Adapted from [45])

References

1. Brenner H (2002) Long-term survival rates of cancer patients achieved by the end of the 20th century: a period analysis. Lancet 360(9340):1131–5
2. Linker C et al (2002) Intensified and shortened cyclical chemotherapy for adult acute lymphoblastic leukemia. J Clin Oncol 20(10):2464–71
3. Richardson PG et al (2005) Bortezomib or high-dose dexamethasone for relapsed multiple myeloma. N Engl J Med 352(24):2487–98
4. O'Brien SG et al (2003) Imatinib compared with interferon and low-dose cytarabine for newly diagnosed chronic-phase chronic myeloid leukemia. N Engl J Med 348(11): 994–1004
5. Coiffier B et al (2002) CHOP chemotherapy plus rituximab compared with CHOP alone in elderly patients with diffuse large-B-cell lymphoma. N Engl J Med 346(4):235–42
6. Bergh J et al (2000) Tailored fluorouracil, epirubicin, and cyclophosphamide compared with marrow-supported high-dose chemotherapy as adjuvant treatment for high-risk breast cancer: a randomised trial. Scandinavian Breast Group 9401 study. Lancet 356(9239):1384–91
7. Chaoui D et al (2004) Incidence and prognostic value of respiratory events in acute leukemia. Leukemia 18(4):670–5
8. Azoulay E et al (1999) Changing use of intensive care for hematological patients: the example of multiple myeloma. Intensive Care Med 25(12):1395–401
9. Kress JP et al (1999) Outcomes of critically ill cancer patients in a university hospital setting. Am J Respir Crit Care Med 160(6):1957–61
10. Soares M et al (2004) Performance of six severity-of-illness scores in cancer patients requiring admission to the intensive care unit: a prospective observational study. Crit Care 8(4):R194–203, Epub 2004 May 24
11. Azoulay E et al (2004) The prognosis of acute respiratory failure in critically ill cancer patients. Medicine (Baltimore) 83(6):360–70
12. Azoulay E et al (2001) Improved survival in cancer patients requiring mechanical ventilatory support: impact of noninvasive mechanical ventilatory support. Crit Care Med 29(3):519–25
13. Meert AP et al (2003) Noninvasive ventilation: application to the cancer patient admitted in the intensive care unit. Support Care Cancer 11(1):56–9, Epub 2002 Jul 19
14. Rabbat A et al (2005) Prognosis of patients with acute myeloid leukaemia admitted to intensive care. Br J Haematol 129(3):350–7

15. Hilbert G et al (2001) Noninvasive ventilation in immunosuppressed patients with pulmonary infiltrates, fever, and acute respiratory failure. N Engl J Med 344(7):481–7
16. Azoulay E, Schlemmer B (2006) Diagnostic strategy in cancer patients with acute respiratory failure. Intensive Care Med 32(6):808–22, Epub 2006 Apr 29
17. Dunagan DP et al (1997) Bronchoscopic evaluation of pulmonary infiltrates following bone marrow transplantation. Chest 111(1):135–41
18. White P, Bonacum JT, Miller CB (1997) Utility of fiberoptic bronchoscopy in bone marrow transplant patients. Bone Marrow Transplant 20(8):681–7
19. Murray PV et al (2001) Use of first line bronchoalveolar lavage in the immunosuppressed oncology patient. Bone Marrow Transplant 27(9):967–71
20. Stover DE et al (1984) Bronchoalveolar lavage in the diagnosis of diffuse pulmonary infiltrates in the immunosuppressed host. Ann Intern Med 101(1):1–7
21. Gruson D et al (1999) Severe respiratory failure requiring ICU admission in bone marrow transplant recipients. Eur Respir J 13(4):883–7
22. Gruson D et al (2000) Utility of fiberoptic bronchoscopy in neutropenic patients admitted to the intensive care unit with pulmonary infiltrates. Crit Care Med 28(7):2224–30
23. Rano A et al (2001) Pulmonary infiltrates in non-HIV immunocompromised patients: a diagnostic approach using non-invasive and bronchoscopic procedures. Thorax 56(5): 379–87
24. Azoulay E et al (2003) Acute monocytic leukemia presenting as acute respiratory failure. Am J Respir Crit Care Med 167(10):1329–33
25. Cordonnier C et al (1987) Evaluation of three assays on alveolar lavage fluid in the diagnosis of cytomegalovirus pneumonitis after bone marrow transplantation. J Infect Dis 155(3):495–500
26. Agusti C et al (1995) Diffuse alveolar hemorrhage in allogeneic bone marrow transplantation. A postmortem study Am J Respir Crit Care Med 151(4):1006–10
27. Afessa B et al (2002) Diffuse alveolar hemorrhage in hematopoietic stem cell transplant recipients. Am J Respir Crit Care Med 166(5):641–5
28. Trof RJ et al (2007) Management of invasive pulmonary aspergillosis in non-neutropenic critically ill patients. Intensive Care Med 33(10):1694–703
29. Castagnola E et al (2008) Incidence of bacteremias and invasive mycoses in children undergoing allogeneic hematopoietic stem cell transplantation: a single center experience. Bone Marrow Transplant 41(4):339–47
30. Patterson TF et al (2000) Invasive aspergillosis. Disease spectrum, treatment practices, and outcomes. I3 Aspergillus Study Group. Med Baltim 79(4):250–60
31. Cordonnier C et al (1986) Pulmonary complications occurring after allogeneic bone marrow transplantation. A study of 130 consecutive transplanted patients. Cancer 58(5): 1047–54
32. Springmeyer SC (1987) The clinical use of bronchoalveolar lavage. Chest 92(5):771–2
33. Milburn HJ, Prentice HG, du Bois RM (1987) Role of bronchoalveolar lavage in the evaluation of interstitial pneumonitis in recipients of bone marrow transplants. Thorax 42(10):766–72
34. Cordonnier C et al (1985) Diagnostic yield of bronchoalveolar lavage in pneumonitis occurring after allogeneic bone marrow transplantation. Am Rev Respir Dis 132(5): 1118–23
35. Akoun GM, Milleron BJ, Mayaud CM (1985) Diagnosis by bronchoalveolar lavage of cause of pulmonary infiltrates in haematological malignancies. Br Med J (Clin Res Ed) 290(6481):1589–90
36. White DA et al (1985) *Pulmonary cell populations in the immunosuppressed patient.* Bronchoalveolar lavage findings during episodes of pneumonitis. Chest 88(3): 352–9
37. Rubenfeld GD, Crawford SW (1996) Withdrawing life support from mechanically ventilated recipients of bone marrow transplants: a case for evidence-based guidelines. Ann Intern Med 125(8):625–33
38. Rabbat A et al (2008) Is BAL useful in patients with acute myeloid leukemia admitted in ICU for severe respiratory complications? Leukemia 22(7):1361–7
39. Murdoch DR (2005) Impact of rapid microbiological testing on the management of lower respiratory tract infection. Clin Infect Dis 41(10):1445–7, Epub 2005 Oct 13
40. Jain P et al (2004) Role of flexible bronchoscopy in immunocompromised patients with lung infiltrates. Chest 125(2):712–22
41. Azoulay E et al (1999) AIDS-related Pneumocystis carinii pneumonia in the era of adjunctive steroids: implication of BAL neutrophilia. Am J Respir Crit Care Med 160(2): 493–9
42. Kovacs JA et al (2001) New insights into transmission, diagnosis, and drug treatment of Pneumocystis carinii pneumonia. JAMA 286(19):2450–60
43. Kovacs JA et al (1984) Pneumocystis carinii pneumonia: a comparison between patients with the acquired immunodeficiency syndrome and patients with other immunodeficiencies. Ann Intern Med 100(5):663–71
44. Ascioglu S et al (2002) Defining opportunistic invasive fungal infections in immunocompromised patients with cancer and hematopoietic stem cell transplants: an international consensus. Clin Infect Dis 34(1):7–14, Epub 2001 Nov 26
45. Caillot D et al (2001) Role of early diagnosis and aggressive surgery in the management of invasive pulmonary aspergillosis in neutropenic patients. Clin Microbiol Infect 7(Suppl 2):54–61
46. Dettenkofer M et al (2005) Surveillance of nosocomial sepsis and pneumonia in patients with a bone marrow or peripheral blood stem cell transplant: a multicenter project. Clin Infect Dis 40(7):926–31, Epub 2005 Mar 4
47. Blazquez RM et al (2005) Sensitivity of urinary antigen test in relation to clinical severity in a large outbreak of Legionella pneumonia in Spain. Eur J Clin Microbiol Infect Dis 24(7):488–91
48. Dominguez J et al (1999) Evaluation of a rapid immunochromatographic assay for the detection of Legionella antigen in urine samples. Eur J Clin Microbiol Infect Dis 18(12):896–8
49. Waterer GW, Baselski VS, Wunderink RG (2001) Legionella and community-acquired pneumonia: a review of current diagnostic tests from a clinician's viewpoint. Am J Med 110(1):41–8

50. Deforges L et al (1999) Case of false-positive results of the urinary antigen test for Legionella pneumophila. Clin Infect Dis 29(4):953–4
51. Mykietiuk A et al (2005) Clinical outcomes for hospitalized patients with Legionella pneumonia in the antigenuria era: the influence of levofloxacin therapy. Clin Infect Dis 40(6):794–9, Epub 2005 Feb 17
52. Dominguez JA et al (1998) Comparison of the Binax Legionella urinary antigen enzyme immunoassay (EIA) with the Biotest Legionella Urin antigen EIA for detection of Legionella antigen in both concentrated and nonconcentrated urine samples. J Clin Microbiol 36(9): 2718–22
53. Wever PC et al (2000) Rapid diagnosis of Legionnaires' disease using an immunochromatographic assay for Legionella pneumophila serogroup 1 antigen in urine during an outbreak in the Netherlands. J Clin Microbiol 38(7):2738–9
54. Yzerman EP et al (2002) Sensitivity of three urinary antigen tests associated with clinical severity in a large outbreak of Legionnaires' disease in The Netherlands. J Clin Microbiol 40(9):3232–6
55. Helbig JH et al (2003) Clinical utility of urinary antigen detection for diagnosis of community-acquired, travel-associated, and nosocomial legionnaires' disease. J Clin Microbiol 41(2):838–40
56. Benson RF, Tang PW, Fields BS (2000) Evaluation of the Binax and Biotest urinary antigen kits for detection of Legionnaires' disease due to multiple serogroups and species of Legionella. J Clin Microbiol 38(7):2763–5
57. Den Boer JW, Yzerman EP (2004) Diagnosis of Legionella infection in Legionnaires' disease. Eur J Clin Microbiol Infect Dis 23(12):871–8
58. Smith MD et al (2003) Rapid diagnosis of bacteremic pneumococcal infections in adults by using the Binax NOW Streptococcus pneumoniae urinary antigen test: a prospective, controlled clinical evaluation. J Clin Microbiol 41(7):2810–3
59. Murdoch DR (2003) Nucleic acid amplification tests for the diagnosis of pneumonia. Clin Infect Dis 36(9):1162–70, Epub 2003 Apr 22
60. Dominguez J et al (2001) Detection of Streptococcus pneumoniae antigen by a rapid immunochromatographic assay in urine samples. Chest 119(1):243–9
61. Murdoch DR et al (2001) Evaluation of a rapid immunochromatographic test for detection of Streptococcus pneumoniae antigen in urine samples from adults with community-acquired pneumonia. J Clin Microbiol 39(10):3495–8
62. Jacobs E, Bennewitz A, Bredt W (1986) Reaction pattern of human anti-Mycoplasma pneumoniae antibodies in enzyme-linked immunosorbent assays and immunoblotting. J Clin Microbiol 23(3):517–22
63. Abele-Horn M et al (1998) Molecular approaches to diagnosis of pulmonary diseases due to Mycoplasma pneumoniae. J Clin Microbiol 36(2):548–51
64. Dorigo-Zetsma JW et al (2001) Molecular detection of Mycoplasma pneumoniae in adults with community-acquired pneumonia requiring hospitalization. J Clin Microbiol 39(3): 1184–6
65. van Elden LJ et al (2002) Polymerase chain reaction is more sensitive than viral culture and antigen testing for the detection of respiratory viruses in adults with hematological cancer and pneumonia. Clin Infect Dis 34(2):177–83, Epub 2001 Dec 4
66. Templeton KE et al (2005) Improved diagnosis of the etiology of community-acquired pneumonia with real-time polymerase chain reaction. Clin Infect Dis 41(3):345–51, Epub 2005 Jun 22
67. van Elden LJ et al (2003) Applicability of a real-time quantitative PCR assay for diagnosis of respiratory syncytial virus infection in immunocompromised adults. J Clin Microbiol 41(9):4378–81
68. van Elden LJ et al (2004) Frequent detection of human coronaviruses in clinical specimens from patients with respiratory tract infection by use of a novel real-time reverse-transcriptase polymerase chain reaction. J Infect Dis 189(4): 652–7, Epub 2004 Jan 28
69. van Kraaij MG et al (2005) Frequent detection of respiratory viruses in adult recipients of stem cell transplants with the use of real-time polymerase chain reaction, compared with viral culture. Clin Infect Dis 40(5):662–9, Epub 2005 Feb 7
70. Martino R et al (2003) Respiratory virus infections in adults with hematologic malignancies: a prospective study. Clin Infect Dis 36(1):1–8, Epub 2002 Dec 9
71. Tanaka Y et al (2002) Monitoring cytomegalovirus infection by antigenemia assay and two distinct plasma real-time PCR methods after hematopoietic stem cell transplantation. Bone Marrow Transplant 30(5):315–9
72. Taplitz RA, Jordan MC (2002) Pneumonia caused by herpesviruses in recipients of hematopoietic cell transplants. Semin Respir Infect 17(2):121–9
73. Druce J et al (2002) Utility of a multiplex PCR assay for detecting herpesvirus DNA in clinical samples. J Clin Microbiol 40(5):1728–32
74. Thomas CF Jr, Limper AH (2004) Pneumocystis pneumonia. N Engl J Med 350(24):2487–98
75. Wakefield AE et al (1991) DNA amplification on induced sputum samples for diagnosis of Pneumocystis carinii pneumonia. Lancet 337(8754):1378–9
76. Arcenas RC et al (2006) A real-time polymerase chain reaction assay for detection of Pneumocystis from bronchoalveolar lavage fluid. Diagn Microbiol Infect Dis 54(3): 169–75, Epub 2006 Jan 19
77. Durand-Joly I et al (2005) Molecular diagnosis of Pneumocystis pneumonia. FEMS Immunol Med Microbiol 45(3): 405–10
78. Alvarez-Martinez MJ et al (2006) Sensitivity and specificity of nested and real-time PCR for the detection of Pneumocystis jiroveci in clinical specimens. Diagn Microbiol Infect Dis 56(2):153–60, Epub 2006 May 4
79. Fischer S et al (2001) The use of oral washes to diagnose Pneumocystis carinii pneumonia: a blinded prospective study using a polymerase chain reaction-based detection system. J Infect Dis 184(11):1485–8, Epub 2001 Nov 13
80. Azoulay E et al (2009) Polymerase chain reaction for diagnosing pneumocystis pneumonia in non-HIV immunocompromised patients with pulmonary infiltrates. Chest 135(3):655–61
81. Ribes JA et al (1997) PCR detection of Pneumocystis carinii in bronchoalveolar lavage specimens: analysis of sensitivity and specificity. J Clin Microbiol 35(4):830–5
82. Maertens J et al (1999) Autopsy-controlled prospective evaluation of serial screening for circulating galactomannan by a sandwich enzyme-linked immunosorbent assay for hematological patients at risk for invasive Aspergillosis. J Clin Microbiol 37(10):3223–8

83. Maertens J et al (2001) Screening for circulating galactomannan as a noninvasive diagnostic tool for invasive aspergillosis in prolonged neutropenic patients and stem cell transplantation recipients: a prospective validation. Blood 97(6):1604–10
84. Maertens J et al (2002) Use of circulating galactomannan screening for early diagnosis of invasive aspergillosis in allogeneic stem cell transplant recipients. J Infect Dis 186(9):1297–306, Epub 2002 Oct 8
85. Maertens J et al (2005) Galactomannan and computed tomography-based preemptive antifungal therapy in neutropenic patients at high risk for invasive fungal infection: a prospective feasibility study. Clin Infect Dis 41(9):1242–50, Epub 2005 Sep 29
86. Borlenghi E et al (2007) Usefulness of the MSG/IFICG/EORTC diagnostic criteria of invasive pulmonary aspergillosis in the clinical management of patients with acute leukaemia developing pulmonary infiltrates. Ann Hematol 86(3):205–10
87. Subira M et al (2003) Clinical applicability of the new EORTC/MSG classification for invasive pulmonary aspergillosis in patients with hematological malignancies and autopsy-confirmed invasive aspergillosis. Ann Hematol 82(2):80–2
88. Bretagne S et al (1997) Serum Aspergillus galactomannan antigen testing by sandwich ELISA: practical use in neutropenic patients. J Infect 35(1):7–15
89. Hohenthal U et al (2005) Bronchoalveolar lavage in immunocompromised patients with haematological malignancy–value of new microbiological methods. Eur J Haematol 74(3):203–11
90. Musher B et al (2004) Aspergillus galactomannan enzyme immunoassay and quantitative PCR for diagnosis of invasive aspergillosis with bronchoalveolar lavage fluid. J Clin Microbiol 42(12):5517–22
91. Francesconi A et al (2006) Characterization and comparison of galactomannan enzyme immunoassay and quantitative real-time PCR assay for detection of Aspergillus fumigatus in bronchoalveolar lavage fluid from experimental invasive pulmonary aspergillosis. J Clin Microbiol 44(7):2475–80
92. MacArthur RD et al (2004) Adequacy of early empiric antibiotic treatment and survival in severe sepsis: experience from the MONARCS trial. Clin Infect Dis 38(2):284–8
93. Xu J et al (2004) Improved laboratory diagnosis of bacterial and fungal infections in patients with hematological malignancies using PCR and ribosomal RNA sequence analysis. Leuk Lymphoma 45(8):1637–41
94. Peters RP et al (2004) New developments in the diagnosis of bloodstream infections. Lancet Infect Dis 4(12):751–60
95. Louie RF et al (2008) Multiplex polymerase chain reaction detection enhancement of bacteremia and fungemia. Crit Care Med 36(5):1487–92
96. Bloos F et al (2010) A multicenter trial to compare blood culture with polymerase chain reaction in severe human sepsis. Intensive Care Med 36(2):241–247
97. Skovbjerg S et al (2009) Optimization of the detection of microbes in blood from immunocompromised patients with haematological malignancies. Clin Microbiol Infect 15(7):680–3
98. Mancini N et al (2008) Molecular diagnosis of sepsis in neutropenic patients with haematological malignancies. J Med Microbiol 57(Pt 5):601–4
99. Mukoyama M et al (1991) Brain natriuretic peptide as a novel cardiac hormone in humans. Evidence for an exquisite dual natriuretic peptide system, atrial natriuretic peptide and brain natriuretic peptide. J Clin Invest 87(4): 1402–12
100. Maisel AS et al (2002) Rapid measurement of B-type natriuretic peptide in the emergency diagnosis of heart failure. N Engl J Med 347(3):161–7
101. Lefebvre A et al (2008) Use of N-terminal pro-brain natriuretic peptide to detect cardiac origin in critically ill cancer patients with acute respiratory failure. Intensive Care Med 34(5):833–9
102. Assicot M et al (1993) High serum procalcitonin concentrations in patients with sepsis and infection. Lancet 341(8844):515–8
103. Kitanovski L et al (2006) Diagnostic accuracy of procalcitonin and interleukin-6 values for predicting bacteremia and clinical sepsis in febrile neutropenic children with cancer. Eur J Clin Microbiol Infect Dis 25(6):413–5
104. Fleischhack G et al (2000) Procalcitonin in paediatric cancer patients: its diagnostic relevance is superior to that of C-reactive protein, interleukin 6, interleukin 8, soluble interleukin 2 receptor and soluble tumour necrosis factor receptor II. Br J Haematol 111(4):1093–102
105. Svaldi M et al (2001) Procalcitonin-reduced sensitivity and specificity in heavily leucopenic and immunosuppressed patients. Br J Haematol 115(1):53–7
106. Perkins GD et al (2005) Safety and Tolerability of Nonbronchoscopic Lavage in ARDS. Chest 127(4): 1358–63
107. Sharma S et al (2005) Pulmonary complications in adult blood and marrow transplant recipients: autopsy findings. Chest 128(3):1385–92
108. Huaringa AJ, Leyva FJ, Signes-Costa J, Morice RC, Raad I, Darwish AA, Champlin RE (2000) Bronchoalveolar lavage in the diagnosis of pulmonary complications of bone marrow transplant patients. Bone Marrow Transplant 25(9):975–979
109. Martin WJ 2nd, Smith TF, Sanderson DR, Brutinel WM, Cockerill FR 3rd, Douglas WW (1987) Role of bronchoalveolar lavage in the assessment of opportunistic pulmonary infections: utility and complications. Mayo Clin Proc 62(7):549–557
110. Xaubet A, Torres A, Marco F, Puig-De la Bellacasa J, Faus R, Agusti-Vidal A (1989) Pulmonary infiltrates in immunocompromised patients. Diagnostic value of telescoping plugged catheter and bronchoalveolar lavage. Chest 95(1):130–135
111. Campbell JH, Raina V, Banham SW, Cunningham D, Soukop M (1989) Pulmonary infiltrates – diagnostic problems in lymphoma. Postgrad Med J 65(770):881–884
112. Pisani RJ, Wright AJ (1992) Clinical utility of bronchoalveolar lavage in immunocompromised hosts. Mayo Clin Proc 67(3):221–227
113. Maschmeyer G, Link H, Hiddemann W, Meyer P, Helmerking M, Eisenmann E, Schmitt J, Adam D (1994) Pulmonary infiltrations in febrile patients with neutropenia. Risk factors and outcome under empirical antimicrobial therapy in a randomized multicenter study. Cancer 73:2296–2304
114. Cazzadori A, Di Perri G, Todeschini G, Luzzati R, Boschiero L, Perona G, Concia E (1995) Transbronchial

biopsy in the diagnosis of pulmonary infiltrates in immunocompromised patients. Chest 107:101–106
115. Pagano L, Pagliari G, Basso A, Marra R, Sica S, Frigieri L, Morace G, Ardito F, Leone G (1997) The role of bronchoalveolar lavage in the microbiological diagnosis of pneumonia in patients with haematological malignancies. Ann Med 29:535–540
116. Heurlin N, Lonnqvist B, Tollemar J, Ehrnst A (1989) Fiberoptic bronchoscopy for diagnosis of opportunistic pulmonary infections after bone marrow transplantation. Scand J Infect Dis 21:359–366
117. Abu-Farsakh HA, Katz RL, Atkinson N, Champlin RE (1995) Prognostic factors in bronchoalveolar lavage in 77 patients with bone marrow transplants. Acta Cytol 39:1081–1088
118. Glazer M, Breuer R, Berkman N, Lossos IS, Kapelushnik J, Nagler A, Naparstek E, Kramer MR, Lafair J, Engelhard D, Or R (1998) Use of fiberoptic bronchoscopy in bone marrow transplant recipients. Acta Haematol 99:22–26

Pleural Effusions and Thoracentesis in Patients with Hematological Malignancies

16

Michael G. Alexandrakis, Paschalis Steiropoulos, and Demosthenes Bouros

Contents

M.G. Alexandrakis
Department of Haematology, Medical School, University of Crete, Heraklion, Greece
e-mail: alexandm@med.uoc.gr

P. Steiropoulos and D. Bouros (✉)
Department of Pneumonology, Medical School, Democritus University of Thrace, 68100 Alexandroupolis, Greece
e-mail: pstirop@med.duth.gr; bouros@med.duth.gr

Pleural effusions are common in patients with malignancies. They can present as an isolated entity or be associated with parenchymal lung abnormalities. Patients with hematological malignancies (HM) can present with pleural effusion at diagnosis or may develop it during the course of their underlying disease [7, 21, 61, 68, 74]. Regarding etiology, various mechanisms can stimulate the accumulation of pleural fluid (Table 16.1) [74, 116]. The disease itself, drug-related pleural toxicity, radiotherapy, infections, secondary malignancies, autoimmunity, extramedullary hematopoiesis and other complications may contribute to the development of pleural effusions in patients with HM [72, 156, 188, 242].

Pleural effusions have been reported in up to 20% of patients with non-Hodgkin's lymphomas (NHL), although effusions are uncommon in the peritoneal and pericardial cavities (Table 16.2) [15, 45, 56, 74, 160, 203]. The second most common condition is bone marrow transplantation (BMT), while acute and chronic leukemias, myelodysplastic syndromes (MDS), multiple myeloma (MM) and other hematological disorders are rarely accompanied by pleural effusions [4, 7, 52, 61, 79, 84, 100, 107, 189, 200, 220, 234].

Routine analysis of the pleural fluid for pH, LDH, protein and cholesterol should be performed, since application of the Light's criteria is useful in distinguishing transudative from exudative pleural effusions (Table 16.3) [140]. Morphological examinations by light microscopy, flow cytometry and in selected cases gene rearrangement studies are useful to document the malignant nature of a pleural effusion [80, 116, 159, 242]. Examination of cytocentrifuged specimens in the hematology laboratory is superior to cytopathological examination for HM [13, 15, 126]. In selected cases of undiagnosed patients, pleural biopsies by needle or thoracoscopy are occasionally indicated [17, 134, 171, 218, 237].

É. Azoulay (ed.), *Pulmonary Involvement in Patients with Hematological Malignancies*,
DOI: 10.1007/978-3-642-15742-4_16, © Springer-Verlag Berlin Heidelberg 2011

Table 16.1 Mechanisms of pleural effusions in patients with hematological malignancies

1. Infiltration by the malignancy (direct invasion with shedding of malignant cells into the pleural space)
2. Compression by the malignancy (impairment of fluid efflux from the pleural space by lymphatic obstruction)
3. Obstruction of the pulmonary and mediastinal lymph nodes and/or thoracic duct obstruction resulting in chylothorax
4. Drug-related pleural toxicity and radiation therapy
5. Infections
6. Pulmonary embolism
7. Bleeding
8. Cardiac insufficiency, hypoalbuminemia from liver or renal insufficencies
9. Capillary-leak syndrome with cytokine production
10. Other complications (secondary malignancies, autoimmunity, extramedullary hematopoiesis in CML, amyloidosis, plasmacytoma, granulocytic sarcoma, veno-occlusive disease and urinothorax, etc.)

Table 16.2 Malignancies associated with pleural effusion

Situations in which pleural effusions are common
• Non-Hodgkin's lymphoma (up to 48% of the patients)
• Hodgkin's disease (about 30% of the cases, most frequently associated with pulmonary involvement)
• Allogeneic and autologous BMT
Situations in which pleural effusions are uncommon
• Acute and chronic leukemias
• Myelodysplastic syndromes
• Multiple myeloma (mostly in IgA myeloma)

Table 16.3 Pleural fluid tests that are useful for the etiological diagnosis of pleural effusion

Always useful (routine tests)
Pleural pH
Pleural LDH and protein rates (Light's criteria)
Morphological examinations by light microscopy in hematological laboratory (with immunophenotyping)
Sometimes useful
Pleural cholesterol
Flow cytometry when cytologic diagnostic is positive (may disclose clonal lymphocytes in the pleural fluid with identical phenotype in case of direct invasion for a lymphoma)
May be useful in selected cases
PCRs to viruses that promote oncogenesis (HHV8, EBC, CMV, etc.)
Gene rearrangement studies
Immunoglobulin and TCR rearrangements
Cytogenetics and molecular studies
Studies of oncogenes expression
Needle pleural biopsies
Pleural biopsy by pleuroscopy or thoracoscopy

Careful evaluation of the pleural effusion to establish its etiology is required to direct therapy [79]. Effusions may result from direct pleural invasion or indirect effects (paraneoplastic effusions), such as impairment of fluid efflux from the pleural space by lymphatic obstruction or pleural effects of cancer radiation or drug therapy. Disease improvement is accompanied by resolution of the effusion [7, 100]. Recurrent resistant effusions may need pleurodesis (e.g., talk, tetracyclines, bleomycin) or local treatment with biological agents (bortezomib or rituximab) [8, 22, 100, 134, 142, 150, 221]. Factors that should be considered prior to chemical pleurodesis include response to therapeutic thoracentesis, the patient's general health, i.e., performance status, pleural space elastance, underlying malignancy and pH of the pleural fluid [100, 200]. When the pleural effusion is due to lung infections, cardiac failure, etc., treatment of the underlying condition usually leads to resolution of the effusion.

16.1 Pleural Effusions in NHL

Pleural effusions are a common complication of NHL, occurring in up to 48% of the patients [7, 21, 61, 74, 75]. Pericardial and peritoneal effusions are much less common complications of malignant lymphomas. In one study, pleural effusions were present in 8.6% of NHL patients, whereas pericardial effusions and ascites occurred in only 0.8% each [62, 233]. The frequency of development of pleural effusions differs among the various sub-types of NHL [45, 62, 97, 110, 152, 180, 239]. Thus, T-cell lymphomas are associated with effusions much more frequently than B-cell lymphomas [35, 63, 88, 115, 230]. Moreover, lymphomatous effusions show substantial age and sex variation [116]. Among malignant pleural effusions, lymphoma/leukemia appears to be more frequent in males (21.1% versus 8% in females) [116]. In a study of malignant pleural effusions in children and young adults, there was a predominance of lymphoma/leukemia cases [98]. In another study, malignant pleural effusions were seen with higher frequency (64.5%) in patients >40 years of age, although lymphoma was the underlying hematological malignancy in only 4.1% of them [194]. Most patients with primary mediastinal B-cell lymphomas have stage I-II disease, yet bulky disease with associated pleural or pericardial effusions occurs in approximately a third of the patients [147]. Diffuse large B-cell lymphoma is the most frequent NHL subtype associated with lymphomatous pleural effusions [86]. Advanced stage III and IV small lymphocytic lymphomas are also associated with pleural effusions due to pleural infiltration [47, 61, 126, 220]. Rarely, pleural effusions have been reported to accompany monocytoid B-cell lymphoma, a low-grade B-cell malignancy that often involves regional lymph nodes and the salivary glands, and rarely the spleen and/or the bone marrow [188, 211]. Pleural effusions can be unilateral or bilateral, while the origin of the monocytoid B-cell lymphocytes obtained by thoracentesis can be confirmed by appropriate immunophenotyping [188]. Although the lung is frequently involved in disseminated lymphomas, isolated primary pulmonary lymphomas occur, but are rare. The most common histological subtype is a pleural low-grade extranodal marginal zone lymphoma of mucosa-associated lymphoid tissue (EMZL/MALT type) [53]. An entire chapter of this book from Wilsez and colleagues is dedicated to this entity. Common presenting features include cough, dyspnea, chest pain, fever and hemoptysis, or it can be an incidental finding on a chest radiograph obtained for other reasons. A safe distinction between EMZL/MALT and lymphoplasmacytic lymphoma (LPL) of the pleura with associated pleural effusion cannot be made based on morphological and immunohistochemicalal characteristics alone, since both are small B-cell proliferations with similar immunohistochemical profiles [153]. At the time of diagnosis, LPL is frequently characterized by infiltration of the bone marrow, lymph nodes and spleen. In contrast, EMZLs usually involve extranodal tissues first [5, 133, 153]. In difficult cases, cell chromosomal analysis and detection of t(14:18) (q32;q21) that involve IGH and MALT 1 are useful in differentiating LPL from MALT [94, 153].

Other types of primary pleural NHL are rare, and available clinical information is based on small observational studies and case reports [126, 220]. In most cases, pleural effusions result from lymphomatous pleural infiltration, while the fluid is typically serous or serosanguinous and located on one or both pleural cavities. Symptoms include dyspnea, cough and chest pain [45, 74, 160]. Rarely, NHL patients with large pleural effusions present with shortness of breath requiring immediate thoracentesis for removal of an adequate amount of fluid prior to initiation of appropriate therapy. In NHL patients with pleural effusion, fluid accumulation can be unilateral or bilateral. T-cell neoplasms, especially lymphoblastic lymphomas, are frequently associated with mediastinal masses and pleural effusions [61]. In rare cases, fluid may be chylous [21, 74]. In rare cases of advanced low-grade lymphomas, pleural effusion can be a transudate due to venous compression, cardiac or renal failure or associated hypoalbuminemia [202].

Recently, a rare case of urinothorax due to ureter obstruction was reported in a patient with NHL [123]. Transudative or exudative reactive pleural effusions have also been observed to accompany lung involvement in lymphomas [12, 184]. Pleural effusions in patients with lymphomas can develop by one or more mechanisms including pleural infiltration with shedding of malignant cells into the pleural space, lymphatic obstruction of the pulmonary and mediastinal lymph nodes, and/or thoracic duct obstruction resulting in chylothorax [21].

Lymphomatous involvement of the pleura is characterized by presence of clonal lymphocytes in the pleural fluid with an identical phenotype to that seen in lymphocytes obtained from affected lymph nodes [15, 45, 96]. On the other hand, in cases of reactive pleural effusions, lymphocytes are polyclonal, small, mature and predominantly of T-cell origin [12, 15, 137]. Difficulties exist in distinguishing neoplastic from reactive lymphocytes in cytopathological specimens, especially in cases of small lymphocytic/lymphoblastic lymphomas [15]. Flow cytometry, immunohistochemistry, immunoglobulin and TCR rearrangements, cytogenetics and studies of oncogenes expression are useful for diagnostic purposes [15, 148, 151, 160].

Cytological evaluation with immunophenotyping of the pleural fluid cells is usually diagnostic of the specific NHL subtype [15]. Various lymphoma subtypes with characteristic cytomorphology have been reported with serous effusions and include Burkitt lymphoma [97], marginal zone lymphoma [58], multilobated type NHL [152], peripheral T-cell NHL [110] including Sézary syndrome [238] and anaplastic large cell lymphoma [115]. Immunological studies define the B- or T-cell origin and degree of maturation. The majority of adults with NHL and pleural effusions have disease of an intermediate grade, a small proportion have low-grade NHL, and an even smaller proportion suffer from high-grade lymphomas [133, 188].

Regarding prognosis, the presence of pleural effusion can influence overall survival depending on the time of diagnosis [74]. In patients with intermediate-grade NHL, the presence of a pleural effusion at the time of presentation does not seem to affect overall survival [74]. On the other hand, the presence of pleural effusion at the time of presentation was associated with extremely poor outcome in a study of 57 patients with primary mediastinal large-cell and immunoblastic lymphomas [130]. In another study of 91 patients with low-grade follicular lymphoma, the presence of pleural effusion was a factor adversely influencing overall survival along with age >70 years, presence of B symptoms, histological subtype of follicular mixed-cell NHL, tumor size >10 cm, >2 extranodal sites of disease, and stage III and IV disease according to the Ann Arbor lymphoma staging system [158].

In a retrospective study, the effects of the biochemical and cytological properties of the pleural fluid on the survival of 284 patients with malignant pleural effusions were determined. Tumor type, as well as some laboratory features of the pleural fluid, such as pH, LDH and protein concentration, influenced survival [22].

Lastly, a retrospective multicenter study analyzed the clinical features and treatment outcomes of B-lymphoblastic lymphoma (B-LBL) and T-lymphoblastic lymphoma (T-LBL) in 55 newly diagnosed patients (45 T-LBL and 10 B-LBL). With the exception of the more frequent involvement in T-LBL, there were no differences in the clinical features between the two subtypes. Clinical outcome of T-LBL versus B-LBL in terms of response and survival was not significantly different, although the presence of pleural effusion was prognostic for overall and progression-free survival [49].

16.2 Pleural Effusions in Hodgkin's Disease

Pleural effusions are common in patients with Hodgkin's disease (HD), whereas pleural effusions occurred in approximately 30% of thoracic HD cases [7]. Although thoracic duct obstruction and impaired lymphatic drainage due to enlarged hilar or mediastinal lymph nodes appear to be the primary mechanism of pleural effusion in HD [61], in some cases fluid accumulation may be due to direct pleural involvement by the tumor [23, 61]. Pulmonary parenchymal disease occurs in 38% of patients with HD and is invariably associated with mediastinal lymphadenopathy and widespread disease [7]. HD rarely affects the pleura alone, and when this happens it is the result of advanced local disease, as demonstrated by thoracic CT scans [23, 183].

Few studies exist regarding immunohistochemistry in the diagnosis of HD associated with serous effusions. Look-a-like of Reed–Stenberg cells (R-S) in pleural effusion cytology can lead to incorrect diagnosis [61, 183]. Hence, in order to avoid these pitfalls, a combination of immunocytochemistry, flow cytometry, cytogenetics and molecular studies should be applied [61, 124, 183].

16.3 Primary Effusion Lymphoma

Primary effusion lymphoma (PEL) is a rare subtype of B-cell lymphomas that presents as pleural, peritoneal and pericardial neoplastic effusions in the absence of a distinct tumor mass or recognizable nodal involvement [32, 39, 42]. This body cavity-based lymphoma is associated with herpesvirus-8 (HHV8) infection, also termed Kaposi sarcoma herpesvirus (KSHV) [31, 39, 40, 44, 167]. HHV8 was initially identified in tissue biopsies of patients with AIDS-related NHL as pleural, peritoneal and pericardial lymphomatous effusions [4, 167, 229, 244].

Nowadays, PEL is considered to be an HHV8-driven malignancy [32, 39, 42]. Viral presence in the neoplastic cells can be demonstrated by immunohistochemical methods using the HHV8 LNA-1 latent protein antibody or other molecular methods [32, 167]. The majority of PEL cases affect HIV-positive patients, although several cases have been described in patients with cancer, cirrhosis or underlying immunosuppression because of solid organ transplantation [40]. In the general population, PEL develops in older individuals living in areas with a high prevalence of HHV8 infection [39, 208]. Few cases of PEL in HIV-negative patients have been reported, and some of them were not associated with HHV8 [40, 90, 108, 212, 229, 244]. The etiological agent(s) responsible for these HHV8-negative cases remain(s) unclear [39].

Most (>90%) HIV-positive cases of PEL also show evidence of EBV infection, suggesting that EBV plays a supportive role in malignant cell transformation [105, 229]. Interestingly, HHV8, like EBV, belongs to the gamma herpesvirus family. HHV8 has also been identified in patients with multicentric Castleman's disease (MCD), as will be discussed next [51, 217].

The mechanism by which HHV8 promotes oncogenesis in PEL is unclear [118]. Nowadays, it is accepted that PEL is a large-cell lymphoma derived from post-germinal center B-cells with an intermediate immunophenotype between immunoblasts and plasma cells [41]. Hence, PEL cells express activation and plasma cell markers such as CD30, CD38 and CD138 [38, 41, 131], whereas routine B-cell (CD19, CD20, CD79a) and T-cell (CD3, CD4, CD8) markers are typically absent [31, 32]. Rarely, PEL cells aberrantly express T-cell markers and rearrangements of the T-cell receptor gene [31, 179, 201]. Regarding PEL prognosis, it is extremely poor, with a median survival of <6 months [215]. Modern antiretroviral treatment appears to improve prognosis [27, 102].

16.4 Castleman's Disease

Castleman's disease (CD) is a rare lymphoid disorder of unknown etiology that is characterized by massive lymphadenopathy, anemia and hypergammaglobulinemia. It is also known as angiofollicular lymphoid hyperplasia, giant lymph node hyperplasia and Castleman's lymphoma.

Three distinct histological variants exist: plasmacytic, hyaline vascular and intermediate [14]. Although CD is most frequently found in the mediastinum, it has also been identified in other anatomical sites such as the neck, pelvis and axilla [191]. Localized CD (or type 2) is usually of the hyaline-vascular type, is located in the mediastinum (79% of cases) and can be cured by surgical excision alone. Pleural effusions in this subtype are due to local compression [14]. Contrary to the benign clinical course of most cases of hyaline-vascular CD, the plasmacytic (type 1) MCD is typically much more aggressive. It usually presents with fever, rash, cytopenias, hypergammaglobulinemia and extensive lymphadenopathy. This form is common in patients with AIDS. HHV8 is causally associated with MCD, since it is present in 95% of HIV-positive patients [91, 191]. Pulmonary symptoms and infiltrates are common, especially in HIV-associated multicentric CD [1, 95, 181]. The most frequent pulmonary manifestation is an acute febrile interstitial pneumonitis typically associated with high fever, weight loss and malaise [95]. The role of various pro-inflammatory cytokines, such as IL-6 and IL-10, has been studied and appears crucial during disease exacerbations [173, 182]. Overproduction of such cytokines is responsible for a nonspecific capillary-leak syndrome, as has been studied in critically ill patients [43, 82].

The extensive angiogenesis seen in CD supports the hypothesis that VEGF participates in the pathophysiology of the disease [43]. Pleural effusions have been described in MCD and are sometimes chylous [26, 228].

16.5 Pyothorax-Associated Lymphoma

Pyothorax-associated lymphoma (PAL) is a distinct type of B-cell NHL that develops in the pleural cavity of patients with chronic pyothorax [87]. It is strongly associated with EBV infection based on the elevated values of serum anti-EBV antibodies, the presence of EBV genomes in the nuclei of tumor cells and the expression of latent infection genes, such as EBNA2, in most patients [122, 170, 178].

HHV8 is not detected in all cases of PAL [176]. Artificial pneumothorax has been found to be a significant risk factor for the development of PAL among chronic pyothorax patients [11]. It is of interest that there are no reports of pleural neoplasia in chronic pyothorax patients after surgical resection of the pyogenic pleural membrane [11, 170]. Repetitive chest radiographs for the artificial pneumothorax may be linked with PAL development due to excessive radiation exposure [104]. Overall prognosis in patients with

PAL is poor. Several factors, such as poor performance status, high levels of ALT and blood urea nitrogen, are associated with worse survival among PAL patients [11, 104]. Recently, a case of PAL of T-cell origin was reported. Tumor was arising from the chest wall, and development followed the therapeutic pneumothorax for pleural tuberculosis [204].

16.6 Multiple Myeloma

MM is a malignant neoplasm of plasma cells that usually invades the bone marrow, but may involve other body sites. Pleural effusions occur in approximately 6% of patients with MM during the course of the disease [187, 199]. The etiology of pleural effusions is multifactorial, and effusions due to pleural myelomatous involvement are rare, occurring in <1% of the cases [7, 199]. The following mechanisms have been implicated in the production of pleural fluid: infiltration of the pleura by malignant plasma cells (i.e., myelomatous pleural effusion), infiltration of the pleural fluid from adjacent affected tissues, renal dysfunction due to infiltration with paraprotein of the renal tubular system with development of glomerular damage, pulmonary embolism, congestive heart failure secondary to amyloidosis, secondary neoplasms and mediastinal lymph node infiltration with accompanying lymphatic obstruction [7, 144, 172, 187]. Among myelomatous pleural effusions, 80% occur in IgA MM, possibly as a result of this type's major tendency to invade extraosseus structures [120, 199, 205]. The remaining cases are IgG MM [199, 205]. Rare cases of IgD MM with associated pleural effusion have also been described [243]. Bence Jones protein type and IgE MM are rarely associated with pleural effusions [243], whereas IgM-type MM is associated with pleural effusions in 5–13% of the cases [9, 112].

Pleural effusion due to MM invasion is rare. When myelomatous effusion is present, outcome is poor with median survival of <4 months. Plasmablastic myeloma is a subtype of MM that is characterized by distinctive morphological features. This subtype is usually associated with renal insufficiency and survival of <6 months [48]. Pleural effusions due to infiltration by malignant plasma cells can occur at any time during the clinical course of the disease, i.e., they can precede clinical diagnosis or develop after treatment's initiation [92, 109].

Although various tests in addition to morphological evaluation have been used in the diagnosis of myelomatous effusions, immunophenotypic analysis of the infiltrating plasma cells is most important for diagnostic purposes [25, 240].

Extramedullary plasmacytoma comprises approximately 4–6% of plasma cell malignancies [169, 186]. Few cases of extramedullary plasmacytoma arising in the mediastinum have been described [186]. Direct extension of the plasmocytoma into the pleural space may result in development of pleural effusion [169]. Amyloidosis, a well-described complication of MM, can in rare cases involve the pleura with resultant transudative or exudative effusions. Diagnosis of pleural amyloidosis by biopsy is important because the disease is usually refractory to conventional treatment and may necessitate pleurodesis [143]. In a retrospective study of 35 patients with biopsy-proven pulmonary amyloidosis, 5 (14%) were found to have associated MM [232].

Waldenstrom's macroglobulinemia (WM) is a relatively rare disorder characterized by lymphoplasmacytic monoclonal proliferation and a high amount of monoclonal serum IgM. In rare cases pleural involvement can occur, and is characterized by identification of lymphoid and plasmacytoid cells in the effusion along with the presence of monoclonal IgM in cell-free suspensions [76].

Pulmonary involvement in WM is relatively rare, occurring in 3–5% of the cases. It usually presents with pulmonary nodules, masses, diffuse infiltrates or pleural effusions [125]. Morphological examination of disease-related small lymphocytes in the pleural effusion is nondiagnostic, rendering flow cytometry and gene rearrangement studies invaluable for accurate diagnosis [125, 146].

In a study of 44 patients with WM with associated pulmonary disease, the authors found that although 15% of the patients had no pulmonary symptoms at diagnosis, two thirds of those with lung disease presented with abnormal findings on chest radiograph. The radiographic findings were initially described as reticulonodular infiltrates, confluent masses or pleural effusions. In 39 patients there was pathologically confirmed lung involvement with WM, a much higher incidence than the 0–5% reported by other groups [196]. In another autopsy study, pathological lung involvement was detected in 16 of 32 patients with WM, despite the absence of respiratory symptoms premortem [241].

Although open lung biopsy can confirm lung and pleural involvement in patients with WM, most cases are diagnosed by transbronchial or pleural biopsy or by thoracentesis [76, 81].

16.7 Pleural Effusions in Acute Leukemia

Pleural effusions in acute myeloid or lymphoblastic leukemia are relatively rare [7], despite the fact that microscopic infiltration of the pleura is a common finding at autopsies of patients with leukemia [71]. Leukemic infiltrates in other tissues were found at autopsy in 10 of 15 patients with acute leukemia who died of an unrelated cause during complete bone marrow remission [207]. Moreover, pleural involvement can accompany bone marrow involvement [71, 197]. In these cases, pleural effusion is typically hemorrhagic or has features of empyema reflecting underlying infections [55, 60, 155, 224]. In other cases, hypoalbuminaemia, cardiac or liver failure contributes to the development of pleural effusion [60]. Cases with pleural involvement at presentation are rare, and the same is true for pleural involvement as the only site of extramedullary relapse [70, 77, 78, 219].

As long-term survival in patients with acute leukemia is increasing, unusual sites of relapse are now more frequently recognized [34, 197]. CNS and testes have long been recognized as the most common sites of extra-medullary relapses in acute leukemia [71, 207]. Granulocytic sarcoma is a solid tumor composed of malignant myeloid cells. It constitutes the solid variant of acute myelogenous leukemia (AML). Primary granulocytic sarcoma of the pleura has been described [71, 77, 207]. Recently, a case of cardiac myeloid sarcoma with associated pericardial and bilateral pleural effusions was described [198]. Most cases reported in the literature concern acute lymphoblastic leukemia (ALL). Typing and differentiation of the cells of the pleural effusion can be difficult. Combined cytomorphology and immunophenotyping lead to correct diagnosis. Rarely, invasive procedures (pleural biopsies) are required for diagnosis [77, 78, 106].

T-LBL is a rare malignancy that accounts for 2–4% of adult NHL [111]. It is much more common in teenage adolescents. At presentation, there is bulky mediastinal involvement frequently associated with pericardial or pleural effusion. In one study, bulky mediastinal involvement with associated pleural effusion was found in about half the patients [138]. In another study, 95% of the 45 patients showed a mediastinal mass at diagnosis, and 40% had concurrent pleural effusion [103]. Unusual cases of pleural effusions with a lymphomatous mediastinal mass of pre-B cell origin and a normal hemogram have been described [189]. According to recent studies, the balance of matrix metalloproteinases plays an important role in the mechanism of leukemic infiltration into extramedullary organs [223]. Other investigators have suggested that the chemokine receptor CXCR4 and its ligand are involved in extramedullary invasion and that VEGFR1 controls the onset of extramedullary disease in ALL [59, 83]. The prognostic significance of pleural effusion at diagnosis in patients with acute leukemia is not well defined. Some investigators claim that it does not affect the rate of hematological remission and survival, while others report a worse prognosis, especially in plasmacytic and hairy cell leukemias [30, 149]. These latter two forms of leukemia can present with pleural effusions that contain typical leukemic cells. In these cases, aggressive treatment is indicated [30, 149].

Pleural effusions in patients with acute leukemia usually disappear quickly after induction chemotherapy. On the other hand, recurrence of pleural exudates is inevitable in those who do not achieve remission. In such cases, respiratory failure due to rapid fluid accumulation can develop, necessitating local treatment with intrapleural chemotherapy, pleurodesis or repeated drainage [2, 33].

16.8 Pleural Effusions in Chronic Lymphocytic Leukemia

Effusions in chronic leukemias, although rare, are more common than in acute leukemias [10, 28, 157, 216]. In chronic lymphocytic leukemia (CLL) the most common cause of pleural effusion is pleural infiltration, a condition that predisposes to transformation to more aggressive lymphoid neoplasms, such as Richter's syndrome or to prolymphocytic transformation [213]. An entire chapter on pulmonary involvement in CLL has been provided by Dr. Wadwha and colleagues in this book. In a large retrospective study of patients with CLL, diverse pulmonary complications were reported in 223/1,000 admissions [6]. Infections were the most frequent complications with the lung as the major site [20, 161, 162]. Pleural involvement by leukemic cells was the second most common complication in 9% of the patients. Studies of patients with CLL show lung involvement in up to 40% of the patients [16, 20]. When the effusion is the result of leukemic pleural infiltration, the fluid is likely to be hemorrhagic and contains malignant lymphocytes that are identical to those found in blood and bone marrow [235].

The differential diagnosis of pleural effusions in patients with CLL includes primary pleural involvement, central lymphatic obstruction, infections, and changes induced by previous radiation or chemotherapy [235]. Immunohistological methods can be used to determine the nature of the pleural effusion [154]. Pleural involvement in B-CLL leads to accumulation of fluid rich in monoclonal B cells, whereas in most reactive pleural effusions, T cells and a small proportion of polyclonal B cells are found. Although the clonality and immunohistochemistry of the lymphocytes that are isolated in the pleural fluid can provide a definitive diagnosis, there are reports showing that lymphocytic infiltration by B-CLL leads to reactive pleural effusions with predominant polyclonal T cells [18, 154]. A high proportion of T cells with monoclonal T-cell receptor rearrangements is characteristic of T-cell neoplasms [154]. Patients with CLL and pleural involvement usually have long-standing disease prior to development of pleural effusion [235]. If tuberculosis is suspected in a patient with known CLL and concurrent pleural effusion, pleural biopsy or thoracoscopy is indicated in order to differentiate tuberculosis from lymphocytic pleural infiltration [225, 235].

16.9 Pleural Effusion in Chronic Myelogenous Leukemia (CML)

The most common cause of pleural effusion in chronic myelogenous leukemia (CML) is extramedullary hematopoiesis, although the pleura are an uncommon site [29, 67]. Frequently, all granulocytic precursors and a few blasts are found in the pleural fluid of patients with CML [157]. Regarding the formation of exudative pleural effusions, there are several possible mechanisms. The first is leukemic infiltration. The fluid is usually hemorrhagic, while pleural infiltration frequently appears shortly before transformation into acute leukemia. In these cases, the pleural fluid contains a greater proportion of blasts [54, 117, 129]. Isolated pleural blast crisis in the absence of medullary transformation is extremely rare [117].

Pleural reaction secondary to intrapleural bleeding is another possible mechanism [113]. Various factors may have a role in hemorrhagic effusions, such as leukostasis and platelet dysfunction. Obstruction of pleural capillaries or infiltration of interstitial lung tissue by leukemic cells during unrestrained leukocytosis along with increased capillary permeability because of cytokine production can also mediate the development of pleural effusion [101, 222]. Infections may play an additional role.

Other chronic myeloproliferative diseases may be associated with pleural effusions, such as systemic mastocytosis, chronic eosinophilic leukemia, myelofibrosis and polycythemia vera. The most common cause of pleuritis in these patients, other than lung infections, is extramedullary hematopoiesis and leukemic transformation with associated infiltration [54]. Pleural effusions can also be reactive. In these cases, they contain a mixture of macrophages, mesothelial cells and T-lymphocytes [168, 192].

16.10 Pleural Effusions in Myelodysplastic Syndromes

Pleural effusions in MDS are rare and usually associated with underlying lung infections. Pleural effusions secondary to leukemic infiltration are a rare initial manifestation of MDS patients [145, 166].

In patients with chronic myelomonocytic leukemia (CMML), pleural effusions are rare and usually respond to appropriate antileukemic therapy [29]. The prognostic significance of extramedullary involvement in patients with CMML has not been well determined. However, most consider it as a sign of advanced disease and recommend aggressive therapy [29, 145] The presence of extramedullary disease in MDS has been well documented in CMML with disease progression [145].

Immunological disorders (defective B-, T- and natural killer-cell function) are frequent in patients with MDS. Increased or decreased levels of immunoglobulins and monoclonal gammopathy may also be found in patients with MDS [121]. Pulmonary vasculitis or eosinophilic infiltrations of the lungs complicated by pleural effusion are additional causes of morbidity and mortality in these patients [24, 165]. MDS patients are also susceptible to pulmonary and disseminated fungal infections because of defective cell-mediated immunity, as shown by a low blood CD4 lymphocyte count [50, 121, 226].

16.11 Pleural Effusions in Bone Marrow Transplantation

Infectious and noninfectious complications occur in 40–60% of all BMT recipients with considerable associated morbidity and mortality [46]. Various factors are thought to play an important role in the manifestation of pulmonary complications including immunological defects secondary to the underlying disease and its treatment, the conditioning regimen and development of graft-versus host disease (GVHD) [119]. Information concerning pleural involvement after BMT is limited. In one study 16% of patients developed pleural effusions within the first 100 days after BMT [175]. Pleural effusions may accompany various potentially life-threatening complications that are associated with BMT, such as infections [175], veno-occlusive disease (VOD) [185], G-CSF toxicity [73], acute and/or chronic GVHD [209], and recurrence of the underlying hematological disease [139]. Multiple effusions appear to be part of the presentation of severe acute or chronic GVHD, often in association with CMV disease in patients who receive allogeneic donor marrow [209, 231].

In these latter cases, CD8+/HLA-DR + lymphocytes expressing CD57 predominate in the pleural fluid [139]. The most common noninfections causes of pleural effusion in BMT recipients are aggressive fluid resuscitation, including use of blood products. Effusions are usually right-sided or bilateral [128]. Other noninfections causes of pleural effusions in BMT recipients include effusions after conditioning with cyclophosphamide and total-body irradiation [164, 175, 190, 206].

In patients with extensive chronic GVHD, isolated effusions have been reported [214]. In these cases, the term serositis has been used to describe the sterile nature of these effusions [139, 206, 214]. Hepatic VOD is a complication of patients treated with chemotherapy and radiation therapy, and pleural effusions have been reported in up to 50% of BMT recipients who develop VOD compared to 3% of BMT recipients without VOD [185]. It is of interest that the affected patients have minimal or no respiratory symptoms.

Post-transplantation lymphoproliferative disorder (PTLD) due to reactivation of EBV has also been occasionally associated with pleural effusions and CD4+ lymphocyte expansion. These patients are frequently resistant to immunosuppressive therapy [139]. PTLD includes a spectrum of lymphoid proliferations ranging from benign reactive lymphoid hyperplasia to high-grade NHL, usually of B-cell immunophenotype, although cases with T or null immunophenotype have also been reported [99, 115, 132].

The pathophysiological mechanism is poorly understood, and the clinical manifestations include in addition to pleural effusions, excessive weight gain, ascites, fever, rash, hypotension and edema associated with kidney and liver abnormalities indicative of a common injury to multiple organs [36, 177]. About 50% of allogeneic or autologous BMT recipients develop noncardiogenic pulmonary edema with or without pleural effusions and half of them have associated hepatic, renal or CNS abnormalities. These observations suggest that circulating leukocytes play an important role in the development of the syndrome [36].

16.12 Pleural Effusions Related to the Treatment of Hematological Malignancies

All-tran-retinoic acid (ATRA) is a potent differentiation agent that is an effective therapy in patients with acute promyelocytic leukemia (APL). Up to 50% of APL patients treated with ATRA may develop a life-threatening complication of uncertain pathogenesis that is characterized by fever, respiratory distress, pulmonary infiltrates, weight gain, pleural and pericardial effusions, renal and cardiac failure, edema and thromboembolic events. Some patients require mechanical ventilation and/or dialysis [136]. Infiltration of the lung parenchyma as well as pleural infiltration by maturing malignant promyelocytes has been implicated in the development of pulmonary capillaritis and pleuritis [37, 64, 65, 174, 227]. Other chemotherapeutic agents, such as high-dose cytarabine, have also been associated with the development of pleural effusions. Pathogenesis remains unclear, but is likely due to direct toxic and immunological mechanisms.

Tyrosine kinase inhibitors (TKIs) (imatinib, nilotinib and dasatinib) have revolutionized the treatment of CML and are increasingly used in other malignancies [89]. Despite the apparent selectivity of these agents, side effects can occur because of off-target kinase inhibition [93, 127]. Clinical consequences are edema, pleural and pericardial effusions. These effusions are mainly associated with dasatinib, occurring much less frequently with imatinib or nilotinib therapy [193].

Regarding dasatinib, the cumulative incidence of pleural effusion at 1 year was 29.5% (95% CI 18.6–43.3%), and pleural effusions occur in 14–35% of CML patients who receive it [66]. Several risk factors have been proposed, but the etiology of the effusions remains unclear. Risk factors are blastic-phase CML, advanced age, previous history of cardiac disease, hypertension, hypercholesterolemia, underlying lung disease, fluid retention, and history of autoimmune diseases and of skin rashes [66, 141]. Pleural effusion was less frequent with once daily dosing than with twice daily dosing (all grades, 18% versus 32%). Dasatinib-induced pleuritis may be related to inhibition of PDGFR-B, which is expressed in pericytes and involved in angiogenesis [114]. Others suggest an immune-mediated mechanism based on the high lymphocyte content of the pleural fluid in these patients, the presence of autoantibodies and the response to corticosteroids [19, 195].

Radiation therapy to the thorax is frequently administered in patients with lymphomas and can be complicated by development of pneumonitis, pleuritis or pericarditis. Pleural effusions as complications of radiation therapy are the result of radiation pleuritis or of lymphatic obstruction from mediastinal fibrosis [135, 163]. Pleural effusions secondary to radiation are usually observed within 6 months following radiotherapy, although some cases occur several years later [163]. Another complication of mediastinal radiation is the development of chylothorax many years after radiotherapy due to radiation-induced fibrosis with resultant alteration of the normal lymphatic flow [85, 236].

16.13 Thoracentesis

Thoracentesis may carry an increased risk for patients with HM because of the presence of numerous comorbidities in these patients, neutropenia and coagulation abnormalities. Unfortunately, published data on the safety of the thoracentesis on this group of patients are sparse.

Bass et al. [17] retrospectively studied 100 (55 males/45 females) patients diagnosed with HM on whom a thoracentesis was performed (ultrasound localization was used in 32% of all cases). Lymphoma was present in 52% of them (46 with non-Hodgkin's lymphoma and 6 with HD), whereas 9 patients were diagnosed with acute myeloid leukemia, 7 with MM, 6 with CLL, 2 with acute lymphocytic leukemia, 1 with CML and 2 with amyloidosis. Bone marrow or stem cell transplants had been performed in 21% of patients, including 14 allogeneic transplants and 7 autologous transplants. The main indications for thoracentesis were exclusion of infection and documentation or diagnosis of malignancy.

At the time of the thoracentesis, neutropenia was observed in 11 patients, a platelet count of <50,000 cells/μL in 13 patients, and coagulopathy with prothrombin time of >15 s and/or a partially activated thromboplastin time of >40 s was present in 14 patients in this study. Prior to the pleural fluid tap, platelet transfusions were performed in 18% of cases, and fresh-frozen plasma was administered in 7% of cases.

Despite possible thrombocytopenia and coagulation defects, complications related to bleeding occurred in only two cases of the study (2%) resulting in hemothorax. Nevertheless, in both cases, no clearly identified coagulation defects were detected (platelet counts and coagulation study findings were normal; one patient though, had an elevated creatinine level of 2.0 mg/dL).

Pneumothorax was also reported in 7% of patients, a rate comparable to that of nonimmunocompromised patients [57, 210], and a tube thoracostomy was required in 4% of patients. In general, all complications were successfully treated.

The evaluation of safety of thoracentesis was the aim of another retrospective study in 50 hematopoietic stem cell transplantation (HSCT) recipients [3]. Of them, 26 patients underwent allogeneic HSCT, while 24 underwent autologous HSCT. Thirty-two patients (68%) in the study had underlying HM, while 17 patients (34%) had solid tumors. The main indications for performing thoracentesis were to exclude infection and document or diagnose malignancy. Before the procedure a platelet transfusion was given if the platelet count was below 50,000 cells/mm^3, and fresh frozen plasma was given if the INR was more than 1.5. The only documented complication was pneumothorax in five patients; three were patients who had the procedure under radiological guidance. A tube thoracostomy was required in 4% of patients. None of the patients developed bleeding or hemothorax secondary to the thoracentesis.

In another report [69] on 22 children with cancer and neutropenia (absolute neutrophil count, <1,500 per mm^3), thoracentesis during febrile episodes in 22 patients revealed infection in 2 patients (9%), both of which were of fungal origin. Eight of the remaining nineteen patients underwent another diagnostic procedure, yielding five additional diagnoses. The procedure was performed with no complications. The authors conclude that thoracentesis is safe and should be considered as a diagnostic test for febrile neutropenic children with pulmonary effusions of presumed infectious etiology, although more invasive tests may be warranted.

In conclusion, thoracentesis seems to be a simple, safe and well-tolerated procedure in patients with HM, with a complication rate that is similar to that reported in other patient populations, either immunocompromised or non-immunocompromised.

References

1. Aaron L, Lidove O, Yousry C, Roudiere L, Dupont B, Viard JP (2002) Human herpesvirus 8-positive Castleman's disease in human immunodeficiency virus-infected patients: the impact of highly active antiretroviral therapy. Clin Infect Dis 35:880–882
2. Aasebo U, Norum J, Sager G, Slordal L (1997) Intrapleurally instilled mitoxantrone in metastatic pleural effusions: a phase II study. J Chemother 9:106–111
3. Adam AK, Zamlut M, Soubani AO (2007) The yield and safety of thoracentesis in hematopoietic stem cell transplantation recipients. Lung 185:257–262
4. Adiguzel C, Bozkurt SU, Kaygusuz I, Uzay A, Tecimer T, Bayik M (2009) Human herpesvirus 8-unrelated primary effusion lymphoma-like lymphoma: report of a rare case and review of the literature. APMIS 117:222–229
5. Ahmad H, Pawade J, Falk S, Morgan JA, Balacumaraswami L (2003) Primary pleural lymphomas. Thorax 58:908–909
6. Ahmed S, Siddiqui AK, Rossoff L, Sison CP, Rai KR (2003) Pulmonary complications in chronic lymphocytic leukemia. Cancer 98:1912–1917
7. Alexandrakis MG, Passam FH, Kyriakou DS, Bouros D (2004) Pleural effusions in hematologic malignancies. Chest 125:1546–1555
8. Alifano M, Guggino G, Gentile M, Elia S, Vernaglia A (1997) Management of concurrent pleural effusion in patients with lymphoma: thoracoscopy a useful tool in diagnosis and treatment. Monaldi Arch Chest Dis 52:330–334
9. Ameis A, Ko HS, Pruzanski W (1976) M components-a review of 1242 cases. Can Med Assoc J 114:889–892, 895
10. Andrieu V, Encaoua R, Carbon C, Couvelard A, Grange MJ (1998) Leukemic pleural effusion in B-cell prolymphocytic leukemia. Hematol Cell Ther 40:275–278
11. Aozasa K, Ohsawa M, Iuchi K, Tajima K, Komatsu H, Shimoyama M (1993) Artificial pneumothorax as a risk factor for development of pleural lymphoma. Jpn J Cancer Res 84:55–57
12. Aquino SL, Chen MY, Kuo WT, Chiles C (1999) The CT appearance of pleural and extrapleural disease in lymphoma. Clin Radiol 54:647–650
13. Awasthi A, Gupta N, Srinivasan R, Nijhawan R, Rajwanshi A (2007) Cytopathological spectrum of unusual malignant pleural effusions at a tertiary care centre in north India. Cytopathology 18:28–32
14. Awotedu AA, Otulana BA, Ukoli CO (1990) Giant lymph node hyperplasia of the lung (Castleman's disease) associated with recurrent pleural effusion. Thorax 45:775–776
15. Bangerter M, Hildebrand A, Griesshammer M (2001) Combined cytomorphologic and immunophenotypic analysis in the diagnostic workup of lymphomatous effusions. Acta Cytol 45:307–312
16. Barcos M, Lane W, Gomez GA et al (1987) An autopsy study of 1206 acute and chronic leukemias (1958 to 1982). Cancer 60:827–837
17. Bass J, White DA (2005) Thoracentesis in patients with hematologic malignancy: yield and safety. Chest 127: 2101–2105
18. Ben-Chetrit E, Assaf Y, Shinar E (1985) Predominant T cells in pleural effusion of a patient with B-cell CLL. Acta Haematol 73:101–103
19. Bergeron A, Rea D, Levy V et al (2007) Lung abnormalities after dasatinib treatment for chronic myeloid leukemia: a case series. Am J Respir Crit Care Med 176:814–818
20. Berkman N, Polliack A, Breuer R, Okon E, Kramer M (1992) Pulmonary involvement as the major manifestation of chronic lymphocytic leukemia. Leuk Lymphoma 8:495–499
21. Berkman N, Breuer R, Kramer MR, Polliack A (1996) Pulmonary involvement in lymphoma. Leuk Lymphoma 20:229–237
22. Bielsa S, Salud A, Martinez M et al (2008) Prognostic significance of pleural fluid data in patients with malignant effusion. Eur J Intern Med 19:334–339
23. Bilgin G, Yilmaz AS, Koksal E et al (2001) Primary chest Hodgkin's disease diagnosed by pleural biopsy: case report. East Afr Med J 78:389–391
24. Billstrom R, Johansson H, Johansson B, Mitelman F (1995) Immune-mediated complications in patients with myelodysplastic syndromes – clinical and cytogenetic features. Eur J Haematol 55:42–48
25. Blade J, Lust JA, Kyle RA (2005) Immunoglobulin D multiple myeloma: presenting features, response to therapy, and survival in a series of 53 cases. J Clin Oncol 12:2398–2404
26. Blankenship ME, Rowlett J, Timby JW, Roth RS, Jones RE (1997) Giant lymph node hyperplasia (Castleman's disease) presenting with chylous pleural effusion. Chest 112: 1132–1133
27. Boulanger E, Gerard L, Gabarre J et al (2005) Prognostic factors and outcome of human herpesvirus 8-associated primary effusion lymphoma in patients with AIDS. J Clin Oncol 23:4372–4380

28. Bourantas KL, Repousis P, Tsiara S, Christou L, Konstantinidou P, Bai M (1998) Chronic myelogenous leukemia terminating in acute megakaryoblastic leukemia. Case report. J Exp Clin Cancer Res 17:243–245
29. Bourantas KL, Tsiara S, Panteli A, Milionis C, Christou L (1998) Pleural effusion in chronic myelomonocytic leukemia. Acta Haematol 99:34–37
30. Bouroncle BA (1987) Unusual presentations and complications of hairy cell leukemia. Leukemia 1:288–293
31. Brimo F, Michel RP, Khetani K, Auger M (2007) Primary effusion lymphoma: a series of four cases and review of the literature with emphasis on cytomorphologic and immunocytochemical differential diagnosis. Cancer 111:224–233
32. Brimo F, Popradi G, Michel RP, Auger M (2009) Primary effusion lymphoma involving three body cavities. CytoJournal 6:21
33. Bronner GM, Baas P, Beijnen JH (1997) Pleurodesis in malignant pleural effusion. Ned Tijdschr Geneeskd 141: 1810–1814
34. Bunin NJ, Pui CH, Hustu HO, Rivera GK (1986) Unusual extramedullary relapses in children with acute lymphoblastic leukemia. J Pediatr 109:665–668
35. Burja IT, Thompson SK, Brown EJ (1997) Cytologic diagnosis of Ki-1 lymphoma in pleural and peritoneal effusions: a case report. Diagn Cytopathol 17:134–137
36. Cahill RA, Spitzer TR, Mazumder A (1996) Marrow engraftment and clinical manifestations of capillary leak syndrome. Bone Marrow Transplant 18:177–184
37. Camacho LH, Soignet SL, Chanel S et al (2000) Leukocytosis and the retinoic acid syndrome in patients with acute promyelocytic leukemia treated with arsenic trioxide. J Clin Oncol 18:2620–2625
38. Carbone A, Gloghini A (2009) AIDS-related lymphomas: from pathogenesis to pathology. Br J Haematol 130: 662–670
39. Carbone A, Gloghini A (2008) KSHV/HHV8-associated lymphomas. Br J Haematol 140:13–24
40. Carbone A, Gloghini A (2008) PEL and HHV8-unrelated effusion lymphomas: classification and diagnosis. Cancer 114:225–227
41. Carbone A, Gloghini A, Larocca LM et al (2001) Expression profile of MUM1/IRF4, BCL-6, and CD138/syndecan-1 defines novel histogenetic subsets of human immunodeficiency virus-related lymphomas. Blood 97:744–751
42. Carbone A, Cesarman E, Gloghini A, Drexler HG (2010) Understanding pathogenetic aspects and clinical presentation of primary effusion lymphoma through its derived cell lines. AIDS 24:479–490
43. Casper C (2005) The aetiology and management of Castleman disease at 50 years: translating pathophysiology to patient care. Br J Haematol 129:3–17
44. Cesarman E, Chang Y, Moore PS, Said JW, Knowles DM (1995) Kaposi's sarcoma-associated herpesvirus-like DNA sequences in AIDS-related body-cavity-based lymphomas. N Engl J Med 332:1186–1191
45. Chaignaud BE, Bonsack TA, Kozakewich HP, Shamberger RC (1998) Pleural effusions in lymphoblastic lymphoma: a diagnostic alternative. J Pediatr Surg 33:1355–1357
46. Chan CK, Hyland RH, Hutcheon MA (1990) Pulmonary complications following bone marrow transplantation. Clin Chest Med 11:323–332
47. Chang H, Sun CF (2008) Detection of B cell lymphoma involvement in T cell-rich serous fluid by immunoglobulin gene rearrangement: a report of two cases. Acta Cytol 52:231–234
48. Chang H, Chou WC, Lee SY, Huang JY, Hung YH (2009) Myelomatous pleural effusion in a patient with plasmablastic myeloma: a case report. Diagn Cytopathol 37:205–207
49. Chang MH, Kim SJ, Kim K et al (2009) Clinical features and treatment outcomes of adult B- and T-lymphoblastic lymphoma: results of multicentre analysis in Korea. Leuk Lymphoma 50:1119–1125
50. Chang WC, Tzao C, Hsu HH et al (2006) Pulmonary cryptococcosis: comparison of clinical and radiographic characteristics in immunocompetent and immunocompromised patients. Chest 129:333–340
51. Chang Y, Cesarman E, Pessin MS et al (1995) Identification of herpesvirus-like DNA sequences in AIDS-associated Kaposi's sarcoma. Science 266:1865–1869
52. Chen YB, Rahemtullah A, Hochberg E (2007) Primary effusion lymphoma. Oncologist 12:569–576
53. Chilosi M, Zinzani PL, Poletti V (2005) Lymphoproliferative lung disorders. Semin Respir Crit Care Med 26:490–501
54. Chubachi A, Wakui H, Miura I et al (1995) Extramedullary megakaryoblastic tumors following an indolent phase of myelofibrosis. Leuk Lymphoma 17:351–354
55. Collet G, Marty P, Le Fichoux Y et al (2004) Pleural effusion as the first manifestation of pulmonary toxoplasmosis in a bone marrow transplant recipient. Acta Cytol 48:114–116
56. Collins J, Muller NL, Leung AN et al (1998) Epstein-Barr-virus-associated lymphoproliferative disease of the lung: CT and histologic findings. Radiology 208:749–759
57. Collins TR, Sahn SA (1987) Thoracocentesis. Clinical value, complications, technical problems, and patient experience. Chest 91:817–822
58. Crapanzano JP, Lin O (2003) Cytologic findings of marginal zone lymphoma. Cancer 99:301–309
59. Crazzolara R, Kreczy A, Mann G et al (2001) High expression of the chemokine receptor CXCR4 predicts extramedullary organ infiltration in childhood acute lymphoblastic leukaemia. Br J Haematol 115:545–553
60. Czader M, Ali SZ (2003) Flow cytometry as an adjunct to cytomorphologic analysis of serous effusions. Diagn Cytopathol 29:74–78
61. Das DK (2006) Serous effusions in malignant lymphomas: a review. Diagn Cytopathol 34:335–347
62. Das DK, Gupta SK, Ayyagari S, Bambery PK, Datta BN, Datta U (1987) Pleural effusions in non-Hodgkin's lymphoma. A cytomorphologic, cytochemical and immunologic study. Acta Cytol 31:119–124
63. Das DK, Chowdhury V, Kishore B, Chachra K, Bhatt NC, Kakar AK (1999) CD-30(Ki-1)-positive anaplastic large cell lymphoma in a pleural effusion A case report with diagnosis by cytomorphologic and immunocytochemical studies. Acta Cytol 43:498–502
64. Davis BA, Cervi P, Amin Z, Moshi G, Shaw P, Porter J (1996) Retinoic acid syndrome: pulmonary computed tomography (CT) findings. Leuk Lymphoma 23:113–117
65. De Botton S, Dombret H, Sanz M et al (1998) Incidence, clinical features, and outcome of all trans-retinoic acid syndrome in 413 cases of newly diagnosed acute promyelocytic leukemia. The European APL Group. Blood 92:2712–2718

66. De Lavallade H, Punnialingam S, Milojkovic D et al (2008) Pleural effusions in patients with chronic myeloid leukaemia treated with dasatinib may have an immune-mediated pathogenesis. Br J Haematol 141:745–747
67. De Renzo A, Micera V, Vaglio S, Luciano L, Selleri C, Rotoli B (1990) Induction of alkaline phosphatase activity in chronic myeloid leukemia cells: in vitro studies and speculative hypotheses. Am J Hematol 35:278–280
68. DeCamp MM Jr, Mentzer SJ, Swanson SJ, Sugarbaker DJ (1997) Malignant effusive disease of the pleura and pericardium. Chest 112:291S–295S
69. Desselle BC, Bozeman PM, Patrick CC (1995) Diagnostic utility of thoracentesis for neutropenic children with cancer. Clin Infect Dis 21:887–890
70. Dettrick AJ, Robertson T, Morris KL (2004) Diagnosis of granulocytic sarcoma on pleural effusion cytology: report of a case. Diagn Cytopathol 31:126–128
71. Dix DB, Anderson RA, McFadden DE, Wadsworth LD (1997) Pleural relapse during hematopoietic remission in childhood acute lymphoblastic leukemia. J Pediatr Hematol Oncol 19:470–472
72. Dunphy CH, Collins B, Ramos R, Grosso LE (1998) Secondary pleural involvement by an AIDS-related anaplastic large cell (CD30+) lymphoma simulating metastatic adenocarcinoma. Diagn Cytopathol 18:113–117
73. Edmonson JH, Hartmann LC, Long HJ et al (1992) Granulocyte-macrophage colony-stimulating factor. Preliminary observations on the influences of dose, schedule, and route of administration in patients receiving cyclophosphamide and carboplatin. Cancer 70:2529–2539
74. Elis A, Blickstein D, Mulchanov I et al (1998) Pleural effusion in patients with non-Hodgkin's lymphoma: a case-controlled study. Cancer 83:1607–1611
75. Essadki O, el Wady N, el Abassi Skalli A (1996) Radiological features of thoracic localizations of lymphomas. Bull Cancer 83:929–936
76. Fadil A, Taylor DE (1998) The lung and Waldenstrom's macroglobulinemia. South Med J 91:681–685
77. Farray D, Al-Masri H, Hattersley E, Smith SE (2005) Megakaryoblastic leukemia with involvement of the pleural fluid. Am J Hematol 79:238–239
78. Fatih T, Selim Y, Mesut A, Demirel YN, Yuksel P (2007) An unusual cause of unilateral pleural effusion in the setting of aortic stenosis: acute myeloid leukemia. Intern Med 46:325–327
79. Ferrer J, Roldan J (2000) Clinical management of the patient with pleural effusion. Eur J Radiol 34:76–86
80. Ferrer J, Villarino MA, Encabo G et al (1999) Diagnostic utility of CYFRA 21-1, carcinoembryonic antigen, CA 125, neuron specific enolase, and squamous cell antigen level determinations in the serum and pleural fluid of patients with pleural effusions. Cancer 86:1488–1495
81. Filuk RB, Warren PW (1986) Bronchoalveolar lavage in Waldenstrom's macroglobulinaemia with pulmonary infiltrates. Thorax 41:409–410
82. Fishel RS, Are C, Barbul A (2003) Vessel injury and capillary leak. Crit Care Med 31:S502–511
83. Fragoso R, Pereira T, Wu Y, Zhu Z, Cabecadas J, Dias S (2006) VEGFR-1 (FLT-1) activation modulates acute lymphoblastic leukemia localization and survival within the bone marrow, determining the onset of extramedullary disease. Blood 107:1608–1616
84. Fragoulis KN, Handrinou E, Papadopoulos V, Dardoufas K, Falagas ME (2006) Delayed effusive pericarditis and recurrent pleural effusion after radiation treatment for Hodgkin's disease responsive to per os doxycycline. Eur J Haematol 76:176–179
85. Franko AJ, Sharplin J (1994) Development of fibrosis after lung irradiation in relation to inflammation and lung function in a mouse strain prone to fibrosis. Radiat Res 140:347–355
86. Fujisawa S, Tanioka F, Matsuoka T, Ozawa T (2005) CD5+ diffuse large B-cell lymphoma with c-myc/IgH rearrangement presenting as primary effusion lymphoma. Int J Hematol 81:315–318
87. Fukayama M, Ibuka T, Hayashi Y, Ooba T, Koike M, Mizutani S (1993) Epstein–Barr virus in pyothorax-associated pleural lymphoma. Am J Pathol 143:1044–1049
88. Funamoto Y, Nagai M, Haba R, Kishida F, Kohno K, Kobayashi S (2002) Hyaluronan synthesis by anaplastic large cell lymphoma with massive lymphomatous effusion. A case report. Acta Cytol 46:864–868
89. Gahler A, Hitz F, Hess U, Cerny T (2003) Acute pericarditis and pleural effusion complicating cytarabine chemotherapy. Onkologie 26:348–350
90. Gaidano G, Carbone A (2001) Primary effusion lymphoma: a liquid phase lymphoma of fluid-filled body cavities. Adv Cancer Res 80:115–146
91. Gillison ML, Ambinder RF (1997) Human herpesvirus-8. Curr Opin Oncol 9:440–449
92. Gogia A, Agarwal PK, Jain S, Jain KP (2005) Myelomatous pleural effusion. J Assoc Physicians India 53:734–736
93. Goldblatt M, Huggins JT, Doelken P, Gurung P, Sahn SA (2009) Dasatinib-induced pleural effusions: a lymphatic network disorder? Am J Med Sci 338:414–417
94. Gomyo H, Kajimoto K, Maeda A et al (2007) t(14;18)(q32;q21)-bearing pleural MALT lymphoma with IgM paraproteinemia: value of detection of specific cytogenetic abnormalities in the differential diagnosis of MALT lymphoma and lymphoplasmacytic lymphoma. Hematology 12:315–318
95. Guihot A, Couderc LJ, Agbalika F et al (2005) Pulmonary manifestations of multicentric Castleman's disease in HIV infection: a clinical, biological and radiological study. Eur Respir J 26:118–125
96. Guzman J, Bross KJ, Costabel U (1991) Malignant lymphoma in pleural effusions: an immunocytochemical cell surface analysis. Diagn Cytopathol 7:113–118
97. Haddad MG, Silverman JF, Joshi VV, Geisinger KR (1995) Effusion cytology in Burkitt's lymphoma. Diagn Cytopathol 12:3–7
98. Hallman JR, Geisinger KR (1994) Cytology of fluids from pleural, peritoneal and pericardial cavities in children. A comprehensive survey. Acta Cytol 38:209–217
99. Hanson MN, Morrison VA, Peterson BA et al (1996) Posttransplant T-cell lymphoproliferative disorders – an aggressive, late complication of solid-organ transplantation. Blood 88:3626–3633
100. Heffner JE (2008) Diagnosis and management of malignant pleural effusions. Respirology 13:5–20
101. Hicsonmez G, Cetin M, Tunc B, Tuncer AM, Gumruk F, Yenicesu I (1998) Dramatic resolution of pleural effusion in children with chronic myelomonocytic leukemia

following short-course high-dose methylprednisolone. Leuk Lymphoma 29:617–623
102. Hocqueloux L, Agbalika F, Oksenhendler E, Molina JM (2001) Long-term remission of an AIDS-related primary effusion lymphoma with antiviral therapy. AIDS 15: 280–282
103. Hoelzer D, Gokbuget N, Digel W et al (2002) Outcome of adult patients with T-lymphoblastic lymphoma treated according to protocols for acute lymphoblastic leukemia. Blood 99:4379–4385
104. Hongyo T, Kurooka M, Taniguchi E et al (1998) Frequent p53 mutations at dipyrimidine sites in patients with pyothorax-associated lymphoma. Cancer Res 58:1105–1107
105. Horenstein MG, Nador RG, Chadburn A et al (1997) Epstein–Barr virus latent gene expression in primary effusion lymphomas containing Kaposi's sarcoma-associated herpesvirus/human herpesvirus-8. Blood 90:1186–1191
106. Horn KD, Penchansky L (1999) Chylous pleural effusions simulating leukemic infiltrate associated with thoracoabdominal disease and surgery in infants. Am J Clin Pathol 111:99–104
107. Hosoki K, Okada S, Ichinohasama R, Yamaguchi M, Uchiyama B, Maeyama T (2007) Angioimmunoblastic T-cell lymphoma developed with lymphocytic pleural effusion. Intern Med 46:739–742
108. Inoue Y, Tsukasaki K, Nagai K, Soda H, Tomonaga M (2004) Durable remission by sobuzoxane in an HIV-seronegative patient with human herpesvirus 8-negative primary effusion lymphoma. Int J Hematol 79:271–275
109. Inoue Y, Chua K, McClure RF et al (2005) Multiple myeloma presenting initially as a solitary pleural effusion later complicated by malignant plasmacytic ascites. Leuk Res 29:715–718
110. Izban KF, Pooley RJ Jr, Selvaggi SM, Alkan S (2001) Cytologic diagnosis of peripheral T-cell lymphoma manifesting as ascites. A case report. Acta Cytol 45:385–392
111. Jabbour E, Koscielny S, Sebban C et al (2006) High survival rate with the LMT-89 regimen in lymphoblastic lymphoma (LL), but not in T-cell acute lymphoblastic leukemia (T-ALL). Leukemia 20:814–819
112. Jancelewicz Z, Takatsuki K, Sugai S, Pruzanski W (1975) IgD multiple myeloma. Review of 133 cases. Arch Intern Med 135:87–93
113. Janckila AJ, Yam LT, Li CY (1985) Immunocytochemical diagnosis of acute leukemia with pleural involvement. Acta Cytol 29:67–72
114. Jayson GC, Parker GJ, Mullamitha S et al (2005) Blockade of platelet-derived growth factor receptor-beta by CDP860, a humanized, PEGylated di-Fab', leads to fluid accumulation and is associated with increased tumor vascularized volume. J Clin Oncol 23:973–981
115. Jimenez-Heffernan JA, Viguer JM, Vicandi B et al (1997) Posttransplant CD30 (Ki-1)-positive anaplastic large cell lymphoma. Report of a case with presentation as a pleural effusion. Acta Cytol 41:1519–1524
116. Johnston WW (1985) The malignant pleural effusion. A review of cytopathologic diagnoses of 584 specimens from 472 consecutive patients. Cancer 56:905–909
117. Jones TI (1993) Pleural blast crisis in chronic myelogenous leukemia. Am J Hematol 44:75–76
118. Judde JG, Lacoste V, Briere J et al (2000) Monoclonality or oligoclonality of human herpesvirus 8 terminal repeat sequences in Kaposi's sarcoma and other diseases. J Natl Cancer Inst 92:729–736
119. Jules-Elysee K, Stover DE, Yahalom J, White DA, Gulati SC (1992) Pulmonary complications in lymphoma patients treated with high-dose therapy autologous bone marrow transplantation. Am Rev Respir Dis 146:485–491
120. Kamble R, Wilson CS, Fassas A et al (2005) Malignant pleural effusion of multiple myeloma: prognostic factors and outcome. Leuk Lymphoma 46:1137–1142
121. Kamiya H, Ishikawa R, Moriya A et al (2008) Disseminated cryptococcosis complicated with bilateral pleural effusion and ascites during corticosteroid therapy for organizing pneumonia with myelodysplastic syndrome. Intern Med 47:1981–1986
122. Kanno H, Yasunaga Y, Ohsawa M et al (1996) Expression of Epstein–Barr virus latent infection genes and oncogenes in lymphoma cell lines derived from pyothorax-associated lymphoma. Int J Cancer 67:86–94
123. Karkoulias K, Sampsonas F, Kaparianos A, Tsiamita M, Tsoukalas G, Spiropoulos K (2007) Urinothorax: an unexpected cause of pleural effusion in a patient with non-Hodgkin lymphoma. Eur Rev Med Pharmacol Sci 11:373–374
124. Katz RL, Raval P, Manning JT, McLaughlin P, Barlogie B (1987) A morphologic, immunologic, and cytometric approach to the classification of non-Hodgkin's lymphoma in effusions. Diagn Cytopathol 3:91–101
125. Kavuru MS, Tubbs R, Miller ML, Wiedemann HP (1992) Immunocytometry and gene rearrangement analysis in the diagnosis of lymphoma in an idiopathic pleural effusion. Am Rev Respir Dis 145:209–211
126. Kawahara K, Sasada S, Nagano T et al (2008) Pleural MALT lymphoma diagnosed on thoracoscopic resection under local anesthesia using an insulation-tipped diathermic knife. Pathol Int 58:253–256
127. Kelly K, Swords R, Mahalingam D, Padmanabhan S, Giles FJ (2009) Serosal inflammation (pleural and pericardial effusions) related to tyrosine kinase inhibitors. Target Oncol 4:99–105
128. Khurshid I, Anderson LC (2002) Non-infectious pulmonary complications after bone marrow transplantation. Postgrad Med J 78:257–262
129. Kim HW, Lee SS, Ryu MH et al (2006) A case of leukemic pleural infiltration in atypical chronic myeloid leukemia. J Korean Med Sci 21:936–939
130. Kirn D, Mauch P, Shaffer K et al (1993) Large-cell and immunoblastic lymphoma of the mediastinum: prognostic features and treatment outcome in 57 patients. J Clin Oncol 11:1336–1343
131. Klein U, Gloghini A, Gaidano G et al (2003) Gene expression profile analysis of AIDS-related primary effusion lymphoma (PEL) suggests a plasmablastic derivation and identifies PEL-specific transcripts. Blood 101:4115–4121
132. Knowles DM, Cesarman E, Chadburn A et al (1995) Correlative morphologic and molecular genetic analysis demonstrates three distinct categories of posttransplantation lymphoproliferative disorders. Blood 85:552–565
133. Kodama K, Yokose T, Takahashi K et al (1999) Low-grade B-cell lymphoma of mucosa-associated lymphoid tissue in

the lung: a report of a case with pleural dissemination. Lung Cancer 24:175–178
134. Kolschmann S, Ballin A, Gillissen A (2005) Clinical efficacy and safety of thoracoscopic talc pleurodesis in malignant pleural effusions. Chest 128:1431–1435
135. Kramer G, Gans S, Rijnders A, Leer J (2000) Long term survival of a patient with malignant pleural mesothelioma as a late complication of radiotherapy for Hodgkin's disease treated with 90yttrium-silicate. Lung Cancer 27: 205–208
136. Larson RS, Tallman MS (2003) Retinoic acid syndrome: manifestations, pathogenesis, and treatment. Best Pract Res Clin Haematol 16:453–461
137. Laurini JA, Garcia A, Elsner B, Bellotti M, Rescia C (2000) Relation between natural killer cells and neoplastic cells in serous fluids. Diagn Cytopathol 22:347–350
138. Le Gouill S, Lepretre S, Briere J et al (2003) Adult lymphoblastic lymphoma: a retrospective analysis of 92 patients under 61 years included in the LNH87/93 trials. Leukemia 17:2220–2224
139. Lechapt-Zalcman E, Rieux C, Cordonnier C, Desvaux D (1999) Posttransplantation lymphoproliferative disorder mimicking a nonspecific lymphocytic pleural effusion in a bone marrow transplant recipient. A case report. Acta Cytol 43:239–242
140. Light RW, Macgregor MI, Luchsinger PC, Ball WC Jr (1972) Pleural effusions: the diagnostic separation of transudates and exudates. Ann Intern Med 77:507–513
141. Lilly MB, Ottmann OG, Shah NP et al (2010) Dasatinib 140 mg once daily versus 70 mg twice daily in patients with Ph-positive acute lymphoblastic leukemia who failed imatinib: Results from a phase 3 study. Am J Hematol 85:164–170
142. Lim ST, Rubin N, Said J, Levine AM (2005) Primary effusion lymphoma: successful treatment with highly active antiretroviral therapy and rituximab. Ann Hematol 84:551–552
143. Maeno T, Sando Y, Tsukagoshi M et al (2000) Pleural amyloidosis in a patient with intractable pleural effusion and multiple myeloma. Respirology 5:79–80
144. Manley R, Monteath J, Patton WN (1999) Co-incidental presentation of IgA lambda multiple myeloma and pleural involvement with IgM kappa non-Hodgkin's lymphoma. Clin Lab Haematol 21:61–63
145. Manoharan A (1999) Malignant pleural effusion in chronic myelomonocytic leukaemia. Thorax 46:461–462
146. Mansoor A, Wagner RP, DePalma L (2000) Waldenstrom macroglobulinemia presenting as a pleural effusion. Arch Pathol Lab Med 124:891–893
147. Martelli M, Ferreri AJ, Johnson P (2008) Primary mediastinal large B-cell lymphoma. Crit Rev Oncol Hematol 68:256–263
148. Matolcsy A, Nador RG, Cesarman E, Knowles DM (1998) Immunoglobulin VH gene mutational analysis suggests that primary effusion lymphomas derive from different stages of B cell maturation. Am J Pathol 153:1609–1614
149. Matyskova M, Krahulcova E, Bulikova A, Novotna H (1995) Pleural effusion in plasmacytic leukemia. Vnitr Lék 41:467–469
150. McConkey D, Nawrocki ST, Andtbacka R (2005) Velcade displays promising activity in primary effusion lymphoma cells. Cancer Biol Ther 4:491–492
151. Mihaescu A, Gebhard S, Chaubert P et al (2002) Application of molecular genetics to the diagnosis of lymphoid-rich effusions: study of 95 cases with concomitant immunophenotyping. Diagn Cytopathol 27:90–95
152. Miller RT, Baker KI, Moga D (1987) Multilobated B-cell lymphoma. Report of a case with immunocytologic diagnosis in pleural fluid. Acta Cytol 31:785–790
153. Mitchell A, Meunier C, Ouellette D, Colby T (2006) Extranodal marginal zone lymphoma of mucosa-associated lymphoid tissue with initial presentation in the pleura. Chest 129:791–794
154. Miyahara M, Shimamoto Y, Sano M, Nakano H, Shibata K, Matsuzaki M (1996) Immunoglobulin gene rearrangement in T-cell-rich reactive pleural effusion of a patient with B-cell chronic lymphocytic leukemia. Acta Haematol 96:41–44
155. Miyake F, Yoshikawa T, Fujita A et al (2006) Pneumonia with marked pleural effusion caused by *Aspergillus* infection. Pediatr Infect Dis J 25:186–187
156. Mizuki M, Ueda S, Tagawa S et al (1998) Natural killer cell-derived large granular lymphocyte lymphoma of lung developed in a patient with hypersensitivity to mosquito bites and reactivated Epstein–Barr virus infection. Am J Hematol 59:309–315
157. Mohapatra MK, Das SP, Mohanty NC, Dash PC, Bastia BK (2000) Haemopericardium with cardiac tamponade and pleural effusion in chronic myeloid leukemia. Indian Heart J 52:209–211
158. Morel P, Dupriez B, Plantier-Colcher I et al (1990) Long-term outcome of follicular low-grade lymphoma. A report of 91 patients. Ann Hematol 66:303–308
159. Moriarty AT, Wiersema L, Snyder W, Kotylo PK, McCloskey DW (1993) Immunophenotyping of cytologic specimens by flow cytometry. Diagn Cytopathol 9:252–258
160. Moriki T, Wada M, Takahashi T, Ueda S, Miyazaki E (2000) Pleural effusion cytology in a case of cytophagic histiocytic panniculitis (subcutaneous panniculitic T-cell lymphoma). A case report. Acta Cytol 44:1040–1044
161. Morrison VA (1998) The infectious complications of chronic lymphocytic leukemia. Semin Oncol 25:98–106
162. Morrison VA, Rai KR, Peterson BL et al (2001) Impact of therapy With chlorambucil, fludarabine, or fludarabine plus chlorambucil on infections in patients with chronic lymphocytic leukemia: Intergroup Study Cancer and Leukemia Group B 9011. J Clin Oncol 19:3611–3621
163. Morrone N, Gama e Silva Volpe VL, Dourado AM, Mitre F, Coletta EN (1993) Bilateral pleural effusion due to mediastinal fibrosis induced by radiotherapy. Chest 104:1276–1278
164. Movsas B, Raffin TA, Epstein AH, Link CJ Jr (1997) Pulmonary radiation injury. Chest 111:1061–1076
165. Mufti GJ, Figes A, Hamblin TJ, Oscier DG, Copplestone JA (1986) Immunological abnormalities in myelodysplastic syndromes. I. Serum immunoglobulins and autoantibodies. Br J Haematol 63:143–147
166. Mufti GJ, Oscier DG, Hamblin TJ, Nightingale A, Darlow S (1984) Serous effusions in monocytic leukaemias. Br J Haematol 58:547–552

167. Nador RG, Cesarman E, Chadburn A et al (1996) Primary effusion lymphoma: a distinct clinicopathologic entity associated with the Kaposi's sarcoma-associated herpesvirus. Blood 88:645–656
168. Nadrous HF, Krowka MJ, McClure RF, Tefferi A, Lim KG (2004) Agnogenic myeloid metaplasia with pleural extramedullary leukemic transformation. Leuk Lymphoma 45:815–818
169. Nagai K, Ando K, Yoshida H et al (1997) Response of the extramedullary lung plasmacytoma with pleural effusion to chemotherapy. Ann Hematol 74:279–281
170. Nakatsuka S, Yao M, Hoshida Y, Yamamoto S, Iuchi K, Aozasa K (2002) Pyothorax-associated lymphoma: a review of 106 cases. J Clin Oncol 20:4255–4260
171. Neragi-Miandoab S (2008) Surgical and other invasive approaches to recurrent pleural effusion with malignant etiology. Support Care Cancer 16:1323–1331
172. Neuman G, Denekamp Y (2009) Dyspnea and pleural effusion as presenting clinical manifestations of multiple myeloma. Isr Med Assoc J 11:118–119
173. Nicholas J, Ruvolo VR, Burns WH et al (1997) Kaposi's sarcoma-associated human herpesvirus-8 encodes homologues of macrophage inflammatory protein-1 and interleukin-6. Nat Med 3:287–292
174. Nicolls MR, Terada LS, Tuder RM, Prindiville SA, Schwarz MI (1998) Diffuse alveolar hemorrhage with underlying pulmonary capillaritis in the retinoic acid syndrome. Am J Respir Crit Care Med 158:1302–1305
175. Noble PW (1989) The pulmonary complications of bone marrow transplantation in adults. West J Med 150: 443–449
176. O'Donovan M, Silva I, Uhlmann V et al (2001) Expression profile of human herpesvirus 8 (HHV-8) in pyothorax associated lymphoma and in effusion lymphoma. Mol Pathol 54:80–85
177. Oeda E, Shinohara K, Kamei S, Nomiyama J, Inoue H (1994) Capillary leak syndrome likely the result of granulocyte colony-stimulating factor after high-dose chemotherapy. Intern Med 33:115–119
178. Ohsawa M, Tomita Y, Kanno H et al (1995) Role of Epstein–Barr virus in pleural lymphomagenesis. Mod Pathol 8:848–853
179. Ohshima K, Ishiguro M, Yamasaki S et al (2002) Chromosomal and comparative genomic analyses of HHV-8-negative primary effusion lymphoma in five HIV-negative Japanese patients. Leuk Lymphoma 43:595–601
180. Okada F, Ando Y, Kondo Y, Matsumoto S, Maeda T, Mori H (2004) Thoracic CT findings of adult T-cell leukemia or lymphoma. AJR Am J Roentgenol 182:761–767
181. Oksenhendler E, Duarte M, Soulier J et al (1996) Multicentric Castleman's disease in HIV infection: a clinical and pathological study of 20 patients. AIDS 10:61–67
182. Oksenhendler E, Carcelain G, Aoki Y et al (2000) High levels of human herpesvirus 8 viral load, human interleukin-6, interleukin-10, and C reactive protein correlate with exacerbation of multicentric castleman disease in HIV-infected patients. Blood 96:2069–2073
183. Olson PR, Silverman JF, Powers CN (2000) Pleural fluid cytology of Hodgkin's disease: cytomorphologic features and the value of immunohistochemical studies. Diagn Cytopathol 22:21–24
184. Ooi GC, Chim CS, Lie AK, Tsang KW (1999) Computed tomography features of primary pulmonary non-Hodgkin's lymphoma. Clin Radiol 54:438–443
185. Ozkaynak MF, Weinberg K, Kohn D, Sender L, Parkman R, Lenarsky C (1991) Hepatic veno-occlusive disease post-bone marrow transplantation in children conditioned with busulfan and cyclophosphamide: incidence, risk factors, and clinical outcome. Bone Marrow Transplant 7: 467–474
186. Pacheco A, Perpina A, Escribano L, Sanz I, Bellas C (1992) Pleural effusion as first sign of extramedullary plasmacytoma. Chest 102:296–297
187. Palmer HE, Wilson CS, Bardales RH (2000) Cytology and flow cytometry of malignant effusions of multiple myeloma. Diagn Cytopathol 22:147–151
188. Patriarca F, Ermacora A, Skert C (1999) Pleural involvement in a case of monocytoid B-cell lymphoma. Haematologica 84:949–950
189. Pei SN, Kuo CY, Ma MC, Wang MC (2009) Mediastinal mass and malignant pleural effusion in an aleukemic case with pre-B acute lymphoblastic leukemia. J Pediatr Hematol Oncol 31:139–141
190. Perry MC, Eaton WL, Propert KJ et al (1987) Chemotherapy with or without radiation therapy in limited small-cell carcinoma of the lung. N Engl J Med 316:912–918
191. Peterson BA, Frizzera G (1993) Multicentric Castleman's disease. Semin Oncol 20:636–647
192. Petit A, Pulik M, Gaulier A, Lionnet F, Mahe A, Sigal M (1995) Systemic mastocytosis associated with chronic myelomonocytic leukemia: clinical features and response to interferon alfa therapy. J Am Acad Dermatol 32:850–853
193. Porkka K, Khoury HJ, Paquette RL, Matloub Y, Sinha R, Cortes JE (2010) Dasatinib 100 mg once daily minimizes the occurrence of pleural effusion in patients with chronic myeloid leukemia in chronic phase and efficacy is unaffected in patients who develop pleural effusion. Cancer 116:377–386
194. Prabhudesai PP, Mahashur AA, Mehta N, Ajay R (1993) Exudative pleural effusions in patients over 40 years of age – an analysis of 76 patients. J Postgrad Med 39:190–193
195. Quintas-Cardama A, Kantarjian H, O'Brien S et al (2007) Pleural effusion in patients with chronic myelogenous leukemia treated with dasatinib after imatinib failure. J Clin Oncol 25:3908–3914
196. Rausch PG, Herion JC (1980) Pulmonary manifestations of Waldenstrom macroglobulinemia. Am J Hematol 9:201–209
197. Rege K, Powles R, Norton J et al (1993) An unusual presentation of acute myeloid leukaemia with pericardial and pleural effusions due to granulocytic sarcoma. Leuk Lymphoma 11:305–307
198. Rigamonti F, Beris P, Sanchez-Pareja A et al (2009) Atypical presentation of acute myeloid leukemia: cardiac myeloid sarcoma. Int J Hematol 89:693–698
199. Rodriguez JN, Pereira A, Martinez JC, Conde J, Pujol E (1994) Pleural effusion in multiple myeloma. Chest 105:622–624
200. Sahn SA (2001) Management of malignant pleural effusions. Monaldi Arch Chest Dis 56:394–399

201. Said JW, Shintaku IP, Asou H et al (1999) Herpesvirus 8 inclusions in primary effusion lymphoma: report of a unique case with T-cell phenotype. Arch Pathol Lab Med 123:257–260
202. Sakemi T, Uchida M, Ikeda Y, Shouno Y (1996) Acute renal failure and nephrotic syndrome in a patient with T-cell lymphoma. Nephron 72:326–327
203. Sandlund JT, Crist WM, Abromowitch M et al (1991) Pleural effusion is associated with a poor treatment outcome in stage III small non-cleaved cell lymphoma. Leukemia 5:71–74
204. Santini M, Fiorello A, Vicidomini G, Busiello L, Baldi A (2009) A surgical case of pyothorax-associated lymphoma of T-cell origin arising from the chest wall in chronic empyema. Ann Thorac Surg 88:642–645
205. Sasser RL, Yam LT, Li CY (1990) Myeloma with involvement of the serous cavities. Cytologic and immunochemical diagnosis and literature review. Acta Cytol 34:479–485
206. Schaap N, Raymakers R, Schattenberg A, Ottevanger JP, de Witte T (1996) Massive pleural effusion attributed to high-dose cyclophosphamide during conditioning for BMT. Bone Marrow Transplant 18:247–248
207. Schmetzer HM, Wilmanns W, Gerhartz HH (1996) Detection of acute myeloid leukemic cells in complete remission and in extramedullary sites by clonal analyses. Acta Haematol 96:83–87
208. Schulz TF (1999) Epidemiology of Kaposi's sarcoma-associated herpesvirus/human herpesvirus 8. Adv Cancer Res 76:121–160
209. Seber A, Khan SP, Kersey JH (1996) Unexplained effusions: association with allogeneic bone marrow transplantation and acute or chronic graft-versus-host disease. Bone Marrow Transplant 17:207–211
210. Seneff MG, Corwin RW, Gold LH, Irwin RS (1986) Complications associated with thoracocentesis. Chest 90:97–100
211. Sheibani K, Burke JS, Swartz WG, Nademanee A, Winberg CD (1988) Monocytoid B-cell lymphoma. Clinicopathologic study of 21 cases of a unique type of low-grade lymphoma. Cancer 62:1531–1538
212. Shimazaki M, Fujita M, Tsukamoto K et al (2003) An unusual case of primary effusion lymphoma in a HIV-negative patient not pathogenetically associated with HHV8. Eur J Haematol 71:62–67
213. Shimoni A, Shvidel L, Shtalrid M, Klepfish A, Berrebi A (1998) Prolymphocytic transformation of B-chronic lymphocytic leukemia presenting as malignant ascites and pleural effusion. Am J Hematol 59:316–318
214. Shulman HM, Sullivan KM, Weiden PL et al (1980) Chronic graft-versus-host syndrome in man. A long-term clinicopathologic study of 20 Seattle patients. Am J Med 69:204–217
215. Simonelli C, Spina M, Cinelli R et al (2003) Clinical features and outcome of primary effusion lymphoma in HIV-infected patients: a single-institution study. J Clin Oncol 21:3948–3954
216. Sivakumaran M, Qureshi H, Chapman CS (1995) Chylous effusions in CLL. Leuk Lymphoma 18:365–366
217. Soulier J, Grollet L, Oksenhendler E et al (1995) Kaposi's sarcoma-associated herpesvirus-like DNA sequences in multicentric Castleman's disease. Blood 86:1276–1280
218. Spector M, Pollak JS (2008) Management of malignant pleural effusions. Semin Respir Crit Care Med 29:405–413
219. Stafford CM, Herndier B, Yi ES, Weidner N, Harrell JH 2nd (2004) Granulocytic sarcoma of the tracheobronchial tree: bronchoscopic and pathologic correlation. Respiration 71:529–532
220. Steiropoulos P, Kouliatsis G, Karpathiou G, Popidou M, Froudarakis ME (2009) Rare cases of primary pleural Hodgkin and non-Hodgkin lymphomas. Respiration 77:459–463
221. Stiksa G, Korsgaard R, Simonsson BG (1979) Treatment of recurrent pleural effusion by pleurodesis with quinacrine. Comparison between instillation by repeated thoracenteses and by tube drainage. Scand J Respir Dis 60:197–205
222. Suh YK, Shin HJ (2000) Fine-needle aspiration biopsy of granulocytic sarcoma: a clinicopathologic study of 27 cases. Cancer 90:364–372
223. Suminoe A, Matsuzaki A, Hattori H, Koga Y, Ishii E, Hara T (2007) Expression of matrix metalloproteinase (MMP) and tissue inhibitor of MMP (TIMP) genes in blasts of infant acute lymphoblastic leukemia with organ involvement. Leuk Res 31:1437–1440
224. Suminoe A, Matsuzaki A, Koga Y, Kusuhara K, Hara T (2007) Human herpesvirus 6 (HHV-6)-associated pleurisy after unrelated cord blood transplantation in children with chemotherapy-resistant malignant lymphoma. J Pediatr Hematol Oncol 29:709–712
225. Swerdlow SH, Zellner DC, Hurtubise PE, Kennealy J (1986) Pleural involvement in B-cell chronic lymphocytic leukemia associated with a T-cell-rich "reactive" pleural effusion. Am Rev Respir Dis 134:172–174
226. Syme RM, Wood CJ, Wong H, Mody CH (1997) Both CD4+ and CD8+ human lymphocytes are activated and proliferate in response to Cryptococcus neoformans. Immunology 92:194–200
227. Tallman MS, Andersen JW, Schiffer CA et al (2000) Clinical description of 44 patients with acute promyelocytic leukemia who developed the retinoic acid syndrome. Blood 95:90–95
228. Ten Hoor T, Hewan-Lowe K, Miller JI, Moss M (1999) A transitional variant of Castleman's disease presenting as a chylous pleural effusion. Chest 115:285–288
229. Terasaki Y, Okumura H, Saito K et al (2008) HHV-8/KSHV-negative and CD20-positive primary effusion lymphoma successfully treated by pleural drainage followed by chemotherapy containing rituximab. Intern Med 47:2175–2178
230. Treaba D, Assad L, Govil H et al (2002) Diagnostic role of fine-needle aspiration of bone lesions in patients with a previous history of malignancy. Diagn Cytopathol 26: 380–383
231. Ueda T, Manabe A, Kikuchi A et al (2000) Massive pericardial and pleural effusion with anasarca following allogeneic bone marrow transplantation. Int J Hematol 71: 394–397
232. Utz JP, Swensen SJ, Gertz MA (1996) Pulmonary amyloidosis. The Mayo Clinic experience from 1980 to 1993. Ann Intern Med 124:407–413
233. Vakar-Lopez F, Yang M (1999) Peripheral T-cell lymphoma presenting as ascites: a case report and review of the literature. Diagn Cytopathol 20:382–384

234. Valdes L, Alvarez D, Valle JM, Pose A, San Jose E (1996) The etiology of pleural effusions in an area with high incidence of tuberculosis. Chest 109:158–162
235. Van den Berge M, Tinga CJ, Bieger R (2001) A 73-year-old man with chronic lymphocytic leukaemia and a haemorrhagic pleural effusion. Ann Hematol 80:183–186
236. Van Renterghem DM, Pauwels RA (1995) Chylothorax and pleural effusion as late complications of thoracic irradiation. Chest 108:886–887
237. Vega F, Padula A, Valbuena JR, Stancu M, Jones D, Medeiros LJ (2006) Lymphomas involving the pleura: a clinicopathologic study of 34 cases diagnosed by pleural biopsy. Arch Pathol Lab Med 130:1497–1502
238. Vernon SE, Rosenthal DL (1979) Sezary cells in ascitic fluid. Acta Cytol 23:408–411
239. Watanabe N, Sugimoto N, Matsushita A et al (2003) Association of intestinal malignant lymphoma and ulcerative colitis. Intern Med 42:1183–1187
240. Xu D (2006) Dual surface immunoglobulin light-chain expression in B-cell lymphoproliferative disorders. Arch Pathol Lab Med 130:853–856
241. Yamaguchi K (1973) Pathology of macroglobulinemia – a review of Japanese cases. Acta Pathol Jpn 23:917–952
242. Yasuda H, Nakao M, Kanemasa H et al (1996) T-cell lymphoma presenting with pericardial and pleural effusion as the initial and primary lesion: cytogenetic and molecular evidence. Intern Med 35:150–154
243. Yokoyama T, Tanaka A, Kato S, Aizaw H (2008) Multiple myeloma presenting initially with pleural effusion and a unique paraspinal tumor in the thorax. Intern Med 47:1917–1920
244. Youngster I, Vaisben E, Cohen H, Nassar F (2006) An unusual cause of pleural effusion. Age Ageing 35:94–96

Diagnostic Yield of BAL Fluid Cytology in Hematologic Malignancies

17

Jean-François Bernaudin and Jocelyne Fleury-Feith

Contents

The lung is one of the most severely affected organs in the course of hematologic malignancies as a result of infection, specific localizations, drug-induced and radiation-induced damage, and pulmonary graft-versus-host disease [59, 67]. As this chapter is specifically devoted to the diagnostic value of analysis of the cells collected by bronchoalveolar lavage (BAL), detection of infectious agents will not be considered apart from certain characteristic cytopathogenic effects related to viral infections.

The lung is a complex organ that can be divided into at least seven compartments [70], and BAL only provides access to the most readily accessible compartment, the bronchoalveolar space. Although BAL has been demonstrated to be very useful for clinical diagnosis, a number of questions remain unresolved on how these cells reflect the pathophysiology of other lung compartments. The use of BAL to investigate the alveolar component of the patient's lung has been widely developed since the mid 1970s [63], and in one of the most frequently cited papers on BAL, published more than 30 years ago, the authors stated that "Over the past 10 years, these techniques have allowed enormous insight into how the human pulmonary inflammatory and immune systems function both in health and disease" [35]. During the 20 years between 1980 and 2000, a very large number of studies reported the value of BAL in the management of various pulmonary diseases, particularly those observed in immunocompromised patients or patients with hematologic malignancies. All data obtained by BAL together with a better understanding of the clinical and radiological features of pulmonary complications associated with hematologic malignancies and the various situations potentially encountered in the everyday care of patients are now fairly well known. According to various hematologists the need for diagnostic BAL is considered to have decreased over the last 10 years. Moreover, with the

J.-F. Bernaudin (✉) and J. Fleury-Feith
Cytopathology Unit, Laboratoire d'Histologie Biologie Tumorale, Université Pierre et Marie Curie Paris 6, Hôpital Tenon APHP, 75020, Paris, France
e-mail: jean-francois.bernaudin@tnn.aphp.fr; jocelyne.fleury@tnn.aphp.fr

É. Azoulay (ed.), *Pulmonary Involvement in Patients with Hematological Malignancies*,
DOI: 10.1007/978-3-642-15742-4_17, © Springer-Verlag Berlin Heidelberg 2011

routine use of prophylaxis, the spectrum of pulmonary complications has evolved, and the value of bronchoscopy is now more controversial [55]. A major question in 2010 is therefore what is the real value of BAL in everyday management of these patients?

In contrast with the recent report by [61] entitled "Is BAL useful in patients with acute myeloid leukemia admitted in ICU for severe respiratory complications?," which concluded that patients with leukemia and lymphoma derived limited benefit from this procedure, we would like to discuss the various areas in which cytological examination of BAL fluid remains a particularly useful diagnostic tool in these patients.

As an overview to this chapter, it should be noted that the diagnosis of pulmonary diseases associated with hematologic malignancies, such as pulmonary hemorrhage and pulmonary alveolar proteinosis, is based on BAL analysis not requiring pathologic examination of tissue samples. In primary lung lymphomas, BAL cytology is a particularly valuable first-line diagnostic procedure, and, in other situations, BAL cytology may make a major contribution to the diagnostic decision.

17.1 Bronchoalveolar Lavage Cytology: Main Technical Points

17.1.1 Routine Cytology

BAL fluid is usually collected by fiberoptic bronchoscopy after instillation of 3×50 mL of saline solution kept at 4°C. The cytologist must take the ratio of recovered-to-instilled fluid into account to assess the significance of the results obtained. In addition to the samples sent to the cytology laboratory, other fluid aliquots are also systematically sent for bacteriologic, virologic and fungal cultures. The first step of the cell analysis procedure is a cell count usually using a hemocytometer grid, then centrifugation (1,200 rpm for 10 min) to obtain a 10^6 mL^{-1} cell concentration. Simple smears and cytospin preparations are obtained [in our practice, at least 4–6 cytospin preparations (100 μL of the 10^6 mL^{-1} cell suspension) are prepared by using a Cytospin Shandon Instrument (500 rpm for 10 min)]. After air-drying, the smears are stained by the May-Grunwald-Giemsa method (other staining methods may be used, such as Papanicolaou's or Diff Quick stain to obtain rapid results). A differential cell count (macrophages, lymphocytes, neutrophils, eosinophils and mast cells) is obtained by counting at least 200 random cells.

A normal BAL cell count is about 130 ± 20 10^3 mL^{-1} cells in non-smokers and 420 ± 50 10^3 mL^{-1} cells in smokers. The normal cell distribution is: lymphocytes $15 \pm 3\%$ (CD3+ T cells >95% with a CD4/CD8 ratio ≈2.5; CD19+ B cells <2%) neutrophils <3% and eosinophils <1%. However, the cell distribution observed on BAL is a snapshot of the intraalveolar cellular milieu, and when interpreting an unusual cell distribution, e.g. lymphocytes, the cytologist must bear in mind that increased numbers of cells in BAL fluid could be due to increased influx, increased local proliferation, reduced apoptosis or decreased efflux or even a combination of all these parameters [51].

17.1.2 Electron Microscopy

For ultrastructural study, a 20-mL aliquot of fresh BAL fluid is immediately fixed in an equal volume of 2.5% glutaraldehyde in 0.1 M cacodylate buffer for 1 h at 4°C. The pellet is then collected by centrifugation (1,500 rpm for 10 min) and processed for transmission electron microscopy as usual [6].

17.1.3 Histochemical and Immunohistochemical Analysis

A smear is systematically stained by Perls' method to detect hemosiderin-laden macrophages. Other histochemical stains may also be useful, such as Periodic-Acid Schiff reaction and Alcian blue for extracellular deposits (see: alveolar proteinosis) or oil red O for intra-macrophage lipid deposits.

Immunocytochemistry that used to be performed on simple smears or cytospin preparations for lymphocyte subtyping has now been replaced by flow cytometry analysis.

17.1.4 Flow Cytometry

Flow cytometry is essential for determination of lymphocyte subpopulations. Aliquots of 5×10^6 mL^{-1} cell suspension are directly incubated with anti-CD45, anti-CD3, anti-CD4 and anti-CD8 for T cells, and anti-CD19 (and/or anti-CD79a) for B cells. In the case of an increase of the CD19-positive cell population or in the presence of lymphoplasmacytic cells or atypical lymphoid cells, BAL cells may be incubated with anti-κ and anti-λ light chain monoclonal antibodies using either the membranous or intracellular staining procedure. Systematic labeling using isotypic controls is performed. Lymphocyte subsets are determined by flow cytometry. Cytometric analysis of BAL cells using standardized procedures with optimum antibody concentrations and gating strategies has been clearly demonstrated to be correlated with immunocytochemical staining [54, 69]. This technique using commercially available antibodies offers a particularly reproducible and less time-consuming method than immunocytochemistry "on slides," with access to a wide range of labeled monoclonal antibodies and using a three- or four-color cytometer.

17.1.5 Molecular Biology Cell Analysis

Most reports concerning molecular biology analysis of BAL cells in hematologic malignancies have concerned the detection of monoclonal populations of B lymphocyte in lymphomas [77] based on the detection of rearrangements of genes encoding the B-cell immunoglobulin receptor using polymerase chain reaction (PCR). For this purpose, fresh or frozen cells are transferred to the molecular biology laboratory for DNA extraction and PCR analysis [56, 77].

17.2 Pulmonary Diseases in Which BAL Cytology is Diagnostic

17.2.1 BAL Cytology and the Diagnosis of Pulmonary Infectious Disease

BAL has been clearly demonstrated to be useful for the diagnosis of pulmonary infectious complications occurring in patients with hematologic malignancies [15,34,48], but should BAL samples still be sent to the cytopathology unit or only to microbiology laboratories?

As discussed in the various chapters of this book, pulmonary opacities in these patients can be due to a wide range of causes, in which BAL can be useful for diagnosis. Characteristic cytopathogenic effects are diagnostic for cytomegalovirus infection (Fig. 17.1) [15,16], and the cellular pattern also provides additional information on detection of the infectious agent itself, as in the case of *Pneumocystis carinii* (PCP) infection (Fig. 17.1).

Acute hypoxemic respiratory failure in patients with chronic lymphoproliferative disease after bone marrow transplantation or chemotherapy should be considered to denote *Pneumocystis* pneumonia until proven otherwise [5].

BAL has been shown to be diagnostic in HIV-negative patients by detecting PCC in 78–87% of patients [9,52]. While in HIV-positive patients PCP is associated with numerous cysts and trophozoites observed on MGG-stained smears, in patients with hematologic malignancies only a few cysts are usually observed, which could make the diagnosis more difficult. Cytologic analysis comparing BAL in HIV-negative and HIV-positive patients with PCP [50] showed no difference for neutrophils, while eosinophils and lymphocytosis >15% were observed significantly more frequently in BAL specimens from HIV-positive patients [28]. However, in BAL from HIV-negative patients, PCP is characterized by lymphocytosis associated with lymphoplasmacytic cell proliferation [27]. Therefore, in the presence of an increase in alveolar lymphocytes associated with a lymphoplasmacytic proliferation, MGG or Gomori-Grocott stained smears must be examined very meticulously to detect rare cysts.

The presence of large numbers of neutrophils is highly suggestive of bacterial infection. Careful examination looking for intracellular bacteria is very important, as it has been demonstrated that the percentage of BAL cells containing intracellular bacteria in nosocomial pneumonia is closely correlated with the total number of bacteria obtained from corresponding lung samples [12] (Fig. 17.1). However, in neutropenic patients, severe neutropenia can be concomitant with decreased cellularity of the alveolar space, particularly affecting alveolar macrophages and neutrophils, and pulmonary bacterial infection may therefore not be associated with an increased number of alveolar neutrophils in BAL fluid [18].

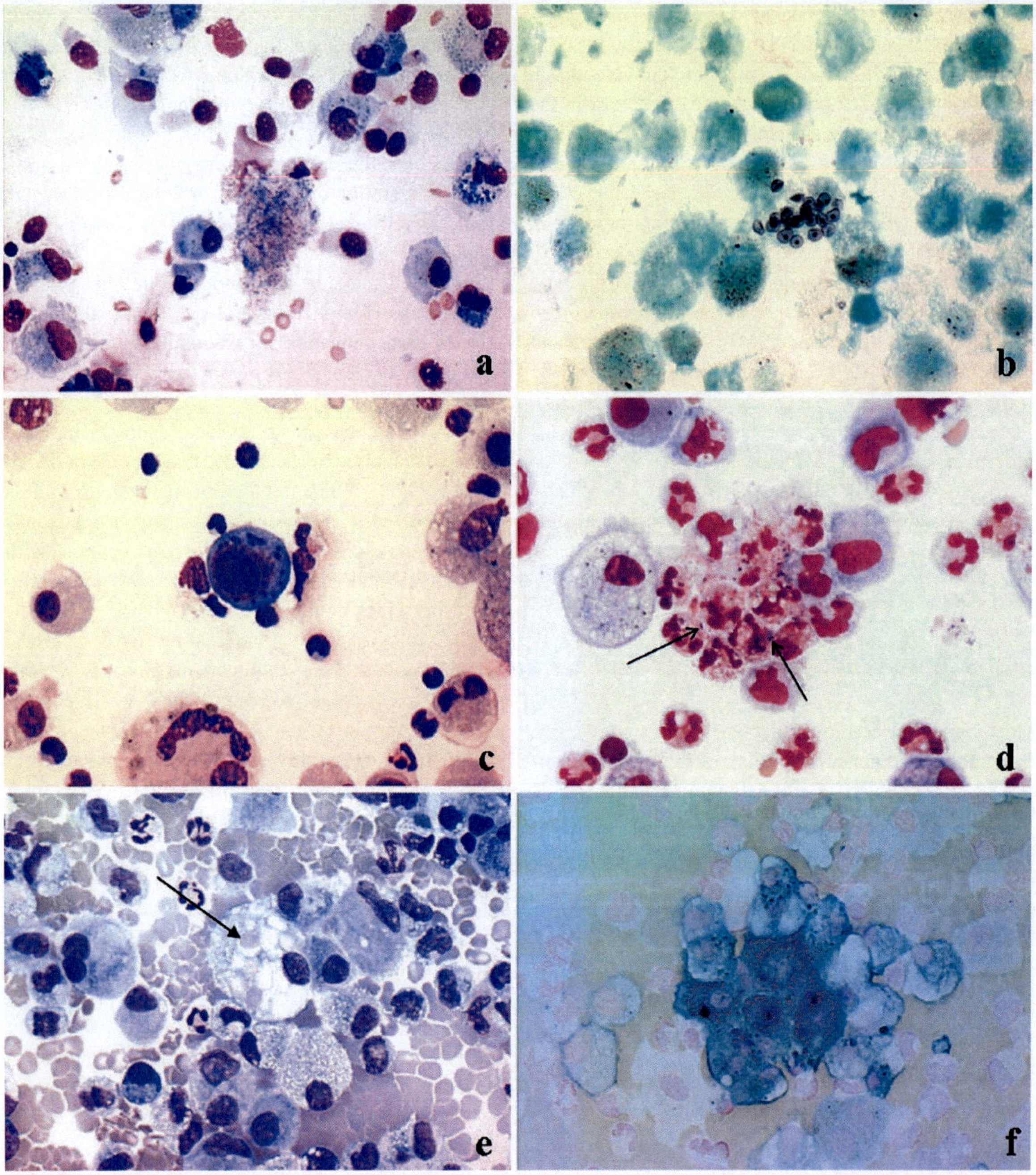

Fig. 17.1 Photographs of cysts of *Pneumocystis carinii* (**a**, **b**), intranuclear and intracytoplasmic inclusions characteristic of CMV infection (**c**), neutrophils containing intracellular bacteria (*arrows*) (**d**), erythrophagocytosis (*arrow*) observed within alveolar macrophages (**e**) and siderophages stained blue by the Perls' reaction (**f**) (Staining method: **a**, **c**–**e**: May–Grunwald–Giemsa; **b**: Grocott; **f**: Perls)

17.2.2 BAL and Diagnosis of Pulmonary Hemorrhage

Pulmonary hemorrhage is a frequent event in patients with hematologic malignancies due to infections as well as blood coagulation disorders [33] or after hematopoietic stem cell transplantation [2, 3, 15].

Diffuse alveolar hemorrhage is the paradigm of the diagnostic value of BAL. Alveolar hemorrhage can be diagnosed by progressively bloodier returns, but the presence of red blood cells in BAL fluid can be related to instrumental trauma, as most of these patients present clotting disorders (thrombocytopenia, etc.), and the appearance of the BAL return is not reliable for diagnosis [2]. The hallmark of alveolar hemorrhage is the presence of siderophages. Siderophages are alveolar macrophages that have phagocytosed red blood cells and digested them in their lysosomal compartment. The remnants of these red blood cells are intracytoplasmic deposits of hemosiderin, which stains dark blue by Prussian blue during Perls' reaction using the ferrocyanide reagent (Fig. 17.1). It may take 33–72 h after acute alveolar hemorrhage for hemosiderin-laden macrophages, i.e., siderophages, to appear in BAL and at least 2–4 weeks for siderophages to clear from the lung and airways [68]. Due to the delayed appearance of siderophages, the absence of Perls' positive siderophages in the BAL fluid does not exclude the possibility of recent (less than 33–48 h) alveolar bleeding (or old bleeding more than 12 days previously, as hemosiderin is cleared after a few days) [68, 3]. When alveolar hemorrhage is strongly suspected on bloody returns of BAL without siderophages, bronchoscopy repeated several days later might show the presence of siderophages [3]. However, if the BAL fluid kept at 4°C has been rapidly sent to the cytopathology unit, the observation of erythrophagocytosis by alveolar macrophages is a valuable criterion for recent intraalveolar bleeding (Fig. 17.1).

Golde DW et al. [30] introduced a ranking score evaluating the hemosiderin load in alveolar macrophages. After staining cytospin preparations for hemosiderin, 200–300 macrophages were counted, and each cell was graded for hemosiderin on a scale from 0 to 4 (0 = no blue color; 1 = faint blue staining of the cytoplasm; 2 = dense blue color in a minor portion of cytoplasm or medium color intensity throughout the cell; 3 = dark blue color in most of the cytoplasm; 4 = dark blue throughout the cytoplasm). A mean score, i.e., the Golde score, for 100 cells was calculated, where zero is the minimum score and 400 is the maximum score. In the initial publication [30], BAL from seven healthy volunteers was used as control, and the observed score was 11 ± 14 (SE). Hemosiderin resorption was therefore considered to be normal when the Golde score ranged from 0 to 20. The presence of alveolar hemorrhage was considered when the score was situated in the medium range from 20 to 70, and therefore associated with so-called occult alveolar hemorrhage, and a score >70 [30] or >100 [37] was highly significant of obvious alveolar hemorrhage. The Golde score has been used to identify pulmonary hemorrhage in various clinical contexts, such as leukemia [30], immunocompromised hosts [37] or pulmonary veno-occlusive disease [62].

More recently, we, as well as other authors [2, 3, 22] have used the presence of 20% or more hemosiderin-laden macrophages as the diagnostic criterion for diffuse alveolar hemorrhage. To obtain such a criterion the Golde score was compared to the percentage of siderophages stained by Prussian blue counted on at least 200 macrophages in 47 BALs from immunocompromised patients [22]. A percentage of siderophages between 20% and 67% was correlated with a Golde score between 20 and 100 and was classified as intermediate by [37], whereas a percentage of siderophages greater than 67% was correlated with a Golde score greater than 100 and was classified as severe by [37]. In normal individuals, the percentage of siderophages was always less than 10% [22]. A percentage of siderophages within the alveolar macrophage population greater than 20% is therefore significant for the presence of alveolar hemorrhage. This method is simpler and faster than the Golde score to establish the diagnosis [2, 3].

17.2.3 BAL and Diagnosis of Secondary Alveolar Proteinosis

Pulmonary alveolar proteinosis (PAP) is a rare disease characterized by deposition in the air spaces of a granular extracellular material composed of proteins and lipids [24]. Secondary PAP develops in association with conditions involving functional impairment or reduced numbers of alveolar macrophages and/or type II pneumocytes, as in some hematologic malignancies [72]. It is associated with different hematologic malignancies particularly acute and chronic myeloid leukemia [16, 17, 36, 53, 67, 71].

PAP is a good example of a lung disease in which BAL is useful for early diagnosis and treatment [17]. Bronchoalveolar lavage fluid in patients with PAP has an opaque and/or milky appearance. Alveolar macrophages are rare and often have a large and foamy, "destroyed" appearance associated with either lymphocytes or neutrophils [17]. In some samples, the differential cell count may not be feasible due to the abundance of extracellular material. The extracellular deposits are the hallmark of the disease and are composed of large acellular bodies in a diffuse background of granules faintly stained by the May-Grunwald or Papanicolaou methods (Fig. 17.2). This proteinaceous material exhibits periodic-acid Schiff (PAS) staining (Fig. 17.2) with no significant Alcian blue staining except when small areas of bronchial mucus are intermixed [43].

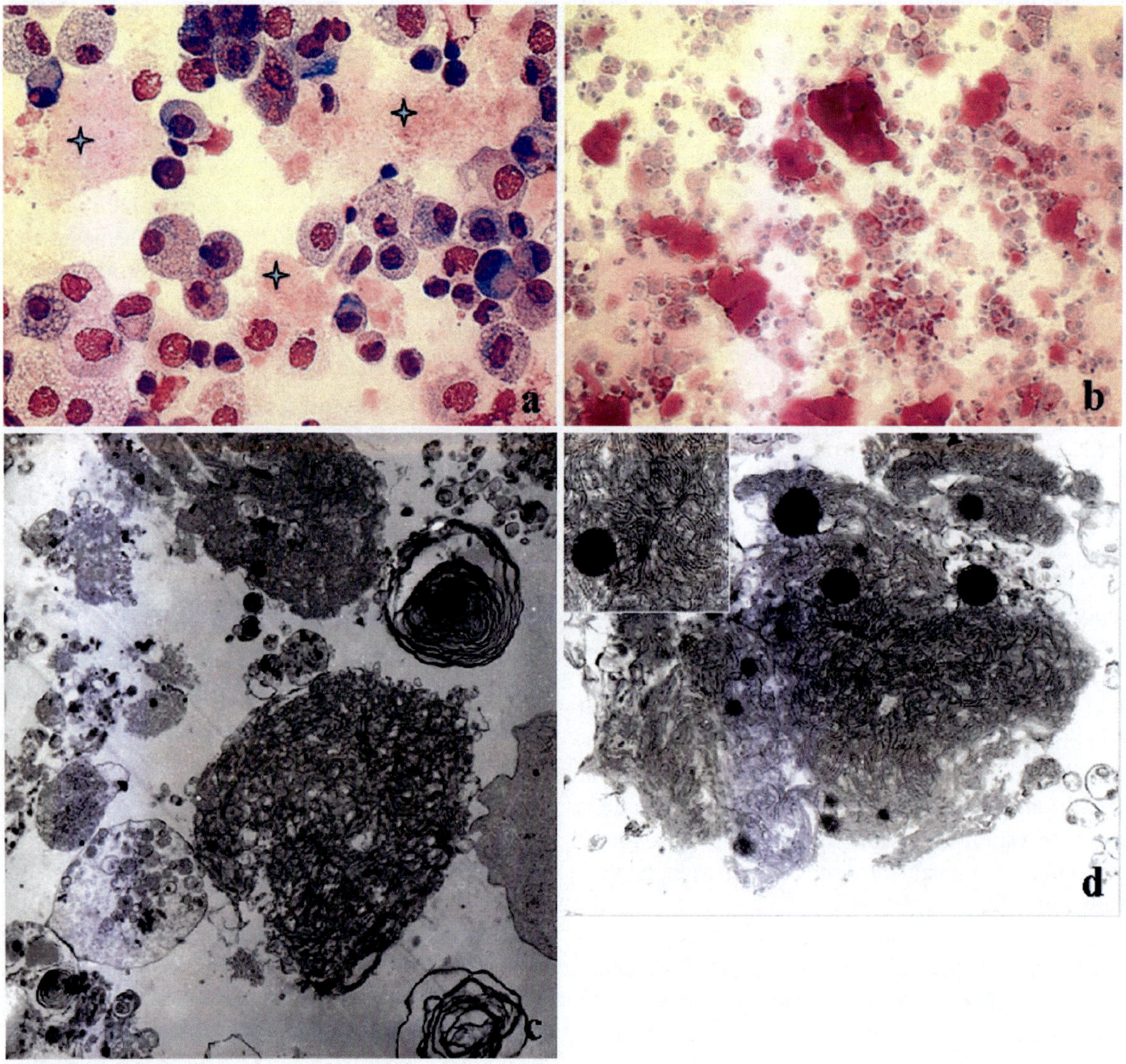

Fig. 17.2 Characteristic features of pulmonary alveolar proteinosis: acellular material (*star*) faintly stained by the May–Grunwald–Giemsa method (**a**) pink-red after periodic-acid Schiff (PAS) staining (**b**). Electron microscopy examination: extracellular material composed of a mixture of electron-dense material and osmiophilic figures (**c**, **d**). Insert in **d** shows the characteristic tubular myelin

On electron microscopy examination, the extracellular material is composed of a mixture of electron-dense granular or amorphous material, osmiophilic amorphous droplets, and regular and concentric myelin-like laminated figures (Fig. 17.2) associated with tubular myelin (Fig. 17.2) characteristic of lipoprotein aggregates and diagnostic of PAP [20]. Ultrastructural studies show that alveolar macrophages contain giant secondary lysosomes filled with the same material that accumulates within the alveoli [31].

17.2.4 BAL and Diagnosis of Pulmonary Lymphoma

In contrast with some authors who have reported that "BAL and bronchial brushings were never diagnostic" in a series of 28 patients with pulmonary AIDS-related non-Hodgkin's lymphoma [25], BAL is a particularly informative investigation that may contribute to the diagnosis of either primary or secondary malignant lymphoproliferative disorders of the lung. For example, a 67% diagnostic yield of BAL has been reported in non-Hodgkin's lymphoma (NHL) [60, 66]. However, the diagnostic yield is particularly good in primary B-cell lymphoma or mucosa-associated lymphoid tissue (MALT) type, but is low in Hodgkin's disease [60].

Lymphomas may involve the lung parenchyma in three ways: (1) hematogenous dissemination of non-Hodgkin's lymphoma or Hodgkin's disease, (2) contiguous invasion from hilar or nodal lymphoma or (3) primary pulmonary involvement [10]. Two different situations may be encountered: firstly, BAL performed to investigate chronic pulmonary opacities suggesting a wide range of diagnoses, particularly primary pulmonary lymphoma [23, 10]; secondly, BAL performed to investigate pulmonary opacities occurring during the course of a known lymphoma, Hodgkin's disease or non-Hodgkin's lymphoma.

17.2.4.1 Primary Pulmonary Lymphoma

Primary pulmonary lymphomas are rare events, representing 3–4% of all extranodal non-Hodgkin's lymphomas, including: (1) low-grade-B cell primary pulmonary lymphoma (PPL-B), the most frequent form (58–87%); (2) high-grade PPL-B and lymphomatoid granulomatosis, a particularly rare disorder [10]. MALT (mucosa-associated lymphoid tissue) lymphomas represent 90% of PPL-B. There is a consensus that it is important to obtain representative tissue for histologic evaluation and classification of lymphomas, but it can be very difficult to obtain such samples. By showing typical lymphomatous cells or a clonal restricted population of lymphocytes, BAL is therefore very useful in this situation. In a series of 13 patients with lymphoma, BAL showed lymphocytosis in every case [23], and, in a more recent study of 20 patients, the mean lymphocytosis in primary and secondary lymphoma was 30% and 36%, respectively (Table 17.1) [77]. BAL is particularly useful in these patients when it shows lymphocytic alveolitis (lymphocytes >20% of total cells) (Fig. 17.3) mainly composed of T lymphocytes [23], but including at least 8–10% of B-lymphocytes [10, 14, 19, 49, 77].

The detection of abnormal lymphoid cells may also be diagnostic (Fig. 17.3). These cells are inconstantly detected [8, 39, 56, 58, 59], whereas in the series by Poletti (1995) [59], 67% of 15 cases of NHL and 3 of the 9 cases of Hodgkin's lymphoma were identified by the presence of characteristic cells, and, in a recent series, they were observed in 9 out of 20 patients (45%) with pulmonary B-NHL [77]. In indolent B-cell lymphoma, lymphomatous cells may have morphological features that do not differ from those of

Table 17.1 Results of BAL cytology in 20 cases of pulmonary non-Hodgkin's lymphoma

	Primary pulmonary NHL ($n=12$)	Secondary pulmonary NHL ($n=8$)
% lymphocytes mean (range)	36 (3–81)	30 (3–61)
Samples with abnormal cells	6	3
Lymphocyte phenotypes n samples studied	7	2
CD3% (range)	58 (27–90)	98–79
CD4% (range)	35 (11–77)	28–21
CD8% (range)	23 (8–56)	71–24
CD19% (range)	37 (9–62)	0–18

Modified according to [77]

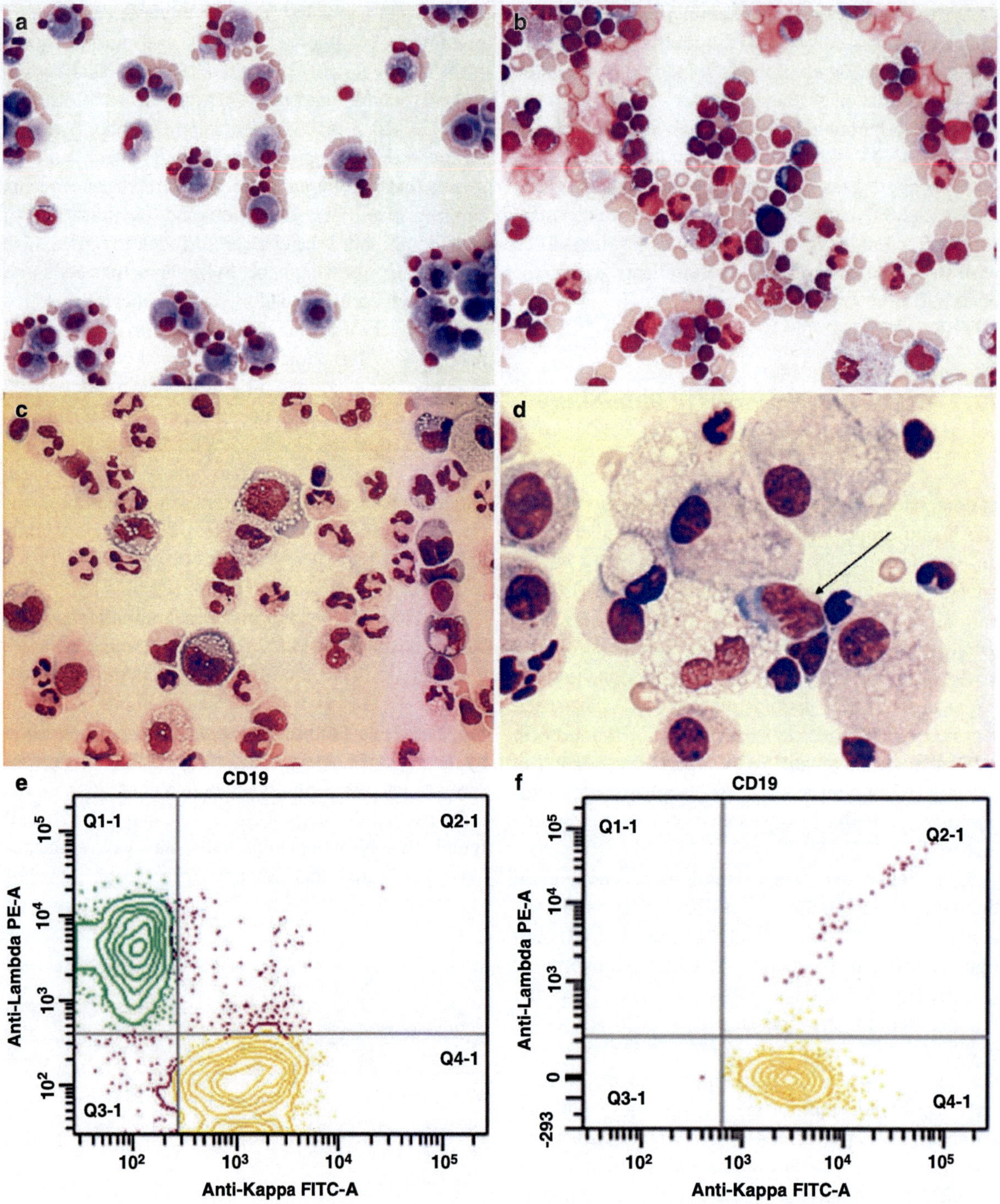

Fig. 17.3 Photographs of normal (**a**) and atypical lymphoplasmacytoid lymphocytes (**b**) and abnormal lymphoid cells from pulmonary non-Hodgkin lymphoma (**c**, **d**) mixed with red blood cells and alveolar macrophages (Staining: May-Grunwald-Giemsa method). Example of flow cytometry analysis of immunoglobulin light chain expression gated on alveolar CD19 lymphocytes (*top* of **e** and **f**) showing a normal distribution of κ and λ light chains (**e**) and a κ light chain restriction demonstrating a B-cell monoclonality (**f**)

normal (Fig. 17.3) or "activated" lymphocytes. Atypical lymphocytes with nuclear membrane irregularities and indentations or lymphoplasmacytoid lymphocytes may be observed, and their presence is suggestive of the diagnosis (Fig. 17.3). As already emphasized, these same morphological features may also be present in non-malignant lymphoproliferative disorders, such as lymphocytic interstitial pneumonia or diffuse Castelman's disease [60]. In high-grade B cell lymphoma, characteristic malignant cells (large cleaved and non-cleaved cells) are suggestive of the diagnosis [60].

As lymphocytes can spread from the lung parenchyma to the alveolar air spaces, the lymphocyte repertoire recovered by BAL reflects the pulmonary infiltration repertoire, and it has been demonstrated that the same dominant B-cell clone is detected in BAL fluid and in lung biopsies of lymphoma [8, 39, 56, 77]. Demonstration of B-cell monoclonality is mandatory for a precise diagnostic report. B-cell monoclonality is demonstrated by immunocytochemistry or flow cytometry assessment of immunoglobulin light chain restriction [39, 49, 58] (Fig. 17.3). Gene rearrangement analysis, i.e., Ig gene clonal rearrangements, using molecular biology, initially Southern blotting, but now usually polymerase chain reaction (PCR) [8, 39, 56, 77], can confirm the results obtained by flow cytometry assessment of immunoglobulin light chain restriction.

Zompi S et al. [77] demonstrated the feasibility of clonality analysis of BAL cells by complementary molecular analysis of lymphocytes in routine practice based on the detection of rearrangements of the gene encoding the B-cell immunoglobulin receptor using PCR [77]. In a series of 106 patients with clinical suspicion of pulmonary NHL, the detection of a strong B-cell clonal population within the BAL cell population was associated with the diagnosis of pulmonary NHL ($p < 0.0001$) with 97% specificity and 95% negative predictive value [77]. However, they noticed that a minor benign B-cell clone can also be detected, particularly in autoimmune and chronic infectious diseases, but its predictive value for the subsequent development of lymphoma remains unclear [77].

A similar approach has been used for pulmonary sites of T-cell CD3–/CD8+ lymphoma by analyzing the clonal rearrangement of the T-cell receptor [39].

17.2.4.2 Other Lymphomas and Hodgkin's Disease

Reports on BAL cytology and the diagnosis of other types of pulmonary lymphomas are rare. BAL may be appropriate for investigating pulmonary parenchymal involvement in Hodgkin's disease, as Reed-Sternberg cells may be observed in BAL [26,74], but reactive large lymphoid cells must not be mistaken for Reed-Sternberg cells, which must meet all of the classical diagnostic criteria. The diagnostic yield of BAL for the diagnosis of Hodgkin's lymphoma seems to be low (33% in [66]), but no large series has been published.

Diffuse myelomatous pulmonary infiltration may be diagnosed by BAL in the presence of monoclonal plasma cells [38].

17.3 Even When BAL Cytology Is Not Definitely Diagnostic, It Can Provide Valuable Clues

17.3.1 Detection of Hematologic Malignant Cells in BAL in Leukemia

Pulmonary leukemic cell infiltrates are found at autopsy in 31–66% of patients dying from leukemia [33], but symptomatic leukemic infiltration of the lung is the least common cause of pulmonary infiltrates [4,60]. However, BAL detection of malignant cells has been reported to be very valuable for the diagnosis of specific pulmonary infiltration, particularly in acute monocytic leukemia [4,65]. Rossi et al. [65] first reported the detection of 20% of monoblastic cells in the BAL of a patient with monocytic leukemia. Azoulay et al. [4] subsequently reported a series of 20 patients admitted for acute respiratory failure due to acute monocytic leukemia and detected monoblastic cells in four cases (20%). The presence of blast cells in BAL fluid may be difficult to interpret when the peripheral blood blast cell count is particularly high, as BAL fluid may be contaminated by peripheral blood cells [4].

When a pulmonary site of a chronic lymphoid leukemia is suspected, similar rearrangements of the gene encoding the B-cell Ig receptor should be observed in BAL and blood lymphocytes, but as these patients usually have a high blood lymphocyte count, the results must be interpreted cautiously.

Reports of the contribution of BAL to the diagnosis of pulmonary leukemic infiltration can therefore be considered to be anecdotal [60].

17.3.2 Other Malignant and Atypical Epithelial Cells in BAL Fluid

Lung cancer may occur in patients with hematologic malignancies, as lung cancer is one of the two most common solid tumors occurring after Hodgkin's disease [1,41] and has been the subject of recent reports after non-Hodgkin's lymphoma (NHL) [21,46,47]. Bronchioloalveolar carcinomas have been rarely reported after treatment for Hodgkin's disease [40] or leukemia, particularly with busulfan [13,45]. It is now widely recognized that BAL cytology provides a major contribution to the diagnosis of peripheral lung carcinoma, particularly adenocarcinomas with a pneumonic pattern in which a diagnostic yield of 66% has been reported [75]. However, numerous non-neoplastic lung diseases may be associated with atypical cells in BAL specimens, raising diagnostic challenges with malignant neoplasms [57,60]. Atypical cells may be seen as single cells or in clusters mimicking cells desquamating from bronchioloalveolar carcinomas (Fig. 17.4). Bone marrow transplant (BMT) recipients have many predisposing factors to the presence of atypical cells in BAL specimens: recent cytoreductive treatment, positive bacterial cultures or graft-versus-host disease [32]. Reactive type II pneumocytes, large cells with a large round nucleus and a dark blue stained cytoplasm after MGG staining, are frequently observed in the case of alveolar damage [60].

17.3.3 Drug-Induced Lung Toxicity

In hematologic patients with acute hypoxemic respiratory failure, BAL is considered to be essential, first to rule out an opportunistic infection, but also to look for evidence of drug-related toxicity [5,11].

The various patterns of infiltrative drug-induced respiratory diseases were reviewed in a recent exhaustive review by Camus P et al. [11]. In nonspecific interstitial pneumonia (NSIP) (caused by methotrexate in the majority of cases, or azathioprine, chlorambucil, cyclophosphamide and rarely vinca alkaloids), BAL fluid usually shows a lymphocytic infiltration. CD4+ and CD8+ lymphocytes have both been shown to contribute to alveolitis [29]. A low CD4+/CD8+ ratio of alveolar lymphocytes is suggestive, but not diagnostic for drug-induced lung disease [11]. Recently pulmonary drug reaction induced by dasatinib treatment for chronic myeloid leukemia has been reported with lymphocytic (25–92%) alveolitis and a CD4/CD8 ratio between 2.9 and 4.8 [7]. Another pattern, consisting of T-cell lymphocytic alveolitis associated with scattered eosinophils, is

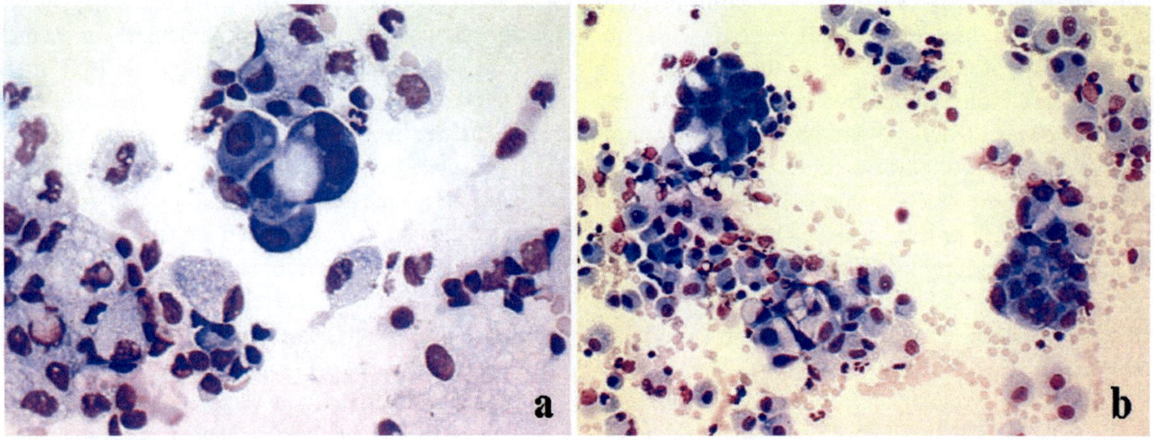

Fig. 17.4 Photographs of alveolar non-malignant atypical cells (**a**) and clusters of malignant cells from bronchioloalveolar carcinoma (**b**). (Staining: May–Grunwald–Giemsa method)

highly suggestive of drug-induced lung damage as observed for methotrexate [59]. True pulmonary eosinophilic pneumonia is rarely observed as an adverse drug reaction in patients with hematologic diseases in contrast with patients in other settings where many drugs may induce this pattern of lung reaction [11]. Organizing pneumonia is a distinctive lung response; increased numbers of lymphocytes, neutrophils or eosinophils may be observed, but there is no distinctive BAL pattern.

17.3.4 Miscellaneous Situations

Acute non-infectious eosinophilic pneumonia not related to adverse drug reaction has been reported after stem cell transplantation [73,76].

The association of alveolar lymphocytosis and GVHD is well known, but the pathogenesis of pulmonary GVHD is still poorly understood. In a mouse model, the acute phase of GVHD appears to be mediated by CD8+ cells, whereas CD4+ cells are associated with the chronic form [60]. However, in patients, late onset of interstitial pneumonitis following allogeneic bone marrow transplantation has been associated with lymphocytic alveolitis with an overall expansion of the CD8+ subset [42]. More recently, a study on BAL fluid cell composition in pediatric bone marrow transplant (BMT) recipients with pulmonary GVHD showed BAL lymphocytosis associated with severe epithelial cell atypia. The authors concluded that this pattern "may suggest the diagnosis" of pulmonary GVHD, but is not diagnostic per se [64].

Other lung diseases not directly associated with hematologic malignancies may be present in these patients. For example, as an illustration of the value of systematic immunophenotyping of lymphocytes, sarcoidosis was demonstrated in a patient with chronic lymphocytic leukemia due to the predominance of CD4+ T cells instead of B lymphocytes in BAL fluid [44].

17.4 Conclusion

The various "cytological" situations most frequently encountered are summarized in Table 17.2.

Table 17.2 Summary of the more frequent "cytological" situations encountered in BAL cytology in hematologic patients

Cytology	Complementary investigation	Diagnosis
Siderophages >20%	None	Alveolar hemorrhage
Abundant extracellular material	PAS; Alcian blue	Secondary PAP
Abnormal cells Lymphoid Myeloid Epithelial	Immunotyping and genotyping Immunotyping (TTF1) and molecular biology (Ras, EGFR mutations)	NHL or Hodgkin's leukemia benign or malignant atypical cells
Lymphocytosis CD4 and/or CD8 T lymphocytes, B lymphocytes >8%	Light chain clonality and IgR rearrangement	Adverse drug reaction, B-cell lymphoma; CLL
Neutrophils >+++	Intracellular bacteria	Bacterial infection; ARDS
Eosinophils >++		Adverse drug reaction

Acknowledgments The authors would like to thank Marie-José Pocholle, Christine Carre, (Unité de Cytopathologie Hôpital Henri Mondor Créteil France), Danièle Cesari, Claudie Prengel and Patricia Roynard (Unité de Cytopathologie Hôpital Tenon Paris France) for their excellent technical assistance in cytopathology and cytometry over all these years and Marie-Claire Pinchon † and Anne Marie Vojtek (Laboratoire de Microscopie Electronique CHIC Creteil France) for their valuable expertise in electron microscopy of BAL.

They would also like to thank Catherine Cordonnier, MD, and Estelle Escudier, MD, from the Hematology Department of Hôpital Henri Mondor Créteil France, with whom we developed our work on BAL 25 years ago, and Anne Fajac, MD, who joined us more recently on this topic.

References

1. Abrahamsen AF, Andersen A, Nome O et al (2002) Long-term risk of second malignancy after treatment of Hodgkin's disease: the influence of treatment, age and follow-up time. Ann Oncol 13:1786–1791
2. Afessa B, Tefferi A, Litzow MR et al (2002) Diffuse alveolar haemorrhage in haematopoietic stem cell transplant recipients. Am J Respir Crit Care Med 166:641–645
3. Afessa B, Tefferi A, Litzow MR et al (2002) Outcome of diffuse alveolar haemorrhage in haematopoietic stem cell transplant recipients. Am J Respir Crit Care Med 166: 1364–1368
4. Azoulay E, Fieux F, Moreau D et al (2003) Acute monocytic leukaemia presenting as acute respiratory failure. Am J Respir Crit Care Med 167:1329–1333
5. Azoulay E, Schlemmer B (2006) Diagnostic strategy in cancer patients with acute respiratory failure. Intensive Care Med 32:808–822
6. Basset F, Soler P, Jaurand MC et al (1977) Ultrastructural examination of bronchoalveolar lavage for diagnosis of pulmonary histiocytosis X. Thorax 32:303–306
7. Bergeron A, Réa D, Levy V et al (2007) Lung abnormalities after dasatinib treatment for chronic myeloid leukemia. Am J Respir Crit Care Med 176:814–818
8. Betsuyaku T, Munakata M, Yamaguchi E et al (1994) Establishing diagnosis of pulmonary malignant lymphoma by gene rearrangement analysis of lymphocytes in bronchoalveolar fluid. Am J Respir Crit Care Med 149:526–529
9. Bollée G, Sarfati C, Thiéry G et al (2007) Clinical picture of Pneumocystis jirovei pneumonia in cancer patients. Chest 132:1305–1310
10. Cadranel J, Wislez M, Antoine M (2002) Primary pulmonary lymphoma. Eur Respir J 20:750–762
11. Camus P, Costabel U (2005) Drug-induced respiratory disease in patients with haematological diseases. Semin Respir Crit Care Med 26:458–481
12. Chastre J, Fagon JY, Bornet-Lecso M et al (1995) Evaluation of bronchoscopic techniques for the diagnosis of nosocomial pneumonia. Am J Respir Crit Care Med 152:231–240
13. Chatte G, Piperno D, Espinouse D et al (1993) Alveolar cell carcinoma following treatment of acute non-lymphocytic leukaemia. Eur J Med 2:444
14. Cordier JF, Chailleux E, Lauque D et al (1993) Primary pulmonary lymphomas. A clinical study of 70 cases in non immunocompromised patients. Chest 103:201–208
15. Cordonnier C, Bernaudin JF, Fleury F et al (1985) Diagnostic yield of bronchoalveolar lavage in pneumonitis occurring after allogeneic bone marrow transplantation. Am Rev Respir Dis 132:1118–1123
16. Cordonnier C, Bernaudin JF, Bierling P et al (1986) Pulmonary complications occurring after allogeneic bone marrow transplantation: a study of 130 consecutive transplanted patients. Cancer 58:1047–1054
17. Cordonnier C, Fleury-Feith J, Escudier E et al (1994) Secondary alveolar proteinosis is a reversible cause of respiratory failure in leukemic patients. Am J Respir Crit Care Med 149:788–794
18. Cordonnier C, Escudier E, Verra F et al (1994) Bronchoalveolar lavage during neutropenic episodes: diagnostic yield and cellular pattern. Eur Respir J 7:114–120
19. Costabel U, Bross KJ, Matthys H (1985) Diagnosis by bronchoalveolar lavage of cause of pulmonary infiltrates in haematological malignancies. Br Med J (Clin Res Ed) 290:1041
20. Costello JF, Moriarty DC, Branthwaite MA et al (1975) Diagnosis and management of alveolar proteinosis: the role of electron microscopy. Thorax 30:121–132
21. De Giacomo T, Martelli M, Venuta F et al (2006) Lung cancer after treatment for non-Hodgkin lymphoma. Minerva Chir 61:467–471
22. De Lassence A, Fleury-Feith J, Escudier E et al (1995) Alveolar haemorrhage: diagnostic criteria and results in 194 immunocompromised hosts. Am J Respir Crit Care Med 151:157–163
23. Drent M, Wagenaar SS, Mulder PHG et al (1994) Bronchoalveolar lavage fluid profiles in sarcoidosis, tuberculosis and non-Hodgkin's and Hodgkin's disease. An evaluation of differences. Chest 105:514–519
24. DuBois RM, McAllister W, Branthwaite MA (1983) Alveolar proteinosis: diagnosis and treatment over a 10-year period. Thorax 38:360–363
25. Eisner MD, Kaplan LD, Herndier B et al (1996) The pulmonary manifestations of AIDS-related non-Hodgkin's lymphoma. Chest 110:729–736
26. Fajac I, Cadranel J, Mariette X et al (2010) Pulmonary Hodgkin's disease in HIV-infected patient. Diagnosis by bronchoalveolar lavage. Chest 1992:1913–1914
27. Fleury J, Escudier E, Pocholle MJ et al (1985) Cell populations obtained by bronchoalveolar lavage in Pneumocystis carinii pneumonitis. Acta Cytol 29:721–726
28. Fleury-Feith J, Tran Van Nhieu J, Picard C et al (1989) Bronchoalveolar lavage eosinophilia associated with Pneumocystis carinii pneumonia in AIDS patients. Comparative study with non-AIDS patients. Chest 95: 1198–1201
29. Fuhrman C, Parrot A, Wislez M et al (2001) Spectrum of CD4 to CD8 ratio in lymphocytic alveolitis associated with methotrexate-induced pneumonitis. Am J Respir Crit Care Med 164:1186–1191

30. Golde DW, Drew WL, Klein HZ et al (1975) Occult pulmonary haemorrhage in leukemia. BMJ 2:166–168
31. Golde DW, Territo M, Finley TN et al (1976) Defective lung macrophages in pulmonary alveolar proteinosis. Ann Intern Med 85:304–309
32. Gulbahce HE, Baker KS, Kumar P et al (2003) Atypical cells in bronchoalveolar lavage specimens from bone marrow transplant recipients. A potential pitfall. Am J Clin Pathol 120:101–106
33. Hildebrand FL, Rosenow EC, Habermann TM et al (1990) Pulmonary complications of leukaemia. Chest 98: 1233–1239
34. Huaringa AJ, Leyva FJ, Signes-Costa J et al (2000) Bronchoalveolar lavage in the diagnosis of pulmonary complications of bone marrow transplant patients. Bone Marrow Transplant 25:975–979
35. Hunninghake GW, Gadek JE, Kawanami O et al (1979) Inflammatory and immune processes in the human lung in health and disease: evaluation by bronchoalveolar lavage. Am J Pathol 97:149–206
36. Inaba H, Jenkins JJ, McCarville MB et al (2008) Pulmonary alveolar proteinosis in pediatric leukemia. Pediatr Blood Cancer 51:66–70
37. Kahn FW, Jones JM, England DM (1987) Diagnosis of pulmonary hemorrhage in the immunocompromised host. Am Rev Respir Dis 136:155–160
38. Kamble R, Rosenzweig T (2006) Diffuse pulmonary parenchymal involvement in multiple myeloma: antemortem diagnosis. Int J Hematol 83:259–261
39. Keicho N, Oka T, Takeuchi K et al (1994) Detection of lymphomatous involvement of the lung by bronchoalveolar lavage. Application of immunophenotypic and gene rearrangement analysis. Chest 105:458–462
40. Kowalski P, Rodziewicz B, Pejcz J et al (1989) Bilateral bronchioloalveolar carcinoma of the lungs in a 7-year-old girl treated for Hodgkin's disease. Tumori 75:449–451
41. Laurie SA, Kris MG, Portlock CS et al (2002) The clinical course of nonsmall cell lung carcinoma in survivors of Hodgkin disease. Cancer 95:119–126
42. Leblond V, Zouabi H, Sutton L et al (1994) Late CD8+ lymphocytic alveolitis after allogeneic bone marrow transplantation and chronic graft-versus-host disease. Am J Respir Crit Care Med 150:1056–1061
43. Martin RJ, Coalson JJ, Rogers RM et al (1980) Pulmonary alveolar proteinosis: the diagnosis by segmental lavage. Am Rev Respir Dis 121:819–825
44. Maruchella A, Epis R, Camerone G et al (1999) Association between chronic lymphocytic leukaemia and sarcoidosis: clinical value of bronchoalveolar lavage. Sarcoidosis Vasc Diffuse Lung Dis 16:101–103
45. Min KW, Györkey F (1968) Interstitial pulmonary fibrosis, atypical epithelial changes and bronchiolar cell carcinoma following busulfan therapy. Cancer 22:1027–1032
46. Moser EC, Noordijk EM, van Leeuwen FE et al (2006) Risk of second cancer after treatment of aggressive non-Hodgkin's lymphoma; an EORTC cohort study. Haematologica 91:1481–1488
47. Mudie NY, Swerdlow AJ, Higgins CD et al (2006) Risk of second malignancy after non-Hodgkin's lymphoma: a British Cohort Study. J Clin Oncol 24:1568–1574
48. Murray PV, O'Brien MER, Padhani AR et al (2001) Use of first line bronchoalveolar lavage in the immunosuppressed oncology patient. Bone Marrow Transplant 27: 967–971
49. Nehashi Y, Nakano M, Utsumi K et al (1993) Primary pulmonary B-cell lymphoma diagnosed by kappa-lambda imaging of broncho-alveolar lavage fluid lymphocytes. Intern Med 32:480–483, 0
50. Nüesch R, Bellini C, Zimmerli W (1999) Pneumocystis carinii pneumonia in human immunodeficiency virus (HIV)-positive and (HIV)-negative immunocompromised patients. Clin Infect Dis 29:1519–1523
51. Pabst R, Tschernig T (1997) Lymphocyte dynamics: caution in interpreting BAL numbers. Thorax 52:1078–1080
52. Pagano L, Fianchi L, Mele L et al (2002) Pneumocystis carinii pneumonia in patients with malignant haematological diseases: 10 years' experience of infection in GIMEMA centres. Br J Haematol 117:379–386
53. Pamuk GE, Turgut B, Vural O et al (2003) Pulmonary alveolar proteinosis in a patient with acute lymphoid leukaemia regression after G-CSF therapy. Leuk Lymphoma 44: 871–874
54. Papiris SA, Kollintza A, Kitsanta P et al (2005) Relationship of BAL and lung tissue CD4+ and CD8+ T lymphocytes and their ratio in idiopathic pulmonary fibrosis. Chest 128:2971–2977
55. Patel NR, Lee PS, Kim JH et al (2005) The influence of diagnostic bronchoscopy on clinical outcomes comparing adult autologous and allogeneic bone marrow transplant. Chest 127:1388–1396
56. Philippe B, Delfau-Larue MH, Epardeau B et al (1999) B-cell pulmonary lymphoma: gene rearrangement analysis of bronchoalveolar lymphocytes by polymerase chain reaction. Chest 115:1242–1247
57. Poletti V, Romagna M, Ka A et al (1995) Bronchoalveolar lavage in the diagnosis of disseminated lung tumors. Acta Cytol 39:472–477
58. Poletti V, Romagna M, Gasponi A et al (1995) Bronchoalveolar lavage in the diagnosis of low-grade, MALT type, B-cell lymphoma of the lung. Monaldi Arch Chest Dis 50:191–194
59. Poletti V, Salvucci M, Zanchini R et al (2000) The lung as a target organ in patients with hematologic disorders. Haematologica 85:855–864
60. Poletti V, Poletti G, Murer B et al (2007) Bronchoalveolar lavage in malignancy. Semin Respir Crit Care Med 28: 534–545
61. Rabbat A, Chaoui D, Lefebvre A et al (2008) Is BAL useful in patients with acute myeloid leukemia admitted in ICU for severe respiratory complications? Leukemia 22:1361–1367
62. Rabiller A, Jaïs X, Hamid A et al (2006) Occult alveolar haemorrhage in pulmonary veno-occlusive disease. Eur Respir J 27:108–113
63. Reynolds HY, Newball HH (1974) Analysis of proteins and respiratory cells obtained from human lungs by bronchoalveolar lavage. J Lab Clin Med 84:559–573
64. Rochat I, Posfay-Barbe KM, Kumar N et al (2008) Bronchoalveolar cytology for diagnosing pulmonary GVHD after bone marrow transplant in children. Pediatr Pulmonol 43:697–702

65. Rossi GA, Balbi B, Risso M et al (1985) Acute myelomonocytic leukaemia: demonstration of pulmonary involvement by bronchoalveolar lavage. Chest 87:259–260
66. Semenzato G, Poletti V (1992) Bronchoalveolar lavage in lung cancer. Respiration 59:44–46
67. Sharma S, Nadrous HF, Peters SG et al (2005) Pulmonary complications in adult blood and marrow transplant recipients: autopsy findings. Chest 128:1385–1392
68. Sherman JM, Winnie G, Thomassen MJ et al (1984) Time course of hemosiderin production and clearance by human pulmonary macrophages. Chest 86:409–411
69. Smith PA, Kohli LM, Wood KL et al (2006) Cytometric analysis of BAL T cells labelled with a standardized antibody cocktail correlates with immunohistochemical staining. Cytometry B Clin Cytom 70:170–178
70. Tschernig T, Pabst R (2009) What is the clinical relevance of different lung compartments? BMC Pulm Med 9:39
71. Tomonari A, Shirafuji N, Iseki T et al (2002) Acquired pulmonary alveolar proteinosis after umbilical cord blood transplantation for acute myeloid leukaemia. Am J Hematol 70: 154–157
72. Trapnell BC, Whitsett JA, Nakata K (2003) Pulmonary alveolar macrophages. N Engl J Med 349:2527–2539
73. Wagner T, Dhedin N, Philippe B et al (2006) Acute eosinophilic pneumonia after allogeneic hematopoietic stem cell transplantation. Ann Hematol 85:202–203
74. Wisecarver J, Ness MJ, Rennard SI et al (1989) Bronchoalveolar lavage in the assessment of pulmonary Hodgkin's disease. Acta Cytol 33:527–532
75. Wislez M, Massiani MA, Milleron B et al (2003) Clinical characteristics of pneumonic-type adenocarcinoma of the lung. Chest 123:1868–1877
76. Yoshimi M, Nannya Y, Watanabe T et al (2009) Acute eosinophilic pneumonia is a non-infectious lung complication after allogeneic hematopoietic stem cell transplantation. Int J Hematol 89:244–248
77. Zompi S, Couderc LJ, Cadranel J et al (2004) Clonality analysis of alveolar B lymphocytes contributes to the diagnostic strategy in clinical suspicion of pulmonary lymphoma. Blood 103:3208–3218

New Methods for Bacterial Diagnosis in Patients with Hematological Malignancies

18

Agnès Ferroni and Jean-Ralph Zahar

Contents

A. Ferroni (✉) and J.-R. Zahar
Laboratoire de Microbiologie,
Assistance Publique-Hôpitaux de Paris,
Hôpital Necker-Enfants Malades and Université René Descartes Paris 5, Faculté de Médecine, 149 Rue de Sèvres, 75015 Paris, France
e-mail: agnes.ferroni@nck.aphp.fr

18.1 Introduction

Determining the etiology of pulmonary infiltrates in patients with hematological malignancies (HM) is challenging, and early empirical treatment with broad-spectrum antimicrobial agents is therefore used when an infection is suspected, with the goal of improving patient outcomes. However, selection of the empirical antibiotics benefits considerably from the early identification of organisms such as *Streptococcus pneumoniae*, *Haemophilus influenzae*, nosocomial bacteria, *Mycoplasma pneumoniae*, *Chlamydophila pneumoniae*, *Legionella pneumophila*, viruses, and fungi.

Traditionally, the identification of causative bacteria rests on blood cultures: sputum cultures for common pathogens and *M. tuberculosis*; serological tests for *C. pneumoniae*, *M. pneumoniae*, and *L. pneumophila*; and cultures of specimens obtained using invasive techniques such as endoscopic bronchial aspiration or bronchoalveolar lavage (BAL). These methods are slow to produce results, lack sensitivity, and are influenced by previous antibiotic therapy. The diagnostic yield of BAL for identifying the cause of pulmonary infiltrates in patients with HM has varied between 31% and 49% [6, 28, 35, 36, 68, 85]. Thus, BAL has a limited impact on early therapeutic decisions. In recent years, noninvasive techniques such as *L. pneumophila* or *S. pneumoniae* antigen detection in urine have proved capable of providing the early etiological diagnosis of infections and, therefore, of allowing the early administration of appropriate antimicrobials. In addition, recent advances in molecular diagnostic technology, such as nucleic acid amplification (PCR), have improved the ability to rapidly identify the cause of pneumonia [46]. PCR detects minute amounts of nucleic acid from potentially all respiratory pathogens and is less affected by prior antimicrobial therapy than

É. Azoulay (ed.), *Pulmonary Involvement in Patients with Hematological Malignancies*,
DOI: 10.1007/978-3-642-15742-4_18, © Springer-Verlag Berlin Heidelberg 2011

are culture-based methods [47]. PCR is probably more sensitive than most comparator culture-based diagnostic tests, as it is affected neither by decreased organism viability associated with specimen transportation nor by previous antibiotic therapy. It must be kept in mind that PCR does not differentiate between viable and nonviable bacteria and that there are no clear data in the literature on DNA decay after the end of antibiotic treatment.

The use of antigen detection in clinical samples and recent advances in real-time amplification systems are discussed here with reference to respiratory bacteria known to cause pneumonia in patients with HM. Unlike the identification of viruses and fungi, for which these new methods have been evaluated in immunocompromised patients [25, 35, 51, 57, 87], the identification of bacteria has been mainly evaluated in patients with community-acquired infections. Table 18.1 lists the methods that can be used in immunocompromised patients with suspected pneumonia.

18.2 PCR

PCR techniques play a major role in the diagnosis of infections that are either very difficult or impossible to diagnose rapidly by other methods. PCR is especially useful for detecting pathogens that are not known to colonize the human respiratory tract (e.g., *Legionella* species), as a positive result strongly suggests infection. To date, PCR methods have been developed for all the major pneumonia-causing pathogens, and commercial assays are available for some of them. However, few studies have compared different assays, and the techniques have not been standardized.

PCR detection involves the extraction of bacterial DNA from the sample (nasopharyngeal aspirate, BAL, sputum, or throat swabs), followed by amplification using primers. Increasingly, real-time PCR techniques, based on fluorescent probes, are superseding the traditional PCR tests in which the products obtained at the end of the amplification cycles are revealed on agarose gel (end-point reaction). The main advantages of real-time PCR are rapidity; safety; ability to quantify bacterial DNA in the specimen; and, given that a single tube is used for all the steps, a reduced risk of cross-contamination.

Cases of culture-positive samples with negative PCR results may be due to DNA degradation, delayed assay performance, or presence of specific inhibitors. Samples, such as sputum or BAL, may include inhibitors, which can cause false-negative results. Therefore, an internal control coextracted with the clinical samples must be used to ensure accurate control of the entire assay [67].

PCR techniques target a single organism (simplex PCR), multiple organisms (multiplex PCR), or all organisms (universal PCR).

18.2.1 Specific PCRs in Respiratory Samples

18.2.1.1 Intracellular Bacteria

Patients with suspected respiratory infections are generally evaluated using PCR tests that target specific organisms to diagnose atypical pneumonia or pneumonia due to fastidious organisms. These organisms are theoretically not found as commensals in the respiratory tract, and qualitative detection is therefore appropriate [79].

M. pneumoniae, C. pneumoniae

M. pneumoniae can be cultured in a routine laboratory on acellular media, but the results are obtained only after 2–3 weeks, and the test is relatively insensitive [19]. *C. pneumoniae* can be cultured only on cell lines in specialized laboratories, which requires 5–10 days. As a result, the diagnosis of these two organisms relied until recently on serological tests, whose disadvantage is that they provide only a retrospective diagnosis. In addition, IgM antibodies to *M. pneumoniae* can persist for years, with levels remaining elevated in asymptomatic individuals [62], particularly healthy children. Furthermore, the variable specificity and sensitivity of current test kits influence the significance of the serological results [5]. Both organisms require treatment with macrolides, tetracyclines, or fluoroquinolones, and therefore sensitive, specific, and fast detection methods available in routine bacteriological practice would be valuable. Real-time PCR is being increasingly used

Table 18.1 New bacterial diagnosis methods potentially applicable in patients with hematological malignancies

Method	Sample type						Time-to-result[a]
	Urine	Serum	Sputum	Bronchoalveolar lavage fluid	Pleural fluid	Throat swab	
Antigen detection (*S. pneumoniae* or *L. pneumophila 1*)	Yes	Yes	No	NE	Yes	No	10 min
PCR targeting atypical bacteria (*M. pneumoniae*, *C. pneumoniae*)	No	No	Yes	Yes	Yes	Yes	3 h
PCR targeting *Legionella*	No	No	Yes	Yes	Yes	No	3 h
PCR ARNr16S	No	NE	No	NE (only onto sterile fluid)	Yes	No	4–8 h
Multiplex PCR	No	NE	NE	NE	Yes	No	3 h
PCR targeting *S. pneumoniae* or *H. influenzae*	No	NE	NE	NE (only quantitative PCR)	Yes	No	3 h
PCR targeting *Mycobacteria*	No	NE	Yes	NE	No	No	3 h

NE not evaluated in patients with hematological malignancies

[a]Time from DNA extraction to availability of the PCR result; however, in most laboratories, PCR and sequencing are not performed every day

for the rapid diagnosis of these organisms [21, 22, 48]. Recently, PCR was found better than serology for confirming *M. pneumoniae* infection in the clinically important first week after pneumonia symptom onset [61]. Nevertheless, in case of late sampling or clearance of the organism following antibiotic treatment, PCR detection may be less sensitive than serology [37]. The targets most commonly used for *M. pneumoniae* are adhesin P1, 16S rRNA, and ATPase operon gene, and for *C. pneumoniae*, the outer membrane protein ompA and ARNr16S. These specific targets can be sought in samples contaminated with commensal flora such as sputum, potentially contaminated BAL, or throat swab containing cells or nasopharyngeal aspirates. Sputum samples have been shown to be more useful than upper respiratory tract samples for PCR identification of *M. pneumoniae* and *C. pneumoniae* [20, 69, 77]. The time-to-result varies across methods from 50 to 90 min. Commercial real-time PCR kits showed variable sensitivities, and their cost was five times higher than that of an in-house assay [81].

Legionella

Legionella species are among the most underdiagnosed causes of pneumonia, due to the major shortcomings of existing diagnostic tests. Isolation of the organism is usually the preferred method but has several limitations, including fastidious growth requirements, extended incubation periods (3–10 days), and overgrowth by other bacteria. Direct *L. pneumophila* detection in clinical specimens by immunofluorescence methods is rapid but lacks sensitivity. Finally, soluble polysaccharide antigen detection in urine detects only *L. pneumophila 1* [73]. PCR for rapid *L. pneumophila* diagnosis, in contrast, detects all *Legionella* species [16, 32, 53, 70, 89]. The most frequently described *Legionella* PCR targets are the mip gene (macrophage infectivity potentiator), a virulence gene present in the majority of *Legionella* species, and the ADNr 5S gene. As *Legionella* does not colonize the human respiratory tract, the specific target genes can be sought in samples contaminated with commensal flora such as sputum or potentially contaminated BAL. PCR can now be considered the test of choice for legionellosis [59], but standardized protocols need to be developed.

18.2.1.2 Common Bacteria (*S. pneumoniae, H. influenzae, Staphylococcus aureus, etc.*)

Pulmonary infections due to common bacteria are underdiagnosed because of the limitations of conventional diagnostic tests. Blood cultures lack sensitivity, particularly in patients who have received previous antibiotic treatment. Isolation of *S. pneumoniae* or *H. influenzae* from sputum or BAL may occur as a result of oropharyngeal contamination. Conversely, isolation may fail because of previous antibiotic therapy, poor transportation conditions, or small inoculum size.

Recently, studies have been carried out on PCRs targeting pyogenic bacteria. However, these tests may be difficult to interpret, as pyogenic bacteria may be present in the commensal flora, making it difficult to distinguish between colonization and infection. These PCRs are therefore feasible in routine practice only on samples that do not contain pyogenic bacteria as commensals, such as pleural fluid or lung biopsies. Preliminary evaluations of PCR applied to pleural fluid indicate good sensitivity for the diagnosis of pneumococcal pneumonia [23, 47]. In theory, BAL fluid and sputum, which are often colonized by *S. pneumoniae* or *H. influenzae*, particularly in children, can be used only if cultures are negative. Nevertheless, a number of investigators have assumed that quantitative PCR may be useful for assessing these contaminated respiratory samples, as the bacterial burden is higher in infection than in colonization [40, 43]. The amount of target nucleic acid in the sample is inversely related to the cycle threshold (Ct) value. This relationship can be used to establish a Ct value cutoff that provides optimal sensitivity and specificity by preventing false-positive results due to colonization with small numbers of organisms. A panel of six real-time PCR assays, including the *lytA* gene of *S. pneumoniae* and the 16S rRNA genes of *H. influenzae* and *S. pyogenes*, were used by Morozumi et al. [56] in a study of 429 clinical samples (sputum, nasopharyngeal aspirates, or throat swabs) from children and adults with pneumonia. Sensitivity and specificity, compared to clinical specimen cultures, were as follows: 96.2% and 93.2% for *S. pneumoniae*, 95.8% and 95.4% for *H. influenzae*, and 100% and 100% for *S. pyogenes*. The Ct values of *S. pneumoniae* and *H. influenzae* showed excellent correlations with the semi-quantitative culture results. All patients with positive PCR and negative culture results for these two pathogens had a history of previous antibiotic therapy.

Another controlled study evaluated the culture-PCR correlation in 235 adults with clinically and biologically confirmed pneumonia. In patients not treated with antibiotics, the PCR-culture correlation was good, whereas in treated patients, PCR improved the etiological diagnostic yield by 10%. However, in the control group, PCR performed on nasopharyngeal aspirates showed the presence of *H. influenzae* and *S. pneumoniae* in 5% and 8% of cases, respectively [78]. Recently, Kumar et al. found S. *pneumoniae* and *S. aureus* in 14% and 8.5% of asymptomatic patients, respectively, underlining the poor specificity of PCR [46]. Specificity can be expected to increase in the near future with improvements in PCR result interpretation, including the determination of Ct cutoffs for quantitative PCR in various pulmonary samples and in well-defined patient populations. Another difficulty in interpreting PCR results stems from the specificity of the target genes used for pneumococcal PCR. The targets used in many pneumococcal PCR assays are the pneumolysin and autolysin genes, but recent evidence casts doubt on their specificity, as these genes, especially pneumolysin, may been found in closely related viridans group *Streptococci* [58, 84, 88]. Recently, the Spn9802 gene fragment compared favorably with quantitative lytA-based real-time PCR in distinguishing patients with pneumonia from control individuals [1].

18.2.1.3 *Mycobacterium tuberculosis* and Atypical *Mycobacteria*

PCR tests perform well on *M. tuberculosis* smear-positive specimens but are less sensitive than culturing. Therefore, PCR is recommended only for smear-positive samples, to determine the species without waiting for the culture result. However, in a study involving routine *M. tuberculosis* PCR in patients with HM, *M. tuberculosis* was found in 2/128 BAL specimens negative by microscopy, which considerably shortened the time to diagnosis [35].

The *M. tuberculosis* PCR uses two main targets: a specific portion of the 16S RNA gene and the insertion sequence IS6110. In recent years, real-time PCR techniques have increasingly superseded conventional PCR [11, 24, 66]. Until recently, very few commercial *M. tuberculosis* PCR kits were available, whereas now many real-time PCR kits are on the market. It is important to keep in mind that a negative PCR result does not rule out tuberculosis. Commercial PCR kits are not currently available for atypical *Mycobacteria*.

18.2.1.4 Multiplex PCR

The multiplex format allows for multiple primer combinations in a single reaction instead of multiple simplex reactions. In addition, the required patient specimen size is smaller. Several studies have evaluated the use of multiplex PCR for detecting atypical organisms or *Mycobacteria* [29, 42, 54, 63], a combination of atypical and common organisms [78], or viral and bacterial pathogens in clinical specimens [46]. In recent years, these in-house assays have tended to be replaced by commercially available products, which are simpler to use in the diagnostic laboratory and allow easier quality assurance compared to in-house assays. Over the last 5 years, these commercial products have been offered mainly for detecting atypical organisms in clinical specimens: *M. pneumoniae* and *C. pneumoniae* [34]; *M. pneumoniae*, *C. pneumoniae*, *L. pneumophila*, *Legionella spp*, *M. pneumoniae*, and *Bordetella pertussis* [27]; *C. pneumoniae*, *Legionella micadadei*, and *B. pertussis* [42]; and *M. pneumoniae*, *Coxiella burnetii*, *C. pneumoniae*, and *Legionella* [12].

Multiplex PCR assays were long described as less sensitive than simplex PCR assays due to competition among primers, but two studies gave identical results with multiplex and simplex PCR tests [27, 34]. In contrast, another study showed higher sensitivity of the simplex PCR nucleic acid sequence-based amplification (NASBA) versus multiplex PCR for detecting *L. pneumophila* [49]. However, the lack of an appropriate reference standard for the quantitative analysis of intracellular pathogens is an obstacle to sensitivity comparisons across assays.

18.2.2 Specific PCR on Blood Samples

The definitive diagnosis of pneumococcal pneumonia in noninvasive respiratory samples requires isolation of the pathogen in a blood sample. However, blood cultures are rarely positive [14]. On the other hand, pneumococcal serology has low sensitivity [8]. Therefore, PCR tests on blood were mainly described for *S. pneumoniae* [15, 55, 59]. A very recent study showed low sensitivity of PCR in plasma for detecting pneumococcal pneumonia (26–35%). However, this test may be useful for the rapid diagnosis in bacteremic patients, as sensitivity reaches 60–70% in this situation. Specificity of ply PCR was low [2].

Recently, a commercial test using multiplex PCR in serum for numerous bacterial pathogens was evaluated in neutropenic patients [82]. However, this test has not been specifically assessed in patients with lung infiltrates.

18.2.3 Universal PCR

Universal PCR detects a gene found in all bacteria, usually the gene coding for 16S ribosomal RNA. The sequence of this gene allows the identification of most bacteria, without a presumptive diagnosis. This sequence includes conserved and variable regions. Universal primers are selected for conserved regions flanking a variable region, which allows differentiation of bacterial species. The amplified product is then sequenced, and the sequence is compared to all bacterial sequences contained in a database (e.g., GenBank). The sensitivity of this PCR varies across bacterial species (10–100 organisms/mL). Universal PCR has been developed chiefly for diseases such as endocarditis, meningitis, and bacteremia. It is useful in case of prior antibiotic treatment, fastidious organisms, or small inoculums. It should be used only for specimens from normally sterile sites, where it can detect only monomicrobial infections, as the presence of two or more organisms produces a mixture of non-interpretable sequences. This technique proved useful for diagnosing pleural empyema in children (40% increase in diagnostic yield compared to culture) and adults (31% increase) [47, 52]. The main organisms detected by universal PCR were *S. pneumoniae*, anaerobic bacteria (*Fusobacterium*, *Prevotella*), *S. aureus*, *H. influenzae*, and *Streptococcus milleri* group. The role for universal PCR in pulmonary samples, which are theoretically contaminated by saprophytic flora, remains to be evaluated. If cultures are negative, then universal PCR is theoretically appropriate. The likelihood of finding a mixture of bacteria by sequencing is not known.

A microarray method has been found promising for the detection and identification of nine bacterial pathogens. For this method, universal primers amplifying a conserved region of the bacterial gyrB/parE gene are used, and the single-stranded PCR products are then characterized by hybridization on an oligonucleotide array. This technique can be used for multibacterial infections, for which PCR products cannot be directly analyzed by DNA sequencing [72].

18.3 Antigen Detection

The diagnosis of pneumonia using antigen detection has made progress in recent years. Commercial antigen detection assays are now widely available for two bacterial pathogens, *L. pneumophila* and *S. pneumoniae*.

18.3.1 Legionella

Urine antigen testing allows the early diagnosis and appropriate antibiotic therapy of legionellosis [41]. The capture antibody technique used in the majority of these assays is considered specific for *L. pneumophila* serogroup 1, which causes most legionellosis cases in humans. However, as many as 40% of cases are related to other serogroups and are missed by the assay. In a recent study on the effectiveness of urine antigen detection, pooled sensitivity was 0.74 (95% CI, 0.68–0.81) and specificity was 0.991 (95% CI, 0.984–0.997) [74].

The antigen detected is a heat-stable component of the lipopolysaccharide portion of the *Legionella* cell wall [44, 86]. It is generally detectable in urine as soon as 3 days after symptom onset and can persist for more than 300 days. In one study, antigen was detected in 88% of patients tested on days 1–3 after symptom onset, 80% on days 4–7, 89% on days 8–14, and 100% after day 14 [45]. The most recent method for detecting antigenuria is the immunochromatographic test (ICT) membrane assay. The ICT assay is similar to a home pregnancy test and is commercially available. The test is simple to perform and does not require special laboratory equipment, and the results are obtained within 15 min. A study found that the ICT assay for *L. pneumophila* serogroup 1 was 80% sensitive and 97% specific [33]. More recently, it was suggested that specificity and sensitivity were higher after 30 min of incubation [17]. The use of concentrated urine samples has been suggested to increase sensitivity [7].

There is still a need for developing antigen capture assays that can diagnose infections with all *Legionella* species and serogroups. Twenty years ago, Tang and Toma developed a broad-spectrum ELISA that detected soluble antigens from numerous *L. pneumophila* serogroups and species by using rabbit antisera from a combination of intradermal, intramuscular, and intravenous inoculations over a period of 8 months [80]. Unfortunately, this test was not commercialized.

18.3.2 *Streptococcus pneumoniae*

The recent development of a rapid ICT assay that detects the C polysaccharide cell wall antigen common to all *S. pneumoniae* strains has renewed interest in antigen detection. The Binax Now test uses a rabbit anti-*S. pneumoniae* antibody that binds to soluble pneumococcal C antigen present in the sample (NOW *Streptococcus pneumoniae* test; Binax, Portland, ME). The resulting complex is immobilized by a band of rabbit anti-*S. pneumoniae* antibodies adsorbed onto a nitrocellulose membrane sample line. A second band of goat antirabbit IgG (control line) captures excess visualizing complex. Usually, a swab is dipped into 200 μL of sample fluid and inserted into the test device. A buffer solution is added, and the device is closed. The result can be read visually after 15 min. A pink to purple color on both the sample and control lines indicates a positive result. Color on the control line only indicates a negative result and absence of color on the control line an invalid test. Pneumococcal pneumonia can be diagnosed using antigen detection in urine, BAL fluid, or pleural fluid.

18.3.2.1 Pneumococcal Antigen Detection in Urine

The reported sensitivity of the ICT assay applied on urine samples ranges from 44.2% to 88.8% [18, 30, 50, 60, 71, 76]. Sensitivity is higher in bacteremic than in nonbacteremic patients and increases when urine samples are concentrated, which is usually achieved by ultracentrifugation and may last for 1–4 h [50, 60, 71]. Several studies of the Binax Now *S. pneumoniae* urine antigen showed good performance for diagnosing bacteremic pneumococcal infections in adults. Sensitivity is good, ranging from 77% to 87% [10, 75, 76]. Specificities of 97–100% were found in studies that used controls with nonpneumococcal bacteremia or noninfectious disorders [75, 76].

Given its excellent specificity, this test can be considered an important tool for detecting *S. pneumoniae* in patients with community-acquired pneumonia of unknown etiology. It provided the diagnosis of pneumococcal pneumonia in one-fourth of cases [26]. It is important to note that the test may remain positive for several weeks after pneumococcal pneumonia [3, 50] and that patients with detectable antigen may have been colonized with *S. pneumoniae.* Indeed, specificity of the ICT urine test has been reported to be low in children due to nasopharyngeal carriage [31]. In adult patients, specificity was 89.7–100%, depending on the reference standard [18, 50, 71]. Antigen-positive results should be interpreted carefully in pneumonia patients with chronic bronchitis, because detectable antigen may be caused by pneumococcal carriage in the lower respiratory tract [9, 10].

In a recent study, pneumococcal urinary antigen detection (Binax Now *S. pneumoniae* Antigen Test) was assessed for diagnosing pneumococcal exacerbations of chronic obstructive pulmonary disease (COPD). Forty-six patients with *S. pneumoniae* in sputum cultures were studied during a stable period and during an exacerbation [4]. During the stable period, the antigen was detected in 10.3% of patients in nonconcentrated urine and in 41.4% of patients in concentrated urine. Corresponding proportions during exacerbations were 17.6% in nonconcentrated urine and 76.5% in concentrated urine. Specificity was evaluated by testing 72 patients whose sputum samples were negative for *S. pneumoniae.* ICT was positive in nonconcentrated urine from one patient and in concentrated urine from nine patients. Factors significantly associated with a positive test on concentrated urine were a history of at least one exacerbation ($P=0.024$), admission for a previous exacerbation ($P=0.027$), and pneumonia within the past year ($P=0.010$). The only factor significantly associated with a positive test on nonconcentrated urine was pneumonia within the past year ($P=0.006$). In conclusion, in COPD patients, a positive pneumococcal urinary antigen test during bronchial exacerbation or pneumonia should be interpreted with caution, as it may reflect a prior *S. pneumoniae* infection [3, 4].

18.3.2.2 Pneumococcal Antigen Detection in Bronchoalveolar Lavage Fluid

Little is known about the use of the ICT assay on BAL fluid samples. However, this test may be useful, as at the time of bronchoscopy most patients are receiving antibiotics, which are known to damage bacterial morphology and prevent growth in cultures. ICT could be used as an adjunct to standard cytological and microbiological studies. However, when the result is positive, the possibility of a mixed flora or superinfecting pathogen should always be considered. In a retrospective study of the Binax Now *Streptococcus pneumoniae* test on BAL fluid samples from patients with suspected pneumonia, 96 BAL fluid samples were tested [38]. Sensitivity was assessed using 20 samples from patients with documented pneumococcal pneumonia. Specificity was tested using BAL fluid samples from patients with nonpneumococcal disease ($n=41$) and in samples containing no respiratory pathogens and a total bacterial count $<10^4$ CFU/mL ($n=35$). Pneumococcal antigen was detected in 29 (30.2%) samples, with 95% sensitivity and 86.8% specificity [38]. An older study of the ICT assay found 50% sensitivity and 100% specificity [39].

18.3.2.3 Pneumococcal Antigen Detection in Pleural Fluid

Pleural empyema rarely complicates community-acquired pneumonia. The rapid identification of the causal agent is required for effective treatment and a good outcome [83]. The classical microbiological technique for the diagnosis of pleural empyema is standard culture and microscopic examination. However, false-negative results related to a small sample volume or previous antibiotic therapy are common. Testing for soluble pneumococcal antigens is a complementary approach, as the results are immediately available, and *S. pneumoniae* can be detected even after antibiotic initiation.

In a recent retrospective study, the ICT Binax Now *Streptococcus pneumoniae* assay was evaluated in adults to determine whether the detection of pneumococcal antigen in pleural fluid was better than conventional microbiological methods for the etiologic diagnosis of pneumonia [65]. In this study, the ICT assay was performed on pleural fluid samples from 34 patients with pneumonia due to *S. pneumoniae*, 89 patients with effusions of nonpneumococcal origin, and 17 patients with pneumonia of unknown etiology. The ICT result was positive in 24 (70.6%) of 34 patients with pneumococcal pneumonia and negative in 83 (93.3%) of 89 patients without pneumococcal pneumonia. The pleural ICT assay was more sensitive than blood cultures (37.5%) and pleural fluid cultures (32.3%), but less sensitive than urine pneumococcal antigen detection (82.1%). However, three patients with pneumococcal pneumonia and negative ICT urine test results had a positive pleural fluid antigen test. Moreover, previous antibiotic exposure did not influence pneumococcal antigen detection in either pleural fluid or urine specimens [65]. In a retrospective study in children, *S. pneumoniae* was identified in 22% of samples by culture and in 69% by the Binax Now assay [64]. This test was positive in all 15 pleural fluid samples that yielded *S. pneumoniae* in culture, two samples that yielded *Streptococcus oralis* and *Streptococcus salivarius* in culture, and 34 culture-negative samples. Fifteen of these 34 culture-negative samples were retrospectively tested by PCR methods, and 14 were shown to contain *S. pneumoniae* DNA [64].

Similar high sensitivity was found in another study in children. Among 60 children with pneumococcal empyema, 17 were diagnosed only by PCR (43%) and 23 by both PCR and culture. Compared to culture and/or PCR, the sensitivity of antigen detection was 90% [47]. More recently, the Binax Now test was evaluated on pleural fluid from 73 children admitted with pleural effusion over a period of 4 years. Sensitivity was 88% and specificity 71%, with a positive predictive value of 96% [13].

18.4 Conclusion

Although these new diagnostic methods have not been specifically evaluated in patients with HM, they seem to hold considerable promise for increasing the performance of current diagnostic strategies. They should be used simultaneously on blood, BAL fluid, sputum, and throat swabs, and compared with conventional cultures. In the near future, molecular methods will complete, rather than replace, culture-based methods for detecting pathogens for which antibiotic resistance is a concern. Antigen detection methods may also have a role. However, a positive *L. pneumophila* test indicates a pulmonary infection due to serogroup 1, but a negative result does not rule out active infection due to other *Legionella species*. For *S. pneumonia,* the interpretation of the urinary antigen test results appears more difficult. A positive test may indicate simple colonization or previous pneumococcal infection, whereas the meaning of a negative test has not been evaluated in patients with HM.

References

1. Abdeldaim GM, Stralin K, Olcen P, Blomberg J, Herrmann B (2008) Toward a quantitative DNA-based definition of pneumococcal pneumonia: a comparison of Streptococcus pneumoniae target genes, with special reference to the Spn9802 fragment. Diagn Microbiol Infect Dis 60: 143–150
2. Abdeldaim G, Herrmann B, Molling P, Holmberg H, Blomberg J, Olcen P, Stralin K (2009) Usefulness of real-time PCR for lytA, ply, and Spn9802, applied to plasma samples to detect pneumococcal pneumonia. Clin Microbiol Infect 16:1135–1141. doi:10.1111/j.1469-0691.2009.03069.x
3. Andreo F, Prat C, Ruiz-Manzano J, Lores L, Blanco S, Cuesta MA, Gimenez M, Dominguez J (2009) Persistence of Streptococcus pneumoniae urinary antigen excretion after pneumococcal pneumonia. Eur J Clin Microbiol Infect Dis 28:197–201
4. Andreo F, Ruiz-Manzano J, Prat C, Lores L, Blanco S, Malet A, Gallardo X, Dominguez J (2009) Utility of pneumococcal urinary antigen detection in diagnosing exacerbations in COPD patients. Respir Med 104:397–403
5. Atkinson TP, Balish MF, Waites KB (2008) Epidemiology, clinical manifestations, pathogenesis and laboratory detection of Mycoplasma pneumoniae infections. FEMS Microbiol Rev 32:956–973
6. Azoulay E, Schlemmer B (2006) Diagnostic strategy in cancer patients with acute respiratory failure. Intensive Care Med 32:808–822
7. Blanco S, Lacoma A, Prat C, Cuesta MA, Fuenzalida L, Latorre I, Dominguez J (2008) Detection of Legionella antigen in nonconcentrated and concentrated urine samples by a new immunochromatographic assay. Eur J Clin Microbiol Infect Dis 27:1249–1251
8. Boersma WG, Lowenberg A, Holloway Y, Kuttschrutter H, Snijder JA, Koeter GH (1991) Pneumococcal capsular antigen detection and pneumococcal serology in patients with community acquired pneumonia. Thorax 46: 902–906
9. Boersma WG, Lowenberg A, Holloway Y, Kuttschrutter H, Snijder JA, Koeter GH (1992) Pneumococcal antigen persistence in sputum from patients with community-acquired pneumonia. Chest 102:422–427
10. Briones ML, Blanquer J, Ferrando D, Blasco ML, Gimeno C, Marin J (2006) Assessment of analysis of urinary pneumococcal antigen by immunochromatography for etiologic diagnosis of community-acquired pneumonia in adults. Clin Vaccine Immunol 13:1092–1097
11. Burggraf S, Reischl U, Malik N, Bollwein M, Naumann L, Olgemoller B (2005) Comparison of an internally controlled, large-volume LightCycler assay for detection of Mycobacterium tuberculosis in clinical samples with the COBAS AMPLICOR assay. J Clin Microbiol 43: 1564–1569
12. Carrillo JA, Gutierrez J, Garcia F, Munoz A, Villegas E, Rojas J, Sorlozano A, Rojas A (2009) Development and evaluation of a multiplex test for the detection of atypical bacterial DNA in community-acquired pneumonia during childhood. Clin Microbiol Infect 15:473–480
13. Casado Flores J, Nieto Moro M, Berron S, Jimenez R, Casal J (2010) Usefulness of pneumococcal antigen detection in pleural effusion for the rapid diagnosis of infection by Streptococcus pneumoniae. Eur J Pediatr 169:581–584
14. Chalasani NP, Valdecanas MA, Gopal AK, McGowan JE Jr, Jurado RL (1995) Clinical utility of blood cultures in adult patients with community-acquired pneumonia without defined underlying risks. Chest 108:932–936
15. Dagan R, Shriker O, Hazan I, Leibovitz E, Greenberg D, Schlaeffer F, Levy R (1998) Prospective study to determine clinical relevance of detection of pneumococcal DNA in sera of children by PCR. J Clin Microbiol 36:669–673
16. Diederen BM, Kluytmans JA, Vandenbroucke-Grauls CM, Peeters MF (2008) Utility of real-time PCR for diagnosis of Legionnaires' disease in routine clinical practice. J Clin Microbiol 46:671–677
17. Diederen BM, Bruin JP, Scopes E, Peeters MF, EP IJ (2009) Evaluation of the Oxoid Xpect Legionella test kit for detection of *Legionella pneumophila* serogroup 1 antigen in urine. J Clin Microbiol 47:2272–2274
18. Dominguez J, Gali N, Blanco S, Pedroso P, Prat C, Matas L, Ausina V (2001) Detection of *Streptococcus pneumoniae* antigen by a rapid immunochromatographic assay in urine samples. Chest 119:243–249
19. Dorigo-Zetsma JW, Zaat SA, Wertheim-van Dillen PM, Spanjaard L, Rijntjes J, van Waveren G, Jensen JS, Angulo AF, Dankert J (1999) Comparison of PCR, culture, and serological tests for diagnosis of *Mycoplasma pneumoniae* respiratory tract infection in children. J Clin Microbiol 37:14–17
20. Dorigo-Zetsma JW, Verkooyen RP, van Helden HP, van der Nat H, van den Bosch JM (2001) Molecular detection of *Mycoplasma pneumoniae* in adults with community-acquired pneumonia requiring hospitalization. J Clin Microbiol 39:1184–1186
21. Dumke R, Jacobs E (2009) Comparison of commercial and in-house real-time PCR assays used for detection of *Mycoplasma pneumoniae.* J Clin Microbiol 47:441–444
22. Dumke R, Schurwanz N, Lenz M, Schuppler M, Luck C, Jacobs E (2007) Sensitive detection of *Mycoplasma pneumoniae* in human respiratory tract samples by optimized real-time PCR approach. J Clin Microbiol 45:2726–2730

23. Falguera M, Lopez A, Nogues A, Porcel JM, Rubio-Caballero M (2002) Evaluation of the polymerase chain reaction method for detection of Streptococcus pneumoniae DNA in pleural fluid samples. Chest 122:2212–2216
24. Flores E, Rodriguez JC, Garcia-Pachon E, Soto JL, Ruiz M, Escribano I, Royo G (2009) Real-time PCR with internal amplification control for detecting tuberculosis: method design and validation. APMIS 117:592–597
25. Frealle E, Decrucq K, Botterel F, Bouchindhomme B, Camus D, Dei-Cas E, Costa JM, Yakoub-Agha I, Bretagne S, Delhaes L (2009) Diagnosis of invasive aspergillosis using bronchoalveolar lavage in haematology patients: influence of bronchoalveolar lavage human DNA content on real-time PCR performance. Eur J Clin Microbiol Infect Dis 28:223–232
26. Genne D, Siegrist HH, Lienhard R (2006) Enhancing the etiologic diagnosis of community-acquired pneumonia in adults using the urinary antigen assay (Binax NOW). Int J Infect Dis 10:124–128
27. Ginevra C, Barranger C, Ros A, Mory O, Stephan JL, Freymuth F, Joannes M, Pozzetto B, Grattard F (2005) Development and evaluation of *Chlamylege*, a new commercial test allowing simultaneous detection and identification of *Legionella*, *Chlamydophila pneumoniae*, and *Mycoplasma pneumoniae* in clinical respiratory specimens by multiplex PCR. J Clin Microbiol 43:3247–3254
28. Gruson D, Hilbert G, Valentino R, Vargas F, Chene G, Bebear C, Allery A, Pigneux A, Gbikpi-Benissan G, Cardinaud JP (2000) Utility of fiberoptic bronchoscopy in neutropenic patients admitted to the intensive care unit with pulmonary infiltrates. Crit Care Med 28:2224–2230
29. Gullsby K, Storm M, Bondeson K (2008) Simultaneous detection of *Chlamydophila pneumoniae* and *Mycoplasma pneumoniae* by use of molecular beacons in a duplex real-time PCR. J Clin Microbiol 46:727–731
30. Gutierrez F, Masia M, Rodriguez JC, Ayelo A, Soldan B, Cebrian L, Mirete C, Royo G, Hidalgo AM (2003) Evaluation of the immunochromatographic Binax NOW assay for detection of *Streptococcus pneumoniae* urinary antigen in a prospective study of community-acquired pneumonia in Spain. Clin Infect Dis 36:286–292
31. Hamer DH, Egas J, Estrella B, MacLeod WB, Griffiths JK, Sempertegui F (2002) Assessment of the Binax NOW Streptococcus pneumoniae urinary antigen test in children with nasopharyngeal pneumococcal carriage. Clin Infect Dis 34:1025–1028
32. Hayden RT, Uhl JR, Qian X, Hopkins MK, Aubry MC, Limper AH, Lloyd RV, Cockerill FR (2001) Direct detection of Legionella species from bronchoalveolar lavage and open lung biopsy specimens: comparison of LightCycler PCR, in situ hybridization, direct fluorescence antigen detection, and culture. J Clin Microbiol 39:2618–2626
33. Helbig JH, Uldum SA, Luck PC, Harrison TG (2001) Detection of *Legionella pneumophila* antigen in urine samples by the BinaxNOW immunochromatographic assay and comparison with both Binax *Legionella* Urinary Enzyme Immunoassay (EIA) and Biotest *Legionella* Urin Antigen EIA. J Med Microbiol 50:509–516
34. Higgins RR, Lombos E, Tang P, Rohoman K, Maki A, Brown S, Jamieson F, Drews SJ (2009) Verification of the ProPneumo-1 assay for the simultaneous detection of *Mycoplasma pneumoniae* and *Chlamydophila pneumoniae* in clinical respiratory specimens. Ann Clin Microbiol Antimicrob 8:10
35. Hohenthal U, Itala M, Salonen J, Sipila J, Rantakokko-Jalava K, Meurman O, Nikoskelainen J, Vainionpaa R, Kotilainen P (2005) Bronchoalveolar lavage in immunocompromised patients with hematological malignancy – value of new microbiological methods. Eur J Haematol 74:203–211
36. Hummel M, Rudert S, Hof H, Hehlmann R, Buchheidt D (2008) Diagnostic yield of bronchoscopy with bronchoalveolar lavage in febrile patients with hematologic malignancies and pulmonary infiltrates. Ann Hematol 87:291–297
37. Hvidsten D, Halvorsen DS, Berdal BP, Gutteberg TJ (2009) Chlamydophila pneumoniae diagnostics: importance of methodology in relation to timing of sampling. Clin Microbiol Infect 15:42–49
38. Jacobs JA, Stobberingh EE, Cornelissen EI, Drent M (2005) Detection of *Streptococcus pneumoniae* antigen in bronchoalveolar lavage fluid samples by a rapid immunochromatographic membrane assay. J Clin Microbiol 43: 4037–4040
39. Jimenez P, Meneses M, Saldias F, Velasquez M (1994) Pneumococcal antigen detection in bronchoalveolar lavage fluid from patients with pneumonia. Thorax 49:872–874
40. Kais M, Spindler C, Kalin M, Ortqvist A, Giske CG (2006) Quantitative detection of *Streptococcus pneumoniae*, *Haemophilus influenzae*, and *Moraxella catarrhalis* in lower respiratory tract samples by real-time PCR. Diagn Microbiol Infect Dis 55:169–178
41. Kashuba AD, Ballow CH (1996) *Legionella* urinary antigen testing: potential impact on diagnosis and antibiotic therapy. Diagn Microbiol Infect Dis 24:129–139
42. Khanna M, Fan J, Pehler-Harrington K, Waters C, Douglass P, Stallock J, Kehl S, Henrickson KJ (2005) The pneumoplex assays, a multiplex PCR-enzyme hybridization assay that allows simultaneous detection of five organisms, *Mycoplasma pneumoniae*, *Chlamydia* (Chlamydophila) *pneumoniae*, *Legionella pneumophila*, *Legionella micdadei*, and *Bordetella pertussis*, and its real-time counterpart. J Clin Microbiol 43:565–571
43. Klugman KP, Madhi SA, Albrich WC (2008) Novel approaches to the identification of *Streptococcus pneumoniae* as the cause of community-acquired pneumonia. Clin Infect Dis 47(Suppl 3):S202–S206
44. Kohler RB, Zimmerman SE, Wilson E, Allen SD, Edelstein PH, Wheat LJ, White A (1981) Rapid radioimmunoassay diagnosis of Legionnaires' disease: detection and partial characterization of urinary antigen. Ann Intern Med 94: 601–605
45. Kohler RB, Winn WC Jr, Wheat LJ (1984) Onset and duration of urinary antigen excretion in Legionnaires disease. J Clin Microbiol 20:605–607
46. Kumar S, Wang L, Fan J, Kraft A, Bose ME, Tiwari S, Van Dyke M, Haigis R, Luo T, Ghosh M, Tang H, Haghnia M, Mather EL, Weisburg WG, Henrickson KJ (2008) Detection of 11 common viral and bacterial pathogens causing community-acquired pneumonia or sepsis in asymptomatic patients by using a multiplex reverse transcription-PCR assay with manual (enzyme hybridization) or automated (electronic microarray) detection. J Clin Microbiol 46: 3063–3072

47. Le Monnier A, Carbonnelle E, Zahar JR, Le Bourgeois M, Abachin E, Quesne G, Varon E, Descamps P, De Blic J, Scheinmann P, Berche P, Ferroni A (2006) Microbiological diagnosis of empyema in children: comparative evaluations by culture, polymerase chain reaction, and pneumococcal antigen detection in pleural fluids. Clin Infect Dis 42:1135–1140
48. Loens K, Ieven M, Ursi D, Beck T, Overdijk M, Sillekens P, Goossens H (2003) Detection of *Mycoplasma pneumoniae* by real-time nucleic acid sequence-based amplification. J Clin Microbiol 41:4448–4450
49. Loens K, Beck T, Ursi D, Overdijk M, Sillekens P, Goossens H, Ieven M (2008) Evaluation of different nucleic acid amplification techniques for the detection of *M. pneumoniae*, *C. pneumoniae* and *Legionella* spp. in respiratory specimens from patients with community-acquired pneumonia. J Microbiol Methods 73:257–262
50. Marcos MA, Jimenez de Anta MT, de la Bellacasa JP, Gonzalez J, Martinez E, Garcia E, Mensa J, de Roux A, Torres A (2003) Rapid urinary antigen test for diagnosis of pneumococcal community-acquired pneumonia in adults. Eur Respir J 21:209–214
51. Maschmeyer G, Beinert T, Buchheidt D, Cornely OA, Einsele H, Heinz W, Heussel CP, Kahl C, Kiehl M, Lorenz J, Hof H, Mattiuzzi G (2009) Diagnosis and antimicrobial therapy of lung infiltrates in febrile neutropenic patients: guidelines of the infectious diseases working party of the German Society of Haematology and Oncology. Eur J Cancer 45:2462–2472
52. Maskell NA, Batt S, Hedley EL, Davies CW, Gillespie SH, Davies RJ (2006) The bacteriology of pleural infection by genetic and standard methods and its mortality significance. Am J Respir Crit Care Med 174:817–823
53. Maurin M, Hammer L, Gestin B, Timsit JF, Rogeaux O, Delavena F, Tous J, Epaulard O, Brion JP, Croize J (2009) Quantitative real-time PCR tests for diagnostic and prognostic purposes in cases of legionellosis. Clin Microbiol Infect 16(4):379–384
54. McDonough EA, Barrozo CP, Russell KL, Metzgar D (2005) A multiplex PCR for detection of *Mycoplasma pneumoniae*, *Chlamydophila pneumoniae*, *Legionella pneumophila*, and *Bordetella pertussis* in clinical specimens. Mol Cell Probes 19:314–322
55. Michelow IC, Lozano J, Olsen K, Goto C, Rollins NK, Ghaffar F, Rodriguez-Cerrato V, Leinonen M, McCracken GH Jr (2002) Diagnosis of *Streptococcus pneumoniae* lower respiratory infection in hospitalized children by culture, polymerase chain reaction, serological testing, and urinary antigen detection. Clin Infect Dis 34:E1–E11
56. Morozumi M, Nakayama E, Iwata S, Aoki Y, Hasegawa K, Kobayashi R, Chiba N, Tajima T, Ubukata K (2006) Simultaneous detection of pathogens in clinical samples from patients with community-acquired pneumonia by real-time PCR with pathogen-specific molecular beacon probes. J Clin Microbiol 44:1440–1446
57. Murali S, Langston AA, Nolte FS, Banks G, Martin R, Caliendo AM (2009) Detection of respiratory viruses with a multiplex polymerase chain reaction assay (MultiCode-PLx Respiratory Virus Panel) in patients with hematologic malignancies. Leuk Lymphoma 50:619–624
58. Murdoch DR (2003) Nucleic acid amplification tests for the diagnosis of pneumonia. Clin Infect Dis 36:1162–1170
59. Murdoch DR (2004) Molecular genetic methods in the diagnosis of lower respiratory tract infections. APMIS 112: 713–727
60. Murdoch DR, Laing RT, Mills GD, Karalus NC, Town GI, Mirrett S, Reller LB (2001) Evaluation of a rapid immunochromatographic test for detection of *Streptococcus pneumoniae* antigen in urine samples from adults with community-acquired pneumonia. J Clin Microbiol 39:3495–3498
61. Nilsson AC, Bjorkman P, Persson K (2008) Polymerase chain reaction is superior to serology for the diagnosis of acute *Mycoplasma pneumoniae* infection and reveals a high rate of persistent infection. BMC Microbiol 8:93
62. Nir-Paz R, Michael-Gayego A, Ron M, Block C (2006) Evaluation of eight commercial tests for *Mycoplasma pneumoniae* antibodies in the absence of acute infection. Clin Microbiol Infect 12:685–688
63. Park H, Kim C, Park KH, Chang CL (2006) Development and evaluation of triplex PCR for direct detection of mycobacteria in respiratory specimens. J Appl Microbiol 100:161–167
64. Ploton C, Freydiere AM, Benito Y, Bendridi N, Mazzocchi C, Bellon G, Vandenesch F (2006) *Streptococcus pneumoniae* thoracic empyema in children: rapid diagnosis by using the Binax NOW immunochromatographic membrane test in pleural fluids. Pathol Biol (Paris) 54:498–501
65. Porcel JM, Ruiz-Gonzalez A, Falguera M, Nogues A, Galindo C, Carratala J, Esquerda A (2007) Contribution of a pleural antigen assay (Binax NOW) to the diagnosis of pneumococcal pneumonia. Chest 131:1442–1447
66. Pounder JI, Aldous WK, Woods GL (2006) Comparison of real-time polymerase chain reaction using the Smart Cycler and the Gen-Probe amplified *Mycobacterium tuberculosis* direct test for detection of *M. tuberculosis* complex in clinical specimens. Diagn Microbiol Infect Dis 54:217–222
67. Raggam RB, Leitner E, Berg J, Muhlbauer G, Marth E, Kessler HH (2005) Single-run, parallel detection of DNA from three pneumonia-producing bacteria by real-time polymerase chain reaction. J Mol Diagn 7:133–138
68. Rantakokko-Jalava K, Marjamaki M, Marttila H, Makela L, Valtonen V, Viljanen MK (2001) LCx *Mycobacterium tuberculosis* assay is valuable with respiratory specimens, but provides little help in the diagnosis of extrapulmonary tuberculosis. Ann Med 33:55–62
69. Raty R, Ronkko E, Kleemola M (2005) Sample type is crucial to the diagnosis of *Mycoplasma pneumoniae* pneumonia by PCR. J Med Microbiol 54:287–291
70. Reischl U, Linde HJ, Lehn N, Landt O, Barratt K, Wellinghausen N (2002) Direct detection and differentiation of *Legionella* spp. and *Legionella pneumophila* in clinical specimens by dual-color real-time PCR and melting curve analysis. J Clin Microbiol 40:3814–3817
71. Roson B, Fernandez-Sabe N, Carratala J, Verdaguer R, Dorca J, Manresa F, Gudiol F (2004) Contribution of a urinary antigen assay (Binax NOW) to the early diagnosis of pneumococcal pneumonia. Clin Infect Dis 38:222–226
72. Roth SB, Jalava J, Ruuskanen O, Ruohola A, Nikkari S (2004) Use of an oligonucleotide array for laboratory diagnosis of bacteria responsible for acute upper respiratory infections. J Clin Microbiol 42:4268–4274
73. Schneeberger PM, Dorigo-Zetsma JW, van der Zee A, van Bon M, van Opstal JL (2004) Diagnosis of atypical

pathogens in patients hospitalized with community-acquired respiratory infection. Scand J Infect Dis 36:269–273
74. Shimada T, Noguchi Y, Jackson JL, Miyashita J, Hayashino Y, Kamiya T, Yamazaki S, Matsumura T, Fukuhara S (2009) Systematic review and metaanalysis: urinary antigen tests for Legionellosis. Chest 2009136:1576–1585
75. Smith MD, Derrington P, Evans R, Creek M, Morris R, Dance DA, Cartwright K (2003) Rapid diagnosis of bacteremic pneumococcal infections in adults by using the Binax NOW *Streptococcus pneumoniae* urinary antigen test: a prospective, controlled clinical evaluation. J Clin Microbiol 41: 2810–2813
76. Smith MD, Sheppard CL, Hogan A, Harrison TG, Dance DA, Derrington P, George RC (2009) Diagnosis of *Streptococcus pneumoniae* infections in adults with bacteremia and community-acquired pneumonia: clinical comparison of pneumococcal PCR and urinary antigen detection. J Clin Microbiol 47:1046–1049
77. Stralin K, Backman A, Holmberg H, Fredlund H, Olcen P (2005) Design of a multiplex PCR for *Streptococcus pneumoniae*, *Haemophilus influenzae*, *Mycoplasma pneumoniae* and *Chlamydophila pneumoniae* to be used on sputum samples. APMIS 113:99–111
78. Stralin K, Korsgaard J, Olcen P (2006) Evaluation of a multiplex PCR for bacterial pathogens applied to bronchoalveolar lavage. Eur Respir J 28:568–575
79. Stralin K, Tornqvist E, Kaltoft MS, Olcen P, Holmberg H (2006) Etiologic diagnosis of adult bacterial pneumonia by culture and PCR applied to respiratory tract samples. J Clin Microbiol 44:643–645
80. Tang PW, Toma S (1986) Broad-spectrum enzyme-linked immunosorbent assay for detection of *Legionella* soluble antigens. J Clin Microbiol 24:556–558
81. Touati A, Benard A, Hassen AB, Bebear CM, Pereyre S (2009) Evaluation of five commercial real-time PCR assays for detection of *Mycoplasma pneumoniae* in respiratory tract specimens. J Clin Microbiol 47:2269–2271
82. von Lilienfeld-Toal M, Lehmann LE, Raadts AD, Hahn-Ast C, Orlopp KS, Marklein G, Purr I, Cook G, Hoeft A, Glasmacher A, Stuber F (2009) Utility of a commercially available multiplex real-time PCR assay to detect bacterial and fungal pathogens in febrile neutropenia. J Clin Microbiol 47:2405–2410
83. Vuori-Holopainen E, Salo E, Saxen H, Hedman K, Hyypia T, Lahdenpera R, Leinonen M, Tarkka E, Vaara M, Peltola H (2002) Etiological diagnosis of childhood pneumonia by use of transthoracic needle aspiration and modern microbiological methods. Clin Infect Dis 34:583–590
84. Whatmore AM, Efstratiou A, Pickerill AP, Broughton K, Woodard G, Sturgeon D, George R, Dowson CG (2000) Genetic relationships between clinical isolates of *Streptococcus pneumoniae*, *Streptococcus oralis*, and *Streptococcus mitis*: characterization of "Atypical" pneumococci and organisms allied to *S. mitis* harboring *S. pneumoniae* virulence factor-encoding genes. Infect Immun 68: 1374–1382
85. White P, Bonacum JT, Miller CB (1997) Utility of fiberoptic bronchoscopy in bone marrow transplant patients. Bone Marrow Transplant 20:681–687
86. Williams A, Lever MS (1995) Characterisation of *Legionella pneumophila* antigen in urine of guinea pigs and humans with Legionnaires' disease. J Infect 30:13–16
87. Williams JV, Martino R, Rabella N, Otegui M, Parody R, Heck JM, Crowe JE Jr (2005) A prospective study comparing human metapneumovirus with other respiratory viruses in adults with hematologic malignancies and respiratory tract infections. J Infect Dis 192:1061–1065
88. Yang S, Lin S, Khalil A, Gaydos C, Nuemberger E, Juan G, Hardick J, Bartlett JG, Auwaerter PG, Rothman RE (2005) Quantitative PCR assay using sputum samples for rapid diagnosis of pneumococcal pneumonia in adult emergency department patients. J Clin Microbiol 43: 3221–3226
89. Yang G, Benson R, Pelish T, Brown E, Winchell JM, Fields B (2010) Dual detection of *Legionella pneumophila* and *Legionella* species by real-time PCR targeting the 23S-5S rRNA gene spacer region. Clin Microbiol Infect 16: 255–261

FDG-PET Imaging in Haematological Patients with Pulmonary Infiltrates

19

Tomohiko Yamane

Contents

T. Yamane
Division of Molecular Imaging, Institute of Biomedical Research and Innovation, 2-2 Minatojima-Minamimachi, Chuo-ku, Kobe 650-0047, Japan
e-mail: yamane@fbri.org

List of Abbreviations

FDG	2-[F-18]-Fluoro-2-deoxy-D-glucose
PET	Positron emission tomography
CT	Computed tomography
MALT	Mucosa-associated lymphoid tissue
IVL	Intravascular large B-cell lymphoma

19.1 FDG-PET

Positron emission tomography (PET) is a diagnostic imaging technique in which the distribution of an injected radioactive tracer substance is imaged, whereby information on the functions and metabolic activity of various organs/tissues of the body is obtained. Many kinds of tracers have been developed for PET, and the most commonly used is a radioactively labelled glucose analogue, 2-[F-18]-fluoro-2-deoxy-D-glucose (FDG) (Fig. 19.1).

Similar to glucose, FDG is also transported into cells by the glucose transporter protein and phosphorylated to FDG-6-phosphate by the enzyme hexokinase.

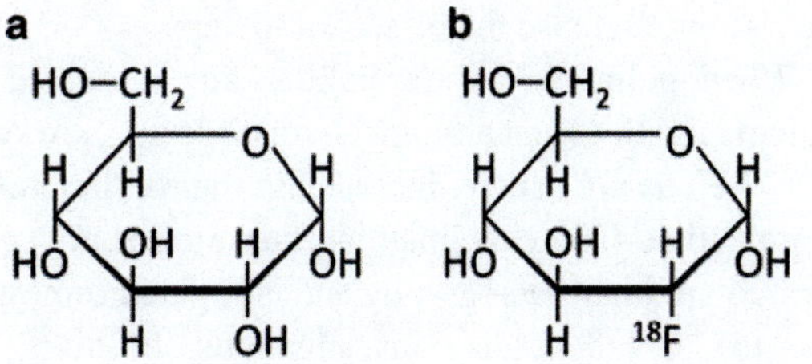

Fig. 19.1 Structures of (**a**) glucose and (**b**) 2-[F-18]-fluoro-2-deoxy-D-glucose

É. Azoulay (ed.), *Pulmonary Involvement in Patients with Hematological Malignancies*,
DOI: 10.1007/978-3-642-15742-4_19,

However, in contrast to glucose-6-phosphate, FDG-6-phosphate does not take part in subsequent reactions of the glycolytic pathway and is retained within the cells.

Malignant cells consume more glucose because of their unlimited capacity for cell division and proliferation as compared to benign cells, and these metabolic differences are exploited for differential diagnosis between these conditions by FDG-PET. Therefore in recent years, FDG-PET has become an established imaging technique for the evaluation of malignant tumours.

FDG also accumulates in inflammatory tissues [1, 2]. This accumulation is considered to reflect the enhanced anaerobic glycolysis that occurs in neutrophils and macrophages infiltrating inflammatory tissues. In addition, increased vessel flow, diffusion, and the proliferative process involved in the formation of granulomas have also been suggested to underlie the FDG accumulation in inflammatory tissues [3, 4].

FDG uptake by inflammatory tissues occasionally leads to false-positive diagnosis of malignant tumours. However, FDG-PET can also be a very useful tool for the diagnosis, evaluation, and follow-up of some inflammatory conditions.

19.2 Lung Lesions of Haematological Malignancies

FDG-PET is an effective tool for the diagnosis of various malignant diseases; among these, it has been reported to be particularly useful for the diagnosis of haematological malignancies, such as malignant lymphoma. Pulmonary infiltrates associated with haematological malignancies can also usually be visualized by FDG-PET, and the technique has been used for the evaluation of these malignancies, the distribution of the lesions, and also the effects of therapy.

When pulmonary abnormalities are suspected in patients with haematological disorders; however, FDG-PET is not usually included in the routine initial examination. The examinations that are usually performed are plain radiography and computed tomography [5] as radiological investigations, followed by bronchoalveolar lavage [6], biopsy [7], and/or biochemical examinations [8].

Thus, FDG-PET is not usually the most commonly employed method for the diagnosis of lung lesions associated with haematological malignancies. However, it is important to understand how lung lesions are visualized on FDG-PET, because they sometimes occur as a component of the systemic disease. In addition, FDG-PET may be effective for selecting the most appropriate biopsy area [9]. FDG-PET findings of lung lesions associated with some haematological diseases are described in the following sections.

19.2.1 Malignant Lymphoma

In relation to haematological disorders, numerous reports have demonstrated the efficacy of FDG-PET for the diagnosis, in particular, of malignant lymphoma [10,11]. Pulmonary lesions of lymphoma, as a component of systemic lymphoma, can also be visualized on FDG-PET. In addition, characteristic lung findings associated with mucosa-associated lymphoid tissue (MALT) lymphoma and intravascular lymphoma have been investigated.

19.2.1.1 MALT Lymphoma

FDG uptake by MALT lymphomas is generally known to be lower as compared with that by other high-grade lymphomas [12–15]. However, some reports have suggested a high sensitivity of FDG-PET for the diagnosis of pulmonary MALT lymphomas [16–18]. MALT lymphomas are most commonly detected in the stomach, where physiological FDG uptake is also frequently observed [19]. Background uptake and tumour morphology have been suggested as some of the factors that might influence the degree of uptake by these gastric tumours; however, the precise nature of their influence is unclear. Pulmonary MALT lymphomas are usually characterized by heterogeneous patterns on FDG-PET, akin to the CT findings, although some cases show a homogenous uptake pattern [18, 20–22]. Further investigations are needed to clarify the mechanisms of FDG uptake and clinical significance of the FDG-PET findings in patients with pulmonary MALT lymphoma.

19.2.1.2 Intravascular Lymphoma

Intravascular large B-cell lymphoma (IVL), classified as a subtype of diffuse large B-cell lymphoma by the World Health Organization [23], is rare and characterized by clonal proliferation of neoplastic lymphoid cells within the capillary lumina of small blood vessels. The major organs involved in IVL are mainly the bone marrow, spleen, liver, central nervous system, skin, and lymph nodes [24,25]. Pulmonary IVL is uncommon and rather difficult to diagnose. Although some articles have described the CT findings of IVL as being characterized by diffuse or patchy interstitial infiltrates [26–28], there have also been cases where final histopathological confirmation of the diagnosis was obtained only at autopsy [29,30]. A case of IVL is reported in the last part of this book by Dr. Darmon and coworkers.

In a case report of pulmonary IVL without any abnormal findings on CT or gallium-67 scintigraphy, only FDG-PET revealed diffuse pulmonary uptake [31]. Physicians tend to hesitate to undertake invasive approaches, such as biopsy, for the diagnosis when CT reveals no abnormalities. Therefore, FDG-PET may play an important role in the diagnosis of pulmonary IVL. Articles dealing with the FDG-PET findings of pulmonary IVL are limited, and the sensitivity and specificity of the technique for the diagnosis of this condition or the characteristic findings of IVL on FDG-PET are unknown. Therefore, further research may provide greater insight regarding the clinical significance of FDG-PET findings in cases with IVL.

19.2.2 Other Haematological Malignancies

There are some reports of the FDG-PET findings in multiple myeloma and plastocytoma [32] and leukaemia [33–35]. However, the effectiveness of FDG-PET for the diagnosis of these diseases has not been fully investigated. Although the use of other tracers that can reflect the cell proliferative activity, such as [F-18]-fluorothymidine, has been discussed for evaluating the therapeutic effect in cases of leukaemia [36], further investigations are necessary. While lung lesions are well known to occur in leukaemia [37–39], the FDG-PET findings have not yet been well characterised. The lung lesions of leukaemia may be expected to be FDG-avid, and the clinical significance of FDG-PET in this disease must be discussed.

19.3 Lung Abnormalities Associated with Haematological Disorders

In patients with haematological disorders, various pulmonary abnormalities such as opportunistic infections or drug-induced disorders may be encountered during the clinical course [6]. These lung disorders can be life threatening, and therefore, immediate diagnosis is essential.

The entire body is usually imaged in FDG-PET, and the imaging is often repeated to evaluate the effect of therapy or for patient follow-up after initial treatment of a malignant tumour. Occasionally, lung abnormalities are unexpectedly detected even in patients without lesions in the lung at the initial examination. Moreover, an integrated PET and CT system has recently been introduced for PET/CT, whereby morphological information can be evaluated simultaneously with functional imaging.

Some diseases that may be diagnosed by FDG-PET during the treatment of haematological disorders are mentioned in the following section.

19.3.1 Infections Associated with the Immunocompromised State

Patients with haematological disorders, especially those in the immunocompromised state during chemotherapy, are at an increased risk of developing various types of infectious diseases. As FDG accumulates in inflammatory tissues, the findings may mimic those of malignant tumours. For example, pneumocystis pneumonia [40,41], tuberculosis [42], cryptococcus infection [43,44], and aspergillus infection [45] have been reported as FDG-avid lung lesions that need to be differentiated from lung malignancy. Diverse uptake patterns can be visualised on FDG-PET, such as diffuse, nodular, and patchy, and it is difficult to diagnose the causative pathogen or differentiate between malignant and inflammatory lesions based on the uptake pattern visualised on FDG-PET alone. Under such circumstances, additional delayed images acquired at 120–160 min post injection of FDG may increase the diagnostic usefulness of FDG-PET [46]. FDG-PET combined with other diagnostic modalities, such as CT, and relevant microbiological and laboratory tests are useful.

19.3.2 Drug-Induced Pneumonitis

Various drug-induced disorders of the lung may be induced during chemotherapy of haematological disorders. Drug-induced pneumonitis caused by chemotherapeutic agents is not uncommon and may occasionally be fatal. Such pneumonitis may be detected as diffuse uptake on FDG-PET, corresponding to the opacity visualised on CT [47–50]. In one case report of diffuse lung uptake of FDG suspected to be caused by drug-induced pneumonitis during chemotherapy for malignant lymphoma [51], chest CT obtained on the same day did not reveal any abnormalities (Fig. 19.2); however, patchy ground-grass opacities on the CT appeared 3 days later; therefore, it appears that FDG-PET may be more sensitive than conventional CT for the early lung changes associated with drug-induced pneumonitis. Therefore, patients with haematological disorders showing diffuse lung

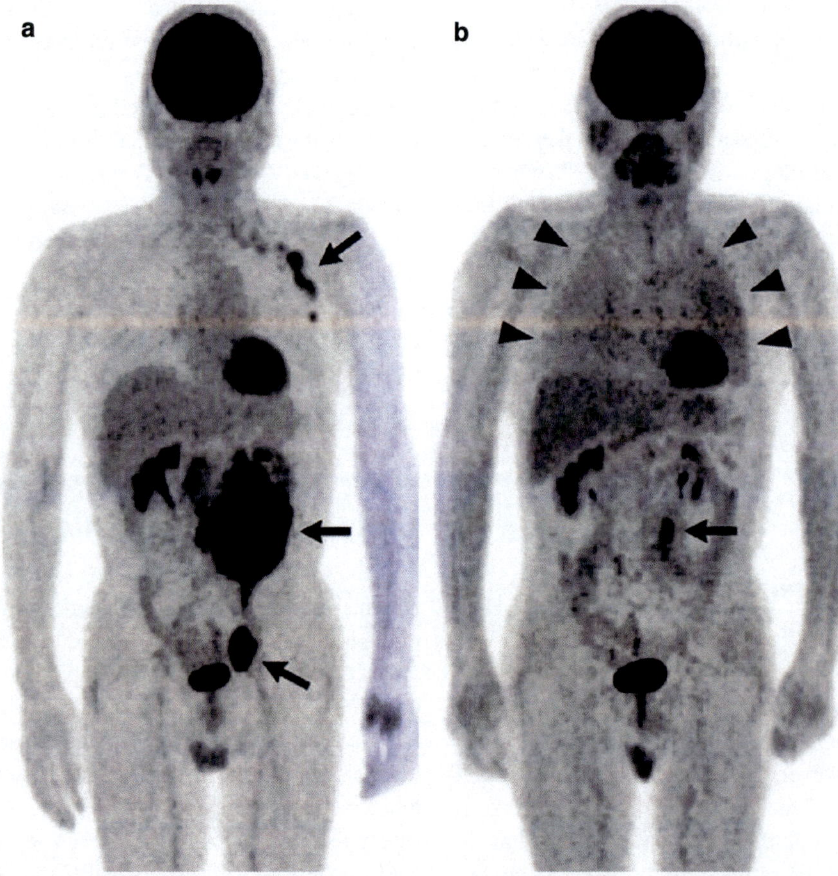

Fig. 19.2 (**a**) Initial FDG-PET image of a diffuse large B-cell lymphoma. Abnormal uptake is observed corresponding to the bulky mass in the left abdomen and in the left axillary, para-aortic, and para-external iliac artery lymph nodes (*arrows*). No increased uptake was observed in the lung. (**b**) FDG-PET after five courses of chemotherapy. Decreased, but persistent uptake by the bulky mass in the left abdomen was observed (*arrow*), whereas the uptake by the other lymph nodes was no longer seen. Although diffuse lung uptake was observed (*arrowheads*), patient did not complain of dyspnea. (**c**) Computed tomography performed after five courses of chemotherapy, immediately after FDG-PET. No abnormal findings are apparent. (**d**) Computed tomography performed 3 days after the initial FDG-PET and CT performed after five courses of chemotherapy. Patchy ground-grass opacities are seen throughout the lung fields (Modified and reprinted with permission of [51])

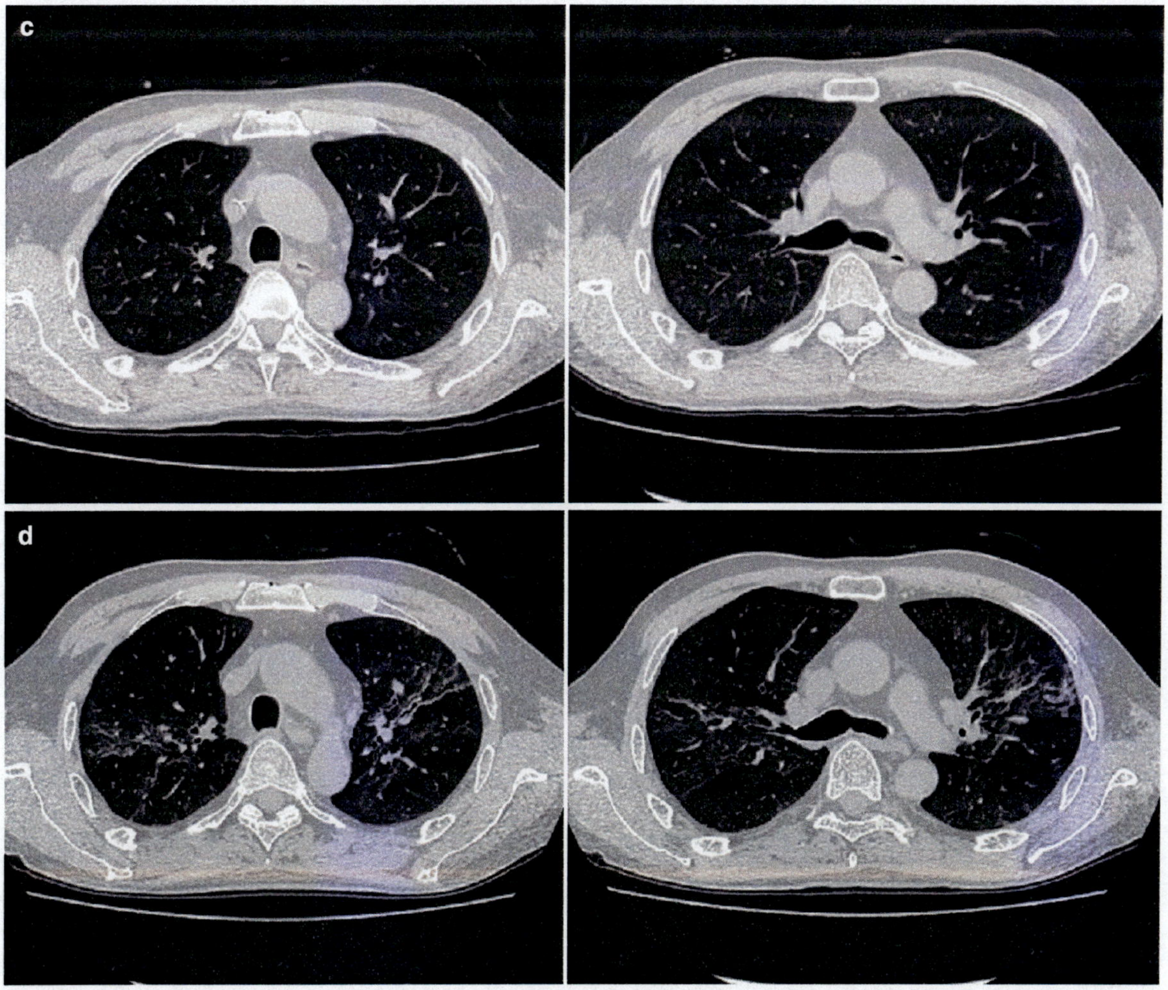

Fig. 19.2 (continued)

uptake on FDG-PET during chemotherapy should be examined carefully, even if the CT reveals no abnormalities.

19.3.3 Other Drug-Induced Diseases

Other complications that might develop during the treatment of haematological disorders are also known, such as sarcoidosis occurring in association with interferon therapy [52] or alveolar proteinosis [53]. Although there are no studies directly comparing the FDG-PET findings in these diseases, they can nevertheless be detected by FDG-PET [54, 55]. FDG-PET may be useful for the diagnosis of these diseases.

19.3.4 Radiation Pneumonitis

One of the major complications of radiation therapy is pneumonitis. FDG is known to accumulate in lesions of radiation pneumonitis, corresponding to the consolidation on CT, and the degree of uptake has been reported to be related to the radiation dose and the clinical symptom severity [56, 57].

19.3.5 Second Malignancies

Occurrence of second malignancy is known in patients treated for malignant lymphoma, and lung cancer is one of the most frequently encountered second

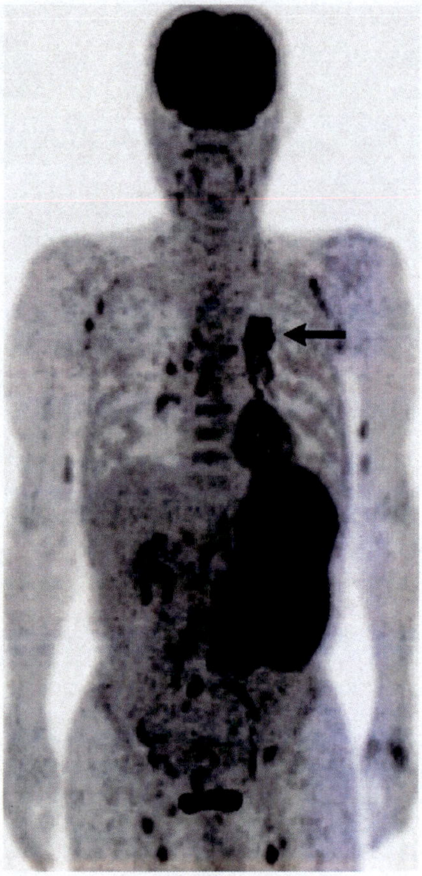

Fig. 19.3 Initial FDG-PET image of a mantle cell lymphoma. Abnormal uptake is observed in the bulky mass in the left abdomen and in the axillary, hilar, and inguinal lymph nodes bilaterally. Higher uptake was observed in left hilar area (*arrow*), which was finally diagnosed as adenocarcinoma of the lung

malignancies [58, 59]. Second malignancies may be difficult to distinguish from the primary haematological disorder on FDG-PET (Fig. 19.3). Differences in the intensity of uptake may be significant for distinguishing between them, but it is important to take into consideration the clinical data and the results of other imaging studies to make a precise diagnosis.

19.4 Conclusion

FDG-PET is an effective tool for the diagnosis of haematological malignancies as well as other malignant tumours. Pulmonary lesions of lymphoma can be visualised on FDG-PET, as a component of systemic lymphoma. Characteristic lung findings may be observed in cases of MALT lymphoma and IVL, and FDG-PET may be useful for the diagnosis of these conditions. In addition, some complications that might occur during the treatment of haematological disorders, such as infectious diseases or drug-induced pneumonitis, may also be detected by FDG-PET. It is possible that subtle changes associated with these conditions may be detected earlier by FDG-PET than by CT; therefore, careful examination of such patients is necessary even if no abnormalities are detected on CT.

References

1. Love C, Tomas MB, Tronco GG et al (2005) FDG PET of infection and inflammation. Radiographics 25:1357–1368
2. Kumar R, Basu S, Torigian D et al (2008) Role of modern imaging techniques for diagnosis of infection in the era of ^{18}F-fluorodeoxyglucose positron emission tomography. Clin Microbiol Rev 21:209–224
3. Yamada S, Kubota K, Kubota R et al (1995) High accumulation of fluorine-18-fluorodeoxyglucose in turpentine-induced inflammatory tissue. J Nucl Med 36:1301–1306
4. Jones HA, Cadwallader KA, White JF et al (2002) Dissociation between respiratory burst activity and deoxyglucose uptake in human neutrophil granulocytes: implications for interpretation of ^{18}F-FDG PET images. J Nucl Med 43:652–657
5. Ninane V (2000) Radiological and invasive diagnosis in the detection of pneumonia in fabrile neutropenia. Int J Antimicrob Agents 16:91–92
6. Azoulay E, Schlemmer B (2006) Diagnostic strategy in cancer patients with acute respiratory failure. Intensive Care Med 32:808–822
7. Gossot D, Girard P, de Kerviler E et al (2001) Thoracoscopy or CT-guided biopsy for residual intrathoracic masses after treatment of lymphoma. Chest 120:289–294
8. Maschmeyer G, Beinert T, Buchheidt D et al (2009) Diagnosis and antimicrobial therapy of lung infiltrates in febrile neutropenic patients: guidelines of the infectious diseases working party of the German Society of Haematology and Oncology. Eur J Cancer Sep 45(14):2462–2472
9. Bauwens O, Dusart M, Pierard P et al (2008) Endobronchial ultrasound and value of PET for prediction of pathological results of mediastinal hot spots in lung cancer patients. Lung Cancer 61:356–361
10. Juweid ME, Stroobants S, Hoekstra OS et al (2007) Use of positron emission tomography for response assessment of lymphoma: consensus of the Imaging Subcommittee of International Harmonization Project in Lymphoma. J Clin Oncol 25:571–578
11. Cheson BD, Pfistner B, Juweid ME et al (2007) Revised response criteria for malignant lymphoma. J Clin Oncol 25:579–586

12. Hoffmann M, Wohrer S, Becherer A et al (2006) ^{18}F-Fluorodeoxy-glucose positron emission tomography in lymphoma of mucosa-associated lymphoid tissue: histology makes the difference. Ann Oncol 17:1761–1765
13. Radan L, Fischer D, Bar-Shalom R et al (2008) FDG avidity and PET/CT patterns in primary gastric lymphoma. Eur J Nucl Med Mol Imaging 35:1424–1430
14. Tsukamoto N, Kojima M, Hasegawa M et al (2007) The usefulness of ^{18}F-fluorodeoxyglucose positron emission tomography (^{18}F-FDG-PET) and a comparison of ^{18}F-FDG-pet with ^{67}gallium scintigraphy in the evaluation of lymphoma: relation to histologic subtypes based on the World Health Organization classification. Cancer 110:652–659
15. Hoffmann M, Kletter K, Diemling M et al (1999) Positron emission tomography with fluorine-18-2-fluoro-2-deoxy-D-glucose (F18-FDG) does not visualize extranodal B-cell lymphoma of the mucosa-associated lymphoid tissue (MALT)-type. Ann Oncol 10:1185–1189
16. Beal KP, Yeung HW, Yahalom J (2005) FDG-PET scanning for detection and staging of extranodal marginal zone lymphomas of the MALT type: a report of 42 cases. Ann Oncol 16:473–480
17. Perry C, Herishanu Y, Metzer U et al (2007) Diagnostic accuracy of PET/CT in patients with extranodal marginal zone MALT lymphoma. Eur J Haematol 79:205–209
18. Bae YA, Lee KS, Han J et al (2008) Marginal zone B-cell lymphoma of bronchus-associated lymphoid tissue: imaging findings in 21 patients. Chest 133:433–440
19. Takahashi H, Ukawa K, Ohkawa N et al (2009) Significance of ^{18}F-2-deoxy-2-fluoro-glucose accumulation in the stomach on positron emission tomography. Ann Nucl Med 23:391–397
20. Enomoto K, Hamada K, Inohara H et al (2008) Mucosa-associated lymphoid tissue lymphoma studied with FDG-PET: a comparison with CT and endoscopic findings. Ann Nucl Med 22:261–267
21. Natsag J, Tomiyama N, Inoue A et al (2005) Pulmonary mucosa-associated lymphoid tissue type lymphoma with increased accumulation of fluorine 18-fluorodeoxyglucose on positron emission tomography. J Comput Assist Tomogr 29:640–643
22. Hara M, Sugie C, Tohyama J et al (2002) Increased $^{(18)}$fluorodeoxyglucose accumulation in mucosa-associated lymphoid tissue-type lymphoma of the lung. J Thorac Imaging 17:160–162
23. Gatter KC, Warnke RA (2001) Intravascular large B-cell lymphoma. In: Jaffe ES, Harris NL HS, Vardiman JW (eds) World Health Organization: pathology and genetics of tumours of haematopoietic and lymphoid tissues. IARC Press, Lyon
24. Murase T, Yamaguchi M, Suzuki R et al (2007) Intravascular large B-cell lymphoma (IVLBCL): a clinicopathologic study of 96 cases with special reference to the immunophenotypic heterogeneity of CD5. Blood 109:478–485
25. Ferreri AJ, Campo E, Seymour JF et al (2004) Intravascular lymphoma: clinical presentation, natural history, management and prognostic factors in a series of 38 cases, with special emphasis on the 'cutaneous variant'. Br J Haematol 127:173–183
26. Martusewicz-Boros M, Wiatr E, Radzikowska E et al (2007) Pulmonary intravascular large B-cell lymphoma as a cause of severe hypoxemia. J Clin Oncol 25:2137–2139
27. Yamagata T, Okamoto Y, Ota K et al (2003) A case of pulmonary intravascular lymphomatosis diagnosed by thoracoscopic lung biopsy. Respiration 70:414–418
28. Walls JG, Hong YG, Cox JE et al (1999) Pulmonary intravascular lymphomatosis: presentation with dyspnea and air trapping. Chest 115:1207–1210
29. Ferry JA, Sohani AR, Longtine JA et al (2009) HHV8-positive, EBV-positive Hodgkin lymphoma-like large B-cell lymphoma and HHV8-positive intravascular large B-cell lymphoma. Mod Pathol 22:618–626
30. Gaul C, Hanisch F, Neureiter D et al (2006) Intravascular lymphomatosis mimicking disseminated encephalomyelitis and encephalomyelopathy. Clin Neurol Neurosurg 108: 486–489
31. Kitanaka A, Kubota Y, Imataki O et al (2009) Intravascular large B-cell lymphoma with FDG accumulation in the lung lacking CT/^{67}gallium scintigraphy abnormality. Hematol Oncol 27:46–49
32. Kim PJ, Hicks RJ, Wirth A et al (2009) Impact of ^{18}F-fluorodeoxyglucose positron emission tomography before and after definitive radiation therapy in patients with apparently solitary plasmacytoma. Int J Radiat Oncol Biol Phys 74:740–746
33. Bruzzi JF, Macapinlac H, Tsimberidou AM et al (2006) Detection of Richter's transformation of chronic lymphocytic leukemia by PET/CT. J Nucl Med 47:1267–1273
34. Endo T, Sato N, Koizumi K et al (2004) Localized relapse in bone marrow of extremities after allogeneic stem cell transplantation for acute lymphoblastic leukemia. Am J Hematol 76:279–282
35. Kuenzle K, Taverna C, Steinert HC (2002) Detection of extramedullary infiltrates in acute myelogenous leukemia with whole-body positron emission tomography and 2-deoxy-2-[^{18}F]-fluoro-D-glucose. Mol Imaging Biol 4:179–183
36. Buck AK, Bommer M, Juweid ME et al (2008) First demonstration of leukemia imaging with the proliferation marker ^{18}F-fluorodeoxythymidine. J Nucl Med 49:1756–1762
37. Kakihana K, Ohashi K, Sakai F et al (2009) Leukemic infiltration of the lung following allogeneic hematopoietic stem cell transplantation. Int J Hematol 89:118–122
38. Wu YK, Huang YC, Huang SF et al (2008) Acute respiratory distress syndrome caused by leukemic infiltration of the lung. J Formos Med Assoc 107:419–423
39. Moore W, Baram D, Hu Y (2006) Pulmonary infiltration from chronic lymphocytic leukemia. J Thorac Imaging 21:172–175
40. Win Z, Todd J, Al-Nahhas A (2005) FDG-PET imaging in Pneumocystis carinii pneumonia. Clin Nucl Med 30: 690–691
41. Sojan SM, Chew G (2005) Pneumocystis carinii pneumonia on F-18 FDG PET. Clin Nucl Med 30:763–764
42. Demura Y, Tsuchida T, Uesaka D et al (2009) Usefulness of ^{18}F-fluorodeoxyglucose positron emission tomography for diagnosing disease activity and monitoring therapeutic response in patients with pulmonary mycobacteriosis. Eur J Nucl Med Mol Imaging 36:632–639
43. Huang CJ, You DL, Lee PI et al (2009) Characteristics of integrated ^{18}F-FDG PET/CT in pulmonary cryptococcosis. Acta Radiol 50:374–378
44. Igai H, Gotoh M, Yokomise H (2006) Computed tomography (CT) and positron emission tomography with [^{18}F]flu-

oro-2-deoxy-D-glucose (FDG-PET) images of pulmonary cryptococcosis mimicking lung cancer. Eur J Cardiothorac Surg 30:837–839
45. Ozsahin H, von Planta M, Muller I et al (1998) Successful treatment of invasive aspergillosis in chronic granulomatous disease by bone marrow transplantation, granulocyte colony-stimulating factor-mobilized granulocytes, and liposomal amphotericin-B. Blood 92:2719–2724
46. Umeda Y, Demura Y, Ishizaki T et al (2009) Dual-time-point ^{18}F-FDG PET imaging for diagnosis of disease type and disease activity in patients with idiopathic interstitial pneumonia. Eur J Nucl Med Mol Imaging 36:1121–1130
47. Morikawa M, Demura Y, Mizuno S et al (2008) FDG positron emission tomography imaging of drug-induced pneumonitis. Ann Nucl Med 22:335–338
48. Kazama T, Faria SC, Uchida Y et al (2008) Pulmonary drug toxicity: FDG-PET findings in patients with lymphoma. Ann Nucl Med 22:111–114
49. Buchler T, Bomanji J, Lee SM (2007) FDG-PET in bleomycin-induced pneumonitis following ABVD chemotherapy for Hodgkin's disease–a useful tool for monitoring pulmonary toxicity and disease activity. Haematologica 92: e120–e121
50. Kirsch J, Arrossi AV, Yoon JK et al (2006) FDG positron emission tomography/computerized tomography features of bleomycin-induced pneumonitis. J Thorac Imaging 21:228–230
51. Yamane T, Daimaru O, Ito S et al (2008) Drug-induced pneumonitis detected earlier by ^{18}F-FDG-PET than by high-resolution CT: a case report with non-Hodgkin's lymphoma. Ann Nucl Med 22:719–722
52. Doyle MK, Berggren R, Magnus JH (2006) Interferon-induced sarcoidosis. J Clin Rheumatol 12:241–248
53. Chung JH, Pipavath SJ, Myerson DH et al (2009) Secondary pulmonary alveolar proteinosis: a confusing and potentially serious complication of hematologic malignancy. J Thorac Imaging 24:115–118
54. Braun JJ, Kessler R, Constantinesco A et al (2008) ^{18}F-FDG PET/CT in sarcoidosis management: review and report of 20 cases. Eur J Nucl Med Mol Imaging 35:1537–1543
55. Hsu CW, Liu FY, Wang CW et al (2009) F-18 FDG PET/CT in pulmonary alveolar proteinosis. Clin Nucl Med 34: 103–104
56. Hart JP, McCurdy MR, Ezhil M et al (2008) Radiation pneumonitis: correlation of toxicity with pulmonary metabolic radiation response. Int J Radiat Oncol Biol Phys 71:967–971
57. Guerrero T, Johnson V, Hart J et al (2007) Radiation pneumonitis: local dose versus [^{18}F]-fluorodeoxyglucose uptake response in irradiated lung. Int J Radiat Oncol Biol Phys 68:1030–1035
58. Andre M, Mounier N, Leleu X et al (2004) Second cancers and late toxicities after treatment of aggressive non-Hodgkin lymphoma with the ACVBP regimen: a GELA cohort study on 2837 patients. Blood 103:1222–1228
59. Sacchi S, Marcheselli L, Bari A et al (2008) Second malignancies after treatment of diffuse large B-cell non-Hodgkin's lymphoma: a GISL cohort study. Haematologica 93: 1335–1342

What Has Been Learned from Postmortem Studies?

20

Stephen M. Pastores, Alina O. Dulu, and Shilpa A. DeSouza

Contents

S.M. Pastores (✉) and S.A. DeSouza
Department of Anesthesiology and Critical Care Medicine, Memorial Sloan-Kettering Cancer Center, Weill Cornell Medical College, 1275 York Avenue C-1179, New York, NY 10065, USA
e-mail: pastores@mskcc.org

A.O. Dulu
Division of Critical Care Medicine, Montefiore Medical Center, Albert Einstein College of Medicine, Bronx, NY, USA

20.1 Introduction

Infectious and noninfectious pulmonary complications occur in 30–60% of patients with hematological malignancy and recipients of hematopoietic stem cell transplantation (HSCT) and are associated with significant morbidity and mortality [1]. In allogeneic HSCT patients who develop respiratory failure requiring mechanical ventilation, the intensive care unit (ICU) and hospital mortality rates often exceed 80% and 85%, respectively [2–5]. The factors that contribute to the development of pulmonary complications in these patients include immunologic defects due to the underlying disease and its treatment, conditioning regimens, development of graft-versus-host disease (GVHD), and the type of HSCT [2, 6, 7]. The spectrum of pulmonary complications in patients with hematological malignancy and HSCT recipients is changing because of recent advances in antineoplastic therapies, such as the use of monoclonal antibodies and other targeted agents, increased application of HSCT for older patients, widespread use of prophylactic antibiotics and novel antimicrobial agents, and advances in supportive care [8].

Prompt investigation and diagnosis of pulmonary complications in patients with hematological malignancies are essential to improving patient survival. Unfortunately, despite the technological advances in diagnostic testing and imaging modalities, obtaining an accurate clinical diagnosis in these patients remains difficult and at times is made only at the time of the postmortem autopsy examination. Autopsy rates in cancer patients are much lower (13–34%) as compared to general medical and surgical patients (53–64%) [7–9]. This probably reflects the unwillingness on the

The authors state that they do not have any conflicts of interest.

É. Azoulay (ed.), *Pulmonary Involvement in Patients with Hematological Malignancies*,
DOI: 10.1007/978-3-642-15742-4_20, © Springer-Verlag Berlin Heidelberg 2011

Table 20.1 Pulmonary findings on postmortem studies in patients with hematologic malignancy including HSCT recipients

Infectious	Non-infectious
Fungal Invasive pulmonary aspergillosis Candida bronchopneumonia Zygomycetes *Trichosporon* spp. *Fusarium* spp. *Chaetomium* spp. *Pneumocystis jiroveci* pneumonia	Diffuse alveolar damage Diffuse alveolar hemorrhage Lymphoma/leukemia Pulmonary thromboembolism Bronchiolitis obliterans organizing pneumonia Bronchiolitis obliterans Pulmonary veno-occlusive disease Pulmonary alveolar proteinosis
Bacterial Vancomycin-resistant enterococci *Legionella* spp. *Stenotrophomonas maltophilia* *Staphylococcus epidermidis* *Staphylococcus aureus* *Streptococcus pneumoniae* *Pseudomonas aeruginosa* *Serratia* spp. Other gram-negative bacilli and streptococcus spp.	
Viral Cytomegalovirus Herpes simplex virus Respiratory syncytial virus Measles virus	
Parasitic Toxoplasmosis	

part of physicians and family members to subject the cancer patient to the same level of scrutiny applied to other major illnesses in determining the primary and contributory causes of death [9]. Additional concerns include legal issues regarding exposition of physicians' errors and non-reimbursement for postmortem examinations [10].

This chapter will review the infectious and noninfectious pulmonary findings that have been described at autopsy in patients with hematological malignancies, including blood and bone marrow transplant recipients. In addition, we discuss the frequently noted diagnostic discrepancies between premortem clinical diagnoses and postmortem autopsy findings in these patients. Finally, we highlight the difficulties in diagnosing many of these conditions antemortem and emphasize the important role of the postmortem examination in accurately establishing the cause of death. Table 20.1 lists the infectious and non-infectious pulmonary disorders reported in autopsy studies of patients with hematologic malignancy, including HSCT recipients.

20.2 Infectious Findings

20.2.1 Invasive Fungal Infections

The incidence of invasive fungal infections in patients with hematologic malignancies has increased steadily over the past three decades [11]. This has been attributed to improvements in the prevention or preemptive treatment of bacterial infections and other opportunistic pathogens, particularly *Candida* and cytomegalovirus; increased administration of chemotherapies with profound and prolonged immunosuppressive effects on T-cell function (e.g., purine nucleoside analogs, anti-T-cell immunoglobulin, and monoclonal antibodies); and the growing number of allogeneic and nonmyeloablative transplantation procedures that carry a higher risk for chronic GVHD [12]. Patients with hematologic malignancies, especially in the neutropenic state after aggressive chemotherapy or HSCT and HSCT recipients with GVHD, are particularly susceptible to invasive fungal infections [13]. Approximately 20–50% of patients with hematological malignancies and HSCT recipients have evidence of invasive fungal infections at autopsy [8]. These include invasive aspergillosis and fungal infections due to *Candida* spp., *Zygomycetes* spp., *Trichosporon* spp., *Fusarium* spp., and various *Chaetomium* species.

In neutropenic patients with acute leukemia, the histopathological pattern of invasive pulmonary aspergillosis (IPA) is characterized by scant inflammation, hyphal angioinvasion with a high fungal burden, and extensive coagulative necrosis [12, 14]. In contrast, among HSCT recipients with GVHD, the histopathological findings consist of severe lung inflammation and less abundant *Aspergillus* burden. Several autopsy studies in HSCT recipients have shown that IPA is frequently not diagnosed antemortem or persistent despite diagnosis by sputum or bronchoalveolar lavage (BAL) cultures or by serum galactomannan assay and treatment with amphotericin B [8, 15–21]. In recent years, treatment of IPA with voriconazole has led to better responses, improved survival rates, and fewer side effects than amphotericin B [22].

Autopsy studies have assisted in describing and confirming the immune reconstitution inflammatory syndrome (IRIS) in patients with IPA who are recovering from the neutropenia [23]. When clinical and radiologic worsening coincides with neutrophil recovery, it is usually assumed that this deterioration is related to progressive aspergillosis, prompting changes in patient management. However, its temporal relation with neutrophil recovery suggests that it may be caused by IRIS. The patients who died during the first month had no evidence of aspergillosis at autopsy. Finally, autopsy studies have proved helpful in documenting the efficacy of systemic antifungal therapy and surgery for IPA [24].

Since the early 1990s, the incidence of invasive candidiasis (candidemia and/or hepatosplenic candidiasis) has continued to decrease due to effective antifungal prophylaxis and empirical treatment of high-risk patients with echinocandins and voriconazole [11]. Mucosal damage is a risk factor for invasive candidiasis among patients receiving antineoplastic therapy. HSCT recipients who received conditioning regimens with total body irradiation and patients treated with chemotherapy regimens containing high-dose cytarabine or an anthracycline have an increased risk of developing invasive disease. In recent years, there has been an increase in bloodstream infections caused by non-albicans Candida species such as *Candida glabrata* and *C. krusei*. The diagnosis of invasive candidiasis is difficult to prove due to the lack of specific clinical features and the low sensitivity of blood cultures to isolate Candida, especially in patients receiving fluconazole prophylaxis [25].

Difficult-to-treat opportunistic molds, such as *Zygomycetes*, *Trichosporon* spp., and various *Chaetomium* spp., including *C. atrobrunneum, C. strumarium, C. globosum, C. perlucidum, and C. cinereus* are being described with increasing frequency on autopsy studies in patients with hematologic malignancies [12, 26–31]. Pulmonary involvement with these mold infections is characterized by tissue necrosis from angioinvasion and subsequent thrombosis. As with many fungal infections, diagnosis of these infections is often not possible until autopsy. Treatment modalities usually involve lipid-based amphotericin B formulations and surgical debulking or debridement in selected cases [32].

20.2.2 Pneumocystis Jiroveci (Formerly Carinii) Pneumonia

Pneumocystis jiroveci pneumonia (PCP) remains a serious infection in patients with acute and chronic leukemias, myelodysplastic syndrome, and HSCT recipients [8]. However, diagnosis of PCP is frequently obtained by bronchoalveolar lavage with or without lung biopsy; thus, the diagnosis is made on autopsy in only a minority of cases.

20.2.3 Bacterial Infections

Bacterial pneumonias caused by *Pseudomonas aeruginosa*, *Streptococcus* spp., *Staphylococcus aureus*, *Serratia* spp., and *Legionella pneumophila* have been described on autopsy studies in patients with hematologic malignancy and HSCT recipients [33]. As the majority of these patients commonly receive empiric antimicrobial therapy during the initial diagnostic workup for infection, very few autopsy studies report unusual bacterial infections. A single center autopsy series of 15 patients with hematological malignancies found multidrug-resistant strains such as *Enterococcus faecium* to be very prevalent [34]. Two coagulase-negative Staphylococcus epidermidis strains were also noted. A few autopsy case reports have also described lethal pulmonary hemorrhage due to *Stenotrophomonas maltophilia* [35].

20.2.4 Viruses

The incidence of autopsy-proven cytomegalovirus (CMV) pneumonia in patients with hematologic malignancy and HSCT recipients has been decreasing in recent years as a result of improvements in early diagnosis and treatment and more effective preventive strategies [36]. However, it is also possible that the declining rate of autopsies may account for the decrease in the number of reported CMV pneumonias. Other etiologies of viral pneumonias that have been described in autopsy reports include infection due to herpes simplex virus, respiratory syncytial virus (RSV) [37], and measles virus [38].

20.2.5 Toxoplasmosis

Reactivation of latent Toxoplasmosis is a rare but well-recognized opportunistic infection in immunocompromised patients. Besides encephalitis, the other common presentation with *Toxoplasma gondii* infection is interstitial pneumonitis. Because of its non-specific clinical and radiological presentation and its lethal outcome, toxoplasmosis is often misdiagnosed and only revealed at autopsy [39]. Toxoplasmic pneumonitis follows the same pathogenetic mechanism, but occurs less frequently than either toxoplasmic encephalitis or other opportunistic pneumonias, such as PCP. Diagnosis is based upon a high degree of clinical suspicion and demonstration of *T. gondii* in BAL fluid and/or lung biopsy specimens. Widely disseminated necrotic areas with numerous cysts of *Toxoplasma gondii* are commonly reported in autopsy cases.

20.3 Noninfectious Pulmonary Findings

Noninfectious pulmonary complications account for up to 70% of autopsy findings in patients with hematologic malignancies, particularly in HSCT recipients. The most common complications are diffuse alveolar damage (DAD) and diffuse alveolar hemorrhage (DAH) [8].

20.3.1 Diffuse Alveolar Damage

Diffuse alveolar damage (DAD) is a nonspecific finding at autopsy often in association with various infectious and noninfectious etiologies, such as shock, aspiration, alveolar hemorrhage, peri-engraftment respiratory distress syndrome, drug toxicity, and radiation therapy. It is characterized by the presence of alveolar injury and the absence of active lower respiratory tract infection. DAD has been reported at autopsy in 63.5% of patients with treated leukemia and lymphoma and close to 50% among HSCT patients [7, 8]. Infections as the cause of DAD are identified on autopsy in only a third of HSCT patients, while approximately 20% have DAH. In over 50% of patients with DAD, no etiology is determined, and these patients are considered as having idiopathic pneumonia syndrome (IPS). It is possible that empirically treated previous infections could have caused the histological changes noted in patients classified as having IPS. Only one third of the cases of DAD are diagnosed antemortem [8]. Given that almost half of the cases of DAD may be secondary to IPS, the role of corticosteroids may need to be furthered studied.

20.3.2 Diffuse Alveolar Hemorrhage

Diffuse alveolar hemorrhage (DAH) is a clinical syndrome characterized by the acute onset of alveolar infiltrates, bloody bronchoalveolar lavage, and hypoxemia in the absence of infection [1, 40]. The incidence of DAH ranges from 1–5% to 3–7% in autologous and allogeneic HSCT recipients, respectively [41–43]. A few case reports have been described in patients with acute leukemia more commonly in association with chemotherapy [44–46]. DAH has also been described in patients undergoing an umbilical cord HSCT [47, 48]. The majority of patients with DAH develop severe respiratory failure with high mortality rates. Vascular damage and inflammation from chemotherapy and radiation therapy used in the conditioning regimen and immune-mediated events including GVHD have been implicated in the pathogenesis of DAH [41, 43, 49]. Wojno et al. reported that 41% of 37 allogeneic HSCT patients who underwent autopsies had extensive pulmonary hemorrhage, which was thought to have led to severe respiratory failure and death [49]. These patients were subdivided into those with significant acute GVHD and those without. Of the patients with acute GVHD, 59% died of acute respiratory failure secondary to DAH compared with 25% of those without GVHD. Pulmonary hemorrhage was also independently found to be associated with pre-transplant total body irradiation. Although pulmonary and systemic infections cause alveolar damage through similar mechanisms [50]. infection-associated alveolar damage has traditionally been excluded from analyses of DAH. Autopsy studies have shown that pulmonary infections are frequently underdiagnosed in HSCT recipients; thus, patients with alveolar hemorrhage and underlying undetected infections can be misclassified as having DAH [7, 8, 51].

Because inflammation is thought to play a role in the pathogenesis of post HSCT-DAH, high-dose steroids have been used for its treatment, based on anecdotal case reports and small retrospective series [52, 53]. Other treatment modalities that have been used for DAH in HSCT recipients include epsilon aminocaproic acid and recombinant factor VIIa [54, 55]. Unfortunately, the mortality from DAH in HSCT recipients remains high because of misdiagnosis and lack of effective treatments.

20.3.3 Lymphomatous or Leukemic Infiltration

Primary pulmonary lymphomas are very uncommon, especially those arising from bronchus-associated lymphoid tissue (BALT) and have a low mortality. They represent 4% of the extranodal non-Hodgkin's lymphomas (NHLs) and only 0.5% of all primary pulmonary malignant neoplasms and less than 1% of lymphomas. Eighty percent of the cases are low-grade B-cell lymphomas, which are slow growing and respond well to therapy. Autopsy case reports suggest that pulmonary BALT lymphoma can remain restrictive to the thorax for long periods before dissemination, but tend to relapse frequently.

Lymphomatous involvement of the lung is common and occurs in 24% and 38%, respectively, of patients with Hodgkin's lymphomas (HL) and NHL [56]. Typical findings in the lung include peribronchial-perivascular, nodular, alveolar, interstitial, and pleural involvement. Peripheral T-cell lymphomas also involve the lung frequently, 20% at diagnosis and a further 20% during the course of the disease. The nodular pattern is a characteristic of lung infiltration in HL, but no differences could be detected in the subtypes.

Pulmonary parenchymal involvement by multiple myeloma cells is very rare and described on autopsy in few case reports. The antemortem diagnosis of lung involvement by myeloma is difficult to make as infections and alveolar hemorrhage can have the same radiologic features.

Leukemic infiltration of the lungs may occur in 20–30% of hyperleucocytic patients with acute myeloid leukemia (AML). Pulmonary infiltrates are usually microscopic and invariably associated with hyperleukocytosis. There are autopsy case reports of pulmonary leukemia as a cause of pulmonary infiltrates, even in non-hyperleukocytosis AML patients with low blast counts. Radiographically, patients present with an airspace disease with a diffuse interstitial reticular pattern in cases of hyperleukocytosis similar to cases of infectious pneumonia.

Pulmonary leukostasis syndrome involves the occlusion of small blood vessels in the lungs and typically occurs with a WBC count of greater than 100,000 per mL. The increased number of WBCs causes blood viscosity to rise due to the decreased deformability of the abnormal leukocytes, resulting in cell clumping and stasis in the microvasculature, leading to severe hypoxemic respiratory failure. Autopsy studies reveal extensive infiltration by leukemic cells in the pulmonary vasculature; pulmonary infarction with hemorrhage is also noted. [57]

Rarely, lung involvement by intravascular large B-cell lymphoma (IVLBCL) is noted on autopsy [58]. Early diagnosis is difficult as neither computed tomography nor 67-gallium scintigraphy can detect lung involvement. However, 18-fluro-deoxyglucose positron tomography (FDG-PET) may be a powerful tool for the early diagnosis of IVLBCL with pulmonary involvement [59].

20.3.4 Pulmonary Thromboembolism

Autopsy studies show that pulmonary thromboembolism (PTE) infrequently complicates the course of patients with acute leukemia and severe thrombocytopenia, and HSCT recipients with an incidence rate ranging from 1% to 6.3% [8]. [60] Patients with acute leukemias commonly have clinically silent haemostatic abnormalities, but some may show clinical manifestations, including venous thromboembolism, pulmonary embolism, disseminated intravascular coagulation, and life-threatening thrombohemorrhagic syndrome. The pathogenesis of PTE is complex and multifactorial and may involve tumor cell-derived procoagulant, fibrinolytic or proteolytic factors, and inflammatory cytokines, which affect clotting activation. Chemotherapy and anti-angiogenic drugs also increase the thrombotic risk in patients with lymphoma, acute leukemia, and multiple myeloma. Infectious complications are another important factor: endotoxins from gram-negative bacteria induce the release of tissue factor (TF), tumor necrosis factor (TNF), and interleukin-1 (IL-1), and gram-positive organisms can release bacterial mucopolysaccharides that directly activate factor XII. Needleman et al. reviewed 80 consecutive autopsies in leukemia patients and found three patients with previously undiagnosed PTE, all of whom had been severely thrombocytopenic. However, Candida forms were abundant in the thromboemboli in all three patients, with some containing septate hyphal forms consistent with *Mucor* or aspergillosis. No vessel wall invasion or necrosis was noted, and fungus was not shown to be present in pulmonary vessels in segments of the lung not involved with thromboembolism [60]. Leukemic patients may also be affected by other prothrombotic factors, including hyperleukocytosis, increased TF expression and activation, and the prothrombotic properties of therapeutic agents, such as all-trans retinoic acid and L-asparaginase, which can induce thrombosis involving multiple organs. A higher index of suspicion may lead to the diagnosis, but the signs and symptoms of PTE in patients with hematologic malignancy are variable and nonspecific as with PTE in other populations.

20.3.5 Bronchiolitis Obliterans with Organizing Pneumonia and Bronchiolitis Obliterans

The majority of patients with hematological malignancies who develop organizing pneumonia (BOOP) have been exposed to various chemotherapeutic agents, including cytarabine and anthracyclines as well as radiation therapy. [61, 62] In one autopsy series, Sharma et al. reported on 71 patients who had undergone HSCT, of whom 3% had BO and 1% had BOOP [8]. Unusual histological variants have also been described, including a case report of acute fibrinous and organizing pneumonia following HSCT in a patient with AML [63] characterized by prominent intraalveolar fibrin deposition and organizing pneumonia. The radiographic presentation revealed patchy consolidation in the lower lobes and a diffuse miliary pattern. Clinically, these cases can have subacute presentations similar to cryptogenic organizing pneumonia or have more rapid progression with clinical features similar to ARDS. BOOP and BO are rare autopsy findings, which may be because infections are being treated aggressively, and often patients not responding to antibiotics and with no clinical evidence of infections are given a trial of corticosteroids.

Yokoi et al. reported bronchiolitis obliterans (BO) on autopsy in 8 of 81 patients who underwent allogeneic BMT with AML or ALL. All patients received conditioning regimens with total body irradiation and cyclophosphamide with or without busulfan or cytosine arabinoside. Immunosuppressive therapies were administered to all patients after BMT, including methotrexate with or without cyclosporine. The onset of respiratory symptoms was 110–430 days after BMT, and the symptoms were non-productive cough, dyspnea, fever, chest pain, and pneumothorax. Seven patients died of progressive respiratory failure and one of relapsed leukemia. Coexistent infections included *CMV*, *varicella zoster*, *Mycobacterium tuberculosis,* and *Aspergillus* [21]. Paz et al. also described two patients who underwent autologous BMT for lymphoma and developed rapidly progressive respiratory insufficiency on post-transplant day 90 and 273. Despite aggressive immunosuppressive therapy, both patients died of respiratory failure. Autopsy studies revealed histological evidence of bronchiolitis obliterans [64].

20.3.6 Pulmonary Veno-occlusive Disease

Pulmonary veno-occlusive disease (PVOD) is a rare cause of pulmonary hypertension that is characterized histopathologically by intimal proliferation and fibrosis of the pulmonary venules and small veins leading to progressive vascular obstruction [65]. The etiology of PVOD remains unclear. It has been reported as an unusual complication of both myeloablative allogeneic, autologous and cord HSCT, suggesting that it might be regimen-related toxicity [65–70]. Surgical lung biopsy provides definitive diagnosis [71]. PVOD carries a poor prognosis, with most reported patients experiencing progressive disease and death within 2 years of diagnosis [72]. Autopsy findings reveal intimal fibrosis of most of the pulmonary veins, with no significant intraluminal thrombi or arterial changes [69]. Treatment recommendations are anecdotal. Steroids and heparin have been reported to possibly improve outcomes [66].

20.3.7 Pulmonary Alveolar Proteinosis

Autopsy studies in patients with hematologic malignancy (particularly with myelodysplastic syndrome) and following HSCT have revealed rare cases of secondary pulmonary alveolar proteinosis (PAP) characterized by intra-alveolar accumulation of surfactant components and cellular debris, with minimal interstitial inflammation or fibrosis [73–75]. Secondary PAP is frequently noted among patients with hematologic malignancies who develop fungal infection, especially pulmonary aspergillosis. KL-6 protein is produced by type II alveolar pneumocytes and can be helpful in establishing an early diagnosis of PAP [74, 76]. The standard therapy for PAP with hematological malignancy has not yet been firmly established. The administration of GM-CSF has been suggested to activate the alveolar macrophages and increase the rate of surfactant clearance [73]. Case reports indicate that the prognosis of PAP with leukemia is very poor because of the high frequency of superinfections in the affected alveoli [73, 75].

20.4 Discrepancies Between Clinical and Postmortem Autopsy Findings

Several autopsy series have reported diagnostic discrepancies between premortem clinical diagnosis and postmortem autopsy findings ranging from 5% to 64% in patients with hematologic malignancy and HSCT recipients (Table 20.2) [15, 77–83]. The Goldman criteria are commonly used to categorize discrepancies between clinical and pathological diagnoses or causes of death [84]. Class 1 discrepancies are defined as missed major diagnoses with potential adverse impact on survival and would have changed management. Class II discrepancies are missed major diagnoses with no potential impact on survival and that would have not changed therapy. Class III discrepancies are defined as missed minor diagnoses related to terminal disease, but not related to the cause of death, and Class IV are other missed minor diagnoses.

Gerain et al. reported a 59% major discrepancy rate in 34 cancer patients who were admitted to a medical oncological ICU over an 11-month period. [77] The majority of major discrepancies were due to complications of the cancer itself or its treatment (such as non-cardiogenic pulmonary edema, acute hemorrhage, and pulmonary embolism) rather than infection. Pastores et al. reported a major missed diagnosis rate of 26% in 86 autopsies performed on cancer patients who died in a medical-surgical ICU [78]. Of the 86 patients, 25 (40%) had undergone HSCT, 18 (29%) had either leukemias or lymphomas, 19 (31%) had solid tumors, and 24 (28%) were surgical cancer patients. Among the patients with discrepancies 54% had class I discrepancies, 32% had class II discrepancies, and 14% had both class I and class II discrepancies. Of the 22 discordant cases, 6 had hematological malignancies and 4 underwent HSCT. Opportunistic infections due to viral, fungal, bacterial, and parasitic organisms and cardiac complications were the most common class I discrepancies. The majority of Class II discrepancies were accounted for by cardiopulmonary complications due to pulmonary embolism and thrombotic endocarditis. The study was limited by the retrospective study design and selection bias that may have occurred as physicians and family members of patients with premortem diagnostic uncertainty would have been more likely to pursue an autopsy. Xavier et al. reported a class I discrepancy rate of 31.3% in 118 autopsies of patients with hematological malignancies or severe aplastic anemia [79]. The most common diagnoses causing these discrepancies were hematological disease, pneumonia, and gastrointestinal hemorrhage. Class I discrepancies were more common in elderly patients (>64 years) and in patients who had not received previous specific treatment for the hematological malignancy, had not been treated with bone marrow or peripheral blood HSCT, or had not been treated in a specialized hematology unit. Seftel et al. reported a discrepancy rate of 64% (34% major, 30% minor) in 48 autopsies of patients who underwent HSCT (blood and bone marrow) [82]. Infectious complications, including pulmonary aspergillosis, candidiasis, and infective endocarditis, accounted for the majority of the major discrepancies. Hoffmeister et al. found a 26% discrepancy rate (4% major, 23% minor) in 111 autopsies of patients who had undergone HSCT [83]. In contrast, Al Saidi et al. found a

Table 20.2 List of selected studies describing discrepancies between premortem and postmortem autopsy diagnoses in patients with hematologic malignancy including HSCT recipients

Al-Saidi et al. 2002 $N=28$	
Class I $n=1$ (3.5%)	Systemic aspergillosis (1)
Class II $n=2$ (7.1%)	Severe GVHD (1)
	Hemorrhagic cecal perforation (1)
Class III $n=6$ (21.4%)	Non infective endocarditis (1)
	Spinal cord demyelination (1)
	CMV pneumonitis (1)
	Bacterial infections (3)
Class IV $n=1$ (3.5%)	Coagulase-negative staphylococcus catheter infection (1)
Pastores et al. 2007 $N=86$	
Class I discrepancies $n=15$ (17.4%)	Opportunistic infections $n=10$
	VRE pneumonia
	Legionella pneumonia
	PCP pneumonia
	Invasive aspergillosis
	Candida empyema
	Varicella-zoster meningoencephalitis
	HSV esophagitis
	CMV pneumonia
	Disseminated necrotizing toxoplasmosis
	Cardiac complications $n=5$
	Ischemic cardiomyopathy (2)
	Thrombotic endocarditis (2)
	Congestive heart failure (1)
Class II discrepancies $n=10$ (11.6%)	Opportunistic infections $n=3$
	Candidemia
	VRE meningitis
	CMV proctitis
	Cardiopulmonary complications $n=7$
	Pulmonary embolism (4)
	Thrombotic endocarditis (2)
	Pulmonary hemorrhage (1)
Seftel et al. (2007) $n=48$	
Class I ($n=16$) (34%)	Candidiasis
	Pulmonary aspergillosis
	Infective endocarditis
	Adenovirus, with no GVHD
	Adenovirus hepatitis
	Relapse of myelodysplasia
	Acetaminophen overdose
	Sepsis with multi-organ failure
	Disseminated Aspergillosis
	Gut perforation
	Pneumonia
	Candida pneumonia
	Myelodysplasia relapse
	CMV adrenalitis; no lymphoma
	Typhlitis relapse leukemia
	Pulmonary lymphoma
	Radiation pneumonia
Class II ($n=14$) (30%)	Cerebral and pulmonary aspergillosis
	Pneumonia; cerebral hemorrhage
	Diffuse alveolar damage
	Congenital absence of kidney
	No pneumonia
	No pneumonia; renal abscess
	No pneumonia; subarachnoid hemorrhage
	No pneumonia; cerebellar hemorrhage
	Hemochromatosis and diffuse alveolar damage
	Idiopathic hepatitis
	Normal colon
	Pulmonary fibrosis
	Sepsis
	Cholestatic liver disease
Xavier et al. (2005) $n=544$	
Class I (8.6%)	Hematological disease – 15
	Pneumonia – 5

Table 20.2 (continued)

	Gastrointestinal hemorrhage, – 3
	Congestive heart failure – 2
	Acute pancreatitis – 2
	Pulmonary embolism – 2
	Invasive pulmonary aspergillosis – 2
	Pulmonary edema – 2
Class II (8.4%)	Pneumonia – 9
	Hematological disease – 5
	Invasive pulmonary aspergillosis – 5
	Pulmonary hemorrhage – 4
	Other forms of aspergillosis – 2
	Pulmonary candidiasis – 2
Class III (18.7%)	Hemosiderosis – 17
	Secondary malignant neoplasm of kidney and renal pelvis – 9
	Pleural effusion in conditions classified elsewhere – 9
	Secondary malignant neoplasm of other unspecified digestive organ – 5
	Pulmonary hemorrhage – 4
Class IV (20.2%)	Pulmonary hemorrhage – 14
	Pulmonary edema – 8
	Gastrointestinal hemorrhage – 7
	Nontraumatic intracerebral hemorrhage – 6
	Pleural effusion in conditions classified elsewhere – 6
	Secondary malignant lung neoplasm – 5
	Chronic tubulo-interstitial nephritis – 5

The Goldman classification of diagnostic discrepancies was applied. Major discrepancies included two categories (class I referred to missed diagnoses that would have led to a change in management with possible increased survival or cure; class II referred to major missed diagnoses that would not have impacted survival because no treatment was available, treatment was given even though the diagnoses was unknown, or the patient refused further treatment). Minor discrepancies included two categories (class III referred to missed minor diagnoses related to the terminal disease process but not directly related to the cause of death, and class IV referred to missed minor diagnoses that did not contribute to the cause of death but ultimately may have been significant had the patient survived the major illness)

significant concordance between the clinical and postmortem diagnoses in 28 critically ill HSCT patients [15]. Ten (36%) of the twenty eight patients had discrepancies uncovered on autopsy; only two discrepancies would have influenced patient management, and none would have altered patient outcome. Most of the unexpected diagnoses were infections, and the rest included non-infective endocarditis, GVHD, and gastrointestinal and neurologic diagnoses. The authors concluded that clinical diagnosis alone might be appropriate for withdrawal of care decision-making in these patients.

20.5 Summary

Infectious and noninfectious pulmonary diseases are commonly found on postmortem autopsy studies in patients with hematological malignancy and HSCT recipients. Despite the technological advances in diagnostic testing and imaging modalities, obtaining an accurate clinical diagnosis remains difficult and is often not possible until autopsy. Major diagnostic discrepancies between clinical premortem diagnoses and postmortem autopsy findings have been reported in patients with hematologic malignancy. The most common missed diagnoses are due to opportunistic infections and cardiopulmonary complications. These findings underscore the importance of enhanced surveillance, monitoring, and treatment of infections and cardiopulmonary disorders in these patients. Autopsies remain important in determining an accurate cause of death and for improved understanding of diagnostic deficiencies, as well as for medical education and quality assurance.

References

1. Yen K, Lee A, Krowka M, Burger C (2004) Pulmonary complications in bone marrow transplantation: a practical approach to diagnosis and treatment. Clin Chest Med 25:189–201
2. Huaringa AJ, Leyva FJ, Giralt SA et al (2000) Outcome of bone marrow transplantation patients requiring mechanical ventilation. Crit Care Med 28:1014–1017
3. Soubani A, Kseibi E, Bander J et al (2004) Outcome and prognostic factors of hematopoietic stem cell transplantation

recipients admitted to a medical ICU. Chest 126: 1604–1611
4. Pene F, Aubron C, Azoulay E et al (2006) Outcome of critically ill allogeneic hematopoietic stem-cell transplantation recipients: a reappraisal of indications for organ failure supports. J Clin Oncol 24:643–649
5. Bach PB, Schrag D, Nierman DM et al (2001) Identification of poor prognostic features among patients requiring mechanical ventilation after hematopoietic stem cell transplantation. Blood 98:3234–3240
6. Jules-Elysee K, Stover DE, Yahalom J et al (1992) Pulmonary complications in lymphoma patients treated with high-dose therapy autologous bone marrow transplantation. Am Rev Respir Dis 146:485–491
7. Roychowdhury M, Pambuccian SE, Aslan DL et al (2005) Pulmonary complications after bone marrow transplantation: an autopsy study from a large transplantation center. Arch Pathol Lab Med 129:366–371
8. Sharma S, Nadrous H, Peters S et al (2005) Pulmonary complications in adult blood and marrow transplant recipients: autopsy findings. Chest 128:1385–1392
9. Kefford RF, Cooney NJ, Woods RL et al (1981) Causes of deaths in an oncology unit. Eur J Cancer Clin Oncol 17: 1117–1124
10. Marwick C (1995) Pathologists request autopsy revival. JAMA 273:1889, 1891
11. Donhuijsen K, Petersen P, Schmid W (2008) Trend reversal in the frequency of mycoses in hematological neoplasias: autopsy results from 1976 to 2005. Deutsches Ärzteblatt Int 105:501–506
12. Chamilos G, Luna M, Lewis R et al (2006) Invasive fungal infections in patients with hematologic malignancies in a tertiary care cancer center: an autopsy study over a 15-year period (1989–2003). Haematologica 91: 986–989
13. Marr K, Carter R, Crippa F et al (2002) Epidemiology and outcome of mould infections in hematopoietic stem cell transplant recipients. Clin Infect Dis 34:909–917
14. Barth PJ, Rossberg C, Koch S, Ramaswamy A (2000) Pulmonary aspergillosis in an unselected autopsy series. Pathol Res Pract 196:73–80
15. Al-Saidi F, Diaz-Granados N, Messner H et al (2002) Relationship between premortem and postmortem diagnosis in critically ill bone marrow transplantation patients. Crit Care Med 30:570–573
16. Bodey G, Bueltmann B, Duguid W et al (1992) Fungal infections in cancer patients: an international autopsy survey. Eur J Clin Microbiol Infect Dis 11:99–109
17. Chandrasekar PH, Weinmann A, Shearer C (1995) Autopsy-identified infections among bone marrow transplant recipients: a clinico-pathologic study of 56 patients. Bone Marrow Transplantation Team. Bone Marrow Transplant 16: 675–681
18. Groll AH, Shah PM, Mentzel C et al (1996) Trends in the postmortem epidemiology of invasive fungal infections at a university hospital. J Infect 33:23–32
19. Hachem R, Sumoza D, Hanna H et al (2006) Clinical and radiologic predictors of invasive pulmonary aspergillosis in cancer patients: should the European Organization for Research and Treatment of Cancer/Mycosis Study Group (EORTC/MSG) criteria be revised? Cancer 106:1581–1586
20. Subir M, Martino R, Rovira M et al (2003) Clinical applicability of the new EORTC/MSG classification for invasive pulmonary aspergillosis in patients with hematological malignancies and autopsy-confirmed invasive aspergillosis. Ann Hematol 82:80–82
21. Yokoi T, Hirabayashi N, Ito M et al (1997) Broncho-bronchiolitis obliterans as a complication of bone marrow transplantation: a clinicopathological study of eight autopsy cases. Nagoya BMT Group. Virchows Arch 431:275–282
22. Herbrecht R, Denning D, Patterson T et al (2002) Voriconazole versus amphotericin B for primary therapy of invasive aspergillosis. N Engl J Med 347:408–415
23. Pagano L, Fianchi L, Mele L et al (2002) Pneumocystis carinii pneumonia in patients with malignant haematological diseases: 10 years' experience of infection in GIMEMA centres. Br J Haematol 117:379–386
24. Buxhofer V, Ruckser R, Kier P et al (2001) Successful treatment of invasive mould infection affecting lung and brain in an adult suffering from acute leukaemia. Eur J Haematol 67:128–132
25. Kami M, Machida U, Okuzumi K et al (2002) Effect of fluconazole prophylaxis on fungal blood cultures: an autopsy-based study involving 720 patients with haematological malignancy. Br J Haematol 117:40–46
26. Barron MA, Sutton DA, Veve R et al (2003) Invasive mycotic infections caused by Chaetomium perlucidum, a new agent of cerebral phaeohyphomycosis. J Clin Microbiol 41: 5302–5307
27. Bethge WA, Schmalzing M, Stuhler G et al (2005) Mucormycoses in patients with hematologic malignancies: an emerging fungal infection. Haematologica 90(Suppl): ECR22
28. Koyanagi T, Nishida N, Osabe S et al (2006) Autopsy case of disseminated Trichosporon inkin infection identified with molecular biological and biochemical methods. Pathol Int 56:738–743
29. Lagrou K, Massonet C, Theunissen K et al (2005) Fatal pulmonary infection in a leukaemic patient caused by Hormographiella aspergillata. J Med Microbiol 54: 685–688
30. Nosari A, Oreste P, Montillo M et al (2000) Mucormycosis in hematologic malignancies: an emerging fungal infection. Haematologica 85:1068–1071
31. Salonen JH (2006) Successful management of cerebral and pulmonary mucormycosis with liposomal amphotericin B in a 28-year-old woman with acute lymphoblastic leukemia. Acta Biomed 77(Suppl 2):28–31
32. Rüping MJGT, Vehreschild J, Cornely O (2008) Patients at high risk of invasive fungal infections: when and how to treat. Drugs 68:1941–1962
33. Ewig S, Torres A, Riquelme R et al (1998) Pulmonary complications in patients with haematological malignancies treated at a respiratory ICU. Eur Respir J 12:116–122
34. Inai K, Iwasaki H, Noriki S et al (2007) Frequent detection of multidrug-resistant pneumonia-causing bacteria in the pneumonia lung tissues of patients with hematological malignancies. Int J Hematol 86:225–232
35. Rousseau A, Morcos M, Amrouche L et al (2004) Lethal pulmonary hemorrhage caused by a fulminant Stenotrophomonas maltophilia respiratory infection in an acute myeloid leukemia patient. Leuk Lymphoma 45: 1293–1296

36. Torres HA, Aguilera E, Safdar A et al (2008) Fatal cytomegalovirus pneumonia in patients with haematological malignancies: an autopsy-based case-control study. Clin Microbiol Infect 14:1160–1166
37. Zaman SS, Seykora JT, Hodinka RL et al (1996) Cytologic manifestations of respiratory syncytial virus pneumonia in bronchoalveolar lavage fluid: a case report. Acta Cytol 40: 546–551
38. Mori S, Maruyama H, Ito I et al (1998) Diagnosis of measles viral pneumonia in a patient with Hodgkin's disease by reverse transcription-polymerase chain reaction of serum. Int J Hematol 68:327–331
39. Duband S, Cornillon J, Tavernier E et al (2008) Toxoplasmosis with hemophagocytic syndrome after bone marrow transplantation: diagnosis at autopsy. Transpl Infect Dis 10: 372–374
40. Specks U (2001) Diffuse alveolar hemorrhage syndromes. Curr Opin Rheumatol 13:12–17
41. Afessa B, Tefferi A, Litzow M et al (2002) Diffuse alveolar hemorrhage in hematopoietic stem cell transplant recipients. Am J Respir Crit Care Med 166:641–645
42. Lewis ID, DeFor T, Weisdorf DJ (2000) Increasing incidence of diffuse alveolar hemorrhage following allogeneic bone marrow transplantation: cryptic etiology and uncertain therapy. Bone Marrow Transplant 26:539–543
43. Weisdorf DJ (2003) Diffuse alveolar hemorrhage: an evolving problem? Leukemia 17:1049–1050
44. Smith LJ, Katzenstein AL (1982) Pathogenesis of massive pulmonary hemorrhage in acute leukemia. Arch Intern Med 142:2149–2152
45. Grigoriyan A, Rishi A, Molina J et al (2007) Diffuse alveolar damage and hemorrhage in acute myelogenous leukemia treated with corticosteroids. Conn Med 71: 201–204
46. Jiang Q, Yang S-M, Jiang B et al (2007) Diffuse alveolar hemorrhage as a complication in patients with hematologic malignancies after chemotherapy: report of two cases and literature review. Zhonghua Xue Ye Xue Za Zhi 28: 230–234
47. Uchiyama M, Ikeda T (2010). Diffuse alveolar hemorrhage after unrelated cord blood transplantation. Bone Marrow Transplant 45(4):789-90. Epub 2009 Aug 31
48. Nuckols JD (1999) Autopsy findings in umbilical cord blood transplant recipients. Am J Clin Pathol 112:335–342
49. Wojno KJ, Vogelsang GB, Beschorner WE et al (1994) Pulmonary hemorrhage as a cause of death in allogeneic bone marrow recipients with severe acute graft-versus-host disease. Transplantation 57:88–92
50. Delclaux C, Azoulay E (2003) Inflammatory response to infectious pulmonary injury. Eur Respir J Suppl 42:10s–14s
51. Agust C, Ramirez J, Picado C et al (1995) Diffuse alveolar hemorrhage in allogeneic bone marrow transplantation. A postmortem study. Am J Respir Crit Care Med 151: 1006–1010
52. Chao NJ, Duncan SR, Long GD et al (1991) Corticosteroid therapy for diffuse alveolar hemorrhage in autologous bone marrow transplant recipients. Ann Intern Med 114: 145–146
53. Metcalf JP, Rennard SI, Reed EC et al (1994) Corticosteroids as adjunctive therapy for diffuse alveolar hemorrhage associated with bone marrow transplantation. University of Nebraska Medical Center Bone Marrow Transplant Group. Am J Med 96:327–334
54. Pastores S, Papadopoulos E, Voigt L et al (2003) Diffuse alveolar hemorrhage after allogeneic hematopoietic stem-cell transplantation: treatment with recombinant factor VIIa. Chest 124:2400–2403
55. Wanko S, Broadwater G, Folz R et al (2006) Diffuse alveolar hemorrhage: retrospective review of clinical outcome in allogeneic transplant recipients treated with aminocaproic acid. Biol Blood Marrow Transplant 12: 949–953
56. Costa MBG, Siqueira SAC, Saldiva PHN et al (2004) Histologic patterns of lung infiltration of B-cell, T-cell, and Hodgkin lymphomas. Am J Clin Pathol 121:718–726
57. Kaminsky DA, Hurwitz CG, Olmstead JI (2000) Pulmonary leukostasis mimicking pulmonary embolism. Leuk Res 24:175–178
58. Murase T, Yamaguchi M, Suzuki R et al (2007) Intravascular large B-cell lymphoma (IVLBCL): a clinicopathologic study of 96 cases with special reference to the immunophenotypic heterogeneity of CD5. Blood 109:478–485
59. Kitanaka A, Kubota Y, Imataki O et al (2009) Intravascular large B-cell lymphoma with FDG accumulation in the lung lacking CT/(67)gallium scintigraphy abnormality. Hematol Oncol 27:46–49
60. Needleman SW, Stein MN, Hoak JC (1981) Pulmonary embolism in patients with acute leukemia and severe thrombocytopenia. Western J Med 135:9–13
61. Daniels C, Myers J, Utz J et al (2007) Organizing pneumonia in patients with hematologic malignancies: a steroid-responsive lesion. Respir Med 101:162–168
62. Mokhtari M, Bach PB, Tietjen PA et al (2002) Bronchiolitis obliterans organizing pneumonia in cancer: a case series. Respir Med 96:280–286
63. Lee S, Park J-J, Sung S et al (2009) Acute fibrinous and organizing pneumonia following hematopoietic stem cell transplantation. Korean J Intern Med 24:156–159
64. Paz HL, Crilley P, Patchefsky A et al (1992) Bronchiolitis obliterans after autologous bone marrow transplantation. Chest 101:775–778
65. Gutman JA, Allen CT, Madtes DK et al (2008) Pulmonary veno-occlusive disease following reduced-intensity cord blood transplantation. Bone Marrow Transplant 42: 559–561
66. Hackman RC, Madtes DK, Petersen FB et al (1989) Pulmonary venoocclusive disease following bone marrow transplantation. Transplantation 47:989–992
67. Kuga T, Kohda K, Hirayama Y et al (1996) Pulmonary veno-occlusive disease accompanied by microangiopathic hemolytic anemia 1 year after a second bone marrow transplantation for acute lymphoblastic leukemia. Int J Hematol 64: 143–150
68. Mukai M, Kondo M, Bohgaki T et al (2003) Pulmonary veno-occlusive disease following allogeneic peripheral blood stem cell transplantation for chronic myeloid leukaemia. Br J Haematol 123:1
69. Troussard X, Bernaudin JF, Cordonnier C et al (1984) Pulmonary veno-occlusive disease after bone marrow transplantation. Thorax 39:956–957
70. Williams LM, Fussell S, Veith RW et al (1996) Pulmonary veno-occlusive disease in an adult following bone marrow

transplantation. Case report and review of the literature. Chest 109:1388–1391
71. Mandel J, Mark EJ, Hales CA (2000) Pulmonary veno-occlusive disease. Am J Respir Crit Care Med 162: 1964–1973
72. Bunte MC, Patnaik MM, Pritzker MR et al (2008) Pulmonary veno-occlusive disease following hematopoietic stem cell transplantation: a rare model of endothelial dysfunction. Bone Marrow Transplant 41:677–686
73. Cordonnier C, Fleury-Feith J, Escudier E et al (1994) Secondary alveolar proteinosis is a reversible cause of respiratory failure in leukemic patients. Am J Respir Crit Care Med 149:788–794
74. Kajiume T, Yoshimi S, Nagita A et al (1999) A case of myelodysplastic syndrome complicated by pulmonary alveolar proteinosis with a high serum KL-6 level. Pediatr Hematol Oncol 16:367–371
75. Watanabe K, Sueishi K, Tanaka K et al (1990) Pulmonary alveolar proteinosis and disseminated atypical mycobacteriosis in a patient with busulfan lung. Acta Pathol Jpn 40: 63–66
76. Kohno N, Inoue Y, Hamada H et al (1994) Difference in sero-diagnostic values among KL-6-associated mucins classified as cluster 9. Int J Cancer Suppl 8:81–83
77. Gerain J, Sculier JP, Malengreaux A et al (1990) Causes of deaths in an oncologic intensive care unit: a clinical and pathological study of 34 autopsies. Eur J Cancer 26: 377–381
78. Pastores SM, Dulu A, Voigt L et al (2007) Premortem clinical diagnoses and postmortem autopsy findings: discrepancies in critically ill cancer patients. Crit Care 11:R48
79. Xavier AC, Siqueira SA, Costa LJ et al (2005) Missed diagnosis in hematological patients – an autopsy study. Virchows Arch 446:225–231
80. Burton EC, Troxclair DA, Newman W III et al (1998) Autopsy diagnoses of malignant neoplasms. How often are clinical diagnoses incorrect? JAMA 280:1245–1248
81. Provencio M, Espana P, Salas C et al (2000) Hodgkin's disease: correlation between causes of death at autopsy and clinical diagnosis. Ann Oncol 11:59–64
82. Seftel MD, Ho M, Pruthi D et al (2007) High rate of discordance between clinical and autopsy diagnoses in blood and marrow transplantation. Bone Marrow Transplant 40: 1049–1053
83. Hofmeister CC, Marinier DE, Czerlanis C et al (2007) Clinical utility of autopsy after hematopoietic stem cell transplantation. Biol Blood Marrow Transplant 13: 26–30
84. Goldman L, Sayson R, Robbins S et al (1983) The value of the autopsy in three medical eras. N Engl J Med 308: 1000–1005

Part IV

Lung Infections in Patients with HM

Common Viral Pneumonia

21

David Schnell, Jérôme Legoff, and Élie Azoulay

Contents

D. Schnell
Hôpital Saint Louis, Service de Réanimation médicale, Université Denis Diderot, 1 avenue Claude Vellefaux, 75010 Paris Cedex, France

J. Legoff
Hôpital Saint Louis, Laboratoire de Virologie, Université Denis Diderot, 1 avenue Claude Vellefaux, 75010 Paris Cedex, France

É. Azoulay (✉)
Service de Réanimation Médicale, Hôpital Saint-Louis, 1 avenue Claude Vellefaux, 75010, Paris, France and Medical Intensive Care Units, Saint-Louis Hospital, Paris 7 University, Paris, France
e-mail: elie.azoulay@sls.aphp.fr

21.1 Introduction

Common respiratory viruses are probably among the leading causes of community-acquired pneumonia [1, 2] but, oddly enough, have long been underrecognised in patients with haematologic malignancies (HMs), perhaps in part due to the lack of rapid and sensitive diagnostic methods and of effective treatments. Over the last 2 decades, the expanding use of high-dose chemotherapy and haematopoietic stem cell transplantation (HSCT) in various malignancies has improved the prognosis of patients with HMs at the cost of increased opportunities for severe infections [3–5]. Combined with the development of new diagnostic methods and introduction of antiviral drugs, this increased infection rate has rekindled interest in the effects of common respiratory viruses in patients with HMs. These viruses are now recognised as true opportunistic respiratory pathogens in immunocompromised hosts.

21.2 Common Respiratory Viruses

There is no clear definition of common respiratory virus. Viruses that consistently produce respiratory manifestations are considered respiratory viruses. These include members of the following families of RNA viruses: Orthomyxoviridae (human influenza viruses), Paramyxoviridae (respiratory syncytial virus [RSV], parainfluenza viruses [PIV], and human metapneumoviruses [MPV]), Coronaviridae (human respiratory coronaviruses), and Picornaviridae (human rhinoviruses). Other viruses that cause respiratory manifestations in many, but not all, patients are considered respiratory viruses because they are often associated

É. Azoulay (ed.), *Pulmonary Involvement in Patients with Hematological Malignancies*,
DOI: 10.1007/978-3-642-15742-4_21, © Springer-Verlag Berlin Heidelberg 2011

with seasonal respiratory events. Examples include Adenoviridae (adenoviruses) and some Picornaviridae (non-poliomyelitic enteroviruses). A separate chapter of this book focuses on newly discovered and emerging respiratory viruses (avian influenza viruses, newly discovered coronaviruses, polyomaviruses KI and WU, human bocavirus, and mimivirus). CMV and Herpes pneumonia will also be addressed by Dr. Chemaly and colleagues in two different chapters in this book.

Human influenza viruses are enveloped, negative-sense, single-stranded RNA viruses. They are classified into three antigenic types, A, B, and C [6]. The envelope of influenza A and B viruses carries two major antigenic proteins, haemagglutinin (HA) and neuraminidase (NA). HA allows the virus to bind to sialic acid-conjugated glycoproteins at the surface of respiratory epithelium cells. NA plays a crucial role in viral dissemination by releasing newly formed virions from host cells. The influenza C envelope supports a unique protein sharing the properties of both HA and NA and known as haemagglutinin-esterase-fusion factor [6]. Influenza B and C viruses can infect humans and some mammalian species, whereas influenza A also infects most avian species [6].

RSV and PIV types 1–4 are enveloped, negative-sense, single-stranded RNA viruses. RSV belongs to the *Paramyxovirus* genus, and PIV 1–4 to the *Pneumovirus* genus, of the Paramyxoviridae family [7]. Their envelopes support two major antigenic surface proteins, one for binding and one for fusion to the cell membrane. Attachment to host cell receptors is mediated by the G protein of RSV and by a haemagglutinin neuraminidase for PIV [7, 8]. The fusion protein F is common to both genera and allows the virus to penetrate within the host cells after binding [8]. Antigenic variations in the G protein determine two major RSV groups, A and B. Antigenic variations also occur in PIV but have less immunological impact [7]. The natural hosts of RSV are humans and chimpanzees, whereas PIV infects only humans [9, 10]. Human MPV is a recently discovered virus belonging to the Paramyxoviridae family [11]. The human MPV genome and structure are very similar to those of RSV, and both viruses display the same surface proteins [12]. Available data indicate that human MPV infects only humans, although this virus is believed to originate from birds [13].

Human rhinoviruses and non-poliomyelitic enteroviruses are non-enveloped, single-stranded RNA viruses belonging to the Picornaviridae family. The *Rhinovirus* genus consists of more than 100 different serotypes divided into three species (A, B, and the newly described C species) based on antigenic variations in the three proteins VP1, VP2, and VP3 found on the capsid surface [14, 15]. Enteroviruses are divided into four species (A, B, C, and D) [16, 17]. They share the same structure as other Picornaviridae. Humans are the only natural host of these viruses [14, 16].

Coronaviruses are enveloped, positive-sense, single-stranded RNA viruses belonging to the Coronaviridae family [18]. Their envelope supports two main proteins, the haemagglutinin-esterase protein and the antigenic protein S [18]. Human coronaviruses 229E and OC43 were the predominant human respiratory coronavirus strains before the recent identification of the new human coronaviruses NL63, HKU1, and SARS [19–21].

Adenoviruses are non-enveloped, double-stranded DNA viruses that form the Adenoviridae family. Six subgenera (A–F) and 51 human serotypes of adenoviruses have been described [22]. Adenoviruses have an icosahedral capsid made of 250 protein subunits called capsomeres [23]. Humans are the only natural hosts of these viruses.

21.3 Epidemiology

Common respiratory viruses are ubiquitous pathogens that share a number of epidemiological features. Most of them are responsible for outbreaks that occur with a remarkable seasonal pattern. These seasonal variations in viral activity occur only in temperate climates and tend to disappear in equatorial zones. This phenomenon is incompletely understood and may involve not only specific viral characteristics, but also seasonal changes in living conditions [6]. Influenza, RSV, human MPV, and Coronavirus activities peak during the winter months [6, 7, 18]. PIV1 and 2 cause outbreaks in the fall [7]. Seasonality is less pronounced for PIV3 and Picornaviridae, which exhibit year-round activity with peaks in the spring for PIV3, spring and fall for human rhinoviruses, and summer and fall for non-poliomyelitic Enteroviruses [7, 14, 16]. Little is known about the epidemiology of PIV4, since this virus is responsible for mild infections and is therefore rarely identified [7].

Common respiratory viruses typically cause infections in early childhood. Influenza C usually causes mild infections that lead to the acquisition of protective antibodies capable of preventing recurrences [24]. Influenza A and B are considerably more common and can cause disease of greater severity, most notably in high-risk groups, such as elderly people and patients with chronic respiratory or cardiovascular conditions, chronic renal failure, diabetes mellitus, or immune deficiencies [6]. It is estimated that about 5% of adults and 20% of children experience an influenza episode every year throughout the world [25]. Although most influenza episodes are mild, the high occurrence rate results in a huge burden of disease that has a severe socioeconomic impact [6]. Influenza viruses are believed to be the seventh cause of death in the USA [26]. Influenza A and B infections start in childhood and continue to occur throughout the life span, because antigenic variations affecting HA and, to a lesser extent NA, hamper the acquisition of protective immunity. Two mechanisms of antigenic variations have been described, antigenic drift and antigenic shift [6]. Antigenic drift probably results from the accumulation of point mutations that occur continuously in influenza viruses, with new variants appearing annually or every few years. These new variants replace pre-existing ones by immunological selection and are only incompletely recognised by immunity resulting from exposure to earlier strains. Antigenic shift is a considerably rarer event that occurs only in influenza A and results in a virus with a completely new HA or NA [6]. The result is an influenza pandemic due to the absence of protective immunity against the new virus. Progressive acquisition of immunity against this new strain attenuates the intensity of the epidemic over the following years. The exact genetic mechanisms of antigenic shift are incompletely known, and the emergence of pandemic strains is not predictable. Pandemic strains originate from the recombination of influenza strains circulating in different animal species, including birds, pigs, and humans [6]. Five pandemics occurred in the twentieth century, and the 2009 "Mexican flu" pandemic due to the new H1N1 influenza virus is the first pandemic in the twenty-first century [6, 27]. RSV and PIV are typically infections of early childhood [7]. RSV and, to a lesser extent, PIV also undergo antigenic changes that lead to recurrences throughout the life span. These recurrences may be severe, especially in patients with chronic respiratory conditions and in the elderly. The burden of RSV-related diseases may be comparable to that of influenza [28].

Few data are available on the specific epidemiological characteristics of common respiratory viruses in patients with HMs. Reported incidence rates vary widely, from 1.8% to 30% [29, 30]. This variability may be explained by disparities in the type of patients enrolled, reasons for screening patients for respiratory viruses and, most importantly, diagnostic methods used. Whatever the exact incidence, one can reasonably assume that attack rates of common respiratory viruses in immunocompromised patients are closely related to the prevalence of respiratory viruses in the community, which serves as the viral reservoir for immunocompromised patients [31]. This has been confirmed in recent studies showing that the occurrence of viral respiratory diseases in the enrolled immunocompromised patients paralleled the concomitant viral activity in the community [32, 33]. Accordingly, influenza viruses and RSV are the viruses most commonly identified in the largest cohorts of HM patients, each accounting for about one-third of viral respiratory events [34–36]. PIV, Picornaviridae, and adenoviruses come next. It must be pointed out that influenza viruses accounted for a much higher proportion (up to 75%) of viral respiratory events in the study by Martino et al. conducted in the setting of a major influenza outbreak in the community [32].

Adenovirus epidemiology in patients with HM deserves special attention. Similar to other common respiratory viruses, adenoviruses cause primary infections in childhood, usually during the first few years of life. Adenoviruses may account for 5% to 10% of viral respiratory infections in children [23], and also cause outbreaks in closed and semi-closed populations of young adults such as the military [37, 38]. A distinctive feature of adenoviruses is the ability to cause chronic latent infection by persisting in lymphoepithelial tissues, most notably in the nasopharynx [23]. The epidemiology of adenoviruses in patients with HM has not been the focus of specific studies. Nevertheless, exogenous contamination, by the respiratory or orofaecal route, may be less important than reactivation of the latent virus [39]. Thus, adenoviral infections in patients with HM may be related chiefly to the level of immunosuppression and, perhaps, to unknown viral factors driving reactivation, rather than to the level of viral activity in the community.

The epidemiologic characteristics of influenza, RSV, and PIV are particularly well known, perhaps in part because infections with these viruses are considerably more common compared to those due to other viruses. However, the availability of simple and rapid diagnostic tools for these three viruses probably played a great role. Since Picornaviridae, Coronaviridae, and the newly discovered human MPV are mainly diagnosed using reverse-transcriptase polymerase-chain-reaction technology (rt-PCR), data on their epidemiology are still limited. Recent studies using rt-PCR detection of respiratory viruses in patients with HM revealed a high incidence of human MPV infections, similar to that of RSV infections [30, 36]. In the near future, studies using molecular biology tools may help to clarify the epidemiology of common respiratory viruses and may lead to a radical change in current concepts.

21.4 Clinical Manifestations

Common respiratory virus infections have been studied chiefly in patients receiving high-dose chemotherapy and haematopoietic stem cell transplantation (HSCT). Compared with immunocompetent patients, several distinctive features have been reported. Viral shedding lasts longer and progression to pneumonia is more common [31]. Late airflow obstruction has been reported in HSCT recipients [40]. Some respiratory viruses are responsible for extra-respiratory manifestations. Although rare in immunocompetent hosts, these manifestations might be more common in patients with HM.

Common respiratory viral infections in patients with HM are characterized by prolonged viral shedding. A median duration of 2 weeks was found in most studies [30, 32, 33, 36]. However, viral shedding may last for months in some cases [41, 42]. In addition, the amount of virus shed per day may be greater in HM patients than in immunocompetent individuals [43]. Similarly to findings in immunocompromised patients, children shed more viruses over a longer period than do adults [31]. This prolonged high-load viral shedding is of critical importance, since it may enhance both viral dissemination [43, 44] and the emergence of resistant strains via prolonged exposure to antiviral drugs [41, 42].

As stated above, common respiratory viruses have long been underrecognised in patients with HM. In the 1990s, the first reports of common respiratory virus infections focused on influenza and RSV [45–50]. In these studies, progression to pneumonia occurred in about 75% of patients infected with influenza viruses and 50% of those infected with RSV, and was associated with mortality rates of 25% for influenza and about 80% for RSV. One possible explanation for these striking observations may be a surge of interest in respiratory viral infections in HM patients that led to the publication of the most severe cases. Not surprisingly, these studies had small numbers of patients and high rates of nosocomial infections.

More recently, studies of large patient cohorts led to better characterization of influenza-related pneumonia in patients with HM [29, 32–34]. About one-third of patients develop lower respiratory tract infection (LRTI). Although less common than in previous reports, influenza-related pneumonia remains a severe condition with a 15–30% mortality rate. As in immunocompetent hosts, upper respiratory tract infection (URTI) is almost always present and often precedes LRTI [32, 49, 51, 52]. URTI can be considered a useful argument supporting the diagnosis of respiratory viral infection in patients with HM investigated for pneumonia [53]. However, the identification of a common respiratory virus does not exclude an associated bacterial or fungal infection. These co-infections are very frequent, occurring in 12–25% of cases of influenza-related pneumonia [32, 34, 50]. There are no reports of extra-respiratory manifestations in patients with HM, although myocarditis, pericarditis, myositis, meningoencephalitis, Guillain-Barré syndrome, and Reye syndrome have been described in immunocompetent patients [6, 54].

RSV-related pneumonia is now believed to complicate about 30–40% of RSV infections in patients with HM [32, 34, 47]. Again, mortality remains high, ranging from 15% to 30%. URTI is a common clinical manifestation. No clear data on the incidence of concomitant bacterial or fungal infections are available in the literature, and RSV-related pneumonia in patients with HM are often ascribed to viral infection [53]. However, bacterial co-infections were present in as many as 30% of patients in a large study of RSV infections in immunocompetent individuals [55]. Bacterial or fungal co-infection may be more common in patients with HM and must be carefully sought. Non-sustained viraemia may accompany RSV infection, and RSV was associated with cardiac arrhythmias and neurological disorders in two case reports [8, 56]. However, no extra-respiratory manifestations of RSV infection have been described in immunocompromised patients.

PIV infections have also been studied in patients with HM [34, 57]. PIV type 3 was the cause in 90% of reported cases. In these studies, PIV-related pneumonia was comparable to influenza-related pneumonia, with about one third of patients being affected, a high rate of concomitant URTI, and a 15–30% mortality rate. Co-infections were found in as many as 53% of the patients studied by Nichols et al. [57]. However, in a recent study using rt-PCR for routine respiratory virus detection in HSCT recipients, PIV was found in respiratory samples of asymptomatic patients [30], whereas influenza, RSV, and human MPV were not detected. This finding suggests that studies using conventional diagnostic methods may have overestimated the true severity of PIV in patients with HM. Some reports suggested a role for PIV3 in the occurrence of neurologic manifestations (such as meningitis, encephalitis, and Guillain-Barré syndrome) and myocarditis [58]. Such manifestations have not been reported in immunocompromised patients.

Case reports suggest that the recently discovered human MPV may induce severe pneumonia in patients with HM [59–61]. To our knowledge, two retrospective cohorts [62, 63] and three prospective cohorts [30, 36, 64] describing human MPV infections in patients with HM have been published. The small number of patients and highly variable results (pneumonia in 0–43% of patients with a 0–40% mortality rate) preclude definitive conclusions about human MPV-related pneumonia in patients with HM. Although debated, the occurrence of asymptomatic viral shedding may suggest lesser severity of human MPV-related pneumonia compared to influenza and RSV [30, 65]. Two cases of encephalitis with human MPV detected in cerebrospinal fluid in immunocompetent paediatric patients have been published [66, 67]. No extra-respiratory manifestations have been reported in patients with HM.

Since the identification of Picornaviridae and Coronaviridae relies chiefly on molecular biology tools, only limited data are available about their contribution to respiratory viral infections in patients with HM. Epidemiological evidence supports an association of human rhinovirus with LRTI in immunocompetent children and elderly people [68, 69]. Despite growing evidence that human rhinovirus is able to replicate in lower respiratory tract cells in vitro and in vivo [70, 71], whether this virus can cause pneumonia remains debated [72]. Several reports in patients with HM link human rhinovirus to LRTI [73–77]. However, these retrospective studies in small patient populations with high rates of pulmonary co-pathogen identification fail to demonstrate a clear role for human rhinovirus in the development of pneumonia. Non-poliomyelitic enteroviruses are chiefly responsible for URTI [16]. Only a few studies with small numbers of patients have focused on these viruses in patients with HM, and no conclusions can be drawn from their results [77–80]. Coronaviridae are also principally responsible for URTI but may occasionally cause pneumonia [81]. No studies have evaluated the role of Coronaviridae in patients with HM, and only two case reports have been published [82, 83].

Although it is now clear that most of the common respiratory viruses are responsible for an increased rate of pneumonia in patients with HM (Table 21.1 and Fig. 21.1–21.3), the exact nature and causative mechanisms of pneumonia in this situation remain unknown. The only risk factor for virus-related pneumonia found consistently in studies is lymphocytopenia, defined

Table 21.1 Clinical manifestations of influenza, respiratory syncytial virus (RSV), parainfluenza virus (PIV), human metapneumovirus (hMPV), and adenovirus in patients with haematological malignancies

	Influenza	RSV	PIV	hMPV	Adenovirus
Pneumonia rate (%)	33	30–40	Up to 30[a]	Up to 40[a]	NA
Coinfection rate (%)	12–25	NA	Up to 50[a]	NA	50
Mortality rate (%)	15–30	15–30	15–30[a]	Up to 40[a]	50–80
Asymptomatic shedding	No	No	Yes	Yes	No

NA not available

[a]The occurrence of asymptomatic viral shedding may indicate lesser severity than previously thought

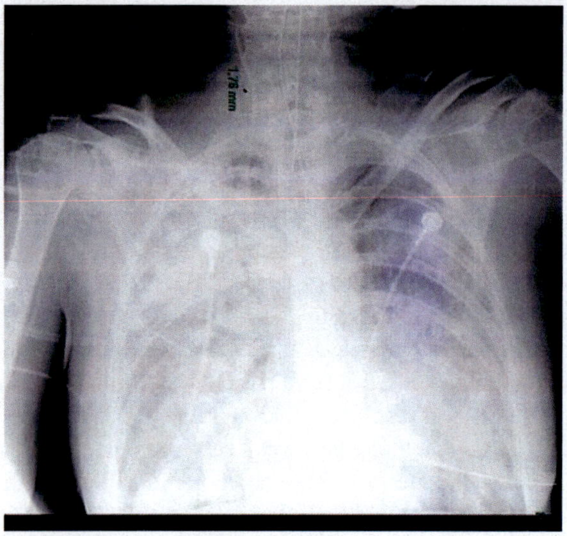

Fig. 21.1 Diffuse alveolo-interstitial pneumonia in a PIV3-infected patient

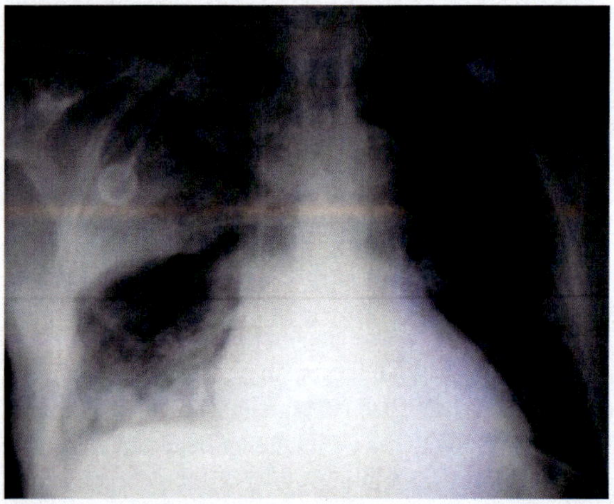

Fig. 21.2 Diffuse alveolar consolidations in a patient co-infected with influenza and *Streptococcus pneumoniae*

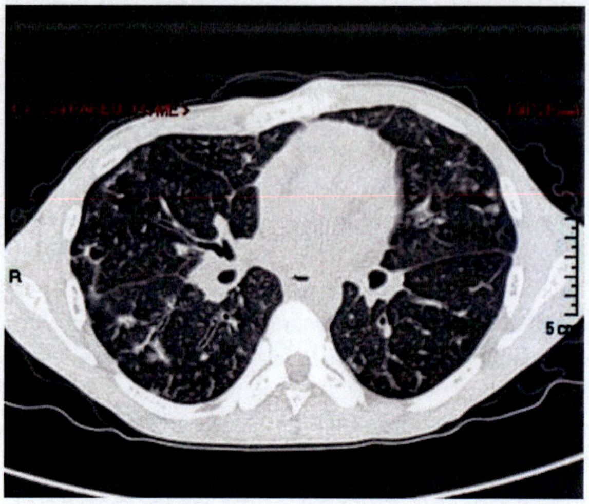

Fig. 21.3 Thoracic CT scan showing bronchiolitis pattern (bronchial wall thickening associated with ground-glass attenuation, interlobular septa thickening and tree-in-bud opacities) in an influenza-infected patient

using a variety of cutoffs [29, 32–34]. One study found that lymphocytopenia (absolute lymphocyte count less than 200 cells/mL) was independently associated with mortality in patients with influenza-related pneumonia [34]. A higher incidence and greater severity of virus-related pneumonia have been noted in HSCT recipients compared with other patients with HM. This finding may reflect deeper lymphocyte depletion. However, in a study by Martino et al., pneumonia rates were comparable in patients with and without lymphocytopenia [32]. The possible higher incidence and greater severity of virus-related pneumonia within the first few days after HSCT, compared with infections occurring later on, may reflect deeper lymphocyte depletion [53]. A similar mechanism may underlie the surprising protective effect of corticosteroid therapy in the study by Nichols et al., since this treatment is often given to treat graft-versus-host disease (GVHD) after lymphoid engraftment [33].

Common respiratory viruses increase mortality in patients with HM mainly by causing severe pneumonia, but they may also contribute to a long-term decline in pulmonary function. RSV, PIV, and influenza infections have been linked to late airflow obstruction in HSCT recipients [40]. In a study focusing specifically on the role of respiratory viruses in late airflow obstruction, PIV LRTI was the strongest risk factor, followed by PIV URTI [84]. Pneumonia caused by RSV was a borderline-significant risk factor. The exact causative mechanisms remain unknown, but inflammation resulting from prolonged viral persistence and pneumonia-induced post-acute-phase inflammation have been suggested as possible factors [84, 85].

A distinctive feature of adenoviruses in HM patients is that they may either be acquired via exogenous respiratory or oro-faecal contamination, or arise via reactivation of latent viruses [39, 86]. Adenoviruses cause a wide spectrum of clinical manifestations ranging from benign conjunctivitis to rapidly fatal disseminated disease. In patients with HM, the risk of severe adenoviral disease seems related to the level of immunosuppression. Adenoviral disease has been reported in 3–27% of HSCT recipients within the first 100 days after transplantation [87–89]. Higher rates may occur in paediatric patients compared with adults [88, 90]. In vivo and ex vivo graft T-cell depletion [86, 87, 91], lymphocytopenia [86], GVHD [87, 89], viral shedding from more than one site [86, 88, 90], and adenovirus viraemia [86, 92–94] have been reported as risk factors for severe adenoviral disease. Adenovirus viraemia consistently preceded viral shedding from more than one site in the study by Chakrabarti et al. [86]. This risk factor is of critical importance since it guides pre-emptive antiviral therapy. Adenoviral disease has been chiefly reported in myeloablative HSCT recipients, but has also been described in non-myeloablative HSCT recipients, autologous transplant recipients, and patients with chronic lymphocytic leukaemia treated with fludarabine combined with CD52 monoclonal antibodies [88, 89]. In allogeneic transplant recipients, the most frequent manifestations of adenoviral infection are gastrointestinal disease and haemorrhagic cystitis [95, 96]. Although haemorrhagic cystitis is a benign localised event, it is associated with high morbidity [90]. It must be pointed out that in a patient with febrile haematuria and adenovirus urinary excretion, the onset of acute renal failure with flank pain may reveal adenovirus nephritis [97]. Gastrointestinal manifestations include gastroenteritis and colitis, which often manifest as febrile haemorrhagic diarrhoea [95, 98]. The most severe manifestations of adenoviral infection are hepatitis, encephalitis, and pneumonia [86, 89, 90]. Adenovirus-related pneumonia occurred in 15 of the 85 patients with adenovirus infection in the study by La Rosa et al. [89]. The pneumonia was isolated in 11 patients and a manifestation of disseminated disease in 4 patients. Bacterial and fungal co-infections were found in 50% of patients, in keeping with other studies [90]. The mortality rate was 73% overall, 50% in patients with isolated pneumonia, and 80% in patients with disseminated disease [89].

21.5 Diagnosis

Respiratory viral infections are the second most common cause of community-acquired pneumonia [2, 99]. They were long considered a simple differential diagnosis, without practical consequences for the patient. Recently, however, the diagnosis of viral respiratory infection has become increasingly relevant for medical care [100, 101]. First, RSV, influenza, PIV, and adenoviruses have been identified as significant causes of community-acquired and nosocomial respiratory infections [29, 102]. Second, new nucleic acid-based assays have been shown to be more sensitive than conventional techniques. Third, specific antiviral drugs are now available for some respiratory viruses, including influenza and adenovirus. Several diagnostic tests have been introduced for the detection of respiratory viruses. The main characteristics of the most widely used assays are shown in Table 21.2.

High-quality clinical specimens are needed to ensure the accurate detection of respiratory viruses. Indeed, respiratory virus detection requires a large number of epithelial cells, since viruses are intracellular pathogens. Nasopharyngeal aspirates and nasopharyngeal washes are recognised to be superior to other sample types for detecting respiratory viruses [103, 104]. Because the collection process is unpleasant and

Table 21.2 Methods for detecting common respiratory viruses

Test	Sensitivity	Specificity	Time to result	Viral targets	Cost
Immunofluorescence staining	++	++	<3 h	<8	15–25 Euros
Rapid antigen testing (immunochromatography)	+	+/++	<1 h	Only available for influenza and RSV	10–15 Euros per test
Cell culture	+	+++	Days to weeks	Depending on the cell lines used	NA
Monoplex NASBA or real-time PCR assay	+++	+++	<12 h	1 or 2 per reaction	10–20 Euros per target
Multiplex molecular assay	+++	++/+++	6 h–24 h	12–20 per reaction in 1 or 2 tubes	50–80 Euros per panel

time-consuming, causes patient discomfort, and requires a suction device, flocked swabs were recently introduced for respiratory sample collection. Flocked swabs were found to improve the collection and release of epithelial cells [105, 106], and were recently recommended for the diagnosis of the new pandemic H1N1 influenza strain. The number of cells collected is lower with flocked swabs than with nasopharyngeal aspirates, but seems sufficient for respiratory virus detection by immunofluorescence [105, 106]. Flocked swab collection is sensitive, specific, easy to use, and better tolerated by patients, and may therefore constitute a good alternative to nasopharyngeal aspiration. Because most respiratory viruses have high replication rates in the upper respiratory tract, nasopharyngeal secretions are usually sufficient to diagnose respiratory viral infections. However, asymptomatic respiratory virus shedding in the upper respiratory tract may occur even in immunocompromised patients, and URTI may be followed by LRTI, particularly during influenza infections. Thus, virus detection in lungs via bronchoalveolar lavage may be useful to assess the causative role for the virus.

Over the past 2 decades, virus isolation and antigen detection have been the mainstay of clinical laboratory testing for respiratory virus infections. Virus isolation required several cell lines and was mainly performed on shell vial cultures. The diagnosis was based on the presence of the cytopathic effect, which requires several days or weeks to develop. To shorten the time to diagnosis, specific monoclonal antibodies were introduced to enable the detection of specific viral antigens within 1–2 days. Direct or indirect fluorescent antibody staining of cells from respiratory specimens (mainly nasopharyngeal swabs or nasopharyngeal aspirates [NPA] and bronchoalveolar lavage fluid) is commonly used to detect viral antigens. In many laboratories, the first-line test is immunofluorescence staining, which requires very little material and provides a result within about 3 h. However commercial monoclonal antibodies are available for a limited number of targets, including influenza A and B; RSV; adenovirus; PIV 1, 2 and 3; and human MPV. Thus, rhinoviruses and coronaviruses, the most frequent causes of URTI and the most recently discovered agents, cannot be detected using monoclonal antibodies.

Nucleic acid amplification tests have been proven to be rapid, very sensitive, and specific. The early tests, including PCR, nucleic acid sequence-based amplification (NASBA), and real-time PCR assays, were developed in monoplex format. Despite the gain in sensitivity and the ability to test for most respiratory viruses, the need to carry out as many PCR tests as targets has limited the use of this method. None of the current PCR assays has sufficiently high throughput to handle large numbers of samples containing multiple targets. Over the last few years, assays have been introduced in multiplex format. Different technologies have been used. In addition, sensitivities may be lower compared to monoplex real-time RT-PCR. Multiplex PCR procedures are difficult to optimise, because each amplification target corresponds to a set of primers characterized by a unique combination of optimal annealing conditions. Multiple primers included in a single tube may also result in primer-primer interference and in nonspecific nucleic acid amplification.

Currently, several multiplex assays can detect up to nine respiratory viruses in a single reaction. Real-time multiplex assays detect up to five targets in a single reaction, depending on the number of channels available in the real-time PCR machine [107–110]. Existing multiplex PCR assays that use agarose gel electrophoresis or capillary electrophoresis as the detection system or multiplex PCR assays combined with an enzyme-linked immunosorbent assay can detect five to nine targets per reaction [111–113].

More recently introduced techniques can detect up to 20 targets in one or two tubes. These include the four techniques detailed below.

1. *Low-density micro-array* based on cDNA spots that are immobilised on a polymer-coated slide and that hybridise with specific DNA sequences previously amplified from the sample using PCR. Hybridisation is detected based on the production of an insoluble product on the microarray at the sites where amplified DNA products are captured by the probes [114].
2. *Multiplex detection based on Luminex* technology. The PCR products are coupled with spectrally distinct fluorescence-labelled micro-beads, which are detected by flow cytometry [115, 116].
3. *Multiplex ligation-dependent probe amplification (MLPA)* involves specific viral amplification followed by amplification after hybridisation and binding of virus-specific probes to the PCR product. Identification is accomplished by PCR fragment size analysis using gel electrophoresis methods [117, 118].

4. *Mass spectrometry* assays for respiratory virus detection are based on the analysis of base compositions in RT-PCR amplicons [119].

Most assays exhibited specificities comparable to those of cell culture and monoplex real-time reverse transcription (RT)-PCR, and sensitivities similar to those of monoplex (RT)-PCR assays.

Although molecular assays, particularly RT-PCR, provide same-day results, they require a nucleic acid extraction step. This step increases the time to results compared to antigen detection by fluorescent staining. Molecular assays should be performed as often as possible to improve patient care by shortening the hospital stay, curtailing or preventing antibiotic therapy, preventing nosocomial spread, and allowing specific antiviral therapy. Therefore, and given the cost of the equipment needed (RT-PCR machine, sequencer, luminex, nucleic acid extractor, DNA chip reader, mass spectrometer), molecular assays will probably be chiefly performed in laboratories receiving large numbers of samples per day.

Few data are available on the exhaustive and sensitive detection of respiratory viruses in HM patients. Recent data show that using molecular assays increases the virus detection rate twofold compared to cultures and fourfold compared to immunofluorescence staining [120]. Two prospective studies of molecular assays in HSCT recipients documented persistent asymptomatic respiratory shedding of PIV and human MPV [30, 65]. These data emphasise the need for prospective studies of the molecular detection of respiratory viruses to elucidate factors associated with symptomatic or asymptomatic respiratory viral infection and to help in the interpretation of positive assays in HM patients.

21.5.1 Antiviral Treatment

A chapter from Dr. Sandherr is dedicated to antiviral therapy in this book. Regarding common viruses, we will briefly describe available treatments on influenza and RSV. Two classes of antiviral drugs are available for the treatment of influenza: M2 ion channel inhibitors and neuraminidase inhibitors. The M2 ion channel inhibitors, amantadine and rimantadine, act by inhibiting the M2 protein needed for viral RNA release within the host cells. They are active only against influenza A strains. Their clinical effect is limited, being not significantly different from that of a placebo [121], and is further hampered by the worldwide emergence of resistant influenza A strains [122]. The neuraminidase inhibitors (Table 21.3), oral oseltamivir and inhaled zanamivir, are sialic acid analogues that competitively inhibit the influenza neuraminidase. Randomised controlled trials

Table 21.3 Antiviral treatments for common viral pneumonia

	Oseltamivir	Zanamivir	Ribavirin	Cidofovir
Therapeutic class	Neuraminidase inhibitor	Neuraminidase inhibitor	Nucleoside analogue	Nucleoside analogue
Route	Oral	Inhaled	Inhaled	Intravenous
Regimen	75 mg *bid*	10 mg *bid*	Up to 2 g *tid*[a]	5 mg/kg weekly[a]
Duration	5 days	5 days	10 days[a]	Variable[b]
Side effects	Rash	Rash bronchospasm	Haemolytic anaemia[d] bronchospasm	Nephrotoxicity[c] myelosuppression retinitis
Indication	Influenza	Influenza	RSV[e]	Adenovirus[e]
Evidence supporting use	Cohort studies	Cohort studies	Cohort studies	Cohort studies

NA not available, *bid* twice daily, *tid* three times daily

[a]The therapeutic regimens are those described in the available literature

[b]Cidofovir is given in a dose of 5 mg/kg weekly for 2 weeks then every 2 weeks according to the clinical response

[c]Hyperhydratation and probenecide may help to prevent cidofovir nephrotoxicity

[d]Haemolytic anaemia may be readily controlled by blood transfusion

[e]These drugs have not been approved by regulating authorities in these indications

showed moderate decreases in symptom intensity and duration with both drugs [123–125]. Neuraminidase inhibitors may also limit bacterial super-infection of the lungs [125, 126]. Early administration of these drugs seems mandatory to obtain a clinical benefit [127]. A more recent cohort study suggested a diminution of 15-day mortality with neuraminidase inhibitors [128]. This result must be interpreted with caution, especially given the study design. There is growing concern about the emergence of oseltamivir-resistant influenza A strains [129]. This phenomenon is not surprising given the high mutation rate in the influenza genome. It should lead clinicians to reconsider the indications of neuraminidase inhibitors and their use as monotherapy to treat influenza [130]. No randomised controlled trials have evaluated the efficacy of neuraminidase inhibitors in patients with HM. The apparently lower mortality in descriptive cohort studies compared with historical studies must be interpreted with caution [33–35, 131]. Many of the patients in these cohorts had bacterial and fungal co-infections, whose specific treatment probably contributed to decreasing mortality. Furthermore, the decision to treat patients was left to clinician discretion, which may have introduced a bias toward selection of patients with greater disease severity. Given both the absence of strong evidence supporting beneficial effects of neuraminidase inhibitor therapy and the rapid emergence of resistant strains, we believe that neuraminidase inhibitor therapy cannot be recommended for HM patients with influenza. Randomised controlled trials are needed to determine the efficacy, safety, and ecological impact of neuraminidase inhibitors in these patients.

Ribavirin is the only available antiviral drug for Paramyxoviridae infection (Table 21.3). The efficacy of aerosolized ribavirin was variable in uncontrolled cohorts of patients with RSV-related pneumonia [34, 46, 132]. Again, the results must be interpreted with caution. Early ribavirin therapy, introduced before the onset of respiratory failure, seemed associated with lower mortality in the study by Whimbey et al. [132]. This observation led some authors to evaluate pre-emptive ribavirin therapy, characterised by ribavirin treatment of RSV URTI to prevent progression to pneumonia [133, 134]. The study by Boeckh et al. is the only randomised controlled trial evaluating pre-emptive ribavirin therapy in patients with RSV infection [133]. Unfortunately, the trial did not enrol a sufficient number of patients to produce conclusions. Intravenous ribavirin has also been evaluated and found unhelpful [29, 135]. Combining ribavirin with intravenous immunoglobulins or RSV-specific immunoglobulins produced variable levels of efficacy in cohort studies [35, 132, 136, 137]. Palivizumab, an RSV-specific monoclonal antibody, was evaluated only in a small cohort [138].

In vitro, ribavirin exhibits mild antiviral activity against PIV [58]. No clear efficacy of aerosolized ribavirin was found in small, uncontrolled cohorts of patients with HM [34, 139]. Early initiation of ribavirin therapy has been proposed to enhance efficacy [140]. No studies have evaluated intravenous immunoglobulins or RSV-specific immunoglobulins, which contain high titres of PIV-specific immunoglobulins.

An in vitro study suggests that ribavirin may be of interest for treating human MPV-related pneumonia, but this drug has not been evaluated in patients with HM [141].

To date, there is no strong evidence supporting the use of ribavirin, either alone or combined with immunoglobulins, to treat Paramyxoviridae-related pneumonia in patients with HM.

No controlled randomised study has evaluated the treatment of adenoviral disease in patients with HM. Ribavirin and cidofovir have been suggested for the treatment of adenoviral infections, but only uncontrolled cohort studies are available to support their use. Intravenous ribavirin therapy failed to demonstrate benefits in available studies [89, 142–147]. Cidofovir therapy (Table 21.3) seemed to result in better outcomes in small, uncontrolled series [148–153]. Ganciclovir and antiretroviral drugs, such as zalcitabine, alovudine, and stavudine, exhibit in vitro activity against adenoviruses, but have not been specifically evaluated in clinical settings [95, 154]. Considering the lack of specific antiviral drugs, decreasing the level of immunosuppression seems to be a rational treatment approach [155]. T-cell therapy has also been reported in some small series [155, 156]. Early cidofovir treatment seems associated with a better outcome [151]. Weekly PCR screening for adenovirus viraemia has been suggested to guide pre-emptive cidofovir therapy [91–94, 153, 157]. The exact threshold above which pre-emptive cidofovir therapy should be initiated is unknown. Randomised controlled trials are needed to better define the optimal viraemia threshold for antiviral therapy and to evaluate the benefits from this treatment.

The greater severity of common respiratory viral infections in HM patients and the lack of clearly proven effective antiviral drugs emphasise the critical importance of preventive strategies.

21.6 Prevention

The occurrence of common respiratory virus infections in patients with HM is closely related to viral activity in the community. However, nosocomial outbreaks have been described in haematologic wards, often within a few days after an outbreak in the community [31, 43, 44, 46, 158–160]. Preventing nosocomial transmission of common respiratory viruses requires a multifaceted approach (Table 21.4) that targets not only the modes of transmission, but also the source of the viruses [43]. Nosocomial outbreaks are believed to originate from infected patients and from infected health-care workers. Infection control measures include screening symptomatic patients for common respiratory viruses, early isolation of infected patients, screening healthcare workers and visitors for respiratory symptoms, and avoiding contact of symptomatic individuals with patients. Most haematologic wards do not allow children to visit patients, as children are highly prone to common respiratory virus infections and may exhibit viral shedding long after symptom resolution [39]. Continual reinforcement of standard hygiene measures, especially hand hygiene before and after contact with patients, is also strongly recommended. Awareness of the usefulness of these measures, and therefore adherence to the measures, are low, but can be enhanced by educational programs [161]. Most of the common respiratory viruses are transmitted by droplets or direct contact of infected secretions with the nasal mucosa or conjunctiva. Indirect transmission via contaminated fomites or devices is also possible, since these viruses may survive several hours on these surfaces [6, 7, 58]. Consequently, contact isolation of infected patients combined with droplet precautions is mandatory [162]. A gown, gloves, and a mask with eye protection must be worn for all contacts with infected patients. Airborne transmission of influenza is suspected [163, 164] but not yet proven, and two recent studies suggest that surgical masks may be as effective in preventing influenza transmission as masks with greater filtration capacity [165, 166]. Infection control measures have not been evaluated in randomised control trials, but a before-and-after study suggests they may help to prevent the transmission of common respiratory viruses [43]. It must be pointed out that asymptomatic viral shedding, when present, limits the effectiveness of infection control measures [30, 65]. The optimal duration of isolation is unknown. Whether isolation should be prolonged in asymptomatic patients with persistent low-titre viral shedding detected only by molecular methods remains unclear. Since adenovirus acquisition is known to result also from endogenous reactivation, adenoviral infections may be chiefly related to the level of immunosuppression [39, 86] and, therefore, may not be effectively prevented by standard infection control measures.

Table 21.4 Infection control measures for common respiratory viruses

Specific infection control measures
Screening patients for respiratory virus infections
Contact isolation with droplet precautions for infected patients
Screening visitors and healthcare workers for URTI symptoms
Prohibiting visits by individuals with URTI symptoms
Prohibiting work for healthcare workers with URTI symptoms
Prohibiting visits by children
Enhanced standard precautions
Reinforced hand hygiene before and after contact with patients
Annual influenza immunisation
Patients with HM
Family contacts of patients
Health-care workers

To date, influenza is the only common respiratory virus for which a vaccine is available. Immunisation remains the cornerstone of influenza prevention [6]. The immunogenicity of the inactivated influenza vaccine is lower in patients with HM compared with immunocompetent controls [167–172]. A second dose of influenza vaccine has been proposed to enhance immunogenicity, but this strategy was not beneficial in an open-label randomised study [169, 170]. The timing of influenza immunisation may be important. Immunogenicity may be improved by giving the vaccine at least 6 months after HSCT or at least 7 days after intensive chemotherapy [168, 171]. The efficacy of influenza immunisation has not been evaluated in randomised control trials. However, a retrospective cohort study suggested benefits from influenza immunisation in HSCT recipients [173]. Influenza immunisation appears safe in patients with HM, and lifelong seasonal administration of the influenza vaccine is therefore recommended in these high-risk patients [174]. Importantly, family contacts should be immunised also to prevent transmission within the household. Of critical importance is the issue of health-care worker immunisation, which is known to prevent nosocomial acquisition of the virus [175].

Pharmacological interventions have been proposed to prevent common respiratory virus infections. Intravenous immunoglobulins and palivizumab have been suggested for RSV infection prevention, but have not been evaluated in patients with HM. Prophylactic post-exposure oseltamivir therapy is currently recommended in patients with HM [176]. This preventive measure has not been evaluated in randomised controlled trials, but seems safe based on a recent retrospective study in HSCT recipients [177]. Considering the lack of proven benefits of oseltamivir therapy and the growing concern about the emergence of oseltamivir-resistant influenza strains, oseltamivir therapy should be carefully evaluated before it is suggested for use on a large scale [130].

Another way to prevent morbidity and mortality related to common respiratory viruses in patients with HM is to limit the risk of progression to pneumonia. The pre-emptive treatment of viral URTI has been discussed above. Given the severity of common respiratory virus pneumonia in patients with HM, it appears logical and prudent to postpone HSCT in patients with documented viral infections. A retrospective cohort study suggested that this measure might prevent RSV-related pneumonia in patients undergoing HSCT [178]. It is unclear whether this measure might be applied to all types of HSCT, to intensive chemotherapy courses, and for all respiratory viruses.

21.7 Conclusion

Common respiratory viruses are now recognised as true opportunistic respiratory pathogens in patients with HM. In these patients, they constitute a common cause of potentially severe pneumonia. However, areas of uncertainty remain, indicating a need for further investigations. The epidemiology of common respiratory virus infections in patients with HM has not been extensively studied. Large epidemiological studies of common respiratory virus infections in patients with HM based on molecular biology tools may lead to radical changes in knowledge. Although it is now clear that common respiratory viruses are responsible for increased pneumonia rates in patients with HM, the exact nature and causative mechanisms of these pneumonia cases remain unknown. Studies are warranted to investigate the role of viruses in the development of these LRTIs. The virus might directly injure alveolar epithelium or promote lung super-infection by causing bronchial epithelium damage. These studies would also help to determine the potential benefit of pre-emptive or curative antiviral therapy. Finally, randomised controlled studies of antiviral therapy in patients with HM are urgently needed.

References

1. File TM (2003) Community-acquired pneumonia. Lancet 362(9400):1991–2001
2. de Roux A et al (2004) Viral community-acquired pneumonia in nonimmunocompromised adults. Chest 125(4):1343–1351
3. Brenner H (2002) Long-term survival rates of cancer patients achieved by the end of the 20th century: a period analysis. Lancet 360(9340):1131–1135
4. Coiffier B et al (2002) CHOP chemotherapy plus rituximab compared with CHOP alone in elderly patients with diffuse large-B-cell lymphoma. N Engl J Med 346(4):235–242
5. Nachman JB et al (1998) Augmented post-induction therapy for children with high-risk acute lymphoblastic leukemia and a slow response to initial therapy. N Engl J Med 338(23):1663–1671
6. Treanor JJ (2005) Influenza virus. In: Mandell G (ed) Principles and practice of infectious diseases, 6th edn. Churchill Livingston, Philadelphia, p 2060
7. Hall CB (2001) Respiratory syncytial virus and parainfluenza virus. N Engl J Med 344(25):1917–1928
8. Falsey AR, Walsh EE (2000) Respiratory syncytial virus infection in adults. Clin Microbiol Rev 13(3):371–384
9. Hall CB, Mccarthy CA (2005) Respiratory syncytial virus. In: Mandell G (ed) Principles and practice of infectious diseases, 6th edn. Churchill Livingstone, Philadelphia, p 2008
10. Wright PF (2005) Parainfluenza viruses. In: Mandell G (ed) Principles and practice of infectious diseases, 6th edn. Churchill Livingstone, Philadelphia, p 1998

11. van den Hoogen BG et al (2001) A newly discovered human pneumovirus isolated from young children with respiratory tract disease. Nat Med 7(6):719–724
12. Kahn JS (2006) Epidemiology of human metapneumovirus. Clin Microbiol Rev 19(3):546–557
13. Falsey AR (2005) Human metapneumovirus. In: Mandell G (ed) Principles and practice of infectious diseases, 6th edn. Churchill Livingstone, Philadelphia, p 2027
14. Greenberg SB (2003) Respiratory consequences of rhinovirus infection. Arch Intern Med 163(3):278–284
15. McErlean P et al (2008) Distinguishing molecular features and clinical characteristics of a putative new rhinovirus species, human rhinovirus C (HRV C). PLoS ONE 3(4): e1847
16. Modlin JF (2005) Introduction to the enteroviruses. In: Mandell G (ed) Principles and practice of infectious diseases. Churchill Livingstone, Philadelphia, p 2141
17. Stanway G (2005) Family Picornaviridae. In: Fauquet CM, Mayo MA, Maniloff J, Desselberger U, Ball LA (eds) Virus taxonomy. Eighth report of the International Committee on Taxonomy of Viruses. Elsevier London, pp 757–778
18. Mcintosh K, Anderson LJ (2005) Coronaviruses, including severe acute respiratory syndrome (SARS)-associated coronavirus. In: Mandell G (ed) Principles and practice of infectious diseases, 6th edn. Churchill Livingstone, Philadelphia, p 1990
19. Kuiken T et al (2003) Newly discovered coronavirus as the primary cause of severe acute respiratory syndrome. Lancet 362(9380):263–270
20. van der Hoek L et al (2004) Identification of a new human coronavirus. Nat Med 10(4):368–373
21. Woo PC et al (2005) Characterization and complete genome sequence of a novel coronavirus, coronavirus HKU1, from patients with pneumonia. J Virol 79(2):884–895
22. Matthews RE (1981) The classification and nomenclature of viruses: summary of results of meetings of the International Committee on taxonomy of viruses in strasbourg, august 1981. Intervirology 16:53
23. Baum SG (2005) Adenovirus. In: Mandell G (ed) Principles and practice of infectious diseases, 6th edn. Churchill Livingstone, Philadelphia, p 1624
24. Matsuzaki Y et al (2006) Clinical features of influenza C virus infection in children. J Infect Dis 193(9):1229–1235
25. Turner D et al (2003) Systematic review and economic decision modelling for the prevention and treatment of influenza A and B. Health Technol Assess 7(35):iii–iv, xi-xiii, 1–170
26. Dushoff J et al (2006) Mortality due to influenza in the United States – an annualized regression approach using multiple-cause mortality data. Am J Epidemiol 163(2): 181–187
27. Dawood FS et al (2009) Emergence of a novel swine-origin influenza A (H1N1) virus in humans. N Engl J Med 360(25):2605–2615
28. Falsey AR et al (2005) Respiratory syncytial virus infection in elderly and high-risk adults. N Engl J Med 352(17): 1749–1759
29. Ljungman P et al (2001) Respiratory virus infections after stem cell transplantation: a prospective study from the Infectious Diseases Working Party of the European Group for Blood and Marrow Transplantation. Bone Marrow Transplant 28(5):479–484
30. Peck AJ et al (2007) Respiratory virus infection among hematopoietic cell transplant recipients: evidence for asymptomatic parainfluenza virus infection. Blood 110(5): 1681–1688
31. Couch RB, Englund JA, Whimbey E (1997) Respiratory viral infections in immunocompetent and immunocompromised persons. Am J Med 102(3A):2–9, discussion 25-6
32. Martino R et al (2003) Respiratory virus infections in adults with hematologic malignancies: a prospective study. Clin Infect Dis 36(1):1–8
33. Nichols WG et al (2004) Influenza infections after hematopoietic stem cell transplantation: risk factors, mortality, and the effect of antiviral therapy. Clin Infect Dis 39(9): 1300–1306
34. Chemaly RF et al (2006) Respiratory viral infections in adults with hematologic malignancies and human stem cell transplantation recipients: a retrospective study at a major cancer center. Medicine (Baltimore) 85(5):278–287
35. Machado CM et al (2003) Low mortality rates related to respiratory virus infections after bone marrow transplantation. Bone Marrow Transplant 31(8):695–700
36. Martino R et al (2005) Prospective study of the incidence, clinical features, and outcome of symptomatic upper and lower respiratory tract infections by respiratory viruses in adult recipients of hematopoietic stem cell transplants for hematologic malignancies. Biol Blood Marrow Transplant 11(10):781–796
37. Kolavic-Gray SA et al (2002) Large epidemic of adenovirus type 4 infection among military trainees: epidemiological, clinical, and laboratory studies. Clin Infect Dis 35(7): 808–818
38. Ryan MA et al (2002) Large epidemic of respiratory illness due to adenovirus types 7 and 3 in healthy young adults. Clin Infect Dis 34(5):577–582
39. Boeckh M (2008) The challenge of respiratory virus infections in hematopoietic cell transplant recipients. Br J Haematol 143(4):455–467
40. Chien JW et al (2003) Airflow obstruction after myeloablative allogeneic hematopoietic stem cell transplantation. Am J Respir Crit Care Med 168(2):208–214
41. Boivin G, Goyette N, Bernatchez H (2002) Prolonged excretion of amantadine-resistant influenza a virus quasi species after cessation of antiviral therapy in an immunocompromised patient. Clin Infect Dis 34(5):E23–E25
42. Weinstock DM, Gubareva LV, Zuccotti G (2003) Prolonged shedding of multidrug-resistant influenza A virus in an immunocompromised patient. N Engl J Med 348(9): 867–868
43. Raad I, Abbas J, Whimbey E (1997) Infection control of nosocomial respiratory viral disease in the immunocompromised host. Am J Med 102(3A):48–52, discussion 53-4
44. Zambon M et al (1998) Molecular epidemiology of two consecutive outbreaks of parainfluenza 3 in a bone marrow transplant unit. J Clin Microbiol 36(8):2289–2293
45. Elting LS et al (1995) Epidemiology of influenza A virus infection in patients with acute or chronic leukemia. Support Care Cancer 3(3):198–202
46. Harrington RD et al (1992) An outbreak of respiratory syncytial virus in a bone marrow transplant center. J Infect Dis 165(6):987–993

47. Khanna N et al (2008) Respiratory syncytial virus infection in patients with hematological diseases: single-center study and review of the literature. Clin Infect Dis 46(3): 402–412
48. Whimbey E et al (1995) Respiratory syncytial virus pneumonia in hospitalized adult patients with leukemia. Clin Infect Dis 21(2):376–379
49. Whimbey E et al (1994) Influenza A virus infections among hospitalized adult bone marrow transplant recipients. Bone Marrow Transplant 13(4):437–440
50. Yousuf HM et al (1997) Influenza among hospitalized adults with leukemia. Clin Infect Dis 24(6):1095–1099
51. Ladisla B (1996) Community respiratory virus infections in hospitalized adult patients with leukemia. In: Abstract of the Infectious Diseases Society of America, 1996, New Orleans, Louisiana, p. Abstract No. 99
52. Whimbey E et al (1996) Community respiratory virus infections among hospitalized adult bone marrow transplant recipients. Clin Infect Dis 22(5):778–782
53. Whimbey E, Englund JA, Couch RB (1997) Community respiratory virus infections in immunocompromised patients with cancer. Am J Med 102(3A):10–18, discussion 25-6
54. Sivadon-Tardy V et al (2009) Guillain-Barre syndrome and influenza virus infection. Clin Infect Dis 48(1):48–56
55. Falsey AR et al (1995) Respiratory syncytial virus and influenza A infections in the hospitalized elderly. J Infect Dis 172(2):389–394
56. Yui I et al (2003) Detection of human respiratory syncytial virus sequences in peripheral blood mononuclear cells. J Med Virol 70(3):481–489
57. Nichols WG, Gooley T, Boeckh M (2001) Community-acquired respiratory syncytial virus and parainfluenza virus infections after hematopoietic stem cell transplantation: the Fred Hutchinson Cancer Research Center experience. Biol Blood Marrow Transplant 7(Suppl):11S–15S
58. Henrickson KJ (2003) Parainfluenza viruses. Clin Microbiol Rev 16(2):242–264
59. Cane PA et al (2003) Human metapneumovirus in a haematopoietic stem cell transplant recipient with fatal lower respiratory tract disease. Bone Marrow Transplant 31(4):309–310
60. Englund JA et al (2006) Brief communication: fatal human metapneumovirus infection in stem-cell transplant recipients. Ann Intern Med 144(5):344–349
61. Pelletier G et al (2002) Respiratory tract reinfections by the new human metapneumovirus in an immunocompromised child. Emerg Infect Dis 8(9):976–978
62. Kamboj M et al (2008) Clinical characterization of human metapneumovirus infection among patients with cancer. J Infect 57(6):464–471
63. Oliveira R et al (2008) Frequency of human metapneumovirus infection in hematopoietic SCT recipients during 3 consecutive years. Bone Marrow Transplant 42(4): 265–269
64. Williams JV et al (2005) A prospective study comparing human metapneumovirus with other respiratory viruses in adults with hematologic malignancies and respiratory tract infections. J Infect Dis 192(6):1061–1065
65. Debiaggi M et al (2007) Long-term study on symptomless human metapneumovirus infection in hematopoietic stem cell transplant recipients. New Microbiol 30(3):255–258
66. Kaida A et al (2006) Seasonal distribution and phylogenetic analysis of human metapneumovirus among children in Osaka City, Japan. J Clin Virol 35(4):394–399
67. Schildgen O et al (2005) Human metapneumovirus RNA in encephalitis patient. Emerg Infect Dis 11(3):467–470
68. Nicholson KG et al (1996) Risk factors for lower respiratory complications of rhinovirus infections in elderly people living in the community: prospective cohort study. BMJ 313(7065):1119–1123
69. Papadopoulos NG (2004) Do rhinoviruses cause pneumonia in children? Paediatr Respir Rev 5(Suppl A):S191–S195
70. Hayden FG (2004) Rhinovirus and the lower respiratory tract. Rev Med Virol 14(1):17–31
71. Papadopoulos NG et al (2000) Rhinoviruses infect the lower airways. J Infect Dis 181(6):1875–1884
72. Kaiser L, Hayden FG (1999) Editorial response: rhinovirus pneumonia–a clinical entity? Clin Infect Dis 29(3):533–535
73. Ghosh S et al (1999) Rhinovirus infections in myelosuppressed adult blood and marrow transplant recipients. Clin Infect Dis 29(3):528–532
74. Gutman JA et al (2007) Rhinovirus as a cause of fatal lower respiratory tract infection in adult stem cell transplantation patients: a report of two cases. Bone Marrow Transplant 40(8):809–811
75. Imakita M et al (2000) Pneumonia caused by rhinovirus. Clin Infect Dis 30(3):611–612
76. Ison MG et al (2003) Rhinovirus infections in hematopoietic stem cell transplant recipients with pneumonia. Clin Infect Dis 36(9):1139–1143
77. Parody R et al (2007) Upper and lower respiratory tract infections by human enterovirus and rhinovirus in adult patients with hematological malignancies. Am J Hematol 82(9):807–811
78. Gonzalez Y et al (1999) Pulmonary enterovirus infections in stem cell transplant recipients. Bone Marrow Transplant 23(5):511–513
79. Gonzalez Y et al (1999) Community respiratory virus infections in patients with hematologic malignancies. Haematologica 84(9):820–823
80. Rabella N et al (1999) Conventional respiratory viruses recovered from immunocompromised patients: clinical considerations. Clin Infect Dis 28(5):1043–1048
81. Kahn JS, McIntosh K (2005) History and recent advances in coronavirus discovery. Pediatr Infect Dis J 24(11 Suppl): S223–S227, discussion S226
82. Folz RJ, Elkordy MA (1999) Coronavirus pneumonia following autologous bone marrow transplantation for breast cancer. Chest 115(3):901–905
83. Pene F et al (2003) Coronavirus 229E-related pneumonia in immunocompromised patients. Clin Infect Dis 37(7): 929–932
84. Erard V et al (2006) Airflow decline after myeloablative allogeneic hematopoietic cell transplantation: the role of community respiratory viruses. J Infect Dis 193(12): 1619–1625
85. Walter MJ et al (2002) Viral induction of a chronic asthma phenotype and genetic segregation from the acute response. J Clin Invest 110(2):165–175
86. Chakrabarti S et al (2002) Adenovirus infections following allogeneic stem cell transplantation: incidence and outcome in relation to graft manipulation, immunosuppression, and immune recovery. Blood 100(5):1619–1627

87. Flomenberg P et al (1994) Increasing incidence of adenovirus disease in bone marrow transplant recipients. J Infect Dis 169(4):775–781
88. Howard DS et al (1999) Adenovirus infections in hematopoietic stem cell transplant recipients. Clin Infect Dis 29(6): 1494–1501
89. La Rosa AM et al (2001) Adenovirus infections in adult recipients of blood and marrow transplants. Clin Infect Dis 32(6):871–876
90. Baldwin A et al (2000) Outcome and clinical course of 100 patients with adenovirus infection following bone marrow transplantation. Bone Marrow Transplant 26(12):1333–1338
91. Lion T et al (2003) Molecular monitoring of adenovirus in peripheral blood after allogeneic bone marrow transplantation permits early diagnosis of disseminated disease. Blood 102(3):1114–1120
92. Echavarria M et al (2001) Prediction of severe disseminated adenovirus infection by serum PCR. Lancet 358 (9279):384–385
93. Erard V et al (2007) Quantitative real-time polymerase chain reaction for detection of adenovirus after T cell-replete hematopoietic cell transplantation: viral load as a marker for invasive disease. Clin Infect Dis 45(8):958–965
94. Schilham MW et al (2002) High levels of adenovirus DNA in serum correlate with fatal outcome of adenovirus infection in children after allogeneic stem-cell transplantation. Clin Infect Dis 35(5):526–532
95. Bruno B et al (2003) Adenovirus infection in hematopoietic stem cell transplantation: effect of ganciclovir and impact on survival. Biol Blood Marrow Transplant 9(5):341–352
96. Hale GA et al (1999) Adenovirus infection after pediatric bone marrow transplantation. Bone Marrow Transplant 23(3):277–282
97. Bruno B et al (2004) Adenovirus nephritis in hematopoietic stem-cell transplantation. Transplantation 77(7):1049–1057
98. Cox GJ et al (1994) Etiology and outcome of diarrhea after marrow transplantation: a prospective study. Gastroenterology 107(5):1398–1407
99. Glezen WP et al (2000) Impact of respiratory virus infections on persons with chronic underlying conditions. JAMA 283(4):499–505
100. Barenfanger J et al (2000) Clinical and financial benefits of rapid detection of respiratory viruses: an outcomes study. J Clin Microbiol 38(8):2824–2828
101. Woo PC et al (1997) Cost-effectiveness of rapid diagnosis of viral respiratory tract infections in pediatric patients. J Clin Microbiol 35(6):1579–1581
102. Singh-Naz N, Brown M, Ganeshananthan M (1993) Nosocomial adenovirus infection: molecular epidemiology of an outbreak. Pediatr Infect Dis J 12(11):922–925
103. Heikkinen T et al (2002) Nasal swab versus nasopharyngeal aspirate for isolation of respiratory viruses. J Clin Microbiol 40(11):4337–4339
104. Stensballe LG et al (2002) Comparison of nasopharyngeal aspirate and nasal swab specimens for detection of respiratory syncytial virus in different settings in a developing country. Trop Med Int Health 7(4):317–321
105. Abu-Diab A et al (2008) Comparison between pernasal flocked swabs and nasopharyngeal aspirates for detection of common respiratory viruses in samples from children. J Clin Microbiol 46(7):2414–2417
106. Daley P et al (2006) Comparison of flocked and rayon swabs for collection of respiratory epithelial cells from uninfected volunteers and symptomatic patients. J Clin Microbiol 44(6):2265–2267
107. Gunson RN, Collins TC, Carman WF (2005) Real-time RT-PCR detection of 12 respiratory viral infections in four triplex reactions. J Clin Virol 33(4):341–344
108. Legoff J et al (2008) Evaluation of the one-step multiplex real-time reverse transcription-PCR ProFlu-1 assay for detection of influenza A and influenza B viruses and respiratory syncytial viruses in children. J Clin Microbiol 46(2): 789–791
109. Markoulatos P, Siafakas N, Moncany M (2002) Multiplex polymerase chain reaction: a practical approach. J Clin Lab Anal 16(1):47–51
110. Templeton KE et al (2004) Rapid and sensitive method using multiplex real-time PCR for diagnosis of infections by influenza a and influenza B viruses, respiratory syncytial virus, and parainfluenza viruses 1, 2, 3, and 4. J Clin Microbiol 42(4):1564–1569
111. Grondahl B et al (1999) Rapid identification of nine microorganisms causing acute respiratory tract infections by single-tube multiplex reverse transcription-PCR: feasibility study. J Clin Microbiol 37(1):1–7
112. Legoff J et al (2005) High prevalence of respiratory viral infections in patients hospitalized in an intensive care unit for acute respiratory infections as detected by nucleic acid-based assays. J Clin Microbiol 43(1):455–457
113. Liolios L et al (2001) Comparison of a multiplex reverse transcription-PCR-enzyme hybridization assay with conventional viral culture and immunofluorescence techniques for the detection of seven viral respiratory pathogens. J Clin Microbiol 39(8):2779–2783
114. Cannon GA et al (2010) A low density oligonucleotide microarray for the detection of viral and atypical bacterial respiratory pathogens. J Virol Methods 163(1):17–24
115. Li H et al (2007) Simultaneous detection and high-throughput identification of a panel of RNA viruses causing respiratory tract infections. J Clin Microbiol 45(7):2105–2109
116. Pabbaraju K et al (2008) Comparison of the Luminex xTAG respiratory viral panel with in-house nucleic acid amplification tests for diagnosis of respiratory virus infections. J Clin Microbiol 46(9):3056–3062
117. Dominguez SR et al (2008) Multiplex MassTag-PCR for respiratory pathogens in pediatric nasopharyngeal washes negative by conventional diagnostic testing shows a high prevalence of viruses belonging to a newly recognized rhinovirus clade. J Clin Virol 43(2):219–222
118. Reijans M et al (2008) RespiFinder: a new multiparameter test to differentially identify fifteen respiratory viruses. J Clin Microbiol 46(4):1232–1240
119. Sampath R et al (2007) Global surveillance of emerging Influenza virus genotypes by mass spectrometry. PLoS ONE 2(5):e489
120. Kuypers J et al (2009) Comparison of conventional and molecular detection of respiratory viruses in hematopoietic cell transplant recipients. Transpl Infect Dis 11(4): 298–303
121. Jefferson TO et al (2002) Amantadine and rimantadine for preventing and treating influenza A in adults. Cochrane Database Syst Rev (3):CD001169

122. Bright RA et al (2006) Adamantane resistance among influenza A viruses isolated early during the 2005-2006 influenza season in the United States. JAMA 295(8): 891–894
123. The MIST (Management of Influenza in the Southern Hemisphere Trialists) Study Group (1998) Randomised trial of efficacy and safety of inhaled zanamivir in treatment of influenza A and B virus infections. Lancet 352(9144):1877–1881
124. Nicholson KG et al (2000) Efficacy and safety of oseltamivir in treatment of acute influenza: a randomised controlled trial. Neuraminidase Inhibitor Flu Treatment Investigator Group. Lancet 355(9218):1845–1850
125. Treanor JJ et al (2000) Efficacy and safety of the oral neuraminidase inhibitor oseltamivir in treating acute influenza: a randomised controlled trial. US Oral Neuraminidase Study Group. JAMA 283(8):1016–1024
126. Monto AS, Webster A, Keene O (1999) Randomized, placebo-controlled studies of inhaled zanamivir in the treatment of influenza A and B: pooled efficacy analysis. J Antimicrob Chemother 44(Suppl B):23–29
127. Aoki FY et al (2003) Early administration of oral oseltamivir increases the benefits of influenza treatment. J Antimicrob Chemother 51(1):123–129
128. McGeer A et al (2007) Antiviral therapy and outcomes of influenza requiring hospitalization in Ontario, Canada. Clin Infect Dis 45(12):1568–1575
129. Hauge SH et al (2009) Oseltamivir-resistant influenza viruses A (H1N1), Norway, 2007-08. Emerg Infect Dis 15(2):155–162
130. Poland GA, Jacobson RM, Ovsyannikova IG (2009) Influenza virus resistance to antiviral agents: a plea for rational use. Clin Infect Dis 48(9):1254–1256
131. Machado CM et al (2004) Use of Oseltamivir to control influenza complications after bone marrow transplantation. Bone Marrow Transplant 34(2):111–114
132. Whimbey E et al (1995) Combination therapy with aerosolized ribavirin and intravenous immunoglobulin for respiratory syncytial virus disease in adult bone marrow transplant recipients. Bone Marrow Transplant 16(3): 393–399
133. Boeckh M et al (2007) Randomized controlled multicenter trial of aerosolized ribavirin for respiratory syncytial virus upper respiratory tract infection in hematopoietic cell transplant recipients. Clin Infect Dis 44(2):245–249
134. Ghosh S et al (2001) Respiratory syncytial virus infections in autologous blood and marrow transplant recipients with breast cancer: combination therapy with aerosolized ribavirin and parenteral immunoglobulins. Bone Marrow Transplant 28(3):271–275
135. Lewinsohn DM et al (1996) Phase I study of intravenous ribavirin treatment of respiratory syncytial virus pneumonia after marrow transplantation. Antimicrob Agents Chemother 40(11):2555–2557
136. DeVincenzo JP et al (2000) Respiratory syncytial virus immune globulin treatment of lower respiratory tract infection in pediatric patients undergoing bone marrow transplantation - a compassionate use experience. Bone Marrow Transplant 25(2):161–165
137. Ghosh S et al (2000) Respiratory syncytial virus upper respiratory tract illnesses in adult blood and marrow transplant recipients: combination therapy with aerosolized ribavirin and intravenous immunoglobulin. Bone Marrow Transplant 25(7):751–755
138. Boeckh M et al (2001) Phase 1 evaluation of the respiratory syncytial virus-specific monoclonal antibody palivizumab in recipients of hematopoietic stem cell transplants. J Infect Dis 184(3):350–354
139. Nichols WG et al (2001) Parainfluenza virus infections after hematopoietic stem cell transplantation: risk factors, response to antiviral therapy, and effect on transplant outcome. Blood 98(3):573–578
140. Chakrabarti S et al (2000) Parainfluenza virus type 3 infections in hematopoetic stem cell transplant recipients: response to ribavirin therapy. Clin Infect Dis 31(6): 1516–1518
141. Wyde PR et al (2003) Comparison of the inhibition of human metapneumovirus and respiratory syncytial virus by ribavirin and immune serum globulin in vitro. Antiviral Res 60(1):51–59
142. Bordigoni P et al (2001) Treatment of adenovirus infections in patients undergoing allogeneic hematopoietic stem cell transplantation. Clin Infect Dis 32(9):1290–1297
143. Chakrabarti S et al (1999) Fulminant adenovirus hepatitis following unrelated bone marrow transplantation: failure of intravenous ribavirin therapy. Bone Marrow Transplant 23(11):1209–1211
144. Gavin PJ, Katz BZ (2002) Intravenous ribavirin treatment for severe adenovirus disease in immunocompromised children. Pediatrics 110(1 Pt 1):e9
145. Liles WC et al (1993) Severe adenoviral nephritis following bone marrow transplantation: successful treatment with intravenous ribavirin. Bone Marrow Transplant 12(4):409–412
146. Mann D et al (1998) Failure of intravenous ribavirin in the treatment of invasive adenovirus infection following allogeneic bone marrow transplantation: a case report. J Infect 36(2):227–228
147. Miyamura K et al (2000) Successful ribavirin therapy for severe adenovirus hemorrhagic cystitis after allogeneic marrow transplant from close HLA donors rather than distant donors. Bone Marrow Transplant 25(5):545–548
148. Hoffman JA et al (2001) Adenoviral infections and a prospective trial of cidofovir in pediatric hematopoietic stem cell transplantation. Biol Blood Marrow Transplant 7(7): 388–394
149. Legrand F et al (2001) Early diagnosis of adenovirus infection and treatment with cidofovir after bone marrow transplantation in children. Bone Marrow Transplant 27(6): 621–626
150. Ljungman P et al (2003) Cidofovir for adenovirus infections after allogeneic hematopoietic stem cell transplantation: a survey by the Infectious Diseases Working Party of the European Group for Blood and Marrow Transplantation. Bone Marrow Transplant 31(6):481–486
151. Neofytos D et al (2007) Treatment of adenovirus disease in stem cell transplant recipients with cidofovir. Biol Blood Marrow Transplant 13(1):74–81
152. Sivaprakasam P et al (2007) Improved outcome from invasive adenovirus infection in pediatric patients after hemopoietic stem cell transplantation using intensive clinical surveillance and early intervention. J Pediatr Hematol Oncol 29(2):81–85

153. Yusuf U et al (2006) Cidofovir for the treatment of adenoviral infection in pediatric hematopoietic stem cell transplant patients. Transplantation 81(10):1398–1404
154. Naesens L et al (2005) Antiadenovirus activities of several classes of nucleoside and nucleotide analogues. Antimicrob Agents Chemother 49(3):1010–1016
155. Chakrabarti S et al (2000) Adenovirus infections following haematopoietic cell transplantation: is there a role for adoptive immunotherapy? Bone Marrow Transplant 26(3): 305–307
156. Feuchtinger T et al (2006) Safe adoptive transfer of virus-specific T-cell immunity for the treatment of systemic adenovirus infection after allogeneic stem cell transplantation. Br J Haematol 134(1):64–76
157. Teramura T et al (2002) Quantitative detection of serum adenovirus in a transplant recipient. Lancet 359(9321): 1945
158. Cortez KJ et al (2001) Outbreak of human parainfluenza virus 3 infections in a hematopoietic stem cell transplant population. J Infect Dis 184(9):1093–1097
159. Kim S et al (2009) Molecular epidemiological investigation of a nosocomial outbreak of human metapneumovirus infection in a pediatric hemato-oncology patient population. J Clin Microbiol 47(4):1221–1224
160. Nichols WG et al (2004) Prolonged outbreak of human parainfluenza virus 3 infection in a stem cell transplant outpatient department: insights from molecular epidemiologic analysis. Biol Blood Marrow Transplant 10(1):58–64
161. Daugherty EL et al (2009) The use of personal protective equipment for control of influenza among critical care clinicians: A survey study. Crit Care Med 37(4):1210–1216
162. Siegel JD et al (2007) 2007 Guideline for Isolation Precautions: Preventing Transmission of Infectious Agents in Health Care Settings. Am J Infect Control 35(10 Suppl 2):S65–S164
163. Blachere FM et al (2009) Measurement of airborne influenza virus in a hospital emergency department. Clin Infect Dis 48(4):438–440
164. Bridges CB, Kuehnert MJ, Hall CB (2003) Transmission of influenza: implications for control in health care settings. Clin Infect Dis 37(8):1094–1101
165. Johnson DF et al (2009) A quantitative assessment of the efficacy of surgical and N95 masks to filter influenza virus in patients with acute influenza infection. Clin Infect Dis 49(2):275–277
166. Loeb M et al (2009) Surgical mask vs N95 respirator for preventing influenza among health care workers: a randomized trial. JAMA 302:1865–1871
167. Brydak LB et al (2006) Humoral response to hemagglutinin components of influenza vaccine in patients with non-Hodgkin malignant lymphoma. Vaccine 24(44–46): 6620–6623
168. Engelhard D et al (1993) Antibody response to a two-dose regimen of influenza vaccine in allogeneic T cell-depleted and autologous BMT recipients. Bone Marrow Transplant 11(1):1–169. Ljungman P, Nahi H, Linde A (2005) Vaccination of patients with haematological malignancies with one or two doses of influenza vaccine: a randomised study. Br J Haematol 130(1):96–98
170. Lo W et al (1993) Antibody response to a two-dose influenza vaccine regimen in adult lymphoma patients on chemotherapy. Eur J Clin Microbiol Infect Dis 12(10): 778–782
171. Ortbals DW et al (1977) Influenza immunization of adult patients with malignant diseases. Ann Intern Med 87(5): 552–557
172. Pauksen K et al (2000) Granulocyte-macrophage colony-stimulating factor as immunomodulating factor together with influenza vaccination in stem cell transplant patients. Clin Infect Dis 30(2):342–348
173. Machado CM et al (2005) The benefit of influenza vaccination after bone marrow transplantation. Bone Marrow Transplant 36(10):897–900
174. Ljungman P et al (2005) Vaccination of stem cell transplant recipients: recommendations of the Infectious Diseases Working Party of the EBMT. Bone Marrow Transplant 35(8):737–746
175. Salgado CD et al (2004) Preventing nosocomial influenza by improving the vaccine acceptance rate of clinicians. Infect Control Hosp Epidemiol 25(11):923–928
176. Groupe de Travail (2005) Taking care of influenza in the context of a pandemic in 2005. Full text. Med Mal Infect 35(Suppl 4):S245–273
177. Vu D et al (2007) Safety and tolerability of oseltamivir prophylaxis in hematopoietic stem cell transplant recipients: a retrospective case-control study. Clin Infect Dis 45(2): 187–193
178. Peck AJ, Corey L, Boeckh M (2004) Pretransplantation respiratory syncytial virus infection: impact of a strategy to delay transplantation. Clin Infect Dis 39(5):673–680

Emerging Viral Infections

22

Oliver Schildgen

Contents

22.1 Introduction

Emerging infectious diseases according to the CDC-hosted journal *Emerging Infectious Diseases* (www.cdc.gov/ncidod/EID/about/background.htm) are defined as diseases "whose incidence in humans has increased in the past two decades or that are expected to have an increased incidence in the near future." These diseases respect no regional, national, or international boarders and include (1) new infections resulting from changes or evolution of existing organisms, (2) known infections spreading to new geographic areas or populations, (3) previously unrecognized infections appearing in areas undergoing ecologic transformation, (4) old infections re-emerging as a result of antimicrobial resistance, and, finally and most importantly for the field of virology, (5) infections caused by newly discovered agents.

After the discovery of the human metapneumovirus (hMPV) in 2001 and the 2002/2003 outbreak of severe acute respiratory syndrome (SARS), the number of known emerging viruses expanded at a fast pace, mainly due to the development of novel virus identification methods and their routine use in patients with suspected infections but negative findings from conventional diagnostic methods. This chapter focuses on these new pathogens and highlights their role in patients with hematological malignancies.

22.2 Human Metapneumovirus

In 2001 the hMPV was described as the third known *Paramyxovirinae* to cause disease in humans, together with the respiratory syncytial virus (RSV) and

O. Schildgen
Kliniken der Stadt Köln gGmbH, Institut für Pathologie, Ostmerheimer Str. 200, 51109 Köln/Cologne, Germany and Private University, Witten/Herdecke, Germany
e-mail: schildgeno@kliniken-koeln.de, oliver.schildgen@freenet.de

É. Azoulay (ed.), *Pulmonary Involvement in Patients with Hematological Malignancies*, DOI: 10.1007/978-3-642-15742-4_22, © Springer-Verlag Berlin Heidelberg 2011

parainfluenza viruses (PIVs), all of which cause respiratory infections [204]. Infections with hMPV and RSV occur worldwide and are associated with a broad clinical spectrum ranging from mild to life-threatening disease. Our group and others have shown that hMPV infections in hospitalized patients or in the elderly are at least as severe as RSV infections [125, 146, 147, 175, 178, 204–206, 218, 220, 221, 229]. Whether hMPV infections cause milder symptoms than RSV infections in otherwise healthy individuals has not yet been systematically investigated. Furthermore, hMPV and RSV often occur as co-pathogens and may then cross-react directly or indirectly [229].

Genetically, hMPV is most closely related to the avian metapneumovirus (APV) [204] and is assumed to have a zoonotic origin, a possibility supported by the fact that it can be transferred to APV-susceptible poultry. Serological and bioinformatic analyses indicate that passage to humans occurred more than 50 years ago [47, 48, 210].

In contrast to RSV, hMPV lacks two genes coding for the nonstructural proteins NS1 and NS2, both of which are assumed to interact with the host's immune response. For this reason, RSV and hMPV may induce different host immune responses [25, 59, 122, 123, 144, 148, 191]. While RSV may be defined as a re-emerging pathogen, at least in some patient cohorts where it was previously underestimated [174], hMPV has been shown to cause a number of severe respiratory events in patients with hematological malignancies. RSV infection and hMPV infection are indistinguishable on clinical grounds alone [229].

In one study including 114 lung transplant recipients, hMPV was detected in bronchoalveolar lavage (BAL) fluid from about 5% of symptomatic patients [45]. Further cases were described after lung and heart–lung transplantation in patients having histological findings of acute pneumonia with diffuse alveolar damage and hyaline membrane formation [112, 192]. In hematopoietic stem-cell transplant recipients, hMPV can cause life-threatening disease. Englund and colleagues described a case series in which the hMPV detection rate by RT-PCR was about 26% among symptomatic patients, and 80% of hMPV-positive patients died from severe infection [63]. Furthermore, in stem-cell transplant recipients, viral shedding and persistence may be prolonged compared to otherwise healthy individuals and may be accompanied by severe infection characterized by rapidly progressive pneumonia with diffuse alveolar hemorrhage [50, 63]. Until now, ribavirin has been the only antiviral agent used to treat severe hMPV infections [28, 85, 93, 165]. Ribavirin was tested in a mouse model and used successfully in two published clinical cases. To date, no other antivirals or vaccines are available.

22.3 Human Bocavirus

Human bocavirus (HBoV) may be an emerging respiratory virus. It was first discovered in 2005 by the Swedish research group led by Tobias Allander at the Karolinska University Hospital in Stockholm [9]. The discovery was made possible by a novel molecular virus screening technique involving DNase treatment, random amplification, cloning, and sequencing. The newly found virus showed up as a possible cause of respiratory disease, particularly acute respiratory tract infections. Clinical symptoms include coughing, fever, and rhinorrhea. It is still unclear whether HBoV is able to trigger disease on its own or occurs only as a co-pathogen [176].

Comparisons of the genomic sequence to other known viruses suggest that HBoV may belong to the *Parvoviridae* family, *Parvovirinae* subfamily, and *Bocavirus* genus. This genus has two other viruses, namely, bovine parvovirus (BPV) and canine minute virus (CnMV). HBoV may be the second *Parvoviridae* known to cause human disease, after parvovirus B19, which belongs to the *Erythrovirus* genus. Several nonpathogenic parvoviruses are also known to infect humans, including the adeno-associated viruses (AAV) of the parvovirus family, *Dependovirus* genus, and, in the same family, parvovirus 4 (PARV4), a possible member of the *Hokovirus* genus [113]. Two new viruses classified as HBoV2 and HBoV3 were discovered recently. HBoV2 has 75% similarity to HBoV, compared to only 18% for HBoV3 and HBoV2 [12, 100]. HBoV2 was detected in children with acute gastroenteritis in England, Pakistan, and Australia, whereas HBoV3 was detected during the course of an HBoV2 surveillance program but could not be associated to any symptoms [12].

HBoV is a non-enveloped single-stranded DNA virus, encapsulated in a simple icosahedral shell with a diameter of 20–26 nm, made up by the arrangement of two proteins. The main genome body containing the open reading frames (ORFs) encoding viral proteins has been sequenced and shown to be 5,309 nt in length [115]. The entire genome length is predicted to be about 6,000 nt [8, 9]. Experiments to directly sequence the virus genome failed and led to faulty data [9, 27]. HBoV is thought to have palindromic hairpin structures flanking the terminal ends, similar to related *Parvoviridae* (e.g., BPV and CnMV). The function of the terminal folds is not fully understood, but it is thought that they act as primers in viral replication and are important for packaging [101]. Until now, it was not possible to decipher the unknown sequences. Attempts to amplify the regions encoding specific enzymes did not reveal the nucleotide sequence [9]. An undetected protein covalent or other protein modification on the HBoV genome may explain this failure, as other parvoviruses (B19, MVM, and H1) possess protein covalents attached to their genomes [39, 51, 168]. Recent findings reveal that the majority (87.5%) of the ssDNA strands packed in the capsid are of negative polarity, independent from their viral subtypes [27]. The genomic composition is as yet unconfirmed, and so far three ORFs have been identified, similar to BPV and CnMV. One of these ORFs encodes for the viral capsid proteins VP1 and VP2, whereas the other two encode for non-structural proteins. The VP2 gene sequence is nested within the VP1 gene sequence. The VP1 sequence, compared to VP2, contains a unique terminal sequence, VP1u [163], which may be required for HBoV genome transfer to the nucleus for replication [236]. The HBoV capsid is composed of 60 proteins, derived from the structural molecule VP1 and its derivative VP2 [9]. The functions of the non-structural proteins NS1 and NP-1 are still equivocal. NS1 may play a role in replication. It generally acts as an initiator protein (for parvoviruses), specifically controlling the process by which several concatemeric intermediates are processed by rolling-hairpin replication [15]. The role for NP-1, located in the middle ORF, is still unclear, but probably also involves parvovirus replication. The transmission route of HBoV is still unknown, but suggested tissue sites for replication are the respiratory and intestinal epithelia, as well as the lymphatic organs. Parvoviruses replicate only in proliferating cells, and the viral proteins are transcribed only during the S-phase. Recently, an in vitro replication system for HBoV using stratified human airway epithelium to imitate the human trachea was successfully established. The cells were inoculated with HBoV-positive material from respiratory tract secretions of hospitalized children. Apical HBoV release from the cells was confirmed using PCR. This study further showed that the transcription model resembled that of both of the other known bocaviruses (BPV and MVC) [52].

Symptoms associated with possible HBoV infection are wheezing, fever, bronchiolitis, and pneumonia [8, 12, 19, 31, 33, 41, 43, 44, 49, 97, 114, 118–121, 124, 126, 141, 176, 177, 179, 183, 195, 198, 203, 213, 219, 226, 235, 237, 239]. However, the presence of HBoV in the respiratory tract does not prove that the virus is the cause of infection. HBoV is often detected concomitantly with other respiratory viruses [41, 216, 226], a fact that adds to the uncertainty regarding the pathogenic potential for HBoV [41, 66, 91, 97, 118, 124, 128, 136, 176, 200, 203, 213, 217, 226, 239]. The symptoms are identical in patients positive for HBoV alone or combined with another virus, but the viral load is higher in mono-infections than in coinfections. Asymptomatic patients can carry the virus. In one study, 43% of tested asymptomatic children were HBoV-positive. These patients were admitted for elective surgery, and the group undergoing mainly ear, nose, and throat surgery had the highest prevalence of asymptomatic HBoV infection [124]. These data suggested that HBoV may persist in the host in the tonsillar lymphoid tissue, contributing to tonsillar hyperplasia [126]. HBoV has been detected in patients with symptoms of gastrointestinal infection, but it is unclear whether the virus is only excreted in stool or is a cause of gastroenteritis. In these studies, HBoV was found concomitantly with a norovirus or other enteric viruses, and HBoV was not directly proven to be a cause of gastrointestinal infection. The virus in suspension in respiratory secretions may be simply swallowed and excreted in stool. The newly discovered HBoV2 and HBoV3 have both been detected in stool samples. HBoV2 was identified in a study involving stool sample screening in children with non-polio acute flaccid paralysis [12, 100, 179], and HBoV2 and HBoV3 were detected in hospitalized children with acute gastroenteritis. More studies on the two new HBoV types are needed to gain a better understanding of their role in gastrointestinal infections. No evidence that HBoV2 and HBoV3 can infect gastrointestinal tissue exists to date. Furthermore, whether detection of these viruses in serum indicates viremia or infection of blood cells is unknown, because there are no currently established methods for detecting HBoV particles. The related parvovirus B19 can infect erythroid progenitor cells in the bone marrow, but no HBoV DNA was detected in bone marrow samples from human immunodeficiency virus (HIV)-positive and -negative individuals, whereas B19 was present in both groups [76, 146]. So far, there is one published report of HBoV associated with severe pneumonia in a pediatric hematopoietic stem cell transplant recipient [172, 173] and one of HBoV infection in an adult with leukemia [109]. However, none of these patients had clinical symptoms different from those caused by other "common cold" pathogens, and no specific antiviral therapy was available.

Since the discovery of HBoV, infections with this virus have been found worldwide. The prevalence of infections in which HBoV may be a causative factor ranges from 1.5% to 19.3%. No seasonal variations have been described. HoBV occurs mainly in pediatric patients aged 6–24 months [4, 5, 9, 10, 12, 16, 17, 37, 40, 42, 44, 61, 74, 77, 86, 91, 95, 99, 103, 116, 127, 132, 143, 149, 158, 160, 162, 166, 167, 179, 187, 189, 194, 214, 219, 226, 235, 238]. Younger children may be protected by maternal antibodies [38]. HBoV-IgG can cross the placental barrier, but it is unclear whether HBoV can be transmitted from the mother to her fetus. Antibodies against HBoV have been found in about 94% of individuals older than 19 years of age [44]. At the moment, only two different genotypes of the single HBoV lineage are known. A simple verification test is available for rapidly differentiating between these two genotypes. Digestion of a 309-bp fragment of the VP1/VP2 gene with BstAPI endonuclease yields two fragments with genotype 1, but induces no cleavage with genotype 2 [54]. Three HBoV2 genotypes have been identified [5], but no information is available for HBoV3.

Despite a large number of clinical studies, the biological background of HBoV is still unknown. The virus can be replicated in a cell line. However, complete genome sequencing is needed to fully understand the virus. As this virus may cause acute respiratory disease, it is crucial to understand the disease process and its causative agent.

22.4 Human Coronaviruses

As of August 2009, five human coronaviruses (CoVs) were known, of which three meet the definition of emerging pathogens. The five human CoVs are OC43 and 229E, two long-known viruses that cause respiratory and/or gastrointestinal disease, and the emerging viruses SARS-CoV [56], NL63 [207], and HKU-1 [233]. SARS-CoV appears to be an archetypical zoonosis responsible for a single outbreak, which was unfortunately accompanied with high mortality and had the potential for a pandemic event. The two other newly detected CoVs, NL63 and HKU-1, occur periodically and infect all age groups worldwide.

After the identification in the 1960s of the first CoVs known to cause human disease, HCoV-229E and HCoV-OC43, and their association with mild respiratory disease [30, 34, 67, 84, 137, 142], little new information emerged in this field until the beginning of the twenty-first century. In 2002/2003, a CoV appeared in the Guangdong province of China, causing severe acute respiratory syndrome (SARS) [56, 108, 156]. SARS was fatal in some patients, although at the time CoVs were believed to cause only mild disease. Strenuous efforts were made to identify and to characterize this new virus and to curb its potential for causing a pandemic.

Among the heterogeneous *Coronaviridae* family, CoV NL63 (HCoV-NL63) was identified in 2004 [207] and CoV HKU1 (HCoV-HKU1) in 2005 [232]. In contrast to SARS-CoV, these newly detected CoV led to clinical symptoms similar to those caused by HCoV-229E and HCoV-OC43. Considerable research has been undertaken to learn more about these viruses, their differences, similarities, and characteristics. This review focuses mainly on SARS-CoV and HCoV-NL63.

Several techniques were employed to characterize and to identify the agent causing SARS. Tests for known respiratory viruses were negative. Patient samples were inoculated onto Rhesus monkey kidney cells (fRhk4) to look for cytopathic effects. Electron microscopy revealed the morphology of the virus and led to characterization of the virus family. Histopathological studies showed mild interstitial inflammation with scattered alveolar pneumocytes. In an immunofluorescence antibody assay, sera from patients had high titers of antibodies against the infected cells. A random RT-PCR assay generated DNA fragments of unknown origin, but with homology to viruses of the *Coronaviridae* family, and confirmed the results of electron microscopy. A few days later, these results were confirmed by two other groups [56, 108, 156].

SARS and its causative agent appeared unexpectedly and spread explosively. The infection was transmitted from palm civets to humans, although it has since been confirmed that bats are the natural reservoir of SARS-CoV. Due to the fast mutation rate of RNA viruses and their resulting genotypic markers, the course of the infection could be reconstituted in great detail. In the early phase of the SARS near pandemic, the very first index patient fulfilling the subsequent WHO definition of SARS resided in Foshan near Guangzhou and was identified on November 16, 2002. One month later, the second case occurred, in Shenzhen, where a man who had regular contact with wild animals was infected and transmitted the disease to his family and to several staff members at the hospital where he was admitted. Similar cases were reported nearby. In January 2003, the second phase of the SARS outbreak started in Guangzhou. Several patients died, and patients were transferred to major hospitals, leading to nosocomial spread of the virus to other patients and health-care workers.

The next and final phase started in mid-February 2003 and heralded the pandemic. A doctor was infected in Guangdong province and took the disease to Hong Kong, where he stayed in a hotel ("hotel M"). He infected 17 other people, who were admitted to different hospitals, where further nosocomial infections occurred. Some of the infected patients transferred the virus via air travel to Vietnam, Singapore, and Toronto, where new cases emerged. A novel CoV was identified on March 21, 2003, and confirmed a few days later. The first strain (Tor2) was fully sequenced on April 12, 2003, and SARS-CoV was proven to be the cause of SARS [134]. In July 2003, the epidemic ended, with no further human-to-human transmissions being reported. In September 2003, a new case was reported at a laboratory in Singapore, and over the next 2 years other accidents occurred in laboratories.

HCoV-NL63 was discovered in a 7-month-old child with bronchiolitis. Diagnostic tests for all known respiratory viruses were negative. Inoculation of a sample on tMK and, later on, LLC-MK2 cell cultures produced a cytopathic effect. In the LLC-MK2 cell culture supernatant, a new virus was identified using the VIDISCA method [161, 207]. Sequence comparisons established that the virus was most closely related to HCoV-229E and, together with PEDV and Bat-CoV, belonged to the coronavirus subgroup 1b. Two further research groups obtained identical results soon afterward [65, 72].

There is some indication in the literature that HCoV-NL63 was detected much earlier. Viruses were described that did not exhibit all the characteristics of HCoV-229E or HCoV-OC43. Unfortunately, these isolates were lost, so that studies could not be done to determine whether one or more of them were identical to HCoV-NL63. SARS-CoV and HCoV-NL63 are both members of the *Coronavirus* genus, *Coronaviridae* family, within the *Nidovirales* order. Both organisms are positive single-stranded RNA viruses with a large genome of about 30 kb. The virus particles are enveloped and possess peculiar spike-shaped proteins on their surface that produce a crown-like appearance. Electron microscopy revealed particles of 80–140 nm located either within the infected cells at the rough endoplasmic reticulum in double-membraned vesicles or outside the cells attached to the plasma membrane.

The genomes of both SARS-CoV and HCoV-NL63 can be roughly divided into two parts. The 5′ two-thirds consists of one large polyprotein (ORF1ab) including several domains with autocatalytic activities, producing nonstructural proteins (NSPs) involved in replication and immune evasion. ORF1ab encodes 16 NSPs in toto in both SARS-CoV and HCoV-NL63.

The last third at the 3′ end of the genome contains the ORFs coding for the functional proteins – spike (S), envelope (E), membrane (M), and nucleocapsid (N) – and for accessory protein genes that vary in number and position across species.

Traditionally, CoVs were classified – due to their antigenic cross-reactivity – into three groups, which were largely confirmed later on by sequence analysis results. Group I and II viruses infect mammals, whereas group III viruses infect only birds. While HCoV-NL63 belongs to group 1b, SARS-CoV and the bat CoVs are considered group 2b viruses, although bat CoVs constitute a newly identified CoV group.

HCoV-NL63 is most closely related to HCoV-229E, and phylogenetic analysis findings suggest that HCoV-NL63 may have diverged from HCoV229E in the twenty-first century. Furthermore, there seem to be two main genetic clusters of HCoV-NL63, and there is evidence that the HCoV-NL63 genome is arranged in a mosaic-like manner.

Patients infected with HCoV-NL63 usually experience only mild symptoms, including cough, rhinitis, rhinorrhea, and pharyngitis, often with a fever. In rare cases, pneumonia can occur, chiefly in children aged 0–3 years, older people, and immunocompromised individuals. Among children with severe lower respiratory tract infection, a substantial number have croup compared to a control group. Croup or laryngotracheobronchitis is characterized by a loud barking cough, inspiratory stridor, and hoarseness. An association with Kawasaki disease has been postulated but not confirmed despite studies by a number of research groups [11, 14, 15, 53, 58, 87, 106, 111, 140, 188, 190, 193, 202, 208].

After the detection of HCoV-NL63 in The Netherlands and, later on, in New Haven, CT, USA, this virus was found in a number of countries, suggesting a worldwide distribution. Except in subtropical regions, HCoV-NL63 was mainly detected in the winter months and often turned up with other co-pathogens, such as influenza, RSV, parainfluenza, and hMPV. The HCoV-NL63 load is attenuated when there is another pathogen. However, and not surprisingly, the infection itself seems more severe in co-infections. As with SARS-CoV, HCoV-NL63 is detectable up to 2 months after recovery from the disease. Seroprevalence studies showed that virtually every adult encounters HCoV-NL63 at least once in a lifetime. Antibodies specific for the S protein are produced and display a neutralizing effect.

People infected with SARS-CoV had a fever, chills, myalgia, rigor, and a nonproductive cough. Clinical symptoms such as rhinorrhea and sore throat were less common. In contrast to HCoV-NL63, SARS-CoV did not infect children, and the disease occurred instead in normal and healthy adults and in the elderly. Of 8,096 infected people, 774 died, demonstrating a nearly 10% mortality rate. SARS-CoV spread to more than 30 countries [26, 29, 35, 94, 186, 227]. The first outbreak occurred in late 2002/early 2003. Seasonality of HCoV-NL63 infection is not known, as the pandemic occurred only once, with the peak in winter. It has been confirmed that SARS-CoV is a zoonosis that originates primarily from bats. Although SARS-CoV was initially spread from civets to humans, the actual transmission route was from humans to humans, most likely by droplets, and probably occurred in health-care facilities, at workplaces, and when using public transportation. The virus was detected not only in the respiratory tract, but also in the gastrointestinal tract, liver, kidney, brain, and other tissues.

Seroprevalence was quite low among the general population, ranging across studies from 0% to 1.81% and being slightly higher in asymptomatic health-care workers. In contrast, a much higher rate (up to 40%) was found in asymptomatic animal handlers, which was not surprising, as these individuals probably acquired immunity via less pathogenic SARS-CoV-like strains that also emerged by zoonotic recombinations. SARS-CoV infection can be accompanied by co-pathogens such as other respiratory viruses (e.g., hMPV) or other CoVs.

The association of SARS-CoV with severe pneumonia in patients with hematological malignancies occurred only during the single outbreak, and studies on the role for NL63 in these high-risk patients are still limited. However, 229E has been detected in hematopoietic stem cell transplant recipients with high fever, cough, and interstitial and alveolar lung disease [157].

22.5 Polyomaviruses

Recently, two novel polyomaviruses were detected in respiratory aspirates. Allander et al. in Sweden discovered a previously unrecognized third human polyomavirus in 6 (1%) of 637 nasopharyngeal aspirates and 1 (0.5%) of 192 fecal samples, and suggested the name KI polyomavirus (KIPyV) [7]. The second newly identified polyomavirus was found by Gaynor et al. in respiratory samples from Bribane, Australia, and St. Louis, MO, USA. This "Washington University" (WU) genome polyomavirus (WUPyV) was amplified and cloned from the nasopharyngeal aspirate of a 3-year-old patient with pneumonia and negative tests for other respiratory viruses. Screening of 2,135 patients with respiratory tract infections identified 43 additional cases [79]. Of note, KIPyV was not named for the Karolinska Institute in Stockholm where it was detected. Since the first description of KIPyV and WUPyV, a number of prevalence studies from various areas have been published, but the association of these viruses with acute respiratory tract infections remains unclear [2, 13, 117].

Prevalence studies of KIPyV and WUPyV showed a worldwide distribution. The prevalence of KIPyV was 1% in Sweden, 1.4% in the United Kingdom, 1.99% in Thailand, and 2.6% in Australia [7, 23, 152, 155]. The prevalence of WUPyV was higher, 7% in South Korea, and 6.29% in Thailand [88, 155]. Australia, the USA, and the UK had WUPyV prevalences of 4.5%, 1.2%, and 1.0%, respectively [23, 79, 152]. The age distribution of KIPyV- and WUPyV-infected patients showed two peaks, in patients younger than 15 years (with the highest rates occurring before 5 years of age) and older than 45 years [3, 150]. Seasonal variations in KIPyV and WUPyV did not appear consistently. KIPyV infections predominated during the winter months in Thailand but not in Australia. In contrast, WUPyV infections were predominantly detected during late winter, peaking in December to early summer in Australia but not in Thailand [23, 24, 155].

KIPyV and WUPyV are frequently associated with other respiratory viruses. High co-detection rates were found in Australia, 74.7% for KIPyV and 79.7% for WUPyV, and the most commonly co-detected viruses were human rhinovirus and HBoV. Co-detection of KIPyV and WUPyV was found in 14 patients, of whom only 1 had no other respiratory virus [23]. Norja et al. detected KIPyV or WUPyV in 19 patients and found a viral coinfection rate of nearly 50% with predominant detection of adenoviruses. The overall frequencies of KIPyV and WUPyV detection were similar in patients with upper respiratory tract infection, lower respiratory tract infection, or no respiratory symptoms, and eight patients were immunosuppressed, although overall the patient groups were not very well described [152].

Data are not available to determine whether KIPyV and WUPyV detection represents a similar phenomenon to JCV and BKV reactivation in immunocompromised patients, or whether KIPyV and WUPyV share the oncogenic potential of other human and animal polyomaviruses, and further studies are needed [242]. However, Koch's modified postulates have not been verified so far, and whether KIPyV and WUPyV are respiratory pathogens or innocent bystanders is still debated. Further studies are required to evaluate the clinical relevance of KIPyV and WUPyV detection in respiratory specimens.

Another newly recognized polyoma virus of interest may be the Merkel cell polyoma virus, MCPyV, recently identified in Merkel cell carcinoma. MCPyV may have oncogenic potential, as it is found mainly in lesional and non-lesional skin from patients with Merkel cell carcinoma and other skin diseases [73]. This oncogenic potential, as well as experience with other oncogenic viruses such as EBV, suggests a high likelihood of MCPyV generating clinical events in patients with hematological malignancies. However, until now, there are more questions than answers regarding this new virus. The role for MCPyV in disease is unclear, and cell-culture and animal models are not yet available [169].

22.6 Picornaviruses

Within the group of picornaviruses, two emerging virus lines were identified recently, namely, rhinovirus X associated with severe respiratory disease and the parechoviruses. The newly identified rhinovirus [105, 129, 171] causes common colds that can progress to fatal infections in high-risk patients. The role for this virus in patients with hematological malignancies is unclear. The number of known parechoviruses is growing rapidly, as novel identification methods have led to the discovery of new variants. Parechoviruses were classified in the *Enterovirus* genus initially, then found to exhibit different biological features, leading to their reclassification in their own genus. Clinically, they cause the same spectrum of disease as enteroviruses. The rodent parechovirus known as Ljungan virus is believed to be associated with greater disease severity [1, 6, 20–22, 55, 68, 90, 96, 107, 151, 170, 199, 209, 212, 223, 230, 231, 234, 240, 241]. As with enteroviruses, parechoviruses deserve careful attention in high-risk patients.

22.7 Reemerging Viruses

22.7.1 Respiratory Syncytial Virus

The RSV has been known for decades and is not believed to be an emerging pathogen. However, recent investigations have demonstrated clearly that RSV infection is underestimated in the elderly and in patients with other malignancies, where it may cause severe to fatal pneumonia [174, 182, 184, 185, 196, 197, 215, 222]. This increasing incidence in some patient groups may define the RSV as a reemerging pathogen, although it is ascribable to the use, for the first time, of molecular RSV diagnostic methods in vulnerable patient groups. In all likelihood, the RSV was present in these groups previously but went unrecognized.

RSV accounts for a large number of infections throughout the treatment of patients with acute lymphoblastic leukemia. In one study, about 57% of patients were positive for RSV at some point in time [102]. RSV is also of clinical significance following allogeneic bone marrow transplantation and has been found in a substantial proportion of patients with lung infections [64, 133]. Furthermore, RSV was responsible for 55% of fatal pneumonia cases in adult immunocompromised patients treated for lymphoma and leukemia in a retrospective study and was a major cause of viral pneumonia in several cohorts of patients with these hematological malignancies [57, 78, 81, 82, 164, 201, 228].

In patients with hematological malignancies, and most notably in hematopoietic stem cell recipients, RSV infection is fatal in up to 80% of cases [89]. In these patients, ribavirin, immunoglobulins, and the RSV-specific humanized monoclonal antibody palivizumab may be used as specific therapy and/or prophylaxis [18, 32, 36, 38, 60, 69, 70, 75, 80, 83, 104, 110, 138, 139, 145, 159, 181, 211, 224, 225]. However, evidence supporting the use of these treatments remains weak at this time.

22.7.2 Parainfluenza Viruses

Clinically, parainfluenza viruses 1–4 cannot be differentiated from RSV or hMPV infection. As they infect the same groups of patients and cause identical symptoms, they require the same attention as other pathogens. They can also be classified among reemerging viruses, as screening was recently introduced. Parainfluenza viruses should be considered in the differential diagnosis of respiratory infection and distinguished from emerging pathogens [98, 154].

22.7.3 Influenza Viruses

Influenza viruses are not emerging viruses, as in theory all potential variants and reassortants are identified based on well-known data on the mode of replication and influenza-associated biological phenomena such as antigen shift. Nevertheless, perhaps due to concern that a lethal variant similar to the Spanish flu may return, or due to the awarding of research grants based on this fear, any "novel" influenza virus variant is estimated to have pandemic potential and is therefore classified as an emerging pathogen (and as an opportunity for the media to generate widespread fear of general social disorganization and massive mortality). The most recent virus classified as an emerging influenza virus was the Mexican H1N1 strain identified in 2009.

Recent developments in the swine-originated H1N1 pandemic indicate that the main target is not the elderly population but, instead, younger adults (www.who.org [153, 180]). The immunosenescence concept suggested that older people would be at greatest risk. The predominant involvement of younger individuals suggests a role for unknown factors that contribute to clinical disease. Alternatively, aging might exert a protective effect. However, it must be hoped that the current wave of H1N1 influenza is not a relatively harmless prelude to a second severe outbreak later in the flu season.

As with any influenza variant, the H1N1 strain warrants close attention in high-risk patients. All influenza variants can cause severe pneumonia in patients with hematological malignancies.

22.7.4 Adenoviruses

Adenoviruses are small naked DNA viruses that occur worldwide and mainly infect children between 0.5 and 5 years of age. The clinical spectrum ranges from mild to severe respiratory diseases to epidemic keratoconjunctivitis ("pink eye"), tonsillopharyngitis, and gastroenteric disorders (vomiting, diarrhea). Adenoviruses occur in over 50 serotypes, affecting all age groups and causing diseases that are usually self-limiting within 14 days or asymptomatic [46, 62, 71, 92, 130, 131, 135]. Importantly, adenoviruses may persist in the infected host [46, 62, 71, 92, 130, 131, 135] and may undergo reactivation in immunosuppressed patients, including those with hematological malignancies. Adenoviruses play a major role in solid-organ transplant recipients but occur less often in stem cell recipients [46, 62, 71, 92, 130, 131, 135], However, novel and more aggressive adenovirus strains may meet the definition for emerging pathogens and may play a future role in patients with hematological malignancies. Consequently, adenoviruses deserve attention. More specifically, shedding may be prolonged in high-risk patients, patient isolation may be required, and no antiviral therapy for adenoviruses is available so far [46, 62, 71, 92, 130, 131, 135].

References

1. Abed Y, Boivin G (2005) Molecular characterization of a Canadian human parechovirus (HPeV)-3 isolate and its relationship to other HPeVs. J Med Virol 77:566–570
2. Abed Y, Wang D, Boivin G (2007) WU polyomavirus in children, Canada. Emerg Infect Dis 13:1939–1941
3. Abedi Kiasari B, Vallely PJ, Corless CE, Al-Hammadi M, Klapper PE (2008) Age-related pattern of KI and WU polyomavirus infection. J Clin Virol 43:123–125
4. Albuquerque MC, Pena GP, Varella RB, Gallucci G, Erdman D, Santos N (2009) Novel respiratory virus infections in children, Brazil. Emerg Infect Dis 15:806–808
5. Albuquerque MC, Rocha LN, Benati FJ, Soares CC, Maranhao AG, Ramirez ML, Erdman D, Santos N (2007) Human bocavirus infection in children with gastroenteritis, Brazil. Emerg Infect Dis 13:1756–1758
6. Alho A, Marttila J, Ilonen J, Hyypia T (2003) Diagnostic potential of parechovirus capsid proteins. J Clin Microbiol 41:2294–2299
7. Allander T, Andreasson K, Gupta S, Bjerkner A, Bogdanovic G, Persson MA, Dalianis T, Ramqvist T, Andersson B (2007) Identification of a third human polyomavirus. J Virol 81: 4130–4136
8. Allander T, Jartti T, Gupta S, Niesters HG, Lehtinen P, Osterback R, Vuorinen T, Waris M, Bjerkner A, Tiveljung-Lindell A, van den Hoogen BG, Hyypia T, Ruuskanen O (2007) Human bocavirus and acute wheezing in children. Clin Infect Dis 44:904–910
9. Allander T, Tammi MT, Eriksson M, Bjerkner A, Tiveljung-Lindell A, Andersson B (2005) Cloning of a human parvovirus by molecular screening of respiratory tract samples. Proc Natl Acad Sci USA 102:12891–12896
10. Arden KE, McErlean P, Nissen MD, Sloots TP, Mackay IM (2006) Frequent detection of human rhinoviruses, paramyxoviruses, coronaviruses, and bocavirus during acute respiratory tract infections. J Med Virol 78:1232–1240
11. Arden KE, Nissen MD, Sloots TP, Mackay IM (2005) New human coronavirus, HCoV-NL63, associated with severe lower respiratory tract disease in Australia. J Med Virol 75: 455–462
12. Arthur JL, Higgins GD, Davidson GP, Givney RC, Ratcliff RM (2009) A novel bocavirus associated with acute gastroenteritis in Australian children. PLoS Pathog 5:e1000391
13. Babakir-Mina M, Ciccozzi M, Dimonte S, Farchi F, Valdarchi C, Rezza G, Perno CF, Ciotti M (2008) Identification of the novel KI polyomavirus in the respiratory tract of an Italian patient. J Med Virol 80:2012–2014
14. Baker SC, Shimizu C, Shike H, Garcia F, van der Hoek L, Kuijper TW, Reed SL, Rowley AH, Shulman ST, Talbot HK, Williams JV, Burns JC (2006) Human coronavirus-NL63 infection is not associated with acute Kawasaki disease. Adv Exp Med Biol 581:523–526
15. Bastien N, Anderson K, Hart L, Van Caeseele P, Brandt K, Milley D, Hatchette T, Weiss EC, Li Y (2005) Human coronavirus NL63 infection in Canada. J Infect Dis 191: 503–506
16. Bastien N, Brandt K, Dust K, Ward D, Li Y (2006) Human Bocavirus infection, Canada. Emerg Infect Dis 12:848–850
17. Bastien N, Chui N, Robinson JL, Lee BE, Dust K, Hart L, Li Y (2007) Detection of human bocavirus in Canadian children in a 1-year study. J Clin Microbiol 45:610–613
18. Bauman J, Eggleston M, Oquist N, Malinoski F (2007) Respiratory syncytial virus: seasonal data for regions of Florida and implications for palivizumab. South Med J 100: 669–676
19. Beder LB, Hotomi M, Ogami M, Yamauchi K, Shimada J, Billal DS, Ishiguro N, Yamanaka N (2009) Clinical and microbiological impact of human bocavirus on children with acute otitis media. Eur J Pediatr 166:1365–1372
20. Benschop KS, Schinkel J, Luken ME, van den Broek PJ, Beersma MF, Menelik N, van Eijk HW, Zaaijer HL, VandenBroucke-Grauls CM, Beld MG, Wolthers KC (2006) Fourth human parechovirus serotype. Emerg Infect Dis 12:1572–1575
21. Benschop KS, Schinkel J, Minnaar RP, Pajkrt D, Spanjerberg L, Kraakman HC, Berkhout B, Zaaijer HL, Beld MG, Wolthers KC (2006) Human parechovirus infections in Dutch children and the association between serotype and disease severity. Clin Infect Dis 42:204–210
22. Benschop K, Thomas X, Serpenti C, Molenkamp R, Wolthers K (2008) High prevalence of human Parechovirus (HPeV) genotypes in the Amsterdam region and identification of specific HPeV variants by direct genotyping of stool samples. J Clin Microbiol 46: 3965–3970
23. Bialasiewicz S, Whiley DM, Lambert SB, Jacob K, Bletchly C, Wang D, Nissen MD, Sloots TP (2008) Presence of the newly discovered human polyomaviruses KI and WU in Australian patients with acute respiratory tract infection. J Clin Virol 41:63–68
24. Bialasiewicz S, Whiley DM, Lambert SB, Wang D, Nissen MD, Sloots TP (2007) A newly reported human polyomavirus, KI virus, is present in the respiratory tract of Australian children. J Clin Virol 40:15–18
25. Bitko V, Shulyayeva O, Mazumder B, Musiyenko A, Ramaswamy M, Look DC, Barik S (2007) Nonstructural proteins of respiratory syncytial virus suppress premature apoptosis by an NF-kappaB-dependent, interferon-independent mechanism and facilitate virus growth. J Virol 81:1 1786–1795
26. Bizri AR, Musharrafieh UM (2003) SARS: the flying death. J Méd Liban 51:148–154
27. Bohmer A, Schildgen V, Lusebrink J, Ziegler S, Tillmann RL, Kleines M, Schildgen O (2009) Novel application for isothermal nucleic acid sequence-based amplification (NASBA). J Virol Methods 158:199–201
28. Bonney D, Razali H, Turner A, Will A (2009) Successful treatment of human metapneumovirus pneumonia using combination therapy with intravenous ribavirin and immune globulin. Br J Haematol 145:667–669

29. Booth CM, Stewart TE (2005) Severe acute respiratory syndrome and critical care medicine: the Toronto experience. Crit Care Med 33:S53–S60
30. Bruckova M, McIntosh K, Kapikian AZ, Chanock RM (1970) The adaptation of two human coronavirus strains (OC38 and OC43) to growth in cell monolayers. Proc Soc Exp Biol Med 135:431–435
31. Calvo C, Garcia-Garcia ML, Blanco C, Santos MJ, Pozo F, Perez-Brena P, Casas I (2008) Human bocavirus infection in a neonatal intensive care unit. J Infect 57:269–271
32. Carbonell-Estrany X, Lazaro y de Mercado P (2009) Health economics and RSV. Paediatr Respir Rev 10(Suppl 1): 12–13
33. Catalano-Pons C, Bue M, Laude H, Cattan F, Moulin F, Menager C, Cosnes-Lambe C, Chalumeau M, Giraud C, Meritet JF, Rozenberg F, Lebon P, Gendrel D (2007) Human bocavirus infection in hospitalized children during winter. Pediatr Infect Dis J 26:959–960
34. Cavallaro JJ, Monto AS (1970) Community-wide outbreak of infection with a 229E-like coronavirus in Tecumseh, Michigan. J Infect Dis 122:272–279
35. Chan-Yeung M (2004) Severe acute respiratory syndrome (SARS) and healthcare workers. Int J Occup Environ Health 10:421–427
36. Chavez-Bueno S, Mejias A, Merryman RA, Ahmad N, Jafri HS, Ramilo O (2007) Intravenous palivizumab and ribavirin combination for respiratory syncytial virus disease in high-risk pediatric patients. Pediatr Infect Dis J 26:1089–1093
37. Chieochansin T, Samransamruajkit R, Chutinimitkul S, Payungporn S, Hiranras T, Theamboonlers A, Poovorawan Y (2008) Human bocavirus (HBoV) in Thailand: clinical manifestations in a hospitalized pediatric patient and molecular virus characterization. J Infect 56:137–142
38. Chirico G, Ravasio R, Sbarigia U (2009) Cost-utility analysis of palivizumab in Italy: results from a simulation model in the prophylaxis of respiratory syncytial virus infection (RSV) among high-risk preterm infants. Riv Ital Pediatr 35:4
39. Chow LT, Broker TR (1994) Papillomavirus DNA replication. Intervirology 37:150–158
40. Chow BD, Huang YT, Esper FP (2008) Evidence of human bocavirus circulating in children and adults, Cleveland, Ohio. J Clin Virol 43:302–306
41. Christensen A, Nordbo SA, Krokstad S, Rognlien AG, Dollner H (2008) Human bocavirus commonly involved in multiple viral airway infections. J Clin Virol 41:34–37
42. Chung JY, Han TH, Kim CK, Kim SW (2006) Bocavirus infection in hospitalized children, South Korea. Emerg Infect Dis 12:1254–1256
43. Chung JY, Han TH, Kim JS, Kim SW, Park CG, Hwang ES (2008) Th1 and Th2 cytokine levels in nasopharyngeal aspirates from children with human bocavirus bronchiolitis. J Clin Virol 43:223–225
44. Costa C, Bergallo M, Cavallo R (2009) Detection of Human Bocavirus in bronchoalveolar lavage from Italian adult patients. J Clin Virol 45:81–82
45. Dare R, Sanghavi S, Bullotta A, Keightley MC, George KS, Wadowsky RM, Paterson DL, McCurry KR, Reinhart TA, Husain S, Rinaldo CR (2007) Diagnosis of human metapneumovirus infection in immunosuppressed lung transplant recipients and children evaluated for pertussis. J Clin Microbiol 45:548–552
46. Darr S, Madisch I, Hofmayer S, Rehren F, Heim A (2009) Phylogeny and primary structure analysis of fiber shafts of all human adenovirus types for rational design of adenoviral gene therapy vectors. J Gen Virol 90:2849–2854
47. de Graaf M, Osterhaus AD, Fouchier RA, Holmes EC (2008) Evolutionary dynamics of human and avian metapneumoviruses. J Gen Virol 89:2933–2942
48. de Graaf M, Schrauwen EJ, Herfst S, van Amerongen G, Osterhaus AD, Fouchier RA (2009) Fusion protein is the main determinant of metapneumovirus host tropism. J Gen Virol 90:1408–1416
49. de Vries JJ, Bredius RG, van Rheenen PF, Smiers FJ, Scholvinck EH, Vossen AC, Claas EC, Niesters HG (2009) Human bocavirus in an immunocompromised child presenting with severe diarrhea. J Clin Microbiol 47: 1241–1243
50. Debiaggi M, Canducci F, Sampaolo M, Marinozzi MC, Parea M, Terulla C, Colombo AA, Alessandrino EP, Bragotti LZ, Arghittu M, Goglio A, Migliavacca R, Romero E, Clementi M (2006) Persistent symptomless human metapneumovirus infection in hematopoietic stem cell transplant recipients. J Infect Dis 194:474–478
51. Deiss V, Ttatschin JD, Weitz M, Siegl G (1990) Cloning of the human parvovirus B19 genome and structural analysis of its palindromic termini. Virology 175:247–254
52. Dijkman R, Koekkoek SM, Molenkamp R, Schildgen O, van der Hoek L (2009) Human bocavirus can be cultured in differentiated human airway epithelial cells. J Virol 83: 7739–7748
53. Dijkman R, van der Hoek L (2009) Human coronaviruses 229E and NL63: close yet still so far. J Formos Med Assoc 108:270–279
54. Ditt V, Viazov S, Tillmann R, Schildgen V, Schildgen O (2008) Genotyping of human bocavirus using a restriction length polymorphism. Virus Genes 36:67–69
55. Drexler JF, Grywna K, Stocker A, Almeida PS, Medrado-Ribeiro TC, Eschbach-Bludau M, Petersen N, Da Costa-Ribeiro H Jr, Drosten C (2009) Novel human parechovirus from Brazil. Emerg Infect Dis 15:310–313
56. Drosten C, Gunther S, Preiser W, van der Werf S, Brodt HR, Becker S, Rabenau H, Panning M, Kolesnikova L, Fouchier RA, Berger A, Burguiere AM, Cinatl J, Eickmann M, Escriou N, Grywna K, Kramme S, Manuguerra JC, Muller S, Rickerts V, Sturmer M, Vieth S, Klenk HD, Osterhaus AD, Schmitz H, Doerr HW (2003) Identification of a novel coronavirus in patients with severe acute respiratory syndrome. N Engl J Med 348:1967–1976
57. Ebbert JO, Limper AH (2005) Respiratory syncytial virus pneumonitis in immunocompromised adults: clinical features and outcome. Respiration 72:263–269
58. Ebihara T, Endo R, Ma X, Ishiguro N, Kikuta H (2005) Detection of human coronavirus NL63 in young children with bronchiolitis. J Med Virol 75:463–465
59. Elliott J, Lynch OT, Suessmuth Y, Qian P, Boyd CR, Burrows JF, Buick R, Stevenson NJ, Touzelet O, Gadina M, Power UF, Johnston JA (2007) Respiratory syncytial virus NS1 protein degrades STAT2 by using the Elongin-Cullin E3 ligase. J Virol 81:3428–3436
60. Emerick K, Cunningham M, Hartnick C (2006) The potential impact of palivizumab on pediatric airway reconstruction. Am J Otolaryngol 27:9–12

61. Endo R, Ishiguro N, Kikuta H, Teramoto S, Shirkoohi R, Ma X, Ebihara T, Ishiko H, Ariga T (2007) Seroepidemiology of human bocavirus in Hokkaido prefecture, Japan. J Clin Microbiol 45:3218–3223
62. Engelmann I, Madisch I, Pommer H, Heim A (2006) An outbreak of epidemic keratoconjunctivitis caused by a new intermediate adenovirus 22/H8 identified by molecular typing. Clin Infect Dis 43:e64–e66
63. Englund JA, Boeckh M, Kuypers J, Nichols WG, Hackman RC, Morrow RA, Fredricks DN, Corey L (2006) Brief communication: fatal human metapneumovirus infection in stem-cell transplant recipients. Ann Intern Med 144: 344–349
64. Escuissato DL, Gasparetto EL, Marchiori E, Rocha Gde M, Inoue C, Pasquini R, Muller NL (2005) Pulmonary infections after bone marrow transplantation: high-resolution CT findings in 111 patients. AJR Am J Roentgenol 185: 608–615
65. Esper F, Weibel C, Ferguson D, Landry ML, Kahn JS (2005) Evidence of a novel human coronavirus that is associated with respiratory tract disease in infants and young children. J Infect Dis 191:492–498
66. Esposito S, Bosis S, Niesters HG, Tremolati E, Sabatini C, Porta A, Fossali E, Osterhaus AD, Principi N (2008) Impact of human bocavirus on children and their families. J Clin Microbiol 46:1337–1342
67. Estola T (1970) Coronaviruses, a new group of animal RNA viruses. Avian Dis 14:330–336
68. Faria NR, de Vries M, van Hemert FJ, Benschop K, van der Hoek L (2009) Rooting human parechovirus evolution in time. BMC Evol Biol 9:164
69. Fitzgerald DA (2009) Preventing RSV bronchiolitis in vulnerable infants: the role of palivizumab. Paediatr Respir Rev 10:143–147
70. Forbes M (2008) Strategies for preventing respiratory syncytial virus. Am J Health Syst Pharm 65:S13–S19
71. Forstmeyer D, Henke-Gendo C, Brocker V, Wildner O, Heim A (2008) Quantitative temporal and spatial distribution of adenovirus type 2 correlates with disease manifestations and organ failure during disseminated infection. J Med Virol 80:294–297
72. Fouchier RA, Hartwig NG, Bestebroer TM, Niemeyer B, de Jong JC, Simon JH, Osterhaus AD (2004) A previously undescribed coronavirus associated with respiratory disease in humans. Proc Natl Acad Sci USA 101:6212–6216
73. Foulongne V, Dereure O, Kluger N, Moles JP, Guillot B, Segondy M (2009) Merkel cell polyomavirus DNA detection in lesional and nonlesional skin from patients with Merkel cell carcinoma or other skin diseases. Br J Dermatol 162:59–63
74. Foulongne V, Olejnik Y, Perez V, Elaerts S, Rodiere M, Segondy M (2006) Human bocavirus in French children. Emerg Infect Dis 12:1251–1253
75. Frogel M, Nerwen C, Boron M, Cohen A, VanVeldhuisen P, Harrington M, Groothuis J (2008) Improved outcomes with home-based administration of palivizumab: results from the 2000-2004 Palivizumab Outcomes Registry. Pediatr Infect Dis J 27:870–873
76. Garbino J, Inoubli S, Mossdorf E, Weber R, Tamm M, Soccal P, Aubert JD, Bridevaux PO, Tapparel C, Kaiser L (2008) Respiratory viruses in HIV-infected patients with suspected respiratory opportunistic infection. AIDS 22:701–705
77. Garcia ML, Calvo C, Pozo F, Perez-Brena P, Vazquez MC, Casas I (2009) Detection of human bocavirus in ill and healthy Spanish children: a 2-year study. Arch Dis Child. 94:249. doi. 10.1136/adc.2007.131045
78. Garcia R, Raad I, Abi-Said D, Bodey G, Champlin R, Tarrand J, Hill LA, Umphrey J, Neumann J, Englund J, Whimbey E (1997) Nosocomial respiratory syncytial virus infections: prevention and control in bone marrow transplant patients. Infect Control Hosp Epidemiol 18:412–416
79. Gaynor AM, Nissen MD, Whiley DM, Mackay IM, Lambert SB, Wu G, Brennan DC, Storch GA, Sloots TP, Wang D (2007) Identification of a novel polyomavirus from patients with acute respiratory tract infections. PLoS Pathog 3:e64
80. Georgescu G, Chemaly RF (2009) Palivizumab: where to from here? Expert Opin Biol Ther 9:139–147
81. Ghosh S, Champlin RE, Englund J, Giralt SA, Rolston K, Raad I, Jacobson K, Neumann J, Ippoliti C, Mallik S, Whimbey E (2000) Respiratory syncytial virus upper respiratory tract illnesses in adult blood and marrow transplant recipients: combination therapy with aerosolized ribavirin and intravenous immunoglobulin. Bone Marrow Transplant 25:751–755
82. Ghosh S, Champlin RE, Ueno NT, Anderlini P, Rolston K, Raad I, Kontoyiannis D, Jacobson K, Luna M, Tarrand J, Whimbey E (2001) Respiratory syncytial virus infections in autologous blood and marrow transplant recipients with breast cancer: combination therapy with aerosolized ribavirin and parenteral immunoglobulins. Bone Marrow Transplant 28:271–275
83. Goddard NL, Cooke MC, Gupta RK, Nguyen-Van-Tam JS (2007) Timing of monoclonal antibody for seasonal RSV prophylaxis in the United Kingdom. Epidemiol Infect 135: 159–162
84. Hambre D, Beem M (1972) Virologic studies of acute respiratory disease in young adults. V. Coronavirus 229E infections during six years of surveillance. Am J Epidemiol 96:94–106
85. Hamelin ME, Prince GA, Boivin G (2006) Effect of ribavirin and glucocorticoid treatment in a mouse model of human metapneumovirus infection. Antimicrob Agents Chemother 50:774–777
86. Hamza IA, Jurzik L, Wilhelm M, Uberla K (2009) Detection and quantification of human bocavirus in river water. J Gen Virol 90:2634–2637
87. Han TH, Chung JY, Kim SW, Hwang ES (2007) Human Coronavirus-NL63 infections in Korean children, 2004–2006. J Clin Virol 38:27–31
88. Han TH, Chung JY, Koo JW, Kim SW, Hwang ES (2007) WU polyomavirus in children with acute lower respiratory tract infections, South Korea. Emerg Infect Dis 13: 1766–1768
89. Harrington RD, Hooton TM, Hackman RC, Storch GA, Osborne B, Gleaves CA, Benson A, Meyers JD (1992) An outbreak of respiratory syncytial virus in a bone marrow transplant center. J Infect Dis 165:987–993
90. Harvala H, Robertson I, McWilliam Leitch EC, Benschop K, Wolthers KC, Templeton K, Simmonds P (2008) Epidemiology and clinical associations of human parechovirus respiratory infections. J Clin Microbiol 46:3446–3453

91. Hindiyeh MY, Keller N, Mandelboim M, Ram D, Rubinov J, Regev L, Levy V, Orzitzer S, Shaharabani H, Azar R, Mendelson E, Grossman Z (2008) High rate of human bocavirus and adenovirus coinfection in hospitalized Israeli children. J Clin Microbiol 46:334–337
92. Hoffmann D, Bayer W, Heim A, Potthoff A, Nettelbeck DM, Wildner O (2008) Evaluation of twenty-one human adenovirus types and one infectivity-enhanced adenovirus for the treatment of malignant melanoma. J Invest Dermatol 128:988–998
93. Hopkins P, McNeil K, Kermeen F, Musk M, McQueen E, Mackay I, Sloots T, Nissen M (2008) Human metapneumovirus in lung transplant recipients and comparison to respiratory syncytial virus. Am J Respir Crit Care Med 178: 876–881
94. Hui DS (2005) An overview on severe acute respiratory syndrome (SARS). Monaldi Arch Chest Dis 63:149–157
95. Jacques J, Moret H, Renois F, Leveque N, Motte J, Andreoletti L (2008) Human Bocavirus quantitative DNA detection in French children hospitalized for acute bronchiolitis. J Clin Virol 43:142–147
96. Joki-Korpela P, Hyypia T (2001) Parechoviruses, a novel group of human picornaviruses. Ann Med 33:466–471
97. Kahn J (2008) Human bocavirus: clinical significance and implications. Curr Opin Pediatr 20:62–66
98. Kahn RE, Clouser DF, Richt JA (2009) Emerging Infections: a tribute to the one medicine, one health concept. Zoonoses Public Health 55:407–428
99. Kaplan NM, Dove W, Abu-Zeid AF, Shamoon HE, Abd-Eldayem SA, Hart CA (2006) Human bocavirus infection among children, Jordan. Emerg Infect Dis 12:1418–1420
100. Kapoor A, Slikas E, Simmonds P, Chieochansin T, Naeem A, Shaukat S, Alam MM, Sharif S, Angez M, Zaidi S, Delwart E (2009) A newly identified bocavirus species in human stool. J Infect Dis 199:196–200
101. Kasamatsu H, Nakanishi A (1998) How do animal DNA viruses get to the nucleus? Annu Rev Microbiol 52:627–686
102. Katsimpardi KPV, Pangalis A, Parcharidou A, Panagiotou JP, Soutis M, Papandreou E, Polychronopoulou S, Haidas S (2006) Infections in a pediatric patient cohort with acute lymphoblastic leukemia during the entire course of treatment. Support Care Cancer 14:277–284
103. Kesebir D, Vazquez M, Weibel C, Shapiro ED, Ferguson D, Landry ML, Kahn JS (2006) Human bocavirus infection in young children in the United States: molecular epidemiological profile and clinical characteristics of a newly emerging respiratory virus. J Infect Dis 194:1276–1282
104. Khanna N, Widmer AF, Decker M, Steffen I, Halter J, Heim D, Weisser M, Gratwohl A, Fluckiger U, Hirsch HH (2008) Respiratory syncytial virus infection in patients with hematological diseases: single-center study and review of the literature. Clin Infect Dis 46:402–412
105. Khetsuriani N, Lu X, Teague WG, Kazerouni N, Anderson LJ, Erdman DD (2008) Novel human rhinoviruses and exacerbation of asthma in children. Emerg Infect Dis 14:1793–1796
106. Koetz A, Nilsson P, Linden M, van der Hoek L, Ripa T (2006) Detection of human coronavirus NL63, human metapneumovirus and respiratory syncytial virus in children with respiratory tract infections in south-west Sweden. Clin Microbiol Infect 12:1089–1096
107. Krogerus C, Egger D, Samuilova O, Hyypia T, Bienz K (2003) Replication complex of human parechovirus 1. J Virol 77:8512–8523
108. Ksiazek TG, Erdman D, Goldsmith CS, Zaki SR, Peret T, Emery S, Tong S, Urbani C, Comer JA, Lim W, Rollin PE, Dowell SF, Ling AE, Humphrey CD, Shieh WJ, Guarner J, Paddock CD, Rota P, Fields B, DeRisi J, Yang JY, Cox N, Hughes JM, LeDuc JW, Bellini WJ, Anderson LJ (2003) A novel coronavirus associated with severe acute respiratory syndrome. N Engl J Med 348:1953–1966
109. Kupfer B, Vehreschild J, Cornely O, Kaiser R, Plum G, Viazov S, Franzen C, Tillmann RL, Simon A, Muller A, Schildgen O (2006) Severe pneumonia and human bocavirus in adult. Emerg Infect Dis 12:1614–1616
110. Kurz H, Herbich K, Janata O, Sterniste W, Bauer K (2008) Experience with the use of palivizumab together with infection control measures to prevent respiratory syncytial virus outbreaks in neonatal intensive care units. J Hosp Infect 70:246–252
111. Lambert SB, Allen KM, Druce JD, Birch CJ, Mackay IM, Carlin JB, Carapetis JR, Sloots TP, Nissen MD, Nolan TM (2007) Community epidemiology of human metapneumovirus, human coronavirus NL63, and other respiratory viruses in healthy preschool-aged children using parent-collected specimens. Pediatrics 120:e929–e937
112. Larcher C, Geltner C, Fischer H, Nachbaur D, Muller LC, Huemer HP (2005) Human metapneumovirus infection in lung transplant recipients: clinical presentation and epidemiology. J Heart Lung Transplant 24:1891–1901
113. Lau SK, Woo PC, Tse H, Fu CT, Au WK, Chen XC, Tsoi HW, Tsang TH, Chan JS, Tsang DN, Li KS, Tse CW, Ng TK, Tsang OT, Zheng BJ, Tam S, Chan KH, Zhou B, Yuen KY (2008) Identification of novel porcine and bovine parvoviruses closely related to human parvovirus 4. J Gen Virol 89:1840–1848
114. Lehmann C, Klar R, Lindner J, Lindner P, Wolf H, Gerling S (2009) Kawasaki disease lacks association with human coronavirus NL63 and human bocavirus. Pediatr Infect Dis J 28:553–554
115. Lin JH, Chiu SC, Lin YC, Chen HL, Lin KH, Shan KH, Wu HS, Liu HF (2009) Clinical and genetic analysis of Human Bocavirus in children with lower respiratory tract infection in Taiwan. J Clin Virol 44:219–224
116. Lin F, Zeng A, Yang N, Lin H, Yang E, Wang S, Pintel D, Qiu J (2007) Quantification of human bocavirus in lower respiratory tract infections in China. Infect Agent Cancer 2:3
117. Lin F, Zheng M, Li H, Zheng C, Li X, Rao G, Wu F, Zeng A (2008) WU polyomavirus in children with acute lower respiratory tract infections, China. J Clin Virol 42:94–102
118. Lindner J, Karalar L, Schimanski S, Pfister H, Struff W, Modrow S (2008) Clinical and epidemiological aspects of human bocavirus infection. J Clin Virol 43:391–395
119. Lindner J, Karalar L, Zehentmeier S, Plentz A, Pfister H, Struff W, Kertai M, Segerer H, Modrow S (2008) Humoral immune response against human bocavirus VP2 virus-like particles. Viral Immunol 21:443–449
120. Lindner J, Modrow S (2008) Human bocavirus–a novel parvovirus to infect humans. Intervirology 51:116–122
121. Lindner J, Zehentmeier S, Franssila R, Barabas S, Schroeder J, Deml L, Modrow S (2008) CD4+ T helper cell responses

against human bocavirus viral protein 2 viruslike particles in healthy adults. J Infect Dis 198:1677–1684
122. Ling Z, Tran KC, Teng MN (2009) The human respiratory syncytial virus nonstructural NS2 protein antagonizes the activation of interferon-{beta} transcription by interacting with RIG-I. J Virol 83:3734–3742
123. Lo MS, Brazas RM, Holtzman MJ (2005) Respiratory syncytial virus nonstructural proteins NS1 and NS2 mediate inhibition of Stat2 expression and alpha/beta interferon responsiveness. J Virol 79:9315–9319
124. Longtin J, Bastien M, Gilca R, Leblanc E, de Serres G, Bergeron MG, Boivin G (2008) Human bocavirus infections in hospitalized children and adults. Emerg Infect Dis 14:217–221
125. Louie JK, Schnurr DP, Pan CY, Kiang D, Carter C, Tougaw S, Ventura J, Norman A, Belmusto V, Rosenberg J, Trochet G (2007) A summer outbreak of human metapneumovirus infection in a long-term-care facility. J Infect Dis 196: 705–708
126. Lu X, Gooding LR, Erdman DD (2008) Human bocavirus in tonsillar lymphocytes. Emerg Infect Dis 14: 1332–1334
127. Ma X, Endo R, Ishiguro N, Ebihara T, Ishiko H, Ariga T, Kikuta H (2006) Detection of human bocavirus in Japanese children with lower respiratory tract infections. J Clin Microbiol 44:1132–1134
128. Mackay IM (2007) Human bocavirus: multisystem detection raises questions about infection. J Infect Dis 196: 968–970
129. Mackay IM, Lambert SB, McErlean PK, Faux CE, Arden KE, Nissen MD, Sloots TP (2008) Prior evidence of putative novel rhinovirus species, Australia. Emerg Infect Dis 14:1823–1824
130. Madisch I, Heim A (2007) Extent of circulation of incorrectly labeled adenovirus 50 and 51 prototype preparations. J Clin Microbiol 45:2092
131. Madisch I, Wolfel R, Harste G, Pommer H, Heim A (2006) Molecular identification of adenovirus sequences: a rapid scheme for early typing of human adenoviruses in diagnostic samples of immunocompetent and immunodeficient patients. J Med Virol 78:1210–1217
132. Maggi F, Andreoli E, Pifferi M, Meschi S, Rocchi J, Bendinelli M (2007) Human bocavirus in Italian patients with respiratory diseases. J Clin Virol 38:321–325
133. Marchiori E, Escuissato DL, Gasparetto TD, Considera DP, Franquet T (2009) "Crazy-paving" patterns on high-resolution CT scans in patients with pulmonary complications after hematopoietic stem cell transplantation. Korean J Radiol 10:21–24
134. Marra MA, Jones SJ, Astell CR, Holt RA, Brooks-Wilson A, Butterfield YS, Khattra J, Asano JK, Barber SA, Chan SY, Cloutier A, Coughlin SM, Freeman D, Girn N, Griffith OL, Leach SR, Mayo M, McDonald H, Montgomery SB, Pandoh PK, Petrescu AS, Robertson AG, Schein JE, Siddiqui A, Smailus DE, Stott JM, Yang GS, Plummer F, Andonov A, Artsob H, Bastien N, Bernard K, Booth TF, Bowness D, Czub M, Drebot M, Fernando L, Flick R, Garbutt M, Gray M, Grolla A, Jones S, Feldmann H, Meyers A, Kabani A, Li Y, Normand S, Stroher U, Tipples GA, Tyler S, Vogrig R, Ward D, Watson B, Brunham RC, Krajden M, Petric M, Skowronski DM, Upton C, Roper RL (2003) The Genome sequence of the SARS-associated coronavirus. Science 300: 1399–1404
135. Mattner F, Sykora KW, Meissner B, Heim A (2008) An adenovirus type F41 outbreak in a pediatric bone marrow transplant unit: analysis of clinical impact and preventive strategies. Pediatr Infect Dis J 27:419–424
136. McIntosh K (2006) Human bocavirus: developing evidence for pathogenicity. J Infect Dis 194:1197–1199
137. McIntosh K, Kapikian AZ, Turner HC, Hartley JW, Parrott RH, Chanock RM (1970) Seroepidemiologic studies of coronavirus infection in adults and children. Am J Epidemiol 91:585–592
138. Meberg A, Bruu AL (2006) Respiratory syncytial virus infections in congenital heart defects–hospitalizations and costs. Acta Paediatr 95:404–406
139. Michaels MG, Fonseca-Aten M, Green M, Charsha-May D, Friedman B, Seikaly M, Sanchez PJ (2009) Respiratory syncytial virus prophylaxis: a survey of pediatric solid organ transplant centers. Pediatr Transplant 13:451–456
140. Minosse C, Selleri M, Zaniratti MS, Cappiello G, Spano A, Schifano E, Lauria FN, Gualano G, Puro V, Campanini G, Gerna G, Capobianchi MR (2008) Phylogenetic analysis of human coronavirus NL63 circulating in Italy. J Clin Virol 43:114–119
141. Miyakis S, van Hal SJ, Barratt J, Stark D, Marriott D, Harkness J (2009) Absence of human Bocavirus in bronchoalveolar lavage fluid of lung transplant patients. J Clin Virol 44:179–180
142. Miyazaki K, Tsunoda A, Kumasaka M, Ishida N (1971) Presence of neutralizing antibody against the 229E strain of coronavirus in the sera of residents of Sendai. Jpn J Microbiol 15:276–277
143. Monteny M, Niesters HG, Moll HA, Berger MY (2007) Human bocavirus in febrile children, The Netherlands. Emerg Infect Dis 13:180–182
144. Moore EC, Barber J, Tripp RA (2008) Respiratory syncytial virus (RSV) attachment and nonstructural proteins modify the type I interferon response associated with suppressor of cytokine signaling (SOCS) proteins and IFN-stimulated gene-15 (ISG15). Virol J 5:116
145. Morris SK, Dzolganovski B, Beyene J, Sung L (2009) A meta-analysis of the effect of antibody therapy for the prevention of severe respiratory syncytial virus infection. BMC Infect Dis 9:106
146. Muller A, Klinkenberg D, Vehreschild J, Cornely O, Tillmann RL, Franzen C, Simon A, Schildgen O (2009) Low prevalence of human metapneumovirus and human bocavirus in adult immunocompromised high risk patients suspected to suffer from Pneumocystis pneumonia. J Infect 58:227–231
147. Muller A, Kupfer B, Vehreschild J, Cornely O, Kaiser R, Seifert H, Viazov S, Tillmann RL, Franzen C, Simon A, Schildgen O (2007) Fatal pneumonia associated with human metapneumovirus (HMPV) in a patient with myeloid leukemia and adenocarcinoma in the lung. Eur J Med Res 12:183–184
148. Munir S, Le Nouen C, Luongo C, Buchholz UJ, Collins PL, Bukreyev A (2008) Nonstructural proteins 1 and 2 of respiratory syncytial virus suppress maturation of human dendritic cells. J Virol 82:8780–8796

149. Naghipour M, Cuevas LE, Bakhshinejad T, Dove W, Hart CA (2007) Human bocavirus in Iranian children with acute respiratory infections. J Med Virol 79:539–543
150. Neske F, Blessing K, Ullrich F, Prottel A, Wolfgang Kreth H, Weissbrich B (2008) WU polyomavirus infection in children, Germany. Emerg Infect Dis 14:680–681
151. Niklasson B, Samsioe A, Papadogiannakis N, Gustafsson S, Klitz W (2009) Zoonotic Ljungan virus associated with central nervous system malformations in terminated pregnancy. Birth Defects Res A Clin Mol Teratol 85:542–545
152. Norja P, Ubillos I, Templeton K, Simmonds P (2007) No evidence for an association between infections with WU and KI polyomaviruses and respiratory disease. J Clin Virol 40:307–311
153. Novel Swine-Origin Influenza A (H1N1) Virus Investigation Team, Dawood FS, Jain S, Finelli L, Shaw MW, Lindstrom S, Garten RJ, Gubareva LV, Xu X, Bridges CB, Uyeki TM (2009) Emergence of a Novel Swine-Origin Influenza A (H1N1) Virus in Humans. N Engl J Med 360:2605–2615
154. Osterhaus AD (2008) New respiratory viruses of humans. Pediatr Infect Dis J 27:S71–S74
155. Payungporn S, Chieochansin T, Thongmee C, Samransamruajkit R, Theamboolers A, Poovorawan Y (2008) Prevalence and molecular characterization of WU/KI polyomaviruses isolated from pediatric patients with respiratory disease in Thailand. Virus Res 135:230–236
156. Peiris JS, Lai ST, Poon LL, Guan Y, Yam LY, Lim W, Nicholls J, Yee WK, Yan WW, Cheung MT, Cheng VC, Chan KH, Tsang DN, Yung RW, Ng TK, Yuen KY (2003) Coronavirus as a possible cause of severe acute respiratory syndrome. Lancet 361:1319–1325
157. Pene F, Merlat A, Vabret A, Rozenberg F, Buzyn A, Dreyfus F, Cariou A, Freymuth F, Lebon P (2003) Coronavirus 229E-related pneumonia in immunocompromised patients. Clin Infect Dis 37:929–932
158. Pierangeli A, Scagnolari C, Trombetti S, Grossi R, Battaglia M, Moretti C, Midulla F, Antonelli G (2008) Human bocavirus infection in hospitalized children in Italy. Influenza Other Respir Viruses 2:175–179
159. Pignotti MS, Catarzi S, Donzelli G (2006) A 4-year survey on palivizumab respiratory syncytial virus (RSV)-prophylaxis: how can compliance be improved? J Matern Fetal Neonatal Med 19:221–224
160. Pozo F, Garcia-Garcia ML, Calvo C, Cuesta I, Perez-Brena P, Casas I (2007) High incidence of human bocavirus infection in children in Spain. J Clin Virol 40:224–228
161. Pyrc K, Dijkman R, Deng L, Jebbink MF, Ross HA, Berkhout B, van der Hoek L (2006) Mosaic structure of human coronavirus NL63, one thousand years of evolution. J Mol Biol 364:964–973
162. Qu XW, Duan ZJ, Qi ZY, Xie ZP, Gao HC, Liu WP, Huang CP, Peng FW, Zheng LS, Hou YD (2007) Human bocavirus infection, People's Republic of China. Emerg Infect Dis 13:165–168
163. Qu XW, Liu WP, Qi ZY, Duan ZJ, Zheng LS, Kuang ZZ, Zhang WJ, Hou YD (2008) Phospholipase A2-like activity of human bocavirus VP1 unique region. Biochem Biophys Res Commun 365:158–163
164. Raad I, Abbas J, Whimbey E (1997) Infection control of nosocomial respiratory viral disease in the immunocompromised host. Am J Med 102:48–52, discussion 53-4
165. Raza K, Ismailjee SB, Crespo M, Studer SM, Sanghavi S, Paterson DL, Kwak EJ, Rinaldo CR Jr, Pilewski JM, McCurry KR, Husain S (2007) Successful outcome of human metapneumovirus (hMPV) pneumonia in a lung transplant recipient treated with intravenous ribavirin. J Heart Lung Transplant 26:862–864
166. Redshaw N, Wood C, Rich F, Grimwood K, Kirman JR (2007) Human bocavirus in infants, New Zealand. Emerg Infect Dis 13:1797–1799
167. Regamey N, Frey U, Deffernez C, Latzin P, Kaiser L (2007) Isolation of human bocavirus from Swiss infants with respiratory infections. Pediatr Infect Dis J 26:177–179
168. Revie D, Tseng BY, Grafstrom RH, Goulian M (1979) Covalent association of protein with replicative form DNA of parvovirus H-1. Proc Natl Acad Sci USA 76: 5539–5543
169. Rockville Merkel Cell Carcinoma Group (2009) Merkel cell carcinoma: recent progress and current priorities on etiology, pathogenesis, and clinical management. J Clin Oncol 27:4021–4026
170. Samsioe A, Papadogiannakis N, Hultman T, Sjoholm A, Klitz W, Niklasson B (2009) Ljungan virus present in intrauterine fetal death diagnosed by both immunohistochemistry and PCR. Birth Defects Res A Clin Mol Teratol 85: 227–229
171. Savolainen-Kopra C, Blomqvist S, Kilpi T, Roivainen M, Hovi T (2009) Novel species of human rhinoviruses in acute otitis media. Pediatr Infect Dis J 28:59–61
172. Schenk T, Huck B, Forster J, Berner R, Neumann-Haefelin D, Falcone V (2007) Human bocavirus DNA detected by quantitative real-time PCR in two children hospitalized for lower respiratory tract infection. Eur J Clin Microbiol Infect Dis 26:147–149
173. Schenk T, Strahm B, Kontny U, Hufnagel M, Neumann-Haefelin D, Falcone V (2007) Disseminated bocavirus infection after stem cell transplant. Emerg Infect Dis 13:1425–1427
174. Schildgen O (2009) The lack of protective immunity against RSV in the Elderly. Epidemiol Infect 137:1687–1690
175. Schildgen O, Geikowski T, Glatzel T, Simon A, Wilkesmann A, Roggendorf M, Viazov S, Matz B (2004) New variant of the human metapneumovirus (HMPV) associated with an acute and severe exacerbation of asthma bronchiale. J Clin Virol 31:283–288
176. Schildgen O, Muller A, Allander T, Mackay IM, Volz S, Kupfer B, Simon A (2008) Human bocavirus: passenger or pathogen in acute respiratory tract infections? Clin Microbiol Rev 21:291–304
177. Schildgen O, Muller A, Simon A (2007) Human bocavirus and gastroenteritis. Emerg Infect Dis 13:1620–1621
178. Schildgen O, Wilkesmann A, Simon A (2006) Wheezing in patients with human metapneumovirus infection. J Allergy Clin Immunol 117:223, author reply 223-4
179. Shan TL, Zhang W, Guo W, Cui L, Yuan CL, Dai XQ, Shen Q, Yang ZB, Zhu JG, Hua XG (2009) The first detection of human bocavirus 2 infections in China. J Clin Virol 46: 196–197
180. Shinde V et al (2009) Triple-Reassortant Swine Influenza A (H1) in humans in United States, 2005–2009. NEJM 360:2616–2625

181. Simoes EA, Groothuis JR, Carbonell-Estrany X, Rieger CH, Mitchell I, Fredrick LM, Kimpen JL (2007) Palivizumab prophylaxis, respiratory syncytial virus, and subsequent recurrent wheezing. J Pediatr 151:34–42, 42 e1
182. Simon A, Ammann RA, Wilkesmann A, Eis-Hubinger AM, Schildgen O, Weimann E, Peltner HU, Seiffert P, Suss-Grafeo A, Groothuis JR, Liese J, Pallacks R, Muller A (2007) Respiratory syncytial virus infection in 406 hospitalized premature infants: results from a prospective German multicentre database. Eur J Pediatr 166: 1273–1283
183. Simon A, Groneck P, Kupfer B, Kaiser R, Plum G, Tillmann RL, Muller A, Schildgen O (2007) Detection of bocavirus DNA in nasopharyngeal aspirates of a child with bronchiolitis. J Infect 54:e125–e127
184. Simon A, Khurana K, Wilkesmann A, Muller A, Engelhart S, Exner M, Schildgen O, Eis-Hubinger AM, Groothuis JR, Bode U (2006) Nosocomial respiratory syncytial virus infection: impact of prospective surveillance and targeted infection control. Int J Hyg Environ Health 209:317–324
185. Simon A, Muller A, Khurana K, Engelhart S, Exner M, Schildgen O, Eis-Hubinger AM, Kamin W, Schaible T, Wadas K, Ammann RA, Wilkesmann A (2008) Nosocomial infection: a risk factor for a complicated course in children with respiratory syncytial virus infection – results from a prospective multicenter German surveillance study. Int J Hyg Environ Health 211:241–250
186. Skowronski DM, Astell C, Brunham RC, Low DE, Petric M, Roper RL, Talbot PJ, Tam T, Babiuk L (2005) Severe acute respiratory syndrome (SARS): a year in review. Annu Rev Med 56:357–381
187. Sloots TP, McErlean P, Speicher DJ, Arden KE, Nissen MD, Mackay IM (2006) Evidence of human coronavirus HKU1 and human bocavirus in Australian children. J Clin Virol 35:99–102
188. Smuts H (2008) Human coronavirus NL63 infections in infants hospitalised with acute respiratory tract infections in South Africa. Influenza Other Respir Viruses 2: 135–138
189. Smuts H, Hardie D (2006) Human bocavirus in hospitalized children, South Africa. Emerg Infect Dis 12: 1457–1458
190. Smuts H, Workman L, Zar HJ (2008) Role of human metapneumovirus, human coronavirus NL63 and human bocavirus in infants and young children with acute wheezing. J Med Virol 80:906–912
191. Spann KM, Tran KC, Collins PL (2005) Effects of nonstructural proteins NS1 and NS2 of human respiratory syncytial virus on interferon regulatory factor 3, NF-kappaB, and proinflammatory cytokines. J Virol 79:5353–5362
192. Sumino KC, Agapov E, Pierce RA, Trulock EP, Pfeifer JD, Ritter JH, Gaudreault-Keener M, Storch GA, Holtzman MJ (2005) Detection of severe human metapneumovirus infection by real-time polymerase chain reaction and histopathological assessment. J Infect Dis 192:1052–1060
193. Suzuki A, Okamoto M, Ohmi A, Watanabe O, Miyabayashi S, Nishimura H (2005) Detection of human coronavirus-NL63 in children in Japan. Pediatr Infect Dis J 24: 645–646
194. Szomor KN, Kapusinszky B, Rigo Z, Kis Z, Rozsa M, Farkas A, Szilagyi A, Berencsi G, Takacs M (2009) Detection of human bocavirus from fecal samples of Hungarian children with acute gastroenteritis. Intervirology 52:17–21
195. Tan BH, Lim EA, Seah SG, Loo LH, Tee NW, Lin RT, Sugrue RJ (2009) The incidence of human bocavirus infection among children admitted to hospital in Singapore. J Med Virol 81:82–89
196. Terrosi C, Di Genova G, Martorelli B, Valentini M, Cusi MG (2009) Humoral immunity to respiratory syncytial virus in young and elderly adults. Epidemiol Infect 137:1684–1686
197. Terrosi C, Di Genova G, Savellini GG, Correale P, Blardi P, Cusi MG (2007) Immunological characterization of respiratory syncytial virus N protein epitopes recognized by human cytotoxic T lymphocytes. Viral Immunol 20: 399–406
198. Terrosi C, Fabbiani M, Cellesi C, Cusi MG (2007) Human bocavirus detection in an atopic child affected by pneumonia associated with wheezing. J Clin Virol 40:43–45
199. Tolf C, Gullberg M, Johansson ES, Tesh RB, Andersson B, Lindberg AM (2009) Molecular characterization of a novel Ljungan virus (Parechovirus; Picornaviridae) reveals a fourth genotype and indicates ancestral recombination. J Gen Virol 90:843–853
200. Tolou H, Buisson Y (2007) Human Bocavirus: a new respiratory pathogen? Med Trop 67:13–14
201. Torres HA, Aguilera EA, Mattiuzzi GN, Cabanillas ME, Rohatgi N, Sepulveda CA, Kantarjian HM, Jiang Y, Safdar A, Raad II, Chemaly RF (2007) Characteristics and outcome of respiratory syncytial virus infection in patients with leukemia. Haematologica 92:1216–1223
202. Vabret A, Mourez T, Dina J, van der Hoek L, Gouarin S, Petitjean J, Brouard J, Freymuth F (2005) Human coronavirus NL63, France. Emerg Infect Dis 11:1225–1229
203. Vallet C, Pons-Catalano C, Mandelcwajg A, Wang A, Raymond J, Lebon P, Gendrel D (2009) Human bocavirus: a cause of severe asthma exacerbation in children. J Pediatr 155:286–288
204. van den Hoogen BG, de Jong JC, Groen J, Kuiken T, de Groot R, Fouchier RA, Osterhaus AD (2001) A newly discovered human pneumovirus isolated from young children with respiratory tract disease. Nat Med 7:719–724
205. van den Hoogen BG, Osterhaus DM, Fouchier RA (2004) Clinical impact and diagnosis of human metapneumovirus infection. Pediatr Infect Dis J 23:S25–S32
206. van den Hoogen BG, van Doornum GJ, Fockens JC, Cornelissen JJ, Beyer WE, de Groot R, Osterhaus AD, Fouchier RA (2003) Prevalence and clinical symptoms of human metapneumovirus infection in hospitalized patients. J Infect Dis 188:1571–1577
207. van der Hoek L, Pyrc K, Jebbink MF, Vermeulen-Oost W, Berkhout RJ, Wolthers KC, Wertheim-van Dillen PM, Kaandorp J, Spaargaren J, Berkhout B (2004) Identification of a new human coronavirus. Nat Med 10: 368–373
208. van der Hoek L, Sure K, Ihorst G, Stang A, Pyrc K, Jebbink MF, Petersen G, Forster J, Berkhout B, Uberla K (2006) Human coronavirus NL63 infection is associated with croup. Adv Exp Med Biol 581:485–491
209. van der Sanden S, de Bruin E, Vennema H, Swanink C, Koopmans M, van der Avoort H (2008) Prevalence of

human parechovirus in the Netherlands in 2000 to 2007. J Clin Microbiol 46:2884–2889
210. Velayudhan BT, Nagaraja KV, Thachil AJ, Shaw DP, Gray GC, Halvorson DA (2006) Human metapneumovirus in turkey poults. Emerg Infect Dis 12:1853–1859
211. Venkatesh MP, Weisman LE (2006) Prevention and treatment of respiratory syncytial virus infection in infants: an update. Expert Rev Vaccines 5:261–268
212. Verboon-Maciolek MA, Groenendaal F, Hahn CD, Hellmann J, van Loon AM, Boivin G, de Vries LS (2008) Human parechovirus causes encephalitis with white matter injury in neonates. Ann Neurol 64:266–273
213. Vicente D, Cilla G, Montes M, Perez-Yarza EG, Perez-Trallero E (2007) Human bocavirus, a respiratory and enteric virus. Emerg Infect Dis 13:636–637
214. Villa L, Melon S, Suarez S, Alvarez-Arguelles ME, Gonzalez D, Morilla A, Boga JA, Rodriguez J, de Ona M (2008) Detection of human bocavirus in Asturias, Northern Spain. Eur J Clin Microbiol Infect Dis 27:237–239
215. Voigt E, Tillmann RL, Schewe JC, Molitor E, Schildgen O (2008) ARDS in an HIV-positive patient associated to respiratory syncytial virus. Eur J Med Res 13:131–132
216. Volz S, Schildgen O, Klinkenberg D, Ditt V, Muller A, Tillmann RL, Kupfer B, Bode U, Lentze MJ, Simon A (2007) Prospective study of Human Bocavirus (HBoV) infection in a pediatric university hospital in Germany 2005/2006. J Clin Virol 40:229–235
217. Volz S, Schildgen O, Muller A, Tillmann RL, Eis-Hubinger AM, Kupfer B, Bode U, Lentze ML, Simon A (2007) The human bocavirus: pathogen in airway infections? Dtsch Med Wochenschr 132:1529–1533
218. von Linstow ML, Eugen-Olsen J, Koch A, Winther TN, Westh H, Hogh B (2006) Excretion patterns of human metapneumovirus and respiratory syncytial virus among young children. Eur J Med Res 11:329–335
219. von Linstow ML, Hogh M, Hogh B (2008) Clinical and epidemiologic characteristics of human bocavirus in Danish infants: results from a prospective birth cohort study. Pediatr Infect Dis J 27:897–902
220. von Linstow ML, Hogh M, Nordbo SA, Eugen-Olsen J, Koch A, Hogh B (2008) A community study of clinical traits and risk factors for human metapneumovirus and respiratory syncytial virus infection during the first year of life. Eur J Pediatr 167:1125–1133
221. von Linstow ML, Larsen HH, Eugen-Olsen J, Koch A, Nordmann Winther T, Meyer AM, Westh H, Lundgren B, Melbye M, Hogh B (2004) Human metapneumovirus and respiratory syncytial virus in hospitalized danish children with acute respiratory tract infection. Scand J Infect Dis 36:578–584
222. von Renesse A, Schildgen O, Klinkenberg D, Muller A, von Moers A, Simon A (2009) Respiratory syncytial virus infection in children admitted to hospital but ventilated mechanically for other reasons. J Med Virol 81:160–166
223. Wakatsuki K, Kawamoto D, Hiwaki H, Watanabe K, Yoshida H (2008) Identification and characterization of two strains of human parechovirus 4 isolated from two clinical cases in Fukuoka City, Japan. J Clin Microbiol 46:3144–3146
224. Wang D, Cummins C, Bayliss S, Sandercock J, Burls A (2008) Immunoprophylaxis against respiratory syncytial virus (RSV) with palivizumab in children: a systematic review and economic evaluation. Health Technol Assess 12:iii, ix–x, 1–86
225. Weisman LE (2009) Respiratory syncytial virus (RSV) prevention and treatment: past, present, and future. Cardiovasc Hematol Agents Med Chem 7:223–233
226. Weissbrich B, Neske F, Schubert J, Tollmann F, Blath K, Blessing K, Kreth HW (2006) Frequent detection of bocavirus DNA in German children with respiratory tract infections. BMC Infect Dis 6:109
227. Wenzel RP, Bearman G, Edmond MB (2005) Lessons from severe acute respiratory syndrome (SARS): implications for infection control. Arch Med Res 36:610–616
228. Whimbey E, Couch RB, Englund JA, Andreeff M, Goodrich JM, Raad V II, Lewis NM, Luna MA, Baxter B et al (1995) Respiratory syncytial virus pneumonia in hospitalized adult patients with leukemia. Clin Infect Dis 21:376–9
229. Wilkesmann A, Schildgen O, Eis-Hubinger AM, Geikowski T, Glatzel T, Lentze MJ, Bode U, Simon A (2006) Human metapneumovirus infections cause similar symptoms and clinical severity as respiratory syncytial virus infections. Eur J Pediatr 165:467–475
230. Williams CH, Panayiotou M, Girling GD, Peard CI, Oikarinen S, Hyoty H, Stanway G (2009) Evolution and conservation in human parechovirus genomes. J Gen Virol 90:1702–1712
231. Wolthers KC, Benschop KS, Schinkel J, Molenkamp R, Bergevoet RM, Spijkerman IJ, Kraakman HC, Pajkrt D (2008) Human parechoviruses as an important viral cause of sepsislike illness and meningitis in young children. Clin Infect Dis 47:358–363
232. Woo PC, Lau SK, Chu CM, Chan KH, Tsoi HW, Huang Y, Wong BH, Poon RW, Cai JJ, Luk WK, Poon LL, Wong SS, Guan Y, Peiris JS, Yuen KY (2005) Characterization and complete genome sequence of a novel coronavirus, coronavirus HKU1, from patients with pneumonia. J Virol 79:884–895
233. Woo PC, Lau SK, Huang Y, Tsoi HW, Chan KH, Yuen KY (2005) Phylogenetic and recombination analysis of coronavirus HKU1, a novel coronavirus from patients with pneumonia. Arch Virol 150:2299–2311
234. Yamamoto M, Abe K, Kuniyori K, Kunii E, Ito F, Kasama Y, Yoshioka Y, Noda M (2009) Epidemic of human parechovirus type 3 in hiroshima city, Japan in 2008. Jpn J Infect Dis 62:244–245
235. Yu JM, Li DD, Xu ZQ, Cheng WX, Zhang Q, Li HY, Cui SX, Miao J, Yang SH, Fang ZY, Duan ZJ (2008) Human bocavirus infection in children hospitalized with acute gastroenteritis in China. J Clin Virol 42:280–285
236. Zadori ZSJ, Lacoste MC, Li Y, Gariepy S, Raymond P, Allaire M, Nabi IR, Tijssen P (2001) A viral phospholipase A2 is required for parvovirus infectivity. Cell Dev 1: 291–302
237. Zhang LL, Tang LY, Xie ZD, Tan XJ, Li CS, Cui AL, Ji YX, Xu ST, Mao NY, Xu WB, Shen KL (2008) Human bocavirus in children suffering from acute lower respiratory tract infection in Beijing Children's Hospital. Chin Med J (Engl) 121:1607–1610
238. Zhao LQ, Qian Y, Zhu RN, Deng J, Wang F, Dong HJ, Sun Y, Li Y (2009) Human bocavirus infections are common in Beijing population indicated by sero-antibody prevalence analysis. Chin Med J (Engl) 122:1289–1292

239. Ziegler S, Tillmann RL, Muller A, Simon A, Schildgen V, Schildgen O (2008) No gastroenteric Bocavirus in high risk patients stool samples. J Clin Virol 43:349–350
240. Zoll J, Erkens Hulshof S, Lanke K, Verduyn Lunel F, Melchers WJ, Schoondermark-van de Ven E, Roivainen M, Galama JM, van Kuppeveld FJ (2009) Saffold virus, a human Theiler's-like cardiovirus, is ubiquitous and causes infection early in life. PLoS Pathog 5:e1000416
241. Zoll J, Galama JM, van Kuppeveld FJ (2009) Identification of potential recombination breakpoints in human parechoviruses. J Virol 83:3379–3383
242. zur Hausen H (2008) Novel human polyomaviruses – re-emergence of a well known virus family as possible human carcinogens. Int J Cancer 123:247–250

Cytomegalovirus Pneumonia in Patients with Hematologic Malignancies

23

Karen J. Vigil and Roy F. Chemaly

Contents

23.1 Introduction

Cytomegalovirus (CMV) is a ubiquitous virus that is found in all geographic locations and infects people from all socioeconomic groups. In the United States, approximately 60% of individuals 6 years of age or older have been infected with CMV; worldwide, the incidence ranges from 60% to 100% [28].

CMV, a DNA virus belonging to the Herpesviridae family, infects more humans than does any other virus. As with other herpesviruses (i.e., Epstein-Barr virus; herpes simplex viruses 1 and 2; varicella-zoster virus; and human herpesviruses 6, 7, and 8), CMV remains latent in the host and has the potential to be reactivated, causing disease. Transmission of CMV occurs from person to person through bodily fluids. Primary CMV disease can cause severe infection when acquired congenitally; however, when acquired postnatally, it usually manifests as a benign mononucleosis-like syndrome.

CMV disease is a frequent complication in patients with hematologic malignancies and may cause significant morbidity and mortality. CMV disease can be caused by reactivation of an endogenous virus or by infection from a transplanted organ or, rarely, a blood product transfusion. CMV infection in immunocompromised patient enhances immune suppression, favoring the development of other opportunistic infections and increasing the incidence of graft failure [5, 24, 29]. The lack of a preserved immune system combined with increased viral activation commonly produces severe systemic disease in these patients, who may develop viremia, pneumonia, gastrointestinal disease, hepatitis, meningoencephalitis, polyradiculopathy, and/or retinitis.

K.J. Vigil (✉)
Division of Infectious Diseases,
The University of Texas Health Science Center at Houston
Medical School, 6431 Fannin, MSB 6.119,
Houston, TX 77030, USA
e-mail: karen.j.vigil@uth.tmc.edu

R.F. Chemaly
Department of Infectious Diseases, Infection Control,
and Employee Health, Unit 402, The University of Texas
M. D. Anderson Cancer Center, 1515 Holcombe Blvd,
Houston, TX 77030, USA
e-mail: rfchemaly@mdanderson.org

É. Azoulay (ed.), *Pulmonary Involvement in Patients with Hematological Malignancies*,
DOI: 10.1007/978-3-642-15742-4_23, © Springer-Verlag Berlin Heidelberg 2011

23.2 Cytomegalovirus Pneumonia

23.2.1 Epidemiologic Characteristics

CMV pneumonia is uncommon in immunocompetent patients. However, immunosuppressed patients are at higher risk of developing CMV pneumonia, which is associated with a high mortality rate even when treated with aggressive antiviral therapy.

A recent study reported an incidence of CMV pneumonia in immunocompromised patients of 3%; of the patients studied, 68% were hematopoietic stem cell transplant (HSCT) recipients, 20% had lymphoma, and 12% had leukemia [25]. In HSCT recipients, CMV pneumonia was one of the most common life-threatening infectious complications with an incidence of 10–30% in allogeneic HSCT recipients compared to 2% in autologous HSCT recipients, who usually develop a less severe form of the disease [31]. The use of preemptive therapy has significantly reduced the incidence rate [12]. However, the development of late CMV disease (>100 days posttransplant) is occurring more frequently and is associated with a high relapse rate and poor outcome [2]. In patients with leukemia, the reported incidence of CMV pneumonia is 2.9% [25]. In patients with lymphoma, CMV pneumonia has an overall incidence of 1.1%, and its incidence is increasing [5]. CMV pneumonia is the most common presentation of CMV disease (82%) and is more common in non-Hodgkin's lymphoma patients (89%) than in other immunocompromised patients [30].

The mean time to onset of CMV pneumonia after HSCT transplant is 45 days (range, 2 weeks to > 2 years) [9]. However, with the use of prophylaxis, time of onset has been delayed to a median of 169 days (range, 96–184 days) [2].

In HSCT recipients, risk factors for developing CMV pneumonia include old age, graft-versus-host disease, positive serology of the HSCT donor, use of granulocyte transfusions from seropositive donors, total body irradiation, depleted antithymocyte globulins, receipt of T-cell-depleted stem cells, and circulating CMV DNA [15, 22]. On the other hand, the use of leukocyte-depleted platelets and CMV-seronegative red blood cells reduce the risk of CMV pneumonitis [3]. In patients with leukemia, use of lymphocytotoxic chemotherapeutic agents has been associated with the development of CMV pneumonia [25]. In patients with lymphoma, more cases occur in patients with B-cell non-Hodgkin's lymphoma (89%), active disease (86%), advanced-stage disease (stage III/IV) (92%), or recurrent disease (55%) [5].

23.2.2 Clinical Presentation

The clinical manifestations of CMV pneumonia in patients with hematologic malignancies are nonspecific. The most common presenting signs and symptoms are fever (80–90%), dry cough (65%), and dyspnea (55%). The disease is severe, and patients frequently require admission to the intensive care unit [5]. Hypoxemia is common and is a poor prognostic sign; patients can progress rapidly to respiratory failure requiring mechanical ventilation, especially if untreated. Severe lymphopenia (<200 lymphocytes/mL) is common and significantly associates with a high mortality [25]. Although not clinical evident, an autopsy-based study demonstrated that 48% of cases had disseminated infection (adrenitis, nephritis, and colitis most commonly).

In HSCT patients, symptomatic disease was described to occur most commonly post engraftment and before day 30 after transplant, when mucosal damage is maximal from chemotherapy. However, with the introduction of ganciclovir prophylaxis and preemptive treatment, CMV disease has been observed more frequently later after transplantation, with a median onset of day 160 [1, 2, 12].

CMV infection can predispose the host to other concomitant infections from opportunistic microbes (i.e., bacterial, fungal, or viral) [5, 29]. In these cases, the role of CMV should not be underestimated.

23.2.3 Diagnosis

Diagnosis is difficult and challenging. An autopsy-based study found that of CMV pneumonia patients with a postmortem diagnosis, only 64% had an antemortem diagnosis, and only 60% of patients with an antemortem diagnosis had received treatment. [29]

The diagnosis of CMV pneumonia requires both clinical and radiographic evidence of pneumonia (Figs. 23.1–23.3) as well as isolation of CMV in bronchoalveolar lavage (BAL) fluid or lung-tissue specimens by culture, cytology, immunohistochemical

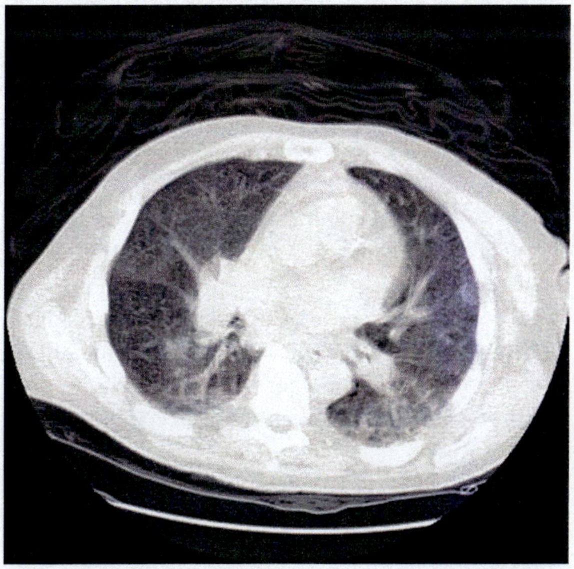

Fig. 23.1 Computerized tomography scan of a 75-year-old patient with chronic lymphocytic leukemia and CMV pneumonia showing areas of ground-glass appearance and interstitial opacities in both lower lobes (*left* more than *right*)

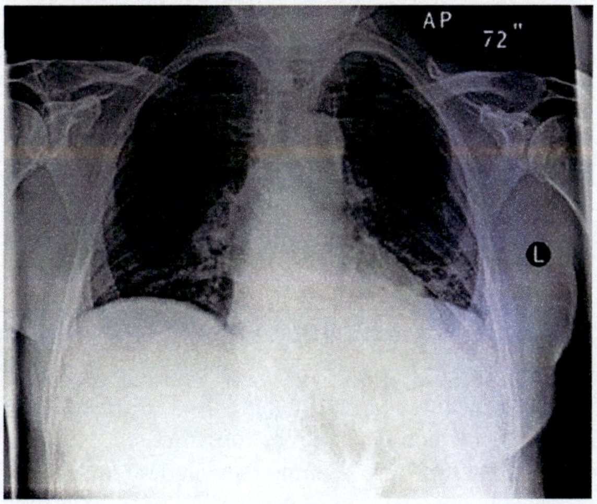

Fig. 23.2 Chest X-ray of a patient with chronic lymphocytic leukemia and CMV pneumonia showing interstitial opacities in both bases

staining, histopathologic examination, or in situ hybridization [20].

23.2.3.1 Radiologic Findings

The radiologic appearances of CMV pneumonia varied widely, with no pattern sufficiently characteristic to allow differentiation of CMV pneumonia from other causes of pneumonia. The most common presentations are bilateral asymmetric ground-glass opacities, airspace opacities, and small centrilobular nodules [16]. However, atypical patterns are not uncommon, and normal chest X-rays have been reported, making it an entity difficult to diagnose on the bases of only imaging [10].

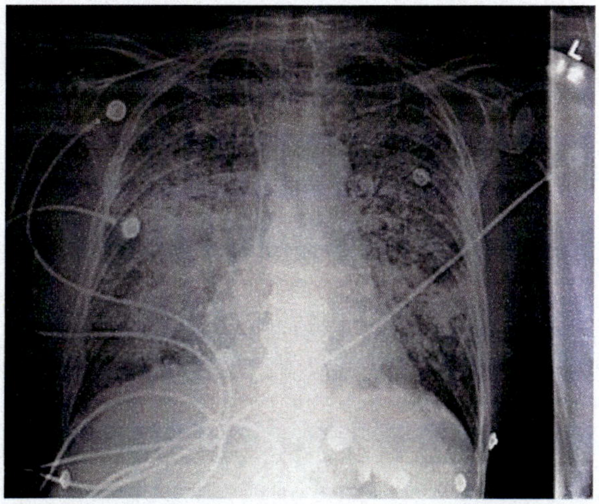

Fig. 23.3 Patients with hematologic malignancies and CMV pneumonia frequently develop superimposed infections. Chest X-ray of a 72-year-old patient with chronic lymphocytic leukemia developed CMV and *Stenotrophomonas maltophilia* pneumonia showing diffuse consolidation in both lungs

Histopathologically, areas of ground-glass attenuation and/or consolidation on CT scans correspond to the areas of alveolar damage that contain cytomegalic cells, hemorrhage, neutrophilic exudates, fibrinous exudates, and hyaline membranes; the lymphocytic interstitial infiltrates that cause alveolar wall or interlobular septal thickening also are seen as ground-glass attenuation. Nodules correspond to inflammatory or hemorrhagic areas or organizing pneumonia, while the centrilobular nodules represent the areas of intralveolar collections of macrophages, red blood cells, and fibrin [18].

23.2.3.2 Lung Biopsy/Cytology

A definitive diagnosis of CMV pneumonia should be based on detection of the virus in lung tissue specimens by immunohistochemical staining, histopathologic evaluation for viral inclusions, or culture (Fig. 23.4). However, lung biopsies are rarely performed in immunocompromised patients because of

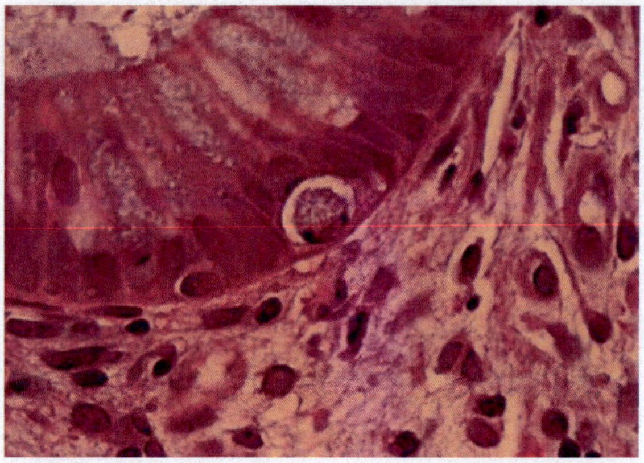

Fig. 23.4 CMV pneumonia. Early owl eye showing nuclear condensation, perinuclear clearing, and typical eosinophilic granules in the cytoplasm (Contribution of Jeffrey J. Tarrand, M.D.)

increased complications, inconsistent diagnosis, and questionable reliability.

Therefore, bronchoalveolar lavage becomes a safe, effective, and rapid method for diagnosing CMV pneumonia in immunocompromised patients. In HSCT recipients, identification of CMV by a rapid centrifugation viral culture of BAL fluid has been shown to be highly correlated with CMV detection in lung tissue specimens [8].

23.2.3.3 Microbiology

Viral cultures are the gold standard for diagnosing CMV infection. However, they have a poor predictive value, lack of quantitation, false-negative results, and long turnaround time (1–6 weeks). Shell vial centrifugation cultures are a modification of conventional culture that has a reduced turnaround time and a high sensitivity that averages between 68% and 100% when compared to conventional viral culture, and are therefore an excellent tool to rapidly diagnose CMV in BAL and tissue specimens [13, 17].

Polymerase chain reaction (PCR) is the most sensitive assay for detecting CMV in BAL fluid. Alveolar cell immunostaining and PCR have a reported sensitivity of 100% for the diagnosis of CMV pneumonitis, whereas viral culture has a sensitivity of only 85.7% [4]. However, diagnosis of CMV pneumonia should not be based exclusively on PCR, as PCR is considered too sensitive and may detect viral shedding without documented disease.

Quantification of CMV has been shown to be useful in differentiating between viral shedding and CMV pneumonia in lung transplant recipients [6, 7]. However, the significance in other immunocompromised patients, including patients with hematologic malignancies, has not been studied.

CMV antigenemia assays are used to monitor CMV infection. The antigenemia assay is based on the detection of the CMV lower matrix protein pp65 in polymorphonuclear leukocytes by immunostaining with monoclonal antibodies. Results are quantified; patients with a high number of antigenemia-positive leukocytes are at a higher risk for developing CMV disease. Researchers have found CMV antigenemia to be a predictor for development of CMV pneumonia [5, 23].

The development of CMV PCR assays has improved efficiency and sensitivity for direct detection of CMV in various specimens, including blood, plasma, urine, CSF, and biopsy material. Because the CMV viral load in blood correlates with the development of CMV disease, determining the CMV DNA viral load during the initial phase of infection and measuring the rate of increase in the viral load may help identify HSCT recipients who are at risk of developing CMV disease [14].

23.2.4 Treatment

23.2.4.1 Treatment Options

Current systemic antiviral agents used to treat CMV infections include ganciclovir, foscarnet, and cidofovir. Therapy for CMV pneumonia includes both ganciclovir and intravenous immunoglobulin. Although this treatment has not been evaluated in a randomized controlled trial and a recent study questioned whether the use of immunoglobulin improves outcome [21], its use is still recommended by experts. The use of ganciclovir is limited by the associated development of neutropenia. Foscarnet is used off-label to treat patients who experience myelosuppression with ganciclovir. However, the use of foscarnet is associated with nephrotoxicity and electrolyte imbalances (i.e., hypokalemia, hypocalcemia, hypomagnesemia, and hypophosphatemia). Cidofovir's side effects include nephrotoxicity and, occasionally, neutropenia (Table 23.1).

Table 23.1 Recommended treatment and prophylaxis doses, side effects, and resistance mechanisms of available antiviral agents with activity against cytomegalovirus

Antiviral agent	Recommended doses	Common side effects	Resistance mechanism
Ganciclovir	Treatment dose: 5 mg/kg IV q 12 h (induction) 5 mg/kg IV q 24 h (maintenance) Prophylaxis dose: 5 mg/kg IV q 24 h	Hematologic toxicities Neurologic toxicity Abnormal liver function Fever Rash	Mutations in *UL97* or *UL54* gene
Foscarnet	Treatment dose: 90 mg/kg IV q 12 h (induction) 90 mg/kg IV q 24 h (maintenance) Prophylaxis dose: 90 mg/kg IV q 24 h	Nephrotoxicity Electrolyte imbalance (hypocalcemia) Seizures Anemia	Mutations in *UL54* gene
Cidofovir	Treatment dose: 1–5 mg/kg/week, followed by maintenance every other week	Nephrotoxicity Hematologic adverse effects	Mutations in *UL54* gene
Valganciclovir	Prophylaxis dose: 900 mg PO daily	Hematologic toxicities Gastrointestinal adverse effects	Mutations in *UL97* or *UL54* gene
Acyclovir	Prophylaxis dose: 500 mg/m^2 IV every 8 h	Acute renal failure Neurologic toxicity	Absence, decrease, or alteration of viral thymidine kinase
Valacyclovir	Prophylaxis dose: 2 g/four times daily	Thrombotic thrombocytopenic purpura	Absence, decrease, or alteration of viral thymidine kinase

DNA deoxyribonucleic acid, *RNA* ribonucleic acid

23.2.4.2 Resistance

Emergence of resistant CMV strains must be considered when choosing a treatment. Resistance to ganciclovir develops from mutations in *UL97* (phosphotransferase), *UL54* (viral DNA polymerase), or both, whereas resistance to cidofovir and foscarnet develops from mutations in *UL54* only. In patients receiving ganciclovir, resistance results exclusively from *UL97* in 90% of patients; however, if use of the drug is continued, *UL54* mutations may develop, precluding the use of cidofovir secondary to cross-resistance, which is uncommon with foscarnet. Similarly, if *UL54*-resistant mutations develop in a patient receiving either ganciclovir or cidofovir, cross-resistance precludes the secondary use of the other drug; however, this is not the case with foscarnet [11].

Although it takes weeks to months for resistance to develop, clinicians should be aware that 66% of patients undergoing treatment for CMV pneumonia may show increased CMV antigenemia or viremia, but this is not associated with resistance [26].

23.2.5 Outcome

Interestingly, the incidence of fatal CMV pneumonia in HSCT recipients has decreased from 4% in 1997 to 0.8% in 2004 [29]. In patients with leukemia, the associated CMV pneumonia mortality rate is 57%; in patients with lymphoma, it is 30% [5, 25]. A high APACHE II score (>16 at onset of CMV pneumonia) and development of toxicity due to the use of antiviral agents have

Table 23.2 Incidence, risk factors, and mortality rates reported in patients with hematologic malignancies and cytomegalovirus pneumonia

	Hematopoietic stem cell transplant recipients	Leukemia patients	Lymphoma patients
Incidence	Allogeneic: 10.0–30.0% autologous: 2.0%	2.9%	1.1%
Risk factors	Old age Graft-versus-host disease Positive serology of the donor Use of granulocyte transfusions from seropositive donors Total-body irradiation Depleted antithymocyte globulins Receipt of T-cell–depleted stem cells Viruria Viremia	Use of lymphocytotoxic chemotherapeutic agents	B-cell non-Hodgkin lymphoma Active disease Advanced-stage disease (stage III/IV) Recurrent disease
Mortality rates (%)	0.8–4.0	57.0	30.0

been shown to be predictors of death in patients with lymphoma and CMV pneumonia [5] (Table 23.2).

23.3 Prevention

One of the main goals in treating immunocompromised patients is the prevention of CMV disease; this goal can be accomplished by early detection of the virus DNA in plasma via PCR assays or CMV antigenemia. Preemptive antiviral therapy, when given immediately after detection of CMV in plasma, can prevent the development of end-organ disease and decrease mortality [19].

However, some clinicians favor the use of prophylactic therapy. Ganciclovir has been shown to be effective at preventing the development of CMV pneumonia in the first 100 days posttransplantation [1]. Valganciclovir, an oral prodrug of ganciclovir that has a tenfold greater bioavailability than oral ganciclovir, is also used as prophylactic therapy in high-risk transplant recipients [27]. Maribavir is a benzimidazole riboside with an unnatural L-sugar moiety that inhibits the UL97 kinase, an early viral gene product involved in viral DNA elongation, DNA packaging, and egress or shedding of capsids from viral nuclei; in a phase II study of prophylactic therapy, maribavir was shown to reduce the incidence of CMV infection without the potential side effect of myelosuppression of ganciclovir [32], providing promising results in the future management of CMV disease. However, preliminary data analysis from a phase III study failed to show any significant difference between maribavir and a placebo in reducing the rate of CMV pneumonia in HSCT recipients within 180 days posttransplantation (unpublished data).

References

1. Boeckh M, Gooley TA, Myerson D et al (1996) Cytomegalovirus pp 65 antigenemia guided early treatment with ganciclovir marrow transplantation: a randomized double blind study. Blood 88:4063–4071
2. Boeckh M, Leisenring WM, Riddell S et al (2003) Late cytomegalovirus disease and mortality in recipients of allogeneic hematopoietic stem cell transplants: importance of viral load and T-cell immunity. Blood 101:407–414
3. Bowden RA, Slichter SJ, Sayers MH et al (1991) Use of leukocyte-depleted platelets and cytomegalovirus-seronegative red blood cells for prevention of primary cytomegalovirus infection after marrow transplant. Blood 78:246–250

4. Cathomas G, Morris P, Pekle K et al (1993) Rapid diagnosis of cytomegalovirus pneumonia in marrow transplant recipients by bronchoalveolar lavage using the polymerase chain reaction, virus culture, and the direct immunostaining of alveolar cells. Blood 81:1909–1914
5. Chemaly RF, Torres HA, Hachem RY et al (2005) Cytomegalovirus pneumonia in patients with lymphoma. Cancer 104:1213–1220
6. Chemaly RF, Yen-Lieberman B, Castilla EA et al (2004) Correlation between viral loads of cytomegalovirus in blood and bronchoalveolar lavage specimens from lung transplant recipients determined by histology and immunohistochemistry. J Clin Microbiol 42:2168–2172
7. Chemaly RF, Yen-Lieberman B, Chapman J et al (2005) Clinical utility of cytomegalovirus viral load in bronchoalveolar lavage in lung transplant recipients. Am J Transplant 5:544–548
8. Crawford SW, Bowden RA, Hackman RC et al (1988) Rapid detection of cytomegalovirus pulmonary infection by bronchoalveolar lavage and centrifugation culture. Ann Intern Med 108:180–185
9. de Medeiros CR, Moreira VA, Pasquini R (2000) Cytomegalovirus as a cause of very late interstitial pneumonia after bone marrow transplantation. Bone Marrow Transplant 26:443–444
10. Demirkazik FB, Akin A, Uzun O et al (2008) CT findings in immunocompromised patients with pulmonary infections. Diagn Interv Radiol 14:75–82
11. Drew WL (2010) Cytomegalovirus resistance testing: pitfalls and problems for the clinician. Clin Infect Dis 50: 733–736
12. Einsele H, Ehninger G, Hebart H et al (1995) Polymerase chain reaction monitoring reduces the incidence of cytomegalovirus disease and the duration and side effects of antiviral therapy after bone marrow transplantation. Blood 86: 2815–2820
13. Emanuel D, Peppard J, Stover D et al (1986) Rapid immunodiagnosis of cytomegalovirus pneumonia by bronchoalveolar lavage using human and murine monoclonal antibodies. Ann Intern Med 104:476–481
14. Emery V, Sabin C, Cope A et al (2000) Application of viral load kinetics to identify patients who developed cytomegalovirus disease after transplantation. Lancet 355:2032–2036
15. Enright H, Haake R, Weisdorf D et al (1993) Cytomegalovirus pneumonia after bone marrow transplantation.Risk factors and response to therapy. Transplantation 55:1339–1346
16. Gasparetto EL, Ono SE, Escuissato D et al (2004) Cytomegalovirus pneumonia after bone marrow transplantation: high resolution CT findings. Br J Radiol 77:724–727
17. Gleaves CA, Smith TF, Shuster EA et al (1985) Comparison of standard tube and shell vial cell culture techniques for the detection of cytomegalovirus in clinical specimens. J Clin Microbiol 21:217–221
18. Kim EA, Lee KS, Primack SL et al (2002) Viral pneumonias in adults: radiologic and pathologic findings. Radiographics 22:S137–S149
19. Ljungman P, Aschan J, Lewensohn-Fuchs I et al (1998) Results of different strategies for reducing cytomegalovirus-associated mortality in allogeneic stem cell transplant recipients. Transplantation 66:1330–1334
20. Ljungman P, Griffiths P, Paya C (2002) Definitions of cytomegalovirus infection and disease in transplant recipients. Clin Infect Dis 34:1094–1097
21. Machado CM, Dulley FL, Boas LS et al (2000) CMV pneumonia in allogeneic BMT recipients undergoing early treatment of pre-emptive ganciclovir therapy. Bone Marrow Transplant 26:413–417
22. Meyers JD, Flournoy N, Thomas ED (1986) Risk factors for cytomegalovirus infection after human marrow transplantation. J Infect Dis 153:478–488
23. Meyers JD, Ljungman P, Fisher LD (1990) Cytomegalovirus excretion as a predictor of cytomegalovirus disease after marrow transplantation: importance of cytomegalovirus viremia. J Infect Dis 162:373–380
24. Nakamura R, Battiwalla M, Solomon S et al (2004) Persisting posttransplantation cytomegalovirus antigenemia correlates with poor lymphocyte proliferation to cytomegalovirus antigen and predicts for increased late relapse and treatment failure. Biol Blood Marrow Transplant 10:49–57
25. Nguyen Q, Estey E, Raad I et al (2001) Cytomegalovirus pneumonia in adults with leukemia: an emerging problem. Clin Infect Dis 32:539–545
26. Nichols WG, Corey L, Gooley T et al (2001) Rising pp 65 antigenemia during preemptive anticytomegalovirus therapy after allogeneic hematopoietic stem cell transplantation: risk factors, correlation with DNA load, and outcomes. Blood 97:867–874
27. Reusser P (2002) Management of viral infections in immunocompromised cancer patients. Swiss Med Wkly 132: 374–378
28. Staras SA, Dollard SC, Radford KW et al (2006) Seroprevalence of cytomegalovirus infection in the United States, 1988-1994. Clin Infect Dis 43:1143–1151
29. Torres HA, Aguilera E, Safdar A et al (2008) Fatal cytomegalovirus pneumonia in patients with hematologic malignancies: an autopsy-based case-control study. Clin Microbiol Infect 14:1160–1166
30. Torres HA, Kontoyiannis DP, Aguilera EA et al (2006) Cytomegalovirus infection in patients with lymphoma: an important cause of morbidity and mortality. Clin Lymphoma Myeloma 6:393–398
31. Wingard JR, Chen DY, Burns WH et al (1988) Cytomegalovirus infection after autologous bone marrow transplantation with comparison to infection after allogeneic bone marrow transplantation. Blood 71:1432–1437
32. Winston DJ, Young JA, Pullarkat V (2008) Maribavir prophylaxis for prevention of cytomegalovirus infection in allogeneic stem cell transplant recipients: a multicenter, randomized, double-blind, placebo-controlled, dose-ranging study. Blood 111:5403–5410

Herpes Simplex Virus Pneumonia in Patients with Hematologic Malignancies

24

Jharna N. Shah and Roy F. Chemaly

Contents

J.N. Shah
Department of Infectious Diseases, Infection Control and Employee Health, The University of Texas M.D. Anderson Cancer Center, 1515 Holcombe Blvd, P.O. Box 402, Houston, TX 77030, USA
e-mail: jharnashah@gmail.com

R.F. Chemaly (✉)
Department of Infectious Diseases, Infection Control and Employee Health, The University of Texas M.D. Anderson Cancer Center, 1515 Holcombe Blvd, P.O. Box 402, Houston, TX 77030, USA
e-mail: rfchemaly@mdanderson.org

24.1 Introduction

Herpes simplex virus (HSV) is known to cause mucocutaneous disease in patients with hematologic malignancies [11, 42]. HSV most commonly leads to orofacial, genital, and esophageal lesions, and less commonly can lead to hepatitis, meningitis, encephalitis, bone marrow suppression, and pneumonia [22, 38, 42]. HSV pneumonia is very rare and has been reported in about 3% of the patients with hematologic malignancies and in about 5% of patients who have undergone hematopoietic stem cell transplant (HSCT) (these patients will be referred to as 'HSCT patients' in the chapter) without prophylaxis [56]. After acyclovir prophylaxis was implemented in patients with a HSCT, the incidence of HSV excretion dropped to 2.5% [49], while HSV pneumonia has been reported in less than 1% of all pneumonias developing after HSCT [16].

Cytomegalovirus (CMV) has been implicated as the most common agent in nonbacterial pneumonias in patients with hematologic malignancies and in patients who have undergone HSCT [33, 46]. However, HSV has been demonstrated as the most common pathogen in bronchial samples of patients with severe respiratory distress who have been treated with assisted ventilation [54]. Before the 1990s, cases of HSV pneumonia were characterized as "idiopathic pneumonia" because of insufficient diagnostic testing or simply lack of awareness of HSV as a causative agent in lower respiratory tract disease [46].

HSV pneumonia is diagnosed most frequently in the setting of severe immunosuppression [14, 16, 17, 27, 60, 64]. Studies involving HSV pneumonia have been conducted frequently in patients who have undergone HSCT and less frequently in other types of immunocompromised patients, such as those with

É. Azoulay (ed.), *Pulmonary Involvement in Patients with Hematological Malignancies*,
DOI: 10.1007/978-3-642-15742-4_24, © Springer-Verlag Berlin Heidelberg 2011

hematologic malignancies, solid tumors, burns, critical illnesses, or acquired immune deficiency syndrome (AIDS) [3, 8, 12, 17, 42, 54]. Respiratory involvement is seen most commonly with herpes simplex virus-1 (HSV-1) [40, 43, 56], but some cases of herpes simplex virus-2 (HSV-2) have been reported [13, 25].

In this chapter, we will focus on incidence and transmission, pathogenesis, risk factors, clinical features, diagnosis, and management for HSV pneumonia in patients with hematologic malignancies and HSCT patients as well as outcome and prognosis. Table 24.1 summarizes the outcomes in studies and

Table 24.1 Studies and case reports on HSV pneumonia

No.	Author, year	No. of cases	Type of immuno-compromised population	Management	Outcome
1	Meyers 1982 [46]	10 Nonbacterial pneumonia.	10 weeks s/p HSCT, GVHD	Not enough information available.	All patients died.
2	Ramsey 1982 [56]	20 Autopsy cases	HM, 2 months s/p HSCT, nonHM; on chemotherapy, radiotherapy	None were on prophylaxis. No treatment given.	All patients died of respiratory failure. Pneumonia to death within 24 days (mean)
3	Ljungman 1990 [40]	3 Acyclovir-resistant HSV-1 pneumonia	Early HSCT period, GVHD	Case 1: Px: ACV 250 mg/m² Q12h × 30 days post-HSCT; Rx: ACV 500 mg/m² Q12h + IV Vidarabine 10 mg/kg	Patient 1: Died on day 70.
				Case 2: Px: ACV 250 mg/m² Q8h × 29 days; Rx: ACV × 250 mg/m² Q8h	Patient 2: Died on day 100.
				Case 3: Px-ACV 500 mg/m² Q8h × 25 days; Rx- Ganciclovir 5 mg/kg Q8h × 19 days, ACV 250 mg/m² Q8h × 39 days	Patient 3: Died on day 131.
5	Schuller 1993 [60]	15 HSV-1 pneumonia	Lymphoma, solid organ transplants, AIDS, SLE	Px- N/A Rx-ACV × 17 days (mean)	33% Died ($n = 5$) from sepsis (2), respiratory failure (2), dehiscence of tracheal anastomosis after lung transplant (1).
9	Ferrari 2005 [23]	1	B-cell ALL on chemotherapy	Px-None Rx-ACV 10 mg/kg Q8h on day 31; later Px- Valacyclovir	Noninvasive ventilation needed→ infection resolved by day 42.
10	Gasparetto 2005 [25]	3 HSV-2 pneumonia	HSCT (two early-phase, one late-phase)	Px- 1 pt on ACV 200 mg Q12h; Rx- ACV 500 mg Q8h	Two patients improved, one died of respiratory failure in 2 weeks
11	Frangoul 2007 [24]	2 ACV-resistant HSV-1 pneumonia	HSCT, GVHD	Px- PO ACV 600 mg/m² Q12h or IV ACV 250 mg/m² Q12h; Rx- IV ACV 250 mg/m² Q8h; Foscarnet 60 mg/kg Q12h – then 90 mg/kg Q12h	Died on day 110 from respiratory failure.
12	Aisenberg 2009 [3]	45 HSV pneumonia (6: proven, 25: probable, 14: possible)	Solid tumors on steroids and radiotherapy	Px-None Rx-ACV ($n = 17$), Valacyclovir ($n = 7$), Famciclovir ($n = 1$) × 13 days (mean)	Ten (22%) died: four treated, six untreated).

ACV Acyclovir, *ALL* acute lymphocytic leukemia, *GVHD* graft-versus-host-disease, *HM* hematologic malignancy, *IV* intravenous, *N/A* not available, *PO* oral, *Px* prophylaxis, *Q8h* every 8 hourly, *Q12h* every 12 hourly, *Rx* treatment, *s/p HSCT* status post-hematopoietic stem cell transplant case reports of patients with HSV pneumonia who have hematologic malignancies and HSCT patients.

24.2 Incidence and Transmission

HSV belongs to the *Herpesviridae* family, which comprises HSV-1, HSV-2, varicella zoster virus, CMV, Epstein-Barr virus, human herpes viruses 6 and 7, and Kaposi's sarcoma-associated herpesvirus (type 8) [37, 66]. HSV (types 1 and 2) belongs to the subfamily *Alphaherpesvirinae* [37, 66].

HSV-1 and -2 are ubiquitous and contagious, and they are transmitted horizontally during close contact with an infected person who is shedding the virus from the skin, saliva, or secretions from the genitals [22, 38]. Asymptomatic viral shedding and transmission are known to occur, especially in HSV-2 infections [38]. HSV-1 is usually acquired orally during childhood, but may also be transmitted sexually [38]. HSV-2 is transmitted primarily by sexual contact [38].

The virus is reactivated secondary to triggers such as psychological stress; fatigue; exposure to heat, cold, or sunlight; menstruation; sexual intercourse; fever; immunosuppression; corticosteroid administration; laser surgery; local tissue trauma; nerve damage; and change in antiviral activity of the saliva [22].

About 80% of adult patients with hematologic malignancies are HSV seropositive [62]. HSV reactivates in about 70–80% of seropositive patients [29]. The incidence of mucocutaneous lesions among seropositive patients with leukemia has been reported to range from 15% (among CLL patients treated with fludarabine) to 90% (in patients with acute leukemia or HSCT) [5, 11, 42, 57, 58]. HSCT patients more commonly show HSV reactivations, especially within the first 4 weeks of the transplant, while primary infections are unusual [45].

24.3 Pathogenesis

24.3.1 Pathogenesis in Humans

HSV is a double-stranded deoxyribonucleic acid (DNA) virus that measures approximately 200 nm in diameter and contains a linear, double-stranded DNA core enclosed within an icosahedral protein capsid, covered by a tegument and a glycoprotein-containing envelope [37, 44, 50, 66, 68].

Initial exposure to herpesviruses often leads to viral invasion of epithelial cells and intracellular replication at the site of primary exposure [50, 66, 68]. Following primary infection, the virus ascends in a retrograde manner through the periaxonal sheath of sensory nerves to the trigeminal, cervical, lumbosacral, or autonomic ganglia of the host's nervous system [50, 66, 68]. The virus replicates and remains dormant for life. The trigeminal and sacral ganglia are the most common locations for HSV-1 and HSV-2 latency, respectively [22].

Pulmonary involvement in patients with hematologic malignancies may be focal or diffuse [56]. Focal disease may begin as mucocutaneous/ororpharyngeal disease and continue down to the lower respiratory tract (contiguous spread), whereas diffuse pneumonia is associated with hematogenous dissemination [56]. Concomitant/preceding HSV in pharynx, urine, liver, or genitals has been reported [27, 52, 56]. HSV-1 pneumonia occurs through aspiration or contiguous spread, and HSV-2 pneumonia is caused by hematogenous spread [44]. HSV pneumonia is an intrabronchial process [27]. Focal or diffuse ulcers in the tracheobronchial epithelium can lead to necrotizing herpetic tracheitis, as was found in autopsy specimens of patients with hematologic malignancies [56].

HSV has been shown to be less replicative than CMV is in alveolar macrophages, thus suggesting the role of altered macrophage function in the development of HSV pneumonia [20]. However, an age-dependent protective role against disseminated HSV disease has also been demonstrated [47].

24.3.2 Animal Models

Studies in animal models have attempted to elucidate the pathogenesis of HSV pneumonia [1, 2, 19]. Reactive oxygen/nitrogen species (RONS) has been implicated in the development of viral pneumonitis [19]. Intranasal infection of mice with HSV-1 resulted in rapid development of pneumonia and decreased lung compliance, and was associated with elevated expression of inducible nitrogen oxide synthase (iNOS) protein and increased nitrotyrosine adduct formation in the lungs of infected mice. When these mice were treated with a NOS inhibitor, pneumonitis was almost completely suppressed, recovery of inflammatory cells from bronchoalveolar lavage fluid was decreased, and both lung compliance and survival were improved [1].

Animal models have also demonstrated that graft-versus-host disease (GVHD) is an important factor in the development of HSV pneumonitis. Allogeneic transplant mice with GVHD developed more severe pneumonitis after intranasal HSV-1 infection than did control mice without GVHD. The former group also showed an enhanced transforming growth factor-1 (TGF-1) production, which was implicated as a more important factor than the pulmonary viral load [2].

24.4 Risk Factors

Several risk factors have been identified that increase the risk of HSV pneumonia in patients with hematologic malignancies. HSV pneumonia is generally a result of reactivation of a latent HSV infection [42, 50, 56, 68]. Several triggers, such as stress, corticosteroid administration, and immunosuppression, may cause reactivation of the virus [22]. HSV affects squamous epithelial cells, and factors promoting squamous metaplasia such as smoking, trauma, burns, and tracheal trauma from intubation may predispose a patient to develop HSV pneumonia [27, 51, 52, 56, 60]. Intubation of a patient with oral herpes can trigger reactivation or cause a lower respiratory tract infection through direct inoculation or aspiration [8, 56]. Thus, intubated patients who fail to be weaned off the ventilator should be evaluated for HSV pneumonia, as it is an often under-recognized cause of nonbacterial pneumonia [46].

Patients with hematologic malignancies who are undergoing aggressive chemotherapy and treatment with corticosteroids are at increased risk of HSV, as impairment of cellular immunity is a risk factor for HSV infections and reactivations [57]. Persistent and severe T-cell depletion is seen after aggressive chemotherapy and after administration of monoclonal antibodies (e.g., anti-CD52 antibody, alemtuzumab) [32, 55] and has been identified as a predictor for HSV infections [15, 17, 64].

HSCT patients are at greater risk of developing HSV infections, as chemotherapy and radiotherapy used before HSCT may damage the normal upper respiratory mucosa and predispose the patient to direct spread of the virus to the lower respiratory tract [56]. These agents may also trigger reactivation of the virus [34]. The use of cyclophosphamide, busulfan, carmustine, and total body irradiation in conditioning regimens has been seen in patients with HSV pneumonia [24, 46]. HSV reactivation occurs most commonly in the first month after HSCT; however, late-onset HSV-associated pneumonia has also been reported [35].

Additionally, patients with hematologic malignancies are often neutropenic [absolute neutrophil count (ANC) <500/mL] secondary to the chemotherapy. Neutropenia has also been observed in patients with hematologic malignancies who have HSV pneumonia [56]. GVHD as a risk factor for HSV disease in HSCT patients and severity of GVHD as a predictor of nonresponsiveness to antiviral therapy has also been reported [16]. In some studies, the immunosuppressive effect of multiple blood transfusions has also been implicated in the development of HSV pneumonia [64]. Patients undergoing solid organ transplant (SOT) are at risk of developing HSV pneumonia. The incidence of HSV pneumonia in SOT patients is about 5%, while mortality of up to 100% has been reported, especially in liver transplant recipients [4, 31, 39].

24.5 Clinical Features

24.5.1 Clinical Manifestations

The clinical manifestations of HSV pneumonia are nonspecific [3, 18, 40, 56]. In HSCT patients, symptomatic disease occurs 2–3 weeks after transplant when mucosal damage is maximal from radiotherapy and chemotherapy [23]. HSV infections can manifest with nonrespiratory symptoms before showing signs of pulmonary involvement [23, 54]. Nonrespiratory manifestations of HSV reactivation infrequently include oral mucocutaneous lesions. Esophagitis and rarely, genital lesions may also precede lower respiratory involvement [54, 56]. Respiratory symptoms of HSV pneumonia include low-grade fever, cough, dyspnea, rales, hypoxemia, tachypnea, intractable wheezing, or chest pain [56]. Hemoptysis may also be present, secondary to tracheitis [63].

Patients with HSV pneumonia may typically either demonstrate worsening respiratory status that is unresponsive to prolonged antibacterial treatment and may require intubation or patients may already be intubated, and may worsen and fail to wean off the ventilator. Persistent low-grade fevers and unimpressive infiltrates on imaging with leukocytosis would indicate a nonbacterial cause. Interstitial lung involvement in HSV pneumonia is characterized by worsening oxygenation [evident from low pO_2 with a high fraction of inspired oxygen (FiO_2)], decrease in diffusing capacity of the lung for carbon monoxide (DLCO), and an increase in alveolar-arterial (A-a) gradient over 30 [18]. HSV pneumonia is often complicated by acute respiratory distress syndrome (ARDS) and respiratory failure, and mechanical ventilation is often needed, especially in untreated patients [56].

24.5.2 Coinfections

Pulmonary coinfections may often be present and may complicate the diagnosis of patients with HSV pneumonia. Up to 65% of the patients with HSV pneumonia may have copathogens, such as CMV, *Candida*, Aspergillus, *Pneumocystis jirovecii*, *mycobacterium avium intracellulare* (MAI), and other bacteria [3, 40, 56]. Patients are often treated preemptively for bacterial pneumonia before diagnosis of HSV has been confirmed, which may lead to a delay in initiation of HSV-specific treatment.

24.5.3 Differential Diagnosis

In an immunocompromised host, the most common infectious cause of pneumonia is bacterial, which presents with acute deterioration and significant hypoxemia. Subacute presentation suggests involvement of atypical bacterial, viral, or fungal organisms, while chronic presentation suggests fungal or mycobacterial infection. *Pneumocystis jirovecii,* CMV, respiratory syncytial virus, and influenza pneumonia are the most important organisms in the differential diagnosis of diffuse bilateral infiltrates, accompanied by significant oxygen defect (A-a gradient >30) [18]. Noninfectious causes may include drug toxicity, pulmonary hemorrhage, GVHD, and heart failure.

24.6 Diagnosis

HSV pneumonia should be suspected in immunocompromised patients who are not on acyclovir prophylaxis, who are intubated with worsening oxygenation, and who have not been weaned off a ventilator despite aggressive management [18, 23, 54].

There are no standardized diagnostic criteria for HSV pneumonia. The definitive diagnosis of HSV pneumonia can be made by isolating the virus from respiratory secretions, bronchoalveolar lavage samples, and lung tissue and by demonstrating viral cytopathic effects on histopathology [18, 42, 56].

24.6.1 Virus Isolation

Shell-vial culture for virus isolation and demonstration of cytopathic effects are methods commonly used to diagnose HSV. The sensitivity of these methods has been reported to be 57%, with a specificity of 100% [10]. The shell-vial culture yields results in 48 h [62].

Rapid antigen detection by direct immunofluorescence is also often employed for early detection of HSV, with sensitivity and specificity of about 80% and 100%, respectively [10].

24.6.2 Gene Amplification

Polymerase chain reaction (PCR) for HSV DNA is more rapid and more sensitive than conventional culture, shell-vial culture, and antigen-detection methods [61]. However, PCR is unable to distinguish between active disease and contamination from oral cavity [61].

Serology is useful for identifying patients with seropositive HSV before induction chemotherapy or before HSCT [62]. Detection of immunoglobulin M (IgM) antibody and demonstration of an increase in immunoglobulin G (IgG) titers can be useful in patients with an active infection [59]. However, it takes several weeks to mount a significant antibody response and depends on a functioning immune system. Thus, serology is less useful with HSV pneumonia when a rapid diagnosis is necessary [30, 59]. Additionally, a fourfold increase in titers is helpful for diagnosing primary HSV infection; however, such an increase may not be observed in recurrent infections [30].

24.6.3 Lung Biopsy/Cytology

Nonspecific fibroproliferative pattern and tissue necrosis are demonstrated on lung biopsy in patients with HSV pneumonia [23]. However, lung biopsy is rarely performed in patients with cancer because of increased complications, inconsistent diagnosis, and questionable reliability [56, 64]. A few scattered ulcers in the trachea or a severe ulcerative process resulting in an obstructed and inflamed tracheobronchial membrane may be evident on direct examination [27].

Parenchymal involvement begins in lungs, adjacent to the terminal and respiratory bronchioles, but may extend throughout the lobule [33, 56]. Diffuse alveolar damage comprising interstitial lymphocyte infiltration, air space hemorrhage, intraalveolar fibrinous exudate, edema, fibroblast proliferation, type 2 hyperplasia, and hyaline membrane formation is often evident [33, 56].

Cytology demonstrates multinucleated giant cells with enlarged, molded, basophilic nuclei of ground-glass appearance or cells with large intranuclear eosinophilic inclusions ("owl-eyes"-Cowdry type A inclusion bodies) in the alveolar or bronchial cells and macrophages obtained in washings or biopsies [56].

24.6.4 Radiology

Radiologic changes in HSV pneumonia are often nonspecific [3, 6, 36, 65]. These changes are similar to those seen in other viral pneumonias and are not different from those seen in immunocompetent patients [65].

Chest x-ray may be near normal early in the disease [18]. In advanced disease, however, focal, multifocal, or diffuse bilateral opacities with predominantly mixed (partly airspace consolidation and partly interstitial) or airspace consolidation is often seen [18, 65]. Less frequently seen are unilateral consolidation, large atelectasis, and pleural effusion [56, 65].

High-resolution computed tomography (CT) scans are used for better delineation of the disease process [25]. HSV-1 shows multifocal, subsegmental, and ground-glass attenuation with consolidation, reticular, and nodular opacities; HSV-2 demonstrates diffuse alveolar damage, small centrilobular nodules, and interstitial pneumonia [6, 25]. Large nodules and pleural effusions are also seen [6, 25].

24.7 Management

24.7.1 Treatment

Acyclovir is the most widely used and effective therapy for HSV pneumonia [11, 68]. However, empiric therapy based on suspicion of HSV pneumonia has not been recommended [18]. HSV-specific treatment of pneumonia has been reported to prevent progression to respiratory failure and mortality in patients with hematologic malignancies and in HSCT patients [23, 25, 35]. Improvement in oxygenation status can be seen in 3–5 days, and patients may be able to be weaned off the ventilator [18]. However, treatment has showed no significant effect on mortality, duration of mechanical ventilation, length of intensive care unit (ICU) stay, or length of hospitalization in a group of immunocompromised patients (patients with lymphoma, with solid-organ transplants, or with AIDS or systemic lupus erythematosus [SLE]) as compared to immunocompetent patients [60].

HSV is susceptible to acyclovir, valacyclovir, famciclovir, foscarnet, cidofovir, and, to a lesser extent, ganciclovir [37]. Table 24.2 shows the mechanisms of action, recommended dosages, and mechanisms of resistance for these drugs.

Foscarnet is used to treat acyclovir-resistant strains. However, strains resistant to foscarnet and acyclovir are now being reported [7]. Cidofovir is the only drug used to treat double-resistant HSV [42], although use of cidofovir is associated with significant renal toxicity [7].

A significant proportion of patients with HSV pneumonia may have concomitant bacterial pneumonia [3, 40, 56]. Thus, empirical broad-spectrum antibiotic therapy that includes an anti-staphylococcal drug can be used in patients with progressive HSV pneumonia who are unresponsive to antiviral therapy.

24.7.2 Prophylaxis

HSV pneumonia accounted for 9% of pneumonias in HSCT patients, prior to acyclovir prophylaxis [56]. Prophylaxis of HSV infection has led to decreased

Table 24.2 Antiviral drugs used in HSV pneumonia

Drug	Susceptibility	Mechanism of action	Doses for pneumonia	Prophylaxis	Side effects	Mechanism of Resistance	FDA-labeled indications	Non-FDA-labeled indications
Acyclovir	Synthetic purine nucleoside analog with in vitro and in vivo inhibitory activity against HSV-1, HSV-2, VZV	Affinity for viral enzyme thymidine kinase (TK) leads to (1) competitive inhibition of viral DNA polymerase, (2) incorporation into and termination of the growing viral DNA chain, and (3) inactivation of the viral DNA polymerase. Metabolized by kidneys.	500 mg/m² or 10 mg/kg IV Q12h × 14–21 days	250 mg/m² or 5 mg/kg IV Q12h, or 200 mg TID to 800 mg BID	Nausea, vomiting, diarrhea, headache, confusion, coma, hematologic dysfunction, liver failure, renal failure, rash	Qualitative and quantitative changes in the viral TK and/or DNA polymerase	Congenital herpes simplex, HSV encephalitis, genital HSV, herpes labialis, mucocutaneous HSV infections, herpes zoster, varicella	Acute retinal necrosis, eczema herpeticum, HSV proctitis, meningitis, hepatitis, respiratory and ophthalmic infections; HZV auricularis and encephalitis; herpetic whitlow; VZV prophylaxis, pneumonia and transverse myelitis, viral encephalitis
Valacyclovir	Same as acyclovir	Same as acyclovir.	500 mg BID × 10 days	500 mg BID	TTP/HUS, neurologic effects, renal impairment	Same as acyclovir	Recurrent genital HSV, herpes labialis, HZV, VZV	Acute retinal necrosis, CMV infection and prophylaxis, nongenital HSV
Famciclovir	Same as acyclovir	The active ingredient is acyclovir. Same as acyclovir, better absorption allows less frequent dosing.	500 mg BID × 10 days	500 mg BID × 3–5 weeks with chemotherapy or after HSCT (longer in children with acute leukemia	Headache, paresthesia, migraine, nausea, vomiting diarrhea, hematologic, liver dysfunction, carcinogenic	Same as acyclovir	HZV, mucocutaneous HSV in HIV, recurrent genital HSV	Acute retinal necrosis, genital HSV, hepatitis B

(continued)

Table 24.2 (continued)

Drug	Susceptibility	Mechanism of action	Doses for pneumonia	Prophylaxis	Side effects	Mechanism of Resistance	FDA-labeled indications	Non-FDA-labeled indications
Foscarnet	Activation (phosphorylation) by thymidine kinase or other kinases NOT required, hence, is active in vitro against HSV TK deficient and CMV UL97 mutants	Selective inhibition at the pyrophosphate-binding site on virus-specific DNA polymerases at concentrations that do not affect cellular DNA polymerases	60 mg/kg IV Q12h, or 40 mg/kg IV Q8h × 7–21 days or until complete healing	N/A	Renal impairment, electrolyte imbalance, seizures, fever, nausea, vomiting, diarrhea, headache, anemia	Resistance due to DNA polymerase mutations have emerged	CMV-retinitis s in AIDS patients, acyclovir-resistant mucocutaneous HSV	Intravitreal use in CMV retinitis, CMV pneumonia, HSV keratitis
Cidofovir	In vitro against CMV, HSV-1, HSV-2	Suppresses CMV replication by selective inhibition of viral DNA synthesis	5 mg/kg once a week × 2 weeks, then once every 2 weeks combined with probenecid and hydration	N/A	Renal impairment, neutropenia, decreased intraocular pressure, anterior uveitis/iritis, metabolic acidosis	Resistance to cidofovir has been selected for in the laboratory setting and occurs through mutations in the viral DNA polymerase. In vivo resistant strains have been reported	CMV retinitis in AIDS	Condyloma acuminatum

AIDS Acquired immune deficiency syndrome, *BID* twice a day, *CMV* cytomegalovirus, *HIV* human immunodeficiency virus, *HSCT* hematopoietic stem cell transplant, *HSV* human herpes simplex virus, *IV* intravenous, *N/A* not available, *Q12h* every 12 hourly, *TID* thrice a day, *TTP/HUS* thrombotic thrombocytopenic purpura, *VZV* Varicella Zoster virus prevalence of HSV pneumonia (less than 2% of HSCT recipients) [9, 41, 49].

Antiviral drug prophylaxis is not recommended in HSV-seronegative leukemic patients during chemotherapy or after SCT, since primary HSV infection in these patients is unusual [62]. In HSV-seropositive patients, antiviral drug prophylaxis has been shown to prevent the development of active HSV disease and to reduce mortality rates [29, 69].

Antiviral drug prophylaxis is part of the standard management at many cancer centers for patients with hematologic malignancies undergoing chemotherapy or for patients undergoing HSCT [62, 63, 67, 69]. Acyclovir has been the most common antiviral drug used [28]. However, newer antivirals such as valaciclovir and famciclovir are also active against HSV and have an oral bioavailability three to five times superior to that of oral acyclovir [53, 62]. Both of these agents are used to prevent HSV reactivation during induction chemotherapy for leukemia or after HSCT [49]. Prophylaxis should be given for 3–5 weeks, after the start of chemotherapy or during the pre-engraftment stage in the first month after HSCT [58, 62, 63, 67]. Children, allogeneic HSCT patients who develop GVHD, or patients who require immunosuppressant treatment should receive prolonged prophylaxis [62].

24.7.3 Resistance to Antivirals

Long-term prophylaxis with acyclovir in HSCT patients appears to prevent the emergence of drug-resistant HSV disease [21]. However, several centers have reported increased incidence of acyclovir-resistant HSV disease, especially in patients who have undergone unrelated HSCT or HLA-mismatched transplant patients with GVHD [16, 40]. Acyclovir resistance is associated with serious morbidity and mortality [7, 16]. Poor response to acyclovir indicates possible resistance, and the patient should be promptly switched to foscarnet or cidofovir [7, 16].

Activation of acyclovir, ganciclovir, valacyclovir, or famciclovir requires initial phosphorylation by viral thymidine kinase (TK) [37]. Resistance to acyclovir can be caused by lack of TK, altered TK, or TK strains with mutations in viral DNA polymerase [37]. TK-negative mutants may cause severe disease in infants and immunocompromised adults [37]. Cross-resistance between acyclovir and foscarnet results from their interaction at the same site on HSV DNA polymerase; however, susceptibility to cidofovir is unaffected by the same viral mutation [26].

24.7.4 Vaccine

There is no licensed effective vaccine for HSV [37].

24.8 Outcome

Patients with HSV pneumonia can require mechanical ventilation and prolonged hospitalization [64]. Mortality in immunocompetent patients has been reported to be about 27% [54]. However, patients with hematologic malignancies and HSCT patients may have high mortality rates (up to 75–100%), if left untreated [46, 56]. Patients with solid tumors and patients with solid-organ transplants have mortality rates that range from 20% to 100%, with a higher percentage of mortality after liver transplants [3, 4, 31].

Severe respiratory distress necessitating mechanical ventilation or worsening respiratory status on a ventilator is often seen in untreated patients with HSV pneumonia, and ARDS or respiratory failure may occur without treatment [54, 56, 64]. Damage to lung function has not been reported in patients that recover from the infection.

24.9 Prognosis

The prognosis of patients with HSV pneumonia depends on the immunologic status of the patient and the type of underlying disease [27]. In immunocompetent hosts, HSV pneumonia is not necessarily a fatal disease [48]. In immunocompromised patients, however, HSV pneumonia can lead to respiratory failure and the need for mechanical ventilation or failure to wean off the ventilator and subsequent mortality [18, 24, 25, 27, 40, 56].

Although rare, HSV pneumonia should be considered in neutropenic hematologic patients undergoing chemotherapy with "suggestive" radiologic findings who have not improved after conventional antibacterial and/or antifungal treatments [18, 24, 25, 27, 40, 56].

References

1. Adler H, Beland JL, Del Pan NC et al (1997) Suppression of herpes simplex virus type 1 (HSV-1)-induced pneumonia in mice by inhibition of inducible nitric oxide synthase (iNOS, NOS2). J Exp Med 185:1533–1540
2. Adler H, Beland JL, Kozlow W et al (1998) A role for transforming growth factor-beta1 in the increased pneumonitis in murine allogeneic bone marrow transplant recipients with graft-versus-host disease after pulmonary herpes simplex virus type 1 infection. Blood 92:2581–2589
3. Aisenberg GM, Torres HA, Tarrand J et al (2009) Herpes simplex virus lower respiratory tract infection in patients with solid tumors. Cancer 115:199–206
4. Allen KA, Markin RS, Rennard SI et al (1989) Bronchoalveolar lavage in liver transplant patients. Acta Cytol 33:539–543
5. Anaissie EJ, Kontoyiannis DP, O'Brien S et al (1998) Infections in patients with chronic lymphocytic leukemia treated with fludarabine. Ann Intern Med 129:559–566
6. Aquino SL, Dunagan DP, Chiles C et al (1998 Sep–Oct) Herpes simplex virus 1 pneumonia: patterns on CT scans and conventional chest radiographs. J Comput Assist Tomogr 22(5):795–800
7. Blot N, Schneider P, Young P et al (2000 Oct) Treatment of an acyclovir and foscarnet-resistant herpes simplex virus infection with cidofovir in a child after an unrelated bone marrow transplant. Bone Marrow Transplant 26(8):903–5
8. Bruynseels P, Jorens PG, Demey HE (2003 Nov 8) Herpes simplex virus in the respiratory tract of critical care patients: a prospective study. Lancet 362(9395):1536–41
9. Burns WH (1999) Advances in the control of cytomegalovirus disease in bone marrow transplant patients. Cancer Treat Res 101:185–201, Review
10. Burrows J, Nitsche A, Bayly B et al (2002 Jun 9) Detection and subtyping of Herpes simplex virus in clinical samples by LightCycler PCR, enzyme immunoassay and cell culture. BMC Microbiol 2:12
11. Bustamante CI, Wade JC (1991 Oct) Herpes simplex virus infection in the immunocompromised cancer patient. J Clin Oncol 9(10):1903–15
12. Byers RJ, Hasleton PS, Quigley A et al (1996 Nov) Pulmonary herpes simplex in burns patients. Eur Respir J 9(11):2313–7
13. Calore EE (2002 Dec) Herpes simplex type 2 pneumonia. Braz J Infect Dis 6(6):305–8
14. Camps K, Jorens PG, Demey HE et al (2002 Oct) Clinical significance of herpes simplex virus in the lower respiratory tract of critically ill patients. Eur J Clin Microbiol Infect Dis 21(10):758–9
15. Chakrabarti S, Pillay D, Ratcliffe D et al (2000) Resistance to antiviral drugs in herpes simplex virus infections among allogeneic stem cell transplant recipients: risk factors and prognostic significance. J Infect Dis 181:2055–8
16. Chen CS, Boeckh M, Seidel K et al (2003 Sep) Incidence, risk factors, and mortality from pneumonia developing late after hematopoietic stem cell transplantation. Bone Marrow Transplant 32(5):515–22
17. Cook CH, Yenchar JK, Kraner TO et al (1998 Oct) Occult herpes family viruses may increase mortality in critically ill surgical patients. Am J Surg 176(4):357–60
18. Cunha BA, Eisenstein LE, Dillard T et al (2007 Jan-Feb) Herpes simplex virus (HSV) pneumonia in a heart transplant: diagnosis and therapy. Heart Lung 36(1):72–8
19. Davis I, Matalon S (2001) Reactive Species in Viral Pneumonitis: Lessons From Animal Models. News Physiol Sci 16:185–190
20. Drew WL, Mintz L, Hoo R et al (1979 Feb) Growth of herpes simplex and cytomegalovirus in cultured human alveolar macrophages. Am Rev Respir Dis 119(2):287–91
21. Erard V, Wald A, Corey L et al (2007 Jul 15) Use of long-term suppressive acyclovir after hematopoietic stem-cell transplantation: impact on herpes simplex virus (HSV) disease and drug-resistant HSV disease. J Infect Dis 196(2):266–70
22. Fatahzadeh M, Schwartz RA (2007 Nov) Human herpes simplex virus infections: epidemiology, pathogenesis, symptomatology, diagnosis, and management. J Am Acad Dermatol 57(5):737–63
23. Ferrari A, Luppi M, Potenza L et al (2005 Nov) Herpes simplex virus pneumonia during standard induction chemotherapy for acute leukemia: case report and review of literature. Leukemia 19(11):2019–21
24. Frangoul H, Wills M, Crossno C et al (2007 Dec) Acyclovir-resistant herpes simplex virus pneumonia post-unrelated stem cell transplantation: a word of caution. Pediatr Transplant 11(8):942–4
25. Gasparetto EL, Escuissato DL, Inoue C et al (2005 May) Herpes simplex virus type 2 pneumonia after bone marrow transplantation: high-resolution CT findings in 3 patients. J Thorac Imaging 20(2):71–3
26. Gilbert C, Bestman-Smith J, Boivin G (2002 Apr) Resistance of herpesviruses to antiviral drugs: clinical impacts and molecular mechanisms. Drug Resist Updat 5(2):88–114
27. Graham BS, Snell JD Jr (1983 Nov) Herpes simplex virus infection of the adult lower respiratory tract. Medicine (Baltimore) 62(6):384–93
28. Guidelines for preventing opportunistic infections among hematopoietic stem cell transplant recipients; recommendations of the CDC, the Infectious Disease Society of America, and the American Society of Blood and Marrow Transplantation. Biol Blood Marrow Transplant 2000;6: 659–734
29. Hann IM, Prentice HG, Blacklock HA et al (1983) Acyclovir prophylaxis against herpes virus infections in severely immunocompromised patients: Randomised double blind trial. Br Med J (Clin Res Ed) 287:384–388
30. Hirsch MS (1995) Herpes simplex virus. In: Mandell GL, Bennett JE, Dolan R (eds) Principles and practice of infectious diseases. Churchill Livingstone, New York, pp 1336–1345
31. Jensen WA, Rose RM, Hammer SM et al (1986) Pulmonary complications of orthotopic liver transplantation. Transplantation 42:484–490
32. Keating MJ, Flinn I, Jain V et al (2002) Therapeutic role of alemtuzumab (Campath-1H) in patients who have failed fludarabine: results of a large international study. Blood 99:3554–3561
33. Kim EA, Lee KS, Primack SL et al (2002) Viral pneumonias in adults: radiologic and pathologic findings. Radiographics Oct;22 Spec No:S137–S49
34. Kingreen D, Nitsche A, Beyer J et al (1997) Herpes simplex infection of the jejunum occurring in the early post-transplantation period. Bone Marrow Transplant 20:989–91

35. Kitabayashi A, Hirokawa M, Horiuchi T et al (2000 Jan) Late-onset herpes simplex virus-associated interstitial pneumonia after allogeneic bone marrow transplantation. Bone Marrow Transplant 25(2):225–6
36. Klainer AS, Oud L, Randazzo J et al (1994 Jul) Herpes simplex virus involvement of the lower respiratory tract following surgery. Chest 106(1 Suppl):8S–14S, discussion 34S-35S
37. Kleymann G (2003) Novel agents and strategies to treat herpes simplex virus infections. Expert Opin 12:165–83
38. Koelle DM, Corey L (2008) Herpes simplex: insights on pathogenesis and possible vaccines. Annu Rev Med 59:381–95
39. Liebau P, Kuse E, Winkler M et al (1996 Mar–Apr) Management of herpes simplex virus type 1 pneumonia following liver transplantation. Infection 24(2):130–5
40. Ljungman P, Ellis MN, Hackman RC et al (1990 Jul) Acyclovir-resistant herpes simplex virus causing pneumonia after marrow transplantation. J Infect Dis 162(1):244–8
41. Ljungman P (2002 Jul) Prevention and treatment of viral infections in stem cell transplant recipients. Br J Haematol 118(1):44–57, Review
42. Ljungman P (2004) Viral infections: current diagnosis and treatment. Hematol J 5(Suppl 3):S63–8
43. Machado CM, Vilas Boas LS, Dulley FL et al (1997 Mar) Herpes Simplex Virus Shedding in Bone Marrow Transplant Recipients During Low-Dose Oral Acyclovir Prohylaxis. Braz J Infect Dis 1(1):27–30
44. Mettenleiter TC, Klupp BG, Granzow H (2006) Herpesvirus assembly: a tale of two membranes. Curr Opin Microbiol 9(4):423–9
45. Meyers JD, Flournoy N, Thomas ED (1980) Infection with herpes simplex virus and cell-mediated immunity after marrow transplant. J Infect Dis 142:338–346
46. Meyers JD, Flournoy N, Thomas ED (1982 Nov–Dec) Nonbacterial pneumonia after allogeneic marrow transplantation: a review of ten years' experience. Rev Infect Dis 4(6):1119–32
47. Mintz L, Drew WL, Hoo R et al (1980 May) Age-dependent resistance of human alveolar macrophages to herpes simplex virus. Infect Immun 28(2):417–20
48. Miyazato A, Kishimoto H, Tamaki K et al (2001 Aug) Herpes simplex virus bronchopneumonia in a non-immunocompromized individual. Intern Med 40(8):836–40
49. Morfin F, Bilger K, Boucher A et al (2004 Aug) HSV excretion after bone marrow transplantation: a 4-year survey. J Clin Virol 30(4):341–5
50. Nadelman CM, Newcomer VD (2000) Herpes simplex virus infections. New treatment approaches make early diagnosis even more important. Postgrad Med 107:189–2000
51. Nash G, Foley FD (1970 Dec) Herpetic infection of the middle and lower respiratory tract. Am J Clin Pathol 54(6):857–63
52. Nash G (1972 Jun) Necrotizing tracheobronchitis and bronchopneumonia consistent with herpetic infection. Hum Pathol 3(2):283–91
53. Orlowski RZ, Mills SR, Hartley EE et al (2004 Nov) Oral valacyclovir as prophylaxis against herpes simplex virus reactivation during high dose chemotherapy for leukemia. Leuk Lymphoma 45(11):2215–9
54. Prellner T, Flamholc L, Haidl S et al (1992) Herpes simplex virus–the most frequently isolated pathogen in the lungs of patients with severe respiratory distress. Scand J Infect Dis 24(3):283–92
55. Rai KR, Freter CE, Mercier RJ et al (2002) Alemtuzumab in previously treated chronic lymphocytic leukemia patients who had also received fludarabine. J Clin Oncol 20:3891–3897
56. Ramsey PG, Fife KH, Hackman RC et al (1982 Dec) Herpes simplex virus pneumonia: clinical, virologic, and pathologic features in 20 patients. Ann Intern Med 97(6):813–20
57. Sandherr M, Einsele H, Hebart H et al (2006) Infectious Diseases Working Party, German Society for Hematology and Oncology. Antiviral prophylaxis in patients with hematological malignancies and solid tumors: Guidelines of the Infectious Disease Working Party (AGIHO) of the German Society of Hematology and Oncology (DGHO). Ann Oncol 17:1051–1059
58. Saral R, Ambinder RF, Burns WH et al (1983 Dec) Acyclovir prophylaxis against herpes simplex virus infection in patients with leukemia. A randomized, double-blind, placebo-controlled study. Ann Intern Med 99(6):773–6
59. Sauerbrei A, Eichhorn U, Schacke M et al (1999 Sep) Laboratory diagnosis of herpes zoster. J Clin Virol 14(1):31–6
60. Schuller D, Spessert C, Fraser VJ et al (1993 Jan) Herpes simplex virus from respiratory tract secretions: epidemiology, clinical characteristics, and outcome in immunocompromised and nonimmunocompromised hosts. Am J Med 94(1):29–33
61. Stránská R, Schuurman R, de Vos M et al (2004 May) Routine use of a highly automated and internally controlled real-time PCR assay for the diagnosis of herpes simplex and varicella-zoster virus infections. J Clin Virol 30(1): 39–44
62. Styczynski J, Reusser P, Einsele H et al (2009 May) Second European Conference on Infections in Leukemia. Management of HSV, VZV and EBV infections in patients with hematological malignancies and after SCT: guidelines from the Second European Conference on Infections in Leukemia. Bone Marrow Transplant 43(10):757–70
63. Taplitz RA, Jordan MC (2002 Jun) Pneumonia caused by herpesviruses in recipients of hematopoietic cell transplants. Semin Respir Infect 17(2):121–9, Review
64. Tuxen DV, Wilson JW, Cade JF (1987 Aug) Prevention of lower respiratory herpes simplex virus infection with acyclovir in patients with the adult respiratory distress syndrome. Am Rev Respir Dis 136(2):402–5
65. Umans U, Golding RP, Duraku S et al (2001) Herpes simplex virus 1 pneumonia: conventional chest radiograph pattern. Eur Radiol 11(6):990–4
66. Villarreal E (2003) Current and potential therapies for the treatment of herpes simplex infections. Prog Drug Res 60:263–307
67. Wade JC, Newton B, Flournoy N et al (1984 Jun) Oral acyclovir for prevention of herpes simplex virus reactivation after marrow transplantation. Ann Intern Med 100(6):823–8
68. Whitley RJ, Roizman B (2001) Herpes simplex virus infections. Lancet 357:1513–8
69. Yahav D, Gafter-Gvili A, Muchtar E et al (2009 Dec) Antiviral prophylaxis in haematological patients: systematic review and meta-analysis. Eur J Cancer 45(18): 3131–48

25 Pneumocystis Pneumonia in Non-AIDS Immunocompromised Patients

Élie Azoulay, Virginie Lemiale, Achille Kouatchet, François Vincent, Antoine Roux, Guillaume Bollée, and Patricia Roux

Contents

25.1 Introduction

Pneumocystis pneumonia (PCP) remains one of the leading causes of morbidity and mortality among AIDS patients all over the world [1–3]. However, PCP is also a life-threatening opportunistic infection that can occur in other immunocompromised patients, mainly in solid organ transplant recipients, patients with cancer disease, hematological malignancy and those treated for autoimmune or inflammatory diseases [1–3].

PCP is caused by *Pneumocystis jirovecii*, a pathogen first identified in the early twentieth century by Chagas and subsequently by Carinii in rat lungs. These authors believed wrongly that they had found a new form of trypanosome. However, several years later, it was established that it was an original species, called *Pneumocystis carinii.* For many decades, pneumocystis was classified as a protozoan, until new phylogenetic studies demonstrated that it was related to the fungi [4]. Pneumocystis organisms have been identified in several mammalians, but in fact, different pneumocystis species with distinct genetic characteristics exist, with each species being host-specific. Thus, the pneumocystis infecting humans was named *Pneumocystis jirovecii* [3].

É. Azoulay (✉), V. Lemiale, A. Roux, and G. Bollée
Service de Réanimation Médicale, Hôpital Saint-Louis, 1 avenue Claude Vellefaux, 75010, Paris, France and Medical Intensive Care Units, Saint-Louis Hospital, Paris 7 University, Paris, France
e-mail: elie.azoulay@sls.aphp.fr

F. Vincent
University, Avicenne Hospital, Paris 13 University

A. Kouatchet
Angers University Hospital

P. Roux
Parasitology-Mycology Department, Saint-Antoine Hospital, Paris 6 University, Paris, France

É. Azoulay (ed.), *Pulmonary Involvement in Patients with Hematological Malignancies,*
DOI: 10.1007/978-3-642-15742-4_25,

Over the last years, advances in hematological treatments (including new drugs, high dose and intensive chemotherapy with bone marrow or stem cell transplantation) and immunomodulation resulted in an increased number of patients with impaired immunity and risk for PCP. This review focuses on practical aspects relevant to risk factors, diagnosis and treatment of PCP, in order to provide to clinicians an actual clinical picture of PCP in non-AIDS patients.

25.2 Transmission

PCP was long thought to result from reactivation of latent infection acquired during childhood. This theory was supported by the seroprevalence of anti-*Pneumocystis* antibodies at a young age, the high rate of PCP among infants with AIDS, the presence of *Pneumocystis jirovecii* in respiratory specimens from patients without immunosuppression and without clinical signs of PCP, and by the characteristics of the organism itself, consistent with long-term carriage [5]. However, several lines of evidence subsequently ruled out the possibility of reactivation of latent infection as the sole mechanism for PCP and found that infection more likely results from environmental exposure or person-to-person transmission [5–7]. In this way, it was shown that *Pneumocystis* DNA was present in the environment, including pond water and various air samples, and that PCP incidence was increased in certain geographic areas. Additional data suggest that *Pneumocystis jirovecii* acquisition could result in a number of cases from airborne transmission from asymptomatic carriers or from patients with PCP [5, 6, 8]. Nevertheless, isolation of patients with PCP is not currently recommended or applied [5].

25.3 Patients at Risk for PCP

Several retrospective studies have led to identification of clinical conditions associated with the occurrence of PCP in HIV-negative immunocompromised patients (Tables 25.1 and 25.2). Fifty years ago, PCP cases were reported in prematurely born and malnourished infants [9]. Nowadays, in rich countries, patients who are the most likely to develop PCP are those suffering from hematological malignancy, solid cancer, inflammatory or autoimmune disease, and solid organ transplant recipients [10–13]. Among those treated for hematological malignancies, five group of patients are at higher risk for PCP [14–16], namely, (1) patients with lymphoproliferative disorders such as lymphoma or acute lymphocytic leukemia (ALL); (2) patients receiving high doses or long-term steroids; (3) recipients of allogeneic but also autologous bone marrow or stem cell transplants; (4) patients treated using anti-CD20 [17] or anti-CD52 antibodies; and (5) patients with deep and prolonged lymphocytopenia after chemotherapy, such as fludarabin. Awareness of patients at risk for PCP is of great importance for clinicians who have to identify the patients requiring prophylaxis and cases where diagnosis of PCP must be considered.

25.3.1 Hematological Malignancies

It has long been established that children with acute lymphoblastic leukemia receiving chemotherapy have a high risk of PCP. In a study by Hugues et al., the attack rate reached 4.1% in this population [18]. Subsequently, PCP cases were reported in almost all hematological malignancies [14, 15]. Although the exact incidence

Table 25.1 Underlying conditions in four series of non-AIDS patients with PCP

	Zahar [49]	Yale [20]	Roblot [48]	Bollée [48]
	n = 39 (%)	*n* = 116 (%)	*n* = 130 (%)	*n* = 56 (%)
Hematological malignancies	28 (71.8)	35 (30.2)	75 (57.7)	44 (78.6)
Solid tumors	7 (17.9)	15 (12.9)	18 (13.8)	9 (16.1)
Solid organ transplantation	0	29 (25)	9 (6.9)	0
Inflammatory diseases	0	26 (22.4)	27 (20.8)	0
Miscellaneous	4 (10.3)	11 (9.5)	1 (0.8)	3 (5.4)

Table 25.2 Incidence of PCP in various types of malignancies (Adapted from [11])

	PCP cases	Patients	Rates (%)
Lymphomas	34	9,907	0.34
Acute lymphocytic leukemia	5	2,929	0.17
Other leukemia	16	5,023	0.32
Solid tumors	30	26,085	0.11
Cerebral tumors	21	3,098	0.68
Bone marrow transplantation	22	1,348	1.63

rate of PCP for each group of hematological malignancies is unknown, the highest incidence seems to occur in lymphoid leukemia and non-Hodgkin's lymphoma, with attack rates being around 0.2–0.5% [11, 14]. Cancer patients who develop PCP have often received chemotherapy. However, in our experience, PCP may also be inaugural of the underlying disease, occurring before any immunosuppressive therapy [16].

Patients undergoing autologous or especially allogeneic hematopoietic stem cell transplantation (HSCT) are also likely to develop PCP. Although older studies showed that PCP occurred in most cases within the first 6 months after allogeneic HSCT, this notion was ruled out by more recent reports. In a recent retrospective study, PCP occurred at a median of 14.5 months after allogeneic HSCT, with the attack rate being 2.5% [19]. Moreover, in most cases, patients were receiving immunosuppressive therapy for chronic graft-versus-host disease or had a relapse of their hematological malignancy [19].

25.4 Immunosuppressive Drugs and Risk of PCP

In HIV-negative patients developing PCP, the immunocompromised state is partly linked to factors related to the underlying disease causing specific immunosuppression, but is also a consequence of treatments such as steroids, cytotoxic drugs and other immunomodulative drugs.

Regardless of the associated underlying disease, steroids have largely been pointed out as a major predisposing factor for PCP in HIV-negative patients. A retrospective analysis of 116 cases of PCP in HIV-negative patients showed that 90.5% were currently receiving steroids when PCP occurred. Median daily dose and median duration of steroids were equivalent to 30 mg and 12 weeks, respectively, and 25% of patients had received as little as 16 mg of prednisone daily [20]. However, patients not taking corticosteroids may also develop PCP. Indeed, in a recent retrospective study by our group of 56 HIV-negative patients with PCP, we observed that 24 patients (42.8%) were not receiving steroids when PCP occurred [16]. This is a crucial issue emphasizing that clinicians have to consider the possibility of PCP occurrence also in patients not receiving corticosteroids.

Risk of PCP in cancer patients has been shown to be associated with the intensity of chemotherapy [18]. The precise role of a particular cytotoxic drug in PCP occurrence is often difficult to establish due to the association of several drugs in most patients. Certain drugs, such as fludarabine, cladribine, cyclophosphamide or methotrexate, have been suspected to be associated with a particularly high risk of PCP; however, these data remain elusive [1, 2, 21, 22].

Among immunosuppressive therapies used after solid organ transplantation, anti-lymphocytes antibodies clearly increase the risk of PCP [23]. PCP risk associated with azathioprine and cyclosporine therapy appears low, whereas it seems higher with tacrolimus [24]. Uncertainties persist regarding the risk associated with mycophenolate-mofenil and sirolimus use. Despite ancecdotal reports, actual risk of PCP related to newer drugs, such as anti-TNFα or anti-CD52 antibodies, has not yet been established.

25.5 CD4+ Lymphocyte Counts in HIV-Negative Patients Developing PCP

PCP has been largely described in HIV-infected patients with a circulating CD4+ T lymphocyte count lower than 200/mm [3]. In other immunocompromised patients, the CD4+ count has also been shown to be related to the risk of PCP. PCP seems more likely to occur in patients with a CD4+ count lower than 300/mm [3]. This suggests that CD4+ counts could be of value to detect patients at risk for PCP and determine those who should receive prophylaxis against PCP. However, the real value of CD4+ count monitoring in

HIV-negative patients remains to be established. The total lymphocyte number should be taken into account.

25.6 Differences in Physiopathology Between Patients with and without AIDS

In a study by Limper et al., bronchoalveolar lavage (BAL) analysis of patients with PCP revealed important differences between patients with and without AIDS. Compared with AIDS patients, each of the other immunocompromised categories (hematological malignancies, solid cancers, solid organs transplantations and steroids therapy) had significantly lower organism numbers and more inflammation, estimated by neutrophil count. Furthermore, inflammation in BAL was inversely correlated with oxygenation and survival [10]. These data explain, at least partly, the differences observed in the clinical presentation of PCP between patients with and without AIDS. Along this line, in HIV infected patients, we previously reported the independent relationship between BAL neutrophilia and severity (hypoxemia) and outcomes (mortality) [25]. This may in part explain how HIV-infected patients with PCP have lower mortality rates compared to non-HIV patients with PCP [26].

25.7 Clinical and Radiological Presentation of PCP in HIV-Negative Patients

25.7.1 Clinical Presentation

HIV-negative patients with PCP typically present with fever in about 60–90% of cases, dyspnea in 75–95% and cough in 50–80%. Although in some cases the evolution is more insidious, fever and respiratory symptoms develop over weeks [16]. Delay from onset of symptoms to diagnosis is rather short, varying from 1 to 14 days in most cases. Clinical examination commonly reveals tachypnea and diffuse crackles at lung auscultation. PaO_2 in room air is usually strongly decreased, around 50–70 mmHg [14–16, 27]. Thus, clinical presentation is typically severe, with rapidly evolving bilateral lung involvement and marked hypoxemia. By comparison with AIDS patients, PCP presents as a more acute and severe disease among HIV negative patients, causing acute respiratory failure and often need for mechanical ventilation [16, 28, 29].

25.7.2 Radiological Presentation

Radiographic features of PCP are similar in patients with and without AIDS [29]. Typically, bilateral or less frequently unilateral interstitial infiltrates are observed (Figs. 25.1–25.3). Rarely, chest radiography may be normal at an early stage. Also, atypical presentations may be misleading (Fig. 25.4). Only few data are specific to non-AIDS patients. Findings from high-resolution CT scans (HRCT) are available to date. A pattern of extensive ground-glass attenuation, which is often distributed in a patchy fashion, with predilection for perihilar regions of the lungs, is the most common feature (Figs. 25.1–25.4). In addition to the infiltrates, atypical HRCT features, such as nodules, nodular components or cavities, may be seen. The presence of these atypical images may be related to granuloma formation in response to PCP (Fig. 25.4), but are more often indicative of a concomitant cancer or infectious disease processes affecting the lungs. Conversely to AIDS patients, cysts related to PCP have not been described in HIV-negative patients with PCP.

25.8 Diagnostic Strategy

25.8.1 Respiratory Samples Collecting Techniques

Owing to the lack of specificity of clinical and radiological presentation, diagnosis of PCP requires microbiological examination from a relevant sample to identify *Pneumocystis jirovecii*. Differences in organism number between patients with and without AIDS have to be borne in mind to address the issue of an adequate diagnostic procedure in non-AIDS immunocompromised patients.

Several procedures are available for obtaining respiratory samples. Induced sputum (IS), a technique

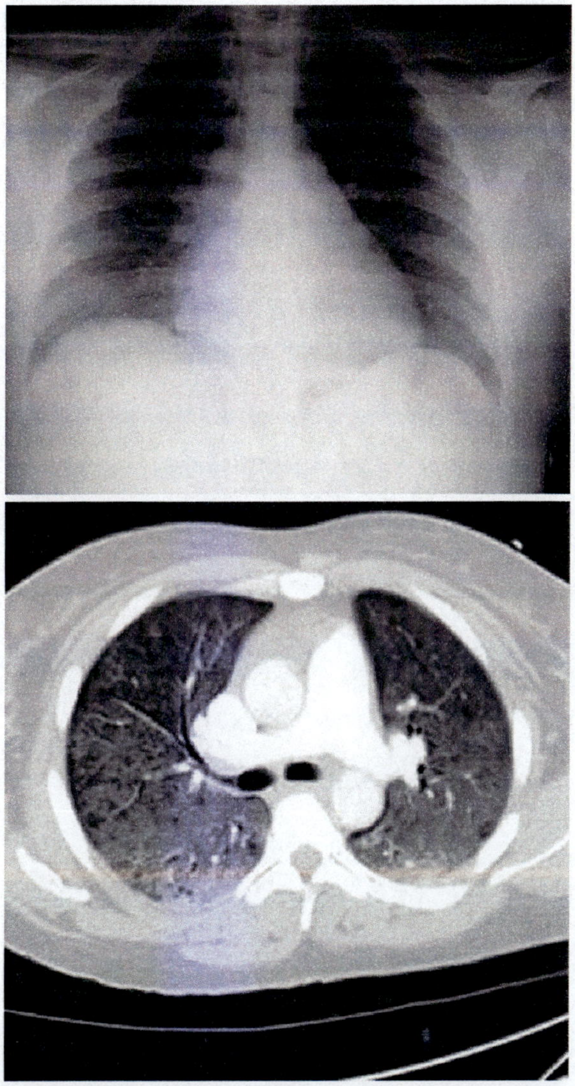

Fig. 25.1 Acute respiratory failure in a chronic lymphocytic leukemia (CLL) patients treated by cyclophosphamide, fludarabine and rituximab. Observance of prophylaxis was hazardous. Induced sputum performed before any antibiotics revealed cystic forms of *Pneumocystis jirovecii*

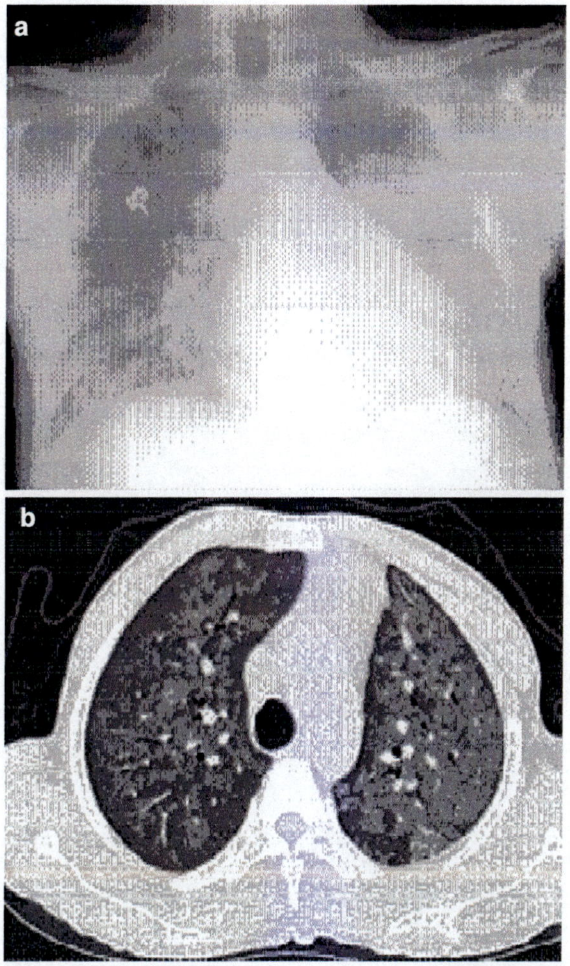

Fig. 25.2 Hypoxemia in a 31-year-old ALL patient treated by long-term steroids. Chest X Ray (*panel a*) and High resolution CT scan (*panel b*) were suggestive of pneumocystis pneumonia. Giemsa staining on BAL fluid analysis was positive

consisting of collection of a sputum specimen by a respiratory therapist after inhalation of nebulized saline for 20 min, has been proven to be a useful technique for the diagnosis of PCP. Bronchospasm may complicate the technique. Also, failure to collect this specimen in hypoxemic patients can be related to non-tolerance of the saline nebulization. Because of concerns about spreading tuberculosis during the procedure, this procedure is not indicated for patients suspected of having TB. Whereas the sensitivity of direct examination on IS from AIDS patients is up to 90% in certain centers, [4] the few available data concerning HIV-negative patients suggest a lower sensitivity of around 50% [30]. Combining a rigorous technique for collecting the sputa and having it done by a trained mycologist clearly make it more sensitive. Bronchoscopy with bronchoalveolar lavage (BAL) represent a more efficient technique for diagnosing PCP [31]. Once again, the sensitivity of direct examination in HIV-negative patients is not well defined, but appears lower than in AIDS patients, around 60–70% [32]. The timing between antibiotic administration and induced sputum or BAL sampling is a key issue. BAL examination samples can be sent to several laboratories, increasing the diagnostic yield. Therefore, concomitant bacterial, viral or

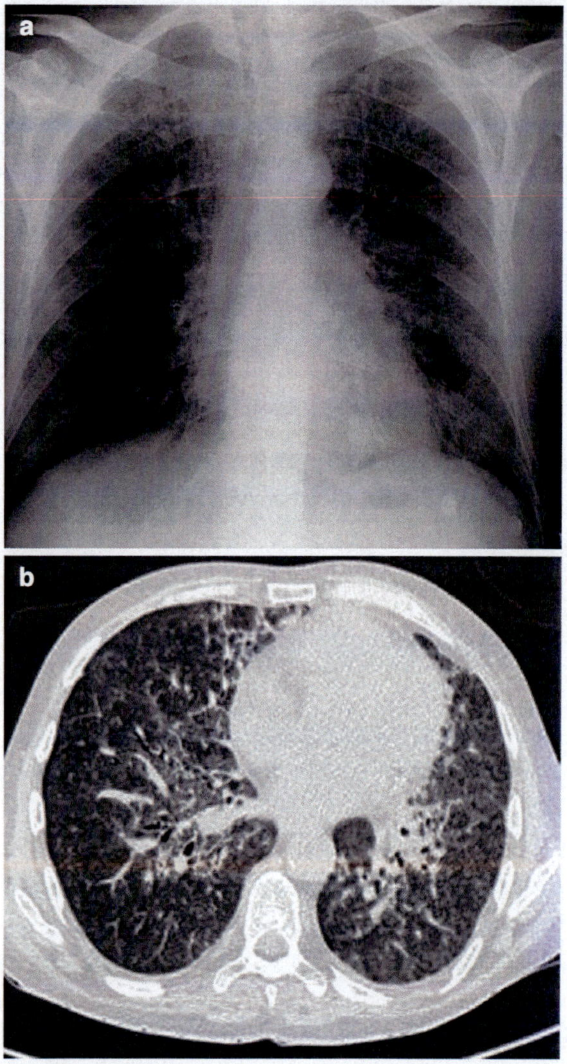

Fig. 25.3 Acute respiratory failure 15 months after allogeneic stem cell transplantation for AML. Prophylaxis was withdrawn at 1 year. Chest X Ray (*panel a*) and High resolution CT scan (*panel b*) were suggestive of *pneumocystis pneumonia*. Induced sputum and BAL were negative for pneumocystis. A positive pneumocystis PCR raised concerns about the negative BAL. Re-examination (on a rescue smear) of BAL revealed trophic forms of pneumocystis

fungal infections can be diagnosed. However, this can also be done using a noninvasive diagnostic strategy [30]. An important limitation of the BAL procedure is the risk of aggravating the respiratory state and the need for mechanical ventilation, which are associated with a high mortality rate [33]. Interestingly, a concomitant pulmonary infection due to viruses, especially cytomegalovirus, bacteria or fungi, is frequently detected by BAL in patients with PCP (Fig. 25.7b) [10]. However, no comparative strategy has demonstrated the benefit of performing BAL, which remains the procedure to perform when IS has failed to identify pneumocystis, concerning mortality or morbidity. Rarely, when less invasive procedures have failed to detect PCP, surgical lung biopsy should be considered [14]. However, the use of polymerase chain reaction (PCR) has made surgical biopsy no longer indicated for PCP patients.

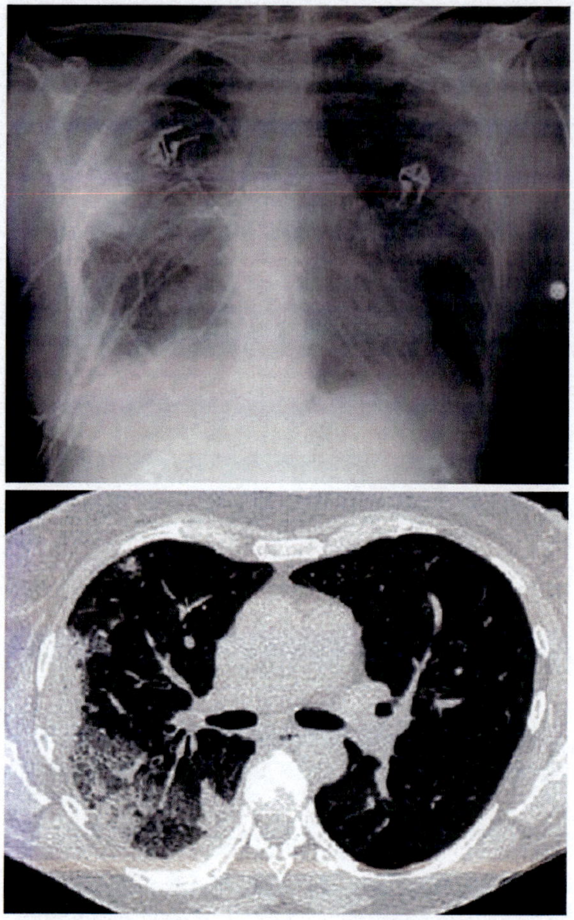

Fig. 25.4 Atypical presentation of *Pneumocystis pneumonia* in a 68-year-old patient with refractory T lymphoma receiving a third-line chemotherapy and anti-CD52 antibodies

25.8.2 Laboratory Diagnosis

A major obstacle to studying and detecting pneumocystis is the impossibility of culturing this organism, despite many attempts [1, 2].

25.8.2.1 Direct Examination

At first, the detection of *Pneumocystis jirovecii* in respiratory samples depends on direct examination, which is based on tinctorial stains and immunofluorescence. Several staining methods, such as calcofluor white, Gomori-Grocott or toluidine blue, only allow detection of cysts, and also mark other fungi (Figs. 25.5a and 25.6) [34]. Other stains, such as Wright–Giemsa (Fig. 25.5b), Diff-Quik and Gram-Weigert, can detect both intracystic bodies (spores) and cysts and trophic forms, but their interpretation may be difficult as they also color other organisms. The development of indirect immunofluorescence using monoclonal antibodies was a significant advance, providing a method that is rapid and more sensitive than conventional stains for detecting *Pneumocystis jirovecii* in respiratory samples (Fig. 25.7a) [35].

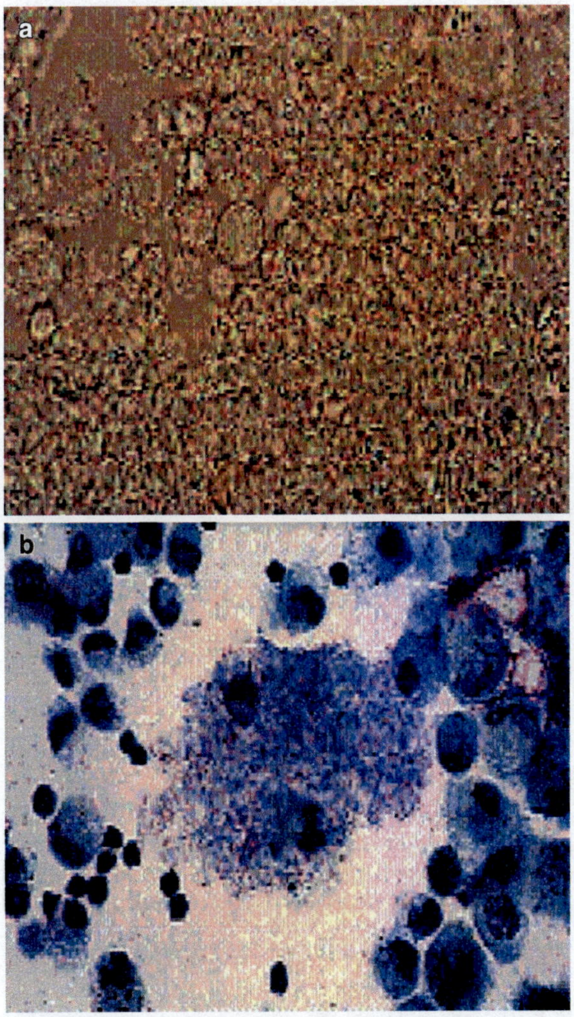

Fig. 25.5 Direct examination of BAL fluid (×1,000, *panel a*). Cluster of *Pneumocystis jirovecii*. Cluster of *Pneumocystis jirovecii* in BAL fluid (Giemsa staining, *panel b*)

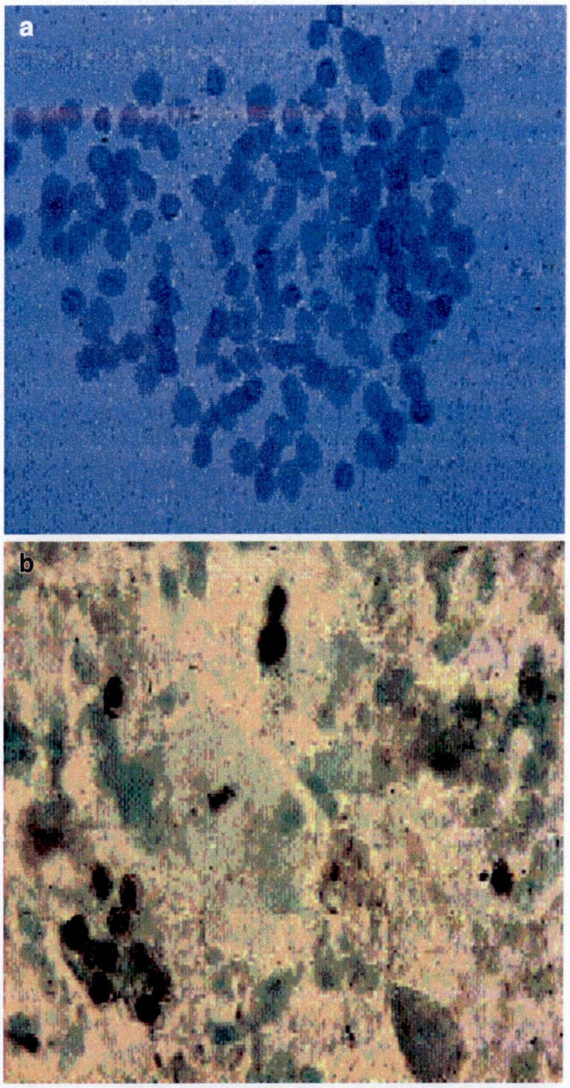

Fig. 25.6 *Pneumocystis jirovecii* cysts in BAL fluid. TBO staining (×1,000, *panel a*). *Pneumocystis jirovecii* cysts in induced sputum. Musto staining (×1,000, *panel b*)

25.8.2.2 Polymerase Chain Reaction as a Significant Advance for Diagnosing PCP

The detection of *Pneumocystis jirovecii* in clinical specimens was greatly improved by the use of

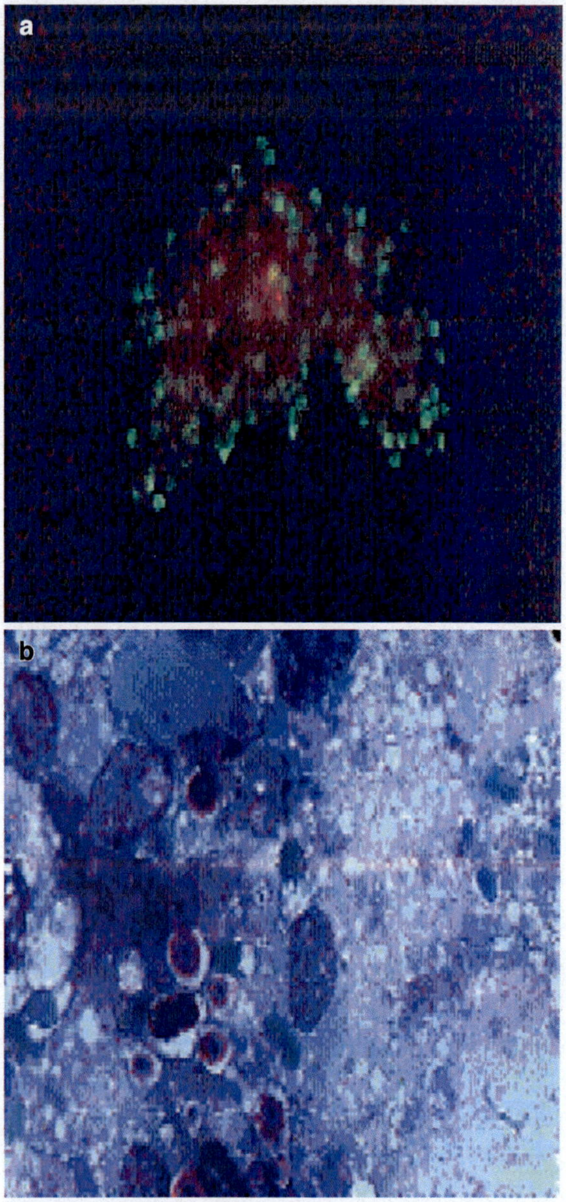

Fig. 25.7 *Pneumocystis jirovecii* cysts in BAL fluid (immunofluorescence, *panel a*). Giemsa staining in induced sputum revealing infection by pneumocystis, Cryptococcus neoformans and colonization by Candida albicans (×1,000, *panel b*)

polymerase chain reactions (PCR). In 1990, Wakefield et al. developed a new technique for DNA amplification specific to pneumocystis using primer sequences for the mitochondrial 5S rRNA gene of *P. carinii* [36]. Subsequent studies highlighted the efficiency of this technique. Principally in AIDS patients, sensitivity was evaluated at 80–100% and 70–85% on BAL and IS specimens, respectively. Specificity appeared also excellent, around 80–100% on BAL and 90–95% on IS [32, 37]. However, since HIV patients have numerous cysts or trophic forms of pneumocystis, the usefulness of PCR remains controversial.

The question about the interpretation of a positive PCR deciding between infection and colonization is often raised. In a study by Sing et al., the PCR value was investigated in different immunocompromised groups. For combined BAL and IS specimens, sensitivity and specificity were respectively calculated to 80% and 100% in AIDS patients, 86% and 97% in transplant recipients, 100% and 95% in cancer patients, and 100% and 98% in other immunocompromised patients [32]. In another study, *Pneumocystis jirovecii* was not detected by direct examination of BAL in 7 of 37 HIV-negative immunocompromised patients with PCP, and PCR was the only microbiological indication of *Pneumocystis jirovecii* in these patients [37]. These data emphasize that routine microbiological evaluation for PCP must involve the use of PCR in all respiratory samples from HIV-negative immunocompromised patients. Nevertheless, this excessively sensitive technique may overestimate PCP diagnosis in patients who are only colonized. In an evaluation by our study group in 448 non-HIV patients, the negative predictive value of pneumocystis PCR was almost 100% [38]. This allows clinicians to rule out the clinical diagnosis of PCP based on the results of PCR, even on induced sputa and without performing BAL. Additional evaluation is warranted. This needs to include (1) actual risk factors for PCP, (2) the level of clinical suspicion of PCP and (3) the results of quantitative PCR, which seem likely to make the difference between colonization and infection.

25.8.2.3 PCR and Colonization

However, a benefit of the PCR technique is the excellent sensitivity allowing the detection of a very low pneumocystis burden related to colonization in asymptomatic patients. Although lung colonization by *Pneumocystis jirovecii* was also reported in immunocompetents patients with various bronchopulmonary diseases [39], immunocompromised patients appear much more likely to be asymptomatic pneumocystis carriers [40]. Long-term steroid use and low CD4+ counts [41] have been shown to be associated with higher colonization rates. In a study by Leigh et al., ISs obtained in 10 immunocompetent patients and 20 solid organ transplant recipients, all asymptomatic, were screened for *Pneumocystis jirovecii* using PCR and immunofluorescence. All 30 specimens were negative for *Pneumocystis jirovecii* using immunofluorescence, and 5 transplant patients but no immunocompetent patients were positive for *Pneumocystis jirovecii* according to PCR alone. One of these patients developed PCP 6 weeks after sputum induction [42]. However, the risk of clinical PCP occurrence in an asymptomatic patient with colonization remains largely uncertain to date. Thus, PCR positivity alone on a respiratory sample may reflect true infection, but also colonization.

25.8.2.4 Real-Time Quantitative PCR

Larsen et al. developed a rapid, sensitive and quantitative Touchdown-PCR (TD-PCR) assay, which constituted another significant improvement in diagnosing PCP and resolved, at least partly, the problem of distinction between true infection and colonization [43]. In a blind retrospective study of respiratory samples obtained in HIV-negative immunocompromised patients, the concentration of pneumocystis DNA measured by using quantitative TD-PCR was significantly higher in patients with PCP than in those with other respiratory disorders. Moreover, application of a cutoff value allowed distinguishing between infection and colonization. Real-time PCR has been demonstrated to be the best technique that avoids contamination, allows quantitation of the fungus copy number and can discriminate between infection and colonization [44].

PCR performed on IS represents an alternative to BAL that may be effective and non-invasive. An oral wash collected after the patient gargles and rinses the mouth with sterile saline appears to be a highly desirable diagnostic specimen, as it can be obtained easily and quickly in a number of patients, including in those unable to sustain invasive procedures. Oral washes do not contain enough organisms to be detected by direct microscopic examination, but PCR may detect pneumocystis DNA in such specimens. Moreover, Larsen et al. demonstrated that quantitative TD-PCR could be used for distinguishing between colonization and infection in oral washes, as in BAL specimens [43]. PCR on oral washes has also been shown to be a useful technique for diagnosing PCP in HIV-negative immunocompromised patients. Helweg-Larsen reported 100% sensitivity and specificity of TD-PCR on 26 oral washes collected in patients with hematological malignancies, with 8 having PCP [45]. Thus, examination of oral washes by TD-PCR is a promising technique to diagnose PCP and should be carried out in increasing numbers of centers for use in the near future.

25.8.2.5 *S*-Adenosylmethionine Plasmatic Concentration Dosage

Pneumocystis is the only cell known to be unable to synthesize *S*-adenosylmethionine, a key intermediary metabolite for all cells. Thus, pneumocystis must extract this compound from its host, resulting in the depletion of the infected animal. It was assessed that plasma *S*-adenosylmethionine was decreased in AIDS patients with PCP, and rapidly increased after recovery [46], suggesting that measurement of plasma *S*-adenosylmethionine could be of great value for diagnosing PCP. However, these promising results will have to be confirmed in the future before being put into use.

25.8.2.6 (1–3)-β-D-Glucan

(1–3)-β-D-Glucan (BG) is present in the cell wall of most medically important fungi (except *Cryptoccoccus* sp. and zygomycetes sp.). In pneumocystis they are localized to the electron-lucent band under the cell membrane of the cysts. Recently, colorimetric assays have been developed (15) to detect BG. The Fungitell test© (Associates of Cape Cod, Inc., Cape Cod, MA) is a chromogenic kinetic test (approved in 2003 by the US Food and Drug Administration) for the presumptive diagnosis of invasive fungal infections. Studies showed that high BG sera levels >500 pg/mL are found during pneumocystosis; [47] they noted that 29/30 confirmed PCP cases were BG positive, and most of them were >500 pg/mL. The median value for the PCP-positive group was in excess of 500 pg/mL. The BG assay is a noninvasive serological test useful for the diagnosis of PCP.

25.9 Prognosis of PCP in HIV-Negative Patients

25.9.1 *Mortality*

Prognosis of PCP is clearly worse in HIV-negative than in AIDS patients, with the mortality rate reported to be around 30–40%. Mortality is even higher in patients requiring mechanical ventilation, reaching 60–75% [14–16, 48].

25.9.2 Prognostic Factors

Many factors associated with mortality in HIV-negative patients with PCP have been described. Unsurprisingly, high respiratory and pulse rates, hypoxemia, involvement of four lung lobes, need for mechanical ventilation or vasopressors, high C reactive protein and lactate dehydrogenase levels, severity scores according to the Simplified Acute Physiology Score II or Organ System Failure score, and concomitant pulmonary infection have been associated with higher mortality [14, 16, 27, 48]. Receiving cancer chemotherapy [27, 49] and long-term steroids [14, 49] is also related to the occurrence of death. Interestingly, high neutrophil counts in BAL specimens are associated with more severe hypoxemia and higher mortality [10, 49], which may support the hypothesis of a beneficial effect of adjuvant high-dose steroids for non-AIDS patients, as previously reported for AIDS patients [50, 51].

25.10 Curative Treatment of PCP

25.10.1 Antimicrobial Therapy

Medications used to treat PCP do not differ between patients with and without AIDS. As the most effective treatment, trimethoprim-sulfamethoxazole (TMP-SMX) given orally or intravenously for 3 weeks must be used as the first-line treatment unless contraindicated. TMP-SMX acts by interfering with folate metabolism: TMP and SMX respectively inhibit dihydrofolate reductase (DHFR) and dihydropteroate synthase (DHPS), which are two integral enzymes of folate synthesis. Emergence of mutations in the DHPS gene related to prophylaxis use has been a concern for several years. However, whether these mutations confer resistance to TMP-SMX remains largely uncertain and controversial. Adverse effects, including fever, rash, cytopenia, hyperkaliemia, hyponatremia, hepatitis and interstitial nephritis, occur less commonly (around 15%) in HIV-negative compared to AIDS patients [52]. The adjunction of folinic acid may lower the risk of neutropenia, but increases the risk for therapeutic failure. Due to the lack of synergy and the risk of occurrence of adverse effects, association with other antimicrobial molecules is not recommended for treating PCP.

In case of intolerance to TMP-SMX, pentamidine should be used as an alternative choice. Pentamidine can be administrated intravenously or by aerosol in mild forms of PCP. The most common adverse drug reaction to pentamidine is renal toxicity, which usually occurs after 2 weeks of treatment and can be prevented by adequate hydration. Other adverse effects, including hypotension (especially in case of rapid infusion), heart arrhythmias, hypo- or hyperglycemia, hypercalcemia, hyperkaliemia, pancreatitis and metallic taste may also occur. Atovaquone, dapsone and clindamycin-primaquine represent other options in the treatment of mild PCP in AIDS patients. However, due to the lack of data, these drugs cannot be recommended for current use in HIV-negative patients with PCP.

25.10.2 Adjuvant Steroids

Steroids are recommended in AIDS patients with PCP who have severe hypoxemia (PaO_2 under 70 mmHg on room air). Indeed, adjuvant steroids have been shown to result in a significant survival improvement by reducing the risk of respiratory failure and mortality [51].

Regarding HIV-negative patients, only a few retrospective studies, including a small number of patients, have investigated the effect of adjuvant steroids. In a study by Delclaux et al., adjuvant steroids were not found to influence the mechanical ventilation requirements and mortality rate [53]. In another study by Pareja et al., adjuvant steroids were associated with a shorter duration of mechanical ventilation, oxygen therapy and stay in the ICU, without decreasing mortality [54]. In our recent study of 56 HIV-negative patients with PCP, we observed a trend toward decreased mortality in patients receiving adjuvant steroids (18.2% vs 42.2%, NS) [16]. Thus, a clear benefit from adjuvant steroids in HIV-negative patients with PCP has not been proved to date. However, considering the results and the limits of these studies, and on the basis of our personal experience, we believe that adjuvant steroids should be advised in HIV-negative patients with severe PCP.

25.11 Prophylaxis of *Pneumocystis pneumonia*

25.11.1 Antimicrobial Drugs Available

Thirty years ago, TMP-SMX was demonstrated to be highly effective and well tolerated in the prevention of PCP among cancer patients [2, 18, 52]. Nowadays, TMP-SMX given orally remains the gold standard for PCP prophylaxis, similarly to curative treatment. Aerosolized pentamidine repeated every month might be an alternative for patients not tolerating TMP-SMX. Although this prophylactic regimen was demonstrated to be less effective than TMP-SMX, aerosolized pentamidine was associated with an increased risk of PCP and other infections, and a higher mortality in bone marrow transplant recipients. Dapsone is another available drug for preventing PCP. Dapsone inhibits DHPS as SMX. However, dapsone alone or associated with pyrimethamine is inferior to TMP-SMX. Moreover, TMP-SMX intolerance often predicts dapsone intolerance. Thus, it is not recommended to replace TMP-SMX by dapsone in case of intolerance [55]. Finally, atovaquone constitutes an effective and well-tolerated alternate choice, also in bone marrow transplant recipients.

25.11.2 Indications for Prophylaxis

Conversely to AIDS patients, no consensus has been reached concerning the indications for prophylaxis against PCP in HIV-negative patients. From our own experience and in view of the risk factors for PCP occurrence, we believe that patients who should receive prophylaxis are:

- Patients with any immunological disorder, including cancer, hematological disease, autoimmune or inflammatory disorders, who are given more than 15 mg of prednisone daily (or the equivalent) for more than 4 weeks.
- Patients with acute leukemia or non-Hodgkin's lymphoma not in remission or receiving chemotherapy.
- Patients undergoing allogenic HSCT; prophylaxis should be maintained for at least 1 year and maintained in patients receiving immunosuppressive drugs, and in those with relapse of their hematological malignancy or with longstanding GVHD.
- Patients undergoing autologous HSCT, for at least 6 months; duration should be extended in patients receiving additional immunosuppressive drugs.
- Solid organ transplant recipients should receive prophylaxis for 6 months after transplantation, except lung transplant recipients, who should have lifelong prophylaxis.

TMP-SMX should be stopped during neutropenia and in patients receiving methotrexate. It remains unclear whether CD4+ monitoring should be used for detecting patients who require prophylaxis. However, a CD4+ count lower than 300/mm [3] should lead to prescribing prophylaxis, especially for patients with malignancies.

25.12 Conclusion

In summary, PCP is a severe opportunistic infection, which may complicate the course of a wide variety of diseases leading to immunosuppression. For clinicians caring for immunocompromised patients, knowledge of conditions associated with PCP is crucial for identifying who should receive prophylaxis and suspecting PCP in order to implement an early, adequate diagnostic and therapeutic strategy. Long-term steroid use is an important but not the only risk factor for PCP patients. In the era of more intensive treatment regimens, new molecules used as cancer chemotherapy or immunomodulation, and extended survival of cancer patients suggest that clinicians need to maintain a high level of suspicion regarding PCP. The development of PCR and noninvasive methods, such as oral washes and β-1–3 glucan detection, constitutes important advances for diagnosing PCP, which should be available in an increased number of centers to allow optimal management of these patients.

References

1. Kovacs JA, Masur H (2009) Evolving health effects of Pneumocystis: 100 years of progress in diagnosis and treatment. JAMA 301(24):2578–2585

2. Thomas CF Jr, Limper AH (2004) Pneumocystis pneumonia. N Engl J Med 350(24):2487–2498
3. Catherinot E, Lanternier F, Bougnoux ME, Lecuit M, Couderc LJ, Lortholary O (2010) Pneumocystis jirovecii Pneumonia. Infect Dis Clin North Am 24(1):107–138
4. Edman JC, Kovacs JA, Masur H, Santi DV, Elwood HJ, Sogin ML (1988) Ribosomal RNA sequence shows Pneumocystis carinii to be a member of the fungi. Nature 334(6182):519–522
5. Morris A, Beard CB, Huang L (2002) Update on the epidemiology and transmission of Pneumocystis carinii. Microbes Infect 4(1):95–103
6. Jacobs JL, Libby DM, Winters RA et al (1991) A cluster of Pneumocystis carinii pneumonia in adults without predisposing illnesses. N Engl J Med 324(4):246–250
7. Yazaki H, Goto N, Uchida K, Kobayashi T, Gatanaga H, Oka S (2009) Outbreak of Pneumocystis jiroveci pneumonia in renal transplant recipients: P. jiroveci is contagious to the susceptible host. Transplantation 88(3):380–385
8. Bensousan T, Garo B, Islam S, Bourbigot B, Cledes J, Garre M (1990) Possible transfer of Pneumocystis carinii between kidney transplant recipients. Lancet 336(8722): 1066–1067
9. Gajdusek DC (1957) Pneumocystis carinii; etiologic agent of interstitial plasma cell pneumonia of premature and young infants. Pediatrics 19(4 Part 1):543–565
10. Limper AH, Offord KP, Smith TF, Martin WJ 2nd (1989) Pneumocystis carinii pneumonia. Differences in lung parasite number and inflammation in patients with and without AIDS. Am Rev Respir Dis 140(5):1204–1209
11. Sepkowitz KA (1992) Pneumocystis carinii pneumonia among patients with neoplastic disease. Semin Respir Infect 7(2):114–121
12. Sepkowitz KA, Brown AE, Telzak EE, Gottlieb S, Armstrong D (1992) Pneumocystis carinii pneumonia among patients without AIDS at a cancer hospital. JAMA 267(6):832–837
13. Sepkowitz KA (1993) Pneumocystis carinii pneumonia in patients without AIDS. Clin Infect Dis 17(Suppl 2):S416–S422
14. Pagano L, Fianchi L, Mele L et al (2002) Pneumocystis carinii pneumonia in patients with malignant haematological diseases: 10 years' experience of infection in GIMEMA centres. Br J Haematol 117(2):379–386
15. Pagano L, Caira M, Fianchi L (2005) Pulmonary fungal infection with yeasts and pneumocystis in patients with hematological malignancy. Ann Med 37(4):259–269
16. Bollee G, Sarfati C, Thiery G et al (2007) Clinical picture of Pneumocystis jiroveci pneumonia in cancer patients. Chest 132(4):1305–1310
17. Katsuya H, Suzumiya J, Sasaki H et al (2009) Addition of rituximab to cyclophosphamide, doxorubicin, vincristine, and prednisolone therapy has a high risk of developing interstitial pneumonia in patients with non-Hodgkin lymphoma. Leuk Lymphoma 50(11):1818–1823
18. Hughes WT, Price RA, Kim HK, Coburn TP, Grigsby D, Feldman S (1973) Pneumocystis carinii pneumonitis in children with malignancies. J Pediatr 82(3):404–415
19. De Castro N, Neuville S, Sarfati C et al (2005) Occurrence of Pneumocystis jiroveci pneumonia after allogeneic stem cell transplantation: a 6-year retrospective study. Bone Marrow Transplant 36(10):879–883
20. Yale SH, Limper AH (1996) Pneumocystis carinii pneumonia in patients without acquired immunodeficiency syndrome: associated illness and prior corticosteroid therapy. Mayo Clin Proc 71(1):5–13
21. Thomas CF Jr, Limper AH (2007) Current insights into the biology and pathogenesis of Pneumocystis pneumonia. Nat Rev Microbiol 5(4):298–308
22. Komano Y, Harigai M, Koike R et al (2009) Pneumocystis jiroveci pneumonia in patients with rheumatoid arthritis treated with infliximab: a retrospective review and case-control study of 21 patients. Arthritis Rheum 61(3):305–312
23. Radisic M, Lattes R, Chapman JF et al (2003) Risk factors for Pneumocystis carinii pneumonia in kidney transplant recipients: a case-control study. Transpl Infect Dis 5(2):84–93
24. Lufft V, Kliem V, Behrend M, Pichlmayr R, Koch KM, Brunkhorst R (1996) Incidence of Pneumocystis carinii pneumonia after renal transplantation. Impact of immunosuppression. Transplantation 62(3):421–423
25. Azoulay E, Parrot A, Flahault A et al (1999) AIDS-related Pneumocystis carinii pneumonia in the era of adjunctive steroids: implication of BAL neutrophilia. Am J Respir Crit Care Med 160(2):493–499
26. Barbier F, Coquet I, Legriel S et al (2009) Etiologies and outcome of acute respiratory failure in HIV-infected patients. Intensive Care Med 35(10):1678–1686
27. Arend SM, Kroon FP, van't Wout JW (1995) Pneumocystis carinii pneumonia in patients without AIDS, 1980 through 1993. An analysis of 78 cases. Arch Intern Med 155(22):2436–2441
28. Nuesch R, Bellini C, Zimmerli W (1999) Pneumocystis carinii pneumonia in human immunodeficiency virus (HIV)-positive and HIV-negative immunocompromised patients. Clin Infect Dis 29(6):1519–1523
29. Kovacs JA, Hiemenz JW, Macher AM, Stover D, Murray HW, Shelhamer J, Lane HC, Urmacher C, Honig C, Longo DL et al (1984) Pneumocystis carinii pneumonia: a comparison between patients with the acquired immunodeficiency syndrome and patients with other immunodeficiencies. Ann Intern Med 100(5):663–671
30. Azoulay E, Mokart D, Rabbat A et al (2008) Diagnostic bronchoscopy in hematology and oncology patients with acute respiratory failure: prospective multicenter data. Crit Care Med 36(1):100–107
31. Rabbat A, Chaoui D, Lefebvre A et al (2008) Is BAL useful in patients with acute myeloid leukemia admitted in ICU for severe respiratory complications? Leukemia 22(7): 1361–1367
32. Sing A, Trebesius K, Roggenkamp A et al (2000) Evaluation of diagnostic value and epidemiological implications of PCR for Pneumocystis carinii in different immunosuppressed and immunocompetent patient groups. J Clin Microbiol 38(4):1461–1467
33. Azoulay E, Schlemmer B (2006) Diagnostic strategy in cancer patients with acute respiratory failure. Intensive Care Med 32(6):808–822, Epub 2006 Apr 29
34. Procop GW, Haddad S, Quinn J et al (2004) Detection of Pneumocystis jiroveci in respiratory specimens by four staining methods. J Clin Microbiol 42(7):3333–3335
35. Kovacs JA, Ng VL, Masur H et al (1988) Diagnosis of Pneumocystis carinii pneumonia: improved detection in

sputum with use of monoclonal antibodies. N Engl J Med 318(10):589–593
36. Wakefield AE, Pixley FJ, Banerji S et al (1990) Detection of Pneumocystis carinii with DNA amplification. Lancet 336(8713):451–453
37. Ribes JA, Limper AH, Espy MJ, Smith TF (1997) PCR detection of Pneumocystis carinii in bronchoalveolar lavage specimens: analysis of sensitivity and specificity. J Clin Microbiol 35(4):830–835
38. Azoulay E, Bergeron A, Chevret S, Bele N, Schlemmer B, Menotti J (2009) Polymerase chain reaction for diagnosing pneumocystis pneumonia in non-HIV immunocompromised patients with pulmonary infiltrates. Chest 135(3): 655–661
39. Sing A, Roggenkamp A, Autenrieth IB, Heesemann J (1999) Pneumocystis carinii carriage in immunocompetent patients with primary pulmonary disorders as detected by single or nested PCR. J Clin Microbiol 37(10):3409–3410
40. Monnet X, Vidal-Petiot E, Osman D et al (2008) Critical care management and outcome of severe Pneumocystis pneumonia in patients with and without HIV infection. Crit Care 12(1):R28
41. Nevez G, Raccurt C, Vincent P, Jounieaux V, Dei-Cas E (1999) Pulmonary colonization with Pneumocystis carinii in human immunodeficiency virus-negative patients: assessing risk with blood CD4+ T cell counts. Clin Infect Dis 29(5): 1331–1332
42. Leigh TR, Gazzard BG, Rowbottom A, Collins JV (1993) Quantitative and qualitative comparison of DNA amplification by PCR with immunofluorescence staining for diagnosis of Pneumocystis carinii pneumonia. J Clin Pathol 46(2): 140–144
43. Larsen HH, Huang L, Kovacs JA et al (2004) A prospective, blinded study of quantitative touch-down polymerase chain reaction using oral-wash samples for diagnosis of Pneumocystis pneumonia in HIV-infected patients. J Infect Dis 189(9):1679–1683, Epub 2004 Apr 16
44. Rohner P, Jacomo V, Studer R, Schrenzel J, Graf JD (2009) Detection of Pneumocystis jirovecii by two staining methods and two quantitative PCR assays. Infection 37(3): 261–265
45. Helweg-Larsen J, Jensen JS, Lundgren B (1997) Non-invasive diagnosis of Pneumocystis carinii pneumonia by PCR on oral washes. Lancet 350(9088):1363
46. Skelly M, Hoffman J, Fabbri M, Holzman RS, Clarkson AB Jr, Merali S (2003) S-adenosylmethionine concentrations in diagnosis of Pneumocystis carinii pneumonia. Lancet 361(9365):1267–1268
47. Koo S, Bryar JM, Page JH, Baden LR, Marty FM (2009) Diagnostic performance of the (1–>3)-beta-D-glucan assay for invasive fungal disease. Clin Infect Dis 49(11): 1650–1659
48. Roblot F, Godet C, Le Moal G et al (2002) Analysis of underlying diseases and prognosis factors associated with Pneumocystis carinii pneumonia in immunocompromised HIV-negative patients. Eur J Clin Microbiol Infect Dis 21(7):523–531, Epub 2002 Jul 13
49. Zahar JR, Robin M, Azoulay E, Fieux F, Nitenberg G, Schlemmer B (2002) Pneumocystis carinii pneumonia in critically ill patients with malignancy: a descriptive study. Clin Infect Dis 35(8):929–934, Epub 2002 Sep 23
50. Gagnon S, Boota AM, Fischl MA, Baier H, Kirksey OW, La Voie L (1990) Corticosteroids as adjunctive therapy for severe Pneumocystis carinii pneumonia in the acquired immunodeficiency syndrome. A double-blind, placebo-controlled trial. N Engl J Med 323(21):1444–1450
51. Bozzette SA, Sattler FR, Chiu J et al (1990) A controlled trial of early adjunctive treatment with corticosteroids for Pneumocystis carinii pneumonia in the acquired immunodeficiency syndrome. California Collaborative Treatment Group. N Engl J Med 323(21):1451–1457
52. Kovacs JA, Hiemenz JW, Macher AM et al (1984) Pneumocystis carinii pneumonia: a comparison between patients with the acquired immunodeficiency syndrome and patients with other immunodeficiencies. Ann Intern Med 100(5):663–671
53. Delclaux C, Zahar JR, Amraoui G et al (1999) Corticosteroids as adjunctive therapy for severe Pneumocystis carinii pneumonia in non-human immunodeficiency virus-infected patients: retrospective study of 31 patients. Clin Infect Dis 29(3):670–672
54. Pareja JG, Garland R, Koziel H (1998) Use of adjunctive corticosteroids in severe adult non-HIV Pneumocystis carinii pneumonia. Chest 113(5):1215–1224
55. Rodriguez M, Fishman JA (2004) Prevention of infection due to Pneumocystis spp. in human immunodeficiency virus-negative immunocompromised patients. Clin Microbiol Rev 17(4):770–782, table of contents

Diagnosis of Invasive Pulmonary Aspergillosis in Patients with Hematologic Diseases

26

Marie-Elisabeth Bougnoux, Fanny Lanternier, Emilie Catherinot, Felipe Suarez, and Olivier Lortholary

Contents

M.-E. Bougnoux (✉)
Unité de Parasitologie-Mycologie, Service de Microbiologie, Université Paris-Descartes. Hôpital Necker Enfants-Malades, 149, rue de Sèvres,
75015, Paris, France
e-mail: marie-elisabeth.bougnoux@nck.aphp.fr

F. Lanternier
Université Paris-Descartes. Hôpital Necker Enfants-Malades, Service de Maladies Infectieuses et Tropicales, Centre d'Infectiologie Necker-Pasteur,
149, rue de Sèvres, 75015, Paris, France

E. Catherinot and F. Suarez
Service d'Hématologie, Université Paris-Descartes. Hôpital Necker Enfants-Malades, Paris, France

O. Lortholary
Service de Maladies Infectieuses et Tropicales, Centre d'Infectiologie Necker-Pasteur,
149, rue de Sèvres, 75015, Paris, France and
Institut Pasteur, Unité de Mycologie Moléculaire, Centre National de Référence Mycologie et Antifongiques, CNRS URA3012, Paris, France

Invasive pulmonary aspergillosis (IPA) is a common infectious complication and a major cause of severe morbidity and mortality in patients with hematologic diseases. It is the leading cause of invasive fungal infections in hematopoietic stem cell transplant (HSCT) patients, accounting for 43% of invasive fungal infections [30]. Despite the availability of new antifungal agents, mortality rates range from 29% to 42% [26, 36, 50]. Several factors, including the severity of immunodeficiency secondary to underlying disease and its treatment, contribute to this extremely poor outcome [13, 16, 48, 67]. However, timely and accurate diagnosis is also of crucial importance for the prognosis [38, 74].

Establishing a definitive diagnosis of IPA remains difficult, and up to 30% of cases are unrecognized antemortem [17]. A substantial delay in establishing an early and accurate diagnosis remains a major impediment to the successful treatment of IPA. Because IPA is the leading cause of infectious deaths in patients with hematologic malignancies and has non-specific clinical presentation, optimized diagnostic procedures are necessary. Here, we will detail the different steps of the diagnosis of IPA in patients with hematologic diseases, focusing on the contribution of new diagnostic tools.

26.1 Risk Factors for Invasive Aspergillosis in Hematology Patients

Recognition of patients at risk for invasive aspergillosis (IA) is crucial to undertake early active diagnostic procedures.

The main defects in host defenses strongly associated with an increased risk for IPA are (1) prolonged

É. Azoulay (ed.), *Pulmonary Involvement in Patients with Hematological Malignancies*,
DOI: 10.1007/978-3-642-15742-4_26, © Springer-Verlag Berlin Heidelberg 2011

neutropenia, (2) qualitative defects in phagocyte function, and (3) deficit in cell-mediated immunity [18, 54, 58, 59]. Absolute neutrophil count <100/mm^3 and a duration >10 days of neutropenia are major risk factors for IPA.

Hematology patients at high risk of IPA include those with prolonged profound neutropenia, i.e., patients receiving cytotoxic chemotherapy for acute leukemia and patients with myelodysplastic syndrome (MSD), and recipients of HSCT. Patients with acute myeloid leukemia (AML) are more frequently affected, with a 10% incidence during post-induction or consolidation neutropenia [49, 51, 54]. Among intensively treated non-allografted patients, those with multiple myeloma are also at high risk of IPA [35]. Increased susceptibility of these patients probably results from the high dose of steroids they received. Finally, ambulatory patients with heavily treated lymphoid malignancies have now emerged as a major subgroup at high risk of invasive aspergillosis among hematology patients [36].

Incidence distribution of IPA is bimodal among allogeneic HSCT recipients. Allogeneic recipients are at increased risk for IPA during the preengraftment phase, when neutropenia is the prevailing risk factor. However, they also experience a second, postengraftment period of vulnerability coincident with the severe cell-mediated immunodeficiency resulting from graft-versus-host disease (GVHD) [23, 41] and its treatment [23, 41].

IPA occurs in 5–15% of allogeneic HSCT, with a higher incidence in recipients of transplants with higher risks for GVHD, i.e., unrelated donor, mismatched transplant, and haploidentical [52]. The incidence of IPA is higher than 10% in patients who benefit from recently discovered procedures such as cord blood transplantation [48]. Of note, a decline in preengraftment aspergillosis has been observed due in part to the reduction of periods of neutropenia and to better measures for minimizing exposure to fungal spores [41, 61]. Nowadays, the majority of IPA occurs after engraftment, and GVHD has emerged as the predominant risk factor [20, 36, 61].

The genetic host factor may modulate the individual risk of IA. Indeed, among allogeneic HSCT recipients from unrelated donors, the donor TLR4 haplotype S4 is associated with an increased risk of invasive aspergillosis [7]. Mannose-binding lectin deficiency is also likely associated with aspergillosis [32].

26.2 Clinical Features

Invasive aspergillosis is mostly confined to the lungs, but sinusitis and central nervous system involvement can also occur [28]. In a recent multicenter study in France among 393 adults, IA was restricted to the lungs in almost 90% of the cases [36]. Fever that persists despite the administration of broad-spectrum antibiotics is suggestive of IPA. Respiratory symptoms and signs may be absent in neutropenic hosts. As the disease progresses, symptoms appear, cough and dyspnea being the most common. Pleuritic chest pain and hemoptysis are less frequent, but suggest pulmonary infarction and the tendency of *Aspergillus* spp. to invade blood vessels. In patients at high risk, these signs and symptoms, although not specific, are suggestive of IPA and drive for appropriate (active diagnostic) investigations, including detailed radiological and mycological evaluation.

26.3 Chest Computed Tomography Scan

High-resolution CT scan is the gold standard imaging technique in IPA [10]. It should be done early when the diagnosis is suspected. Single or multiple nodules are the most common finding in early IPA in neutropenic and HSCT recipients. The "halo sign," which is a mass-like infiltrate surrounded by ground-glass opacity, is considered an early and transient sign of IPA (Fig. 26.1a). It reflects hemorrhages or edema around the nodule and is a characteristic chest CT feature of the angioinvasive organisms. In a recent study reviewing 235 patients with IPA, 94% of them had at least one macro-nodular lesion, and 61% had a halo sign [22]. Other CT aspects include consolidations, infarct-shaped nodules, cavitation and air-crescent sign. The air-crescent sign, defined as a crescentic pocket of gas surmounting a sequestrum within a nodule, indicates central necrosis of a nodular lesion, and it usually occurs late in the course of the disease at the time of neutrophil recovery (Fig. 26.1b). Of note, patients with suggestive signs, such as halo and air-crescent signs, have a better prognosis [22].

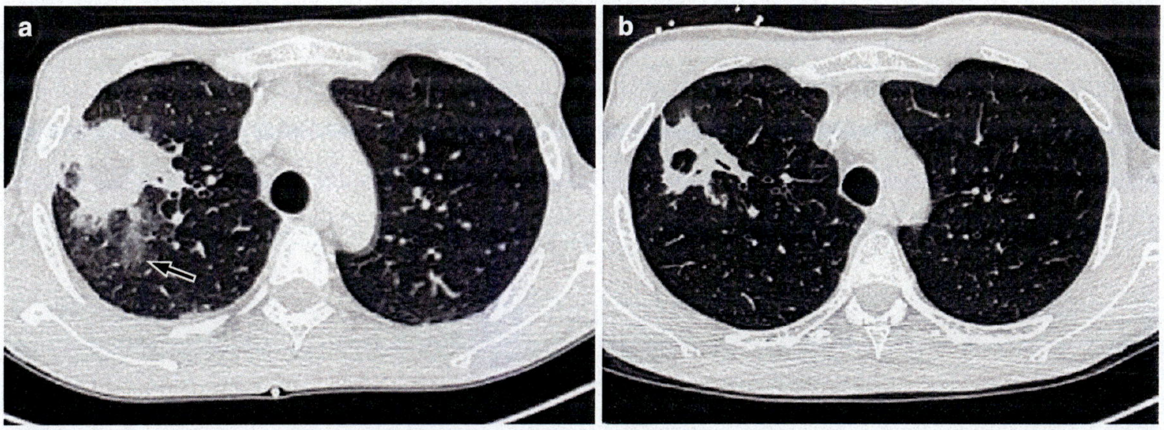

Fig. 26.1 CT scan appearance of invasive pulmonary aspergillosis in a 35-year-old patient undergoing chemotherapy for acute myeloid leukemia secondary to myelodysplasia. (**a**) Peripheral nodular consolidation and halo sign (*arrow*). (**b**) Ten-day evolution after recovery from neutropenia, showing cavitation with air crescent sign

26.4 Laboratory Diagnosis

Clinical and radiological IPA presentation is similar to other mold/dimorphic (zygomycosis or endemic mycosis) and bacterial infections (tuberculosis, *Pseudomonas aeruginosa*). Therefore, microbiological diagnosis is of primary importance. If noninvasive tests are negative, bronchoscopy with bronchoalveolar lavage (BAL) or CT-guided needle biopsy should be performed when possible [33].

26.4.1 Mycological Microscopy and Culture

Respiratory specimens, including sputum, fluid obtained by endotracheal aspiration or BAL, as well as lung biopsies, i.e., CT-guided lung biopsy and open-lung biopsy, should be obtained for microscopy and fungal culture.

26.4.1.1 Direct Microscopy

Direct microscopic examination has to be performed for all clinical respiratory samples and biopsies. Several procedures are currently being used by mycology laboratories. They include (1) wet mount examination of the sample after addition of chlorazol black, a chitin stain that aids in the visualization of the hyphal elements, and (2) staining with Grocott-Gomori silver and Giemsa stain of the microscope slides prepared from touch preparation of the biopsy specimen, or from cytospin of fluid samples. Fluorescent dyes, such as Calcofluor® white, which selectively binds polysaccharides within fungal cell walls, improve direct examination of the specimens. *Aspergillus* spp. typically appears as slender, septate hyphae that exhibit angular dichotomous branching. Sensitivity of direct microscopy is approximately 30% for sputum samples, 50% for BAL fluid, 70% for CT-guided lung biopsy, and 90% for open-lung biopsy [29, 74]. Detection of fungal elements can provide a presumptive diagnosis in less than 1 h; its diagnostic value depends of the origin of the sample. Visualization of fungal elements morphologically compatible with *Aspergillus* spp. in a lung biopsy allows definite diagnosis of invasive fungal infection (IFI), but does not prove IPA. In BAL samples, their presence has a higher predictive value for the diagnosis than in sputum samples. In a recent multicenter study in France, direct examination was performed in 325/393 (83%) patients with the lowest rate in the acute leukemia group (95/135 = 70%). The global yield of direct examination was 56% (182/325), with a significantly lower rate in the allo-HSCT group [36].

26.4.1.2 Fungal Culture

Isolation of *Aspergillus* strain by culture of fluid and tissue specimens is essential in IPA because it (1) confirms microscopic findings and the diagnostic of IPA, (2) allows an accurate identification of *Aspergillus* species and testing of the antifungal susceptibility of the strain. Cultures are best performed on Sabouraud dextrose agar with the addition of antibiotic agents at both 30°C and 35°C. The growth is visible after between 48 h to several days, depending on the fungal load in the analyzed specimen and on the *Aspergillus* species involved. In a recent multicenter study, samples processed for mycological culture were available in 324/393 (82%) patients. When performed, culture was positive for 76% (245/324), from 53% (50/95) for acute leukemia and 68% (45/66) for AlloHSCT to >86% for the other groups [36].

26.4.1.3 Identification of *Aspergillus* spp.

The choice of appropriate antifungal therapy is strongly influenced by the inherent resistance phenotype of each *Aspergillus* species, and correct identification is therefore of paramount clinical importance [46, 75]. Current identification of the species of *Aspergillus* is based on macroscopic and microscopic morphological characteristics, such as color, shape, ornamentation, and recognition of asexual or sexual stages. Sometimes conventional phenotypic methods are not sufficient to provide accurate identification, and molecular identification is used as second-line for species identification.

Aspergillus fumigatus is the leading etiological agent of IPA followed by *Aspergillus flavus*, *Aspergillus niger*, *Aspergillus terreus*, and *Aspergillus nidulans* [75]. When positive (245/324 – 75.6%), cultures mainly yielded *A. fumigatus* (84%) in a recent French study [36].

For these common species, a conventional approach routinely provides an adequate level of identification. For the new species of *Aspergillus* spp. recently reported as responsible for cases of IPA, such as *Aspergillus lentulus*, *Neosartorya fischeri* [34], *N. pseudofischeri* [66], *N. hiratsukae* [24], *N. udagawae* [72], *A. insuetus* [21], *A. calidoustus* [55, 70], or *A. niveus* [3], phenotypic methods do not allow a correct identification, and the use of molecular identification is strongly recommended to obtain accurate species identification.

Molecular identification of *Aspergillus* species is based on the partial sequencing of genes coding for beta-tubulin, calmodulin, or actin [5]. This approach has been included in recent guidelines [46, 76].

26.4.1.4 Antifungal Susceptibility Testing

Antifungal drug resistance of some *Aspergillus* spp. is now well established [53, 62, 68, 71]. Some of the newly described species responsible for IPA have decreased susceptibility to antifungal drugs. Therefore, the determination of the in vitro susceptibility of the strains is necessary. However, there is no formal recommendation for the method to use.

26.4.2 Histopathology

Different patterns of tissue injury can be observed in the lung tissues of hematology patients with IPA. In patients with profound neutropenia, but also in HSCT recipients, histopathologic patterns are characterized by angioinvasion, defined by the presence of hyphal structure within the wall or lumen of arteries or veins, and intra-alveolar hemorrhage. In non-neutropenic patients, histopathologic patterns characterized by inflammatory necrosis and granulomas are more prevalent [64].

26.4.3 Detection of Circulating Surrogate Markers

Biologic markers, including fungal antigens or DNA released by the *Aspergillus* hyphae during growth in host tissues, are used as early indicators of disease. Their diagnostic value has been evaluated in adult and pediatric hematological patients. Standardized assays allowing detection of galactomannan and β-1–3-d-glucan antigens are now included in the EORTC/MSG criteria for the diagnosis of IA [15]. As of today, molecular methods for detection of *Aspergillus* DNA in clinical specimens are not included, because the techniques have not been standardized yet.

26.4.3.1 Detection of Galactomannan Antigen

Galactomannan (GM) is a polysaccharide cell wall component of *Aspergillus* species released in blood by fungal hyphae during growth in tissues in IA. The commercially available sandwich enzyme-linked immunosorbent assay (ELISA) (Platelia® *Aspergillus*, BioRad, Marnes-La-coquette, France) detects approximately 1 ng/mL GM [69]. GM detection can be performed in different biologic specimens, including serum, BAL fluids, CSF, and urine. However, the assay has only been formally evaluated in BAL and serum.

Serum Aspergillus GM Detection

The usefulness of the GM detection for diagnosis of IA has been clearly demonstrated both in adult and pediatric patients with hematologic disorders [39, 63]. The threshold for positivity when the assay is performed in serum is an index of >0.5 [40]. Screening for circulating GM twice weekly during high-risk susceptibility periods in hematology patients (patients with prolonged neutropenia after chemotherapy or HSCT, and patients receiving high doses of corticosteroid) reduces the time to diagnosis of IPA [9, 39]. Sensitivity, specificity, and positive and negative predictive values of GM for IA were 88.2%, 95.8%, 75%, and 98.3 %, respectively, in high-risk adult hematology patients [65]. However, the reported predictive values of the GM detection have been highly variable, depending on the population, i.e., pediatric or adult, non-neutropenic hematology patients, and prevalence of IA related to the type of hematology disorders in the tested patients [12, 43]. In the recent French study, galactomannan tests were more often positive (>68%) for acute leukemia and AlloHSCT than for the others (<42%) [36].

Major Causes of Variable Test Performances

High Variations of GM Levels in Serum Conditions

The *Aspergillus* species involved and the neutrophil counts modify the serum GM levels and therefore the performance of GM detection for IPA [12, 25]. GM levels have been reported to be lower in non-neutropenic hematology patients than in patients with profound neutropenia (<100 PMN/mm^3) [12]. Higher GM levels in neutropenic patients could reflect a higher *Aspergillus* burden because of more extensive lesions. Indeed, in an autopsy study, histological patterns were different between non-neutropenic HSCT recipients and neutropenic patients, the latter having a higher *Aspergillus* burden and more angio-invasive lesions but less inflammation [11]. Last, GM levels may be higher in patients with angioinvasive aspergillosis than in those with airway IA [27].

False-Positive Detection

Several causes of false-positivity of the GM Platelia ELISA have been reported, including cross reactivity with several non-*Aspergillus* molds [14], presence of GM-like material in fluids for intravenous hydratation, such as plasmalyte, solutions for parenteral nutrition, or some antibiotic agents, such as piperacillin/tazobactam [4, 73] and more recently saccharose containing therapeutic immunoglobulins [8]. In addition, high rates of false positivity have also been reported in allogeneic HSCT recipients during the first 100 days after transplantation or in those with gastrointestinal GVHD [1, 2]. Passage of dietary GM through injured mucosa is the favored hypothesis of false positivity in these patients.

GM as a Marker of Aspergillosis Outcome

The outcome of patients with IA appears strongly correlated with the serum GM index. Indeed, persistent GM index positivity is associated with failure and death, whereas normalization of the GM index is associated with survival in neutropenic patients and in non-neutropenic onco-hematology adult patients [47, 77].

BAL Aspergillus GM Detection

GM assay performed in BAL fluids is a valuable adjunctive diagnostic tool to other conventional microbiological tests, i.e., mycological examination and culture [19, 56]. A recent study in neutropenic and non-neutropenic hematology patients found that BAL

GM testing performed better than conventional methods for the microbiological diagnosis of IA in hematology patients when an index cutoff of >1 was used [37]. GM detection in BAL had a sensitivity of 57.6% (95% CI, 40.8–72.8%) and a specificity of 95.6% (95% CI, 87.8–98.5%) in a recent study performed in St. Louis Hospital in Paris [6].

26.4.3.2 Detection of Beta-1-3-D-Glucan Antigen

Beta-1-3-D-glucan antigen (BG) is a fungal cell wall component circulating in the blood of patients with invasive fungal infections (IFI), i.e., IA, invasive candidiasis, *Pneumocystis* pneumonia, and other invasive fungal diseases. However, its detection does not differentiate among the various fungal etiologic agents. The assay has been recently included in the EORTC/MSG criteria for the diagnosis of IFI [15]. Two commercial kits are available (Fungitec G-test® and Fungitell®). Several causes of false-positivity have been reported, including intravenous immunoglobulin or albumin use, and hemodialysis with cellulose membrane [31]. False-positive results have also been reported in bacteremic patients and in those treated with fungus-derived antibiotics such as amoxicillin–clavulanic acid [44, 45, 57]. Therefore, the BG assay must be used and interpreted cautiously in such patients. Although a recent study has reported the usefulness of BG monitoring for early diagnosis of IFI in patients with acute leukemia, studies in larger groups of hematology patients are still needed to define the place of this test in the diagnosis strategy of IPA [60].

26.4.3.3 DNA Detection by PCR

Screening for circulating DNA of *Aspergillus* spp. by PCR has shown potential in the definitive diagnosis of IA [42]. However, a major concern is the lack of standardization of the PCR procedures. Marked differences are observed between studies in the type of the samples tested (whole blood vs serum), the volume of sample to analyze (large vs small), the DNA extraction procedures, and the targets used for amplification. Currently, no consensus has been reached about an optimal methodology [76]. Nevertheless, DNA detection should be quickly validated. Indeed, it appeared from the result of a recent large meta-analysis that a single PCR-negative result is sufficient to exclude a diagnosis of proven or probable IA [42]. In addition, the excellent performances of weekly PCR screening of circulating DNA on large serum volumes in high-risk patients with hematological malignancies have also been clearly demonstrated [65].

The European Organization for Research and Treatment of Cancer/Mycosis study group (EORTC/MSG) has published criteria to define possible, probable, and proven fungal infections [15]. Criteria for IPA, which are summarized in Tables 26.1 and 26.2, can help to undertake active diagnostic procedures in patients with a high suspicion index.

Diagnosing IPA relys on the association of compatible host factors and clinical presentation combined with non-invasive diagnostic tests. Whereas galactomanann antigen use is well established, β-D-glucan suffers from a lack of specificity and PCR from a lack of standardization. When these tests cannot lead to a diagnosis of probable aspergillosis, invasive procedures such as BAL and/or CT-guided needle biopsy should be undertaken to confirm diagnosis, even though those patients are often cytopenic. However, diagnostic procedures should not delay antifungal treatment as soon as IPA is suspected.

Table 26.1 Criteria required for proven, probable, or possible invasive pulmonary aspergillosis (Adapted from [15])

IPA	Criteria
Proven	Histopathologic, cytopathologic, or direct microscopic examination of a specimen obtained by needle aspiration or biopsy in which hyphae forms are seen accompanied by evidence of associated tissue damage
	Isolation of *Aspergillus* strain by culture of a specimen obtained by needle aspiration or biopsy, excluding bronchoalveolar lavage fluid
Probable	A host factor, a clinical criterion, and a mycological criterion[a]
Possible	A host factor and a clinical criterion[a]

[a]See Table 26.2

Table 26.2 Host factors, clinical and mycological criteria for invasive pulmonary aspergillosis in patients with hematological disorders (Adapted from [15])

Type of criteria	Criteria
Host factors	Recent history of neutropenia (<0.5 × 10^9 neutrophils/L (<500 neutrophils/mm^3) for >10 days) temporally related to the onset of fungal disease
	Receipt of an allogeneic stem cell transplant
	Prolonged use of corticosteroids at a mean minimum dose of 0.3 mg kg^{-1} day^{-1} of prednisone equivalent for >3 weeks
	Treatment with other recognized T cell immunosuppressants, such as cyclosporine, TNF-α blockers, specific monoclonal antibodies (such as alemtuzumab), or nucleoside analogues during the past 90 days
	Inherited severe immunodeficiency (such as chronic granulomatous disease or severe combined immunodeficiency)
Clinical	Presence of one of the following three signs on CT: Dense, well-circumscribed lesions(s) with or without a halo sign, air-crescent sign, cavity
Mycological	
Direct test (cytology, direct microscopy, or culture)	Presence of fungal elements morphologically compatible with *Aspergillus* spp. in BAL, sputum, bronchial brush, and/ or isolation of *Aspergillus* strain in these respiratory specimens
Indirect tests	Galactomannan antigen detected in plasma, serum, bronchoalveolar lavage fluid, or CSF
	β-D-glucan detected in serum

References

1. Asano-Mori Y (2010) Fungal infections after hematopoietic stem cell transplantation. Int J Hematol 91 (4):576–587
2. Asano-Mori Y, Kanda Y, Oshima K, Kako S, Shinohara A, Nakasone H, Kaneko M, Sato H, Watanabe T, Hosoya N, Izutsu K, Asai T, Hangaishi A, Motokura T, Chiba S, Kurokawa M (2008) False-positive Aspergillus galactomannan antigenaemia after haematopoietic stem cell transplantation. J Antimicrob Chemother 61(2):411–416
3. Auberger J, Lass-Flörl C, Clausen J, Bellmann R, Buzina W, Gastl G, Nachbaur D (2008) First case of breakthrough pulmonary Aspergillus niveus infection in a patient after allogeneic hematopoietic stem cell transplantation. Diagn Microbiol Infect Dis 62(3):336–339
4. Aubry A, Porcher R, Bottero J, Touratier S, Leblanc T, Brethon B, Rousselot P, Raffoux E, Menotti J, Derouin F, Ribaud P, Sulahian A (2006) Occurrence and kinetics of false-positive Aspergillus galactomannan test results following treatment with beta-lactam antibiotics in patients with hematological disorders. J Clin Microbiol 44(2):389–394
5. Balajee SA, Borman AM, Brandt ME, Cano J, Cuenca-Estrella M, Dannaoui E, Guarro J, Haase G, Kibbler CC, Meyer W, O'Donnell K, Petti CA, Rodriguez-Tudela JL, Sutton D, Velegraki A, Wickes BL (2009) Sequence-based identification of Aspergillus, fusarium, and mucorales species in the clinical mycology laboratory: where are we and where should we go from here? J Clin Microbiol 47(4): 877–884
6. Bergeron A, Belle A, Sulahian A, Lacroix C, Chevret S, Raffoux E, Arnulf B, Socie G, Ribaud P, Tazi A (2010) Contribution of galactomannan antigen detection in bronchoalveolar lavage to the diagnosis of invasive pulmonary aspergillosis in patients with hematologic malignancies. Chest 137(2):410–415
7. Bochud PY, Chien JW, Marr KA, Leisenring WM, Upton A, Janer M, Rodrigues SD, Li S, Hansen JA, Zhao LP, Aderem A, Boeckh M (2008) Toll-like receptor 4 polymorphisms and aspergillosis in stem-cell transplantation. N Engl J Med 359(17):1766–1777
8. Bougnoux ME, Coignard H, Alanio A, Lanternier F, Charlier C, Suarez F, Catherinot E, Frange P, Debré M, Clement R, Ben Soltana M, Lecuit M, Bourget P, Lortholary O. Saccharose-stabilized intravenous immune globulin as a cause of false positive Aspergillus galactomannan assay in patients. In: ESCMID (ed) 20th European congress of clinical microbiology and infectious diseases, Vienna, Austria, 2010
9. Busca A, Locatelli F, Barbui A, Limerutti G, Serra R, Libertucci D, Falda M (2006) Usefulness of sequential Aspergillus galactomannan antigen detection combined with early radiologic evaluation for diagnosis of invasive pulmonary aspergillosis in patients undergoing allogeneic stem cell transplantation. Transplant Proc 38(5):1610–1613
10. Caillot D, Casasnovas O, Bernard A, Couaillier JF, Durand C, Cuisenier B, Solary E, Piard F, Petrella T, Bonnin A, Couillault G, Dumas M, Guy H (1997) Improved management of invasive pulmonary aspergillosis in neutropenic patients using early thoracic computed tomographic scan and surgery. J Clin Oncol 15(1):139–147
11. Chamilos G, Luna M, Lewis RE, Bodey GP, Chemaly R, Tarrand JJ, Safdar A, Raad II, Kontoyiannis DP (2006) Invasive fungal infections in patients with hematologic malignancies in a tertiary care cancer center: an autopsy study over a 15-year period (1989-2003). Haematologica 91(7):986–989
12. Cordonnier C, Botterel F, Ben Amor R, Pautas C, Maury S, Kuentz M, Hicheri Y, Bastuji-Garin S, Bretagne S (2009) Correlation between galactomannan antigen levels in serum and neutrophil counts in haematological patients with invasive aspergillosis. Clin Microbiol Infect 15(1):81–86
13. Cordonnier C, Ribaud P, Herbrecht R, Milpied N, Valteau-Couanet D, Morgan C, Wade A (2006) Prognostic factors for death due to invasive aspergillosis after hematopoietic stem cell transplantation: a 1-year retrospective study of

consecutive patients at French transplantation centers. Clin Infect Dis 42(7):955–963
14. Cummings JR, Jamison GR, Boudreaux JW, Howles MJ, Walsh TJ, Hayden RT (2007) Cross-reactivity of non-Aspergillus fungal species in the Aspergillus galactomannan enzyme immunoassay. Diagn Microbiol Infect Dis 59(1): 113–115
15. De Pauw B, Walsh TJ, Donnelly JP, Stevens DA, Edwards JE, Calandra T, Pappas PG, Maertens J, Lortholary O, Kauffman CA, Denning DW, Patterson TF, Maschmeyer G, Bille J, Dismukes WE, Herbrecht R, Hope WW, Kibbler CC, Kullberg BJ, Marr KA, Munoz P, Odds FC, Perfect JR, Restrepo A, Ruhnke M, Segal BH, Sobel JD, Sorrell TC, Viscoli C, Wingard JR, Zaoutis T, Bennett JE (2008) Revised definitions of invasive fungal disease from the European Organization for Research and Treatment of Cancer/Invasive Fungal Infections Cooperative Group and the National Institute of Allergy and Infectious Diseases Mycoses Study Group (EORTC/MSG) Consensus Group. Clin Infect Dis 46(12):1813–1821
16. Del Bono V, Mikulska M, Viscoli C (2008) Invasive aspergillosis: diagnosis, prophylaxis and treatment. Curr Opin Hematol 15(6):586–593
17. Denning DW (2000) Early diagnosis of invasive aspergillosis. Lancet 355(9202):423–424
18. Denning DW (1998) Invasive aspergillosis. Clin Infect Dis 26(4):781–803, quiz 804-805
19. Desai R, Ross LA, Hoffman JA (2009) The role of bronchoalveolar lavage galactomannan in the diagnosis of pediatric invasive aspergillosis. Pediatr Infect Dis J 28(4):283–6
20. Garcia-Vidal C, Upton A, Kirby KA, Marr KA (2008) Epidemiology of invasive mold infections in allogeneic stem cell transplant recipients: biological risk factors for infection according to time after transplantation. Clin Infect Dis 47(8):1041–1050
21. Gené J, Azón-Masoliver A, Guarro J, De Febrer G, Martínez A, Grau C, Ortoneda M, Ballester F (2001) Cutaneous infection caused by Aspergillus ustus, an emerging opportunistic fungus in immunosuppressed patients. J Clin Microbiol 39(3):1134–1136
22. Greene RE, Schlamm HT, Oestmann JW, Stark P, Durand C, Lortholary O, Wingard JR, Herbrecht R, Ribaud P, Patterson TF, Troke PF, Denning DW, Bennett JE, de Pauw BE, Rubin RH (2007) Imaging findings in acute invasive pulmonary aspergillosis: clinical significance of the halo sign. Clin Infect Dis 44(3):373–379
23. Grow WB, Moreb JS, Roque D, Manion K, Leather H, Reddy V, Khan SA, Finiewicz KJ, Nguyen H, Clancy CJ, Mehta PS, Wingard JR (2002) Late onset of invasive aspergillus infection in bone marrow transplant patients at a university hospital. Bone Marrow Transplant 29(1):15–19
24. Guarro J, Kallas EG, Godoy P, Karenina A, Gené J, Stchigel A, Colombo AL (2002) Cerebral aspergillosis caused by Neosartorya hiratsukae, Brazil. Emerging Infect Dis 8(9): 989–991
25. Hachem RY, Kontoyiannis DP, Chemaly RF, Jiang Y, Reitzel R, Raad I (2009) Utility of galactomannan enzyme immunoassay and (1, 3) beta-D-glucan in diagnosis of invasive fungal infections: low sensitivity for Aspergillus fumigatus infection in hematologic malignancy patients. J Clin Microbiol 47(1):129–133
26. Herbrecht R, Denning DW, Patterson TF, Bennett JE, Greene RE, Oestmann JW, Kern WV, Marr KA, Ribaud P, Lortholary O, Sylvester R, Rubin RH, Wingard JR, Stark P, Durand C, Caillot D, Thiel E, Chandrasekar PH, Hodges MR, Schlamm HT, Troke PF, de Pauw B (2002) Voriconazole versus amphotericin B for primary therapy of invasive aspergillosis. N Engl J Med 347(6):408–415
27. Hidalgo A, Parody R, Martino R, Sanchez F, Franquet T, Gimenez A, Blancas C (2009) Correlation between high-resolution computed tomography and galactomannan antigenemia in adult hematologic patients at risk for invasive aspergillosis. Eur J Radiol 71(1):55–60
28. Jantunen E, Piilonen A, Volin L, Parkkali T, Koukila-Kahkola P, Ruutu T, Ruutu P (2000) Diagnostic aspects of invasive Aspergillus infections in allogeneic BMT recipients. Bone Marrow Transplant 25(8):867–871
29. Kim K, Lee MH, Kim J, Lee KS, Kim SM, Jung MP, Han J, Sung KW, Kim WS, Jung CW, Yoon SS, Im YH, Kang WK, Park K, Park CH (2002) Importance of open lung biopsy in the diagnosis of invasive pulmonary aspergillosis in patients with hematologic malignancies. Am J Hematol 71(2):75–79
30. Kontoyiannis DP, Marr KA, Park BJ, Alexander BD, Anaissie EJ, Walsh TJ, Ito J, Andes DR, Baddley JW, Brown JM, Brumble LM, Freifeld AG, Hadley S, Herwaldt LA, Kauffman CA, Knapp K, Lyon GM, Morrison VA, Papanicolaou G, Patterson TF, Perl TM, Schuster MG, Walker R, Wannemuehler KA, Wingard JR, Chiller TM, Pappas PG (2010) Prospective surveillance for invasive fungal infections in hematopoietic stem cell transplant recipients, 2001-2006: overview of the Transplant-Associated Infection Surveillance Network (TRANSNET) Database. Clin Infect Dis 50(8):1091–1100
31. Koo S, Bryar JM, Page JH, Baden LR, Marty FM (2009) Diagnostic performance of the (1–>3)-beta-D-glucan assay for invasive fungal disease. Clin Infect Dis 49(11):1650–1659
32. Lambourne J, Agranoff D, Herbrecht R, Troke PF, Buchbinder A, Willis F, Letscher-Bru V, Agrawal S, Doffman S, Johnson E, White PL, Barnes RA, Griffin G, Lindsay JA, Harrison TS (2009) Association of mannose-binding lectin deficiency with acute invasive aspergillosis in immunocompromised patients. Clin Infect Dis 49(10):1486–1491
33. Lass-Florl C, Resch G, Nachbaur D, Mayr A, Gastl G, Auberger J, Bialek R, Freund MC (2007) The value of computed tomography-guided percutaneous lung biopsy for diagnosis of invasive fungal infection in immunocompromised patients. Clin Infect Dis 45(7):e101–114
34. Lonial S, Williams L, Carrum G, Ostrowski M, McCarthy P (1997) Neosartorya fischeri: an invasive fungal pathogen in an allogeneic bone marrow transplant patient. Bone Marrow Transplant 19(7):753–755
35. Lortholary O, Ascioglu S, Moreau P, Herbrecht R, Marinus A, Casassus P, De Pauw B, Denning DW (2000) Invasive aspergillosis as an opportunistic infection in nonallografted patients with multiple myeloma: a European Organization for Research and Treatment of Cancer/ Invasive Fungal Infections Cooperative Group and the Intergroupe Francais du Myelome. Clin Infect Dis 30(1):41–46
36. Lortholary O, Gangneux JP, Sitbon K, Lebeau B, de Maubrisson F, Dromer F, Coignard B, Bretagne S. Prospective surveillance of invasive aspergillosis in 4 French regions: 2005–2007. In: ESCMID (ed) 19th European

congress of clinical microbiology and infectious diseases, Helsinski, Finland, 2009
37. Maertens J, Maertens V, Theunissen K, Meersseman W, Meersseman P, Meers S, Verbeken E, Verhoef G, Van Eldere J, Lagrou K (2009) Bronchoalveolar lavage fluid galactomannan for the diagnosis of invasive pulmonary aspergillosis in patients with hematologic diseases. Clin Infect Dis 49(11):1688–1693
38. Maertens J, Theunissen K, Verhoef G, Verschakelen J, Lagrou K, Verbeken E, Wilmer A, Verhaegen J, Boogaerts M, Van Eldere J (2005) Galactomannan and computed tomography-based preemptive antifungal therapy in neutropenic patients at high risk for invasive fungal infection: a prospective feasibility study. Clin Infect Dis 41(9):1242–1250
39. Maertens J, Van Eldere J, Verhaegen J, Verbeken E, Verschakelen J, Boogaerts M (2002) Use of circulating galactomannan screening for early diagnosis of invasive aspergillosis in allogeneic stem cell transplant recipients. J Infect Dis 186(9):1297–1306
40. Maertens JA, Klont R, Masson C, Theunissen K, Meersseman W, Lagrou K, Heinen C, Crepin B, Van Eldere J, Tabouret M, Donnelly JP, Verweij PE (2007) Optimization of the cutoff value for the Aspergillus double-sandwich enzyme immunoassay. Clin Infect Dis 44(10):1329–1336
41. Marr KA, Carter RA, Boeckh M, Martin P, Corey L (2002) Invasive aspergillosis in allogeneic stem cell transplant recipients: changes in epidemiology and risk factors. Blood 100(13):4358–4366
42. Mengoli C, Cruciani M, Barnes RA, Loeffler J, Donnelly JP (2009) Use of PCR for diagnosis of invasive aspergillosis: systematic review and meta-analysis. Lancet Infect Dis 9(2):89–96
43. Mennink-Kersten MA, Donnelly JP, Verweij PE (2004) Detection of circulating galactomannan for the diagnosis and management of invasive aspergillosis. Lancet Infect Dis 4(6):349–357
44. Mennink-Kersten MA, Ruegebrink D, Verweij PE (2008) Pseudomonas aeruginosa as a cause of 1, 3-beta-D-glucan assay reactivity. Clin Infect Dis 46(12):1930–1931
45. Mennink-Kersten MA, Warris A, Verweij PE (2006) 1, 3-beta-D-glucan in patients receiving intravenous amoxicillin-clavulanic acid. N Engl J Med 354(26):2834–2835
46. Meunier F, Lukan C (2008) The First European Conference on Infections in Leukaemia - ECIL1: a current perspective. Eur J Cancer 44(15):2112–2117
47. Miceli MH, Grazziutti ML, Woods G, Zhao W, Kocoglu MH, Barlogie B, Anaissie E (2008) Strong correlation between serum aspergillus galactomannan index and outcome of aspergillosis in patients with hematological cancer: clinical and research implications. Clin Infect Dis 46(9):1412–1422
48. Mikulska M, Raiola AM, Bruno B, Furfaro E, Van Lint MT, Bregante S, Ibatici A, Del Bono V, Bacigalupo A, Viscoli C (2009) Risk factors for invasive aspergillosis and related mortality in recipients of allogeneic SCT from alternative donors: an analysis of 306 patients. Bone Marrow Transplant 44(6):361–370
49. Muhlemann K, Wenger C, Zenhausern R, Tauber MG (2005) Risk factors for invasive aspergillosis in neutropenic patients with hematologic malignancies. Leukemia 19(4): 545–550
50. Neofytos D, Horn D, Anaissie E, Steinbach W, Olyaei A, Fishman J, Pfaller M, Chang C, Webster K, Marr K (2009) Epidemiology and outcome of invasive fungal infection in adult hematopoietic stem cell transplant recipients: analysis of Multicenter Prospective Antifungal Therapy (PATH) Alliance registry. Clin Infect Dis 48(3):265–273
51. Pagano L, Caira M, Candoni A, Offidani M, Fianchi L, Martino B, Pastore D, Picardi M, Bonini A, Chierichini A, Fanci R, Caramatti C, Invernizzi R, Mattei D, Mitra ME, Melillo L, Aversa F, Van Lint MT, Falcucci P, Valentini CG, Girmenia C, Nosari A (2006) The epidemiology of fungal infections in patients with hematologic malignancies: the SEIFEM-2004 study. Haematologica 91(8):1068–1075
52. Pagano L, Caira M, Nosari A, Van Lint MT, Candoni A, Offidani M, Aloisi T, Irrera G, Bonini A, Picardi M, Caramatti C, Invernizzi R, Mattei D, Melillo L, de Waure C, Reddiconto G, Fianchi L, Valentini CG, Girmenia C, Leone G, Aversa F (2007) Fungal infections in recipients of hematopoietic stem cell transplants: results of the SEIFEM B-2004 study–Sorveglianza Epidemiologica Infezioni Fungine Nelle Emopatie Maligne. Clin Infect Dis 45(9):1161–1170
53. Panackal AA, Imhof A, Hanley EW, Marr KA (2006) Aspergillus ustus infections among transplant recipients. Emerg Infect Dis 12(3):403–408
54. Patterson TF, Kirkpatrick WR, White M, Hiemenz JW, Wingard JR, Dupont B, Rinaldi MG, Stevens DA, Graybill JR (2000) Invasive aspergillosis. Disease spectrum, treatment practices, and outcomes. I3 Aspergillus Study Group. Medicine (Baltimore) 79(4):250–260
55. Pavie J, Lacroix C, Hermoso DG, Robin M, Ferry C, Bergeron A, Feuilhade M, Dromer F, Gluckman E, Molina JM, Ribaud P (2005) Breakthrough disseminated Aspergillus ustus infection in allogeneic hematopoietic stem cell transplant recipients receiving voriconazole or caspofungin prophylaxis. J Clin Microbiol 43(9):4902–4904
56. Penack O, Rempf P, Graf B, Blau IW, Thiel E (2008) Aspergillus galactomannan testing in patients with long-term neutropenia: implications for clinical management. Ann Oncol 19(5):984–989
57. Pickering JW, Sant HW, Bowles CA, Roberts WL, Woods GL (2005) Evaluation of a (1->3)-beta-D-glucan assay for diagnosis of invasive fungal infections. J Clin Microbiol 43(12):5957–5962
58. Segal BH (2009) Aspergillosis. N Engl J Med 360(18): 1870–1884
59. Segal BH, Walsh TJ (2006) Current approaches to diagnosis and treatment of invasive aspergillosis. Am J Respir Crit Care Med 173(7):707–717
60. Senn L, Robinson JO, Schmidt S, Knaup M, Asahi N, Satomura S, Matsuura S, Duvoisin B, Bille J, Calandra T, Marchetti O (2008) 1, 3-Beta-D-glucan antigenemia for early diagnosis of invasive fungal infections in neutropenic patients with acute leukemia. Clin Infect Dis 46(6):878–885
61. Singh N (2003) Impact of current transplantation practices on the changing epidemiology of infections in transplant recipients. Lancet Infect Dis 3(3):156–161
62. Snelders E, van der Lee HA, Kuijpers J, Rijs AJ, Varga J, Samson RA, Mellado E, Donders AR, Melchers WJ, Verweij PE (2008) Emergence of azole resistance in Aspergillus fumigatus and spread of a single resistance mechanism. PLoS Med 5(11):e219

63. Steinbach WJ, Addison RM, McLaughlin L, Gerrald Q, Martin PL, Driscoll T, Bentsen C, Perfect JR, Alexander BD (2007) Prospective Aspergillus galactomannan antigen testing in pediatric hematopoietic stem cell transplant recipients. Pediatr Infect Dis J 26(7):558–564
64. Stergiopoulou T, Meletiadis J, Roilides E, Kleiner DE, Schaufele R, Roden M, Harrington S, Dad L, Segal B, Walsh TJ (2007) Host-dependent patterns of tissue injury in invasive pulmonary aspergillosis. Am J Clin Pathol 127(3):349–355
65. Suarez F, Lortholary O, Buland S, Rubio MT, Ghez D, Mahe V, Quesne G, Poiree S, Buzyn A, Varet B, Berche P, Bougnoux ME (2008) Detection of circulating Aspergillus fumigatus DNA by real-time PCR assay of large serum volumes improves early diagnosis of invasive aspergillosis in high-risk adult patients under hematologic surveillance. J Clin Microbiol 46(11):3772–3777
66. Summerbell RC, de Repentigny L, Chartrand C, St Germain G (1992) Graft-related endocarditis caused by Neosartorya fischeri var. spinosa. J Clin Microbiol 30(6):1580–1582
67. Upton A, Kirby KA, Carpenter P, Boeckh M, Marr KA (2007) Invasive aspergillosis following hematopoietic cell transplantation: outcomes and prognostic factors associated with mortality. Clin Infect Dis 44(4):531–540
68. Verweij PE, Mellado E, Melchers WJ (2007) Multiple-triazole-resistant aspergillosis. N Engl J Med 356(14): 1481–1483
69. Verweij PE, Rijs AJ, De Pauw BE, Horrevorts AM, Hoogkamp-Korstanje JA, Meis JF (1995) Clinical evaluation and reproducibility of the Pastorex Aspergillus antigen latex agglutination test for diagnosing invasive aspergillosis. J Clin Pathol 48(5):474–476
70. Verweij PE, van den Bergh MF, Rath PM, de Pauw BE, Voss A, Meis JF (1999) Invasive aspergillosis caused by Aspergillus ustus: case report and review. J Clin Microbiol 37(5):1606–1609
71. Verweij PE, Varga J, Houbraken J, Rijs AJ, Verduynlunel FM, Blijlevens NM, Shea YR, Holland SM, Warris A, Melchers WJ, Samson RA (2008) Emericella quadrilineata as cause of invasive aspergillosis. Emerg Infect Dis 14(4):566–572
72. Vinh DC, Shea YR, Sugui JA, Parrilla-Castellar ER, Freeman AF, Campbell JW, Pittaluga S, Jones PA, Zelazny A, Kleiner D, Kwon-Chung K, Holland SM (2009) Invasive aspergillosis due to Neosartorya udagawae. Clin Infect Dis 49(1):102–111
73. Viscoli C, Machetti M, Cappellano P, Bucci B, Bruzzi P, Van Lint MT, Bacigalupo A (2004) False-positive galactomannan platelia Aspergillus test results for patients receiving piperacillin-tazobactam. Clin Infect Dis 38(6):913–916
74. von Eiff M, Roos N, Schulten R, Hesse M, Zuhlsdorf M, van de Loo J (1995) Pulmonary aspergillosis: early diagnosis improves survival. Respiration 62(6):341–347
75. Walsh TJ, Anaissie EJ, Denning DW, Herbrecht R, Kontoyiannis DP, Marr KA, Morrison VA, Segal BH, Steinbach W, Stevens DA, van Burik JA, Wingard JR, Patterson TF (2008) America IDSo. Treatment of aspergillosis: clinical practice guidelines of the Infectious Diseases Society of America. Clin Infect Dis 46(3):327–360
76. White PL, Bretagne S, Klingspor L, Melchers WJ, McCulloch E, Schulz B, Finnstrom N, Mengoli C, Barnes RA, Donnelly JP, Loeffler J (2010) Aspergillus PCR: one step closer to standardization. J Clin Microbiol 48(4):1231–1240
77. Woods G, Miceli MH, Grazziutti ML, Zhao W, Barlogie B, Anaissie E (2007) Serum Aspergillus galactomannan antigen values strongly correlate with outcome of invasive aspergillosis: a study of 56 patients with hematologic cancer. Cancer 110(4):830–834

Emerging Fungal Infections

27

Marcia Garnica and Marcio Nucci

Contents

27.1 Introduction

Invasive fungal disease (IFD) represents a major complication in patients with cancer, especially patients with hematological malignancies, and hematopoietic stem cell transplant (HCT) recipients [69]. While *Aspergillus* species remain the most frequent agent of IFD, other fungi have emerged, including *Fusarium* spp., Zygomycetes, the agents of phaeohyphomycosis [37, 63], and non-*fumigatus Aspergillus* spp. [31].

The term emerging infection (Table 27.1) may be used to denote an infection that has newly appeared in the population, is rapidly increasing in incidence or geographic range, a new clinical presentation of an infection caused by a known pathogen or even a new antifungal susceptibility pattern of a known pathogen [43]. These infections are a major challenge for clinicians because they frequently carry a poor prognosis as a consequence of various factors: clinicians may not be aware of that clinical presentation or the new pathogen, and this may result in a delay in establishing the diagnosis; a good laboratory is mandatory to appropriately identify the agent and to perform antifungal susceptibility tests; the emerging pathogens are usually resistant to various antifungal drugs; and these emerging infections are more likely to occur in severely immunosuppressed patients. In this chapter we will discuss the epidemiology, clinical presentation, radiology, diagnostic tools and treatment options for pulmonary infections caused by these emerging fungal pathogens in patients with hematological diseases. The following agents will be discussed: non-*fumigatus Aspergillus*, *Fusarium* spp., Zygomycetes, and the agents of phaeohyphomycosis.

M. Garnica and M. Nucci (✉)
Department of Internal Medicine, Hematology Unit and Mycology Laboratory, University Hospital, Universidade Federal do Rio de Janeiro. Rua Professor Rodolpho Paulo Rocco, 255 Sala 4A, 12 21941-913, Rio de Janeiro, Brazil
e-mail: mnucci@hucff.ufrj.br

É. Azoulay (ed.), *Pulmonary Involvement in Patients with Hematological Malignancies*,
DOI: 10.1007/978-3-642-15742-4_27, © Springer-Verlag Berlin Heidelberg 2011

Table 27.1 Definition of emerging fungal infections

Emerging fungal infections[a]
Non-*fumigatus Aspergillus* spp.
Fusarium spp.
Zygomycetes
The agents of phaeohyphomycosis

[a]The term emerging infection may be used to denote an infection that has newly appeared in the population, is rapidly increasing in incidence or geographic range, a new clinical presentation of an infection caused by a known pathogen, or even a new antifungal susceptibility pattern of a known pathogen [43]

27.2 The Host

Host factors are probably the most important determinants of the emergence of fungal infections caused by unusual pathogens. These emerging fungi are usually nonpathogenic in the normal host (and even in less severely immunosuppressed patients), but emerge in patients with severe immunosuppression. Immunocompromised patients at high risk for IFD are those with prolonged neutropenia and/or severe T-cell immunodeficiency.

Several chemotherapeutic agents impair T-cell defenses and hence may increase the risk of IFD. These include the purine analogs fludarabine, cladribine and deoxycorfomycin, and monoclonal antibodies alemtuzumab, infliximab and daclizumab [1, 8, 22, 23, 34, 35]. Indeed, cases of IFD have been increasingly reported in patients with lymphoproliferative diseases treated with some of these agents [24, 60, 62]. In addition to the use of specific immunosuppressive agents, changes in treatment strategies resulting in cumulative immunosuppression have also resulted in the emergence of IFD. This is the case of multiple myeloma in which the treatment evolved from the classical regimen of oral melphalan and prednisone, with minimal impact on the immune system, to strategies that include one or two autologous HCTs, high-dose corticosteroids, bortezomib and others [41].

In the context of HCT, practices that increase the risk and severity of graft versus host disease (GVHD) have a potential to increase the risk for IFD [54, 68]. These include: peripheral blood instead of bone marrow as the source of stem cells, increasing upper age limit, transplants with HLA-mismatched or unrelated donors, non-myeloablative transplants, and the use of donor lymphocyte infusions. In addition, patients submitted to multiple transplants and those receiving transplants with T-cell depletion are at increased risk for these infections, probably because the immune reconstitution in such transplants is delayed [10].

The association of severe GVHD and mold infections is due to the combination of the immunodeficiency of GVHD itself, associated with the immunodeficiency caused by its treatment, and the reactivation of immunomodulatory viruses, such as cytomegalovirus. Severe GVHD requires the use of high-dose corticosteroids and, if refractory, other immunosuppressive agents that per se may increase the risk for mold infections. For example, in a study, the use of infliximab (an antitumor necrosis factor alpha) for the treatment of severe or refractory acute GVHD was associated with a higher risk for mold infections (aspergillosis and zygomycosis) by multivariate analysis [33].

Non-myeloablative transplants are associated with a higher frequency of mold infections [16, 21]. In a retrospective single-center study, mold infections occurred in 25 out of 163 patients submitted to non-myeloablative transplants (four due to Zygomycetes and one due to *Fusarium* sp.). Risk factors for these infections by multivariate analysis included severe acute GVHD, chronic extensive GVHD and cytomegalovirus disease [12].

Risk factors for infection caused by *Fusarium* and Zygomycetes in HCT recipients have been assessed in a single-center retrospective study [32]. Underlying multiple myeloma and mismatched or unrelated transplants were associated with fusariosis (hazard ratios of 6.9 and 2.7, respectively), whereas underlying myelodysplastic syndrome (hazard ratio 4.1) and acute GVHD (hazard ratio 3.1) were predictors of zygomycosis. As pointed out, treatment of myeloma is associated with a cumulative and severe T-cell-mediated immunodeficiency [41].

The time of occurrence of the emerging fungal infections varies according to the agent. While scedosporiosis is more likely to occur before engraftment (during neutropenia), infection by Zygomycetes occurs later (>day + 90 after transplantation) in the setting of GVHD and its treatment [32]. By contrast, fusariosis has a trimodal distribution following HCT, with the first peak at a median of 16 days posttransplantation, a second peak between day + 61 and day + 80 (median day + 64), and a third peak after day + 360. A remarkable finding in the cases of late fusariosis is that they occurred in the context of chronic GVHD and no patient was neutropenic [44].

27.3 The Fungi

Most of the emerging fungal pathogens are common soil saprophytes, and the main mechanism of acquisition is the inhalation of conidia, with subsequent pneumonia and/or sinusitis in a process similar to that of invasive aspergillosis. Nevertheless, some of these infections occur as a result of penetrating trauma (phaeohyphomycosis, fusariosis) or at sites of skin breakdown (fusariosis).

While *Aspergillus fumigatus* is by far the most frequent species causing invasive aspergillosis, in recent years, the incidence of infection due to non-*fumigatus* species has also increased [31]. In a series of 40 cases of aspergillosis in patients with cancer from 1998 to 2001, 70% were caused by non-*fumigatus Aspergillus*. Among the 28 non-*fumigatus Aspergillus* spp., *Aspergillus flavus* was identified in 13 cases, *Aspergillus terreus* in 11, *Aspergillus niger* in 3, and *Aspergillus nidulans* in 1 case [59].

Aspergillus terreus is an important emerging agent of aspergillosis [15]. The reasons for the emergence of this species in particular are not clear, but may be related to local epidemiologic characteristics (including the environment and patient populations), since its incidence varies among different institutions: *A. terreus* was responsible for 30% of cases of invasive aspergillosis at a center in Vienna, Austria [25], 1% of 1,477 cultures positive for *Aspergillus* spp. from 24 US centers in a 1-year period [48], and 7% of cases of invasive aspergillosis enrolled in a large worldwide clinical trial [17].

Aspergillus ustus is frequently found in foods, soil and indoor environments, and has been increasingly reported as cause of invasive disease, mostly in severely immunosuppressed patients [46, 53, 61]. Breakthrough infection in patients receiving voriconazole and caspofungin has been reported [19, 47, 56].

Infections caused by a recently recognized species of *Aspergillus* have been reported [4, 5]. The organism, which, according to classical morphological typing methods, is typically identified as *A. fumigatus*, clusters as a unique species with multilocus sequence typing [4], supporting the proposed designation of *Aspergillus lentulus*.

Fusarium is a plant pathogen and a soil saprophyte that causes a broad spectrum of infections in humans, including superficial, locally invasive and disseminated infection. The most frequent species causing infection in humans are *Fusarium solani*, *Fusarium oxysporum* and *Fusarium moniliforme* [36, 39]. Fusariosis emerged as an important and frequently fatal infection in immunosuppressed patients, the majority of cases occurring in patients with acute leukemia developing prolonged and profound neutropenia [42]. More recently, cases of fusariosis occurring in patients without neutropenia but with severe T-cell immunodeficiency have been reported, underscoring the importance of the immunity on the emergence of opportunistic fungal infections [44].

Zygomycetes is a class of filamentous fungi that is subdivided into two orders: Mucorales and Entomorphthorales. Most infections in humans are caused by the Mucorales. The spectrum infection caused by Zygomycetes ranges from cutaneous to disseminated disease, and the most frequent clinical form of the disease in neutropenic patients is pneumonia [13].

The genus *Scedosporium* contains two medically important species: *Scedosporium apiospermum* and *Scedosporium prolificans*. *Scedosporium apiospermum* has a sexual form called *Pseudallesceria boydii*. In immunocompromised patients, *S. apiospermum* causes deeply invasive infections such as pneumonia, sinusitis and brain abscess [7, 66], and most cases occur in the setting of severe neutropenia. Pulmonary involvement is common in HCT recipients: in a series of ten cases, nine had lung disease, frequently with sinusitis (six cases). *Scedosporium prolificans* causes disseminated infection in neutropenic patients [52].

Agents of phaeohyphomycosis have been increasingly reported as causes of systemic infection in immunocompromised patients. A report of infection at a cancer center from 1989 to 2008 showed that the incidence of phaeohyphomycosis increased in this period, from 1.0 to 3.1 cases per 100,000 patient-days. Lungs, skin (38% each) and sinuses (36%) were the most frequently involved organs.

27.4 Clinical Manifestation

Lung involvement is frequent in most of the emerging fungal infections. While their clinical presentation may overlap, some features are characteristic of specific pathogens and may therefore be of help in establishing the correct diagnosis (Table 27.2). In addition,

Table 27.2 Diagnostic characteristics of invasive pulmonary mold infections in neutropenic patients

	Aspergillosis	Fusariosis	Zygomycosis	Scedosporiosis	Phaeohyphomycosis
Clinical picture	Fever, cough, pleuritic chest pain	Similar to aspergillosis + metastatic skin lesions (70%)	Similar to aspergillosis	Similar to aspergillosis; *S. prolificans*: metastatic skin lesions	Similar to aspergillosis
Radiologic pattern	Angioinvasion, nodules +/- halo sign	Similar to aspergillosis	Similar to aspergillosis, >10 nodules and pleural effusion more frequent	Similar to aspergillosis	Similar to aspergillosis
Blood culture	Negative	Positive (60%)	Negative	*S. prolificans*: positive (70%)	May be positive
Serum galactomannan	Sensitivity 70%; specificity 92%. Good at ruling out the diagnosis	Positive results reported in *F. solani* and *F. oxysporum*	Negative	Negative	Positive results reported with some species
Serum 1,3-beta-D-glucan	Positive	Positive	Negative	May be positive	May be positive

a major determinant of the clinical form of fungal pneumonia is the immune status of the host. One side of the spectrum is represented by patients with severe (<100/mm^3) and prolonged (>15 days) neutropenia, mostly patients with acute leukemia receiving induction remission, and allogeneic HCT recipients in the early post-transplant period. In these patients, infection is characterized by angioinvasion, with intra-alveolar hemorrhage and pulmonary infarction. The second group is represented by non-neutropenic allogeneic HCT recipients. In these patients, pneumonia occurs in the context of severe T-cell immunodeficiency caused by GVHD and its treatment. Although angioinvasion may be observed, it is less frequent than in severely neutropenic patients. However, although the number of neutrophils is normal, there is a paucity of inflammatory cells in lung tissue, indicating that these patients are functionally neutropenic [58].

The most frequent clinical presentation of pneumonia caused by emerging molds in neutropenic patients is that of persistent or recurrent fever in patients with prolonged neutropenia, associated with signs of pulmonary infarction: dry cough and pleuritic chest pain. By contrast, in non-neutropenic allogeneic HCT recipients, the clinical manifestations are subtle and non-specific. Fever is frequently absent.

In a series of 84 patients with fusariosis and an underlying hematologic disease, lung infiltrates (presumed to be due to fusariosis) were present in 54% of patients and, like in aspergillosis, consisted of non-specific alveolar or interstitial infiltrates, nodules and cavities. The clinical presentation was non-specific, with some presenting with a clinical picture similar to invasive aspergillosis, with dry cough, pleuritic chest pain and shortness of breath [42].

Among 294 cases of fusariosis reported in the literature until 2002, lung involvement was present in 114 (39%) and was more common among immunocompromised (109 cases, 42%) than immunocompetent patients (5 cases, 16%; $p=0.004$). Risk factors for fusarial pneumonia include a diagnosis of acute leukemia, prolonged neutropenia and HCT. Pneumonia as the sole manifestation of fusariosis was reported in 14 cases (11 in immunocompromised patients). The most frequent radiological pattern was alveolar infiltrates (46%), pulmonary nodules and interstitial infiltrates (9% each), and cavities (4%). Nodular and cavitary lesions were more common among patients with isolated lung involvement (6 of 14, 43% vs 18 of 100, 18%; $p=0.04$). A confirmation of lung involvement was obtained in 60 cases (53%). The most frequent pulmonary material that contributed to the diagnosis was lung tissue obtained from autopsy (63%), followed by sputum (17%), bronchial aspirate (8%), lung biopsy (7%) and bronchoalveolar lavage (BAL 5%). Patients with fusarial pneumonia were more likely to die compared to those without lung involvement (77% vs 59%, $p < 0.001$), even after controlling for status of the host defenses and neutropenia [40].

In another study, 61 cases of fusariosis in HCT recipients (including some previously reported cases) were identified in nine centers. Infection occurred in 54 allogeneic and 7 autologous HCT recipients. Similar to the other reports, the most frequent clinical picture was disseminated infection (75%), with positive blood cultures (43%) and/or metastatic skin lesions (54%). Other patterns of infection included pneumonia and sinusitis. Neutropenia was present in 46% of allogeneic and in 71% of autologous HSCT recipients, and neutropenic patients were more likely to have disseminated disease ($p = 0.001$). Acute and chronic GVHD was present in 57% and 20% of patients, respectively.

A remarkable characteristic of invasive fusariosis that distinguishes it from aspergillosis is the high frequency of positive blood cultures and metastatic disseminated skin lesions (Fig. 27.1). This is because *Fusarium* spp. produces yeast-like structures (adventitious sporulation) that facilitate dissemination and growth in the blood. Patients with disseminated disease typically have multiple erythematous papular or nodular and painful lesions, frequently with central necrosis giving the lesions an echtyma gangrenosum-like appearance. Fusarial skin lesions involve practically any site, with predominance in the extremities, and evolve rapidly, usually over a few days (range 1–5 days). Lesions at different stages of evolution (papules, nodules and necrotic lesions) and concomitant myalgias (suggesting muscle involvement) are frequently present [39]. Some patients present cellulitis at the site of onychomycosis, local trauma or intertrigus. These lesions may be the primary site of disseminated infection.

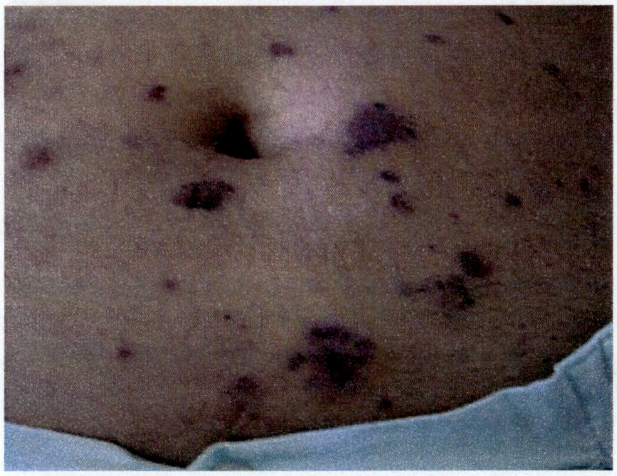

Fig. 27.1 Typical metastatic erythematous skin lesions in a patient with disseminated fusariosis

Pneumonia is the most frequent clinical presentation of zygomycosis in patients with hematological malignancies and in HCT recipients, as opposed to the typical rhinocerebral form that affects diabetic patients [2, 3, 20, 26–28, 55, 64, 65]. The clinical presentation is similar to that of invasive pulmonary aspergillosis, but the radiologic picture may differ (see below). Most cases develop as breakthrough infections if treatment with antifungal agents effective against *Aspergillus* spp. is administered [9].

In immunocompromised patients, *S. apiospermum* causes deeply invasive infections, such as pneumonia, sinusitis and brain abscess [7, 66]. The clinical presentation is similar to aspergillosis. Neutropenia and organ transplantation represent the most frequent underlying conditions. The most frequent clinical finding in sinopulmonary infection caused by *Scedosporium* spp. is fever, followed by dyspnea and pleuritic chest pain. By the time of diagnosis of *Scedosporium* pneumonia, signs of disseminated disease are usually present, including maculo-papular or nodular skin lesions, myalgias and focal neurologic signs.

Similar to fusariosis, infection due to *S. prolificans* (but not *S. apiospermum*) is frequently associated with positive blood cultures and metastatic skin lesions [29]. In a review of 25 cases of scedosporiosis in cancer patients, 3 were HCT recipients. All had positive blood cultures and two had skin lesions [29]. In a review of 72 cases of disseminated phaeohyphomycosis, the most frequent agent was *S prolificans*, accounting for 30 cases. Five of these patients were HCT recipients, all with neutropenia [52].

27.5 Radiology

Computed tomography (CT) of the chest is an important diagnostic tool of pneumonia caused by the emerging fungal pathogens. The chest X-ray is not useful, especially if the patient is neutropenic. It is often abnormal, but the appearance is nonspecific, with patchy segmental or lobar consolidations [9].

The radiologic features in severely neutropenic patients reflect the angioinvasive nature of the disease.

Nodular opacities, with or without a ground-glass opacity surrounding the nodule (halo sign), are the most typical lesions. They represent pulmonary edema and hemorrhage surrounding an area of coagulative necrosis. The halo sign is not specific to aspergillosis and has been described in pneumonia caused by other fungi, including *Fusarium* spp., *Scedosporium* spp. and Zygomycetes (Fig. 27.2). The halo sign may also be present in a variety of non-infectious (such as Wegener granulomatosis, Kaposi sarcoma and hemorrhagic metastases) and infectious conditions (such as viral pneumonias and tuberculosis). Other findings in the CT scan include nodules, consolidations, ground-glass opacities, mass, air bronchogram, effusions and cavitation (Figs. 27.3–27.5).

In non-neutropenic allogeneic HCT recipients, mold infections may be characterized by angioinvasion (like in neutropenic patients) or airway invasion. In the later form, the radiologic picture is that of a bronchopneumonia. The X-ray shows patchy air space consolidation, with or without small nodules (Fig. 27.6), and the CT scan exhibits air space consolidations or nodules.

The radiologic manifestations of fusarial pneumonia are indistinguishable from those caused by *Aspergillus* spp., with alveolar infiltrates, pulmonary nodules, interstitial infiltrates and cavities [42, 44]. By contrast radiologic manifestations of Zygomycosis may differ. A study compared the radiologic aspects of pulmonary Zygomicosis and aspergillosis. Zygomycosis was more likely to present with multiple (>10) nodules and pleural effusion [9].

Radiologic manifestations in phaeohyphomycosis were mostly pulmonary nodules, with or without halo sign and nonspecific pulmonary infiltrates. Pleural effusion and cavitary lesions seem to be less frequent [6].

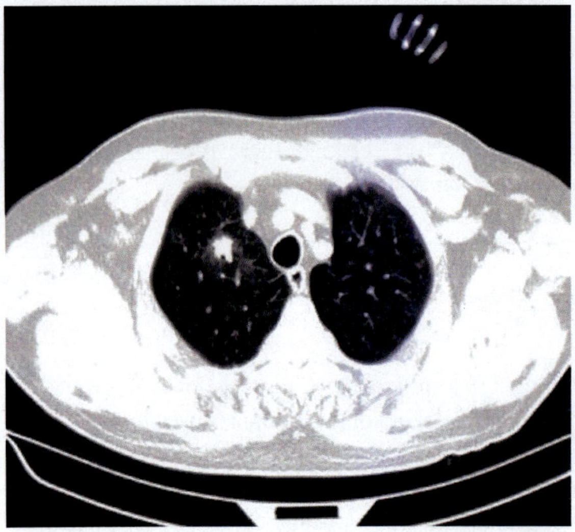

Fig. 27.2 Chest CT showing nodule with ground-glass opacity surrounding the nodule (halo sign) in a neutropenic patient with invasive fusariosis

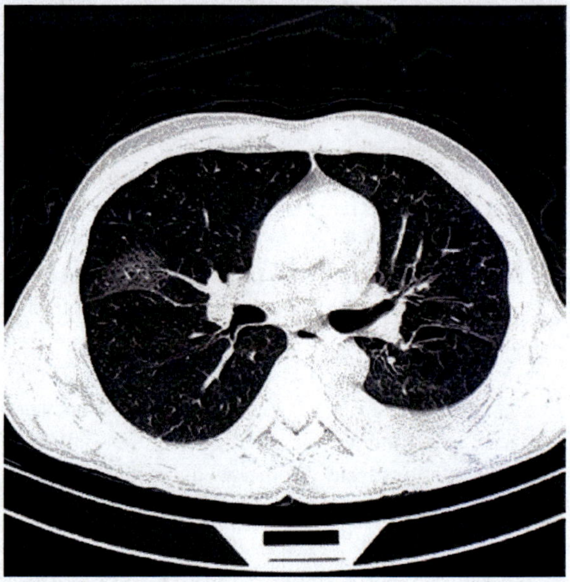

Fig. 27.3 Chest CT showing ground-glass infiltrates and pleural effusion in a non-neutropenic hematopoietic stem cell transplant recipient with invasive fusariosis

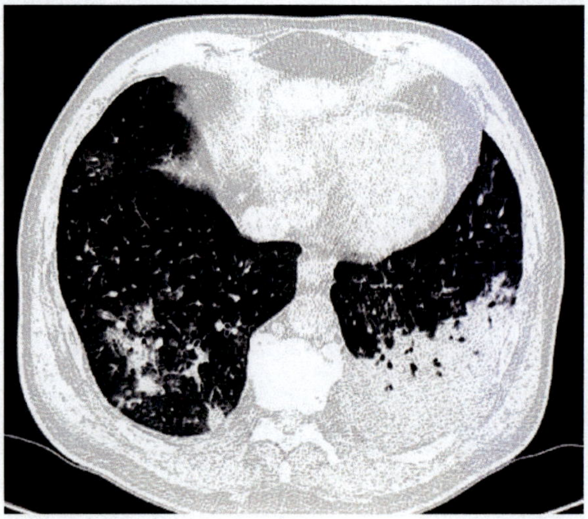

Fig. 27.4 Chest CT showing alveolar infiltrates and nodule in a neutropenic patient with invasive fusariosis

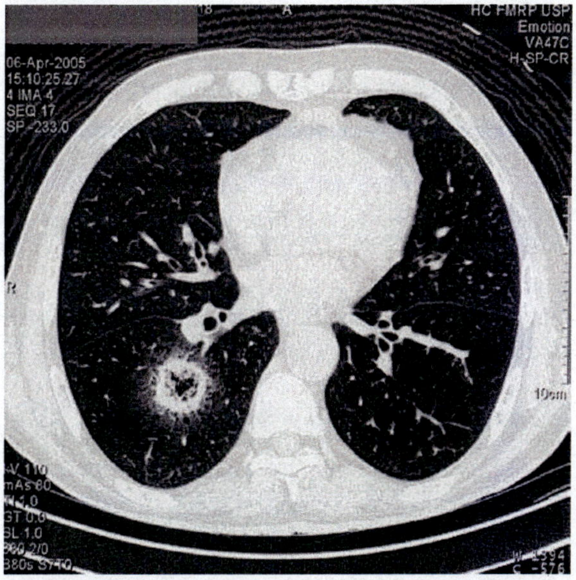

Fig. 27.5 Chest CT showing nodule with cavity and ground-glass opacity surrounding the nodule in a neutropenic patient with zygomycosis (Courtesy of Belinda P. Simões, University of São Paulo, Ribeirão Preto, Brazil)

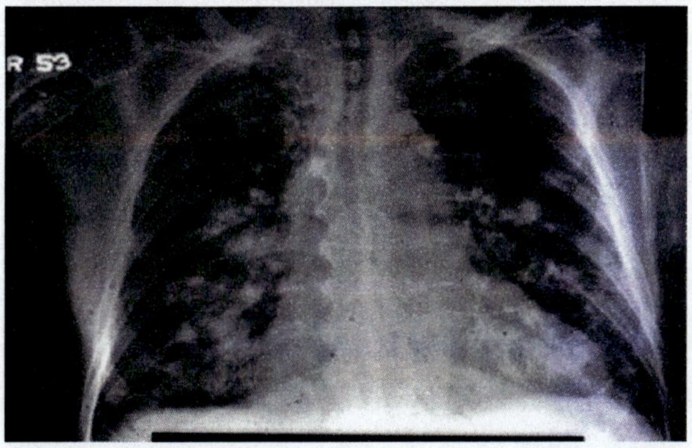

Fig. 27.6 Chest X-ray showing bilateral patchy infiltrates in a neutropenic patient with invasive fusariosis

27.6 Other Diagnostic Tools

The mainstay of the diagnosis of invasive fungal infections is the demonstration of tissue invasion by fungal elements and the growth of the organism from tissue culture. Unfortunately, in the majority of cases this is not achieved because clinical conditions preclude lung biopsy. Since the appearance of most hyaline and black molds is similar in tissue (hyalohyphomycosis and phaeohyphomycosis), culture of tissue is critical. Indeed, it is practically impossible to distinguish infection with *Aspergillus* spp. from infection by any of the angioinvasive molds such as *Fusarium* and *Scedosporium* spp., or the dematiaceous fungi such as *Bipolaris*, *Exserohilum* and *Alternaria* spp. and to a lesser extent infections caused by the agents of zygomycosis. For the diagnosis of phaeohyphomycosis, the Fontana-Masson stain for melanin is important and reveals the typical pigmentation of hyphae.

Culture of respiratory secretions is an alternative, but the interpretation of fungal growth may be difficult. Fungi may colonize the airways, and many of the emerging fungal pathogens are frequent contaminants in the laboratory. The isolation of several colonies from the same specimen or the same fungus from different specimens is highly suggestive of a true growth, whereas the isolation of a single colony from only one biological sample should raise the question if it is a contamination. When interpreting the result of a mycological examination, a positive direct examination of the biological material in addition to isolation of the fungus in culture provides a more reliable diagnosis. However, the sensitivity of detection by smear examination is low. Therefore, the clinical significance of a single positive culture with a negative direct smear is difficult to determine. Potassium-hydroxide concentrated smears prepared from sedimented remains of clinical specimens may be useful to differentiate between contamination and infection [70].

In addition to culture-based diagnostics, serologic tests have been developed. The Bio-Rad Platelia™ sandwich ELISA for the detection of *Aspergillus* antigens in blood has good sensitivity for the early diagnosis of aspergillosis [50]. The test has excellent performance characteristics in profoundly neutropenic patients provided it is performed at least two or three times a week and supported by chest CT scan findings. Although considered specific for the diagnosis of aspergillosis, the test may be positive in infections caused by emerging pathogens, such as *Fusarium solani*, *Fusarium oxysporum*, *Paecilomyces* spp., *Acremonium* spp. and *Alternaria* spp. Limitations of the test include reduced sensitivity during receipt of mold-active antifungal agents and false-positive results with the use of some semi-synthetic β-lactam antibiotics, including ampicillin, amoxicillin-clavulanate and piperacillin-tazobactam [51]. The galactomannan assay may also be performed in BAL fluid [30].

Detection of 1,3-beta-D-glucan in the serum is another tool that has been developed for the early diagnosis of IFD. It can detect a much broader spectrum of fungal species than the Platelia™ sandwich ELISA, including *Candida*, *Aspergillus*, *Fusarium* and others [45]. False-positive readings may result from the use of albumin or immunoglobulins, exposure to glucan-containing gauze, hemodialysis and some antimicrobial preparations (amoxicillin-clavulanate).

27.7 Treatment

As pointed out, the management of emerging fungal infections is challenging (Table 27.3). The first step is to make all efforts to perform the correct diagnosis, including isolation of the agent and its identification to species level. Antifungal susceptibility tests may be of help in selecting the appropriate antifungal agent, although a good correlation between minimal inhibitory concentration and clinical outcome has not been established.

The typical antifungal susceptibility profile of *Fusarium* spp. is that of relative resistance to most antifungal agents. However, different species may have different patterns of susceptibility. *F. solani* and *Fusarium verticillioides* are usually resistant to azoles and exhibit higher MICs for amphotericin B than other *Fusarium* spp. [38]. By contrast, *F. oxysporum*, and *F. moniliforme* may be susceptible to voriconazole and posaconazole. The relevance of these in vitro data is not clear, because there are not enough data documenting a correlation between MIC values and the clinical outcome. Because of the lack of clinical trials and the critical role of immune reconstitution in outcome of fusariosis, the optimal treatment strategy for patients with severe fusarial infection remains unclear. However, taking the results of in vitro susceptibility tests, it seems more prudent to start treatment of systemic fusariosis with a lipid preparation of amphotericin B. The response rate to a lipid formulation of amphotericin B appeared superior to that of deoxycholate amphotericin B (46% vs 32%, respectively) in a series of 84 cases in patients with hematological malignancies [42]. Other options for the treatment are voriconazole and posaconazole [38].

The prognosis of invasive fusariosis has been poor regardless of the underlying disease. In a series of 84 patients with hematological malignancies and fusariosis, 33 of which were HCT recipients, only 21% of patients were alive 90 days after the diagnosis of fusariosis. Multivariate predictors of poor outcome were persistent neutropenia and the use of corticosteroids [42]. In HCT, the mortality rate was 89% among 61 cases reported in the literature and 87% in a series of patients from 9 centers [44]. In this later series, the actuarial survival at 90 days postdiagnosis of fusariosis was only 13%, with a median survival of 13 days after diagnosis. The single variable associated with poor outcome was persistent neutropenia.

The clinical presentation of infection due to *A. terreus* is not different from aspergillosis caused by other species. The most important difference is in susceptibility to antifungal agents. MIC_{50} of voriconazole (0.25 μg/mL) and itraconazole (0.062 μg/mL) tested in 43 *A. terreus* isolates was not different from *A. fumigatus* (0.25 and 0.25 μg/mL, respectively. By contrast, MIC_{50} of amphotericin B was 2 μg/mL for *A. terreus* and 1 μg/mL for *A. fumigatus* [11]. Accordingly, a retrospective analysis of 83 cases of infection due to *A. terreus* showed higher mortality rates if patients received a preparation of amphotericin B compared to patients receiving voriconazole, and by multivariate analysis, the single variable significantly associated with better outcome was receipt of voriconazole [57]. *A. terreus* exhibits variable susceptibility to antifungal agents. In a report of six cases in HCT recipients, four out of six isolates exhibited MICs for amphotericin B of 2 μg/mL. MICs for voriconazole were also high (4 μg/mL in two isolates and 8 μg/mL in four isolates) [46].

S. apiospermum is susceptible to the antifungal triazoles, but not to amphotericin B, whereas *S. prolificans* is resistant to all antifungal agents [11]. In a series of eight pediatric patients with scedosporiosis, all six *S. apiospermum* infections responded to voriconazole, but not the two patients infected with *S. prolificans* [67]. In another study, response to voriconazole was also observed in two of six patients with *S. apiospermum* infection and in one of four with *S. prolificans* infection [49].

Zygomycosis usually has a very devastating clinical course, especially the rhinocerebral form. Therefore, early diagnosis is paramount. Indeed, the prognosis of such infections has improved in recent years because of improvements in early diagnosis [13]. Like in the other mycoses, the prognosis of infection is also

Table 27.3 Therapeutic management in emerging fungal infections

	Aspergillus terreus	Fusariosis	Zygomycosis[a]	Scedosporiosis
Azoles		In vitro resistance for *Fusarium solani* and *verticillioides*		
Voriconazole	Variable susceptibility Optimal first line therapy	*F. oxysporum* and *F. moniliforme* may be susceptible in vitro Acceptable alternative to polyenes		*S. apiospermum* is sensitive, but *S.* prolificans is resistant Optimal first line therapy
Posaconazole			*Posaconazole* is a salvage therapy	
Lipid preparation of amphotericin B	Increased MIC_{50} compared to Fumigatus (2 μg/mL)	Higher MICs for *Fusarium solani* and *verticillioides* Optimal first line therapy	Optimal first line therapy High doses are recommended	*S. apiospermum* and *S. prolificans* are resistant

[a]Combined medical and surgical treatment

influenced by the clinical form of disease, with a better prognosis for localized forms and death in most patients with disseminated infection [20]. Another aspect of zygomycosis is that a combined surgical and medical treatment seems to be crucial. A study showed cure or improvement occurred in 7 of 11 transplant recipients with zygomycosis who were treated with amphotericin B colloidal dispersion. All cured patients had been submitted to a surgical procedure in addition to antifungal treatment [18]. Amphotericin B is considered the drug of choice for the treatment of zygomycosis, and high doses are recommended [13]. In addition, posaconazole has been studied as salvage therapy with fair response rates [14, 42]. However, concerns regarding the use of posaconazole in the primary treatment of zygomycosis include its low in vitro activity against some of the most frequent agents of zygomycosis and the lack of an intravenous formulation.

27.8 Conclusions

The emergence of fungal pathogens is a consequence of the dynamic interaction between the host, the environment and the pathogen. Although some fungal infections seem to have emerged as a result of selective pressure of the widespread use of prophylactic antifungal agents, the large majority of fungal infections emerge because of severe immunosuppression. Therefore, as the number and categories of immunosuppressed patients expand, it is not surprising that the list of emerging fungal infections is increasing. Clinicians must be aware of new pathogens, new clinical entities and clinical presentations in order to make a prompt and accurate diagnosis. Mycology laboratories must be prepared to establish the diagnosis to the species level, and this may require the availability of molecular tests. Finally, antifungal susceptibility tests should also be available to select the most adequate antifungal drug.

Acknowledgment: Financial support: Pro Vita, Rio de Janeiro (M.G.) and Conselho Nacional de Desenvolvimento Científico e Tecnológico (CNPq), Brazil, Grant 200425/2009-9 (M.N.)

References

1. Anaissie EJ, Kontoyiannis DP, O'Brien S, Kantarjian H, Robertson L, Lerner S, Keating MJ (1998) Infections in patients with chronic lymphocytic leukemia treated with fludarabine. Ann Intern Med 129:559–566
2. Asai K, Suzuki K, Takahashi T, Ito Y, Kazui T, Kita Y (2003) Pulmonary resection with chest wall removal and reconstruction for invasive pulmonary mucormycosis during antileukemia chemotherapy. Jpn J Thorac Cardiovasc Surg 51:163–166
3. Bakshi NA, Volk EE (2001) Pulmonary mucormycosis diagnosed by fine needle aspiration cytology. A case report. Acta Cytol 45:411–414
4. Balajee SA, Gribskov JL, Hanley E, Nickle D, Marr KA (2005) *Aspergillus lentulus* sp. nov., a new sibling species of *A. fumigatus*. Eukaryot Cell 4:625–632

5. Balajee SA, Weaver M, Imhof A, Gribskov J, Marr KA (2004) *Aspergillus fumigatus* variant with decreased susceptibility to multiple antifungals. Antimicrob Agents Chemother 48:1197–1203
6. Ben-Ami R, Lewis RE, Raad II, Kontoyiannis DP (2009) Phaeohyphomycosis in a tertiary care cancer center. Clin Infect Dis 48:1033–1041
7. Bouza E, Munoz P (2004) Invasive infections caused by *Blastoschizomyces capitatus* and *Scedosporium* spp. Clin Microbiol Infect 10(Suppl 1):76–85
8. Bulpa P, Dive A, Sibille Y (2007) Invasive pulmonary aspergillosis in patients with chronic obstructive pulmonary disease. Eur Respir J 30:782–800
9. Chamilos G, Marom EM, Lewis RE, Lionakis MS, Kontoyiannis DP (2005) Predictors of pulmonary zygomycosis versus invasive pulmonary aspergillosis in patients with cancer. Clin Infect Dis 41:60–66
10. Daly A, McAfee S, Dey B, Colby C, Schulte L, Yeap B, Sackstein R, Tarbell NJ, Sachs D, Sykes M, Spitzer TR (2003) Nonmyeloablative bone marrow transplantation: infectious complications in 65 recipients of HLA-identical and mismatched transplants. Biol Blood Marrow Transplant 9:373–382
11. Espinel-Ingroff A, Johnson E, Hockey H, Troke P (2008) Activities of voriconazole, itraconazole and amphotericin B in vitro against 590 moulds from 323 patients in the voriconazole Phase III clinical studies. J Antimicrob Chemother 61:616–620
12. Fukuda T, Boeckh M, Carter RA, Sandmaier BM, Maris MB, Maloney DG, Martin PJ, Storb RF, Marr KA (2003) Risks and outcomes of invasive fungal infections in recipients of allogeneic hematopoietic stem cell transplants after nonmyeloablative conditioning. Blood 102:827–833
13. Gonzalez CE, Rinaldi MG, Sugar AM (2002) Zygomycosis. Infect Dis Clin North Am 16:895–914, vi
14. Greenberg RN, Mullane K, van Burik JA, Raad I, Abzug MJ, Anstead G, Herbrecht R, Langston A, Marr KA, Schiller G, Schuster M, Wingard JR, Gonzalez CE, Revankar SG, Corcoran G, Kryscio RJ, Hare R (2006) Posaconazole as salvage therapy for zygomycosis. Antimicrob Agents Chemother 50:126–133
15. Hachem RY, Kontoyiannis DP, Boktour MR, Afif C, Cooksley C, Bodey GP, Chatzinikolaou I, Perego C, Kantarjian HM, Raad II (2004) *Aspergillus terreus*: an emerging amphotericin B-resistant opportunistic mold in patients with hematologic malignancies. Cancer 101: 1594–1600
16. Hagen EA, Stern H, Porter D, Duffy K, Foley K, Luger S, Schuster SJ, Stadtmauer EA, Schuster MG (2003) High rate of invasive fungal infections following nonmyeloablative allogeneic transplantation. Clin Infect Dis 36:9–15
17. Herbrecht R, Denning DW, Patterson TF, Bennett JE, Greene RE, Oestmann JW, Kern WV, Marr KA, Ribaud P, Lortholary O, Sylvester R, Rubin RH, Wingard JR, Stark P, Durand C, Caillot D, Thiel E, Chandrasekar PH, Hodges MR, Schlamm HT, Troke PF, de Pauw B (2002) Voriconazole versus amphotericin B for primary therapy of invasive aspergillosis. N Engl J Med 347:408–415
18. Herbrecht R, Letscher-Bru V, Bowden RA, Kusne S, Anaissie EJ, Graybill JR, Noskin GA, Oppenheim BA, Andres E, Pietrelli LA (2001) Treatment of 21 cases of invasive mucormycosis with amphotericin B colloidal dispersion. Eur J Clin Microbiol Infect Dis 20:460–466
19. Imhof A, Balajee SA, Fredricks DN, Englund JA, Marr KA (2004) Breakthrough fungal infections in stem cell transplant recipients receiving voriconazole. Clin Infect Dis 39: 743–746
20. Jahagirdar BN, Morrison VA (2002) Emerging fungal pathogens in patients with hematologic malignancies and marrow/stem-cell transplant recipients. Semin Respir Infect 17:113–120
21. Junghanss C, Marr KA, Carter RA, Sandmaier BM, Maris MB, Maloney DG, Chauncey T, McSweeney PA, Storb R (2002) Incidence and outcome of bacterial and fungal infections following nonmyeloablative compared with myeloablative allogeneic hematopoietic stem cell transplantation: a matched control study. Biol Blood Marrow Transplant 8: 512–520
22. Keating MJ, Flinn I, Jain V, Binet JL, Hillmen P, Byrd J, Albitar M, Brettman L, Santabarbara P, Wacker B, Rai KR (2002) Therapeutic role of alemtuzumab (Campath-1 H) in patients who have failed fludarabine: results of a large international study. Blood 99:3554–3561
23. Labbe AC, Su SH, Laverdiere M, Pepin J, Patino C, Cohen S, Kiss T, Lachance S, Sauvageau G, Busque L, Roy DC, Roy J (2007) High incidence of invasive aspergillosis associated with intestinal graft-versus-host disease following nonmyeloablative transplantation. Biol Blood Marrow Transplant 13:1192–1200
24. Laros-van Gorkom BA, Huisman CA, Wijermans PW, Schipperus MR (2007) Experience with alemtuzumab in treatment of chronic lymphocytic leukaemia in the Netherlands. Neth J Med 65:333–338
25. Lass-Florl C, Griff K, Mayr A, Petzer A, Gastl G, Bonatti H, Freund M, Kropshofer G, Dierich MP, Nachbaur D (2005) Epidemiology and outcome of infections due to *Aspergillus terreus*: 10-year single centre experience. Br J Haematol 131:201–207
26. Lee DG, Choi JH, Choi SM, Yoo JH, Kim YJ, Min CK, Lee S, Kim DW, Shin WS, Kim CC (2002) Two cases of disseminated mucormycosis in patients following allogeneic bone marrow transplantation. J Korean Med Sci 17: 403–406
27. Losee JE, Selber J, Vega S, Hall C, Scott G, Serletti JM (2002) Primary cutaneous mucormycosis: guide to surgical management. Ann Plast Surg 49:385–390
28. MacKenzie KM, Baumgarten KL, Helm BM, McFadden PM, Deduska NJ, Loss GE Jr, Eason JD (2002) Innovative medical management with resection for successful treatment of pulmonary mucormycosis despite diagnostic delay. J La State Med Soc 154:82–85
29. Maertens J, Lagrou K, Deweerdt H, Surmont I, Verhoef GE, Verhaegen J, Boogaerts MA (2000) Disseminated infection by Scedosporium prolificans: an emerging fatality among haematology patients. Case report and review. Ann Hematol 79:340–344
30. Maertens J, Maertens V, Theunissen K, Meersseman W, Meersseman P, Meers S, Verbeken E, Verhoef G, Van EJ, Lagrou K (2009)) Bronchoalveolar lavage fluid galactomannan for the diagnosis of invasive pulmonary aspergillosis in patients with hematologic diseases. Clin Infect Dis 49: 1688–1693

31. Marr KA, Carter RA, Boeckh M, Martin P, Corey L (2002) Invasive aspergillosis in allogeneic stem cell transplant recipients: changes in epidemiology and risk factors. Blood 100:4358–4366
32. Marr KA, Carter RA, Crippa F, Wald A, Corey L (2002) Epidemiology and outcome of mould infections in hematopoietic stem cell transplant recipients. Clin Infect Dis 34:909–917
33. Marty FM, Lee SJ, Fahey MM, Alyea EP, Soiffer RJ, Antin JH, Baden LR (2003) Infliximab use in patients with severe graft-versus-host disease and other emerging risk factors of non-Candida invasive fungal infections in allogeneic hematopoietic stem cell transplant recipients: a cohort study. Blood 102:2768–2776
34. Meersseman W, Lagrou K, Maertens J, Van WE (2007) Invasive aspergillosis in the intensive care unit. Clin Infect Dis 45:205–216
35. Nath DS, Kandaswamy R, Gruessner R, Sutherland DE, Dunn DL, Humar A (2005) Fungal infections in transplant recipients receiving alemtuzumab. Transplant Proc 37:934–936
36. Nelson PE, Dignani MC, Anaissie EJ (1994) Taxonomy, biology, and clinical aspects of Fusarium species. Clin Microbiol Rev 7:479–504
37. Nucci M (2003) Emerging moulds: *Fusarium*, *Scedosporium* and *Zygomycetes* in transplant recipients. Curr Opin Infect Dis 16:607–612
38. Nucci M, Anaissie E (2007) Fusarium infections in immunocompromised patients. Clin Microbiol Rev 20:695–704
39. Nucci M, Anaissie E (2002) Cutaneous infection by *Fusarium* species in healthy and immunocompromised hosts: implications for diagnosis and management. Clin Infect Dis 35:909–920
40. Nucci M, Anaissie E (2006) Emerging fungi. Infect Dis Clin North Am 20:563–579
41. Nucci M, Anaissie E (2009) Infections in patients with multiple myeloma in the era of high-dose therapy and novel agents. Clin Infect Dis 49:1211–1225
42. Nucci M, Anaissie EJ, Queiroz-Telles F, Martins CA, Trabasso P, Solza C, Mangini C, Simoes BP, Colombo AL, Vaz J, Levy CE, Costa S, Moreira VA, Oliveira JS, Paraguay N, Duboc G, Voltarelli JC, Maiolino A, Pasquini R, Souza CA (2003) Outcome predictors of 84 patients with hematologic malignancies and Fusarium infection. Cancer 98: 315–319
43. Nucci M, Marr KA (2005) Emerging fungal diseases. Clin Infect Dis 41:521–526
44. Nucci M, Marr KA, Queiroz-Telles F, Martins CA, Trabasso P, Costa S, Voltarelli JC, Colombo AL, Imhof A, Pasquini R, Maiolino A, Souza CA, Anaissie E (2004) Fusarium infection in hematopoietic stem cell transplant recipients. Clin Infect Dis 38:1237–1242
45. Odabasi Z, Mattiuzzi G, Estey E, Kantarjian H, Saeki F, Ridge RJ, Ketchum PA, Finkelman MA, Rex JH, Ostrosky-Zeichner L (2004) Beta-D-glucan as a diagnostic adjunct for invasive fungal infections: validation, cutoff development, and performance in patients with acute myelogenous leukemia and myelodysplastic syndrome. Clin Infect Dis 39:199–205
46. Panackal AA, Imhof A, Hanley EW, Marr KA (2006) *Aspergillus ustus* infections among transplant recipients. Emerg Infect Dis 12:403–408
47. Pavie J, Lacroix C, Hermoso DG, Robin M, Ferry C, Bergeron A, Feuilhade M, Dromer F, Gluckman E, Molina JM, Ribaud P (2005) Breakthrough disseminated *Aspergillus ustus* infection in allogeneic hematopoietic stem cell transplant recipients receiving voriconazole or caspofungin prophylaxis. J Clin Microbiol 43: 4902–4904
48. Perfect JR, Cox GM, Lee JY, Kauffman CA, de Repentigny L, Chapman SW, Morrison VA, Pappas P, Hiemenz JW, Stevens DA (2001) The impact of culture isolation of *Aspergillus* species: a hospital-based survey of aspergillosis. Clin Infect Dis 33:1824–1833
49. Perfect JR, Marr KA, Walsh TJ, Greenberg RN, Dupont B, de la Torre-Cisneros J, Just-Nubling G, Schlamm HT, Lutsar I, Espinel-Ingroff A, Johnson E (2003) Voriconazole treatment for less-common, emerging, or refractory fungal infections. Clin Infect Dis 36:1122–1131
50. Pfeiffer CD, Fine JP, Safdar N (2006) Diagnosis of invasive aspergillosis using a galactomannan assay: a meta-analysis. Clin Infect Dis 42:1417–1427
51. Racil Z, Kocmanova I, Lengerova M, Winterova J, Mayer J (2007) Intravenous PLASMA-LYTE as a major cause of false-positive results of platelia *Aspergillus* test for galactomannan detection in serum. J Clin Microbiol 45: 3141–3142
52. Revankar SG, Patterson JE, Sutton DA, Pullen R, Rinaldi MG (2002) Disseminated phaeohyphomycosis: review of an emerging mycosis. Clin Infect Dis 34:467–476
53. Saracli MA, Mutlu FM, Yildiran ST, Kurekci AE, Gonlum A, Uysal Y, Erdem U, Basustaoglu AC, Sutton DA (2007) Clustering of invasive *Aspergillus ustus* eye infections in a tertiary care hospital: a molecular epidemiologic study of an uncommon species. Med Mycol 45:377–384
54. Schutt P, Brandhorst D, Stellberg W, Poser M, Ebeling P, Muller S, Buttkereit U, Opalka B, Lindemann M, Grosse-Wilde H, Seeber S, Moritz T, Nowrousian MR (2006) Immune parameters in multiple myeloma patients: influence of treatment and correlation with opportunistic infections. Leuk Lymphoma 47:1570–1582
55. Singh N (2002) Imaging findings in invasive zygomycosis. Liver Transpl 8:306–307
56. Siwek GT, Pfaller MA, Polgreen PM, Cobb S, Hoth P, Magalheas-Silverman M, Diekema DJ (2006) Incidence of invasive aspergillosis among allogeneic hematopoietic stem cell transplant patients receiving voriconazole prophylaxis. Diagn Microbiol Infect Dis 55:209–212
57. Steinbach WJ, Benjamin DK Jr, Kontoyiannis DP, Perfect JR, Lutsar I, Marr KA, Lionakis MS, Torres HA, Jafri H, Walsh TJ (2004) Infections due to *Aspergillus terreus*: a multicenter retrospective analysis of 83 cases. Clin Infect Dis 39:192–198
58. Stergiopoulou T, Meletiadis J, Roilides E, Kleiner DE, Schaufele R, Roden M, Harrington S, Dad L, Segal B, Walsh TJ (2007) Host-dependent patterns of tissue injury in invasive pulmonary aspergillosis. Am J Clin Pathol 127: 349–355
59. Torres HA, Rivero GA, Lewis RE, Hachem R, Raad II, Kontoyiannis DP (2003) Aspergillosis caused by non-fumigatus *Aspergillus* species: risk factors and in vitro susceptibility compared with *Aspergillus fumigatus*. Diagn Microbiol Infect Dis 46:25–28

60. Tsiodras S, Samonis G, Boumpas DT, Kontoyiannis DP (2008) Fungal infections complicating tumor necrosis factor alpha blockade therapy. Mayo Clin Proc 83:181–194
61. Vagefi PA, Cosimi AB, Ginns LC, Kotton CN (2008) Cutaneous *Aspergillus ustus* in a lung transplant recipient: emergence of a new opportunistic fungal pathogen. J Heart Lung Transplant 27:131–134
62. Van Den NE, Michaux L, Layios N, Costantini S, Francart J, Lambert C, Sonet A, Andre M, Robert A, Ferrant A (2004) High incidence of complications after 2-chloro-2'-deoxyadenosine combined with cyclophosphamide in patients with advanced lymphoproliferative malignancies. Ann Hematol 83:356–363
63. Varkey JB, Perfect JR (2008) Rare and emerging fungal pulmonary infections. Semin Respir Crit Care Med 29:121–131
64. Vera A, Hubscher SG, McMaster P, Buckels JA (2002) Invasive gastrointestinal zygomycosis in a liver transplant recipient: case report. Transplantation 73:145–147
65. Virgili A, Zampino MR, Mantovani L (2002) Fungal skin infections in organ transplant recipients. Am J Clin Dermatol 3:19–35
66. Walsh TJ, Groll A, Hiemenz J, Fleming R, Roilides E, Anaissie E (2004) Infections due to emerging and uncommon medically important fungal pathogens. Clin Microbiol Infect 10(Suppl 1):48–66
67. Walsh TJ, Lutsar I, Driscoll T, Dupont B, Roden M, Ghahramani P, Hodges M, Groll AH, Perfect JR (2002) Voriconazole in the treatment of aspergillosis, scedosporiosis and other invasive fungal infections in children. Pediatr Infect Dis J 21:240–248
68. Wingard JR (1999) Opportunistic infections after blood and marrow transplantation. Transpl Infect Dis 1:3–20
69. Wingard JR (2007) New approaches to invasive fungal infections in acute leukemia and hematopoietic stem cell transplant patients. Best Pract Res Clin Haematol 20: 99–107
70. Yuen KY, Woo PC, Ip MS, Liang RH, Chiu EK, Siau H, Ho PL, Chen FF, Chan TK (1997) Stage-specific manifestation of mold infections in bone marrow transplant recipients: risk factors and clinical significance of positive concentrated smears. Clin Infect Dis 25:37–42

Candida Pneumonia in Patients with Hematological Neoplasia

28

Carlos Carvajal, Jordi Rello, and Jeffrey Lipman

Contents

C. Carvajal
Critical Care Department, Hospital Pablo Tobon Uribe, Calle 78B #69-240 Medellín (Antioquia),
Colombia - Suramérica, 43007 Tarragona, Spain
e-mail: cabetus@yahoo.com.ar

J. Rello (✉)
Critical Care Department,
Hospital Vall d'Hebron, CIBERES,
Vall D'Hebron Institut Recerca (VHIR),
Universitat Autonoma de Barcelona,
Ps Vall d'Hebron 119-129
08035 Barcelona, Spain
e-mail: jrellohi23.ics@gencat.cat

J. Lipman
Department of Intensive Care Medicine, Intensive Care Unit, Royal Brisbane and Women's Hospital, Herston Road, Brisbane, Australia and
Burns, Trauma, Critical Care Research Centre,
University of Queensland, Australia
e-mail: j.lipman@uq.edu.au

28.1 Introduction

Advances in the management of hematological malignancies have resulted in marked improvements in life expectancy and the quality of patients' lives. However, patients with malignancies are rendered highly susceptible to infection by virtue of their underlying diseases and their associated therapies, including chemotherapy, radiation therapy, and surgery.

Traditionally, infection has accounted for up to 75% of deaths in patients with hematologic neoplasia. However, advances in prevention and treatment have decreased infectious-related death to about 50% [1, 2]. Infectious complications represent a major death risk during neutropenia; the lung is the most frequently involved site. Pneumonia is the most frequent life-threatening infectious complication occurring during the course of neutropenia in patients with cancer. Lung infection can be caused by a variety of pathogens, including bacteria, viruses, protozoa, and fungi. *Candida* is the most frequent causative agent of invasive fungal infections in immunocompromised hosts.

Candida is part of the normal human microbial flora localized in the skin, mucous membranes, digestive tract, and urogenital tract. In immunocompromised hosts such as patients with hematologic neoplasia, *Candida* can be an opportunistic pathogen causing life-threatening disseminated infections [3]. The ability of the *Candida* to alter its morphology between yeast and true hyphal growth forms is thought to contribute to its pathogenicity. The skin and mucosal surfaces are the first barriers in the host defense against fungal invasion, followed by neutrophil and macrophage activation,

Supported in part by CIBERES 06/06/0036, AGAUR 09/SGR/920

DOI: 10.1007/978-3-642-15742-4_28,

factors usually preventing fungal dissemination [3]. Candida infection is not common in immunocompromised patients without neutropenia [4].

Although neutropenia is the most important predisposing factor for invasive candidiasis, other mechanisms that have been implicated are deficiencies in humoral and cellular immunity, impairments in mucosal defensive mechanisms, and functional alterations of neutrophils [5]. In these patients bloodstream infections and catheter-related infections are the most common types of *Candida* infections, and pneumonia is *extremely uncommon*. Invasive candidiasis has been associated with severe sepsis, septic shock, and multiorgan failure with clinical characteristics resembling those caused by bacterial pathogens [6].

28.2 Epidemiology

Fungal infections have increased dramatically during the last decades. *Candida* has evolved as a prominent cause of infection in ICU patients. However *Candida* infection can easily be overestimated (Fig. 28.1), as the diagnosis of invasive candidiasis is difficult. With the exception of candidemia, diagnosis requires histological confirmation. For this reason, epidemiological data on *Candida* pneumonia are scarce and often unreliable [7].

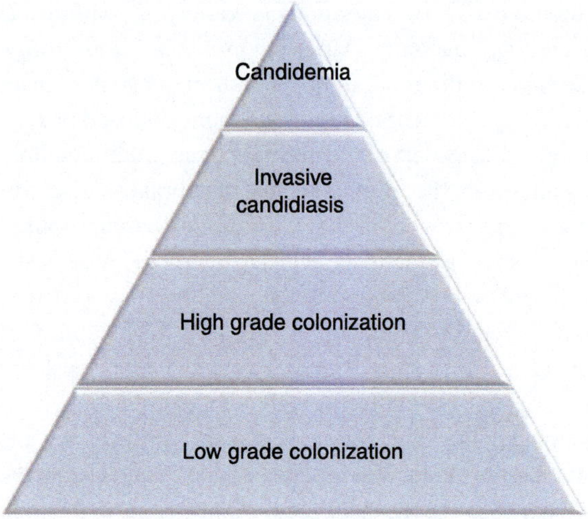

Fig. 28.1 The spectrum of disease caused by *Candida*. Candidemia is the top of the iceberg. Invasive candidiasis includes *Candida* pneumonia. Colonization (high and low grade) is determined by number of sites with positive cultures

The incidence of infection and/or fungal colonization in critically ill patients has increased over recent decades. In the United States, sepsis related to fungal infections has multiplied by threefold, from over 5,000 cases in 1979 to more than 16,000 in 2000 [8, 9]. This involves a significant increase of candidemia.

Candida pneumonia was first described in 1771 by Rosen Von Rosenstein; later Castellani reported *Candida* pneumonia in tea tasters in Ceylon. Since then, there have been only scattered reports [10]. *Candida* pneumonia is rare, and it occurs most often in patients receiving immunosuppressive or broad-spectrum antibiotic therapy. Haron et al. [11], found an incidence of 0.4% among 7,725 patients, which is similar to Masur's findings some years before (0.23%) [12]. In a search of the PubMed database (http://www.ncbi.nlm.nih.gov/pubmed accessed 14 May 2009), 91 cases of *Candida* pneumonia (Table 28.1) confirmed by histopathology [2, 10, 11, 13–15] were identified.

Although *non-albicans* species have emerged as significant pathogens in critically ill patients, *Candida albicans* continues causing the largest number of infections, representing more than half of all isolates in *Candida* pneumonia, followed by *Candida tropicalis* and *Candida glabrata*. Other species, such as *Candida krusei* and *Candida parapsilosis*, are less frequently isolated [2, 10, 11, 15].

With the exception of candidemia, the impact of invasive *Candida* infections, in terms of morbidity and mortality, has not been studied in great detail. *Candida* endophthalmitis is associated with a mortality rate estimated at 80% [16], and primary *Candida* pneumonia has a mortality rate up 70% [2, 11].

There are few identified factors associated with mortality in *Candida* pneumonia. Intubation and need for mechanical ventilation because of respiratory failure are associated with 90% mortality. Additionally, when antifungal therapy was started later (>10 days), mortality rose above 70% ($p<0.05$) [2].

28.3 Risk Factors for Invasive Pulmonary Candidiasis

Previous colonization by *Candida* in nonsterile sites has been identified as a risk factor for invasive infection [17]. Indeed, about 90% of patients with invasive *Candida* infection showed previous colonization of the

Table 28.1 Cases confirmed by histopathology of *Candida* pneumonia

Study	Patient type	Prior broad-spectrum antibiotics	Prior steroids/immunosuppressive treatment	Organism	Cases	Mortality
Schröter et al. [13]	After liver transplantation	–	–	–	7	–
Mohsenifar et al. [10]	Primary malignant	20	16	20 *C. albicans*	20	–
Buff et al. [14]	Hematological malignancies	–	11	–	20	–
Haron et al. [11]	Primary malignant	28	15	11 *C. albicans* 2 *C. tropicalis* 1 *C. parapsilosis* 18 not reported	31	84%
von Eiff et al. [2]	Hematological malignancies	12	6	6 *C. albicans* 1 *C. glabrata*	12	–
Petrocheilou-Paschou et al. [15]	After heart transplantation	1	1	1 *C. krusei*	1	1

respiratory tract by the same type of *Candida* [18, 19]. Risk factors for colonization are underlying disease, central venous catheterization, parenteral nutrition, exposure to broad-spectrum antimicrobials, acute pancreatitis, abdominal surgery, and gastrointestinal fistulas.

Candida albicans pneumonia can originate in one of two ways. True Candida pneumonia is a hematogenously disseminated pulmonary infection along with involvement of other organs, often resulting in fungal emboli in the lung. The other form is rare and occurs after aspiration of oropharyngeal material, causing primary pneumonia. Although the lungs have innate mechanisms of defense that render them very resistant to tissue invasion by *Candida sp.*, this is not so for nonfilamentous fungi, such as *Aspergillus* sp.

Non-albicans Candida species are also an important cause of *Candida* pneumonia [2, 11, 15]. Fluconazole has been identified as a risk factor for the emergence of non-*albicans Candida* [20]. From a practical point of view, it is important to predict when *Candida* infection may be caused by species potentially resistant to fluconazole, i.e., *C. glabrata* or *C. krusei*. However *C. glabrata* or *C. krusei* infection also may occur in patients without previous exposure to this antimicrobial.

28.4 Diagnosis

In the evaluation of acutely ill, immunocompromised patients with suspected pneumonia, a meticulous and thorough history and physical examination must be performed. Diagnosis confirmation and identification of underlying microorganisms is essential for appropriate therapy.

Even though patients with advanced hematologic disease are at higher risk of developing pneumonia, this complication frequently affects patients with hematologic diseases at their onset. The diagnosis of *Candida* pneumonia can be difficult for a number of reasons: an impaired inflammatory response can reduce clinical or radiological signs; an etiological diagnosis is difficult to obtain because of the risk of hemorrhage due to thrombocytopenia. As a result, a considerable proportion of pulmonary fungal infections are not diagnosed *ante mortem* in cancer patients [21].

Several procedures are recommended for the identification of *Candida* infection: (1) clinical presentation and imaging, (2) culture of respiratory samples, (3) detection of circulating antigens, (4) detection of specific antibodies, (5) detection of metastatic seeds, and (5) histopathologic confirmation (Fig. 28.2).

All the above-mentioned methods have their drawbacks: The clinical presentation is not specific; only

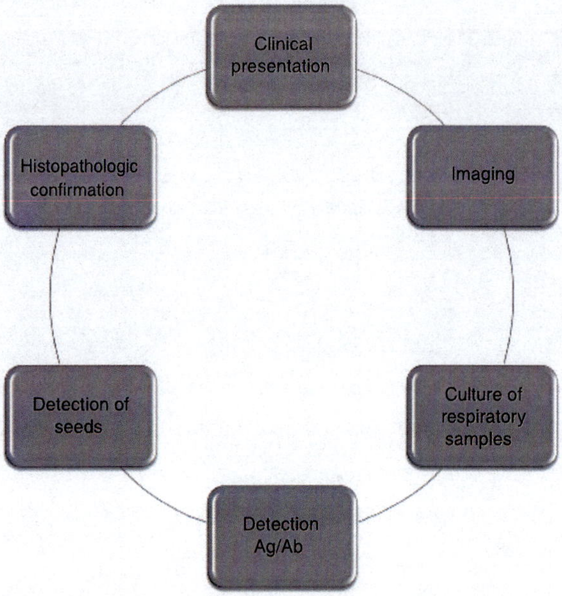

Fig. 28.2 Procedures for reliable identification of *Candida* infection. Antigens (*Ag*), antibodies (*Ab*)

50% of blood cultures are positive in patients with systemic candidiasis [22], and detection methods for antigens have low sensitivity [18, 23, 24]. Similarly, the detection of antibodies against *Candida* also has limited value, because patients are immunosuppressed and therefore present with an impaired immune response, and finally there is an excess of false-positive results [25].

Clinical presentation is characterized by cough, expectoration of purulent secretions, occasional hemoptysis and invariably hypoxemia [10]. Fever and progressive shortness of breath (and concomitant tachypnea) tend to be common symptoms, although in the neutropenic patient all these signs and symptoms are likely to be unimpressive or even absent. Fever appears in 80% of cases and leukocytosis in 50% (although there are patients with neutropenia), endophthalmitis in 9–15%, and cutaneous lesions or septic arthritis in less than 1% [26] (Fig. 28.3).

Chest radiographs (CXR) should be obtained promptly in the patient with suspected pneumonia. However, the diagnostic yield of conventional CXR is poor, and compared with computer tomography (CT), conventional CXR manifests often too late to be the correct trigger for the start of therapy [27] (Table 28.2). CT scan increases the accuracy of diagnosing and typing of the pneumonia. If the pneumonic infiltrates are located in the upper and lower lobes of the lungs or the lingula, there is a real risk that the pneumonia may be missed when CXR is performed. This obviously may lead to an erroneous treatment decision [28].

Heussel et al. [27], found in a series of neutropenic patients with fever of unknown origin and normal CXR that 60% of CT studies were indicative of pneumonia. In 54% of these studies, either clinical (chest radiography) or microbiologic documentation of pulmonary infiltration was possible. Sensitivity of CT was 87% (88% in transplant recipients), specificity was 57% (67%), and the negative predictive value was 88% (97%). Moreover, a time gain of 5 days using CT in comparison with the exclusive use CXR has been found.

The primary diagnostic challenge is the differentiation of fungal colonization from fungal infection. The isolation of *Candida* from the respiratory tract samples ranges from 11% [29] to 52% [18], increasing its rate in mechanically ventilated patients up to 70% [30, 31]. Isolation of *Candida* in the bronchial tree reflects colonization, but in many occasions this "benign" *Candida* colonization may be unfairly categorized as *Candida* pneumonia. This reflects the extremely difficult confirmation of diagnosis of *Candida* pneumonia. The value of quantitative cultures of respiratory samples for yeasts is unknown [32].

Histological confirmation is the gold standard for diagnosis of *Candida* pneumonia. However, biopsy is difficult to perform, and autopsy studies aimed to estimate the incidence are biased by the refusal of next of kin to give the informed consent. For this reason it is still a matter of debate whether *Candida* is able to cause pneumonia in immunosuppressed but non-neutropenic patients [4].

28.5 Treatment

Treatment of *Candida* pneumonia in neutropenic patients should be essentially the same as in non-neutropenic patients. The decision to initiate intensive care treatment has to take into account the prognosis of the underlying disease. Mortality in patients with hematological malignancies admitted to an ICU with *Candida* pneumonia is 70% [2, 11]. Treatment must be started immediately to improve tissue oxygenation, restore cardiovascular function, and improve other organ functions [33, 34].

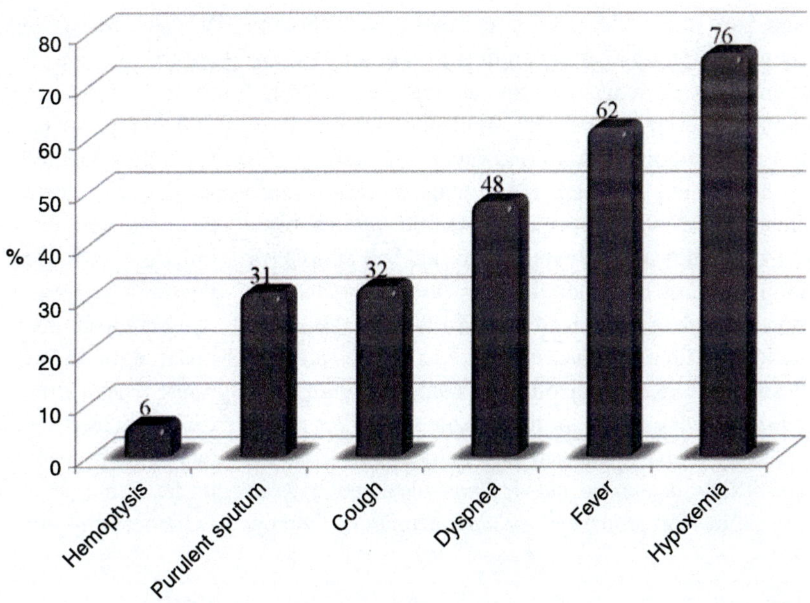

Fig. 28.3 Clinical presentation in pneumonia by *Candida* in four series [2, 10, 11, 15]

Table 28.2 Radiographic findings in *Candida* pneumonia

Radiographic findings	% Patients			
	Mohseni far [10]	Haron [11]	Petrocheilou Paschou [15]	Buff [14]
Diffuse bilateral infiltrates with confluent areas of air space consolidation	16/20	15/31	–	8/20
Localized pneumonia (1 or more lobes)	4/20	16/31	1/1	12/20
Effusion pleural	5/20	–	–	5/20

Although targeted treatment is the best therapy for *Candida* pneumonia, there are four approaches to antimycotic therapy: prophylaxis, preemptive treatment, empiric treatment, and targeted treatment [26].

Targeted treatment requires positive cultures and directed antifungal therapy. Currently, there are several antifungal drugs available for the treatment of *Candida* infections in general and, in particular, in high-risk subjects such as the critically ill. These include deoxycholate preparation and lipid-based formulations of amphotericin B, azoles like fluconazole, itraconazole or voriconazole, and echinocandins. Unfortunately, amphotericin deoxycholate plus flucytosine are the only option with clinical evidence [2].

Conventional deoxycholate amphotercin B (AmB-d) is an effective drug in treating systemic fungal infections. Nevertheless, it can produce a wide variety of severe adverse events such as renal failure. Because of this, it should not be used in critically ill patients [35]. Nephrotoxicity is the most common serious adverse effect associated with AmB-d therapy, resulting in acute renal failure in up to 50% of recipients [36, 37]. However, continuous infusions (24 h) of amphotericin B are significantly better tolerated and can reduce nephrotoxicity and side effects without increasing mortality [38], although one prospective study by Ellis et al. concluded that infusion rates for 4 h did not modify amphotericin B toxicity [39]. Lipid-based formulations of amphotericin B (LF-AmB) have been developed and approved for use in humans. There are three formulations commercially available. These agents possess the same spectrum of activity as AmB-d with less nephrotoxicity [36, 37].

The new azoles, fluconazole in particular, offer a form of treatment that is less toxic than AmB-d and equally effective, provided that they are used at adequate doses (Table 28.3) and that it is possible to identify high-risk patients requiring "empiric" treatment [26]. Fluconazole can be chosen for initial empiric therapy in clinically stable patients who have not received prior azoles. However, if *C. glabrata* is isolated, the patient should be started on high-dose fluconazole (>12 mg/kg/day or >800 mg/day for a 70-kg patient) or switched to echinocandins or amphotericin B, although, there are few data supporting this recommendation [40]. On the other hand, certain *non-albicans Candida* species are less susceptible to fluconazole, and some *Candida albicans* can be resistant to fluconazole.

There are other azoles with activity against *Candida* species. Posaconazole and voriconazole do not have an indication for primary *Candida* pneumonia therapy. Voriconazole is effective for both mucosal and invasive candidiasis, but it has not been proven in clinical trials. Its clinical use has been primarily for step-down oral therapy in patients with infection due to *C. krusei* and fluconazole-resistant, voriconazole-susceptible *C. glabrata.* However, drug-drug interactions are common with voriconazole and should be considered when initiating and discontinuing treatment with this compound [41].

Echinocandins, caspofungin, anidulafungin, and micafungin are available only as parenteral preparations. These drugs have fungicidal activity against *Candida* targeting the fungal cell wall. The absence of this target in mammalian cells probably contributes to its favorable safety profile with few adverse effects. Echinocandins are at least as effective as amphotericin

Table 28.3 Antifungal agents approved for invasive candidiasis treatment

Antifungal	Loading doses	Maintenance doses	Comments
Polyenes			
Deoxycholate amphotericin B	1 mg/kg/day	1 mg/kg/day	It can cause renal insufficiency
Amphotericin B lipid complex	5 mg/kg/day	5 mg/kg/day	Dosage should be adjusted in renal insufficiency
Amphotericin B liposomal	6 mg/kg/day	6 mg/kg/day	Dosage should be adjusted in renal insufficiency
Amphotericin B colloidal dispersion	4–6 mg/kg/day	4–6 mg/kg/day	Dosage should be adjusted in renal insufficiency
Azoles			
Fluconazole	800 mg × 1 doses	400 mg/day	Dosage should be adjusted in renal or hepatic insufficiency
	12 mg/kg	6 mg/kg/day	
Itraconazole	200 mg/kg/12 h	200 mg/kg/12 h	Dosage should be adjusted in renal or hepatic insufficiency
	3 mg/kg/12 h	3 mg/kg/12 h	
Voriconazole	400 mg/day × 2 doses	200 mg/12 h	Dosage should be adjusted in renal or hepatic insufficiency
	6 mg/kg/day × 2 doses	3 mg/kg/12 h	
Echinocandins			
Caspofungin	70 mg/day × 1 doses	50 mg/day	Dosage reduction for patients with moderate to severe hepatic dysfunction.
			No required dosage adjustment for renal insufficiency or dyalisis
Anidulafungin	200 mg/day × 1 doses	100 mg/day	No required dosage adjustment for renal insufficiency or dyalisis
Micafungin	100 mg/day	100 mg/day	No required dosage adjustment for renal insufficiency or dyalisis

B for the treatment of invasive candidiasis and even more so for candidemia [41, 42]. The minimal inhibitory concentrations (MICs) of the echinocandins are low for a broad spectrum of *Candida* species, as they retain activity against isolates with resistance to azoles or polyenes [41, 42]. However, clinical trials of echinocandins treatment in *Candida* pneumonia have not been done yet (Table 28.3).

Flucytosine demonstrates broad antifungal activity against most *Candida* species, with the exception of *C. krusei.* However, flucytosine is rarely administered as a single agent, but is usually given in combination with AmB for patients with pneumonia by *Candida* [10, 11].

28.6 Conclusion

Infectious complications are common and represent a major death risk during neutropenia. Pneumonia is extremely uncommon, but associated with high mortality. Isolation of *Candida* from the respiratory tract samples reflects colonization of the bronchial tree (or sample contamination from oropharynx). Therefore, diagnosis of pneumonia by *Candida* should require histological confirmation. Finally, if documented, antifungal agents for treatment of pneumonia by *Candida* should essentially be the same as for invasive candidiasis.

Competing Interests: The authors declare that they have no competing interests.

References

1. Daly JS, Finberg RW (2008) Acute infection in the immunocompromised host. In: Irwin RS, Rippe JM (eds) Irwin and Rippe's intensive care medicine, 6th edn. Lippincott Williams & Wilkins, Philadelphia
2. von Eiff M, Roos N, Fegeler W et al (1996) Hospital-acquired candida and aspergillus pneumonia – diagnostic approaches and clinical findings. J Hosp Infect 32:17–28
3. Galvan B, Mariscal F (2006) Epidemiologia de la candidemia en UCI. Rev Iberoam Micol 23:12–15
4. Vélez L, Correa LT, Maya MA et al (2007) Diagnostic accuracy of bronchoalveolar lavage samples in immunosuppressed patients with suspected pneumonia: analysis of a protocol. Respir Med 101:2160–2167
5. Rossini F, Verga M, Pioltelli P et al (2000) Incidence and outcome of pneumonia in patients with acute leukemia receiving first induction therapy with anthracycline-containing regimens. Haematologica 85:1255–1260
6. Pappas PG, Rex JH, Sobel JD (2004) Infectious diseases Society of America. Guidelines for treatment of candidiasis. Clin Infect Dis 38:161–189
7. Kishikawa H, Tojima H, Tokudome T (1997) Microscopic polyangiitis and pulmonary fibrosis in a patient who died of Candida pneumonia and intra-alveolar hemorrhage. Nihon Kyobu Shikkan Gakkai Zasshi 35:915–920 [Japanese – Abstract]
8. Martin GS, Mannino DM, Eaton S et al (2003) The epidemiology of sepsis in the United States from 1979 through 2000. N Engl J Med 348:1546–1554
9. Trick WE, Fridkin SK, Edwards JR et al (2002) National Nosocomial Infections Surveillance System. Secular trend of hospital-acquired candidemia among intensive care unit patients in the united states during 1989–1999. Clin Infect Dis 35:627–630
10. Mohsenifar Z, Chopra SK, Johnson BL et al (1979) Candida pneumonia: experience with 20 patients. West J Med 131: 196–200
11. Haron E, Vartivarian S, Anaissie E et al (1993) Primary Candida pneumonia. Experience at a large cancer center and review of the literature. Medicine (Baltimore) 72:137–142
12. Masur H, Rosen PP, Armstrong D (1977) Pulmonary disease caused by Candida species. Am J Med 63:914–925
13. Schröter GP, Hoelscher M, Putnam CW et al (1977) Fungus infections after liver transplantation. Ann Surg 186: 115–122
14. Buff SJ, McLelland R, Gallis HA et al (1982) Candida albicans pneumonia: radiographic appearance. AJR Am J Roentgenol 138:645–648
15. Petrocheilou-Paschou V, Georgilis K, Kontoyannis D et al (2002) Pneumonia due to Candida krusei. Clin Microbiol Infect 8:806–809
16. Menezes AV, Sigesmund DA, Demajo WA et al (1994) Mortality of hospitalized patients with Candida endophthalmitis. Arch Intern Med 154:2093–2097
17. Pittet D, Monod M, Suter PM et al (1994) Candida colonization and subsequent infections in critically ill surgical patients. Ann Surg 220:751–758
18. Bär W, Hecker H (2002) Diagnosis of systemic Candida infections in patients of the intensive care unit. Significance of serum antigens and antibodies. Mycoses 45:22–28
19. Voss A, Hollis RJ, Pfaller MA et al (1994) Investigation of the sequence of colonization and candidemia in nonneutropenic patients. J Clin Microbiol 32:975–980
20. Almirante B, Rodríguez D, Park BJ, Barcelona Candidemia Project Study Group et al (2005) Epidemiology and predictors of mortality in cases of Candida bloodstream infection: results from population-based surveillance, barcelona, Spain, from 2002 to 2003. J Clin Microbiol 43: 1829–1835
21. Sickles EA, Greene WH, Wiernik PH (1975) Clinical presentation of infection in granulocytopenic patients. Arch Intern Med 135:715–719 [Abstract]
22. Vincent JL, Anaissie E, Bruining H et al (1998) Epidemiology, diagnosis and treatment of systemic Candida infection in surgical patients under intensive care. Intensive Care Med 24:206–216

23. Yeo SF, Zhang Y, Schafer D et al (2000) A rapid, automated enzymatic fluorometric assay for determination of D-arabinitol in serum. J Clin Microbiol 38:1439–1443
24. Allaouchiche B, Coronel B, Gagnieu MC et al (2004) Cytokine levels in bronchoalveolar lavage fluid and blood of neutropenic patients with pneumonia. Bull Cancer 91: 77–80
25. Petri MG, König J, Moecke HP, Paul-Ehrlich Society for Chemotherapy, Divisions of Mycology and Pneumonia Research et al (1997) Epidemiology of invasive mycosis in ICU patients: a prospective multicenter study in 435 non-neutropenic patients. Intensive Care Med 23:317–325
26. De Bellis P, Bonfiglio M, Gerbi G et al (2003) High-dose fluconazole therapy in intensive care unit. Minerva Anestesiol 69:145–152
27. Heussel CP, Kauczor HU, Heussel GE et al (1999) Pneumonia in febrile neutropenic patients and in bone marrow and blood stem-cell transplant recipients: use of high-resolution computed tomography. J Clin Oncol 17:796–805
28. Syrjälä H, Broas M, Suramo I et al (1998) High-resolution computed tomography for the diagnosis of community-acquired pneumonia. Clin Infect Dis 27:358–363
29. Weinberger M, Sacks T, Sulkes J et al (1997) Increasing fungal isolation from clinical specimens: experience in a university hospital over a decade. J Hosp Infect 35:185–195
30. Azoulay E, Timsit JF, Tafflet M et al (2006) Candida colonization of the respiratory tract and subsequent pseudomonas ventilator-associated pneumonia. Chest 129:110–117
31. El-Ebiary M, Torres A, Fàbregas N et al (1997) Significance of the isolation of Candida species from respiratory samples in critically ill, non-neutropenic patients. An immediate postmortem histologic study. Am J Respir Crit Care Med 156:583–590
32. Rello J, Esandi ME, Díaz E et al (1998) The role of Candida sp isolated from bronchoscopic samples in nonneutropenic patients. Chest 114:146–149
33. Penack O, Beinert T, Buchheidt D, German Society of Hematology and Oncology et al (2006) Management of sepsis in neutropenia: guidelines of the infectious diseases working party (AGIHO) of the German Society of Hematology and Oncology (DGHO). Ann Hematol 85: 424–433
34. Benoit DD, Vandewoude KH, Decruyenaere JM et al (2003) Outcome and early prognostic indicators in patients with a hematologic malignancy admitted to the intensive care unit for a life-threatening complication. Crit Care Med 31: 104–112
35. Garnacho-Montero J, Díaz-Martín A, Cayuela-Dominguez A (2008) Management of invasive Candida infections in non-neutropenic critically ill patients: from prophylaxis to early therapy. Int J Antimicrob Agents 32(Suppl 2): S137–S141
36. Deray G (2002) Amphotericin B nephrotoxicity. J Antimicrob Chemother 49(Suppl 1):37–41
37. White MH, Bowden RA, Sandler ES et al (1998) Randomized, double-blind clinical trial of amphotericin B colloidal dispersion vs. amphotericin B in the empirical treatment of fever and neutropenia. Clin Infect Dis 27:296–302
38. Eriksson U, Seifert B, Schaffner A (2001) Comparison of effects of amphotericin B deoxycholate infused over 4 or 24 hours: randomised controlled trial. BMJ 322:579–582
39. Ellis ME, al-Hokail AA, Clink HM et al (1992) Double-blind randomized study of the effect of infusion rates on toxicity of amphotericin B. Antimicrob Agents Chemother 36: 172–179
40. Chen H, Suda KJ, Turpin RS et al (2007) High- versus low-dose fluconazole therapy for empiric treatment of suspected invasive candidiasis among high-risk patients in the intensive care unit: a cost-effectiveness analysis. Curr Med Res Opin 23:1057–1065
41. Pappas PG, Kauffman CA, Andes D et al (2009) Infectious Diseases Society of America. Clinical practice guidelines for the management of candidiasis: 2009 update by the Infectious Diseases Society of America. Clin Infect Dis 48:503–535
42. Mora-Duarte J, Betts R, Rotstein C, Caspofungin Invasive Candidiasis Study Group et al (2002) Comparison of caspofungin and amphotericin B for invasive candidiasis. N Engl J Med 347:2020–2029

Parasitic Lung Infections

29

Jean-François Timsit, Jean-Paul Brion, and Hervé Pelloux

Contents

J.-F. Timsit (✉)
Medical Polyvalent ICU, Albert Michallon University Hospital, BP 217, 38043, Grenoble Cedex 09, France and
Inserm U 823, Team 11: Epidemiology of Cancer and Critical Illnesses, Grenoble, France
e-mail: jftimsit@chu-grenoble.fr

J.-P. Brion
Infectious Diseases Department, Albert Michallon University Hospital, Grenoble, France
e-mail: jpbrion@chu-grenoble.fr

H. Pelloux
Department of Mycology, Albert Michallon University Hospital, Grenoble, France
e-mail: hpelloux@chu-grenoble

Pulmonary involvement with eukaryotic parasites in patients with hematological malignancies is less common than infections by bacteria or other eukaryotic pathogens such as fungi (mainly *Pneumocystis*, *Aspergillus*, and *Candida*). However, parasitic infections in immunocompromised patients are associated with a high morbidity and mortality rates if not prevented or diagnosed and treated in time [1–4]. These infections are rare or restricted to specific geographic areas in patients with hematological malignancies. One of the main features of parasitic infections is dissemination, which may be confused with another opportunistic infection, resulting in diagnostic delays. Two parasitic lung infections are sufficiently frequent to be described in detail, namely, toxoplasmosis and stongyloidiasis.

29.1 Host–Parasite Interaction

The complexity of host–parasite interactions can explain, to some extent, the difficulties encountered in preventing, diagnosing, and treating parasitic infections in severely immunocompromised patients. These interactions vary widely across parasites, as these pathogens differ in their life cycles and structures, and induce host responses that do not involve the same pathways and mechanisms. The two parasites that deserve special attention in patients with hematological malignancies are the protozoan *Toxoplasma gondii* and the nematode *Stongyloides stercoralis*. Here, we describe the main characteristics of the host–parasite interactions that explain the clinical and biological features observed in hematological malignancy patients infected by these parasites.

É. Azoulay (ed.), *Pulmonary Involvement in Patients with Hematological Malignancies*,
DOI: 10.1007/978-3-642-15742-4_29, © Springer-Verlag Berlin Heidelberg 2011

29.1.1 Toxoplasmosis

The relationship between *T. gondii* and its host is very complex [5, 6]. In immunocompetent patients, the host and parasite reach an equilibrium, as shown by the fact that chronic asymptomatic *T. gondii* infection is found in 50% of individuals in France. However, when the host immune responses are depressed (e.g., by AIDS or a hematological malignancy), the reactivation of latent parasite forms (bradyzoites) from quiescent cysts to virulent parasites (tachyzoites, Figs. 29.1 and 29.2) can lead to serious lesions in the brain, lungs, or other organs. The reactivated parasites may occur locally or disseminate via the bloodstream. Globally, host–parasite interactions depend on several factors, related both to the parasite and to the patient. Among parasite-related factors, the population structure of *T. gondii* allows the differentiation of three main lineages (types I, II, and III strains) and of nonarchetypal and highly virulent strains found mainly in South America [7]. These virulent strains can cause clinical lesions in immunocompetent patients that are as serious as those seen immunocompromised patients with disseminated type-II strain disease. Type II strains are found in more than 90% of the toxoplasmosis cases in western countries. Pathogenicity of type II strains occurs almost only in immunocompromised individuals and patients with congenital toxoplasmosis. Among patient-related factors, chronic infection is the main source of clinical toxoplasmosis in patients with hematological malignancies, and new infections are very rare. The decrease in host immune control leads to cyst rupture (in the brain and muscles), conversion from bradyzoites to tachyzoites, and development of local abscesses and/or hematogenous dissemination. Briefly, in immunocompetent patients, the process that leads to parasite encystation is driven by both innate and adaptive immune processes, with the balance between pro- and antiinflammatory cytokines being of paramount importance in reaching the equilibrium necessary for both host and parasite survival. The encysted quiescent parasites are protected from the immune response of the host. Taken as a whole, cellular immunity, macrophages, T lymphocytes, NK cells, and associated cytokines (mainly IFNγ) are the main immune elements involved in controlling *T. gondii* infection. However, not all T-cell-deficient patients contract clinical toxoplasmosis, as the genetic background of the patient and parasite also plays a role. Therefore, the probability of clinical toxoplasmosis occurring cannot be predicted in the individual patient.

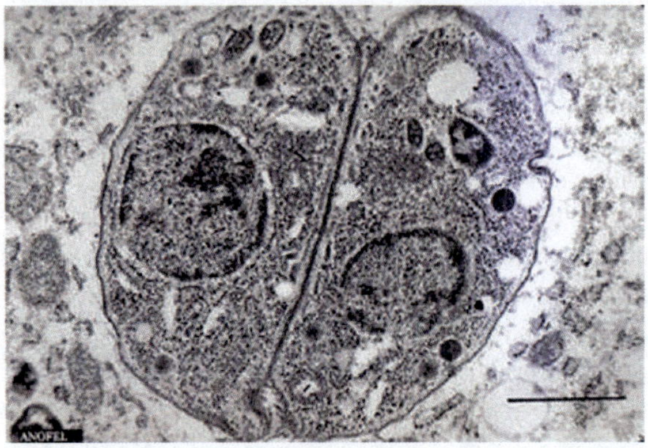

Fig. 29.1 Dividing *T. gondii* tachyzoites (endodyogeny). Electronic microscopy (Photograph H. Pelloux, E. Brambilla for ANOFEL, with permission)

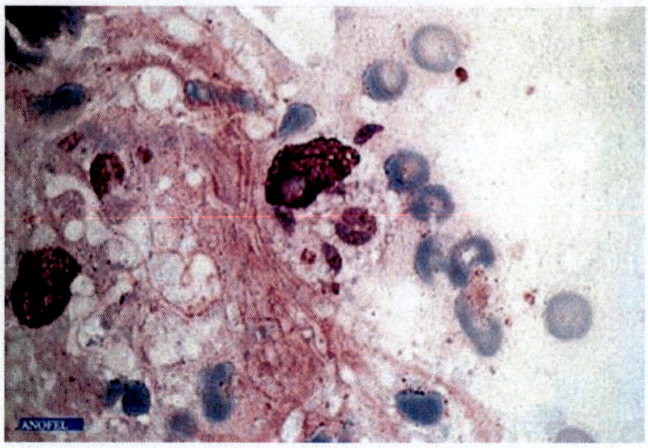

Fig. 29.2 *Toxoplasma gondii*. Tachyzoite (May-Grünwald-Giemsa) in bronchoalveolar lavage fluid (Photograph P. Marty for ANOFEL, with permission)

In immunocompromised patients with hematological malignancies, lung involvement is due to hematogenous dissemination of the parasites, as pulmonary tissues are not known to harbor chronic *Toxoplasma* cysts. Recent data indicate that patients with hematological malignancies may experience *T. gondii* parasitemia without patent clinical symptoms [8, 9]. This possibility should be considered in patients known to be seropositive for *T. gondii* before the onset of the hematological malignancy and is of importance for interpreting laboratory tests used to diagnose toxoplasmosis in these patients. Immune reconstitution after bone marrow transplantation or remission of the malignancy leads to the development of a new host–parasite equilibrium and removes the risk of cyst reactivation.

29.1.2 Strongyloidiasis

S. stercoralis is an intestinal nematode with a highly complex life cycle. It can persist in humans for decades and can lead to a fulminant hyperinfection syndrome if the host becomes immunosuppressed [3]. Thus, the main risk for patients with hematological malignancies in western countries is progression of chronic strongyloidiasis that was present before onset of the malignancy. Primary infection, transmission via an allogeneic transplant, and nosocomial transmission are exceedingly rare [10]. The chronic nature of strongyloidiasis, which is unique among nematodes, is due to the fact that *S. stercoralis* larvae can cause autoinfection: the eggs hatch in the intestine, releasing larvae that penetrate the intestinal wall and follow the normal infective cycle if the host is immunocompetent. This mechanism can lead to decades-long infection without re-infection in endemic areas. The normal life cycle includes a pulmonary step in which the filariform larvae are carried to the alveolar spaces via the circulatory system, then reach the pharynx and are swallowed to reach the intestine. In immunocompetent patients, the pulmonary step is most often asymptomatic. Furthermore, incomplete host–parasite equilibrium, less perfect than that seen in *T. gondii* infection, is induced, and the number of parasitic larvae is controlled to some extent. The infection cycle is not stopped, but its importance is limited. The widespread use of immunosuppressive therapy and the chronicity of strongyloidiasis make hyperinfection a clinically important problem even in nonendemic countries where migrant people live. Risk factors for hyperinfection and disseminated disease include impaired cell-mediated immunity, chronic corticosteroid therapy, hematopoietic stem cell transplantation, hematological malignancies such as lymphoma, human T-lymphotropic virus type 1 infection, hypogammaglobulinemia, and solid organ transplantation [11]. The most common risk factor is corticosteroid use, which results in eosinopenia, hampering the eosinophil-specific immune response against *S. stercoralis.*

Of note, despite the overlap in endemic regions between HIV infection and strongyloidiasis, the incidence of strongyloidiasis is not higher than in the non-HIV-infected population. Eosinophils and interleukin-5 are known to be important components of the immune response to *S. stercoralis* infection. Activated eosinophils kill helminthic parasites in vitro, and interleukin-5-knockout CB57BL/6 mice exhibit increased susceptibility to stronglyoidiasis [12]. In patients with hematological malignancies, immunosuppression leads to loss of the host-parasite equilibrium with a marked increase in the activity of the normal life cycle that considerably augments the number of larvae disseminating into the body. The number of larvae in the lung and alveolar space leads to pulmonary function impairments that can progress to respiratory failure and death. *S. stercoralis* hyperinfection after solid organ transplantation can coincide with corticosteroid use to prevent graft rejection and usually manifests between 1 and 3 months after transplantation. However, *S. stercoralis* hyperinfection manifests earlier in hematopoietic stem cell transplant recipients, owing to their profound immunosuppression [4].

29.2 Toxoplasmosis

Pulmonary toxoplasmosis is a well-known entity [13] that has been reported in immunocompetent patients, but chiefly affects the rapidly growing number of immunocompromised patients with cell-mediated immune deficiencies. In the 1990s, most of the patients with pulmonary toxoplasmosis had AIDS and a history of other AIDS-related infections. Patients with *T. gondii* pneumonia had a higher mortality rate than did patients with extra-pulmonary disease, with a median survival of 150 days after the diagnosis [14].

As progress was made in means of controlling HIV infection, the populations chiefly affected with pulmonary toxoplasmosis became organ transplantation recipients and patients with hematological malignancies. Allogeneic hematopoietic stem cell transplant recipients are at very high risk, whereas toxoplasmosis is rare in autologous stem cell transplant recipients. In bone marrow transplant recipients, the incidence of pulmonary toxoplasmosis varies markedly, from 0.28% to 4% of patients [15]. The infection rate is highest in countries where the prevalence of toxoplasmosis is high in the general population. However, when only seropositive recipients are considered, the incidence ranges from 1.9% to 5.7% [16]. The main risk factors are pretransplantation seropositivity of the recipient, allogeneic transplant, and graft versus host disease (requiring intensified immunosuppressive therapy) [2]. Myeloablative conditioning and conditioning with high-dose total body irradiation increase the risk of *T. gondii* reactivation [17]. Of note, alentuzumab, a new agent to treat lymphoproliferative disorders, might increase the risk of opportunistic infections via lysis of lymphocytes and other CD52-expressing cells through complement activation and antibody-dependent cell-mediated toxicity [18, 19]. In a review of 81 allogeneic stem cell transplant recipients with toxoplasmosis [16], the median time to disease onset was 2 months after transplantation. Fewer than 10% of cases occurred during the first month and fewer than 15–20% after day 100.

In bone marrow transplant recipients, disseminated toxoplasmosis carries a poorer prognosis than does cerebral toxoplasmosis, with a 5.28-fold increase in the odds of dying [20]. Of 55 patients with disseminated toxoplasmosis after bone marrow transplantation, only four survived, yielding a 93% mortality rate. This poor prognosis emphasizes the need for appropriate primary prevention in individuals at risk for the disease. Pulmonary toxoplasmosis is usually related to dissemination from another site rather than as the only disease location.

29.2.1 Clinical Presentation

The clinical presentation is relatively nonspecific. Fever is usually present, and dyspnea and cough are reported in one-third of cases. Chest roentgenographs generally show diffuse interstitial infiltrates (see Sect. 19.6.4), but micronodular or nodular infiltrates are common also. Less common findings include cavitary infiltrates, lobar pneumonia, and pleural effusion [21].

High-resolution CT usually shows bilateral ground-glass opacities with superimposed septal thickening and intralobular linear opacities [21].

Since the central nervous system is the most typical target of toxoplasmosis, neurological abnormalities are common, although nonspecific. They may include mental status changes and seizures with or without focal deficits [20]. Chorioretinitis may occur also.

The clinical picture is frequently associated with multiple organ failure, in particular acute respiratory distress syndrome, shock, and severe acute thrombocytopenia due to disease dissemination [22, 23] or hemophagocytic syndrome [1].

The first step of the diagnosis of toxoplasmosis in patients with hematological malignancies takes place before the development of deep immunosuppression. Since clinical toxoplasmosis usually results from reactivation of chronic infection, a serological test for *T. gondii* should be performed. Seropositive patients are at risk for reactivation, while seronegative patients are not, as they have no cysts in their brain and muscles [16]. Although primary prophylaxis with sulfamethoxazole/trimethoprim is not always effective in preventing toxoplasmosis, absence of such prophylaxis after bone marrow transplantation supports a diagnosis of toxoplasmosis. Proof of chronic infection consists in the detection of specific anti-*T. gondii* IgG in peripheral blood.

When pulmonary toxoplasmosis is suspected in a previously seropositive patient with a hematological malignancy, the responsibility of *T. gondii* in the lung lesions must be confirmed. Extremely high levels of serum lactate dehydrogenase have been reported in patients with severe *T. gondii* pneumonia or disseminated disease and should prompt specific diagnostic procedures. The demonstration of tachyzoites by microscopic examination of the sputum [24], bronchoalveolar lavage fluid, or bone marrow aspirates remains the simplest means of establishing the diagnosis. Now, the diagnosis can also be made using real-time PCR on blood, cerebrospinal fluid, or, more invasively, from fluid recovered after fiberoptic bronchoscopy and bronchoalveolar lavage [24, 25]. The most efficient technique to date for *T. gondii* detection is PCR [16, 23]. PCR is sufficiently sensitive to detect very small amounts of parasite, and quantitative real-time techniques can estimate the parasite load in lungs and help to monitor treatment efficacy, although no validated reference standard exists for interpreting the results. Thus, whatever the technique used, the presence of *T. gondii* in pulmonary samples from a patient with a hematological malignancy constitutes proof of pulmonary toxoplasmosis. However, the diagnosis of toxoplasmosis is often more complex in these patients. Lung involvement with *T. gondii* can also be strongly suspected when suggestive clinical and imaging signs are present and PCR in the peripheral blood or antibody titer changes over time indicate parasite dissemination [8].

29.3 Strongyloidiasis

Strongyloidiasis is present in temperate, tropical, and subtropical climates. It is endemic in sub-Saharan Africa, the West Indies, South America, Southeast Asia, Bangladesh, Pakistan, and the southeastern United States, as well as in eastern European countries such as Romania and the Mediterranean countries [3, 4]. The global prevalence of strongyloidiasis is unclear and varies between 30 million and 100 million people infected [3]. The overall rate of *S. stercoralis* infection was 1 per 10,000 patients with newly diagnosed cancer in the United States [26, 27].

Hyperinfection occurs when immune suppression develops in a patient who has chronic strongyloidiasis. Although malnutrition remains the major secondary cause worldwide, in the developed world iatrogenic immune suppression is an important precipitant.

Transplant recipients are at risk for developing *S. stercoralis* hyperinfection syndrome related to chronic intestinal *S. stercoralis* infection, acquisition of primary *S. stercoralis* infection in endemic areas, or transmission via an allogeneic transplant. Progression of chronic intestinal infection present before transplantation appears to be the most common mechanism. The low rate of strongyloidiasis after hematopoietic stem cell transplantation can be explained by routine screening for the parasite and the use of prophylactic treatment before transplantation.

As with toxoplasmosis, the detection of chronic *S. stercoralis* infection before deep immunosuppression develops is crucial to prevent reactivation of the parasitic disease [3, 28]. Screening for chronic strongyloidiasis involves careful history-taking with attention to all trips to possibly endemic areas and to clinical symptoms consistent with strongyloidiasis. Laboratory screening involves serological testing for specific IgG antibodies, as peripheral eosinophilia may be intermittent [29, 30]. An enzyme-linked immunosorbent assay (ELISA) for detecting serum immunoglobulin G (IgG) against filariform *S. stercoralis* larvae has 95% sensitivity and negative predictive value. However, the *S. stercoralis* antibody test can show cross-reactivity with other helminth infections, such as filariasis, ascariasis, and schistosomiasis, leading to poor specificity of the test. In addition, *S. stercoralis* antibody testing cannot discriminate between past and current strongyloidiasis [12]. Finally, *S. stercoralis* antibody testing can be falsely negative in immunocompromised patients.

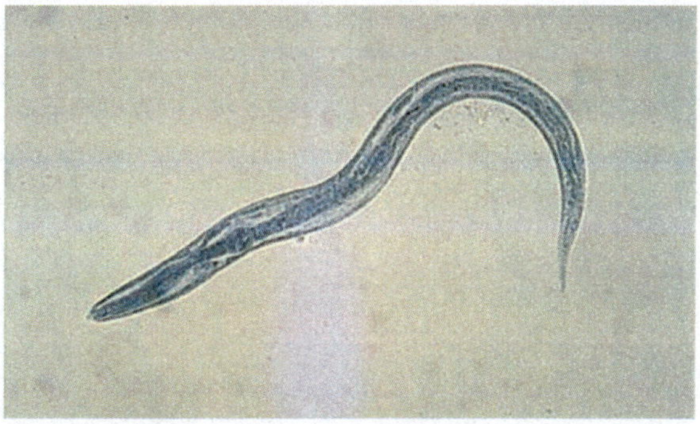

Fig. 29.3 Rhabditoid larvae of *Strongyloides stercoralis* in stool (Photograph P. Le Pape for ANOFEL, with permission)

The detection of parasite larvae in stool samples remains of main importance, although sensitivity is low if a single sample is tested. Detection relies chiefly on microscopy in routine practice, but molecular techniques are being developed and have produced promising results [31]. Stool sample examination (ideally three different samples) should be repeated if possible in an expert laboratory, as this increases sensitivity to 60–70% and perhaps higher in immunocompromised patients, which is worth the additional time needed. Concentration techniques such as the Baermann technique and stool culture technique must be used to increase the sensitivity of the test (Fig. 29.3).

29.3.1 Clinical Presentation

The first step is careful history-taking for a history of stays in endemic regions and of *S. stercoralis* infestation. More than 50% of patients infected with *S. stercoralis* are asymptomatic, and 75% have fluctuating mild (5–15%) eosinophilia [32]. Other rare but classical symptoms involve the skin, gastrointestinal tract, and respiratory system. The typical skin lesion is a migratory, serpiginous, urticarial rash (larva currens or creeping larvae) due to larvae invading the skin, particularly of the buttocks, trunk, and inguinal regions. A history of intermittent hypereosinophilia, especially before immunosuppressive treatment initiation, should be sought carefully.

Hyperinfection syndrome develops when immunosuppression allows intensification of the normal life cycle of the parasite, causing massive increases in the amounts of larvae produced. The larvae proliferate massively in the duodenum, migrate through the bowel wall, and travel through the venous system to the lungs and back to the small bowel.

This can produce worsening pulmonary function impairments that start with wheezing and, in some patients, progress to acute respiratory distress syndrome, frequently accompanied by intra-alveolar hemorrhage leading to intractable respiratory failure and death. Gastrointestinal symptoms, such as dyspepsia, diarrhea, constipation, severe ileus, and gastrointestinal bleeding, may occur concomitantly. Hyperinfection syndrome is frequently accompanied with gram-negative enteric bacteremia caused by larvae migrating from the bowel through the venous system. *S. stercoralis* dissemination through the venous system to other locations in the body may also result in bacterial translocation to other organs, causing meningitis, cholecystitis, or liver abscesses. The presence of gram-negative sepsis is in itself life-threatening and may obscure the presence of disseminated *S. stercoralis* infection. When hyperinfection syndrome is suspected, the diagnosis must be made without delay. In this situation, there is usually no eosinophilia. The chest X-ray shows diffuse alveolar infiltrate consistent with intraalveolar hemorrhage. The presence of concurrent bacterial or fungal sepsis complicates the diagnosis of strongyloidiasis. The medical biologist must be informed of the suspected diagnosis. The techniques used are very simple and easy to perform, as the larval lung burden is high. Direct microscopic examination of wet mount preparations of sputum or bronchoalveolar lavage fluid is sufficient to establish the diagnosis and can be performed in any medical laboratory.

29.4 Treatment of Strongyloidiasis and Toxoplasmosis

Acute disseminated infections caused by these two parasites require the prompt administration of antiparasitic drugs and the discontinuation or reduction of the immunosuppressive treatments if possible. Empiric or preemptive treatment is often needed before the diagnosis is confirmed. In this situation, the antiparasitic treatment is usually combined with an antibiotic or antiviral agent.

29.5 Toxoplasmosis

The currently recommended anti-*T. gondii* drugs act against the tachyzoites and therefore do not eradicate the encysted forms. Consequently, secondary prophylaxis is required. Extensive studies in patients with AIDS have evaluated the treatment of toxoplasmosis, most notably manifesting as encephalitis or brain abscesses. This experience has been extrapolated to other immunodeficient patients.

The treatment combines either sulfadiazine or clindamycin with pyrimethamine. Pyrimethamine is a folic acid antagonist whose main common side effect is dose-related bone marrow suppression. Folinic acid should be administered concomitantly and blood cell counts checked twice a week. An oral 200-mg loading dose is recommended followed by 50 (<60 kg) to 70 mg (>60 kg) per day orally. No intravenous form is available.

Pyrimethamine should be combined with sulfadiazine or clindamycin. Sulfadiazine acts synergistically with pyrimethamine as a folic acid antagonist. Crystalluria and oliguria with renal failure should be prevented by hyperhydratation. Skin rash is the most common side effect and may be life threatening. Desensitization protocols have been successful in allergic patients who required sulfadiazine. The dosage is 1,000 mg (<60 kg) to 1,500 mg (>60 kg) orally every 6 h. No intravenous form is available. Clindamycin is an antibiotic that inhibits protein synthesis and seems to act by targeting translation in the *T. gondii* apicoplast. The main adverse reactions to clindamycin include rash, nausea, vomiting, and diarrhea, which may be associated with *Clostridium difficile*. Clindamycin can be administrated orally or intravenously. The dosage is 600 mg every 6 h by either route.

29.5.1 Possible Alternative Regimens

Trimethoprim-sulfamethoxazole can be used as an alternative to pyrimethamine.

Other drugs such as atovaquone (1,500 mg orally twice a day), dapsone (100 mg orally once a day), azithromycin (900–1,200 mg once a day), or clarithromycin (500 mg every 12 h) can be used in combination with pyrimethamine. These combinations are less effective than pyrimethamine plus sulfadiazine or clindamycin.

29.5.2 Management of Pulmonary Toxoplasmosis in Hematopoietic Stem Cell Transplant Recipients

Due to the diagnostic difficulties and considerable mortality related to disseminated toxoplasmosis, preemptive treatment must be initiated at symptom onset. Thus, PCR monitoring of *T. gondii* is extremely useful in these patients. In their review, Sing et al. [25] showed that about half the patients died within 3 days after pulmonary symptom onset.

No data are available to determine the optimal drug combination for treating pulmonary toxoplasmosis. Extrapolating from previous experience supports the use of pyrimethamine plus sulfadiazine. In the most severe forms, if gastrointestinal absorption may be impaired, intravenous clindamycin should used instead of oral sulfadiazine. Adjunctive corticosteroid therapy needs further evaluation. The time to clinical response remains to be evaluated. The changes at the end of the first week are of crucial importance; ideally, the patient should be clinically improved, with negative PCT tests in blood and bronchoalveolar lavage fluid and fading of the radiographic infiltrates. The optimal treatment duration is unknown, and the drugs are often given for 6–8 weeks.

After successful primary treatment, maintenance therapy or secondary prophylaxis is required with lower drug doses (half the initial dosage for pyrimethamine, sulfadiazine or clindamycin). The duration of the maintenance therapy depends on many factors, such as immune recovery of the patient, engraftment, graft-versus-host-disease prevention or treatment with immunosuppressive drugs, and whether the immunosuppressive drug regimen was interrupted. After toxoplasmosis treatment, hematopoietic stem cell recipients should continue to receive suppressive doses of trimethoprim-sulfamethoxazole or an alternative regimen for the duration of their immunosuppression (bone-marrow transplant guidelines). Intolerance to the treatment is frequent and may lead to poor patient adherence to maintenance therapy.

29.5.3 Primary Prophylaxis

Prophylaxis with trimethoprim-sulfamethoxazole has been proven effective against *T. gondii* reactivation in AIDS patients and can be used after allogeneic bone marrow transplantation. High trimethoprim-sulfamethoxazole dosages may be more effective than low dosages [33]. In part because trimethoprim-sulfamethoxazole may depress hematopoiesis, *T. gondii* prophylaxis is rarely used now in bone marrow transplant recipients, even those at highest risk, and there is no evidence to support such prophylaxis. Nevertheless, clinical observation shows that disseminated toxoplasmosis may develop in patients who do not receive chemoprophylaxis, in keeping with data on AIDS. Thus, routine chemoprophylaxis in high-risk patients may effectively prevent toxoplasmosis reactivation in bone marrow transplant recipients [34].

In practice, because reactivation of chronic infection is the most common cause of toxoplasmosis after allogeneic hematopoietic stem cell transplantation, patients who are seropositive should receive prophylaxis (Table 29.1). Post-transplantation serological testing is not helpful in this group of patients because the results may be affected by the use of intravenous immunoglobulins or by hypogammaglobulinemia. Therefore, pre-transplantation serological testing is crucial.

Very few cases of toxoplasmosis related to transmission by the donor have been reported. Serological tests ensure the early diagnosis, allowing early preemptive therapy.

29.6 Strongyloidiasis

All people infected with *S. stercoralis* should be treated to eradicate the infection.

Three drugs are available, ivermectin, 200 μg/kg once daily; thiabendazole, 25 mg/kg twice daily; and albendazole, 400 mg twice daily.

Table 29.1 Toxoplasmosis prophylaxis among seropositive allogeneic hematopoietic stem cell transplant (HSCT) recipients

Indication	First Choice	Alternatives
Prophylaxis among seropositive allogeneic HSCT recipients	Trimethoprim-sulfamethoxazole	Clindamycin plus pyrimethamine plus leucovorin
Note: Start after engraftment and administer as long as patients remain on immunosuppressive therapy (i.e., generally, until 6 months after HSCT)	Adults/adolescents:	Adults/adolescents
	One double-strength (160/800 mg) tablet orally once daily; or	Clindamycin: 300–450 mg orally every 6–8 h; plus pyrimethamine: 25–75 mg orally once daily; plus leucovorin: 10–25 mg orally once daily
	One single-strength (80/400 mg) tablet orally once daily; or	
	One double-strength tablet orally three times/week	
	Pediatrics:	Pediatrics:
	150 mg trimethoprim/750 mg sulfamethoxazole/m^2/day by mouth with any of the following schedules: two divided doses three times/week on consecutive days; or a single dose orally three times/week on consecutive days; or two divided doses daily for 7 days; or two divided doses three times/week on alternate days	Clindamycin: 20–30 mg/kg/day by mouth, in four divided doses; plus pyrimethamine: 1 mg/kg orally daily; plus leucovorin: 5 mg orally every 3 days

29.6.1 Management of Hyperinfection or Disseminated Infection

Ivermectin 200 μg/kg orally once a day is the most efficient drug. The treatment must be continued for at least 7 days until the larvae are no longer detected in stool, sputum, and urine. Broad-spectrum antibiotics with activity against enteric organisms should be given also.

Paralytic ileus may impair the absorption of ivermectin, even after nasogastric tube administration. Subcutaneous injections of veterinary preparations have been successful, whereas oral therapy has failed.

The combination of ivermectin and albendazole has been used successfully to treat disseminated strongyloidiasis.

The treatment must be repeated if the infection is not eradicated (presence of larvae in stool 2 weeks after treatment completion).

29.6.2 Preventive Therapy

Candidates for allogeneic or autologous hematopoietic stem cell transplantation should avoid contact with soil, beaches, or other surfaces that might be contaminated by human feces. Health-care workers (in hospitals or institutions) should wear gloves when working with patients or in areas with possible fecal contamination.

29.6.3 Preventing Disease and Disease Recurrence

Candidates for allogeneic hematopoietic stem cell transplantation or immunosuppressive chemotherapy should be screened for *S. stercoralis* using serological tests and eosinophil counts, especially those who have visited or lived in endemic areas or who have HTLV1 infection (which impairs the Th2 immune response). The same recommendations apply to autologous hematopoietic stem cell transplantation, although strongyloidiasis is rarely reported in association with this procedure.

Empiric treatment with ivermectin (200 μg/kg/day orally for 2 consecutive days then repeat after 2 weeks) is required even if multiple stool examinations are negative. Alternative treatments consist of albendazole 400 mg orally twice daily for 7 days and thiabendazole 25 mg/kg (maximum 3 g/day) orally bid for 2 days. A total of three stool examinations is required if the serologic tests are negative and strongyloidiasis is suspected clinically.

To prevent recurrences, parasite clearance should be controlled by performing three or more stool examinations. Chemoprophylaxis is not recommended after hematopoietic stem cell transplantation to prevent strongyloidiasis recurrence, because data are lacking.

29.6.4 Clinical Vignette

29.6.4.1 Disseminated Toxoplasmosis

A 40-year-old women with a history of idiopathic medullary aplasia received an HLA-identical peripheral blood stem cell transplant on October 25 (day 0) after conditioning with fludarabine (52.5 mg), cyclophosphamide (3,720 mg), and anti-CD52 antibodies (30 mg) (chest X-ray A).

She received cyclosporine and mycophenolate for prevention of graft-versus-host disease. The pretransplant IgG anti-*T. gondii* titer for toxoplasmosis was 8 IU/mL (positive if >7 IU/mL), with no IgM antibodies. Aerosolized pentamidine was given for *Pneumocystis* pneumonia prophylaxis because of a

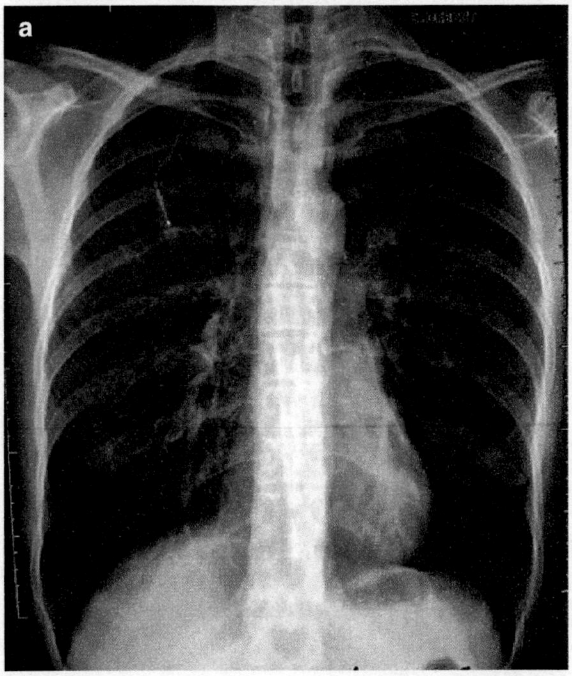

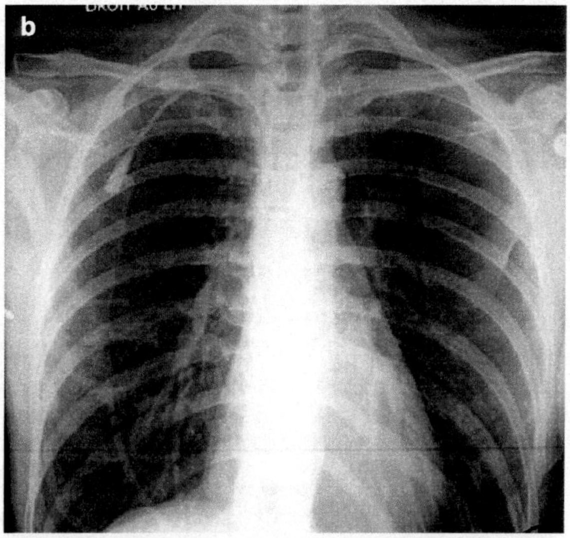

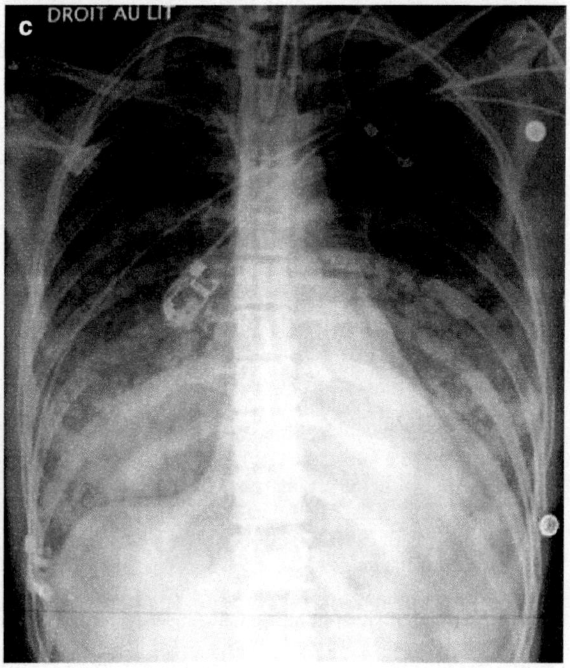

previous cutaneous reaction to sulfonamides. On day 18, her blood leukocyte count reached 2,000/mm^3. On day 20, a fever developed and persisted despite broad-spectrum antimicrobials. On day 22, she had a blood leukocyte count of only 500/mm^3 with thrombocytopenia. A skin reaction consistent with graft-versus-host disease prompted intensification of the corticosteroid therapy. Cytomegalovirus antigenemia was positive (19 cells), and she was given the antiviral gancyclovir.

The chest X-ray (B) was considered unchanged. A fever of 38°C persisted without any other findings except persistent cytomegalovirus antigenemia.

On day 30, rapid onset of severe tachypnea and hypoxia required ICU admission and noninvasive mechanical ventilation. The chest X-ray (C) showed bilateral alveolar infiltrates. The echocardiogram disclosed a moderate pericardial effusion and diffuse hypokinesia.

On day 31, she had two episodes of seizures and required intubation. All microbiological tests were negative. The Giemsa stain on bronchoalveolar lavage fluid was negative. A second bronchoalveolar lavage performed on day 42 because of clinical deterioration showed *T. gondii* tachyzoites.

Retrospective PCR analysis of bronchoalveolar lavage fluid obtained on day 31 was positive. Tests for IgM antibodies were negative.

Treatment with pyrimethamine and clindamycin was started, but the patient died on day 59 from multiple organ failure and fungal superinfection.

References

1. Duband S, Cornillon J, Tavernier E, Dumollard JM, Guyotat D, Peoc'h M (2008) Toxoplasmosis with hemophagocytic syndrome after bone marrow transplantation: diagnosis at autopsy. Transpl Infect Dis 10(5):372–374
2. Edvinsson B, Lappalainen M, Anttila VJ, Paetau A, Evengard B (2009) Toxoplasmosis in immunocompromised patients. Scand J Infect Dis 41(5):368–371
3. Roxby AC, Gottlieb GS, Limaye AP (2009) Strongyloidiasis in transplant patients. Clin Infect Dis 49(9):1411–1423
4. Wirk B, Wingard JR (2009) Strongyloides stercoralis hyperinfection in hematopoietic stem cell transplantation. Transpl Infect Dis 11(2):143–148
5. Darde ML (2008) Toxoplasma gondii, "new" genotypes and virulence. Parasite 15(3):366–371
6. Maubon D, Ajzenberg D, Brenier-Pinchart MP, Darde ML, Pelloux H (2008) What are the respective host and parasite contributions to toxoplasmosis? Trends Parasitol 24(7): 299–303
7. Ajzenberg D, Yera H, Marty P et al (2009) Genotype of 88 Toxoplasma gondii isolates associated with toxoplasmosis in immunocompromised patients and correlation with clinical findings. J Infect Dis 199(8):1155–1167
8. Fricker-Hidalgo H, Bulabois CE, Brenier-Pinchart MP et al (2009) Diagnosis of toxoplasmosis after allogeneic stem cell transplantation: results of DNA detection and serological techniques. Clin Infect Dis 48(2):e9–e15
9. Martino R, Bretagne S, Einsele H et al (2005) Early detection of Toxoplasma infection by molecular monitoring of Toxoplasma gondii in peripheral blood samples after allogeneic stem cell transplantation. Clin Infect Dis 40(1): 67–78
10. Sugiyama K, Hasegawa Y, Nagasawa T, Hitomi S (2006) Exposure of medical staff to Strongyloides stercolaris from a patient with disseminated strongyloidiasis. J Infect Chemother 12(4):217–219
11. Siddiqui AA, Berk SL (2001) Diagnosis of Strongyloides stercoralis infection. Clin Infect Dis 33(7):1040–1047
12. Keiser PB, Nutman TB (2004) Strongyloides stercoralis in the immunocompromised population. Clin Microbiol Rev 17(1):208–217
13. Pomeroy C, Filice GA (1992) Pulmonary toxoplasmosis: a review. Clin Infect Dis 14(4):863–870
14. Rabaud C, May T, Lucet JC, Leport C, Ambroise-Thomas P, Canton P (1996) Pulmonary toxoplasmosis in patients infected with human immunodeficiency virus: a French National Survey. Clin Infect Dis 23(6):1249–1254
15. de Medeiros BC, de Medeiros CR, Werner B, Loddo G, Pasquini R, Bleggi-Torres LF (2001) Disseminated toxoplasmosis after bone marrow transplantation: report of 9 cases. Transpl Infect Dis 3(1):24–28
16. Derouin F, Pelloux H (2008) Prevention of toxoplasmosis in transplant patients. Clin Microbiol Infect 14(12): 1089–1101
17. Meers S, Lagrou K, Theunissen K et al (2010) Myeloablative conditioning predisposes patients for Toxoplasma gondii reactivation after allogeneic stem cell transplantation. Clin Infect Dis 50:1127–1134
18. Peleg AY, Husain S, Kwak EJ et al (2007) Opportunistic infections in 547 organ transplant recipients receiving alemtuzumab, a humanized monoclonal CD-52 antibody. Clin Infect Dis 44(2):204–212
19. Martin SI, Marty FM, Fiumara K, Treon SP, Gribben JG, Baden LR (2006) Infectious complications associated with alemtuzumab use for lymphoproliferative disorders. Clin Infect Dis 43(1):16–24
20. Mele A, Paterson PJ, Prentice HG, Leoni P, Kibbler CC (2002) Toxoplasmosis in bone marrow transplantation: a report of two cases and systematic review of the literature. Bone Marrow Transplant 29(8):691–698
21. Escuissato DL, de Aguiar RO, Gasparetto EL, Muller NL (2004) Disseminated toxoplasmosis after bone marrow transplantation: high-resolution CT appearance. J Thorac Imaging 19(3):207–209
22. Montoya JG, Liesenfeld O (2004) Toxoplasmosis. Lancet 363(9425):1965–1976
23. Ortonne N, Ribaud P, Meignin V et al (2001) Toxoplasmic pneumonitis leading to fatal acute respiratory distress syndrome after engraftment in three bone marrow transplant recipients. Transplantation 72(11):1838–1840
24. Laibe S, Ranque S, Curtillet C, Faraut F, Dumon H, Franck J (2006) Timely diagnosis of disseminated toxoplasmosis by sputum examination. J Clin Microbiol 44(2):646–648
25. Sing A, Leitritz L, Roggenkamp A et al (1999) Pulmonary toxoplasmosis in bone marrow transplant recipients: report of two cases and review. Clin Infect Dis 29(2):429–433
26. Dulley FL, Costa S, Cosentino R, Gamba C, Saboya R (2009) Strongyloides stercoralis hyperinfection after allogeneic stem cell transplantation. Bone Marrow Transplant 43(9):741–742

27. Safdar A, Malathum K, Rodriguez SJ, Husni R, Rolston KV (2004) Strongyloidiasis in patients at a comprehensive cancer center in the United States. Cancer 100(7):1531–1536
28. Orlent H, Crawley C, Cwynarski K, Dina R, Apperley J (2003) Strongyloidiasis pre and post autologous peripheral blood stem cell transplantation. Bone Marrow Transplant 32(1):115–117
29. Roman-Velez JM, Martinez-Camacho RN, Alayon-Laguer D et al (2009) An unusual presentation of alveolar hemorrhage. Prim Care Respir J 18(4):337–339
30. Schaffel R, Portugal R, Maiolino A, Nucci M (2004) Strongyloidiasis pre and post autologous peripheral blood stem cell transplantation. Bone Marrow Transplant 33(1):117
31. ten Hove RJ, van Esbroeck M, Vervoort T, van den Ende J, van Lieshout L, Verweij JJ (2009) Molecular diagnostics of intestinal parasites in returning travellers. Eur J Clin Microbiol Infect Dis 28(9):1045–1053
32. Segarra-Newnham M (2007) Manifestations, diagnosis, and treatment of Strongyloides stercoralis infection. Ann Pharmacother 41(12):1992–2001
33. Roemer E, Blau IW, Basara N et al (2001) Toxoplasmosis, a severe complication in allogeneic hematopoietic stem cell transplantation: successful treatment strategies during a 5-year single-center experience. Clin Infect Dis 32(1):E1–8
34. Martino R, Cordonnier C (2003) Toxoplasmosis following allogeneic hematopoietic stem cell transplantation. Bone Marrow Transplant 31(7):617–618, author reply 9

30 Pulmonary Mycobacterial Infections in Patients with Hematological Malignancies

Khalid A. Al-Anazi and Asma M. Al-Jasser

Contents

K.A. Al-Anazi (✉)
Section of Adult Hematology and Hematopoietic Stem Cell Transplantation, Oncology Centre, King Fahad Specialist Hospital, P.O. Box 15215, Dammam 31444, Saudi Arabia
e-mail: kaa_alanazi@yahoo.com

A.M. Al-Jasser
Central Laboratory, Ministry of Health, P.O. Box 61734, Riyadh 11575, Saudi Arabia
e-mail: asjass2007@gmail.com

30.1 Introduction

Patients with hematological malignancies are at increased risk for infection with *Mycobacterium tuberculosis* and nontuberculous mycobacteria (NTM), which usually (but not consistently) manifest as pulmonary disease [1, 4, 9, 21, 93, 98]. Tuberculosis (TB) may be either active or latent. Latent TB is clinically silent and is not contagious, but can undergo reactivation when the malignancy or treatment causes immunosuppression [23]. Patients should be evaluated and sometimes treated for latent TB infection when they are diagnosed with immunosuppressive conditions or before starting treatment with immunosuppressive agents such as corticosteroids or monoclonal antibodies [67]. Both TB and NTM infection may progress rapidly to severe disseminated disease in immunocompromised patients, making the early diagnosis crucial, as specific antimicrobial agents must be given [40, 47, 96, 107, 110].

30.2 Incidence and Risk Factors of Tuberculosis in Patients with Hematological Malignancies

The incidence of mycobacterial infections in patients with hematological malignancies largely depends on the background incidence in the community and ranges from ninefold to 22-fold of that in the general population [10, 56, 97]. TB prevalence in these patients ranges from less than 1% to more than 10% [93]. Reactivation of latent TB is common and often causes severe disseminated disease [96]. When TB occurs as a complication of diagnosed hematological malignancies, the mean time from chemotherapy completion to development of

É. Azoulay (ed.), *Pulmonary Involvement in Patients with Hematological Malignancies*,
DOI: 10.1007/978-3-642-15742-4_30,

TB is 3–20 months [1, 4, 56]. TB does not usually delay chemotherapy and, once treated, rarely flares up during subsequent chemotherapy cycles [65].

Among hematological malignancies, acute leukemia has the strongest association with TB [56, 65]. A high index of suspicion should be maintained in patients with acute leukemia living in areas of TB endemicity [4, 97]. In adults, TB is more common in acute myeloid leukemia than in acute lymphoblastic leukemia, despite the use of steroids and radiotherapy to treat this disease. TB is also common in patients with hairy cell leukemia, chronic myelogenous leukemia, chronic lymphocytic leukemia, multiple myeloma, Hodgkin's and non-Hodgkin's lymphoma, and myelodysplastic syndrome [1, 4, 38, 56, 64, 69, 93, 97]. Among lymphomas, nodular sclerotic Hodgkin's disease has the strongest association with TB [62]. Tyrosine kinase inhibitors and monoclonal antibodies used to treat hematological malignancies have been associated with TB (Table 30.1) [9, 18]. In chronic TB, CD8+ T-cells assist macrophages in controlling the intracellular mycobacteria via a mechanism orchestrated by the T-cell receptor. The tyrosine kinase inhibitor imatinib affects T-cell receptor signal transduction, suggesting a mechanism by which imatinib might increase the risk of TB reactivation [18]. Also, in areas of TB endemicity, patients scheduled to receive the monoclonal antibody alemtuzumab should undergo a careful initial evaluation to determine whether prophylactic anti-TB therapy is in order [9].

Table 30.1 Risk factors for mycobacterial infections in patients with hematologic malignancy

1. The primary disease causing reduced immunity; particularly in relapse
2. Old age
3. Cytotoxic chemotherapy
4. Corticosteroid therapy
5. Radiotherapy
6. Other immunosuppressive therapies, e.g., monoclonal antibodies, tyrosine kinase inhibitors, etc.
7. Other comorbidities, e.g., diabetes mellitus, malnutrition, weight loss, etc.
8. Hematopoietic stem cell transplant:
(a) Graft-versus-host disease; acute and chronic
(b) T-cell depletion
(c) Matched unrelated allografts
(d) Total body irradiation and cyclophosphamide conditioning
(e) Bronchiolitis obliterans

Identification of risk factors for TB may be useful for TB prevention and earlier TB diagnosis. Risk factors for TB in patients with hematological malignancies include malnutrition; age older than 50 years; corticosteroid therapy; cytotoxic agents, particularly fludarabine; radiotherapy, a history of active TB; and residing in an endemic area (Table 30.1) [4, 6, 93]. Intravenous cytotoxic chemotherapy is associated with earlier and more disseminated TB infection compared to oral cytotoxic chemotherapy [4]. Routine screening of patients for latent TB infection and exclusion of active disease prior to cancer chemotherapy initiation may be discussed in endemic areas [17, 67]. Prophylactic anti-TB treatment of patients with a history of TB should help to minimize the risk of TB reactivation [4, 10, 96]. Chemotherapy solutions may undergo contamination with the BCG when prepared under biosafety hoods also used to prepare BCG solutions for bladder cancer treatment [111].

30.3 Clinical Presentations of Tuberculosis in Patients with Hematological Malignancies

Although the lungs are involved in 70–90% of TB cases in patients with hematological malignancies [1, 93], dissemination to other sites is common [19, 46, 69]. Disseminated TB with miliary lung densities and pleural effusions develops in 10–15% of patients [1, 44, 46]. Risk factors for disseminated TB include advanced age, female sex, immunosuppression, diabetes mellitus, and weight loss (Table 30.1) [29, 107]. Disseminated TB may produce a variety of nonspecific symptoms, such as fever of unknown origin, anorexia, malaise, weight loss, cough, night sweats, headache, neck stiffness, choroid tubercles, altered mental status, abdominal pain, and hepatosplenomegaly [29, 63, 69]. Therefore, a high index of suspicion should be maintained so that appropriate investigations are conducted promptly. Disseminated TB is curable provided the diagnosis is made early and the treatment initiated promptly [4, 29, 63, 69, 107]. Specific treatment of macrophage activation syndrome may help to prevent associated organ dysfunction. In patients with advanced hematological malignancies, 27% of cases of disseminated TB are diagnosed at autopsy [29].

Pulmonary TB may manifest as TB pneumonia or cavitation. In a study in hematopoietic stem cell transplant (HSCT) recipients, the most common presenting symptom was a fever in TB pneumonia and hemoptysis in TB cavitation. Cavitation was often located in the upper lobes and diagnosed early, whereas TB pneumonia was randomly distributed and often diagnosed late [54]. TB infection shares similar clinical and radiological features to those seen in infections due to NTM [10].

30.4 Diagnosis of Active Tuberculosis

30.4.1 Clinical Manifestations

The early diagnosis of TB is particularly important in patients with hematological malignancies, given the high risk of severe and rapidly progressive disseminated disease [107]. Careful attention should be given to clinical symptoms such as persistent cough, pyrexia, night sweats, dyspnea, hemoptysis, or chest pain [41, 42, 93]. However, these symptoms are not specific and may overlap with those of the hematological malignancy, and the immunodeficiency may attenuate the symptoms of TB. Therefore, a high level of suspicion is crucial [2, 19, 93, 97].

30.4.1.1 First-Line Investigations

Sputum smear examination is the mainstay of the diagnosis of pulmonary TB, but is often negative in immunocompromised patients. Furthermore, staining does not differentiate *M. tuberculosis* from NTMs [90, 100].

Once TB is suspected, a chest radiograph should be obtained [19]. Findings vary widely and may include areas of consolidation consistent with pneumonia, fine reticulonodular shadows consistent with pulmonary fibrosis, calcification, pleural effusions, lymph node enlargement, basal atelectasis, cavity formation, and miliary shadows (Figs. 30.1, 30.2 and 30.4). However, the chest radiograph is normal in a substantial proportion of patients [4, 44, 63, 69, 102].

Routine laboratory tests may show a variety of abnormalities. Anemia is common and is usually mild and responsive to anti-TB treatment, although a hemolytic or immune mechanism may be involved [55, 72, 94]. Other hematological abnormalities may include leukocytosis, neutrophilia, lymphocytosis, lymphocytopenia, monocytosis, monocytopenia, thrombocytosis, and thrombocytopenia [4, 55, 66, 70, 94]. Immune thrombocytopenic purpura, thrombotic thrombocytopenic purpura, and hemophagocytic syndrome have been reported [72, 106]. Hematological abnormalities may be associated with a poor prognosis [35, 37]. Other abnormalities reported in patients with TB and possibly mediated by macrophage activation syndrome include elevated erythrocyte sedimentation rate; high serum levels of ferritin, vitamin B_{12}, alkaline phosphatase, and lactic dehydrogenase; low serum levels of albumin, sodium, and calcium; hypoxemia; and hyponatremia. Another possible feature is liver dysfunction, mainly in the form of hepatic transaminase elevation [29, 37, 58, 63, 69, 70, 109].

The tuberculin skin test (TST) may be positive in about one-third of cases, although this may indicate infection with other mycobacterial species or vaccination with the BCG [18, 63]. Two interferon-gamma release assays (IGRAs) intended for use on blood samples have emerged as alternatives to the TST [13, 52, 82]. In patients with TB, interferon-gamma [INF-γ] is released from T-cells after stimulation with specific TB antigens (ESAT-6 and CFP-10) that are highly specific for *M. tuberculosis* but absent from the BCG and most NTMs [13, 19, 52, 81, 82]. A positive result indicates a cellular immune response to *M. tuberculosis*. Although IGRAs were designed to detect latent TB, they may assist in the diagnosis of active TB in immunocompromised individuals. However, a negative result does not rule out active TB [19].

30.4.1.2 Other Investigations

CT of the chest may rapidly provide valuable clues to the diagnosis of TB and allows an accurate assessment of the extent, pattern, and sites of TB infection, and provides information on complications such as cavities, bronchogenic spread, bronchiectasis, and aspergillomas (Fig. 30.2) [51, 102]. Serial CT scans are helpful in monitoring disease progression [51]. However, CT of the lung may lack

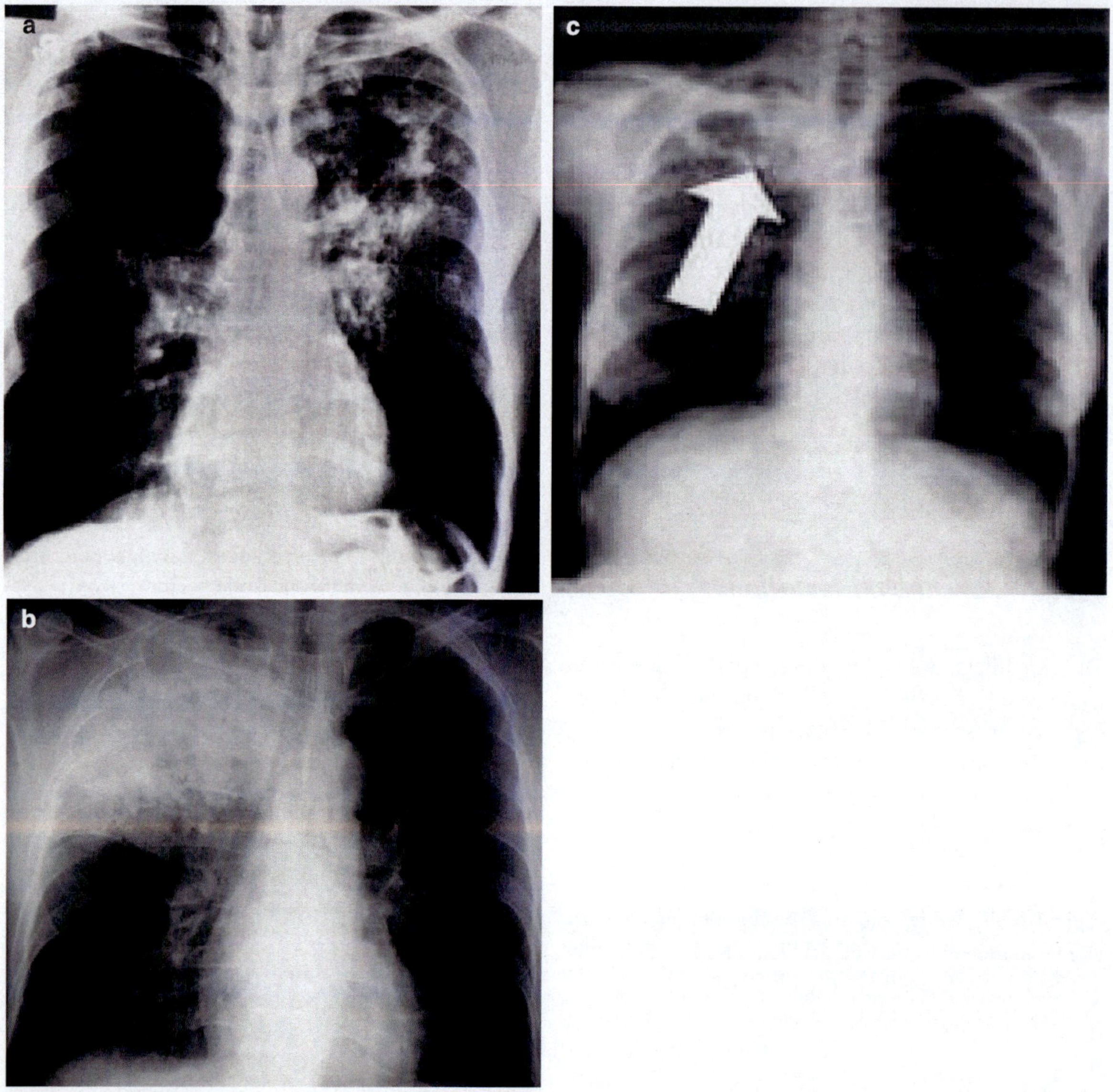

Fig. 30.1 (**a**) Bilateral hilar lymphadenopathy and scarring of upper lobe of left lung. (**b**) Tuberculous consolidation involving right upper lobe. (**c**) Cavitation of upper lobe of the right lung due to tuberculosis. Figure 30.1 shows various radiological appearances of pulmonary tuberculosis

accuracy in febrile immunocompromised patients because of the absence of the typical cavitary consolidations of TB [22]. On positron emission tomography (PET) scans, pulmonary tuberculomas are commonly visible as foci of increased uptake. Therefore, in regions of TB endemicity, positive PET scan results may indicate TB rather than lung involvement by the malignancy [32].

In patients with pulmonary TB, cultures of sputum and bronchoalveolar lavage (BAL) fluid may recover the organism. BAL is a good alternative to more invasive investigations that are risky in these frail patients [15, 73]. When the infection is disseminated, blood and bone marrow cultures may be positive, and histological examination of biopsies from lymph nodes, bone marrow, and/or the liver may show the organism and/or granulomas [63, 69]. Thus, bone marrow examination usually shows decreased iron stores, histiomonocytosis, granulomas without giant cells, a positive Ziehl–Neelsen stain, and positive cultures (Fig. 30.3) [35, 58, 63, 69].

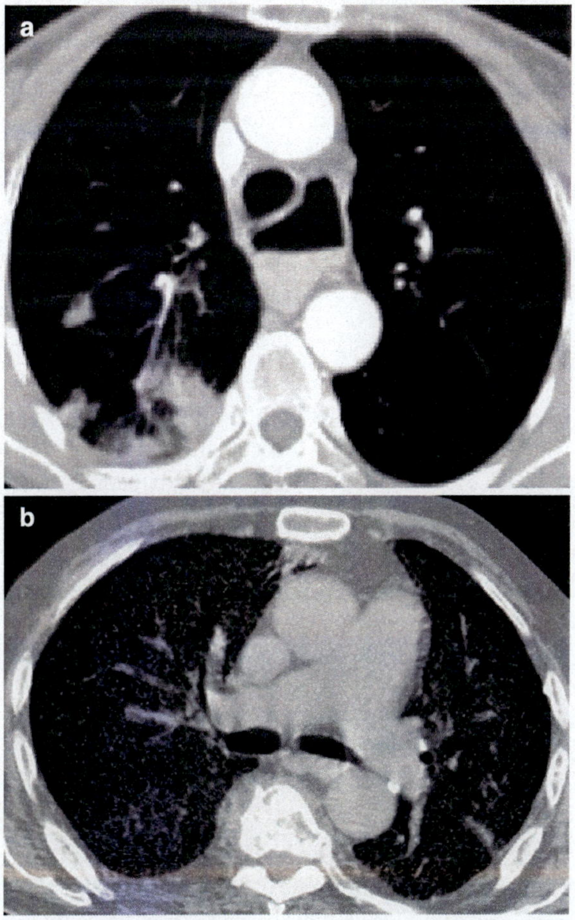

Fig. 30.2 (**a**) CAT scan showing upper lobe consolidation and a solitary nodule. (**b**) CAT scan of lungs showing diffuse miliary micronodular shadows. Figure 30.2 shows various CAT scan appearances in pulmonary tuberculosis

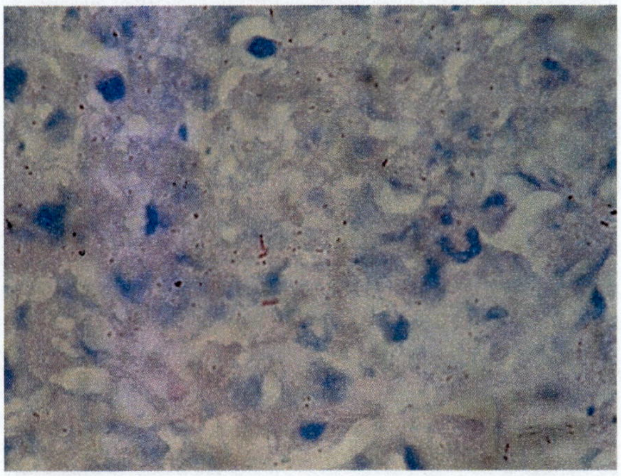

Fig. 30.3 Shows Ziehl-Nelsen stain for acid-fast bacilli on a lung biopsy specimen

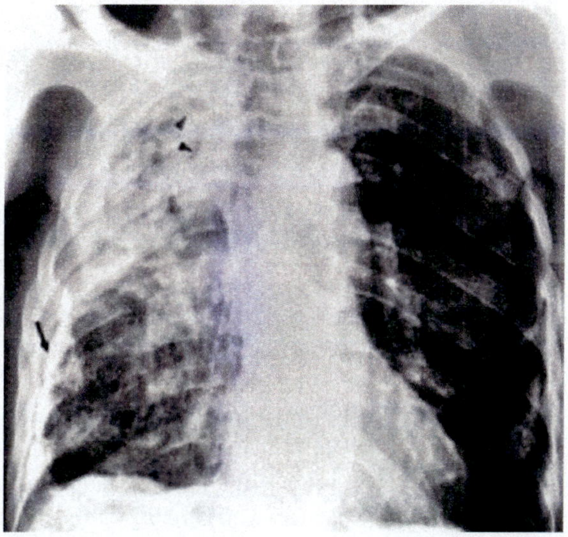

Fig. 30.4 Shows an *Aspergillus* ball in a tuberculous cavity on a chest X-ray

Axial mediastinoscopy may deserve consideration in selected patients with lesions in the axial mediastinum, given its good yield, low cost, and few contraindications. A large retrospective study of axial mediastinoscopy in patients with various mediastinal lesions, including TB and lymphoma, showed that global sensitivity, global specificity, accuracy, and mortality were 94%, 100%, 95%, and 0.0%, respectively [80].

Recent studies have shown that elevated CA-125 levels are found in several infections, including TB. The CA-125 level can serve as a marker of the treatment response and as an indicator of disease activity [113].

30.4.1.3 New Tests for Tuberculosis

Many tests for TB have low sensitivity and specificity, and cultures require at least 3 weeks to become positive. Therefore, the development of new rapid tests has generated considerable interest. New versions of nucleic acid amplification (NAA) assays, immune-based assays, a skin patch test, and rapid culture systems have been introduced [76]. NAA assays are 80% sensitive but are highly specific, particularly with respiratory specimens [19]. Their sensitivity is too low and too variable to rule out TB in the event of a negative result, especially in paucibacillary disease with negative smears [30, 57, 74]. Nested PCR-restriction fragment length polymorphism analysis focusing on the *hsp 65* gene performed well on 204 smear-positive and culture-positive sputum specimens [114]. The new molecular techniques are expected to complement rather than to replace conventional diagnostic tools. Further studies are needed to assess performance and to standardize assay procedures. Then guidelines will have to be developed on how best to use the new tools. Cost-effectiveness and economic constraints will have to be evaluated, particularly in low-income countries [100].

Serological (antibody-mediated) tests have been available for many years, although no guidelines recommend their use for diagnosing TB [19]. Published data on commercial serological tests provide inconsistent estimates of sensitivity and specificity. Combinations of carefully selected peptides derived from highly immunogenic proteins are being evaluated for use in immunodiagnostic tests for TB [90].

New tests are being developed for use in the laboratory. For instance, nucleic acid probes can be used to identify cultured organisms. Several new tests assist in detecting drug resistance [77, 100].

30.4.1.4 Therapeutic Trial

Despite recent improvements in clinical and laboratory methods, the diagnosis of mycobacterial infections may still take weeks [10]. Microbiological studies may be negative in one-half to three-fourths of patients, and histological specimens may fail to show acid-fast bacilli (AFB) and typical epithelioid-cell granulomas with caseation necrosis [4, 19, 46, 62]. Thus, many patients receive a presumptive diagnosis of TB based on the clinical and radiological manifestations. In this situation, a trial of anti-TB therapy may be justified [19, 41]. In patients with TB, the response to anti-TB medications is usually prompt and dramatic despite the immune system suppression [4, 38, 41, 46, 62, 65, 97]. If no clinical or radiological improvement is achieved within 2 months, the use of empirical therapy should be reevaluated [19].

30.5 Outcomes and Treatment of Tuberculosis in Patients with Hematological Malignancies

30.5.1 Antituberculous Drug Therapy

30.5.1.1 Antituberculous Drugs

Early appropriate anti-TB treatment is effective [76]. However, a fatal outcome has been reported in 5%–10% of cases, and in patients who are diagnosed late and who have disseminated TB the mortality rate may reach 62.5% [2, 4, 46, 62, 65, 93]. Attributable mortality of TB in patients with hematological malignancies has ranged from 21% to 62.5% [4, 21, 93]. Postmortem examinations in these patients should include bacteriological and histological studies to establish the correct diagnosis [84].

The standard short-course therapy for TB recommended by the World Health Organization (WHO) is based on a four-drug regimen that must be strictly followed to prevent the acquisition of drug resistance. Direct observation of patient compliance is provided to ensure effective treatment. *M. tuberculosis* mutants resistant to any single drug are naturally present in any large bacterial population, irrespective of exposure to drugs. The frequency of mutants resistant to rifampin and INH is relatively high, and therefore the large extracellular population of actively metabolizing and rapidly growing tubercle bacilli in cavitary lesions contains organisms that are resistant to a single drug. The concomitant administration of multiple drugs is consequently crucial to avoid selecting drug-resistant mutants [24].

Immunocompromised patients with TB should be treated for 9–12 months with INH and rifampin combined initially with ethambutol, streptomycin, or pyrazinamide [4, 95]. However, the treatment may need to be prolonged if the response is slow, and patients should be followed up carefully after the treatment to detect early relapses [95].

The current resurgence of TB, which is mainly ascribable to the development of multidrug resistant (MDR) and extensively drug-resistant (XDR) strains, has increased the need for studies into the molecular mechanisms of drug effects and drug resistance, which should provide valuable information for developing new compounds [24]. Unfortunately, since the introduction of rifampin 40 years ago, only two anti-TB drugs have been marketed, rifabutin and rifapentine [104]. Nonclinical and clinical studies are focusing on the development of new and faster-acting anti-TB compounds, e.g., moxifloxacin, nitroimidazole, oxazolidinones, diarylquinoline, and rifamycin derivatives [104, 105]. Unfortunately, the development of adjuvant immunotherapy for TB is not progressing [104].

30.5.1.2 Compliance and Tolerance

Noncompliance with anti-TB treatment regimens increases morbidity and mortality rates, perpetuates transmission, and generates bacterial resistance. Data on the incidence and risk factors of noncompliance are needed to design interventions. Risk factors for noncompliance include treatment required for more than 2 months, low socioeconomic status, age between 21 and 30 years, and a history of skipping more than two doses. Direct observation of treatment may be needed to ensure adequate compliance. Another strategy consists of providing support to the family and intervening immediately in the event of missed doses [12].

Although *M. tuberculosis* is eradicated rapidly during therapy in some patients with pulmonary TB, it may persist for many months in others. Tolerance to anti-TB medications emerges after prolonged drug exposure and may be an important determinant of the outcome of TB therapy [112].

30.5.1.3 Side Effects

Major adverse reactions to anti-TB drugs can cause significant morbidity and limit the use of anti-TB medications. Risk factors include female sex, age older than 60 years, and birthplace in Asia [116]. The incidence of major side effects from first-line anti-TB agents was highest with pyrazinamide and lowest with ethambutol. More specifically, the rates of hepatotoxicity and rash were substantially higher with pyrazinamide than with other first-line anti-TB drugs and higher than previously reported [116].

Anti-TB drug-induced hepatotoxicity is not uncommon and is significantly more frequent in patients with pre-existing liver disease, low basal metabolic index, and extensive or open pulmonary TB. Early diagnosis and treatment is crucial, particularly in developing countries where both TB and liver disease are common [60]. INH-induced hepatitis is uncommon, but when it occurs it resolves completely if the drug is stopped early enough. Fatal forms of hepatitis are extremely rare if the patients are monitored closely. The overall mortality rate from INH hepatotoxicity is less than 0.01% [17, 88].

Agranulocytosis (pancytopenia) has been reported in patients receiving anti-TB treatment. It usually develops 1–3 months after starting treatment and is allergic in nature [92]. Leukopenia may develop during anti-TB treatment, but does not require immediate treatment discontinuation, as the leukocyte count recovers spontaneously or remains stable during treatment in most instances. Patients who develop leukopenia due to anti-TB drugs may have weaker natural or acquired immunological responses to TB infection and greater vulnerability of bone marrow and hepatic cells to anti-TB agents [68].

30.5.1.4 Corticosteroid Therapy

Patients with hematological malignancies often receive corticosteroid therapy as part of their anticancer regimen [14]. In patients with TB infection, corticosteroid therapy is indicated in some forms of extrapulmonary disease such as pleurisy, meningitis, pericarditis, and adrenal gland infection. Other indications include endobronchial disease, hypersensitivity reactions to drugs or infection, and severe systemic manifestations due to pulmonary or extrapulmonary infection [7, 14, 28].

The usual prednisone dose is 40–60 mg/day orally for 4–6 weeks depending on the system involved, after which the dose is tapered gradually [7]. Randomized, placebo-controlled studies are required to determine the role for corticosteroids in the standard therapy of TB [7, 14]. Corticosteroids may interact with other medications, e.g., oral contraceptives and rifampin [7].

30.5.1.5 Surgery

In patients with malignant hematological disorders and tuberculomas or localized tuberculous pulmonary cavitations, surgical resection of the involved segment or lobe may be essential not only to eradicate pulmonary TB, especially if the infection is caused by an MDR organism, but also to prevent the development of further complications such as aspergilloma (Fig. 30.3) after further immune depression occurs due to disease progression or cytotoxic chemotherapy [6, 99, 101].

30.6 Multidrug Resistant Tuberculosis

The emergence of MDR-TB and, more recently, of XDR-TB is a major threat to TB control and eradication. The prevalences of MDR-TB and XDR-TB are inversely proportional to the quality of TB control and of second-line anti-TB drug utilization [61]. For some MDR-TB and XDR-TB strains, no curative treatment is available. Concern that these strains may spread around the world is prompting active research into new diagnostic tools, anti-TB drugs, and TB vaccines [77]. The risk of uncontrollable MDR-TB and XDR-TB outbreaks is real considering the current levels of financing and commitment to care [61]. Global risk factors for MDR-TB include a history of anti-TB treatment and a known contact with a person having drug-resistant TB [33].

Traditional laboratory methods for detecting drug resistance are slow and not generally available outside specialized laboratories [33]. Rapid molecular methods are increasingly used in well-resourced settings, and simple cheap alternatives are being developed for resource-limited settings [33, 64]. Line-probe assays, bacteriophage-based assays, molecular beacons, and the microscopic-observation drug-susceptibility assay can assist in detecting drug resistance [76, 77, 100].

The prevention of drug-resistant TB rests on optimizing compliance with anti-TB therapy and promptly detecting resistant strains [33]. Few data are available to guide the drug treatment of resistant TB. Well-designed regimens based largely on second-line anti-TB drugs can considerably improve cure rates [61]. However, new drugs free of cross-resistance with known antimycobacterial agents are urgently needed [105].

30.7 Latent Tuberculosis

30.7.1 Diagnosis of Latent Tuberculosis

Identifying and treating patients with latent TB infection are crucial to prevent reactivation [23, 81]. Until recently, the diagnosis of latent TB infection relied solely on the century-old TST, which has a number of limitations [13, 52]. In immunocompromised individuals, an induration of 5 mm or more is considered positive [17, 67]. The TST results may be falsely negative due to drug therapy or to anergy related to the malignancy [17]. Two-step testing may increase the TST yield [67]. The introduction of two IGRAs (T-SPOT. TB and QuantiFERON-TB gold) is a major advance [13, 52, 67, 82]. Immunosuppression does not affect the performance of these tests, which can identify a large proportion of TB-infected patients with anergy to tuberculin [13, 19, 49, 52, 67, 75, 79, 81, 82]. However, the QuantiFERON-TB gold test may produce negative or indeterminate results in immunocompromised patients [49]. IGRAs may be particularly helpful in regions where widespread BCG vaccination limits the usefulness of the TST [13, 19, 49, 52, 67, 75, 79, 81, 82]. IGRAs may decrease the unnecessary use of anti-TB drugs in patients with positive TSTs because of BCG vaccination [52, 75].

The Canadian Tuberculosis Committee on IGRAs for diagnosing latent TB infection in immunocompromised individuals has issued the following recommendations: (1) TST should be used first; (2) if the TST is positive, a diagnosis of latent TB infection is given; (3) if the TST is negative and the clinician is still concerned about the possibility of latent TB infection, an IGRA test may be performed; (4) if the IGRA result is positive, the person may be considered to have latent TB infection; and (5) if the IGRA result is indeterminate, the test should be repeated to rule out laboratory error [13].

30.7.1.1 Tuberculosis Chemoprophylaxis in Patients with Hematological Malignancies

Immunosuppressive therapy and leukemia increase the risk of progression to active TB. INH chemoprophylaxis has been recommended in some groups of immunocompromised patients, including patients with hematological malignancies and/or iatrogenic immunosuppression. The usual dosage is 300 mg/day for 6–12 months [17, 71, 88, 115]. Patients with evidence of latent TB who require prolonged high-dose corticosteroid therapy (more than 10 mg/day of prednisolone) should receive chemoprophylaxis [115]. New guidelines recommend INH treatment for 6–9 months or rifampin for 4 months or with rifampin plus pyrazinamide for 2 months [17].

30.8 Nontuberculous Mycobacterial Infections

30.8.1 Diagnosis of NTM Nontuberculous Mycobacterial Infections

NTM infection is not a communicable disease, although health care-associated outbreaks have been reported. *M. avium* complex (MAC) is the main NTM responsible for disease in humans [78, 103]. Lung involvement with a chronic productive cough, dyspnea, and hemoptysis is the most common presentation, although any organ can be affected [78]. NTMs are often difficult to identify, but repeated culturing of various sources including bone marrow may help to establish the diagnosis early [40]. When cultures are negative but serum alkaline phosphatase is elevated, a liver biopsy should be considered. Early diagnosis and prompt therapy are important, as NTM infection in patients with hematological malignancies may manifest as severe disseminated disease. Among hematological malignancies, hairy cell leukemia and chronic myelogenous leukemia may predispose patients more particularly to disseminated NTM infection [36, 47, 110].

NTM infection may be difficult to differentiate from colonization. Treatment of NTM pulmonary infection requires 18–24 months of treatment with multiple drugs selected based on the infecting species. This drug treatment is expensive, frequently noncurative, and associated with substantial side effects. Therefore, it is warranted only in patients with sufficient NTM-related pathology. The likelihood of infection as opposed to colonization is greater in patients receiving intensive cytotoxic chemotherapy and in those with previous pulmonary involvement by the malignancy. Clinicians must cooperate with microbiologists, pathologists, and radiologists to improve treatment outcomes [50, 78, 83].

M. kansasii may cause pulmonary or disseminated infection in patients with hematological malignancies. A single isolation of the organism may not be clinically significant, and the diagnosis can only be established after a second isolation unless the clinical situation strongly supports infection. Lung cavitation is the main radiological presentation [25, 27]. In a study of 12 patients with the slow-growing NTM *M. lentiflavum*, 11 (92%) patients had a hematological malignancy [86]. However, slow-growing NTMs are very rarely a probable cause of infection. Risk factors for infections due to slow-growing mycobacteria are severe lymphocytopenia, systemic steroids, and acute graft-versus-host disease (GvHD) in hematopoietic stem-cell transplant (HSCT) recipients (Table 30.1) [86]. Rapidly growing mycobacteria cause colonization about eight times more often than they cause true infection. Nevertheless, infection with these organisms should be considered in patients with pulmonary infiltrates, particularly those treated with intensive chemotherapeutic regimens [83].

30.8.1.1 Treatment of Nontuberculous Mycobacterial Infections

NTM infections are usually difficult to treat, as they do not respond to traditional anti-TB agents. At least three effective drugs are usually required for at least 12 months after sputum cultures become negative [50, 78]. Novel antimicrobial agents including clarithromycin and azithromycin were effective in three pediatric patients with acute lymphoblastic leukemia and NTM infection [98].

The new macrolides have shown limited effectiveness in patients with MAC disease [87]. Patients with macrolide-resistant MAC isolates have higher mortality rates than patients with macrolide-susceptible isolates. Since the advent of the new macrolides, no substantial progress has been made in the treatment of MAC lung disease or NTM infections in general. First-line treatment offers the best opportunity for a cure, and protection against the emergence of macrolide-resistant MAC isolates is crucial [34]. MAC isolates are usually susceptible to clofazidime, cycloserine, and ansamycin and resistant to isoniazid, streptomycin, ethambutol, rifampin, and ethionamide [47].

The pulmonary diseases caused by certain types of NTM such as *M. kansasii* or *M. szulgai* are usually treated with rifampin, ethambutol, and isoniazid, i.e., the same regimens that generally lead to satisfactory results in patients with TB [87]. Although rifampin-based conventional and combined chemotherapy is usually effective in the treatment of *M. kansasii* infections, persistence and recurrence develop in 11% and 7% of patients, respectively [25, 27, 43]. On the other hand, *M. lentiflavum* is usually susceptible to isoniazid, ethambutol, clarithromycin, and amikacin, but resistant to rifampin [87].

In patients infected with NTM, the main indications for surgical resection are continuous hemoptysis, continuous productive cough, exacerbation of CXR features, and localized disease that fails medical management [78, 87].

30.9 Mycobacterial Infections in Stem-Cell Transplant Recipients

Cell-mediated immunity is severely impaired in allogeneic HSCT recipients due to pre-transplant conditioning regimens, immunosuppressive therapy, and GvHD. These patients have a 10- to 40-fold increase in the mycobacterial infection rate compared to the general population [11, 20, 26, 48].

The incidence of mycobacterial infections varies considerably according to the type of HSCT, type of infective mycobacteria, and incidence in the local general population [3–5, 8, 16, 20, 21, 26, 39, 53, 91, 117]. In allogeneic HSCT recipients, it ranges from 0.49% to 9.7% [4, 5, 11, 16, 21, 26, 31, 39, 53, 59, 85]. The incidence of NTM infections in allogeneic HSCT recipients is approximately 1.9% [8]. Among allogeneic HSCT recipients, those with acute or chronic myelogenous leukemia or myelodysplastic syndrome are at highest risk for mycobacterial infections. Other risk factors include the use of total body irradiation, cyclophosphamide, and busulphan in the conditioning regimen; acute or chronic extensive GvHD; corticosteroid therapy; T-cell depletion in allografts; mismatched allografts or matched unrelated donor grafts; and previous history of TB infection (Table 30.1) [4, 5, 16, 20, 26, 39, 53]. Factors selectively associated with NTM infections in HSCT recipients include leukemia relapse, mismatched allografts or matched unrelated donor grafts, acute GvHD, and bronchiolitis obliterans (Table 30.1) [8].

Mycobacterial infections develop within 45–365 days after allograft transplantation [4, 5, 11, 16, 20, 39, 53, 59]. The lungs are involved in 50%–100% of patients [4, 5, 8, 11, 20, 39]. Clinical manifestations include unexplained pyrexia, cough, dyspnea, and pleuritic chest pain. Imaging studies may show air-space consolidation, diffuse reticulonodular shadows predominating in the upper lobe, tree-in-bud appearance, ground-glass opacities, cavity formation, and hilar and mediastinal lymphadenopathy (Figs. 30.1, 30.2 and 30.4). In the absence of prompt treatment, rapid dissemination may occur, with severe pyrexia, adult respiratory distress syndrome (ARDS), hypotension, hypoxia, sepsis, multiorgan failure, and death [4, 16, 20, 21, 39, 48, 85, 91, 108]. Furthermore, dissemination with prominent extrapulmonary manifestations is a feature at presentation in at least one-third of cases [4, 21, 31, 48, 53, 59, 91]. Osteomyelitis and central venous catheter or tunnel infections have been reported in HSCT recipients with NTM infection [85].

The NTMs most often responsible for infections in HSCT recipients are *M. fortuitum*, *M. chelonae*, *M. gordonnae*, *M. scrofolaceum*, and *M. avium intracellular* [8]. Positive microbiological studies for NTM indicate severe immunosuppression and a poor prognosis. NTM may coexist with other pathogens such as *Aspergillus*. Colonization may be difficult to distinguish from infection, despite the development of elaborate but empirical clinical, radiological, and microbiological criteria. The threshold for starting therapy is unclear. However, invasive NTM infections require prolonged therapy [8].

In umbilical cord blood transplant (UCBT) recipients, mycobacterial infections may develop as early as day 45 after transplantation [59]. The risk is greatest in patients with acute myelogenous leukemia, mismatched grafts, T-cell depletion, GvHD, and residence in an area of TB endemicity (Table 30.1). Patients present with pyrexia, a cough, chest pain, and evidence of pneumonia [21, 91]. UCBT recipients may have higher incidences of disseminated mycobacterial infections and reactivation of previous mycobacterial MTB infection compared to other allogeneic HSCT recipients. Lung lesion histology usually shows caseous necrosis without granuloma formation. Combination anti-TB drug therapy is usually of limited efficacy [59].

The diagnosis of mycobacterial infections is challenging in HSCT recipients, who often have mild nonspecific symptoms and no granulomas in histological specimens [21]. In HSCT recipients with diffuse reticulonodular shadows, miliary TB should be suspected, as open lung biopsy shows this condition in 9% of cases. Respiratory failure and acute GvHD are the main events of adverse prognostic significance, and mortality may reach 50% in these patients [45]. Mycobacterial infections in HSCT recipients usually respond well to anti-TB treatment, particularly if the diagnosis is made early [4, 20]. The response rate may reach 90–100% with early treatment, compared to 50% or less when treatment is delayed [4, 20, 89, 107]. No excessive side effects of anti-TB medications have been reported [4, 39]. However, TB in HSCT recipients may complicate the post-transplant management, as anti-TB drugs frequently decrease the serum levels of cyclosporine-A, thus worsening GvHD [20].

INH prophylaxis has been used successfully to prevent TB reactivation in HSCT recipients [4]. However, the possible benefits of routine TB chemoprophylaxis in patients with positive TST results and normal CXR findings should be balanced against the risk of hepatotoxicity in HSCT recipients [5]. Therefore, INH prophylaxis should not be given routinely, but close follow-up and monitoring for reactivation of latent infection are recommended [16]. In patients who have received BCG immunotherapy and in those with inadequately treated TB, a TST should be performed and, when this test is positive, TB chemoprophylaxis should be considered [5]. Furthermore, in countries where TB is endemic, tests for latent TB should be performed before transplantation, chemoprophylaxis considered, and follow-up provided after transplantation [11].

References

1. Adzic T (2004) Pulmonary tuberculosis in patients with hematological malignancies. Med Pregl 57(1):65–68
2. Aisenberg GM, Jacobson K, Chemaly RF, Rolston KV, Raad II, Safdar A (2005) Extrapulmonary tuberculosis active infection misdiagnosed as cancer. Cancer 104(12): 2882–2887
3. Akan H, Arslan O, Akan OA (2006) Tuberculosis in stem cell transplant patients. J Hosp Infect 62(4):421–426
4. Al-Anazi KA, Al-Jasser AM, Evans DAP (2007) Infections caused by *Mycobacterium tuberculosis* in patients with hematological disorders and in recipients of hematopoietic stem cell transplant: a 12 year retrospective study. Ann Clin Microbiol Antimicrob 6:16
5. Aljurf M, Gyger M, Alrajhi A, Sahovic E, Chaudhri N, Musa M, Ayoub O, Seth P, Alsam M, Al-Fiar F (1999) *Mycobacterium tuberculosis* infection in allogeneic bone marrow transplant patients. Bone Marrow Transplant 24: 551–554
6. Al-Kattan K, Ashour M, Hajjar W, Salah El Din M, Fouda M, Al Bakry A (2001) Surgery for pulmonary aspergilloma in post-tuberculous vs. immuno-compromised patients. Eur J Cardiothorac Surg 20:728–733
7. Alzeer AH, FitzGerald JM (1993) Corticosteroids and tuberculosis: risks and use as adjunct therapy. Tuber Lung Dis 74(1):6–11
8. Au WY, Cheng VCC, Ho PL, Yuen KY, Hung I, Ma SY, Lie AKW, Kwong YL (2003) Nontuberculous mycobacterial infections in Chinese hematopoietic stem cell transplantation recipients. Bone Marrow Transplant 32:709–714
9. Au WY, Leung AY, Tse EW, Cheung WW, Shek TW, Kwong YL (2008) High incidence of tuberculosis after alemtuzumab treatment in Hong Kong Chinese patients. Leuk Res 32(4):547–551
10. Brown ST, Almenoff PL (1992) Pulmonary mycobacterial infections associated with neoplasia. Semin Respir Infect 7(2):104–113
11. Budak-Alpdogan T, Tangün Y, Kalayoglu-BesisiK S, Ratip S, Akan H, Baslar Z, Soysal T, Bayik LA, Koc H (2000) The frequency of tuberculosis in adult allogeneic stem cell transplant recipients in Turkey. Biol Blood Marrow Transplant 6(4):370–374
12. Caceres FdM, Orozco LC (2007) Incidence of and factors for non-compliance to antituberculous treatment. Biomedica 27: 498–504
13. Canada Communicable Disease Report, an Advisory Committee Statement [Canadian Tuberculosis Committee] (2008) Updated recommendations on interferon gamma release assays for latent tuberculosis infection. Public Health Agency of Canada 34(6):1–13
14. Cisneros JR, Murray KM (1996) Corticosteroids in tuberculosis. Ann Pharmacother 30(11):1298–1303
15. Cordani S, Manna A, Vignali M, Tascini C (2008) Bronchoalveolar large as a diagnostic tool in patients with hematological malignancies and pneumonia. Le Infezioni In Medicina 4:209–213
16. Cordonnier C, Martino R, Trabasso P, Held TK, Akan H, Ward MS, Fabian K, Ullmann AJ, Wulffraat N, Ljungman P, Alessandrino EP, Pretnar J, Gmür J, Varela R, Vitek A, Sica S, Rovira M, for the European Blood and Marrow Transplant Group Infectious Diseases Working Party (2004) Mycobacterial infections: a difficult and late diagnosis in stem cell transplant recipients. Clin Infect Dis 38: 1229–1236
17. Curley C (2003) New guidelines: what to do about an unexpected positive tuberculin test. Cleve Clin J Med 70(1): 49–55
18. Daniels JM, Vonk-Noordegraaf A, Janssen JJ, Postmus PE, van Altena R (2009) Tuberculosis complicating imatinib treatment for chronic myeloid leukemia. Eur Respir J 33(3):670–672

19. Davies PDO, Pai M (2008) The diagnosis and misdiagnosis of tuberculosis. Int J Tuberc Lung Dis 12(11):1226–1234
20. de la Camara R, Martino R, Granados E, Rodriguez-Salvanës FJ, Rovira M, Caberera R, Löpez J, Parody R, Sierra J, Fernandez Ranada JM, Carreras E, for the Spanish Group on Infections Complication in Hematopoietic Transplantation (2000) Tuberculosis after hematopoietic stem cell transplantation: incidence, clinical characteristics and outcome. Bone Marrow Transplant 26:291–298
21. De La Rosa GR, Jacobson KL, Rolston KV, Raad II, Kontoyiannis DP, Safdar A (2004) *Mycobacterium tuberculosis* at a comprehensive cancer centre: active disease in patients with underlying malignancy during 1990–2000. Clin Microbiol Infect 10(8):749–752
22. Demirkazik FB, Akin A, Uzun O, Akpinar MG, Ariyürek MO (2008) CT findings in immunocompromized patients with pulmonary infections. Diagn Interv Radiol 14:75–82
23. Dinnes J, Deeks J, Kunst H, Gibson A, Cummins E, Waugh N, Drobniewski F, Lavlani A (2007) A systemic review of rapid diagnostic tests for the detection of tuberculosis infection. Health Technol Assess 11(3):1–178
24. Ducati RG, Ruffino-Netto A, Basso LA, Santos DS (2006) The resumption of consumption – a review on tuberculosis. Mem Inst Oswaldo Cruz 101(7):697–714
25. Echevarria MP, Martin G, Pérez J, Urkijo JC (1994) Pulmonary infection of *Mycobacterium Kansasii*. Presentation of 27 cases (1988–1992). Enferm Infecc Microbiol Clín 12(6): 280–284
26. Erdstein AA, Daas P, Bradstock KF, Robinson T, Hertzberg MS (2004) Tuberculosis in allogeneic stem cell transplant recipients: still a problem in the 21st century. Transpl Infect Dis 6(4):142–146
27. Etxebarrieta M, Rodrigo A, Martin C, Ojer M, Ruz A, Dorronsoro I (2002) Clinical importance of *Mycobacterium Kansasii* and evaluation of the need to identify nontuberculous mycobacteria. Enferm Infecc Microbiol Clin 20(3): 113–116
28. Evans DJ (2008) The use of adjunctive corticosteroids in the treatment of pericardial, pleural and meningeal tuberculosis: do they improve outcome? Respir Med 102(6): 793–780
29. Funada H, Machi T, Matsuda T (1991) Disseminated mycobacteriosis in patients with severe hematologic disorders. Kansenshogaku Zasshi 65(10):1297–1303
30. Fusegawa H, Miyachi H, Ohshima T, Arimori S, Ando Y (1992) Rapid diagnosis of tuberculosis by amplification of mycobacterial DNA in blood diseases. Rihsho Ketsueki 33(4):418–422
31. George B, Mathews V, Srivastava V, Srivastava A, Chandy M (2001) Tuberculosis among allogeneic bone marrow transplant recipients in India. Bone Marrow Transplant 27: 973–975
32. Goo JM, Im J-G, Do K-H, Yeo JS, Seo JB, Kim HY, Chung J-K (2000) Pulmonary Tuberculoma evaluated by means of FDG PET: findings in 10 cases. Radiology 216:117–121
33. Grant A, Gothard P, Thwaites G (2008) Managing drug resistant tuberculosis. Br Med J (Middle East) 15:80–85
34. Griffith DE (2007) Therapy of nontuberculous mycobacterial disease. Curr Opin Infect Dis 20(2):198–203
35. Hakawi AM, Alrajhi AA (2006) Tuberculosis of the bone marrow: clinico-pathological study of 22 cases from Saudi Arabia. Int J Tuberc Lung Dis 10(9):1041–1044
36. Han XY, Tarrand JJ, Infante R, Jacobson KL, Troung M (2005) Clinical significance and epidemiologic analyses of *Mycobacterium avium* and *Mycobacterium intracellular* among patients without AIDS. J Clin Microbiol 43(9): 4407–4412
37. Hasibi M, Rasoulinejad M, Hosseini SM, Davari P, Sahebian A, Khashayar P (2008) Epidemiological, clinical, laboratory findings and outcomes of disseminated tuberculosis in Tehran, Iran. South Med J 101(9):910–913
38. Ibrahim EM, Uwaydah A, al-Mulhim FA, Ibrahim AM, el-Hassan AY (1989) Tuberculosis in patients with malignant disease. Indian J Cancer 26(2):53–57
39. Ip SMS, Yuen KY, Woo PCY, Luk WK, Tsang KWT, Lam WK, Liang RHS (1998) Risk factors for pulmonary tuberculosis in bone marrow transplant recipients. Am J Respir Crit Care Med 158:1173–1177
40. Itoh M, Oida E, Iwai K, Okazaki T, Tashima M, Uchiyama T (2001) Disseminated atypical mycobacteriosis in a patient with chronic myelogenous leukemia. Rinsho Ketsueki 42(3):209–215
41. Iuldasheva NE, Karachunskii MA, Pivnik AV (2002) Various approaches to tuberculosis diagnosis in patient with hemoblastosis. Ter Arkh 74(4):35–38
42. Iuldasheva NE, Karachunskii MA, Pivnik AV (2004) Clinical picture of tuberculosis with concomitant hemoblastoses. Ter Arkh 76(3):49–51
43. Jacobson KL, Teira R, Libshitz HI, Raad I, Rolston KV, Terrand J, Whimbey E (2000) *Mycobacterium kansasii* infections in patients with cancer. Clin Infect Dis 31(2): 628–631
44. Jin S-M, Lee HJ, Park E-A, Lee HY, Lee S-M, Yang S-C, Yoo C-G, Kim YW, Han SK, Shim Y-S, Yim J-J (2008) Frequency and predictors of miliary tuberculosis in patients with miliary pulmonary nodules in South Korea: a retrospective cohort study. BMC Infect Dis 8:160
45. Jung JI, Lee DG, Kim YJ, Yoon HK, Kim CC, Park SH (2009) Pulmonary tuberculosis after hematopoietic stem cell transplantation: radiologic findings. J Thorac Imaging 24(1):10–16
46. Karachunskii MA, Pivnik AV, Iuldasheva NE (2002) Tuberculosis in patients with hemoblastoses. Probl Tuberk 5:24–27
47. Kiehn TE, Edwards FF, Brannon P, Tsang AY, Maio M, Gold JWM, Whimbey E, Wong B, McClatchy JK, Armstrong D (1985) Infections caused by *Mycobacterium avium* complex in immunocompromized patients: diagnosis by blood culture and fecal examination, antimicrobial susceptibility tests, and morphological and seroagglutination characteristics. J Clin Microbiol 21(2):168–173
48. Kindler T, Schindel C, Brass U, Fischer T (2001) Fatal sepsis due to *Mycobacterium tuberculosis* after allogeneic bone marrow transplantation. Bone Marrow Transplant 27: 217–218
49. Kobashi Y, Mouri K, Yagi S, Obase Y, Fukuda M, Miyashita N, Oka M (2008) (2008) Usefulness of the QuantiFERON TB-2G test for the differential diagnosis of pulmonary tuberculosis. Intern Med 47(4):237–243
50. Koh W-J, Kwon OJ, Lee KS (2005) Diagnosis and treatment of nontuberculous mycobacterial pulmonary diseases: a Korean perspective. J Korean Med Sci 20: 913–925

51. Kublman JE, Deutsch JH, Fishman EK, Siegelman SS (1990) CT features of thoracic mycobacterial disease. Radiographics 10:413–431
52. Lavlani A (2007) Diagnosing tuberculosis infection in the 21st century. Chest 131:1898–1906
53. Lee J, Lee MH, Kim WS, Kim K, Park SH, Lee SH, Lee KE, Park JO, Jung CW, Im YH, Kang WK, Park K (2004) Tuberculosis in hematopoietic stem cell transplant recipients in Korea. Int J Hematol 79(2):185–188
54. Lee KM, Choe KH, Kim SJ (2006) Clinical investigations of cavitary tuberculosis and tuberculous pneumonia. Korean J Intern Med 21:230–235
55. Lee SW, Kang YA, Yoon YS, Um S-W, Lee SM, Yoo C-G, Kim YW, Han SK, Shim Y-S, Yim J-J (2006) The prevalence and evolution of anemia associated with tuberculosis. J Korean Med Sci 21:1028–1032
56. Libshitz HI, Pannu HK, Elting LS, Cooksley CD (1997) Tuberculosis in cancer patients: an update. J Thorac Imaging 12(1):41–46
57. Ling DI, Flores LL, Riley LW, Pai M (2008) Commercial nucleic acid amplification tests for diagnosis of pulmonary tuberculosis in respiratory specimens: meta-analysis and meta-regression. PLoS ONE 3(2):e1536
58. Lombard EH, Mansvelt EP (1993) Hematological changes associated with miliary tuberculosis of the bone marrow. Tuber Lung Dis 74(2):131–135
59. Maeda T, Kusumi E, Kami M, Kawabata M, Le Pavoux A, Hara S, Chizuka A, Murashige N, Tanimoto TE, Matsumura T, Kuji Ko, Wake A, Miyakoshi S, Morinaga S, Taniguchi S, for the Tokyo Stem Cell transplant (SCT) Consortium (2005) Disseminated tuberculosis following reduced-intensity cord blood transplantation for adult patients with hematological diseases. Bone Marrow Transplant 35: 91–97
60. Makhlouf HA, Helmy A, Fawzy E, El-Attar M, Rashed HAG (2008) A prospective study of antituberculous drug-induced hepatotoxicity in an area endemic for liver disease. Hepatol Int 2:353–360
61. Matteelli A, Migliori GB, Cirillo D, Centis R, Girard E, Raviglion M (2007) Multidrug-resistant and extensively drug-resistant *Mycobacterium tuberculosis*: epidemiology and control. Expert Rev Anti Infect Ther 5(5):857–871
62. Melero M, Gennaro O, Dominguez C, Sanchez Avalos JC (1992) Tuberculosis in patients with lymphoma. Medicina (B Aires) 52(4):291–295
63. Mert A, Bilir M, Tabak F, Ozaras R, Ozturk R, Senturk H, Aki H, Seyhan N, Karayel T, Aktuglu Y (2001) Miliary tuberculosis: clinical manifestations, diagnosis and outcome in 38 adults. Respirology 6(3):217–224
64. Migliori GB, Matteelli A, Cirillo D, Pai M (2008) Diagnosis of multidrug-resistant tuberculosis and extensively drug-resistant tuberculosis: current standards and challenges. Can J Infect Dis Med Microbiol 19(2):169–172
65. Mishra P, Kumar R, Mahapatra M, Sharma S, Dixit A, Chaterjee T, Choudhry DR, Saxena R, Choudhry VP (2006) Tuberculosis in acute leukemia: a clinico-hematological profile. Hematology 11(5):335–340
66. Morris CD, Bird AR, Nell H (1989) The hematological and biochemical changes in severe pulmonary tuberculosis. Q J Med 73(272):1151–1159
67. Munsiff S, Nilsen D, Dworkin F (2005) Guidelines for testing and treatment of latent tuberculosis infection. NYC Department of Health and Mental Hygiene. Bureau of Tuberculosis Control, New York, pp 1–12
68. Nagayama N, Shishido Y, Masuda K, Baba M, Tamura A, Nagai H, Akagawa S, Kawabe Y, Machida K, Kurashima A, Komatsu H, Yotsumoto H (2004) Leucopenia due to antituberculous chemotherapy including rifampicin and isoniazid. Kekkaku 79(5):341–348
69. Neonakis IK, Alexandrakis MG, Gitti Z, Tsirakis G, Krambovitis E, Spandidos DA (2008) Miliary tuberculosis with no pulmonary involvement in myelodysplastic syndrome: a curable, yet rarely diagnosed disease: case report and review of the literature. Ann Clin Microbiol Antimicrob 7:8
70. Olaniyi JA, Aken'Ova YA (2003) Hematological profile of patients with pulmonary tuberculosis in Ibadan, Negeria. Afr J Med Med Sci 32(3):239–242
71. Ortona L, Fantoni M (1998) Tuberculin skin test and chemoprophylaxis of tuberculosis. Rays 23(1):218–224
72. Ozkalemkas F, Ali R, Ozkan A, Ozcelik T, Ozkocaman V, Kunt-Uzaslan E, Bahadir-Erdogan B, Akalin H (2004) Tuberculosis presenting presenting as immune thrombocytopenic purpura. Ann Clin Microbiol Antimicrob 3:16
73. Pagano L, Pagliari G, Basso A, Marra R, Sica S, Frigieri L, Morace G, Ardito F, Leone G (1997) The role of bronchoalveolar lavage in the microbiological diagnosis of pneumonia in patients with hematological malignancies. Ann Med 29(6):535–540
74. Pai M, Flores LL, Hubbard A, Riley LW, Colford JM Jr (2004) Nucleic acid amplification tests in the diagnosis of tuberculous pleuritis: a systemic review and meta-analysis. BMC Infect Dis 4:6
75. Pai M, Kalantri S, Dheda K (2006) New tools and emerging technologies for the diagnosis of tuberculosis: Part I. Latent tuberculosis. Expert Rev Mol Diagn 6(3):413–422
76. Pai M, Kalantri S, Dheda K (2006) New tools and emerging technologies for the diagnosis of tuberculosis: Part II. Active tuberculosis and drug resistance. Expert Rev Mol Diagn 6(3):423–432
77. Palomino JC (2005) Nonconventional and new methods in the diagnosis of tuberculosis: feasibility and applicability in the field. Eur Respir J 26:339–350
78. Parrish SC, Myers J, Lazarus A (2008) Nontuberculous mycobacterial pulmonary infections in non-HIV patients. Postgrad Med 120(4):78–86
79. Piana F, Codecasa LR, Cavallerio P, Ferrarese M, Migliori GB, Barbarano L, Morra E, Cirillo DM (2006) Use of a T-cell-based test for detection of tuberculosis infection among immunocompromized patients. Eur Respir J 28:31–34
80. Porte H, Roumilhac D, Eraldi L, Cordonnier C, Puech P, Wurtz A (1998) The role of mediastinoscopy in the diagnosis of mediastinal lymphadenopathy. Eur J Cardiothorac Surg 13(2):196–199
81. Richeldi L (2006) An update on the diagnosis of tuberculosis infection. Am J Respir Crit Care Med 174: 736–742
82. Richeldi L, Luppi M, Losi M, Luppi F, Potenza L, Roversi P, Cerri S, Millington KA, Ewer K, Fabbri LM, Torelli G, Lalvani A (2006) Diagnosis of occult tuberculosis in hematological malignancy by enumeration of antigen-specific T cells. Leukemia 20(2):379–381

83. Rolston KV, Jones PG, Fainstein V, Bodey GP (1985) Pulmonary disease caused by rapidly growing mycobacteria in patients with cancer. Chest 87(4):503–506
84. Rosenthal T, Pitlik S, Michaeli D (1975) Fatal undiagnosed tuberculosis in hospitalized patients. J Infect Dis 131: S 51–S 56
85. Roy V, Weisdorf D (1997) Mycobacterial infections following bone marrow transplantation: a 20 year retrospective review. Bone Marrow Transplant 19:467–470
86. Safdar A, Han XY (2005) *Mycobacterium lentiflavum*, a recently identified slow-growing mycobacterial species: clinical significance in immunocompromised cancer patients and summary of reported cases of infection. Eur J Clin Microbiol Infect Dis 24(8):554–558
87. Sakatani M, Nakajima Y (2006) Treatment of non-tuberculous pulmonary mycobacteriosis. Kekkaku 81(1):35–50
88. Salpeter S (1992) Tuberculosis chemoprophylaxis. West J Med 157:421–424
89. Sharma S, Nadrous HF, Peters SG, Tefferi A, Litzow MR, Aubry M-C, Afessa B (2005) Pulmonary complications in adult blood and marrow transplant recipients. Chest 128: 1385–1392
90. Shen G, Behera D, Bhalla M, Nadas A, Laal S (2009) Peptide-based antibody detection for tuberculosis diagnosis. Clin Vaccine Immunol 16(1):49–54
91. Shima T, Yoshimoto G, Miyamoto T, Yoshida S, Kamezaki K, Takenaka K, Iwasaki H, Harada N, Nagafuji K, Teshima T, Shimono N, Akashi K (2009) Disseminated tubeculosis following second unrelated cold blood transplantation for acute myelogenous leukemia. Transpl Infect Dis 11(1): 75–77
92. Shishido Y, Nagayama N, Masuda K, Baba M, Tamura A, Nagai H, Akagawa S, Kawabe Y, Machida K, Kurashima A, Komatsu H, Yotsumoto H (2003) Agranulocytosis due to anti-tuberculous drugs including isoniazid (INH) and rifampicin (RFP) – a report of four cases and review of the literature. Kekkaku 78(11):683–689
93. Silva FA, Matos JO, de Q Mello FC, Nucci M (2005) Risk factors for and attributable mortality from tuberculosis in patients with hematologic malignancies. Haematologica 90(8):1110–1115
94. Singh KJ, Ahluwalia G, Sharma SK, Saxena R, Chaudhary VP, Anant M (2001) Significance of hematological manifestations in patients with tuberculosis. J Assoc Physicians India 49(788):790–794
95. Snider DE Jr, Cohn DL, Davidson PT, Harshfield ES, Smith MH, Sutton FD Jr (1985) Standard therapy for tuberculosis 1985. Chest 87:117S–124S
96. Sos G, Arvieux C, Cazalets C, Cador B, Belaval P, Michelet C (2005) Factors of immunosuppression in patients with tuberculosis. Presse Méd 34(6):420–424
97. Stefan DC, Kruis AL, Schaaf HS, Wessels G (2008) Tuberculosis in oncology patients. Ann Trop Paediatr 28(2): 111–116
98. Suryanarayan K, Campbell J, Eskenazi AE (2002) Nontuberculous mycobacterial infections in pediatric acute leukemia. J Pediatr Hematol Oncol 24(7):558–560
99. Suzuki T, Kawashiro T (2004) Pulmonary infection in immunocompromized hosts. Nippon Geka Gakkai Zasshi 105(12):734–736
100. Su WJ (2002) Recent advances in the molecular diagnosis of tuberculosis. J Microbiol Immunol Infect 35: 209–214
101. Tanabe S, Yamada T, Tsukuura T, Tomiyama J, Tanaka T, Adachi Y (1990) Indications for surgery in a patient with tuberculoma accompanied by chronic myeloid leukemia. Kyoba Geka 43(12):1009–1011
102. Tanaka N, Matsumoto T, Miura G, Emoto T, Matsunaga N (2002) HRCT findings of chest complications in patients with leukemia. Eur Radiol 12(6):1512–1522
103. Tartaglione T (1997) Treatment of nontuberculous mycobacterial infections: role of clarithromycin and azithromycin. Clin Ther 19(4):626–638
104. Tomioka H, Namba K (2006) Development of anti-tuberculous drugs: current status and future prospects. Kekkaku 81(12):753–774
105. Tomioka H (2006) Current status of some antituberculous drugs and the development of new antituberculous agents with special reference to their in vitro and in vivo antimicrobial activities. Curr Pharm Des 12(31): 4047–4070
106. Tongyoo S, Vilaichone W, Sukpanichnant S, Auewarakul C, Chaiprasert A, Ratanarat R, Permpikul C (2003) Thrombocytopenic purpura associated with miliary tuberculosis. J Med Assoc Thai 86(10):976–980
107. Uetake T, Sakamaki T, Onozawa Y, Kimura H, Fukayama M (1990) Clinicopathological study of miliary tuberculosis in patients with hematologic disease. Kekkkaku 65(4): 273–283
108. Ullah K, Raza S, Ahmed P, Satti TM, Ikram A, Chaudhry QU, Kamal MK, Akhtar FM (2007) Pulmonary tuberculosis in allogeneic stem cell transplant recipients. J Pak Med Assoc 57(11):567–569
109. Undar L, Karpuzoğlu G, Karadoganan I, Gelen T, Artvinli M (1996) Tuberculosis associated hemophagocytic syndrome: a report of two cases and a review of the literature. Acta Haematol 96(2):73–78
110. Vejlgaard TB, Haar V, Peterslund NA (1997) Atypical mycobacteria. Disseminated infection in patients with hematologic diseases. Ugeskr Laeger 159(36): 5362–5367
111. Waecker NJ Jr, Stefanova R, Cave MD, Davis CE, Dankner WM (2000) Nosocomial transmission of *Mycobacterium bovis* Bacille Calmette-Guerin to children receiving cancer therapy and to their health care providers. Clin Infect Dis 30:356–362
112. Wallis RS, Patil S, Cheon S-H, Edmonds K, Philips M, Perkins MD, Joloba M, Namale A, Johnson JL, Teixeira L, Dietze R, Siddiqi S, Mugerwa RD, Eisenach K, Ellner JJ (1999) Drug tolerance in *Mycobacterium tuberculosis*. Antimicrob Agents Chemother 43(11): 2600–2606
113. Wani AM, Akhtar M (2008) CA-125: a marker for diagnosis and follow-up of pleuroperitoneal and lymph node tuberculosis. Ann Saudi Med 28(2):142–143
114. Wu T-L, Chia J-H, Kuo A-J, Su L-H, Wu T-S, Lai H-C (2008) Rapid identification of mycobacteria from smear-positive sputum samples by nested PCR-restriction fragment length polymorphism analysis. J Clin Microbiol 46(11):3591–3594

115. Yamaghishi F (2003) Measures for tuberculosis in compromised hosts – mainly on chemoprophylaxis. Kekkaku 78(10):661–667
116. Yee D, Valiquette C, Pelletier M, Parisien I, Rocher I, Menzies D (2003) Incidence of serious side effects from first-line antituberculous drugs among patients treated for active tuberculosis. Am J Respir Crit Care Med 167: 1472–1477
117. Yuen KY, Woo PC (2001) Tuberculosis in blood and marrow transplant recipients. Hematol Oncol 20(2): 51–62

Part V

Noninfectious Pulmonary Involvement in Patients with HM

Pleuropulmonary Changes Induced by Drugs in Patients with Hematologic Diseases

31

Philippe Camus

Contents

P. Camus
Department of Pulmonary Disease and Intensive Care, University Medical Center Le Bocage & Medical School at the Université de Bourgogne, F-21079, Dijon, France
e-mail: ph.camus@chu-dijon.fr, phil.camus@orange.fr, www.pneumotox.com

31.1 Introduction

Patients with hematologic diseases who are being treated with therapy drugs, or receive radiation therapy or blood transfusions may develop a host of potentially fatal infectious and noninfectious pulmonary complications [1]. The increased complexity of multimodality and high-dose treatment regimens with the intended benefit of augmented antineoplastic efficacy and prolonged disease-free survival, the use of a panel of novel drugs to treat malignant and nonmalignant hematologic conditions (e.g., azacytidine, bortezomib, cladribine, dasatinib, fludarabine, imatinib, lenalidomide, rituximab, and thalidomide), total body irradiation (TBI) and hematopietic stem cell transplantation (HSCT) have increased the incidence of severe sometimes life-threatening pulmonary complications.

As the incidence of infectious complications has decreased as a result of improved diagnostic methods

É. Azoulay (ed.), *Pulmonary Involvement in Patients with Hematological Malignancies*,
DOI: 10.1007/978-3-642-15742-4_31, © Springer-Verlag Berlin Heidelberg 2011

and effective prophylaxis, noninfectious, iatrogenic radiation- and drug-induced pulmonary complications have emerged as a major cause of early and late pulmonary morbidity, which may claim the lives of long-term survivors of hematologic malignancies. Toxic pneumonitis may account for 16% of all pulmonary events in this setting [2], and long-term adverse effects of treatments require prolonged follow-up in regard to the development of nonneoplastic and neoplastic conditions in heart and lung [3]. Noninfectious pulmonary complications represent a real challenge to the practitioner who needs be wary of the multitude of drug-, radiation- and procedure-induced adverse effects. Drug-induced respiratory disease in hematology patients may manifest acutely or subacutely by hypersensitivity reactions (bronchospasm, anaphylaxis), pulmonary edema, acute lung injury (ALI), an adult respiratory distress syndrome (ARDS) picture, diffuse alveolar hemorrhage, interstitial lung disease (ILD) with or without tissue eosinophilia, pleural effusion or pulmonary vasculopathy.

The diagnosis of iatrogenic disease is complex, and it is by exclusion. The diagnosis is made against [1] pulmonary involvement from the underlying benign (e.g., sickle cell disease, myelodysplastic syndrome, *polycythemia vera*) or malignant hematologic condition (e.g., acute and chronic leukemias, Hodgkin's and non-Hodgkin's lymphoma, multiple myeloma), [2] alveolar hemorrhage, [3] circulatory overload, left ventricular dysfunction and [4] an opportunistic viral, bacterial, fungal or protozoan infection with few reliable clinical or imaging discriminators to separate these entities. To complicate matters, there is often little time for establishing the diagnosis and initiating appropriate therapy before the patient's condition deteriorates irreversibly. Patients who require mechanical ventilatory support have an ominous outcome. There is almost no specific pattern of drug-induced lung involvement on pathology. Thus, the lung biopsy is mainly used to rule out diagnoses other than drugs, and patients suspected of having drug-induced lung disease may be managed conservatively using bronchoalveolar lavage (BAL), transbronchial lung biopsy (TBLB) and microbiological tests as the main diagnostic tools. Drug discontinuance followed by resolution of symptoms is a simple test that may aid in the recognition of drug-induced disease.

The diagnosis of DIRD can be straightforward in patients with a benign underlying hematologic condition who are being treated with a compatible drug as a solo agent, and drug discontinuance is followed by remission of symptoms. Drug-induced disease is more complex to diagnose in patients with a background of hematologic malignancy who received several potentially pneumotoxic drugs, each having different times for drug-induced disease to present, and/or who have received radiation therapy, blood transfusions or have a history of exposure to oxygen or corticosteroids. Such patients are likely to be severely immunocompromised under the combined influence of underlying illness, drugs used to treat their condition, corticosteroid and radiation therapy, and an opportunistic lung infection is a strong consideration [4]. Diagnosing drug-induced disease is even more complex in recipients of hematopoietic stem cell transplants, who in addition to the above complications, may develop several distinctive post-transplant manifestations, including engraftment syndrome, pulmonary edema, bronchiolitis obliterans organizing pneumonia (BOOP), diffuse alveolar hemorrhage (DAH) and late-onset noninfectious pulmonary complications including idiopathic pulmonary syndrome (IPS) [5, 6]. In rare instances, pulmonary complications develop in hematopoietic stem cell donors in the form of pulmonary infiltrates during colony-stimulating factor-(CSF)-induced stem cell mobilization [7].

The older literature is replete with cases of pulmonary toxicity induced by drugs such as busulfan, BCNU or other nitrosoureas, bleomycin, chlorambucil, cyclophosphamide, hydroxyurea or melphalan when patients with varied hematologic conditions were exposed to these drugs as a solo agent. Sometimes, the pattern of pulmonary involvement from these drugs is distinctive and can still be detected even though the drug is part of a multiagent chemotherapy or conditioning regimen. Establishing which drug in the regimen causes the lung injury is useful, for it may enable withholding the specific drug instead of all drugs in the regimen. Diagnosing drug-induced lung disease is not of pure academic interest. An important practical consequence is selective drug withdrawal while other nonpneumotoxic drugs are continued to the benefit of the patient. Although rechallenge was once considered hazardous and still is with many drugs, rechallenge and steroid-supported rechallenge can be attempted with vital drugs such as imatinib or dasatinib.

Here we review the pulmonary complications induced by drugs, blood transfusion and radiation therapy.

Drug-induced opportunistic infections, respiratory manifestations in recipients of bone marrow and stem cell transplant and iatrogenic complications of chest tubes and central venous access are covered elsewhere [8, 9].

31.2 Diagnostic Criteria for Drug-Induced Respiratory Disease

Criteria for diagnosis include the following [10]:

1. Correct identification of the drug [11]

Dose and duration of treatment with each drug taken in isolation or in a chemotherapy regimen should be reviewed. Causality is more difficult to assess when several pneumotoxic drugs were received concomitantly or in sequence. The likelihood and delay time for drug-induced disease to present vary with drug, dosage, whether the drug was coadministered with other pneumotoxic drugs and the patient. Patients of Asian descent may be at increased risk for certain drug-induced pulmonary complications. It is also necessary to compute exposure to G/GM-CSF, blood and blood components (e.g., fresh frozen plasma, whole blood-derived platelets), anesthetic agents, oxygen, parenteral nutrition and nonhematologic drugs, for all of these may effectuate lung injury [11].

2. Temporal eligibility

Respiratory signs and symptoms should follow (not predate) the onset of treatment with the suspected drug. Time to onset of the respiratory reaction varies with drug, host, schedule of administration and pattern of involvement. The shorter the latency period is, the easier the suggestion of the drug etiology. Longer delay times increase the likelihood that the drug etiology goes unrecognized. Drug-induced- bronchospasm, anaphylaxis, pulmonary edema (e.g., gemcitabine- or acaytine-induced), acute lung injury (e.g., transfusion-related acute lung injury or TRALI), acute respiratory distress syndrome (ARDS) and alveolar hemorrhage tend to develop shortly after exposure to the causal agent, with a time to onset of minutes to hours or at most a few days. Instead, it may take weeks, months or years for drug- (viz. methotrexate, azathioprine or thalidomide) induced cellular interstitial pneumonia to develop. Drug- and radiation-induced pulmonary fibrosis develops after months or years into treatment or after termination of treatment. For instance, patients who received busulfan, cyclophosphamide, nitrosoureas or radiation therapy in the past may be diagnosed with iatrogenic pulmonary fibrosis or the idiopathic pulmonary syndrome many years later [12, 13].

3. Drug singularity

Assessment of causality is problematic if patients were exposed to several pneumotoxic drugs. This creates confusion about which drug is responsible for the lung reaction, and it may at times be impossible to sort this out. In patients treated with several chemotherapy agents, drug toxicity may develop at dosages of each drug that are lower than the threshold above which drug toxicity develops when the drug is taken in isolation. Weighing the responsibility of each drug taken separately is critical regarding future management of the underlying hematologic disease. Identification of the causal drug may enable selective cessation of the culprit drug. A review on nonhematology drugs is indicated, as many drugs can injure the lung [11]

4. Whether the pulmonary reaction is appropriate for the particular drug

The pattern of involvement from some drugs can be suggestive, owing to the close temporal relationship of exposure versus onset of respiratory symptoms (e.g., the swift development of pulmonary infiltrates following treatments with anti-thymocyte globulin, gemcitabine, ATRA, cytarabine or blood transfusion (TRALI) [14]. For other drugs it is because the clinical, imaging, BAL and/or pathologic pattern of involvement is distinctive [e.g., bleomycin and bibasilar shadowing or multiple lung nodules, cyclophosphamide and severe pleuropulmonary involvement, imatinib or dasatinib and pleural effusion, methotrexate and an acute hypersensitivity pneumonitis with a granulomatous pattern of involvement, rituximab and ARDS; retinoic acid (ATRA) and diffuse alveolar hemorrhage (DAH), of BCNU/CCNU or busulfan with otherwise unexplained pulmonary fibrosis].

It is difficult to predict the pathologic background of drug-induced reactions using HRCT data alone [15], and in one study of 20 patients [16], imaging and pathology were concordant in only nine cases (45%). A confirmatory lung biopsy (open or transbronchial) can be necessary in selected cases mainly to discard etiologies other than drugs rather than to prove the drug etiology. Any attempt at deducing pathology from imaging as done in some studies [17] should be viewed with caution.

5. Exclusion of other causes

There are many diagnostic contenders to consider when pulmonary infiltrates develop in patients with hematologic disease treated with drugs. These include the pulmonary manifestations of the native benign or malignant hematologic condition (for instance, pulmonary involvement from malignant lymphoma [15] or acute leukemia [18], extramedullary hematopoiesis [19], multiple myeloma [20–22], interstitial lung disease including pulmonary alveolar proteinosis that may occur in association with untreated hematologic diseases [23]), capillary leak, tumor lysis syndrome, cardiac pulmonary edema, an opportunistic viral, bacterial, fungal or protozoan infections including *Pneumocystis jiroveci* pneumonia, a common encounter in hematology patients [24–28], and a graft-versus-host reaction [29]. All of these can produce similar patterns of involvement on imaging. The BAL and TBLB with appropriate sample staining, culture and molecular techniques should be routinely performed to help exclude an infection [2]. Heart ultrasonography and diuresis may also aid in the recognition of drug-induced vs. cardiogenic pulmonary edema.

6. Remission of signs and symptoms with removal of the drug

Signs and symptoms typically clear after drug removal. However, fulminate iatrogenic reactions to drugs (e.g., drug-induced pulmonary edema, TRALI, methotrexate pneumonitis, bleomycin lung) may progress despite removal. Similarly, pulmonary fibrosis induced by drugs or that develops as a late consequence of conditioning regimens often is an irreversible process that may not respond to drug discontinuance. Corticosteroid therapy is often given to patients with severe drug-induced lung disease to accelerate recovery. However, this is at the expense of drug causality assessment.

7. Recurrence with rechallenge

Rechallenge followed by recurrence is central to the diagnosis of any drug-induced disease [10], but seldom is performed intentionally because of risks [30]. Of note, drug-induced pleuropulmonary reactions to imatinib [31], dasatinib [32] or antithymocyte globulin [33] were shown not to relapse in all patients upon reexposure, enabling continued treatment of the underlying hematologic disease. Rechallenge is reserved for cases where the drug is vital, there is no alternative efficacious drug to treat the underlying condition, and it is given in small incremental doses of the drug and corticosteroid therapy.

8. Tests may support the diagnosis of DILD

BAL is instrumental in ruling out an infection and may show an increased percentage of lymphocytes, eosinophils or neutrophils depending on which drug caused the reaction (for a review, see [14]).

Studies of peripheral or BAL lymphocyte activation or migration following in vitro challenge with the suspected drug have produced inconsistent results, and overall, evidence for the usefulness of this test is low, and there is a lack of consensus about the appropriateness of these tests inasmuch as in a recent series, there was no correlation of lymphocyte stimulation with the clinical result effect of rechallenge with the drug [34].

KL-6 has been found to be elevated in some patients with drug-induced fibrosis. However, this marker remained normal in cases of pulmonary toxicity from rituximab, methotrexate and radiation therapy. Similarly, time-related changes in plasma or BAL TGF-ß1 and IL1 in patients receiving chemotherapy and/or radiation therapy yielded inconsistent results, and there is no consensus regarding their measurements in routine.

Areas of drug-, radiation- and talc-induced reactions can be tracer-avid on FDG-PET scans [35].

31.3 Patterns of Reactions to Drugs and Radiation

31.3.1 Interstitial-Infiltrative Lung Diseases (ILD)

ILD is a group of conditions characterized by pulmonary infiltrates, restrictive physiology, impaired gas exchange, shifts in BAL cells percentages (lymphocytes, eosinophils or neutrophils) and pathologic evidence of parenchymal inflammation. Fever, a nonproductive cough and dyspnea are common presenting symptoms. Diagnosis of drug-induced ILD is supported by BAL, a negative workup for lung infection and reversal of the symptom following drug removal. Tissue sampling is not always required. Severity of ILD ranges from mild transient pulmonary infiltrates and the asymptomatic state to diffuse shadowing or dense consolidation with the gas exchange features of ALI or ARDS [36]. Histological findings are dominated by interstitial inflammation with or without tissue eosinophilia or a granulomatous pattern of involvement, organizing pneumonia, pulmonary edema, diffuse alveolar damage (DAD) or alveolar hemorrhage. The lung architecture is retained [37].

31.3.1.1 Cellular or Nonspecific Interstitial Pneumonia

Drug-induced cellular interstitial pneumonia, also known as alveolitis or hypersensitivity pneumonitis, is a common pattern of pulmonary reaction to drugs [11]. Drugs causing cellular interstitial pneumonia in hematology include azacytidine, azathioprine, chlorambucil, 2-chlorodeoxyadenosine (cladribine), cyclophosphamide, cytarabine, dasatinib, floxuridine, fludarabine, GM-CSF, gemtuzumab, hydroxurea, imatinib, interferon alpha and beta, lenalidomide, methotrexate, procarbazine, rituximab, thalidomide, vinca alkaloids and chest radiation therapy [11]. Time to onset is a few days to several years into treatment and is unpredictable as serial pulmonary function is not capable of predicting development of this complication. Onset of the disease may be insidious over a few days or weeks, with moderate fever followed by the development of cough and breathlessness. Methotrexate lung is known to accelerate, causing rapidly progressive respiratory failure. Radiographic studies indicate bilateral, usually symmetrical interstitial or alveolar ground-glass opacities, mosaic attenuation or consolidation. The infiltrates may predominate in the lung bases and mid-lung zones, or they can be diffuse. Radiographic attenuation can be a discrete haze, ground-glass, inter- or intralobular septal thickening, a crazy-paving, mosaic appearance or dense bilateral consolidation with air bronchograms [38–42]. A miliary pattern, pleural effusions and mediastinal lymph node enlargement are occasional features of methotrexate lung [36, 43]. Imaging features may not enable the separation of ILD due to drugs from infectious pneumonia or from the manifestations of the underlying hematologic condition [26, 44, 45]. Pulmonary function indicates restrictive physiology and impaired gas exchange [36]. Physiology tends to correlate with the extent of involvement on imaging [46] except in azathioprine pneumonitis and bleomycin lung [47, 48]. Fiberoptic bronchoscopy and BAL are indicated to rule out an infection. The BAL usually shows a lymphocyte predominance [49]. The contribution of lymphocyte typing is unclear, because increases in both CD4+ or CD8+ subsets have been observed depending on time from onset of pneumonitis and whether the patient has received corticosteroid therapy [50]. A low ratio of CD4+ to CD8+ lymphocytes is suggestive for the drug etiology, but this is not a specific finding. Other BAL patterns include neutrophilia or a pattern of lymphocytosis and neutrophilia or eosinophilia. BAL samples should be processed with special stains, cultures and molecular techniques for the detection of bacteria, fungi and protozoa and viruses, including the recently recognized metapneumovirus and H1N1 [51]. A lung biopsy may be required in selected cases, since drug-induced lung disease may be a mimic of *Pneumocystis* pneumonia [52] and other opportunistic infections [53]. The TBLB approach can document interstitial pneumonia although sample size may be an issue. Histopathological features include interstitial inflammation, edema and a cellular interstitial infiltrate. Less common findings include granulomas during treatments with methotrexate [43], interferon [54] or lenalidomide [55], organizing pneumonia with rituximab or thalidomide, and interstitial fibrosis [43]. Alveolar edema or hemorrhage may be found as a manifestation of severe ILD [43, 56].

Management includes drug removal and supportive care. This may suffice in benign cases [57]. Corticosteroids are indicated in severe cases once an infection has been reasonably ruled out. Oral prednisolone or i.v. methylprednisolone daily for a few days is indicated depending on severity, followed by a tapering dosage of oral corticosteroid therapy. Mega-doses of methylprednisolone of 1 g/day are given to patients in some countries, with no documented benefit compared to a standard dose regimen. Fatalities have been reported in patients with severe disease, particularly if corticosteroids were not given in time and in patients rechallenged with the drug [30]. Lung fibrosis following recognition and treatment of this problem is seldom seen. Although rechallenge with the drug may not be followed with relapse [32, 58], this should be discussed on an individual basis. Patients and caregivers should be instructed to avoid unjustified reexposure to the drug or to a congener.

31.3.1.2 Eosinophilic Pneumonia

The association of pulmonary infiltrates with blood and/or tissue eosinophilia defines eosinophilic pneumonia. This is an uncommon pattern of lung response to drugs used in hematology, contrasting with nonsteroidal antiinflammatory drugs and minocycline. Causal hematology drugs include bleomycin, chlorambucil, cladribine, cotrimoxazole, fludarabine, GM-CSF, interferon, inhaled or parenteral pentamidine, procarbazine and radiocontrast media. More common causal agents include nonsteroidal antiinflammatory drugs or minocycline [11]. Adverse reactions to methotrexate or blood transfusion can be accompanied by mild peripheral eosinophilia, but the BAL and pathologic features are not those of eosinophilic pneumonia. Onset of the condition is unpredictable. Acute eosinophilic pneumonia may produce acute respiratory failure. Unusual PIE cases present with rash and internal involvement, and this has been aptly coined DRESS for drug-rash and eosinophilia with systemic symptoms. A few DRESS cases were described with the use of azathioprine, bortezomib, hydroxyurea and imatinib [59]. On imaging, PIE is in the form of the photographic negative of pulmonary edema, or it is disseminated with faint shadowing, discreet ground-glass, Kerley "B" lines, or dense and diffuse infiltrates. An increase in blood, BAL and/or lung tissue eosinophils is diagnostic. The lung biopsy rarely is required and shows an interstitial infiltrate of eosinophils admixed with mononuclear cells. Drug discontinuance is indicated. Corticosteroids are reserved for severe cases. Outcome is good.

31.3.1.3 Interstitial Lung Disease with a Granulomatous Component

Granulomatosis has been reported in a few patients after treatment of non-Hodgkin's disease in the form of reticulo-nodular infiltrates and/or medisatinal lymphadenopathy [60, 61]. Most cases of drug-induced granulomatosis with or without extrathoracic organ involvement and hypercalcemia are related to treatments with interferon alpha or beta. Methotrexate and lenalidomide can also produce a granulomatous pulmonary reaction (see below under interferon and methotrexate).

31.3.1.4 Organizing Pneumonia

Organizing pneumonia (OP/BOOP) is a distinctive pattern of lung response to a few drugs and to hematopoietic stem cell transplantation as well, which is best defined by the pathologic finding of alveolar and ductal buds of connective tissue or fibrosis. Strictly speaking, organizing pneumonia is best diagnosed when a large sample of lung tissue is available for review to make sure BOOP is not an incidental finding among other more distinctive pathologic features. Claimed cases of BOOP without pathologic evidence are equivocal. This is not trivial, for pulmonary aspergillosis and BOOP can be indistinguishable on imaging [53]. Causal drugs used to treat hematologic conditions include bleomycin, busulfan (mostly the acute busulfan lung), cyclophosphamide, interferon, lenalidomide, rituximab, thalidomide and chemotherapy [11, 62]. At any rate, the diagnosis of drug-induced BOOP is against the background of BOOP, which can occur as a late noninfectious pulmonary complication in hematopoietic stem cell transplant recipients [5]. BOOP can manifest with chest pain, dyspnea and areas of consolidation or without respiratory failure [63], or it is discovered incidentally on imaging [64]. Nodular organizing pneumonia is a distinctive pattern of bleomycin pulmonary toxicity and is in the form of round-shaped areas of consolidation that may localize in lung bases and simulate metastatic lung disease [65]. A lung biopsy may be required to exclude this possibility [66], although clinical reasoning and observation coupled to 18F-dideoxyglucose PET scanning may suffice [67]. There is no BAL pattern that is characteristic of this condition. The percentage of lymphocytes and/or of neutrophils or eosinophils can be increased. If a lung biopsy is contemplated, the video-assisted approach is preferred as a larger sample lends greater support to the diagnosis. Histology reveals interstitial inflammation, superimposed on the dominant background of alveolar and ductal fibrosis [68]. Some patients present with overlapping features of organizing and eosinophilic pneumonia [66]. Drug discontinuation with corticosteroid therapy in severe cases is followed by improvement.

31.3.1.5 Diffuse Alveolar Damage and the Chemotherapy Lung

The treatment of hematologic malignancies with chemotherapy agents, particularly alkylating agents but not exclusively so, may induce a pattern of lung derangements termed the "chemotherapy lung," a wide-ranging term [14, 69]. Patients treated for leukemia, particularly patients with high blast counts during remission induction [70], Hodgkin's disease or non-Hodgkin's lymphoma and recipients of bone marrow or stem cell transplant are at risk. The entity refers to non-hemodynamic, noninfectious and nonneoplastic pulmonary complications, which develop in a variable proportion of patients (<1–60% in some phase I or II studies) following administration of single-agent (e.g., BCNU or other nitrosoureas, bleomycin, bortezomib, busulfan, chlorambucil, cyclophosphamide, docetaxel, gemcitabine, melphalan, methotrexate, procarbazine, vinblastine) or multi-agent chemotherapy, particularly when drugs were used at elevated dosages or there is an association of several lung-toxic drugs with or without radiation therapy in the treatment schedule [71–73]. Substitution of one agent in a chemotherapy regimen can markedly alter the safety profile. For instance, in patients with de novo-treated Hodgkin's disease, the substitution of gemcitabine with dacarbazine in the ABVD regimen [doxorubicin, bleomycin, vinblastin, gemcitabine instead of dacarbazine (ABVG)] resulted in an unacceptable 42% incidence rate of pulmonary toxicity [74]. Likewise, in a phase I/II dose-escalation study in 27 patients with advanced-stage Hodgkin's disease, the substitution of gemcitabine for etoposide in the escalated BEACOPP regimen (bleomycin, doxorubicin, cyclophosphamide, vincristine, procarbazine, prednisone and gemcitabine instead of etoposide) resulted in pulmonary toxicity in 29.6% of the patients [75]. Crucially, the disease needs be separated from an infection, mainly pneumonia due to *Pneumocystis jiroveci* or viral agents [76], acute heart failure and an acute transfusion reaction [77, 78]. If investigation of the sputum, BAL, blood and other fluids is unrevealing, especially on two consecutive evaluations for an infection, the diagnosis of chemotherapy lung is entertained further. It is challenging to assess the specific responsibility of each drug in the regimen to the syndrome if patients have received several pneumotoxic agents concomitantly or in sequence. Assessing causality is important though, for identification of the causal drug may allow selective drug discontinuation rather than withdrawal of all drugs in the chemotherapy regimen. It may be possible to discern methotrexate or bleomycin pulmonary toxicity when it occurs in patients receiving a multi-agent chemotherapy regimen. For instance, non-Hodgkin's lymphoma patients who received m-BACOD or m-ACOD regimens developed a picture similar to methotrexate lung, whereas no pulmonary infiltrates were observed in patients receiving the CHOP regimen, which does not include methotrexate [79]. Similarly, the different incidence of pulmonary events in two arms of a therapeutic regimen that differed by only one drug (for instance with or without bleomycin, BCNU, CSF, gemcitabine, or radiation therapy) or by the dosage of one particular drug (e.g., low vs. high BCNU) enabled deducing which drug was exactly causing the reaction [80]. The likelihood of developing chemotherapy lung is increased when radiation therapy to the chest, TBI, oxygen, and possibly CSFs are given concomitantly. The term 'chemotherapy lung' is not ideal, because non-chemotherapy agents such as ATRA, IL-2 and imatinib, oxygen, transfusion of blood or proteins including IVIG, infusion of stem cells, radiation therapy and nonchemo agents can also cause the syndrome [11].

In addition to the intrinsic risk attendant to specific drugs, with busulfan carrying an extra risk compared to other chemotherapeutic agents [81], other factors include advanced age, current smoking, drug dosage and intensity of the conditioning regimen [myeloablative vs. nonmyeloablative, multi-agent combination chemotherapy, abrupt corticosteroid withdrawal, the type of stem cell transplantation (allogeneic vs. autologous, T-cell depleted) and a background of graft-vs.-host reaction in transplant recipients].

Time to onset of the chemotherapy lung is variable from shortly after the first administration of low doses of the drug [70, 82] to months into treatment or after termination of treatment. Usual doses of oral corticosteroids may not prevent the condition from developing. Depending on patient and time of diagnosis, the chemotherapy lung may have overlapping features with, and be difficult to distinguish clinically and on imaging from acute pulmonary edema, diffuse alveolar hemorrhage, accelerated pulmonary fibrosis or dense interstitial pneumonias. The main histopathological feature of chemotherapy lung is diffuse alveolar damage (DAD) with, characteristically, hyaline membranes and fibrin deposits lining the alveolar border, dysplasia of type II cells, free alveolar fibrin, cells and debris in alveolar spaces, and various stages of interstitial edema and alveolar inflammation and organization [83–85]. Reactive type II pneumocytes are sometimes present in BAL mounts [86]. The term idiopathic pneumonia syndrome (IPS) or delayed pulmonary toxicity syndrome (PTS) is used in recipients of stem cell transplant [5] to denote late lung changes that may result from previously inflicted insult collectively induced by chemotherapeutic agents, conditioning regimens and total body irradiation [87, 88].

The clinical imaging expression of chemo- or chemo-radiotherapy lung is wide ranging [38–40, 89]. At one end of the spectrum, patients present with isolated dyspnea and a progressive decrease in the diffusing capacity as the only manifestation of toxicity [90]. Others present with bilateral interstitial and/or alveolar shadowing, which abates after discontinuation of the drugs and/or corticosteroid therapy [91]. Yet other patients with severe presentation progress to respiratory failure and respiratory death despite drug discontinuation [92]. The HRCT discloses scattered ground-glass haze, inter- and/or intralobular septal thickening or areas of condensation [40]. If patients are able to withstand the test, pulmonary function is restrictive, and hypoxemia is present. The diffusing capacity is decreased, and typically the decrease predates the onset of symptoms or the development of radiographic abnormalities. The changes are progressive or can be reactivated with further treatment with the causal drug, notably bleomycin or rituximab, and careful follow-up is needed before any further administration of the drug is contemplated [73, 90]. The BAL indicates an increase in neutrophils, or neutrophils and activated lymphocytes [93].

A lung biopsy is reserved for patients with an atypical presentation or those who do not improve on empiric antibiotic and steroid treatment [94]. Judicious use of lung biopsy may help to diagnose an infection and tailor treatment accordingly [2, 85]. However, the critical condition of these patients often precludes this option, as the procedure is associated with increased mortality when it is done in patients with significant respiratory impairment. In the setting of chemotherapy, the respective benefit of a minimally invasive approach with drug removal, empiric treatment with antibiotics and corticosteroids [95] as opposed to the more invasive approach remains unclear [96]. A fraction of patients respond favorably to drug discontinuation and corticosteroid drugs, especially if the condition is recognized early. For instance, in a series of 65 patients with hematologic malignancies who received a carmustine-based conditioning regimen prior to bone marrow transplantation, 17 (26%) developed pulmonary infiltrates thought to be drug-induced. Of these, 15 responded to corticosteroids [97]. One patient died of pneumonitis [97]. Corticosteroids should be tapered carefully to avoid catastrophic respiratory failure [98, 99]. Despite occasional success with immunosuppressive drugs [100], the response to treatment and the prognosis of this condition when it is advanced, when corticosteroids fail or when ventilatory support is required are disappointing. Chemotherapy-induced lung toxicity may also negatively impact on the management of the underlying hematologic disease, as a change in therapy may be required toward less efficacious or more toxic drugs.

In patients who recover from chemotherapy lung, mild reduction of vital capacity and/or the diffusing capacity may persist in the long term [101], and the likelihood of permanent physiologic impairment is greater in smokers [102]. Patients who receive alkylating agents for Hodgkin's disease or non-Hodgkin's lymphoma should be discouraged from smoking, as persistent smoking greatly increases the likelihood of developing lung cancer later in life [103, 104].

The high incidence, severity and unpredictability of pulmonary complications from chemotherapy raise the question of whether early detection is meaningful using pulmonary function tests or imaging. Deterioration of indices of pulmonary function is common in patients exposed to chemotherapeutic agents [105, 106], including conditioning regimens for hematopoietic stem cell transplantation [107]. Changes cannot be predicted on an individual basis and occur more in patients who receive TBI in addition to drugs. Corticosteroids may mitigate or reverse these changes [107]. In the majority of patients, though, these subclinical changes do not predict the development of overt disease. In contrast, exposure to methotrexate does not alter lung functions [108]. Some investigators believe it is prudent to discontinue chemotherapy once the diffusing capacity has decreased to <50% of pretherapy values, while others do not rely on this measurement since it is their belief that the diffusing capacity does not equate to and may not predict toxicity, and there is the risk of unnecessarily withdrawing an effective chemotherapy [109]. An abrupt fall in the monthly measurement of the diffusing capacity may indicate impending toxicity. When radiation therapy is planned after administration of chemotherapeutic agents, it is advisable to wait for any chemotherapy-induced decrease in the diffusing capacity to stabilize or show a trend toward improvement, before the patient undergoes radiation therapy [90]. Although changes on imaging are common in patients receiving bleomycin or rituximab, it is impractical to rely on imaging to detect changes consistent with pulmonary toxicity of chemotherapeutic agents. Patients on chemotherapy may develop new opacities on CT although they never develop symptomatic disease [110]. There is no current agreement as to how patients on chemotherapy should be followed to reliably and cost-effectively detect meaningful therapy-induced pulmonary complications. However, many treating physicians have a chest radiograph, PFT and diffusing capacity measured serially during treatment, particularly if patients are being treated with bleomycin.

31.3.1.6 Cell Lysis Pneumopathy

A subset of patients with acute leukemia and high blast counts may develop acute pulmonary complications during induction of remission in the form of diffuse pulmonary infiltrates and an ARDS picture with or without alveolar hemorrhage [111, 112]. This was coined cell lysis pneumonopathy [111] because the pathology indicates blasts in pulmonary capillaries and cell remnants or debris on a background of diffuse alveolar damage. [113]. In a recent study, pulmonary failure developed acutely (within 2 weeks of the initiation of chemotherapy) in 8% of 1,541 patients during remission induction. Male sex, acute promyelocytic leukemia, poor performance status, lung infiltrates at diagnosis and increased creatinine were risk factors for the development of this syndrome. Seventy-three percent of the patient died [70].

31.3.1.7 Drug-Induced and Iatrogenic Pulmonary Fibrosis

The condition mostly develops in hematology patients treated with BCNU, bleomycin, busulfan, chlorambucil, cyclophosphamide, melphalan and/or radiation therapy/TBI. Less often, drug-induced fibrosis complicates treatments with gemcitabine, mercaptopurine, methotrexate and rituximab [11]. Drug-induced fibrosis may develop during treatment with drugs or it is diagnosed after termination of treatment. Imaging prior to onset of treatment with the drug helps confirm the time course of lung changes with respect to exposure to the drug or drugs, and enables separation from fibrosis of other causes. Early disease is in the form of linear or streaky opacities and loss of volume. Honeycombing is a late and inconsistent finding. For those patients who are still on the causal drug, drug removal may not be followed by improvement, and the response to steroids is often not gratifying. On histology, there is interstitial fibrosis, and the lung structure may not be retained. A reactive epithelium is suggestive of but not specific to exposure to alkylating agents and/or radiation therapy. In children or adults who have received cyclophosphamide for the treatment of hematologic malignancy, pleural and subpleural fibrosis can develop in addition to the more classic changes of pulmonary fibrosis [114]. This results in encasing of the lung, anteroposterior narrowing of the chest and severe restrictive physiology causing respiratory failure. It is unfortunate when the syndrome develops in a child, while the basic disease is cured. A few patients who received chlorambucil or methotrexate develop accelerated pulmonary fibrosis in the form of acute interstitial pneumonia [115, 116]. The outcome of pulmonary fibrosis is poor, despite drug withdrawal and institution of high-dose corticosteroids. Lung transplantation has been an option in a few patients.

31.3.1.8 Drug-Induced Pulmonary Edema

Noncardiac pulmonary edema (NCPE) shows a classic pattern of response to several chemotherapeutic agents used to treat hematologic conditions. NCPE is due to the loss of integrity of the endothelial barrier and consequent fluid leakage. NCPE is characterized by the rapid or sudden onset of dyspnea, hypoxemia and alveolar infiltrates, with no evidence of left ventricular dysfunction or iatrogenic circulatory overload [although drugs used to treat malignancies may cause deterioration of cardiac function and cardiogenic pulmonary edema [117–121]. There is often close temporal association of exposure to the drug, onset of dyspnea and the development of pulmonary infiltrates. Chemotherapeutic agents associated with NCPE include ATG, cytosine arabinoside, all-transretinoic acid (ATRA), amphotericin-B, arsenic trioxide (As_2O_3), bleomycin, blood and blood components, carmustine, CSF, cyclophosphamide, deferoxamine, docetaxel, doxorubicine, fludarabine, gemcitabine, interleu-kin-2, methotrexate, mitomycin, radiocontrast agents, rituximab, vinorelbine and vinblastine and several multiagent chemotherapy regimens [11, 122]. Most patients present with NCPE as an isolated finding, but in a few, weight gain, lower extremity or more diffuse edema and pleural and/or pericardial effusions suggest capillary leak [122, 123]. Pathology indicates bland pulmonary edema, with proteinaceous fluid filling most alveolar spaces and sometimes diffuse alveolar damage with little or no inflammation [37]. Severe cases can be fatal, but in most the infiltrates resolve with supportive care and corticosteroid therapy.

31.3.1.9 Diffuse Alveolar Hemorrhage

DAH is a unusual pattern of response to drugs in hematology patients [124]. This condition is on the background of DAH as a manifestation of the underlying disease with or without thrombocytopenia. Alemtuzumab, anticoagulants, ATRA, cytosine arabinoside and CSFs can produce this condition [11]. DAH can also occur with induction of remission in leukemia [125] and as a complication of hematopoietic stem cell transplantation [5, 29, 126, 127]. DAH is characterized by dyspnea, recent anemia, bilateral infiltrates and hypoxemia. The diagnosis is by BAL, which shows increased blood staining in sequential aliquots. DAH can be fatal [127].

31.3.2 Pulmonary Nodules

Single or multiple nodules with the features of BOOP or circumscribed fibrosis on pathology may develop in children and in adults following treatments with aracytine, bleomycin, bleomycin *and* cyclophosphamide, and vinblastine [66, 67, 128–130]. Nodules can pose a difficult challenge in a patient with a history of malignancy, particularly when they assume a round shape. A critical review of other etiologies is necessary [131]. Close follow-up including imaging and 18F-dideoxyglucose PET scan is indicated. A lung biopsy may be required to confidently exclude malignancy. A patient with chronic lymphatic leukemia developed multiple shaggy lung nodules during treatment with fludarabine [132]. The nodules corresponded to sterile aggregates of mononuclear cells on pathology. They disappeared after drug withdrawal and corticosteroid therapy.

Hematopoietic stem cell recipients may develop multiple pulmonary nodules in the context of fever a few months after infusion. Histological studies indicate sterile necrotic aggregates of leukocytes and a disrupted endothelium. The lesions have been coined pulmonary cytolytic thrombi [133].

Careful exclusion of malignancy and an infection is required in all cases, for infection due to *Pneumocystis jiroveci*, *Aspergillus* sp. and other fungi, HSP, *Rhodococcus*, *Mucor*, *Cryptococcus*, *Fusarium* and tuberculosis can manifest with lung nodules.

31.3.3 Acute Chest Pain

White et al. reported on 12 episodes of severe chest pain during infusions of bleomycin, suggesting the diagnosis of acute cardiac or pulmonary events [134]. Incidence of the syndrome was 2.8% of the patients being treated with the drug. Electrocardiographic changes suggestive of pericarditis were found in two cases and radiographic evidence of a small pleural effusion in one. The syndrome was self-limited or relieved with analgesics, and improvement was seen when the infusions were stopped. Further courses of bleomycin did not lead to recurrent episodes. There were no long-term sequelae. Substernal pain or pressure also was described during treatments with high-dose etoposide [135, 136] and methotrexate [137]. The lupus syndrome induced by drugs (for instance interferon) may manifest with acute chest pain [138]. Infusions of 5-fluorouracil or etoposide can produce acute coronary spasm and consequent chest pain [136]. Chest pain is a recognized adverse event in stem cell donors during mobilization [139].

31.3.4 Bronchospasm

Wheezing and bronchospasm are common symptoms in patients receiving antineoplastic drugs including monoclonal antibody therapy such as alemtuzumab or rituximab [140, 141]. Wheezing may be part of the "infusion reaction," a constellation of symptoms including dyspnea, cough, facial flushing, skin rash or urticaria, pruritus, chest tightness and malaise. There is relapse upon rechallenge, except if pretreatment is given or the dose is reduced.

Bronchospasm has been reported with the use of amphotericin B, l-asparaginase, amphotericin B, campath-1H, etoposide, GM-CSF, methotrexate, procarbazine, vinca alkaloids and corticosteroid drugs [11]. The excipients and solvents dimethylsulfoxide [142] and cremophor [143] have also been implicated. There is a close temporal relation of drug administration and wheezing, and in most patients symptoms are mild to moderate. Patients with bronchospasm could be successfully rechallenged using slower doses or infusion rate, or following premedication with antihistamines and corticosteroids.

Some patients develop anaphylaxis, a life-threatening reaction with upper airway obstruction, severe bronchospasm, abdominal cramps and shock [144]. Drugs including antibiotics, anesthetic agents, oxaliplatin and blood can cause this condition [145, 146].

31.3.5 Pleural Involvement

Pleural effusion can be present on imaging in patients with pulmonary reactions to methotrexate, procarbazine or ATRA, especially if the reaction is severe [11, 147]. Bleomycin, cyclophosphamide, IL-2, IVIG, methotrexate, ATRA and radiation therapy can produce lone exudative pleural effusions [11, 148]. Pleural thickening and retraction is a form of late cyclophosphamide toxicity [114, 149]. Pneumothorax can complicate fibrosis induced by BCNU, cyclophosphamide or bleomycin [150]. Radiation-induced pleural changes are mentioned below.

31.3.6 Late Changes

Mild drug-induced reduction of vital capacity and/or diffusing capacity may persist for a few months in patients treated for hematologic malignancies. The likelihood of permanent physiological impairment is greater in smokers [102]. Follow-up of patients is required, especially in those who received a stem cell transplant, to monitor progressive changes (although their incidence is lower than it used to be [151]) and to detect post-treatment lymphoproliferative disease and other malignancies.

31.3.7 Drug-Induced Lymphoma and Second Cancers

As basic disease-related mortality has decreased with time in patients with Hodgkin's disease and non-Hodgkin's lymphoma once remission is obtained, therapy-related mortality increases with time and is becoming the most prevalent cause of late deaths [152]. Although a downward trend in mortality has been noted in more recent years (1980–1995) compared to the prior treatment era (1962–1980), second cancers and cardiovascular complications still account for 20% and 14% of late deaths, respectively [152]. The risk of second or higher-order lung cancer in Hodgkin's disease and non-Hodgkin's lymphoma is increased [153], and it correlates with the dose of radiation delivered to the lung, amount of chemotherapeutic agents received and whether the patient is a smoker. In one study, the relative risk of lung cancer in patients who received ≥9.6 Gy was 9.6 compared to <1 Gy. Patients who had smoked >10 pack-years after the diagnosis of Hodgkin's disease had a further sixfold increase in risk, compared with patients who smoked <1 pack-year. A positive interaction on a multiplicative scale was observed between the carcinogenic effects of smoking and radiation [103]. Studies have found a positive interaction between treatment with MOPP (mechlorethamine, vincristine, procarbazine and prednisone), the number of cycles and the risk of lung cancer [154]. Radiation therapy added to the risk [155]. In another study, treatment with MOPP was associated with a greater risk of lung cancer, compared to chlorambucil, vinblastine, procarbazine and prednisone [156]. Since tobacco use appears to synergize the risks from treatments and increase lung cancer risk more than 15- to 20-fold, physicians treating these patients need to be wary of the risk and should make a special effort to dissuade patients with Hodgkin's disease from smoking after receiving chemotherapy and radiotherapy. Smoking cessation is a vital part of long-term management of such patients.

Incidence of pleural mesothelioma increases post-radiation therapy in malignant lymphoma survivors [157]

31.4 Drugs Causing Pleuropulmonary Toxicity in Hematology

31.4.1 Amphotericin B

Not uncommonly, infusions of amphotericin B produce wheezing and bronchospasm [11, 158]. Rarely, amphotericin evokes an anaphylactic reaction with or without upper airway obstruction [159]. Not all manifestations will return upon rechallenge, and there are guidelines to reexpose patients to the drug [160].

Wright et al. described 14 patients who developed pulmonary infiltrates and acute respiratory failure shortly after infusion of amphotericin B and granulocytes [161]. Lung biopsy and autopsy studies disclosed DAH and pulmonary edema. Other studies failed to confirm an association. The possibility of a TRALI syndrome induced by coadministered granulocytes is a possibility. No further case has appeared in the literature.

Infusion of liposomal amphotericin B or amphotericin in 20% intralipid can produce dyspnea, chest tightness, pulmonary infiltrates and pulmonary edema [162]. Histopathological studies in a fatal case evidenced fat embolism with lipid material in pulmonary capillaries [163].

31.4.2 Anti-thymocyte Globulin

Transient pulmonary infiltrates thought to represent mild pulmonary edema or, less often, an ARDS picture have been described following anti-thymocyte globulin (ATG) infusion [164]. Rechallenge was followed by recurrence of pulmonary infiltrates [164]. In one recent report, steroid-supported rechallenge was not followed by relapse [33].

31.4.3 All-trans-Retinoic Acid (ATRA) and Arsenic Trioxide As_2O_3

All-*trans*-retinoic acid or ATRA, the active metabolite of vitamin A, and arsenic trioxide (As_2O_3) have emerged as important agents to induce remission in newly diagnosed or relapsed acute promyelocytic leukemia [165], where these agents accelerate the differentiation and maturation of normal promyelocytic cells, which quenched the life-threatening hemorrhagic complications of the disease at its onset. The administration of ATRA during induction of remission is often followed in a few days by a sharp increase in the number of circulating myeloid cells and neutrophils. This is temporally associated in some patients with the development of fever, weight gain, pleuritic chest pain, pleural or pericardial effusion, lower extremity edema, dyspnea, pulmonary infiltrates, pulmonary edema, alveolar hemorrhage, or an ARDS picture [166–169]. This aggregate of symptoms developed an average of 8 days after initiation of treatment and is grouped under the eponym "retinoic acid- or ATRA syndrome" [166]. Similar manifestations are observed in patients who receive As_2O_3 in up to 31% in one study [170], causing respiratory death [171]. The condition is also referred to as ATRA or retinoic acid syndrome. Onset of ATRA syndrome can be heralded by an increase in circulating neutrophils. Patients with neutrophil counts above 10,000/μL are considered at risk of developing the syndrome, while the condition is considered unusual in leukopenic patients [166]. ATRA syndrome is thought to result from the sequestration of activated neutrophils in pulmonary capillaries, leading to acute lung injury and vascular leakage. Radiographic studies indicate ill-defined infiltrates, ground-glass opacities, lung nodules that may progress to diffuse alveolar shadows, and pleural effusions [172]. Blasts and promyelocytes containing Auer rods were evidenced in the BAL in one case [173]. Postmortem studies indicate maturing and mature myeloid cells within the pulmonary interstitium [166]. Capillaritis and diffuse alveolar hemorrhage have been reported once [174]. Patients improve on drug removal and high-dose corticosteroids [166]. Prophylactic corticosteroids have decreased both the severity and incidence of ATRA syndrome down to about 8% [175]. Mortality from ATRA syndrome is about 8% or 1% of all patients treated with these agents. In most cases, ATRA therapy can be reinstituted once the syndrome has resolved [176], although at 75% of the initial dosage [177]. ATRA may also cause venous thromboembolism and infarction in several end organs, including the lung [178]. As_2O_3 may also cause adverse cardiac effects [179].

31.4.4 Azacytidine

The DNA hypomethylating agent azacitidine was approved for treatment of myelodysplastic syndrome. A few cases report the association of treatments with the drug and episodes of ILD, BOOP, or reversible ARDS [180–182]

31.4.5 Bis-Chlororethyl Nitrosourea Carmustine

The bis-chlororethyl nitrosourea (BCNU, carmustine) drug derives from the vesicant chemical warfare mustard. BCNU is an alkylating agent introduced in 1963 in the treatment of malignant brain tumors because of its low molecular weight. Currently, BCNU is used for the treatment of high-risk breast carcinoma and as a conditioning regimen for bone marrow and stem cell transplantation along with busulfan or cyclophosphamide and total body irradiation (TBI). BCNU and TBI are thought to play a crucial role in the pathogenesis of chemotherapy lung and idiopathic pulmonary syndrome (see above). The lower incidence of idiopathic pulmonary complications with nonmyeloablative as opposed to myeloablative preconditioning regimens supports the causal role of the intensity of the conditioning regimen in its development. The pulmonary complications of BCNU when the drug was used as a solo agent have been described in children and in adults, and BCNU has caused pulmonary toxicity more often than the other nitrosoureas CCNU (lomustine), DCNU (chlorozotocin), methyl-CCNU, streptozotocine, fotemustine, and estramustine. Carmustine lung damage is dose-related, and the incidence is between 1% and 10%. BCNU pulmonary toxicity is one form of chemotherapy lung, and it resembles clinically, pathologically and on imaging the pneumonitis induced by bleomycin, busulfan, chlorambucil, cyclophosphamide, melphalan, and vinblastine. A total dose of 1,000–1,200 mg/m^2 of BCNU is considered the threshold above which the incidence of pulmonary toxicity increases steeply when the drug is used as a single agent [183]. Incidence of BCNU toxicity increases about tenfold when cyclophospamide or irradiation is given concomitantly. Up to two thirds of patients treated with high-dose chemotherapy and BCNU develop clinical and physiological evidence of pulmonary toxicity [184]. An attempt to reduce pulmonary toxicity in a modified CBV regimen using CCNU instead of BCNU followed by autologous hematopoietic cell transplantation in 16 patients with relapsed or refractory Hodgkin's disease or non-Hodgkin's lymphoma was associated with a 63% incidence of interstitial pneumonitis, and 6 of 16 affected patients died of interstitial pneumonitis [185].

Early disease presents subacutely, a form of BCNU lung toxicity that is more amenable to corticosteroid therapy, thereby having an improved prognosis [107, 184]. Late BCNU toxicity is characterized by pulmonary fibrosis [186] and progressive respiratory failure [187]. The histopathological appearances of BCNU pneumonitis are similar to those from other alkylating agents with interstitial edema, diffuse alveolar damage, a reactive epithelium, and interstitial fibrosis [188–190]. Less common features include pleural fibrosis [189], vascular thrombosis, venoocclusive disease, or pulmonary alveolar proteinosis [187]. Long-term follow-up indicates that a fraction of patients with hematologic malignancies may die late from nitrosourea-related respiratory failure [191].

31.4.6 Bleomycin

In the 1960s, bleomycin was one of the first drugs recognized as a cause of lung disease [192]. Bleomycin pulmonary toxicity (BPT) is common [193, 194] and there are recent reports in patients who received the drug with other antineoplastic agents for the treatment of malignant lymphoma [195, 196] or solid tumors [197, 198]. Many therapy-related pneumonitis cases that occur in patients receiving chemotherapy regimens containing bleomycin (e.g., ABVD, BACOD) are reported as BPT [196].

Onset of BPT is not as acute as that of methotrexate lung. BPT can be severe, but this form of toxicity may be less debilitating than busulfan, nitrosoura, or myleran lung. The characteristics of BPT may be discernible even though bleomycin is given along with other chemotherapeutic agents [193]. Even though early reports warned of the possibility of BPT after low cumulative dosages of the drug [199], for many years it was believed that bleomycin caused pulmonary toxicity only above 500 mg. In fact, although the incidence of BPT is dose-dependent [193], BPT can occur with as little as 20 or 34 mg bleomycin [200, 201]. Renal failure places patients at higher risk of developing BPT [79, 202], owing to decreased clearance of the drug. Slow as opposed to rapid i.v. infusion and intramuscular administration of bleomycin lessen the risk of BPT. Previous use of bleomycin should be considered in those patients requiring retreatment, as there is cumulative toxicity. In some but not all studies, advancing age was a risk factor for BPT. Concomitant or recent irradiation [203, 204], treatments with cyclophosphamide [205], and exposure to high concentrations of oxygen add to the risk and may trigger the onset of BPT [206]. Although not everyone will agree [207], it is prudent to request that anesthetists use the lowest possible fractional concentration of oxygen when patients with a history of exposure to bleomycin undergo any surgical procedure. In some but not all studies, a history of BPT negatively impacts overall survival of patients with malignant lymphoma [196, 208].

Incidence of BPT was once estimated to be 2–3% [209, 210], but recent figures are around 10–15% [196, 197, 202]. Recently, a 11.5% incidence of BPT was reported when bleomycin was administered with vincristine and cisplatin every 10 days [197]. Mortality is about 10%, and overall mortality was 2.3% in a study of 194 patients treated for germ cell tumors with this agent [202]. Mortality is higher in older patients, in those with renal failure [202], and in those with severe BPT, where mortality can be as high as 60% [209].

Clinically, BPT presents acutely or subacutely with dyspnea, and sometimes chest pain [134, 194, 210]. Some chest discomfort may be present at some point before BPT is suspected, representing early BPT that went unrecognized [210]. Crackles on auscultation may precede the radiographic changes of BPT. Imaging studies indicate the predominant involvement of the lung bases as opposed to the apices, costophrenic angles, and subpleural regions, and there is often generalized loss of lung volume [193, 211]. A retrospective review of chest films may show the gradual development of these changes, and it is easy to miss the actual onset of BPT. On HRCT in mild cases, a diffuse ill-defined ground-glass pattern or haze is present. Later, patients develop discrete subpleural crescent-like opacities, streaky opacities along the bronchovascular bundles, alveolar infiltrates, alveolar densities, consolidation, or the clinical-radiographic picture of ARDS [48, 194, 212, 213]. Changes on imaging correlate poorly with impairment of the diffusing capacity [48]. Some patients present with masses on imaging that may about the pleura [48, 214]. Pleural thickening or an effusion is an unusual finding. Several of the above mild HRCT findings are common (up to 80%) in asymptomatic patients during treatments with bleomycin [193]. However, they do not necessarily indicate toxicity, and drug discontinuance is not always required. In one study, such changes occurred in 15 out of 18 patients [215], none of which developed clinically recognizable disease. Thus, serial HRCT may not be a practical test to ensure early detection of BPT, which is best monitored using history, clinical examination, pulmonary function, and the chest radiograph.

On pulmonary function tests a restrictive defect, hypoxemia, and a reduction in the diffusing capacity are present. A low diffusing capacity does not equate toxicity and may predate onset of overt toxicity by weeks. The BAL pattern is neutrophilic [216]. Pathologic features of BPT resemble those seen with the other alkylating agents such as busulfan, chlorambucil, cyclophosphamide, melphalan, and nitrosoureas. Tissue eosinophilia is uncommon and has been reported in patients with the diffuse [198, 217] and nodular (BOOP) [66] form of the disease. The development of parenchymal lung nodules in patients receiving bleomycin is almost unique to this compound, and it can be problematical [218], raising the possibility of parenchymal involvement from the underlying hematologic malignancy [66]. The area's BPT can be tracer-avid on PET scan [35, 219]. Previous imaging, time course of disease markers, earlier PET scan, and response to chemotherapy will dictate whether watchful waiting is indicated or a lung biopsy is necessary so separate these entities. Nodular BPT corresponds to the histological pattern of BOOP with or without eosinophilia in the tissue. Nodular BPT may shrink or clear in a few weeks.

Overall, the prognosis of BPT is less dismal than with the other alkylating agents. A sizable fraction of patients with BPT have reversible disease [194], even though there was evidence for fibrosis on pathology [220]. Corticosteroids are the mainstay of treatment, and, although no controlled study is available, there is clinical evidence for benefit of this form of treatment in mild or moderate BPT. Corticosteroid therapy can be without an effect in severe BPT [197]. It is considered that if patients survive the initial episode of BPT, they are likely to recover gradually [194]. Early or abrupt withdrawal of corticosteroids is discouraged, as this may lead to a severe relapse of BPT [209], and a slow taper is recommended. Some patients develop irreversible bleomycin-induced pulmonary fibrosis [221] with, ultimately, honeycomb lung and clubbing, and die from the condition [209].

The question of whether serial pulmonary function testing is useful in identifying patients who will develop BPT was assessed in 59 men with non-seminomatous testicular carcinoma (the findings probably apply to hematology patients as well) [110]. Patients received a three-course regimen consisting of vinblastine, bleomycin, and platinum. The average bleomycin dose was 555.5 units. Pulmonary physiology was serially evaluated prior to each treatment course. The diffusing capacity fell significant by 11.8% with bleomycin treatment. However, the diffusing capacity failed to predict which patients would develop clinical toxicity. The reduction in the total lung capacity had a better correlation with clinical toxicity [110]. Despite the inability of the diffusing capacity to detect patients who will develop clinical toxicity [110, 222], serial measurement of lung volumes and of diffusing capacity are still routinely performed in this population also for medical-legal reasons [223]. The diffusing capacity decreases in up to 75% of the patients treated with bleomycin, and in only a few will clinical toxicity develop [223]. Any asymptomatic impairment of the DLCO is likely to improve slowly upon termination of treatment. The lung of patients exposed to bleomycin in the remote past should be considered vulnerable, as suggested by occasional reports of unexpected ARDS after minor insults years after termination of treatment with this agent [224].

31.4.7 Blood and Blood Products: Transfusion-Related Acute Lung Injury

TRALI is a potentially devastating complication defined by hypoxemic respiratory failure within 6 h of transfusion, once other causes are excluded. To some extent, TRALI is avoidable and can be prevented. By definition, acute lung injury is defined by a PaO_2/FIO_2 ratio <300, hence the term TRALI. However, some severe TRALI cases would deserve the eponym TR-ARDS, for the PaO_2/FIO_2 ratio in those cases is <200. TRALI is a noncardiogenic pulmonary edema that is temporally and mechanistically related to transfusion of blood and/or blood components. TRALI occurs within 6 h of transfusion. TRALI results from the sequestration of primed and activated neutrophils in the pulmonary circulation, thereby causing endothelial injury and consequent fluid leakage. TRALI is more common in ICU patients [225], and the condition adversely affects outcome. TRALI has a 10% attendant mortality and is the leading cause for transfusion-related deaths [78, 225–231]. Although all blood components have been implicated in TRALI, those that contain a significant amount of plasma, namely fresh frozen plasma and whole blood-derived platelet concentrates, are exposed to a higher risk, compared to red blood cells or whole blood [230, 232]. Plasma-rich components carry a greater risk of containing a substantial quantity of antibody from a donor, which in the majority of cases is the cause of TRALI. Whole blood, immunoglobulins, stem cells, or, rarely, autologous blood have also been implicated [230, 232].

TRALI results from the transfusion of an anti-HLA I, -HLA AII, or human neutrophil alloantigen (HNA-3a-(5b)) antibody from one donor in the pool into patients whose leukocytes express the corresponding cognate antigens [230]. Such antibodies are found in 60–85% of cases. The case for a relationship is more compelling if concordance between the antigen specificity of the leukocyte antibodies in the donor plasma and the corresponding antigen on the cells of the affected recipient is demonstrated [233]. This is found in about 50% of cases. The antibody-antigen interaction causes complement-mediated activation and sequestration of neutrophils in the pulmonary circulation and intravascular cholesterol crystal formation [234], endothelial damage, vascular leakage, and consequent pulmonary edema [230, 234, 235]. Antibodies are more prevalent in women with a history of pregnancies, and the antibody titer increases with the number of pregnancies. Antibody prevalence is lowest in men and in nulliparous women. Although this antibody-antigen hypothesis is attractive, there are antibody negative TRALI cases, TRALI can occur in neutropenic patients, and there is one cause of TRALI following auto-transfusion. Understanding and recognizing TRALI are important. The responsible donor, generally a multiparous woman with high titers of antibody, should be identified. Laboratory investigations should be undertaken in donors to identify the antibody and in the recipient to determine whether his leukocytes bear the cognate antigen. Then the TRALI case can be classified into immune or nonimmune TRALI, the blood bank should be notified to quarantine other components from the same donation until the diagnosis is confirmed, and the implicated donor is identified. The implicated donor should be deferred from further blood donation or their blood diverted to prepare plasma-poor products, not whole blood, FFP, or platelets [232].

TRALI is poorly known [236], and it is underreported [237]. Incidence of TRALI is about 1 in 5,000 transfusions in the US (between 0.08% and 0.16% of all blood transfusions) and is less in Europe. Incidence is higher in ICU patients and in patients with a history of recent bypass surgery, recent infection, in patients with hematologic diseases, and in those who received CSF. This is consistent with a two-hit hypothesis for TRALI, whereby pulmonary endothelial cells are first activated, and PMN are primed and sequester in the pulmonary circulation. Then, transfusion of a biologic response modifier such as anti-granulocyte antibody or biologically active lipids activates adherent neutrophils resulting in endothelial damage vascular leakage and TRALI [238].

By definition, the symptoms of TRALI develop within 6 h of the transfusion in the form of abrupt respiratory failure with rigors, dyspnea, tachypnea, cyanosis, hypotension, leukopenia, mild eosinophilia "whiteout" of the lungs [239], and evidence for fluid leakage [240]. Severe cases are heralded by a protein-rich exudate at the mouth or in ventilator tubings [241]. Sudden intraoperative hypoxemia during blood transfusion or infusion of FFP should raise the suspicion of TRALI [242, 243]. Transient hypoxemia following blood transfusion in patients on the respirator may correspond to TRALI [238]. The main competing diagnoses include transfusion-associated circulatory overload or TACO (both conditions can coexist), transfusion-related sepsis, anaphylaxis, and hemolytic reactions [244]. Imaging studies and measurement of BNP levels may aid in separating TACO from TRALI [245], and an important distinction for diuretics is contraindicated in TRALI [230]. Once TRALI is suspected, laboratory investigation should be undertaken on the remains of transfused products, in the recipient, and in donors whose blood or component were given within 6 h prior to the development of TRALI for the presence of antibodies [226]. Retrospective investigation can evidence an antibody in one donor in the pool in up 89% of cases [246], and a cognate antigen-antibody correlation was identified in 14 of 16 TRALI cases in one study [247].

Underrecognition and underreporting of TRALI may have detrimental consequences. A lookback investigation following a fatal case of TRALI indicated that administration of blood from the implicated donor had produced 15 previous adverse reactions in 14 patients, of which eight were severe [226]. Only two were reported to the regional blood collection facility, and the donor was not deferred from blood donation [226]. Other less common mechanisms for TRALI include antileukocyte antibody in the recipient that react with donor's leukocytes [248] and shelf aging of blood products, leading to accumulation of lipid-derived biologic response modifiers.

Management of TRALI is supportive and includes judicious fluid management, oxygen, and mechanical ventilation in severe cases. Approximately three quarters of patients with TRALI need ventilatory support. The effect of corticosteroid drugs is controversial. Diuretics should be used with caution as TRALI often is associated with fluid leakage, and diuretic therapy may aggravate hemodynamic instability [249]. Diuretics are reserved for cases with documented fluid overload and/or left ventricular failure [244, 249]. Most TRALI cases will recover within 96 h.

Prevention of TRALI relies on parsimonious use of blood transfusion, particularly of plasma rich blood components and in the ICU. Other measures include blood washing to remove biologically active substances, the use of solvent-detergent plasma, improved donor selection, male predominant or male only policy, which is associated with a reduction in the incidence of TRALI, and minimization of shelf life of blood products. Awareness, proper recognition, and reporting of TRALI are essential. Screening blood donors or testing donors with a history of pregnancy or transfusion is a logical and cost-effective TRALI prevention strategy. However, this may not meet with success, as not all blood components with antibodies will produce TRALI in the clinic.

31.4.8 Bortezomib

Treatments with the proteasome inhibitor bortezomib have been associated with the development of pulmonary infiltrates [250–253]. The incidence is 3% in Japan and is less in the West. The highest recorded incidence was 31% [254]. Corticosteroid therapy may prevent the development of bortezomid-associated pulmonary infiltrates. The condition needs be separated from the pulmonary manifestations of multiple myeloma, which include plasma cell infiltrates and crystal-storing histiocytosis, and from an infection [20, 22].

31.4.9 Busulfan (Myleran)

Most cases of busulfan lung were described in the 1960s and 1970s [255], when the drug was used as a single-agent for the treatment of chronic myelogenous leukemia [256]. Nowadays, busulfan is mainly used in conditioning prior to hematopoietic stem cell transplantation, where busulfan pulmonary toxicity is enhanced by drug dosage as seen in recipients of autologous stem cell transplant [257] and by concomitant irradiation [257]. Time to onset of busulfan lung is from a few weeks to 10 years. Administration of other chemotherapy agents increases the risk of developing the condition. Busulfan lung is notable for hugely reactive alveolar cells in the lung and in other epithelia [258], pulmonary fibrosis [259], and, less commonly, a pattern of organizing pneumonia [260], or pulmonary alveolar proteinosis [261]. Long-term exposure to busulfan may produce a brownish discoloration of the skin simulating Addison's disease [256]. Although the incidence of busulfan lung is relatively high, with figures up to 6%, the disease is difficult to predict as pulmonary function of unaffected patients may remain unchanged during treatment [262]. Although reports of pure busulfan lung have decreased in the past years, busulfan pulmonary toxicity continues to afflict patients with hematologic malignancies or breast carcinoma who receive chemotherapy regimens including this drug, although the lung illness in these cases is not coined busulfan lung any longer [257].

31.4.10 Chlorambucil

Chlorambucil is prescribed primarily for the treatment of chronic lymphatic leukemia and low-grade lymphomas. The clinical imaging presentation and pathologic features of chlorambucil pulmonary toxicity are not dissimilar to those described in other alkylating agent-induced pulmonary toxicity [263–265]. Notably, there are atypical changes in alveolar lining cells. A handful of cases of seemingly cellular interstitial lung disease have been reported, with recovery following drug discontinuance and corticosteroid therapy [265]. One recent case report of focal BOOP is thought to reflect chlorambucil pulmonary toxicity [266].

31.4.11 Colony-Stimulating Factors

Colony-stimulating factors (G & GM-CSF) stimulate the production of neutrophils from committed hematopoietic progenitor cells. These agents are used to restore neutrophil counts in patients who are receiving myeloablative chemotherapy or have aplastic anemia, and to mobilize progenitor cells in stem cell donors. A few case reports described pulmonary infiltrates in patients receiving G-CSF monotherapy [7, 267, 268]. Most cases described pulmonary infiltrates or ARDS in patients who were being treated with chemotherapeutic agents (bleomycin, busulfan, methotrexate, or TBI) in conjunction with G- or GM-CSF [208, 269]. In a series of 36 patients with non-Hodgkin's lymphoma receiving a BACOP regimen, 12 received recombinant G-CSF. Out of these 12, four developed respiratory complications (3 died), as opposed to 1 of 24 unexposed patients [270]. Other reports reported fatal respiratory distress in patients receiving CSF for hematologic malignancies [271] or nonneoplastic conditions [271].

Experimental evidence indicates that G-CSF leads to sequestration of activated neutrophils in lung [272] and enhances the damage from bleomycin [273].

However, a randomized study in patients with germ cell tumors failed to demonstrate an increase in incidence of BPT in patients who were exposed G-CSF compared to bleomycin controls [274]. In several patients, but not in all, pulmonary infiltrates developed concomitant with CSF-induced peak in circulating neutrophils [275]. A few cases were described in patients who had persistently low neutrophil counts.

Clinical severity ranged from transient subclinical hypoxemia [276] to diffuse pulmonary infiltrates or an ARDS picture [276]. Lymphocytosis was found in the BAL in one case [277]. CSF-associated infiltrates cleared in a few days or they persisted for weeks. Mortality is about 20%, and prognosis is improved on corticosteroid therapy [275]. Rechallenge may not lead to relapse of the pulmonary infiltrates [275].

CSF-induced mobilization in donors can also induce pulmonary complications. These range from a subclinical drop in PaO_2 with a widened A-a oxygen gradient [278] to pulmonary infiltrates, ARDS, or capillary leak and pleuropericardial effusion [7, 268, 278, 279].

31.4.12 Corticosteroids

Long-term corticosteroid therapy leads to mediastinal lipomatosis, a radiographic curiosity in most patients and a cause for cough or mediastinal hemorrhage in a few [280, 281].

Corticosteroids may induce respiratory muscle weakness, with consequent restrictive lung dysfunction [282].

Allergy and anaphylaxis are rare [283–285].

Corticosteroids exert a broad range of immunosuppressive activities [286], and patients on corticosteroids long-term run the risk of developing opportunistic pulmonary infections, including *Pneumocystis jiroveci* pneumonia [8].

31.4.13 Cyclophosphamide

Like busulfan and nitrosoureas, cyclophosphamide is an alkylating agent used in the treatment of various forms of leukemias and lymphomas and as a conditioning agent prior to stem cell transplantation. Cyclophosphamide may produce early or late pleuropulmonary toxicity [114].

Early cyclophosphamide pulmonary toxicity resembles that of other alkylating agents, is associated with BAL lymphocytosis [287], and is reversible upon removal of the drug, except in patients who develop early ARDS [288]. The prognosis of early cyclophosphamide pulmonary toxicity exceeds that for the nitrosoureas and busulfan, and if diagnosed early, this form of cyclophosphamide pulmonary toxicity is largely reversible upon removal of the drug and institution of corticosteroid therapy. It is important to rule out an infection [289], especially *Pneumocystis jiroveci* pneumonia, which is difficult to differentiate from, and can coexist with cyclophosphamide pneumonitis [290].

Late cyclophosphamide pulmonary toxicity mostly follows chronic oral exposure [114, 291], occurring with up to 13 years of treatment [292]. Chronic cyclophosphamide pneumonitis takes the form of progressive pulmonary fibrosis with respiratory failure, and sometimes digital clubbing is present [293]. The peculiar feature in a subset of patients with late cyclophosphamide toxicity is a pattern of pleuropulmonary fibroelastosis that involves the upper and lateral aspects of the pleura, which is thickened, in addition to more conventional changes of pulmonary fibrosis of the underlying lung [114, 149, 294, 295]. Progressive narrowing of the anteroposterior aspect of the thorax may develop in children, contributing the restrictive physiology, which is progressive with time [149, 296]. Pneumothorax may complicate this form of late cyclophosphamide pleuropulmonary toxicity, and it is difficult to treat as the underlying fibrotic lung reexpands poorly. Chronic cyclophosphamide pneumonitis is irreversible, even with drug withdrawal and institution of corticosteroid therapy [114].

31.4.14 Cytosine-Arabinoside (Ara-C)

Treatments with high-dose Ara-C can be complicated by transient pulmonary infiltrates or pulmonary edema [297–299]. The condition develops in close temporal association with administration of the drug [299, 300]. In a series of 181 autopsies of patients with leukemia, unexplained massive proteinaceous pulmonary edema correlated with recent administration of Ara-C [297]. Pathology discloses bland alveolar flooding by proteinaceous material, suggesting acute fluid leakage [301]. Little or no inflammation is present. Less severe cases show diffuse alveolar damage [85]. Several case histories are consistent with a beneficial effect of corticosteroid therapy in aracytine-induced pulmonary edema.

Recently, acute pulmonary edema and bilateral pleural effusion were diagnosed in a patient who received methotrexate 1,000 mg/m^2 daily and cytarabine 3,000 mg/m^2 twice a day on day 2 and 3 and G-CSF [302]. A patient who received 10 mg/m^2 mitoxantrone daily for 6 days and 3 g/m^2 IV ARA-C developed histologically documented BOOP. Chagnon et al. described transient centrilobular nodules in six patients with acute myelogenous leukemia and treatment-induced neutropenia [303]. These abnormalities of uncertain background and significance were thought to represent drug toxicity.

31.4.15 Dasatinib

Dasatanib is a multitargeted inhibitor of bcr-abl and SRC family tyrosine kinases that is approved for rescue therapy in patients with imatinib-resistant chronic myelogenous leukemia, and it is also used when imatinib induces adverse effects. The drug is known to cause pleural effusions in 10–35% of patients who receive it [304, 305]. The effusion was an exudate in 78% of the assessable cases [306]. Dasatinib may also cause lung injury in the form of pulmonary infiltrates [32]. In 40 patients on dasatinib, 6 had a lymphocyte predominant pleural exudates, and 7 had parenchymal ground-glass or alveolar opacities or septal thickening [32]. Lymphocytes represented up to 92% of the cells in the BAL, and lymphocytes were confirmed in pleural tissue in one case. Upon dasatinib discontinuance (with corticosteroid therapy in one patient), manifestations of the disease abated or resolved in all nine cases. Interestingly, no relapse occurred in three of four rechallenged patients [32], enabling resumption of treatment with this often vital drug. Lymphocyte-rich effusions (bilateral in one case) were also reported in two patients [304]. Chylous fluid was present in one patient. The authors suggested that the effusions were the result of PDGFR inhibition [304].

Dasatinib 100 mg once daily instead of the classic 70 mg twice daily retains efficacy and reduces toxicity with reduced incidence of pleural effusions from 16% to 7% [307]. With the better delineation of dasatinib-induced pleuropulmonary toxicity, noninvasive diagnosis and management should enable cost containment of this adverse effect [308].

31.4.16 Deferoxamine

Deferoxamine is used to treat iron overload in transfusion-dependent thalassemia. When given in high dosages or over more than 24 h, deferoxamine may cause diffuse alveolar damage or pulmonary edema [309]. IgE-coated mast cells were evidenced in lung tissue [310]. Rarely, deferoxamine triggers an anaphylactic reaction [311]. No recent case has been published.

31.4.17 Etoposide

The podophylotoxin derivative etoposide (VP16-213) is part of conditioning regimens for stem cell transplantation, and the drug is used in the management of refractory Hodgkin's lymphoma. Pulmonary reactions are of the hypersensitivity type, with suggestive chronology, facial flushing, wheezing, and hypotension [141]. Prudent rechallenge with the drug can be attempted and was successful in up to three quarters of cases [135]. Very few patients with presumed etoposide pneumonitis have been described. The histopathological features may include diffuse alveolar damage, alveolar hemorrhage, and type II cells reactive changes [312].

31.4.18 Fludarabine

Fludarabine monophosphate, the 2-fluoro, 5′ phosphate derivative of 9-beta-D-arabinofuranosyl adenine (ara-A), is a purine analogue used in the treatment of a variety of hematologic malignancies, including chronic lymphatic leukemia, other low-grade non-Hodgkin's lymphoma resistant to alkylating agents, and acute leukemias. Acute interstitial pneumonitis due to fludarabine was first described in 1987 [313]. The disease improved on high-dose steroids, recurred with steroid withdrawal, and abated with further steroid therapy [313]. Fludarabine pneumonitis can occur as early as

7 days into treatment, with an incidence rate of 1–8.6% [314]. Patients with a background of chronic lymphatic leukemia and preexisting interstitial pulmonary opacities may be at higher risk of developing pulmonary toxicity [315, 316]. On pathology, cellular interstitial pneumonia, eosinophilic pneumonia, granulomas, BOOP, and DAD with reactive type II cell changes have been described [316, 317]. Fludarabine pneumonitis can occasion severe symptoms and can be fatal [318]. In most cases, symptoms abate with drug removal and corticosteroid therapy. Rechallenging the patient leads to recurrence of manifestations of the disease [316, 318].

31.4.19 Gemcitabine

Gemcitabine (2,2-difluorodeoxycytidine) is a deoxycytidine analog with structural similarities to cytosine arabinoside. The drug is to treat several hematologic and nonhematologic malignancies, including malignant lymphoma and lung cancer. The first description of gemcitabine pulmonary toxicity was in 1997 in the form of noncardiac pulmonary edema, ARDS, and alveolar hemorrhage in three patients, and corticosteroid therapy was effective in reversing symptoms [92]. Thirty-one reports of gemcitabine pulmonary toxicity were available in the literature in 2006, and there were 147 other unpublished reports gathered in the RADAR project [319].

The incidence of gemcitabine pulmonary toxicity is 0.02–3% [122, 320, 321]. Gemcitabine pulmonary toxicity may develop after one or several courses with the drug, with a mean time to onset of 48 days (range 1–529 days). Drugs that cause pulmonary injury such as bleomycin or docetaxel may synergize gemcitabine pulmonary toxicity [319]. The incidence of gemcitabine pulmonary toxicity was 22% when the drug was added to bleomycin, doxorubicine, and vinblastine in a phase I/II trial in end-stage Hodgkin's disease [75]. Combining gemcitabine and docetaxel induced a 37% incidence rate of pneumonitis [322]. In yet another study where gemcitabine was added to doxorubicin, bleomycin and vinblastine for the treatment of de novo Hodgkin disease, the incidence of pulmonary toxicity was 41.7% [74]. In a recent study, gemcitabine given with the anti-CD30 antibody VGN-30 was associated in a 31% rate of pulmonary toxicity [323]. Whether and to what extent pulmonary toxicity in these studies is due to gemcitabine or to the coadministered drugs is unclear. Gemcitabine potentiates the adverse effects of radiation therapy [324].

Gemcitabine pulmonary toxicity manifests with cough, dyspnea, and fever in the context of diffuse bilateral ground-glass or denser shadowing with or without pleural effusion. Features consistent with capillary leak such as weight gain and lower extremity or generalized edema can be present [122]. On HRCT, the appearances of gemcitabine pulmonary toxicity include inter- and intralobular thickening, ground-glass opacities, and pleural effusions. Histopathological appearances include alveolar edema, hyaline membranes, diffuse alveolar damage, and accelerated lung fibrosis, whereas alveolar hemorrhage, interstitial pneumonia, and reactive type II cells are less common features [92, 325–327]. Corticosteroids were used with benefit in several cases. Mortality is about 20% [328]. Rechallenge with the drug produces relapse of symptoms [329] and may occasion fatal respiratory failure [92].

Gemcitabine pulmonary toxicity may also manifest in the form of the hemolytic and uremic syndrome (HUS). Presenting features include systemic hypertension, anemia, thrombocytopenia, hematuria, renal failure, and circulating schizocytes. The incidence is up to 2.2%, and 35 cases were reviewed [330]. Subclinical HUS has been described, and monitoring of hemoglobin, creatinine, and circulating schizocytes is advised in patients who have received the drug.

31.4.20 Hydroxyurea

Eleven cases of hydroxyurea-induced pneumonitis were reviewed in 2003 [331]. The pulmonary reaction developed after 3–12 weeks on the drug in the form of fever and bilateral reticular or nodular infiltrates, and a small pleural effusion was present in five cases. Rechallenge with the drug was followed by recurrence. Outcome is good [331].

31.4.21 Interferon

Interferon (IFN) alpha and beta are a therapeutic option in patients with chronic myelogenous leukemia, myeloma, and myelofibrosis, in addition to their established use for the treatment of chronic hepatitis C virus infection and multiple sclerosis. Interferon gamma has been used experimentally as a salvage therapy of corticosteroid-resistant pulmonary toxicity syndrome following BCNU-based chemotherapy and met with limited success in the treatment of pulmonary fibrosis. The respiratory complications from IFN (mostly alpha 2b [332]) may be dose-dependent and occur more commonly following the use of pegylated IFN, and may develop regardless of the underlying disease for which IFN is given. However, most reports are in patients with hepatitis C virus infection [333]. The most distinctive adverse effect of IFN alpha and beta is a picture indistinguishable from naturally occurring sarcoidosis. After a few months into treatment, patients develop *de novo* sarcoidosis or there is reactivation of previously diagnosed quiescent sarcoidosis. The lung, liver, heart, central nervous system, and skin can be involved [333], and hypercalcemia has been reported [334]. On imaging, IFN-induced sarcoidosis-like disease is in the form of hilar or mediastinal lymphadenopathy, ground-glass shadowing, micronodular infiltrates, or thickening along the bronchovascular bundles [335]. Increased lymphocytes, generally of the CD8+ phenotype, are present in the BAL [335, 336], and this is at variance with the findings in naturally occurring sarcoidosis. Eighty-five percent of patients stabilize or improve, 15% develop chronic stable disease, and a third require corticosteroid treatment [333].

Interferons can induce other forms of ILD. Interferon therapy may induce volume loss with a disproportionate decrease of diffusing capacity for CO and no discernible pulmonary opacities [337, 338], cellular interstitial pneumonia, ARDS [339], desquamative interstitial pneumonia [340], pulmonary fibrosis [340], eosinophilic pneumonia [341], and BOOP [342]. The latter condition may manifest with diffuse infiltrates [343, 344] or a mass [64]. Most cases of IFN-induced interstitial lung disease respond to diminution of drug dosage, drug removal, and corticosteroid therapy [336]. A recent review of 25 published cases showed onset of the disease after 23 days to 10 months into treatment [332]. There was one fatality [332].

Other adverse effects of IFN include lone dyspnea, chronic cough [345], exacerbation of asthma [346], pleural effusion [347], pulmonary hypertension [348], and drug-induced lupus [349].

31.4.22 Imatinib

Imatinib is a protein kinase inhibitor that downregulates the Bcr-Abl protein kinase generated by the Philadelphia chromosome in chronic myelogenous leukemia. Pneumonitis [17, 350], fluid retention, and pleural effusion [351] have been reported during treatments of chronic myelogenous leukemia with the drug. A series of 27 interstitial pneumonitis cases (with a preponderance of males) was published in 2006 [17]. Onset of the disease was after a median of 49 days into treatment with no evidence that drug dosage was playing a role. Clinical presentation included dyspnea and hypoxemia. Histopathological findings included interstitial inflammation, fibrosis, organizing pneumonia, and eosinophilic pneumonia, and a reactive epithelium [17]. Drug lymphocyte stimulation test was negative in all nine patients so tested [17]. The drug was withdrawn in all patients, and most patients received corticosteroid therapy to alleviate symptoms. The condition resolved in seven patients and improved in 16. In the 11 patients who were rechallenged, the disease relapsed in only 4, an important consideration regarding the management of the native hematologic malignancy. One patient was successfully rechallenged while receiving 60 mg of prednisolone [352]. At least seven cases of imatinib-induced pneumonitis with or without fluid retention and pleural effusion have been reported in the interim of the above report [17]. One case of eosinophilic pneumonia ascribed to this agent is available [353], and pulmonary alveolar proteinosis developed in another patient [354].

31.4.23 Lenalidomide

Three cases of lenalidomide-induced pneumonitis have been reported in patients with multiple myeloma. Lymphocytes were increased in the BAL two cases. Pathology disclosed interstitial pneumonia and granulomas and BOOP in one case each [55, 355–358].

31.4.24 Melphalan

Meplhalan produces epithelial changes in the lung that resemble those of other alkylating agents [359]. There are not many well-documented cases of melphalan-induced pneumonitis [360–362]. The condition typifies the chemotherapy lung. In early cases, the disease is acute and reverses with drug withdrawal and corticosteroid therapy [361]. Later cases present with the features of late chemotherapy lung, i.e., lung fibrosis and reactive type II cell changes [363]. Corticosteroids are indicated and have reversed late melphalan toxicity [362].

31.4.25 Methotrexate

Methotrexate lung can complicate treatments of various neoplastic and nonneoplastic conditions (mainly rheumatoid arthritis nowadays) in 0.86–6.9% of patients on the drug [364]. Risk factors in rheumatoid arthritis include prior ILD, advanced age, diabetes mellitus, and low serum albumin. A previous episode of methotrexate pneumonitis is the strongest risk factor for relapse, should the patient be reexposed to the drug. The first report of methotrexate pneumonitis dates back 41 years [365]. Acute pulmonary disease developed in seven children in clinical remission from their hematologic malignancy. The disease was life threatening in six. Open lung biopsy showed interstitial pneumonitis with granuloma formation. Cessation of the drug and corticosteroid therapy were effective with a return to normal in 10–40 days. Methotrexate could be continued in some patients.

In 2000, 123 cases of methotrexate lung in hematology and rheumatology patients were summarized [43]. Methotrexate pneumonitis can develop after treatment of leukemia, solid tumors, rheumatoid arthritis, psoriasis, primary biliary cirrhosis, asthma, or molar or ectopic pregnancy [36]. The majority of patients (62%) are women. Methotrexate pneumonitis develops after doses of the drug ranging from 2.5 to 1,400 mg/week. Duration of treatment was from single exposure to 5 years, although half of the patients developed the disease within the first 32 weeks of treatment [366]. The development of methotrexate pneumonitis is unpredictable. There is no correlation between dose and time to onset, or clinical severity. Fatal methotrexate pneumonitis can occur with the low-dosage regimen of methotrexate used in the treatment of rheumatoid arthritis. All routes of administration including the oral, parenteral, and intrathecal ones expose the patient to the risk. The majority of patients are on the drug at the time of pneumonitis, with rare cases of delayed onset of the condition [367]. Methotrexate lung is annunciated by the insidious onset of a dry cough for days or a few weeks, contrasted with unchanged chest radiograph. Then, the disease accelerates with cough in 81% of the patients, fever in 76%, shortness of breath in 82%, dense ILD on imaging, and hypoxemia. Mild peripheral eosinophilia is present in about 40% of patients [368]. Radiographic studies indicate diffuse symmetrical interstitial lung shadowing, and in severe cases dense bilateral alveolar opacities with air bronchograms and volume loss [369]. HRCT discloses dense, patchy, widespread, or diffuse septal lines, geographic ground-glass or alveolar densities [370]. Pulmonary physiology is restrictive, with a low diffusing capacity and significant hypoxemia. Unusual patterns of methotrexate pulmonary toxicity include a subacute presentation, eosinophilic pneumonia, pulmonary fibrosis, and acute chest pain. The BAL is best done in the ICU where provision is made to correct the hypoxemia that almost invariably occurs with the procedure. The BAL discloses increased cellularity with a percentage of lymphocytes averaging 58% vs. 10% in normals [371]. Interindividual differences in lymphocyte counts and/or CD4+ or CD8+ subtype percentages are likely to be the result of when into the disease the BAL is performed and whether corticosteroids have been given [50]. Rare cases show eosinophilia in the BAL.

The condition must be separated from an opportunistic infection, mainly *Pneumocystis pneumonia*, which methotrexate pneumonitis can resemble mainly when a granulomatous pattern of reaction is present, with no reliable clinical or radiological discriminators. The arsenal of tools to diagnose *Pneumocystis jiroveci* in BAL specimens should be used, for *Pneumocystis* is not detected in all cases on direct stains of BAL fluid, and sputum examination may be unrewarding. A lung biopsy may be needed to separate these entities. Methotrexate lung must also be separated from other opportunistic infections due to *Cytomegalovirus*, *Cryptococcus*, *Herpes zoster* and *Nocardia*, which have been described as a complication of chronic treatments with methotrexate [8], especially but not exclusively so when blood CD4+ cells are <150/μL or cumulated doses of methotrexate are above 700 mg.

Histological findings in methotrexate lung include interstitial inflammation, fibrosis, granuloma formation, and increased tissue eosinophils in 71%, 59%,

35%, and 18% of the cases, respectively [43]. Granulomas in methotrexate pneumonitis are typically small and ill-defined, with sterile necrosis being an unusual feature [43]. In patients with predominantly granulomatous methotrexate lung, the disease is patchy with intervening areas of normal lung tissue or tissue showing mild cellular inflammation [43]. Type II cell hyperplasia is an occasional feature in methotrexate lung. Alveolar edema, diffuse alveolar damage, hyaline membranes, and DAH are unusual findings that denote severe cases. Rare appearances include a DIP pattern, a sarcoid-like reaction, and acute interstitial pneumonia [43, 115]. Although the differential diagnosis of methotrexate lung is complex, the clinical-pathologic pattern of an acute granulomatous pneumonitis with no evidence of infection and mild blood eosinophilia is distinctive compared to any other chemotherapeutic agent [43].

Methotrexate pneumonitis responds to drug discontinuation. Corticosteroid therapy is indicated in severe cases. A few cases responded to corticosteroid therapy even though treatment with methotrexate was continued [43]. Dose and duration of corticosteroid treatment have not been determined precisely and are guided by clinical, physiologic, and radiographic response. It is estimated that 85% of patients with methotrexate pneumonitis recover. Mortality is 15%, mainly from progressive respiratory failure [372]. Pulmonary fibrosis following the diagnosis of this condition is unusual [43]. Rechallenge with methotrexate will not lead to recurrence in all patients. However, the disease relapses in up to two thirds of the patients, so tested with a 50% mortality rate in those patients who relapse [30].

Pulmonary function has been prospectively evaluated in patients on methotrexate long-term, in an attempt to detect methotrexate lung at an earlier stage than when the condition is diagnosed clinically [364]. As opposed to alkylating agents, nearly all studies found no deterioration of lung function or imaging that would enable early detection of methotrexate lung [108]

31.4.26 Procarbazine

Procarbazine is one drug in the MOPP regimen. The drug was mostly used to treat Hodgkin's disease and other malignant lymphomas. Eight cases of procarbazine pulmonary toxicity have been described [373]. Typically, procarbazine lung manifests acutely with fever, cough, and dyspnea. Pulmonary infiltrates may be discreet. Pleural effusion [374] and mild peripheral eosinophilia [375] were present in one case each. Procarbazine pulmonary toxicity can be fatal [376, 377]. Symptoms decline upon drug discontinuance and corticosteroid therapy. There is no recent case in the literature.

31.4.27 Rituximab

Rituximab is a chimeric monoclonal antibody directed against the CD20-receptor on B cells. The drug is mainly used to treat malignant lymphomas of B cell lineage, post-transplantation lymphoproliferative disorders, bullous pemphigoid, and rheumatoid arthritis. Incidence of pulmonary toxicity is 0.03–8% [378]. Most patients were receiving rituximab in association with CHOP, CEOP, or CVP and had increased incidence of pulmonary toxicity compared to the pre-rituximab era [379]. Bitzan et al. reviewed 30 cases of rituximab-associated lung disease. Seventy-one percent of the patients received concomitant chemotherapy. Time to onset from the last rituximab dose was 14 days. Eleven of 31 patients required mechanical ventilatory support, and nine died (29%). High-dose glucocorticoid therapy did not improve survival or prevent the development of severe lung disease or death [380]. Forty-five cases of rituximab-associated pulmonary injury were reviewed [381]. The most common presentation in 37 of the 45 cases was in the form of acute or subacute BOOP and respiratory failure within 2 weeks after the fourth course of treatment, resolving (in most cases with corticosteroid therapy. A CD4+-predominant lymphocytosis (up to 90% of all cells) was found in the BAL. Five patients developed early acute pneumonitis, DAD, or ARDS within a few hours after the first infusion of the drug, a pattern consistent with acute cell lysis pneumopathy or cytokine release. Two of these five patients died. Three patients developed macronodules of organizing pneumonia, a form of toxicity that responded successfully to corticosteroid therapy. Mortality was 18%. Pulmonary infiltrates relapsed in about 2/3 of the patients rechallenged with the drug. Two cases of DAH have from this agent have also been reported [11].

31.4.28 Thalidomide

Thalidomide was approved in 2006 for the treatment of multiple myeloma, myelodysplastic syndrome, and graft-vs.-host disease. The first cases of thalidomide-associated pneumonitis was from Spain [382, 383] in the form of ILD, which improved with drug removal and corticosteroid therapy. Two cases had excess lymphocytes in the BAL [384, 385], and eosinophilia was present in another case [386]. One case of BOOP has been reported [387]. Rechallenge with the drug was followed by relapse [384]. A patient was switched to lenalidomide after an episode of thelidomide pulmonary toxicity and did not experience relapse of the interstitial pneumonia [356]. Other adverse effects of thalidomide include pulmonary hypertension [388] and venous thromboembolism [389, 390]. The risk of thromboembolic events is higher when thalidomide is given in association with darpoietin-alpha [390].

31.4.29 Vinca Alkaloids

Treatments with vinca alcaloids (vinblastine, vinorelbine) alone or in combination with mitomycin C in lung cancer patients can be complicated by wheezing, bronchospasm, abrupt dyspnea, or pulmonary infiltrates that correspond to pulmonary edema or diffuse alveolar damage on pathology [391]. Ventilatory support is required is some patients. Incidence of acute shortness of breath and pulmonary infiltrates is 4–6%. On PFTs, there is deterioration of gas exchange and of the diffusing capacity. In several patients, rechallenge with the drug was followed by recurrence of symptoms. Approximately 60 percent of the patients experienced residual chronic respiratory impairment, in the form of restrictive lung function impairment with or without hypoxemia, and residual pulmonary opacities that only respond incompletely to corticosteroid therapy [391].

31.5 Adverse Effects of Radiation Therapy to the Chest

For those patients who receive in-field radiation therapy to the chest, the clinical imaging picture of radiation pneumonitis includes classic radiation pneumonitis, which typically develops 1–2 months after the onset of treatment in the form of a discrete haze, ill-defined patchy opacities, or an area of condensation predominantly in the radiation field. Radiation metrics (area, beam trajectory, fractionation, mean lung dose, and volume of the lung that receives >20 Gy) are used to monitor the risk of radiation pneumonia. A lymphocyte-predominant BAL accompanies these changes, and, interestingly, the lymphocytic reaction also involves the contralateral lung. These changes usually reverse within 6 months, or slowly progress towards a demarcated area of fibrosis and distortion, with volume loss and later bronchiectasis [392, 393]. Late complications of this form of radiation scar are unusual, and include pneumothorax or colonization by *Aspergillus* sp. Although patients with early radiation pneumonitis usually respond well to the administration of corticosteroids, these drugs are not required in all cases, and the dosage and duration of treatment are guided by the severity of symptoms. In rare instances, infiltrates of radiation pneumonitis extend outside the radiation field to involve the lung diffusely or both lungs bilaterally. This is associated with significant clinical symptoms, and, in some patients, respiratory failure or an ARDS picture develops [394]. Most patients respond satisfactorily to the administration of corticosteroids. Acute diffuse radiation/chemoradiation pneumonitis may develop in stem cell transplant recipients following the administration of a conditioning regimen followed by TBI. Whether or not TBI is given and the amount of radiation (>12 Gy) influence the likelihood of developing diffuse pulmonary toxicity, a detrimental prognostic indicator [392].

Most chronic complications from radiation therapy that are now seen are the result of methods, indications, and equipment used in the past [13]. Radiation therapy is not given any longer to patients who achieve complete response after ABVD, and extended field radiation therapy has been supplanted by newer conformal techniques, which spare more of the normal lung. Due to the anatomical complexity and intricateness of multiple organs in the chest, there are a multitude of early or late complications that may cause severe impairment [13]. Depending on the radiation dose and beam, long-term progressive changes following chest radiation therapy may injure the lung, airways, pleura, heart valves, myocardium, pericardium, coronary arteries, mediastinum, lymphatics, esophagus, and cranial nerves, imparting varied clinical and imaging expressions to late radiation-induced injury [13, 395, 396]. A restrictive lung dysfunction can be found in up to a third of patients who received radiation therapy in childhood or adolescence [397]. A fraction of patients (about 3%) develop progressive restrictive lung dysfunction, impacting the quality of life. Paramediastinal sharply demarcated opacities of fibrosis and architectural distortion are present in the previously irradiated area. These changes are greater in patients previously exposed to bleomycin [204]. Fibrosis localizes in the bilateral apices, and paramediastinal and parahilar areas following mantle irradiation. However, these changes are not found in every patient, and the presence and severity of the fibrosis are influenced by the area and size of the radiation fields, particularly with regard to the volume of the irradiated lung, and on whether or not in-field coverage of the hilum or lung was required. The "amount" of chemotherapy, and particularly the dose of bleomycin or other alkylating agents, also may influence the expression of radiation-induced changes in the lung [204]. In severe cases, a distinctive, Y-shaped pattern of fibrotic changes is present on frontal chest films. Severe restriction or encasing of mediastinal structures may ensue. Pleural effusion and chylothorax [13, 398] and the "dropped head syndrome" may be present [13]. Lymphoma survivors must also be evaluated and monitored using auscultation, cardiac ultrasonography, and cardiac stress regarding the frequent development of valvular incompetence/regurgitation, coronary disease, atrioventricular block, or other late cardiac complications of radiation therapy (e.g., heart failure, pericardial thickening/effusion, and pulmonary vein compression), phrenic nerve, or left vocal cord palsy [13, 397, 399, 400].

Patients must also be explored regarding esophageal dysmotility and cranial nerve dysfunction, which may cause chronic aspiration and inflict further lung damage. Late patients also need to be followed up carefully, because second and higher order cancers may occur years after irradiation, including lung cancer, which accounts for one fifth of all lung cancers in lymphoma survivors. Of note, late fibrotic changes in the chest when present may hamper optimal management of lung cancer. Since radiation and antineoplastic drugs synergize the effect of smoking, smoking cessation is an essential step in long-term management and follow-up of patients with a history of cured hematologic malignancy.

References

1. Carver JR, Shapiro CL, Ng A, Jacobs L, Schwartz C, Virgo KS, Hagerty KL, Somerfield MR, Vaughn DJ (2007) American Society of Clinical Oncology Clinical Evidence Review on the ongoing care of adult cancer survivors: cardiac and pulmonary late effects. J Clin Oncol 25(25): 3991–4008
2. Mulabecirovic A, Gaulhofer P, Auner HW, Popper H, Krause R, Hesse C, Sill H (2004) Pulmonary infiltrates in patients with haematologic malignancies: transbronchial lung biopsy increases the diagnostic yield with respect to neoplastic infiltrates and toxic pneumonitis. Ann Hematol 83:420–422
3. Liles A, Blatt J, Morris D, Wardrop R, Sharma A, Sznewajs A, Goldsby R (2008) Monitoring pulmonary complications in long-term childhood cancer survivors: guidelines for the primary care physician. Clev Clin J Med 75:531–539
4. Chemaly RF, Ghosh S, Bodey GP, Rohatgi N, Safdar A, Keating MJ, Champlin RE, Aguilera EA, Tarrand JJ, Raad II (2006) Respiratory viral infections in adults with hematologic malignancies and human stem cell transplantation recipients – a retrospective study at a major cancer center. Medicine (Baltimore) 85:278–287
5. Tanaka N, Matsumoto T, Miura G, Emoto T, Matsunaga N (2002) HRCT findings of chest complications in patients with leukemia. Eur Radiol 12:1512–1522
6. Kotloff RM, Ahya VN, Crawford SW (2004) Pulmonary complications of solid organ and hematopoietic stem cell transplantation. Am J Respir Crit Care Med 170:22–48
7. Arimura K, Inoue H, Kukita T, Matsushita K, Akimot M, Kawamata N, Yamaguchi A, Kawada H, Ozak A, Arima N, Te C (2005) Acute lung injury in a healthy donor during mobilization of peripheral blood stem cells using granulocyte-colony stimulating factor alone. Haematologica 90: ECR10
8. White DA (2004) Drug-induced pulmonary infection. Clin Chest Med 25:179–188
9. Plataki M, Bouros D (2004) Iatrogenic and rare pleural effusion. In: Bouros D (ed) Pleural disorders. Marcel Dekker, New York, pp 897–913
10. Naranjo CA, Busto U, Sellers EM, Sandor P, Ruiz I, Roberts EA (1981) A method for estimating the probability of adverse drug reactions. Clin Pharmacol Ther 30:239–245
11. Pneumotox® Website: 1997. Producers: P Foucher – Ph Camus: Last update: June 4, 2010, http://www.pneumotox.com
12. O'Driscoll BR, Hasleton PS, Taylor PM, Poulter LW, Gattamaneni HR, Woodcock AA (1990) Active lung fibrosis up to 17 years after chemotherapy with carmustine (BCNU) in childhood. N Engl J Med 323:378–382
13. Cabot RC, Harris NL, Shepard J-A O, Rosenberg ES, Cort AM, Ebeling SH, Peters CC, Ng AK, Abramson JS, Digumarthy SR, Reingold JS, Stone JR (2010) Case records of the Massachusetts General Hospital. Case 24 – 2010. A 56-year-old woman with a history of Hodgkin's lymphoma and sudden onset of dyspnea and shock. N Engl J Med 363:664–675
14. Camus P, Rosenow EC III (2010) Drug-induced and iatrogenic lung disease. Hodder Arnold, London

15. Vargas HA, Hampson FA, Babar JL, Shaw AS (2009) Imaging the lungs in patients treated for lymphoma. Clin Radiol 64:1048–1055
16. Cleverley JR, Screaton NJ, Hiorns MP, Flint JD, Müller NL (2002) Drug-induced lung disease: high-resolution CT and histological findings. Clin Radiol 57:292–299
17. Ohnishi K (2006) Twenty-seven cases of drug-induced interstitial lung disease associated with imatinib mesylate. Leukemia 20:1162–1164
18. Tanaka N, Newell JD, Brown KK, Cool CD, Lynch DA (2004) Collagen vascular disease-related lung disease. High-resolution computed tomography findings based on the pathologic classification. J Comput Assist Tomogr 28:351–360
19. Bajwa AA, Usman F, Wolfson D, Laos LF, Cury JD (2010) A 62-year-old woman with dyspnea, leukocytosis, and diffuse ground-glass opacities. Chest 137:1470–1473
20. Kintzer JS Jr, Rosenow EC III, Kyle RA (1978) Thoracic and pulmonary abnormalities in multiple myeloma. A review of 958 cases. Arch Intern Med 138:727–730
21. Chantranuwat C (2007) Noncrystallized form of immunoglobulin-storing histiocytosis as a cause of chronic lung infiltration in multiple myeloma. Ann Diagn Pathol 11:220–222
22. Todd WU, Drabick JJ, Benninghoff MG, Frauenhoffer EE, Zander DS (2009) Pulmonary crystal-storing histiocytosis diagnosed by computed tomography-guided fine-needle aspiration. Diagn Cytopathol 38(4):274–278
23. Chung JH, Pipavath SJ, Myerson DH, Godwin D (2009) Secondary pulmonary alveolar proteinosis: a confusing and potentially serious complication of hematologic malignancy. J Thorac Imaging 24:115–118
24. Roychowdhury M, Pambuccian SE, Aslan DL, Jessurun J, Rose AG, Manivel JC, Gulbahce E (2005) Pulmonary complications after bone marrow transplantation. An autopsy study from a large transplantation center. Arch Pathol Lab Med 129:366–371
25. Franquet T, Muller NL, Lee KS, Gimenez A, Flint JD (2005) High-resolution CT and pathologic findings of noninfectious pulmonary complications after hematopoietic stem cell transplantation. AJR Am J Roentgenol 184:629–637
26. Franquet T (2006) High-resolution computed tomography (HRCT) of lung infections in non-AIDS immunocompromised patients. Eur Radiol 16:707–718
27. Franquet T, Rodriguez S, Martino R, Gimenez A, Salinas T, Hidalgo A (2006) Thin-section CT findings in hematopoietic stem cell transplantation recipients with respiratory virus pneumonia. AJR Am J Roentgenol 187:1085–1090
28. Marchiori E, Escuissato DL, Gasparetto TD, Considera DP, Franquet T (2009) "Crazy-paving" patterns on high-resolution CT scans in patients with pulmonary complications after hematopoietic stem cell transplantation. Korean J Radiol 10:21–24
29. Coy DL, Ormazabal A, Godwin JD, Lalani T (2005) Imaging evaluation of pulmonary and abdominal complications following hematopoietic stem cell transplantation. Radiographics 25:305–317, discussion 318
30. Kremer JM, Alarcon GS, Weinblatt ME, Kaymakcian MV, Macaluso M, Cannon GW, Palmer WR, Sundy JS, St Clair EW, Alexander RW, Walker-Smith GJ, Axiotis CA (1997) Clinical, laboratory, radiographic, and histopathologic features of methotrexate-associated lung injury in patients with rheumatoid arthritis. Arthritis Rheum 40:1829–1837
31. Grimison P, Goldstein D, Schneeweiss J, Murray N (2005) Corticosteroid-responsive interstitial pneumonitis related to imantinib mesylate with successful rechallenge, and potential causative mechanisms. Intern Med J 35:136–137
32. Bergeron A, Rea D, Levy V, Picard C, Meignin V, Tamburini J, Bruzzoni-Giovanelli H, Calvo F, Tazi A, Rousselot P (2007) Lung abnormalities after dasatinib treatment for chronic myeloid leukemia: a case series. Am J Respir Crit Care Med 176:814–818
33. Goligher EC, Cserti-Gazdewich C, Balter M, Gupta V, Brandwein JE (2009) Acute lung injury during antithymocyte globulin therapy for aplastic anemia. Can Respir J 16:e3–e5
34. Hirata S, Hattori N, Kumagai K, Haruta Y, Yokoyama A, Kohno N (2009) Lymphocyte transformation test is not helpful for the diagnosis of methotrexate-induced pneumonitis in patients with rheumatoid arthritis. Clin Chim Acta 407:25–29
35. Kirsch J, Arrossi AV, Yoon JK, Wu G, Neumann DR (2006) FDG positron emission tomography/computerized tomography features of bleomycin-induced pneumonitis. J Thorac Imaging 21:228–230
36. Zisman DA, McCune WJ, Tino G, Lynch JPI (2001) Drug-induced pneumonitis: the role of methotrexate. Sarcoidosis Vasc Diffuse Lung Dis 18:243–252
37. Flieder DB, Travis WD (2004) Pathologic characteristics of drug-induced lung disease. Clin Chest Med 25:37–46
38. Rossi SE, Erasmus JJ, McAdams P, Sporn TA, Goodman PC (2000) Pulmonary drug toxicity: radiologic and pathologic manifestations. Radiographics 5:1245–1259
39. Erasmus JJ, McAdams HP, Rossi SE (2002) Drug-induced lung injury. Semin Roentgenol 37:72–81
40. Erasmus JJ, McAdams HP, Rossi SE (2002) High-resolution CT of drug-induced lung disease. Radiol Clin North Am 40:61–72
41. Lindell RM, Hartman TE (2004) Chest imaging in iatrogenic respiratory disease. Clin Chest Med 25:15–24
42. Mellot F, Scherrer A (2005) Imaging features of drug-induced lung diseases. J Radiol 86:550–557
43. Imokawa S, Colby TV, Leslie KO, Helmers RA (2000) Methotrexate pneumonitis: review of the literature and histopathological findings in nine patients. Eur Respir J 15:373–381
44. Chong S, Lee KS, Yi CA, Chung MJ, Kim TS, Han JH (2006) Pulmonary fungal infection: imaging findings in immunocompetent and immunocompromised patients. Eur J Radiol 59:371–383
45. Washington L, Palacio D (2007) Imaging of bacterial pulmonary infection in the immunocompetent patient. Semin Roentgenol 42:122–145
46. Akira M, Ishikawa H, Yamamoto S (2002) Drug-induced pneumonitis: thin-section CT findings in 60 patients. Radiology 224:852–860
47. Rubin G, Baume P, Vandenberg R (1972) Azathioprine and acute restrictive lung disease. Aust NZ J Med 3:272–274
48. Bellamy EA, Nicholas D, Husband JE (1987) Quantitative assessment of lung damage due to bleomycin using computed tomography. Br J Radiol 60:1205–1209

49. Costabel U, Uzaslan E, Guzman J (2004) Bronchoalveolar lavage in drug-induced lung disease. Clin Chest Med 25:25–36
50. Fuhrman C, Parrot A, Wislez M, Prigent H, Boussaud V, Bernaudin JF, Mayaud C, Cadranel J (2001) Spectrum of CD4 to CD8 T-cell ratios in lymphocytic alveolitis associated with methotrexate-induced pneumonitis. Am J Respir Crit Care Med 164:1186–1191
51. Joos L, Chhajed PN, Wallner J, Battegay M, Steiger J, Gratwohl A, Tamm M (2007) Pulmonary infections diagnosed by BAL: a 12-year experience in 1066 immunocompromised patients. Respir Med 101:93–97
52. Wondergem MJ, Grunberg K, Wittgen BP, Sonneveld P, Zweegman S (2009) Interstitial pneumonitis caused by *Pneumocystis jirovecii* pneumonia (PCP) during bortezomib treatment. Histopathology 54(5):631–633
53. Forghieri F, Potenza L, Morselli M, Maccaferri M, Pedrazzi L, Barozzi P, Vallerini D, Riva G, Zanetti E, Quadrelli C, Rossi G, Rivasi F, Messino M, Rumpianesi F, Grottola A, Venturelli C, Pecorari M, Codeluppi M, Torelli G, Luppi M (2010) Organizing pneumonia mimicking invasive fungal disease in leukaemic patients. Eur J Haematol 85(1):76–82
54. Marzouk K, Saleh S, Kannass M, Sharma OP (2004) Interferon-induced granulomatous lung disease. Curr Opin Pulm Med 10:435–440
55. Lerch E, Gyorik S, Feilchenfeldt J, Mazzucchelli L, Quadri F (2010) A case of lenalidomide-induced hypersensitivity pneumonitis. Onkologie 33:249–252
56. Stetter M, Schmidli M, Krapf R (1994) Azathioprine hypersensitivity mimicking Goodpasture's syndrome. Am J Kidney Dis 23:874–877
57. Berkani K, Bayle JY, Perol M, Bejui-Thivolet F, Perrot D, Guérin JC (2003) "Spontaneous" resolution of two severe methotrexate-induced pneumonias. Rev Pneumol Clin 59:301–305
58. Fehr T, Jacky E, Bachli EB (2003) Successful reintroduction of methotrexate after acute, pneumonitis in a patient with acute lymphoblastic leukemia. Ann Hematol 82:193–196
59. Ben m'rad M, Leclerc-Mercier S, Blanche P, Franck N, Rozenberg F, Fulla Y, Guesmi M, Rollot F, Dehoux M, Guillevin L, Moachon L (2009) Drug-induced hypersensitivity syndrome: clinical and biologic disease patterns in 24 patients. Medicine (Baltimore) 88:131–140
60. Hirschi S, Lange F, Battesti JP, Lebargy F (1998) Pulmonary sarcoid-like granulomatosis associated with Hodgkin's disease and complicated by bleomycin-induced pulmonary nodules. Ann Med Interne (Paris) 149:164–166
61. Kornacker M, Kraemer A, Leo E, Ho AD (2002) Occurrence of sarcoidosis subsequent to chemotherapy for non-Hodgkin's lymphoma: report of two cases. Ann Hematol 81:103–105
62. Egerer G, Witzens M, Spaeth A, Breitbart A, Moller P, Goldschmidt H, Ho AD (2001) Successful treatment of bronchiolitis obliterans organizing pneumonia with low-dose methotrexate in a patient with Hodgkin's disease. Oncology 61:23–27
63. Kalambokis G, Stefanou D, Arkoumani E, Kitsanou M, Bourantas K, Tsianos EV (2004) Fulminant bronchiolitis obliterans organizing pneumonia following 2 days of treatment with hydroxyurea, interferon-alpha and oral cytarabine ocfosfate for chronic myelogenous leukemia. Eur J Haematol 73:67–70
64. Ferriby D, Stojkovic T (2001) Bronchiolitis obliterans with organizing pneumonia during interferon ß-1a treatment. Lancet 357:751
65. Gehl HB, Hauptmann S, Sohn M, Bohndorf K (1992) Late pulmonary changes following bleomycin administration in computed tomography. Nodular fibrosis mimicking a seminoma metastasis. Radiologe 32:80–82
66. Santrach PJ, Askin FB, Wells RJ, Azizkhan RG, Merten DF (1989) Nodular form of bleomycin-related pulmonary injury in patients with osteogenic sarcoma. Cancer 64:806–811
67. Weyl Ben-Arush M, Roguin A, Zamir E, Et-Hassid R, Pries D, Gaitini D, Dale A, Postovsky S (1997) Bleomycin and cyclophosphamide toxicity simulating metastatic nodules to the lungs in childhood cancer. Pediatr Hematol Oncol 14:381–386
68. Drakopanagiotakis F, Polychronopoulos V, Judson MA (2008) Organizing pneumonia. Am J Med Sci 335:34–39
69. Limper AH (2004) Chemotherapy-induced lung disease. Clin Chest Med 25:53–64
70. Al Ameri A, Koller C, Kantarjian H, Ravandi F, Verstovsek S, Borthakur G, Pierce S, Mattiuzzi G (2010) Acute pulmonary failure during remission induction chemotherapy in adults with acute myeloid leukemia or high-risk myelodysplastic syndrome. Cancer 116:93–97
71. Roig J, Domingo C, Gea E (2006) Pulmonary toxicity caused by cytotoxic drugs. Clin Pulmonary Med 13:53–62
72. Vahid B, Marik PE (2008) Pulmonary complications of novel antineoplastic agents for solid tumors. Chest 133:528–538
73. Herishanu Y, Polliack A, Leider TL, Grieff Y, Metser U, Naparstek E (2006) Fatal interstitial pneumonitis related to rituximab-containing regimen. Clin Lymphoma Myeloma 6:407–409
74. Friedberg JW, Neuberg D, Kim H, Miyata S, McCauley M, Fisher DC, Takvorian T, Canellos GP (2003) Gemcitabine added to doxorubicin, bleomycin, and vinblastine for the treatment of de novo Hodgkin disease. Unacceptable acute pulmonary toxicity. Cancer 98:978–982
75. Bredenfeld H, Franklin J, Nogova L, Jesting A, Fries S, Mailander V, Oertel J, Diehl V, Engert A (2004) Severe pulmonary toxicity in patients with advanced-stage Hodgkin's disease treated with a modified bleomycin, doxorubicin, cyclophosphamide, vincristine, procarbazine, prednisone, and gemcitabine (BEACOPP) regimen is probably related to the combination of gemcitabine and bleomycin: a report of the German Hodgkin's lymphoma Study Group. J Clin Oncol 22:2424–2429
76. Vento S, Cainelli F, Ternesgen Z (2008) Lung infections after cancer chemotherapy. Lancet Oncol 9:982–992
77. Sokolovic M, Pastores SM (2010) Transfusion therapy and acute lung injury. Expert Rev Respir Med 4:387–393
78. Sihler KC, Napolitano LM (2010) Complications of massive transfusion. Chest 137:209–220
79. Hoskin PJ, Lowry L, Horwich A, Jack A, Mead B, Hancock BW, Smith P, Qian W, Patrick P, Popova B, Pettitt A, Cunningham D, Pettengell R, Sweetenham J, Linch D, Johnson PW (2009) Randomized comparison of the Stanford V regimen and ABVD in the treatment of advanced Hodgkin's lymphoma: United Kingdom National Cancer Research Institute Lymphoma Group Study ISRCTN 64141244. J Clin Oncol 27:5390–5396

80. Moormeier JA, Williams SF, Kaminer LS, Garner M, Bitran JD (1990) High-dose tri-alkylator chemotherapy with autologous stem cell rescue in patients with refractory malignancies. J Natl Cancer Inst 82:29–34
81. Rubio C, Hill ME, Milan S, O'Brien MER, Cunningham D (1997) Idiopathic pneumonia syndrome after high dose chemotherapy for relapsed Hodgkin's disease. Br J Cancer 75:1044–1048
82. Quigley M, Brada M, Heron C, Horwich A (1988) Severe lung toxicity with a weekly low dose chemotherapy regimen in patients with non-Hodgkin's lymphoma. Hematol Oncol 6:319–324
83. Flieder DB, Koss MN (2004) Nonspecific interstitial pneumonia: a provisional category of idiopathic interstitial pneumonia. Curr Opin Pulm Med 10:441–446
84. Leslie KO (2009) My approach to interstitial lung disease using clinical, radiological and histopathological patterns. J Clin Pathol 62:387–401
85. Parambil JG, Myers JL, Aubry MC, Ryu JH (2007) Causes and prognosis of diffuse alveolar damage diagnosed on surgical lung biopsy. Chest 132:50–57
86. Linssen KC, Jacobs JA, Poletti VE, van Mook W, Cornelissen EI, Drent M (2004) Reactive type II pneumocytes in bronchoalveolar lavage fluid. Acta Cytol 48:497–504
87. Wong CC, Brown D, Howling SJ, Parker NE (2003) Hydroxyurea-induced pneumonitis in a patient with chronic idiopathic myelofibrosis after prolonged drug exposure. Eur J Haematol 71:388–390
88. Patriarca F, Poletti V, Costabel U, Battista M, Sperotto A, Medeot M, Toffoletti E, Fanin R (2009) Clinical presentation, outcome and risk factors of late-onset non-infectious pulmonary complications after allogeneic stem cell transplantation. Curr Stem Cell Res Ther 4:161–167
89. Boiselle PM, Morrin MM, Huberman MS (2000) Gemcitabine pulmonary toxicity: CT features. J Comput Assist Tomogr 24:977–980
90. Lind PA, Marks LB, Jamieson TA, Carter DL, Vredenburgh JJ, Folz RJ, Prosnitz LR (2002) Predictors for pneumonitis during locoregional radiotherapy in high-risk patients with breast carcinoma treated with high-dose chemotherapy and stem-cell rescue. Cancer 94:2821–2829
91. Wilczynski SW, Erasmus JJ, Petros WP, Vredenburgh JJ, Folz RJ (1998) Delayed pulmonary toxicity syndrome following high-dose chemotherapy and bone marrow transplantation for breast cancer. Am J Respir Crit Care Med 157:565–573
92. Pavlakis N, Bell DR, Millward MJ, Levi JA (1997) Fatal pulmonary toxicity resulting from treatment with gemcitabine. Cancer 80:286–291
93. Bhalla KS, Wilczynski SW, Abushamaa AM, Petros WP, McDonald CS, Loftis JS, Chao NJ, Vredenburgh JJ, Folz RJ (2000) Pulmonary toxicity of induction chemotherapy prior to standard or high-dose chemotherapy with autologous hematopoietic support. Am J Respir Crit Care Med 161:17–25
94. Dai MS, Lee SC, Ho CL, Chen YC, Kao WY, Chao TY (2001) Impact of open lung biopsy for undiagnosed pulmonary infiltrates in patients with hematological malignancies. Am J Hematol 68:87–90
95. Chap L, Shpiner R, Levine M, Norton L, Lill M, Glaspy J (1997) Pulmonary toxicity of high-dose chemotherapy for breast cancer: a non-invasive approach to diagnosis and treatment. Bone Marrow Transplant 20:1063–1067
96. White DA, Wong PW, Downey R (2000) The utility of open lung biopsy in patients with hematologic malignancies. Am J Respir Crit Care Med 161:723–729
97. Alessandrino EP, Bernasconi P, Colombo A, Caldera D, Martinelli G, Vitulo P, Malcovati L, Nascimbene C, Varettoni M, Volpini E, Klersy C, Bernasconi C (2000) Pulmonary toxicity following carmustine-based preparative regimens and autologous peripheral blood progenitor cell transplantation in hematological malignancies. Bone Marrow Transplant 25:309–313
98. Richter JE, Hastedt R, Dalton JF, Marshall D, Raymond LW (1979) Pulmonary toxicity of bischloronitrosourea. Report of a case with transient response to corticosteroid therapy. Cancer 43:1607–1612
99. White DA, Orenstein M, Godwin TA, Stover DE (1984) Chemotherapy-associated pulmonary toxic reactions during treatment for breast cancer. Arch Intern Med 144:953–956
100. Zappasodi P, Dore R, Castagnola C, Astori C, Varettoni M, Mangiacavalli S, Lazzarino M, Corso A (2007) Rapid response to high-dose steroids of severe bortezomib-related pulmonary complication in multiple myeloma. J Clin Oncol 25:3380–3381
101. Bossi G, Cerveri I, Volpini E, Corsico A, Baio A, Corbella F, Klersy C, Arico M (1997) Long-term pulmonary sequelae after treatment of childhood Hodgkin's disease. Ann Oncol 8:19–24
102. Jensen BV, Carlsen NLT, Groth S, Nissen NI (1990) Late effects on pulmonary function of mantle-field irradiation, chemotherapy or combined modality therapy for Hodgkin's disease. Eur J Haematol 44:165–171
103. van Leeuwen FE, Klokman WJ, Stovall M, Hagenbeek A, van den Belt-Dusebout AW, Noyon R, Boice JD Jr, Burgers JMV, Somers R (1995) Roles of radiotherapy and smoking in lung cancer following Hodgkin's disease. J Natl Cancer Inst 87:1530–1537
104. Tward JD, Wendland MM, Shrieve DC, Szabo A, Gaffney DK (2006) The risk of secondary malignancies over 30 years after the treatment of non-Hodgkin lymphoma. Cancer 107:108–115
105. Rivera MP, Detterbeck FC, Socinski MA, Moore DT, Edelman MJ, Jahan TM, Ansari RH, Luketich JD, Peng G, Monberg M, Obasaju CK, Gralla RJ (2009) Impact of preoperative chemotherapy on pulmonary function tests in resectable early-stage non-small cell lung cancer. Chest 135:1588–1595
106. Yumuk PF, Kefeli U, Ceyhan B, Dane F, Eroglu BT, Gumus M, Cabuk D, Basaran G, Abacioglu U, Turhal NS (2009) Pulmonary toxicity in patients receiving docetaxel chemotherapy. Med Oncol. Dec 25. [Epub ahead of print)
107. Kalaycioglu M, Kavuru M, Tuason L, Bolwell B (1995) Empiric prednisone therapy for pulmonary toxic reaction after high-dose chemotherapy containing carmustine. Chest 107:482–487
108. Dawson JK, Graham DR, Desmond J, Fewins HE, Lynch MP (2002) Investigation of the chronic pulmonary effects of low-dose oral methotrexate in patients with rheumatoid arthritis: a prospective study incorporating HRCT scanning and pulmonary function tests. Rheumatology (Oxford) 41: 262–267

109. Bell MR, Meredith DJ, Gill PG (1985) Role of carbon monoxide diffusing capacity in the early detection of major bleomycin-induced pulmonary toxicity. Aust NZ J Med 15:235–240
110. Wolkowicz J, Sturgeon J, Rawji M, Chan CK (1992) Bleomycin-induced pulmonary function abnormalities. Chest 101:97–101
111. Tryka AF, Godleski JJ, Fanta CH (1982) Leukemic cell lysis pneumonopathy. A complication of treated myeloblastic leukemia. Cancer 50:2763–2770
112. Azoulay E, Fieux F, Moreau D, Thiery G, Rousselot P, Parrot A, LeGall JR, Dombret H, Schlemmer B (2003) Acute monocytic leukemia presenting as acute respiratory failure. Am J Respir Crit Care Med 167:1329–1333
113. Dombret H, Hunault M, Faucher C, Dombret MC, Degos L (1992) Acute lysis pneumopathy after chemotherapy for acute myelomonocytic leukemia with abnormal marrow eosinophils. Cancer 69:1356–1361
114. Malik SW, Myers JL, DeRemee RA, Specks U (1996) Lung toxicity associated with cyclophosphamide use. Two distinct patterns. Am J Respir Crit Care Med 154: 1851–1856
115. Bedrossian CWM, Miller WC, Luna MA (1979) Methotrexate-induced diffuse interstitial pulmonary fibrosis. South Med J 72:313–318
116. Attar EC, Ervin T, Janicek M, Deykin A, Godleski J (2000) Acute interstitial pneumonitis related to gemcitabine. J Clin Oncol 18:697–698
117. Trigg ME, Finlay JL, Bozdech M, Gilbert E (1987) Fatal cardiac toxicity in bone marrow transplant patients receiving cytosine arabinoside, cyclophosphamide, and total body irradiation. Cancer 59:38–42
118. Singal PK, Iliskovic N (1998) Doxorubicin-induced cardiomyopathy. N Engl J Med 339:900–905
119. Chanan-Khan A, Srinivasan S, Czuczman MS (2004) Prevention and management of cardiotoxicity from antineoplastic therapy. J Support Oncol 2:251–256, discussion 259–261, 264–256
120. Hayek ER, Speakman E, Rehmus E (2005) Acute doxorubicin cardiotoxicity. N Engl J Med 352:2456–2457
121. Yahalom J, Portlock CS (2008) Long-term cardiac and pulmonary complications of cancer therapy. Hematol Oncol Clin North Am 22:305–318, VII
122. Briasoulis E, Pavlidis N (2001) Noncardiogenic pulmonary edema: an unusual and serious complication of anticancer therapy. Oncologist 6:153–161
123. Schwartz RN, Stover L, Dutcher J (2002) Managing toxicities of high-dose interleukin-2. Oncology (Williston Park) 16:11–20
124. Schwarz MI, Fontenot AP (2004) Drug-induced diffuse alveolar hemorrhage syndromes and vasculitis. Clin Chest Med 25:133–140
125. Salvucci M, Zanchini R, Molinari AL, Zuffa E, Poletti V, Poletti G, Zaccaria A (2000) Lung toxicity following fludarabine, cytosine arabinoside and mitoxantrone (FLAN) treatment for acute leukemia. Haematologica 85: 769–770
126. Ben-Abraham R, Paret G, Cohen R, Szold O, Cividalli G, Toren A, Nagler A (2003) Diffuse alveolar hemorrhage following allogeneic bone marrow transplantation in children. Chest 124:660–664
127. Terrabuio AA Jr, Parra ER, Farhat C, Capelozzi VL (2007) Autopsy-proven causes of death in lungs of patients immunocompromised by secondary interstitial pneumonia. Clinics (Sao Paulo) 62:69–76
128. Glasier CM, Siegel MJ (1981) Multiple pulmonary nodules: unusual manifestation of bleomycin toxicity. AJR Am J Roentgenol 137:155–156
129. Franchi F, Seminara P, Gualdi GF (1984) Lung pseudometastases due to vinblastine toxicity. Klin Wochenschr 62:1047–1048
130. Scharstein R, Johnson JF, Cook BA, Stephenson SR (1987) Bleomycin nodules mimicking metastatic osteogenic sarcoma. Am J Pediatr Hematol Oncol 9:219–221
131. Boitsios G, Bankier AA, Eisenberg RL (2010) Diffuse pulmonary nodules. AJR Am J Roentgenol 194:W354–W366
132. Garg S, Garg MS, Basmaji N (2002) Multiple pulmonary nodules: an unusual presentation of fludarabine pulmonary toxicity: Case report and review of literature. Am J Hematol 70:241–245
133. Gulbahce HE, Pambuccian SE, Jessurun J, Woodard P, Steiner ME, Manivel JC, Hite S, Ramsay NKC, Baker KS (2004) Pulmonary nodular lesions in bone marrow transplant recipients. Impact of histologic diagnosis on patient management and prognosis. Am J Clin Pathol 121:205–210
134. White DA, Schwartzberg LS, Kris MG, Bosl GJ (1987) Acute chest pain syndrome during bleomycin infusions. Cancer 59:1582–1585
135. Hudson MM, Weinstein HJ, Donaldson SS, Greenwald C, Kun L, Tarbell NJ, Humphrey WA, Rupp C, Marina NM, Wilimas J et al (1993) Acute hypersensitivity reactions to etoposide in a VEPA regimen for Hodgkin's disease. J Clin Oncol 11:1080–1084
136. Yano S, Shimada K (1996) Vasospastic angina after chemotherapy by with carboplatin and etoposide in a patient with lung cancer. Jpn Circ J 60:185–188
137. Urban C, Nirenberg A, Caparros B, Anac S, Cacavio A, Rosen G (1983) Chemical pleuritis as the cause of acute chest pain following high-dose methotrexate treatment. Cancer 51:34–37
138. Rubin RL (2005) Drug-induced lupus. Toxicology 209: 135–147
139. Pulsipher MA, Chitphakdithai P, Miller JP, Logan BR, King RJ, Rizzo JD, Leitman SF, Anderlini P, Haagenson MD, Kurian S, Klein JP, Horowitz MM, Confer DL (2009) Adverse events among 2408 unrelated donors of peripheral blood stem cells: results of a prospective trial from the National Marrow Donor Program. Blood 113:3604–3611
140. Shepherd GM (2003) Hypersensitivity reactions to chemotherapeutic drugs. Clin Rev Allergy Immunol 24:253–262
141. Syrigou E, Makrilia N, Koti I, Saif MW, Syrigos KN (2009) Hypersensitivity reactions to antineoplastic agents: an overview. Anticancer Drugs 20:1–6
142. Santos NC, Figueira-Coelho J, Martins-Silva J, Saldanha C (2003) Multidisciplinary utilization of dimethyl sulfoxide: pharmacological, cellular, and molecular aspects. Biochem Pharmacol 65:1035–1041
143. Price KS, Castells MC (2002) Taxol reactions. Allergy Asthma Proc 23:205–208
144. Ferrucci PF, Martinoni A, Cocorocchio E et al (2002) Evaluation of acute toxicities associated with autologous

peripheral blood progenitor cell reinfusion in patients undergoing high-dose chemotherapy. Bone Marrow Tranplant 25:173–177

145. Shen Y, Li L, Grant J, Rubio A, Zhao Z, Zhang X, Zhou L, Fowler D (2009) Anaphylactic deaths in Maryland (United States) and Shanghai (China): a review of forensic autopsy cases from 2004 to 2006. Forensic Sci Int 186(1–3):1–5
146. Worth A, Soar J, Sheikh A (2010) Management of anaphylaxis in the emergency setting. Expert Rev Clin Immunol 6:89–100
147. Camus P (2004) Drug-induced pleural disease. In: Bouros D (ed) Pleural disorders. Marcel Dekker, New York, pp 317–352
148. Camus P (2010) Drug-induced pleural diseases. In: Bouros D (ed) Lung biology in health and disease: pleural diseases, 2nd edn. Marcel Dekker, New York, Basel, p 843
149. Becker CD, Gil J, Padilla ML (2008) Idiopathic pleuroparenchymal fibroelastosis: an unrecognized or misdiagnosed entity? Mod Pathol 21:784–787
150. Jain TP, Thulkar S, Saha S, Bakhshi S, Dominic J (2005) Extensive pneumothorax, pneumomediastinum and surgical emphysema as a complication of bleomycin therapy. Pediatr Radiol 35:1227–1229
151. Fanfulla F, Locatelli F, Zoia MC, Giorgiani G, Bonetti F, Spagnolatti L, Cerveri I (1997) Pulmonary complications and respiratory function changes after bone marrow transplantation in children. Eur Respir J 10:2301–2306
152. Hoppe RT (1997) Hodgkin's disease: complications of therapy and excess mortality. Ann Oncol 8:115–118
153. Moser EC, Noordijk EM, van Leeuwen FE, Baars JW, Thomas J, Carde P, Meerwaldt JH, van Glabbeke M, Kluin-Nelemans HC (2006) Risk of second cancer after treatment of aggressive non-Hodgkin's lymphoma; an EORTC cohort study. Haematologica 91:1481–1488
154. Travis LB, Gospodarowicz M, Curtis RE, Clarke EA, Andersson M, Glimelius B, Joensuu T, Lynch CF, van Leeuwen FE, Holowaty E, Storm H, Glimelius I, Pukkala E, Stovall M, Fraumeni JF, Boice JD, Gilbert E (2002) Lung cancer following chemotherapy and radiotherapy for Hodgkin's disease. J Natl Cancer Inst 94:182–192
155. Gilbert ES, Stovall M, Gospodarowicz M, van Leeuwen FE, Andersson M, Glimelius B, Joensuu T, Lynch CF, Curtis RE, Holowaty E, Storm H, Pukkala E, van't Veer MB, Fraumeni JE, Boice JD, Clarke EA, Travis LB (2003) Lung cancer after treatment for Hodgkin's disease: focus on radiation effects. Radiat Res 159:161–173
156. Swerdlow AJ, Schoemaker MJ, Allerton R, Horwich A, Barber JA, Cunningham D, Lister TA, Rohatiner AZS, Hudson GV, Williams MV, Linch DC (2001) Lung cancer after Hodgkin's disease: a nested case-control study of the relation to treatment. J Clin Oncol 19:1610–1618
157. De Bruin ML, Burgers JA, Baas P, vantVeer MB, Noordijk EM, Louwman MW, Zijlstra JM, van den Berg H, Aleman BM, van Leeuwen FE (2009) Malignant mesothelioma following radiation treatment for Hodgkin's lymphoma. Blood 113(16):3679–3681
158. Spitzer TR, Creger RJ, Fox RM, Lazarus HM (1989) Rapid infusion amphotericin B: effective and well-tolerated therapy for neutropenic fever. Pharmatherapeutica 5:305–311
159. Lowery MM, Greenberger PA (2003) Amphotericin-induced stridor: a review of stridor, amphotericin preparations, and their immunoregulatory effects. Ann Allergy Asthma Immunol 91:460–466
160. Collazos J, Martinez E, Mayo J, Ibarra S (2001) Pulmonary reactions during treatment with amphotericin B: review of published cases and guidelines for management. Clin Infect Dis 33:E75–E82
161. Wright DG, Robichaud KJ, Pizzo PA, Deiseroth AB (1981) Lethal pulmonary reactions associated with the combined use of amphotericin B and leukocyte transfusions. N Engl J Med 304:1185–1189
162. Arning M, Heer-Sonderhoff AH, Wehmeir A, Schneider W (1995) Pulmonary toxicity during infusion of liposomal amphotericin B in two patients with acute leukemia. Eur J Clin Microbiol Infect Dis 14:41–43
163. Tolentino LF, Tsai SF, Witt MD, French SW (2004) Fatal fat embolism following amphotericin B lipid complex injection. Exp Mol Pathol 77:246–248
164. Maillard N, Foucher P, Caillot D, Durand C, Sgro C, Camus P (1999) Transient pulmonary infiltrates during treatment with anti-thymocyte globulin. Respiration 66:279–282
165. Castaigne S, Chomienne C, Daniel MT, Ballerini P, Berger R, Fenaux P, Degos L (1990) All-trans retinoic acid as a differentiation therapy for acute promyelocytic leukemia. I: Clinical results. Blood 76:1704–1709
166. Frankel SR, Eardley A, Lauwers G, Weiss M, Warrell RP Jr (1992) The "retinoic acid syndrome" in acute promyelocytic leukemia. Ann Intern Med 117:292–296
167. Su YC, Dunn P, Shih LY, Kuo MC, Chang H, Wu JH, Lin TL, Wang PN, Tang TC, Hung YS (2009) Retinoic acid syndrome in patients following the treatment of acute promyelocytic leukemia with all-trans retinoic acid. Chang Gung Med J 32:535–542
168. Zimmerman JJ (2007) Understanding another acute respiratory distress syndrome. Crit Care Med 35:974–975
169. Schreiber J, Kachel R, Florschutz A (2007) ATRA-syndrome. Pneumologie 61:226–227
170. Camacho LH, Soignet SL, Chanel S, Ho R, Heller G, Scheinberg DA, Ellison R, Warrell RP Jr (2000) Leukocytosis and the retinoic acid syndrome in patients with acute promyelocytic leukemia treated with arsenic trioxide. J Clin Oncol 18:2620–2625
171. Beer TM, Tangen CM, Nichols CR, Margolin KA, Dreicer R, Stephenson WT, Quinn DI, Raghavan D, Crawford ED (2006) Southwest Oncology Group phase II study of arsenic trioxide in patients with refractory germ cell malignancies. Cancer 106:2624–2629
172. Davis BA, Cervi P, Amin Z, Moshi G, Shaw P, Porter J (1996) Retinoic acid syndrome: pulmonary computed tomography (CT) findings. Leuk Lymphoma 23:113–117
173. Maloisel F, Petit T, Kessler R, Oberling F (1996) Cytologic examination of broncho-alveolar fluid during the retinoic acid syndrome. Eur J Haematol 56:319–320
174. Nicolls MR, Terada LS, Tuder RM, Priniville SA, Schwarz MI (1998) Diffuse alveolar hemorrhage with underlying pulmonary capillaritis in the retinoic acid syndrome. Am J Respir Crit Care Med 158:1302–1305
175. Wiley JS, Firkin FC (1995) Reduction of pulmonary toxicity by prednisolone prophylaxis during all-trans retinoic acid treatment of acute promyelocytic leukemia. Leukemia 9:774–778

176. Koenig SM (2007) Drug-induced respiratory disease: "the great mimicker". South Med J 100:863–864
177. Ahmed Z, Shaikh MA, Raval A, Mehta JB, Byrd RP Jr, Roy TM (2007) All-trans retinoic acid syndrome: another cause of drug-induced respiratory failure. South Med J 100:899–902
178. Goldschmidt N, Gural A, BenYehuda D (2003) Extensive splenic infarction, deep vein thrombosis and pulmonary emboli complicating induction therapy with all-trans-retinoic acid (ATRA) for acute promyelocytic leukemia. Leuk Lymphoma 44:1433–1437
179. Raghu KH, Yadav GK, Singh R, Prathapan A, Sharma S, Bhadauria S (2009) Evaluation of adverse cardiac effects induced by arsenic trioxide, a potent anti-APL drug. J Environ Pathol Toxicol Oncol 28:241–252
180. Gryn J, Zeigler ZR, Shadduck RK, Lister J, Raymond JM, Sbeitan I, Srodes C, Meisner D, Evans C (2002) Treatment of myelodysplastic syndromes with 5-azacytidine. Leuk Res 26:893–897
181. Adams CD, Szumita PM, Baroletti SA, Lilly CM (2005) Azacitidine-induced interstitial and alveolar fibrosis in a patient with myelodysplastic syndrome. Pharmacotherapy 25:765–768
182. Hueser CN, Patel AJ (2007) Azacitidine-associated hyperthermia and interstitial pneumonitis in a patient with myelodysplastic syndrome. Pharmacotherapy 27:1759–1762
183. Aronin PA, Mahaley MSJ, Rudnick SA, Dudka L, Donohue JF, Selker RG, Moore P (1980) Prediction of BCNU pulmonary toxicity in patients with malignant gliomas: an assessment of risk factors. N Engl J Med 303:183–188
184. Cao TM, Negrin RS, Stockerl-Goldstein KE, Johnston LJ, Shizuru JA, Taylor TL, Rizk NW, Wong RM, Blume KG, Hu WW (2000) Pulmonary toxicity syndrome in breast cancer patients undergoing BCNU-containing high-dose chemotherapy and autologous hematopoietic cell transplantation. Biol Blood Marrow Transplant 6:387–394
185. Stuart MJ, Chao NS, Horning SJ, Wong RM, Negrin RS, Johnston LJ, Shizuru JA, Long GD, Blume KG, Stockerl-Goldstein KE (2001) Efficacy and toxicity of a CCNU-containing high-dose chemotherapy regimen followed by autologous hematopoietic cell transplantation in relapsed or refractory Hodgkin's disease. Biol Blood Marrow Transplant 7:552–560
186. Tucci E, Verdiani P, Di Carlo S, Sforza V (1986) Lomustine (CCNU)-induced pulmonary fibrosis. Tumori 72:95–98
187. Massin F, Coudert B, Foucher P, Lombard JN, Reybet-Degat O, Jeannin L, Camus P (1992) Nitrosourea-induced pneumonitis. Rev Mal Respir 9:575–582
188. Mitsudo SM, Greenwald ES, Banerji B, Koss LG (1984) BCNU (1 3-bis-(2-chloroethyl)-1-nitrosourea) lung. Drug-induced pulmonary changes. Cancer 54:751–755
189. Parish JM, Muhm JR, Leslie KO (2003) Upper lobe pulmonary fibrosis associated with high-dose chemotherapy containing BCNU for bone marrow transplantation. Mayo Clin Proc 78:630–634
190. Skorupski KA, Durham AC, Duda L, Sorenmo KU (2008) Pulmonary fibrosis after high cumulative dose nitrosourea chemotherapy in a cat. Vet Comp Oncol 6:120–125
191. Lohani S, O'Driscoll BR, Woodcock AA (2004) 25-Year study of lung fibrosis following carmustine therapy for brain tumor in childhood. Chest 126:1007
192. Ishizuka M, Takayama H, Takeuchi T, Umezawa H (1967) Activity and toxicity of bleomycin. J Antibiot (Tokyo) 20:15–24
193. Balikian JP, Jochelson MS, Bauer KA, Skarkin AT, Garnick MB, Canellos GP, Smith EH (1982) Pulmonary complications of chemotherapy regimens containing bleomycin. AJR Am J Roentgenol 139:455–461
194. Sleijfer S (2001) Bleomycin pneumonitis. Chest 120: 617–624
195. Godoy MCB, Nonaka D, Raphael BG, Vlahos I (2008) Diffuse ground-glass opacities in a patient with Hodgkin lymphonia and progressive respiratory failure. Chest 134:207–212
196. Ngeow J, Tan IB, Kanesvaran R, Tan HC, Tao M, Quek R, Lim ST (2010) Prognostic impact of bleomycin-induced pneumonitis on the outcome of Hodgkin's lymphoma. Ann Hematol. Jul 31. (Epub ahead of print)
197. Ki KD, Lee JM, Lee SK, Tong SY, Huh CY, Ryu JK, Kim KY (2010) Pulmonary toxicity after a quick course of combinatorial vincristine, bleomycin, and cisplatin neoadjuvant chemotherapy in cervical cancer. J Korean Med Sci 25:240–244
198. Hapani S, Chu D, Wu S (2010) Eosinophilic pneumonia associated with bleomycin in a patient with mediastinal seminoma: a case report. J Med Case Rep 4:126
199. Iacovino JR, Leitner J, Abbas AK, Lokich JJ, Snider GL (1976) Fatal pulmonary reaction from low doses of bleomycin: an idiosyncratic tissue response. JAMA 235:1253–1255
200. Bechard DE, Fairman RP, DeBlois GG, Via CT (1987) Fatal pulmonary fibrosis from low-dose bleomycin therapy. South Med J 80:646–649
201. Real E, Roca MJ, Vinuales A, Pastor E, Grau E (1999) Life threatening lung toxicity induced by low doses of bleomycin in a patient with Hodgkin's disease. Haematologica 84:667–668
202. Simpson AB, Paul J, Graham J, Kaye SB (1998) Fatal bleomycin pulmonary toxicity in the west of Scotland 1991–95: a review of patients with germ cell tumours. Br J Cancer 78:1061–1066
203. Einhorn L, Krause M, Hornbarck N, Furnas B (1976) Enhanced pulmonary toxicity with bleomycin and radiotherapy in oat cell lung cancer. Cancer 37:2414–2416
204. Loyer E, Fuller L, Libshitz HI, Palmer JL (2000) Radiographic appearance of the chest following therapy for Hodgkin disease. Eur J Radiol 35:136–148
205. Krous HF, Hamlin WB (1973) Pulmonary toxicity due to bleomycin. Report of a case. Arch Pathol 95:407–410
206. Toledo CH, Ross WE, Hood CI, Block ER (1982) Potentiation of bleomycin toxicity by oxygen. Cancer Treat Rep 66:359–362
207. Donat SM, Levy DA (1998) Bleomycin associated pulmonary toxicity: is perioperative oxygen restriction necessary? J Urol 160:1347–1352
208. Martin WG, Ristow KM, Habermann TM, Colgan JP, Witzig TE, Ansell SM (2005) Bleomycin pulmonary toxicity has a negative impact on the outcome of patients with Hodgkin's lymphoma. J Clin Oncol 23:7614–7620
209. White DA, Stover DE (1984) Severe bleomycin-induced pneumonitis. Clinical features and response to corticosteroids. Chest 86:723–728

210. Kawai K, Akaza H (2003) Bleomycin-induced pulmonary toxicity in chemotherapy for testicular cancer. Expert Opin Drug Saf 2:587–596
211. Daba MH, El-Tahir KE, Al-Arifi MN, Gubara OA (2004) Drug-induced pulmonary fibrosis. Saudi Med J 25: 700–706
212. Bellamy EA, Husband JE, Blaquiere RM, Law MR (1985) Bleomycin related lung damage: CT evidence. Radiology 156:155–158
213. Müller NL, White DA, Jiang H, Gemma A (2004) Diagnosis and management of drug-associated interstitial lung disease. Br J Cancer 91:S24–S30
214. Mills P, Husband J (1990) Computed tomography of pulmonary bleomycin toxicity. Semin Ultrasound CT MR 11:417–422
215. Rimmer MJ, Dixon AK, Flower CDR, Sikora K (1985) Bleomycin lung: computed tomographic observations. Br J Radiol 58:1041–1045
216. White DA, Kris MG, Stover DE (1987) Bronchoalveolar lavage cell populations in bleomycin lung toxicity. Thorax 42:551–552
217. Yousem SA, Lifson JD, Colby TV (1985) Chemotherapy-induced eosinophilic pneumonia. Relation to bleomycin. Chest 88:103–106
218. Trump DL, Bartel E, Pozniak M (1988) Nodular pneumonitis after chemotherapy for germ cell tumors. Ann Intern Med 109:431–432
219. Morikawa M, Demura Y, Mizuno S, Ameshima S, Ishizaki T, Okazawa H (2008) FDG positron emission tomography imaging of drug-induced pneumonitis. Ann Nucl Med 22:335–338
220. O'Neill TJ, Kardinal CG, Tierney LM (1975) Reversible interstitial pneumonitis associated with low-dose bleomycin. Chest 68:265–267
221. Tashiro M, Izumikawa K, Yoshioka D, Nakamura S, Kurihara S, Sakamoto N, Seki M, Kakeya H, Yamamoto Y, Yanagihara K, Mukae H, Hayashi T, Fukushima K, Tashiro T, Kohno S (2008) Lung fibrosis 10 years after cessation of bleomycin therapy. Tohoku J Exp Med 216:77–80
222. Lewis BM, Izbicki R (1980) Routine pulmonary function tests during bleomycin therapy. Tests may be ineffective and potentially misleading. JAMA 243:347–351
223. Maher J, Daly PA (1993) Severe bleomycin lung toxicity: reversal with high dose corticosteroids. Thorax 48:92–94
224. Schaaf W, Vogel H, Kresuer E, Demandt M (2003) Postoperative ARDS as a possible consequence of bleomycin therapy performed 7 years ago: a case study. Anästhesiol Intensivmed 44:436–440
225. Li G, Kojicic M, Reriani MK, Perez ERF, Thakur L, Kashyap R, Van Buskirk CM, Gajic O (2010) Long-term survival and quality of life after transfusion-associated pulmonary edema in critically ill medical patients. Chest 137:783–789
226. Kopko PM, Marshall CS, MacKenzie MR, Holland PV, Popovsky MA (2002) Transfusion-related acute lung injury. Report of a clinical look-back investigation. JAMA 287:1968–1971
227. Vlaar AP, Schultz MJ, Juffermans NP (2009) Transfusion-related acute lung injury: a change of perspective. Neth J Med 67:320–326
228. Moiz B, Sharif H, Bawany FA (2009) Transfusion related acute lung injury-TRALI: an under diagnosed entity. JPMA J Pak Med Assoc 59:39–41
229. Federico A (2009) Transfusion-related acute lung injury. J Perianesth Nurs 24:35–37, quiz 38–40
230. Silliman CC, Fung YL, Ball JB, Khan SY (2009) Transfusion-related acute lung injury (TRALI): current concepts and misconceptions. Blood Rev 23:245–255
231. Kopko PM (2010) Transfusion-related acute lung injury. J Infus Nurs 33:32–37
232. Popovsky MA (2008) Transfusion-related acute lung injury: incidence, pathogenesis and the role of multicomponent apheresis in its prevention. Transfus Med Hemother 35:76–79
233. Curtis BR, McFarland JG (2006) Mechanisms of transfusion-related acute lung injury (TRALI): anti-leukocyte antibodies. Crit Care Med 34:S118–S123
234. Jensen HM, Galante JM, Kysar PE, Tolstikov VV, Reddy KJ, Holland PV (2010) TRALI is due to pulmonary venule damage from leucocytes with cholesterol crystal formation. Vox Sang. Feb;98(2):130–137
235. Popovsky MA (2001) Transfusion and lung injury. Transfus Clin Biol 8:272–277
236. Kram R, Loer SA (2005) Transfusion-related acute lung injury: lack of recognition because of unawareness of this complication? Eur J Anaesthesiol 22:369–372
237. Vlaar AP, Wortel K, Binnekade JM, van Oers MH, Beckers E, Gajic O, Schultz MJ, Juffermans NP (2010) The practice of reporting transfusion-related acute lung injury: a national survey among clinical and preclinical disciplines. Transfusion. Feb;50(2):443–451
238. Silliman CC, McLaughlin NJD (2006) Transfusion-related acute lung injury. Blood Rev 20:139–159
239. Droog W, van Thiel SW, Visser SJ, Rhemrev JP (2009) Complications due to transfusion-related acute lung injury. Obstet Gynecol 113:560–563
240. Carilli AD, Ramamurthy MV, Chang Y-S, Shin D, Sehti V (1978) Noncardiogenic pulmonary edema following blood transfusion. Chest 74:310–312
241. Djalali AG, Moore KA, Kelly E (2005) Report of a patient with severe transfusion-related acute lung injury after multiple transfusions, resuscitated with albumin. Resuscitation 66:225–230
242. Dubois M, Lotze MT, Diamond WJ, Kim YD, Flye MW, MacNamara TE (1980) Pulmonary shunting during leukoagglutinin-induced noncardiac pulmonary edema. JAMA 244:2186–2189
243. Yost CS, Matthay MA, Gropper MA (2001) Etiology of acute pulmonary edema during liver transplantation. Chest 119:219–223
244. Popovsky MA (2004) Transfusion and the lung: circulatory overload and acute lung injury. Vox Sang 87:62–65
245. Zhou L, Giacherio D, Cooling L, Davenport RD (2005) Use of B-natriuretic peptide as a diagnostic marker in the differential diagnosis of transfusion-associated circulatory overload. Transfusion 45:1056–1063
246. Gajic O, Moore SB (2005) Transfusion-retaled acute lung injury. Mayo Clin Proc 80:766–770
247. Kopko PM, Paglieroni TG, Popovsky MA, Muto KN, MacKenzie MR, Holland PV (2003) TRALI: correlation of

antigen-antibody and monocyte activation in donor-recipient pairs. Transfusion 43:177–184
248. Knop S, Bux J, Kroeber SM, Bader P, Hebart H, Kanz L, Einsele H (2004) Fatal immune-mediated pancytopenia and a TRALI-like syndrome associated with high titers of recipient-type antibodies against donor-derived peripheral blood cells after allogeneic bone marrow transplantation following dose reduced conditioning. Haematologica 89:ECR12
249. Levy GJ, Shabot MM, Hart ME, Mya WW, Goldfinger D (1986) Tranfusion-associated noncardiogenic pulmonary edema. Report of a case and a warning regarding treatment. Transfusion 26:278–281
250. Boyer JE, Batra RB, Ascensao JL, Schechter GP (2006) Severe pulmonary complication after bortezomib treatment for multiple myeloma. Blood 108:1113
251. Chew E, Filshie R, Wei A (2007) Development of fatal bortezomib induced acute lung injury despite concurrent therapy with high-dose dexamethasone. Leuk Lymphoma 48:212–213
252. Pitini V, Arrigo C, Altavilla G, Naro C (2007) Severe pulmonary complications after bortezomib treatment for multiple myeloma: an unrecognized pulmonary vasculitis? Leuk Res 31:1027–1028
253. Zhou X, Sun C, Wang J, Mao J, Guo H (2010) Rapid fatal pulmonary complications in a chinese patient after bortezomib treatment for ALK-negative anaplastic large-cell lymphoma. Clin Lymphoma Myeloma Leuk 10:152–154
254. Narimatsu H, Hori A, Matsumura T, Kodama Y, Takita M, Kishi Y, Hamaki T, Yuji K, Tanaka Y, Komatsu T, Kami M (2008) Cooperative relationship between pharmaceutical companies, academia, and media explains sharp decrease in frequency of pulmonary complications after bortezomib in Japan. J Clin Oncol 26:5820–5823
255. Oliner H, Schwartz R, Rubio F Jr, Dameshek W (1961) Interstitial pulmonary fibrosis following busulfan therapy. Am J Med 31:134–139
256. Massin F, Fur A, Reybet-Degat O, Camus P, Jeannin L (1987) Busulfan-induced pneumonitis. Rev Mal Respir 4:3–10
257. Kalaycio M, Pohlman B, Kuczkowski E, Rybicki L, Andresen S, Sobecks R, Bolwell B (2006) High-dose busulfan and the risk of pulmonary mortality after autologous stem cell transplant. Clin Transplant 20:783–787
258. Nelson BM, Andrews GA (1964) Breast cancer and cytologic dysplasia in many organs after Busulfan. Am J Clin Pathol 42:37–44
259. Anonymous (1997) Case records of the Massachusetts General Hospital – Case 25-1997. N Engl J Med 337: 480–489
260. Kirschner RH, Esterly JR (1971) Pulmonary lesions associated with busulfan therapy of chronic myelogenous leukemia. Cancer 27:1074–1080
261. Aymard JP, Gyger M, Lavallee R, Legresley LP, Desy M (1984) A case of pulmonary alveolar proteinosis complicating chronic myelogenous leukemia. A peculiar pathologic aspect of busulfan lung ? Cancer 53:954–956
262. Littler WA, Ogilvie C (1970) Lung function in patients receiving busulphan. Br Med J ii:530–532
263. Giles FJ, Smith MP, Goldstone AH (1990) Chlorambucil lung toxicity. Acta Haematol 83:156–158
264. Mohr M, Kingreen D, Rühl H, Huhn D (1993) Interstitial lung disease: an underdiagnosed side-effect of chlorambucil? Ann Hematol 67:305–307
265. Khong HT, McCarthy J (1998) Chlorambucil-induced pulmonary disease: a case report and review of the literature. Ann Hematol 77:85–87
266. Kalambokis G, Stefanou D, Arkoumani E, Tsianos E (2004) Bronchiolitis obliterans organizing pneumonia following chlorambucil treatment for chronic lymphocytic leukemia. Eur J Haematol 73:139–142
267. Ruiz-Argüelles GJ, Arizpe-Bravo D, Sanchez-Sosa S, Rojas-Ortega S, Moreno-Ford V, Ruiz-Argüelles A (1999) Fatal G-CSF-induced pulmonary toxicity. Am J Hematol 60:82–83
268. Halter J, Kodera Y, Ispizua AU, Greinix HT, Schmitz N, Favre G, Baldomero H, Niederwieser D, Apperley JF, Gratwohl A (2009) Severe events in donors after allogeneic hematopoietic stem cell donation. Haematologica 94:94–101
269. Azoulay E, Attalah H, Harf A, Schlemmer B, Delclaux C (2001) Granulocyte colony-stimulating factor or neutrophil-induced pulmonary toxicity: myth or reality? Systematic review of clinical case reports and experimental data. Chest 120:1695–1701
270. Lei KIK, Leung WT, Johnson PJ (1994) Serious pulmonary complications in patients receiving recombinant granulocyte colony-stimulating factor during BACOP chemotherapy for agressive non-Hodgkin's lymphoma. Br J Cancer 70:1009–1013
271. Gertz MA, Lacy MQ, Bjornsson J, Litzow MR (2000) Fatal pulmonary toxicity related to the administration of granulocyte colony-stimulating factor in amyloidosis: a report and review of growth factor-induced pulmonary toxicity. J Hematother Stem Cell Res 9:635–643
272. Gatti E, Scagliotti GV, Ferrari G, Mutti L, Pozzi E, Stacchini A, Fubini L, Aglietta M (1995) Blood cell redistribution in the lung after administration of recombinant human granulocyte-macrophage colony-stimulating factor. Eur Respir J 8:1566–1571
273. Azoulay E, Herigault S, Levame M et al (2003) Effect of granulocyte colony-stimulating factor on bleomycin-induced acute lung injury and pulmonary fibrosis. Crit Care Med 31:1442–1448
274. Saxman SB, Nichols CR, Einhorn LH (1997) Pulmonary toxicity in patients with advanced-stage germ cell tumors receiving bleomycin with and without granulocyte colony stimulating factor. Chest 111:657–660
275. Yokose N, Ogata K, Tamura H, An E, Nakamura K, Kamikubo K, Kudoh S, Dan K, Nomura T (1998) Pulmonary toxicity after granulocyte colony stimulating factor-combined chemotherapy for non-Hodgkin's lymphoma. Br J Cancer 77:2286–2290
276. Schilero GJ, Oropello J, Benjamin E (1995) Impairment in gas exchange after granulocyte colony stimulating factor (G-CSF) in a patient with the adult respiratory distress syndrome. Chest 107:276–278
277. Philippe B, Couderc LJ, Balloul-Delclaux E, Janvier M, Caubarrère I (1994) Pulmonary toxicity of chemotherapy and GM-CSF. Respir Med 88:715
278. Yoshida I, Matsuo K, Teshima T, Hashimoto D, Tanimoto Y, Harada M, Tanimoto M (2006) Transient respiratory

disturbance by granulocyte-colony-stimulating factor administration in healthy donors of allogeneic peripheral blood progenitor cell transplantation. Transfusion 46: 186–192
279. de Azevedo AM, Tabak DG (2001) Life-threatening capillary leak syndrome after G-CSF mobilization and collection of peripheral blood progenitor cells for allogeneic transplantation. Bone Marrow Transplant 28:311–312
280. Sorhage F, Stover DE, Mortazavi A (1996) Unusual etiology of cough in a woman with asthma. Chest 110: 852–854
281. Taillé C, Fartoukh M, Houël R, Kobeiter H, Rémy P, Lemaire F (2001) Spontaneous hemomediastinum complicating steroid-induced mediastinal lipomatosis. Chest 120:311–313
282. Decramer M, de Bock V, Dom R (1996) Functional and histologic picture of steroid-induced myopathy in chronic obstructive pulmonary disease. Am J Respir Crit Care Med 153:1958–1964
283. Kilpiö K, Hannuksela M (2003) Corticosteroid allergy in asthma. Allergy 58:1131–1135
284. Erdmann SM (2005) Anaphylaxis induced by glucocorticoids. J Am Board Fam Pract 18:143–146
285. Nahum A, Garty BZ, Marcus N, Shoenfeld T, Levy Y (2009) Severe hypersensitivity reactions to corticosteroids in children. Pediatr Emerg Care 25:339–341
286. Lionakis MS, Kontoyiannis DP (2003) Glucocorticoids and invasive fungal infections. Lancet 362:1828–1838
287. Cuguillière A, Bérard H, N'Guyen G, Miltgen J, Martert G, Eskandari J, Bonnet D (1999) Pneumopathie interstitielle liée au cyclophosphamide. Rev Pneumol Clin 55:100–104
288. Woolley RJ (1993) Salicylate-induced pulmonary edema: a complication of chronic aspirin therapy. J Am Board Fam Pract 6:399–401
289. Kulke MH, Vance EA (1997) Pneumocystis carinii pneumonia in patients receiving chemotherapy for breast cancer. Clin Infect Dis 25:215–218
290. Anonymous (1984) Case records of the Massachusetts General Hospital - Case 35-1984. N Engl J Med 311:585–593
291. Burke DA, Stoddart JC, Ward MK, Simpson CGB (1982) Fatal pulmonary fibrosis occurring during treatment with cyclophosphamide. Br Med J 285:696
292. Karim FWA, Ayash RE, Allam C, Salem PA (1983) Pulmonary fibrosis after prolonged treatment with low-dose cyclophosphamide. Oncology 40:174–176
293. Topilow AA, Rothenberg SP, Cottrell TS (1973) Interstitial pneumonia after prolonged treatment with cyclophosphamide. Am Rev Respir Dis 108:114–117
294. Hamada K, Nagai S, Kitaichi M, Jin G, Shigematsu M, Nagao T, Sato A, Mishima M (2003) Cyclophosphamide-induced late-onset lung disease. Intern Med 42:82–87
295. Frankel SK, Cool CD, Lynch DA, Brown KK (2004) Idiopathic pleuroparenchymal fibroelastosis: description of a novel clinicopathologic entity. Chest 126:2007–2013
296. Tucker AS, Newman AJ, Alvorado C (1977) Pulmonary, pleural and thoracic changes complicating chemotherapy. Radiology 125:805–809
297. Haupt HM, Hutchins GM, Moore GW (1981) Ara-C lung: non-cardiogenic pulmonary edema complicating cytosine arabinoside therapy of leukaemia. Am J Med 70:256–261
298. Jehn U, Göldel N, Rienmüller R, Wilmanns W (1988) Non-cardiogenic pulmonary edema complicating intermediate and high-dose Ara C treatment for relapsed acute leukemia. Med Oncol Tumor Pharmacother 5:41–47
299. Kopterides P, Lignos M, Mentzelopoulos S, Armaganidis A, Pappa V (2005) Cytarabine-induced lung injury: case report. Anticancer Drugs 16:743–745
300. Shearer P, Katz J, Bozeman P, Jenkins J, Laver J, Krance R, Hurwitz C, Mahmoud N, Mirro J (1994) Pulmonary insufficiency complicating therapy with high dose cytosine arabinoside in five pediatric patients with relapsed acute myelogenous leukemia. Cancer 74:1953–1958
301. Andersson BS, Luna BS, Yee C, Hui KK, Keating MJ, McCreadie KB (1990) Fatal pulmonary failure complicating high-dose cytosine arabinoside therapy in acute leukemia. Cancer 65:1079–1084
302. Yegin ZA, Aki S, Sucak G, Yagci M (2007) Cytarabine induced noncardiogenic pulmonary edema in a case of acute lymphoblastic leukemia. Int J Lab Hematol 29:482–483
303. Chagnon K, Boissel N, Raffoux E, Dombret H, Tazi A, Bergeron A (2009) A new pattern of cytosine-arabinoside-induced lung toxicity. Br J Haematol
304. Goldblatt M, Huggins JT, Doelken P, Gurung P, Sahn SA (2009) Dasatinib-induced pleural effusions: a lymphatic network disorder? Am J Med Sci 338:414–417
305. Kantarjian H, Shah NP, Hochhaus A, Cortes J, Shah S, Ayala M, Moiraghi B, Shen Z, Mayer J, Pasquini R, Nakamae H, Huguet F, Boque C, Chuah C, Bleickardt E, Bradley-Garelik MB, Zhu C, Szatrowski T, Shapiro D, Baccarani M (2010) Dasatinib versus imatinib in newly diagnosed chronic-phase chronic myeloid leukemia. N Engl J Med 362:2260–2270
306. Quintás-Cardama A, Kantarjian H, O'Brien S, Borthakur G, Bruzzi J, Munden R, Cortes J (2007) Pleural effusion in patients with chronic myelogenous leukemia treated with dasatinib after imatinib failure. J Clin Oncol 25: 3908–3914
307. Shah NP, Kantarjian HM, Kim DW, Rea D, Dorlhiac-Llacer PE, Milone JH, Vela-Ojeda J, Silver RT, Khoury HJ, Charbonnier A, Khoroshko N, Paquette RL, Deininger M, Collins RH, Otero I, Hughes T, Bleickardt E, Strauss L, Francis S, Hochhaus A (2008) Intermittent target inhibition with dasatinib 100 mg once daily preserves efficacy and improves tolerability in imatinib-resistant and -intolerant chronic-phase chronic myeloid leukemia. J Clin Oncol 26:3204–3212
308. Stephens J, Carpiuc KT, Botteman M (2010) The burden of managing pleural effusions in patients with chronic myelogenous leukemia post-imatinib failure: a literature-based economic analysis. Int J Gen Med 3:31–36
309. Tenenbeim M, Kowalski S, Sienko A, Bowden DH, Adamson IYR (1992) Pulmonary toxic effects of continuous desferrioxamine administration in acute iron poisoning. Lancet 399:699–701
310. Freedman MH, Grisaru D, Olivieri N, McLusky I, Thorner PS (1990) Pulmonary syndrome in patients with thalassemia major receiving intravenous deferoxamine infusions. Am J Dis Child 144:565–569
311. Miller KB, Rosenwasser LJ, Bessette JAM, Beer DJ, Rocklin RE (1981) Rapid desensitization for desferrioxamine anaphylactic reaction. Lancet 1:1059

312. Fassas A, Gojo I, Rapoport A, Cottler-Fox M, Meisenberg B, Papadimitriou JC, Tricot G (2001) Pulmonary toxicity syndrome following CDEP (cyclophosphamide, dexamethasone, etoposide, cisplatin) chemotherapy. Bone Marrow Transplant 28:399–403
313. Hurst PG, Habib MP, Garewal H, Bluestein M, Paquin M, Greenberg BR (1987) Pulmonary toxicity associated with fludarabine monophosphate. Invest New Drugs 5:207–210
314. Solal-Celigny P, Brice P, Brousse N, Caspard H, Bastion Y, Haioun C, Bosly A, Tilly H, Bordessoule D, Sebban C, Harousseau JL, Morel P, Dupas B, Plassart F, Vasile N, Fort N, Leporrier M (1996) Phase II trial of fludarabine monophosphate as first-line treatment in patients with advanced follicular lymphoma: a multicenter study by the Groupe d'Etude des Lymphomes de l'Adulte. J Clin Oncol 14:514–519
315. Cervantes F, Salgado C, Montserrat E, Rozman C (1990) Fludarabine for prolymphocytic leukaemia and risk of interstitial pneumonitis. Lancet 336:1130
316. Helman DL Jr, Byrd JC, Ales NC, Shorr AF (2002) Fludarabine-related pulmonary toxicity. A distinct clinical entity in chronic lymphoproliferative syndromes. Chest 122:785–790
317. Trojan A, Meier R, Licht A, Taverna C (2002) Eosinophilic pneumonia after administration of fludarabine for the treatment of non-Hodgkin's lymphoma. Ann Hematol 81: 535–537
318. Ales NC, Helman DL, Shorr AF, Byrd JC (2000) Fludarabine associated pulmonary toxicity in chronic in lymphoproliferative disoders: a case series. Blood 96:756a–757a
319. Belknap SM, Kuzel TM, Yarnold PR, Slimack N, Lyons EA, Raisch DW, Bennett CL (2006) Clinical features and correlates of gemcitabine-associated lung injury-Findings from the RADAR project. Cancer 106:2051–2057
320. Tamiya A, Endo M, Shukuya T, Igawa S, Tsuya A, Nakamura Y, Murakami H, Takahashi T, Boku N, Yamamoto N (2009) Features of gemcitabine-related severe pulmonary toxicity: patients with pancreatic or biliary tract cancer. Pancreas 38:838–840
321. Hiraya D, Kagohashi K, Sakamoto N, Kondo T, Satoh H (2010) Gemcitabine-induced pulmonary toxicity in a patient with pancreatic cancer. Jop 11:186–188
322. Esteban E, Villanueva N, Muniz I, Fernandez Y, Fra J, Luque M, Jimenez P, Llorente B, Capelan M, Vieitez JM, Estrada E, Buesa JM, Jimenez LA (2008) Pulmonary toxicity in patients treated with gemcitabine plus vinorelbine or docetaxel for advanced non-small cell lung cancer: outcome data on a randomized phase II study. Invest New Drugs 26:67–74
323. Blum KA, Jung SH, Johnson JL, Lin TS, Hsi ED, Lucas DM, Byrd JC, Cheson BD, Bartlett NL (2010) Serious pulmonary toxicity in patients with Hodgkin's lymphoma with SGN-30, gemcitabine, vinorelbine, and liposomal doxorubicin is associated with an Fc{gamma}RIIIa-158 V/F polymorphism. Ann Oncol. Nov;21(11):2246–2254
324. Arrieta O, Gallardo-Rincon D, Villarreal-Garza C, Michel RM, Astorga-Ramos AM, Martinez-Barrera L, de la Garza J (2009) High frequency of radiation pneumonitis in patients with locally advanced non-small cell lung cancer treated with concurrent radiotherapy and gemcitabine after induction with gemcitabine and carboplatin. J Thorac Oncol 4:345–352
325. Marruchella A, Fiorenzano G, Merizzi A, Rossi G, Chiodera PL (1998) Diffuse alveolar damage in a patient treated with gemcitabine. Eur Respir J 11:504–506
326. Maniwa K, Tanaka E, Inoue T, Kato T, Sakuramoto M, Minakuchi M, Maeda Y, Noma S, Kobashi Y, Taguchi Y (2003) An autopsy case of acute pulmonary toxicity associated with gemcitabine. Intern Med 42:1022–1025
327. Galvao FH, Pestana JO, Capelozzi VL (2010) Fatal gemcitabine-induced pulmonary toxicity in metastatic gallbladder adenocarcinoma. Cancer Chemother Pharmacol Feb;65(3):607–610
328. Barlési F, Villani P, Doddoli C, Gimenez C, Kleisbauer JP (2004) Gemcitabine-induced severe pulmonary toxicity. Fundam Clin Pharmacol 18:85–91
329. Sauer-Heilborn A, Kath R, Schneider CP, Hoeffken K (1999) Severe non-haematological toxicity after treatment with gemcitabine. J Cancer Res Clin Oncol 125:637–640
330. Desramé J, Duvic C, Bredin C, Bechade D, Artru P, Brezault C, Defuentes G, Poirier JM, Dourthe LM, Coutant G, Chaussade S, de Gramont A, Algayres JP (2005) Hemolytic uremic syndrome as a complication of gemcitabine treatment: report of six cases and review of the literature. Rev Med Interne (Paris) 26:179–188
331. Schwonzen M, Spangenberger H, Spengler M (2003) Hydroxyurea-induced pneumonitis. Med Klin (Munich) 98:394–397
332. Slavenburg S, Heijdra YF, Drenth JP (2010) Pneumonitis as a consequence of (Peg)-interferon-ribavirin combination therapy for hepatitis C: a review of the literature. Dig Dis Sci 55:579–585
333. Ramos-Casals M, Mana J, Nardi N, Brito-Zeron P, Xaubet A, Sanchez-Tapias JM, Cervera R, Font J (2005) Sarcoidosis in patients with chronic hepatitis C virus infection: analysis of 68 cases. Medicine (Baltimore) 84:69–80
334. Weyer P, Cummings OW, Knox KS (2005) A 49-year-old woman with hepatitis, confusion, and abnormal chest radiograph findings. Chest 128:3076–3079
335. Ishizaki T, Sasaki F, Ameshima S, Shiozaki K, Takahashi H, Abe Y, Ito S, Kuriyama M, Nakai T, Kitagawa M (1996) Pneumonitis during interferon and/or herbal drug therapy in patients with chronic active hepatitis. Eur Respir J 9:2691–2696
336. Moriya K, Yasuda K, Koike K, Ichinose Y, Yotsuyanagi H, Kurokawa K, Iino S (1994) Induction of interstitial pneumonitis during interferon treatment for chronic hepatitis C. J Gastroenterol 29:514–517
337. Anderson P, Höglund M, Rödjer S (2003) Pulmonary side effects of interferon-a therapy in patients with hematological malignancies. Am J Hematol 73:54–58
338. Hillier AE, Mand J, Raza A, Markov M, Nadir A (2006) Consensus interferon induced interstitial pneumonitis in a patient with HCV. Am J Gastroenterol 101:200–202
339. Vartany E, Caldwell CA, Trow TK (2008) Adult respiratory distress syndrome after treatment with pegylated interferon alpha-2a and ribavirin. Heart Lung 37:153–156
340. Kamisako T, Adachi Y, Chihara J, Yamamoto T (1993) Interstitial pneumonitis and interferon-alfa. Br Med J 306:896
341. Hoffman SD, Hammadeh R, Shah N (2003) Eosinophilic pneumonitis secondary to pegylated interferon alpha-2b and/or ribavirin. Am J Gastroenterol 98:S152

342. Oymak FS, Demirbas HM, Mavili E, Akgun H, Gulmez I, Demir R, Ozesmi M (2005) Bronchiolitis obliterans organizing pneumonia. Clinical and roentgenological features in 26 cases. Respiration 72:254–262
343. Ogata K, Koga T, Yagawa K (1994) Interferon-related bronchiolitis obliterans organizing pneumonia. Chest 106:612–613
344. Kumar KS, Russo MW, Esposito S, Borczuk A, Jacobson I et al (2001) Severe pulmonary toxicity of interferon and ribavirin therapy in chronic hepatitis C. Am J Gastroenterol 96:127
345. Pileire G, Leclerc P, Hermant P, Meeus E, Camus P (1999) Toux chronique isolée pendant un traitement par interféron. Presse Méd 28:913
346. Krasnowska M, Malolepszy J, Liebhart E (1992) Interferon as a bronchospastic factor in patients with bronchial asthma. Pneumonol Alergol Pol 60:22–25
347. Takeda A, Ikegame K, Kimura Y, Ogawa H, Kanazawa S, Nakamura H (2000) Pleural effusion during interferon treatment for chronic hepatitis C. Hepato-gastroenterology 47:1431–1435
348. Fruehauf S, Steiger S, Topaly J, Ho AD (2001) Pulmonary artery hypertension during interferon-alpha therapy for chronic myelogenous leukemia. Ann Hematol 80:308–310
349. Price EJ, Venables PJ (1995) Drug-induced lupus. Drug Saf 12:283–290
350. Bergeron A, Bergot E, Vilela G, Ades L, Devergie A, Esperou H, Socie G, Calvo F, Gluckman E, Ribaud P, Rousselot P, Tazi A (2002) Hypersensitivity pneumonitis related to imatinib mesylate. J Clin Oncol 20: 4271–4272
351. Goldsby R, Pulsipher M, Adams R, Coffin C, Albritton K, Wagner L (2002) Unexpected pleural effusions in 3 pediatric patients treated with STI-571. J Pediatr Hematol Oncol 24:694–695
352. Ma CX, Hobday TJ, Jett JR (2003) Imatinib mesylate-induced interstitial pneumonitis. Mayo Clin Proc 78: 1578–1579
353. Yokoyama T, Miyazawa K, Kurakawa E, Nagate A, Shimamoto T, Iwaya K, Akata S, Aoshima M, Serizawa H, Ohyashiki K (2004) Interstitial pneumonia induced by imatinib mesylate: pathologic study demonstrates alveolar destruction and fibrosis with eosinophilic infiltration. Leukemia 18:645–646
354. Wagner U, Staats P, Moll R, Feek U, Vogelmeier C, Groneberg DA (2003) Imatinib-associated pulmonary alveolar proteinosis. Am J Med 115:674
355. Thornburg A, Abonour R, Smith P, Knox K, Twigg HL 3rd (2007) Hypersensitivity pneumonitis-like syndrome associated with the use of lenalidomide. Chest 131:1572–1574
356. Pretz J, Medeiros BC (2009) Thalidomide-induced pneumonitis in a patient with plasma cell leukemia: no recurrence with subsequent lenalidomide therapy. Am J Hematol 84:698–699
357. Chen Y, Kiatsimkul P, Nugent K, Raj R (2010) Lenalidomide-induced interstitial lung disease. Pharmacotherapy 30:325
358. Kortuem M, Einsele H (2010) Lenalidomide-induced hypersensitivity pneumonitis. Onkologie 33:219
359. Taetle R, Dickman PS, Feldman PS (1978) Pulmonary histopathologic changes associated with melphalan therapy. Cancer 42:1239–1245
360. Mufti GJ, Hamblin TJ, Gordon J (1983) Melphalan-induced pulmonary fibrosis in osteosclerotic myeloma. Acta Haematol 69:140–141
361. Lioté H, Gauthier JF, Prier A, Gauthier-Rahman S, Kaplan G, Akoun G (1989) Acute, reversible, interstitial pneumopathy induced by melphalan. Rev Mal Respir 6:461–464
362. Akasheh MS, Freytes CO, Vesole DH (2000) Melphalan-associated pulmonary toxicity following high-dose therapy with autologous hematopoietic stem cell transplantation. Bone Marrow Transplant 26:1107–1109
363. Major PP, Laurin S, Bettez P (1980) Pulmonary fibrosis following therapy with melphalan: report of two cases. Can Med Assoc J 123:197–202
364. Cottin V, Tébib J, Massonnet B, Souquet PJ, Bernard J-P (1996) Pulmonary function in patients receiving long-term low-dose methotrexate. Chest 109:933–938
365. Clarysse AM, Cathey WJ, Cartwright GE, Wintrobe MM (1969) Pulmonary disease complicating intermittent therapy with methotrexate. JAMA 209:1861–1864
366. Kremer JM, Joong KL (1986) The safety and efficacy of the use of methotrexate in long term therapy for rheumatoid arthritis. Arthritis Rheum 29:822–831
367. Pourel J, Guillemin F, Fener P, Webanck L, Bene M-C, Delorme N (1991) Delayed methotrexate pneumonitis in rheumatoid arthritis. J Rheumatol 18:303–304
368. Sostman HD, Matthay RA, Putman CE, Smith GJW (1976) Methotrexate-induced pneumonitis. Medicine (Baltimore) 55:371–388
369. Everts CS, Wescott JL, Bragg DG (1973) Methotrexate therapy and pulmonary disease. Radiology 107:539–543
370. Arakawa H, Yamasaki M, Kurihara Y, Yamada H, Nakajima Y (2003) Methotrexate-induced pulmonary injury: serial CT findings. J Thorac Imaging 18:231–236
371. Schnabel A, Richter C, Bauerfeind S, Gross WL (1997) Bronchoalveolar lavage cell profile in methotrexate induced pneumonitis. Thorax 52:377–379
372. Newman ED, Harrington TM (1988) Fatal methotrexate pneumonitis in rheumatoid arthritis. Arthritis Rheum 31:1585–1586
373. Mahmood T, Mudad R (2002) Pulmonary toxicity secondary to procarbazine. Am J Clin Oncol 25:187–188
374. Jones SE, Moore M, Blank N, Castellino RA (1972) Hypersensitivity to procarbazine (Matulane) manifested by fever and pleuropulmonary reaction. Cancer 29:498–500
375. Ecker MD, Jay B, Keohane MF (1978) Procarbazine lung. AJR Am J Roentgenol 131:527–528
376. Horton LWL, Chappell AG, Powell DEB (1977) Diffuse interstitial pulmonary fibrosis complicating Hodgkin's disease. Br J Dis Chest 71:44–48
377. Rosenow EC (1980) Chemotherapeutic drug-induced pulmonary disease. Semin Respir Med 2:89–96
378. Liu X, Hong XN, Gu YJ, Wang BY, Luo ZG, Cao J (2008) Interstitial pneumonitis during rituximab-containing chemotherapy for non-Hodgkin lymphoma. Leuk Lymphoma 49:1778–1783
379. Katsuya H, Suzumiya J, Sasaki H, Ishitsuka K, Shibata T, Takamatsu Y, Tamura K (2009) Addition of rituximab to cyclophosphamide, doxorubicin, vincristine, and prednisolone therapy has a high risk of developing interstitial pneumonia in patients with non-Hodgkin lymphoma. Leuk Lymphoma 50:1818–1823

380. Bitzan M, Ouahed JD, Carpineta L, Bernard C, Bell LE (2010) Cryptogenic organizing pneumonia after rituximab therapy for presumed post-kidney transplant lymphoproliferative disease. Pediatr Nephrol. Jun;25(6):1163–1167
381. Lioté H, Lioté F, Seroussi B, Mayaud C, Cadranel J (2010) Rituximab-induced lung disease: a systematic literature review. Eur Respir J 35:681–687
382. Carrion Valero F, Bertomeu Gonzalez V (2002) Lung toxicity due to thalidomide. Arch Bronconeumol 38:492–494
383. Garcia BD, de Gafas AP, Alvarez MJF (2003) Lung toxicity due to thalidomide. Arch Bronconeumol 39:240
384. Onozawa M, Hashino S, Sogabe S, Haneda M, Horimoto H, Izumiyama K, Kondo T, Aldana LP, Hamada K, Asaka M (2005) Thalidomide-induced interstitial pneumonitis. J Clin Oncol 23:2425–2426
385. Buttin BM, Moore MJ (2008) Thalidomide-induced reversible interstitial pneumonitis in a patient with recurrent ovarian cancer. Gynecol Oncol. Dec;111(3):546–548
386. Iguchi T, Sakoda M, Chen CK, Yokoyama K, Hattori Y, Ikeda Y, Okamoto S (2004) Interstitial pneumonia during treatment with thalidomide in a patient with multiple myeloma. Rinsho Ketsueki 45:1064–1066
387. Feaver AA, McCune DE, Mysliwiec AG, Mysliwiec V (2006) Thalidomide-induced organizing pneumonia. South Med J 99:1292–1294
388. Younis TH, Alam A, Paplham P, Spangenthal E, McCarthy P (2003) Reversible pulmonary hypertension and thalidomide therapy for multiple myeloma. Br J Haematol 123:563
389. Bennett CL, Schumock GT, Desai AA, Kwaan HC, Raisch DW, Newlin R, Stalder W (2002) Thalidomide-associated deep vein thrombosis and pulmonary embolism. Am J Med 113:603–606
390. Steurer M, Sudmeier I, Stauder R, Gastl G (2003) Thromboembolic events in patients with myelodysplastic syndrome receiving thalidomide in combination with darbepoietin-alpha. Br J Haematol 121:101–103
391. Rivera MP, Kris MG, Gralla RJ, White DA (1995) Syndrome of acute dyspnea related to combined mitomycin plus vinca alkaloid chemotherapy. Am J Clin Oncol 18:245–250
392. Movsas B, Raffin TA, Epstein AH, Link CJ (1997) Pulmonary radiation injury. Chest 111:1061–1076
393. Abratt RP, Onc FR, Morgan GW, Silvestri G, Willcox P (2004) Pulmonary complications of radiation therapy. Clin Chest Med 25:167–177
394. Goldman AL, Enquist R (1975) Hyperacute radiation pneumonitis. Chest 67:613–615
395. Park KJ, Chung JY, Chun MS, Suh JH (2000) Radiation induced lung disease and the impact of radiation methods on imaging features. Radiographics 20:83–98
396. Choi YW, Munden RF, Erasmus JJ, Park KJ, Chung WK, Jeon SC, Park CK (2004) Effects of radiation therapy on the lung: radiologic appearances and differential diagnosis. Radiographics 24:985–997, discussion 998
397. Bölling T, Konemann S, Ernst I, Willich N (2008) Late effects of thoracic irradiation in children. Strahlentherapie Und Onkologie 184:289–295
398. Deist TJ, Freytag A (2001) Therapy of abdominal and thoracic chylous effusions 18 years after radiation therapy. Z Gastroenterol 39:523–527
399. Crestanello JA, McGregor CGA, Danielson GK, Daly RC, Dearani JA, Orszulak TA, Mullany CJ, Puga FJ, Zehr KJ, Schleck C, Schaff HV (2004) Mitral and tricuspid valve repair in patients with previous mediastinal radiation therapy. Ann Thorac Surg 78:826–831
400. Prosnitz RG, Chen YH, Marks LB (2005) Cardiac toxicity following thoracic radiation. Semin Oncol 32:S71–S80

Cardiovascular Complications of Cancer and Radiation Therapy

32

Callie S. Kwartler and Aarif Y. Khakoo

Contents

C.S. Kwartler
Department of Internal Medicine,
University of Texas Health Science Center at Houston,
Houston, TX, 77030

A.Y. Khakoo (✉)
Department of Cardiology,
University of Texas MD Anderson Cancer Center,
Houston, TX, 77030
e-mail: aykhakoo@mdanderson.org

32.1 Introduction

As the number of cancer survivors increases, more attention must be paid to secondary illnesses and side effects that arise as a result of cancer or its treatment. Cardiovascular disease is a leading cause of death in the general population and is also a growing issue for cancer survivors. The risk of cardiovascular disease is approaching, and in some cases overtaking, the risk of cancer recurrence as the primary health concern of cancer survivors [1]. The pathogenesis and treatment of cardiovascular disease can be affected by cancer or cancer treatments such that it is difficult for clinicians to manage.

Cancer and its therapies can cause a wide range of cardiovascular effects including pericardial disease, thromboembolism, heart failure, valve disease, and vessel stenosis [2]. Because the same diseases can occur in the general population, especially in older patients who have accumulated cardiovascular risk factors, because some cancers themselves predispose patients to these conditions, and because most patients are on treatment regimens containing many different anticancer therapies that alone or in combination can cause cardiovascular complications, it can be extremely difficult to pin down the actual cause of the disease [3].

The aim of this chapter is to describe the cardiovascular complications that can arise as a result of cancer or radiation treatment. Clinicians need to be aware of the possible implications of cancer and its treatments on the heart and vasculature because early detection of toxic effects may reduce cardiac damage.

É. Azoulay (ed.), *Pulmonary Involvement in Patients with Hematological Malignancies*,
DOI: 10.1007/978-3-642-15742-4_32, © Springer-Verlag Berlin Heidelberg 2011

32.2 Cardiovascular Complications of Cancer

32.2.1 Primary Cardiac Tumors

Although rare, primary cardiac tumors do exist. Most are benign, with about half of all cases being myxomas. Myxomas are endocardial-based masses that can cause heart failure-like symptoms, embolic phenomena, valvular obstruction, or arrhythmias [4]. Myxomas can be sporadic or familial, sometimes associated with a rare familial syndrome called "Carney complex" where cardiac myxomas occur in conjunction with skin lesions, myxoid fibroadenomas of the breast or other secondary tumors, and endocrinopathy [5, 6]. Mutations in the PRKAR1α gene, encoding a regulatory subunit of protein kinase A, have been reported to cause a majority of Carney complex cases [5] and have rarely been associated with nonsyndromic familial myxomas [7]. Most centers report a higher prevalence of disease in women [6, 8, 9].

In many cases, myxomas occur with a variety of immunologic symptoms, including fever, malaise, weight loss, and myalgias [7]. Several studies have found increased serum levels of IL-6 secreted by the tumor [10–12], and patients with higher IL-6 levels have more intense constitutional symptoms [7]. Multiple studies have also found a correlation between tumor size and serum levels of IL-6 or α1-globulin [7, 13], and it has been suggested that IL-6 may be important in tumor recurrence [14].

Myxomas most commonly present in the left atrium, with about 15% in the right atrium, and rare biatrial or ventricular tumors [6, 8, 9]. Diagnosis can be achieved with careful auscultation for the characteristic "plop" caused by the tumor moving in and out of the mitral valve planes. Diagnosis is confirmed with transthoracic, or occasionally transesophageal, echocardiography [8]. The tumors are generally polyploid, often pedunculated, and can vary in color, size, and texture. Gelatinous lobated tumors, tumors in the left atrium, and tumors causing a nonsinus rhythm may be more likely to result in embolism. Treatment is by immediate surgical resection and is curative in a majority of sporadic cases. Incomplete resection or embolization of the tumor can cause recurrence. Additionally, multifocal tumors are most likely to recur, explaining the increased rates of recurrence of familial myxomas.

Other benign heart tumors include papillary fibroelastomas, which are fibrous connective tissue tumors lined with endothelial cells [15]. No clear risk factors are associated with development of this tumor type, and they predominantly occur on the surface of the heart valves [16]. The tumor typically has an "anemone" or "flower-like" shape, and is often highly mobile. The most common clinical presentation is transient ischemic attack or stroke due to an embolus in the cerebral arteries, but myocardial infarction, angina, embolism in other arteries, and sudden death are also possible presentations [16]. Asymptomatic tumors are often diagnosed accidentally during routine echocardiography of the heart, but transesophogeal imaging is usually required for complete diagnosis [17]. Anticoagulant therapy may be used until surgery can be performed, but surgery is the treatment of choice for papillary fibroelastoma [16, 18]. No recurrence of this tumor type has been reported.

Rhabdomyomas are the most common cardiac tumor type in pediatric patients; they primarily occur in conjunction with tuberous sclerosis [19]. This tumor type can be diagnosed in utero by fetal ultrasound [20] or in older children by echocardiography. They consist of smooth muscle tissue in hamartomas and can occur in any area of the heart. Arrhythmias, heart failure, and intrauterine or sudden death have been associated with rhabdomyomas, but about 50% are asymptomatic [21]. Although in many cases these tumors have been reported to regress spontaneously [19, 21, 22], surgical resection is recommended if the tumor is causing cardiac symptoms.

Other benign tumors occur even more rarely. Fibromas are fibroblast-rich tumors mostly seen in infants, which may cause heart failure, arrhythmia, or sudden death [4]. Hemangiomas are caused by proliferation of vascular endothelial cells and occur most frequently in children and adolescents [23]. Hemangiomas are classified as cavernous, capillary, or arteriovenous based on histology, and cardiac tumors can be a combination of types [24]. They are frequently asymptomatic and most often diagnosed incidentally during routine echocardiography. Lipomas are adipose tissue tumors that are usually asymptomatic, and teratomas are germ cell tumors that can occur rarely in the heart. All of these tumor types are preferentially treated by surgical resection wherever possible.

Even more rare are malignant primary cardiac tumors. Primary cardiac lymphoma is rare, but can occur and lead to rapidly progressing heart failure, arrhythmias, cardiac tamponade, or superior vena cava syndrome. Cardiac involvement in disseminated lymphoma is fairly common, occurring in 10–20% of patients. Unlike typical lymphomas, primary cardiac cases occur at a higher rate in immunocompromised patients. Prognosis is poor for this tumor type due to a typically late diagnosis. Chemotherapy and radiation treatments may prolong survival [25, 26]. Various types of sarcomas can also exist in the heart; histology is extremely variable, and patients can present with a wide variety of cardiac symptoms. Patients with cardiac sarcomas have an extremely poor prognosis with limited chances of survival beyond 1 year. Aggressive surgical treatment can prolong survival and provide relief of symptoms, but risk of early metastasis or recurrence remains high.

32.2.2 Venous Thromboembolism

Venous thromboembolism (VTE) is an important cause of morbidity and mortality in patients with cancer [27]. Here we provide the reader with a brief overview of several of the key issues regarding VTE in cancer patients. For a more detailed treatment of this topic, the reader is referred to more detailed reviews [28, 29]. Although an increased risk of VTE is seen in most patients with cancer, the cancers most associated with VTE, when adjusted with disease prevalence, are those of the pancreas, ovary, and brain [30]. Multiple pathogenic factors contribute to the increased risk of VTE in the cancer patient, including hypercoagulability, vessel wall injury, venous stasis (particularly in bedbound patients or patients undergoing surgery), and the presence of long-term, indwelling central venous catheters.

Despite a 15% incidence of clinically apparent VTE in patients with cancer, VTE in the cancer patient is likely to be significantly underdiagnosed, since autopsy studies of cancer patients suggest that the incidence of VTE approaches 50% [31]. Unilateral upper or lower extremity swelling is the most common sign on physical examination, although exam findings are not terribly reliable. Compression duplex venography represents the best initial test for suspected upper extremity or lower extremity deep vein thrombosis, with magnetic resonance venography reserved for those patients in whom duplex venography is inconclusive [32]. The utility of D-dimer testing in ruling out the presence of DVT in cancer patients is unclear [33].

Clinical symptoms of new-onset chest pain or shortness of breath without another clear cause warrants investigation for possible pulmonary embolism (PE) in the cancer patient. In addition, up to 10% of patients presenting with PE will experience syncope as their initial presenting sign [34]. The most common electrocardiographic finding in a patient with PE is the presence of sinus tachycardia, and can often be accompanied by ST segment/T wave changes in the early precordial leads. The identification of a new onset atrial arrhythmia, such as atrial fibrillation or atrial flutter, should raise suspicion of acute PE in the cancer patient [35]. Elevations of cardiac biomarkers, such as troponin I and B-type natriuretic peptide (BNP), can be seen in patients with acute PE and may identify a subgroup of patients with poor prognoses [36].

Anticoagulation represents the mainstay of treatment of patients with VTE. Low molecular weight heparin (LMWH) appears to be superior to unfractionated heparin in the therapy of patients with DVT, with lower bleeding rates and decreased mortality in the acute setting. Furthermore, LMWH appears to be safe and efficacious in the initial therapy of patients with suspected or clinically confirmed PE. In patients with catheter-related VTE, removal of the catheter in addition to anticoagulation should be considered [37]. The treatment of patients with cancer with VTE can be particularly challenging due to the presence of cancer-related or treatment-related thrombocytopenia. There are no current studies available to guide therapy in a cancer patient with thrombocytopenia and VTE, and the treatment must be individualized to the risk/benefit ratio for the individual patient. Patients with primary or metastatic CNS malignancies who develop VTE represent another challenging patient group. Recent studies suggest that systemic anticoagulation for the treatment of brain tumor patients with VTE is warranted in the absence of a history of intracranial hemorrhage or the presence of profound thrombocytopenia [38].

Because of the high risk of recurrence of VTE in patients with cancer, strong consideration should be given to lifelong anticoagulation in a cancer patient with a history of VTE [39]. The optimal agent for the long-term treatment of patients with VTE is unclear. Traditionally, patients were treated with unfractionated or LMWH initially, and then were subsequently transitioned to oral anticoagulant therapy (e.g., coumadin). However, a retrospective analysis revealed that patients with cancer and a history of VTE who were treated with coumadin had a much higher likelihood of recurrent thrombotic events and major bleeding compared with noncancer patients [39]. A subsequent study reinforced these findings, with a VTE recurrence rate of 20% over 12 months in cancer patients with VTE despite oral anticoagulation with warfarin [40]. Building upon these findings, the LMWH dalteparin was compared with warfarin in a randomized trial for the treatment of cancer patients with a history of VTE. Patients treated with dalteparin had a 9% incidence of recurrent thromboembolism over a 6-month period, whereas warfarin-treated patients had a 17% incidence over the same timeframe, a difference that was highly statistically significant. There was no difference in major bleeding between the two groups. Based upon these findings, some authors have suggested LMWHs as the treatment of choice for long-term treatment of cancer patients with a history of VTE [40, 41].

Cancer patients undergoing major surgery are among the highest risk group for the development of VTE in the postoperative period, with an incidence of VTE approaching 50% in the absence of any prophylactic therapy [40]. Current guidelines recommend that cancer patients undergoing surgery receive a thromboprophylaxis regimen consisting of a LMWH and intermittent pneumatic compression devices, and that treatment with LMWH be continued for up to 1 month post-discharge [42]. Similarly, hospitalized cancer patients should receive multimodality DVT prophylaxis in the absence of contraindications because of their high risk of developing VTE. Little evidence supports the use of prophylactic anticoagulation to prevent VTE in cancer patients with no history of prior VTE in the outpatient setting. In particular, although low dose warfarin is often utilized to prevent thrombosis in patients with indwelling central venous catheters, several studies have found no demonstrable benefit of this approach [28].

32.2.3 Pericardial Disease

Many of the primary cardiac tumors detailed above can have pericardial involvement or cause pericardial symptoms. Additionally, pericardial mesothelioma is a rare primary pericardial tumor type arising from the mesothelial cells of the pericardium [43]. These tumors are highly aggressive, and pallative care may be the only option for treatment [44]. Diagnosis can be challenging as the tumor presents similarly to pericardial effusion, and can even be indistinguishable on echocardiogram [45]. Surgical excision may be attempted in some patients, along with treatment of symptoms of pericardial disease (described in detail below), but in most cases a cure is impossible and survival expectancy is merely months.

In addition to primary cardiac tumors, metastases to the heart are sometimes observed, and up to 70% of heart metastases include involvement of the pericardium [46]. The most frequent cancer types that metastasize to the pericardium are breast cancers, lung cancers, leukemias, and lymphomas [46]. Invasion of the pericardium by malignant tumors can cause pericardial effusions that may rapidly accumulate and lead to life-threatening cardiac tamponade [47]. In cancer patients with pericardial involvement, pericardial disease significantly worsens prognosis and may itself significantly contribute to cancer-related mortality.

Cardiac tamponade presents clinically as dyspnea and chest pain, with possible symptoms of low systemic arterial pressure, low pulse pressure, and tachycardia [48]. Because the most common presenting symptoms are respiratory, pericardial involvement is often missed or mistaken for progression of pulmonary metastases. Many patients show abnormal pulsus paradoxus or elevated jugular venous pressure. Diagnosis of cardiac tamponade and evaluation of the level of hemodynamic compromise, and thus the urgency of treatment, should be confirmed by echocardiography. Echocardiography is useful to assess the size of the effusion and its accessibility for percutaneous drainage. When considering the need for percutaneous drainage, attention should be given not only to the size of the effusion, but also to the degree to which it is causing hemodynamic compromise, assessed by quantifying the degree of respirophasic variation of flow across the mitral and tricuspid valves, indicative of the intraventricular dependence and tamponade physiology [49].

Pericardiocentesis is often the first procedure attempted to drain the fluid from the pericardium, as it is quick and generally effective. Echocardiographic guidance is often employed, aiding in accessing the effusion through a subxiphoid approach. In selected patients, an echocardiographically guided anterior approach yields the best results, but care must be taken to avoid puncture of the left internal mammary artery [50]. In effusions localized to the posterior aspect of the heart, drainage via a CT-guided approach is optimal [51]. Pericardiocentesis alone also results in an approximately 40% recurrence rate [46], which can be reduced substantially by placement of a pericardial drain at the time of pericardiocentesis for extended drainage [52].

After pericardiocentesis is performed, injection of sclerosing agents into the pericardium may reduce the incidence of recurrent effusions. There are a few options for preventing reaccumulation of fluid. Tetracycline has been most successfully used for this purpose [53], but its usage has been limited by the development of severe chest discomfort in patients receiving such treatments. More recently, the use of the antineoplastic agent thiotepa delivered to the pericardial space has shown promise in preventing recurrence of pericardial effusions with little or no patient discomfort [54]. Further long-term studies are needed to verify the safety and efficacy of this approach.

In cases in which pericardiocentesis is unsuccessful or in which recurrence of the effusion occurs after extended drainage, surgical options are available [55]. Pericardectomy, or the surgical removal of a large portion of the pericardium, should be used in extreme cases only. Although recurrence is virtually zero after this procedure, operative risks are high (17–30% periprocedural mortality in some series) [46]. A more commonly used surgical approach is the formation of a pericardial window. This can be done surgically using a subxiphoid route, by anterior thoracotomy, or by thoracoscopy. This procedure still requires general anesthesia, but is generally well tolerated and is effective to prevent recurrence of disease [46, 56].

32.3 Radiation Therapy-Induced Cardiovascular Disease

Cardiovascular complications of radiation therapy have long been recognized. Radiation treatments directed at the breasts, mediastinum, or neck are particularly dangerous for long-term risks of cardiovascular disease. Although improved knowledge and improved techniques for radiation delivery have limited the area and dose of radiation to sensitive areas, the risks of radiation-induced disease are still very real for cancer patients.

32.3.1 Pericardial Disease

Pericardial disease, characterized by fibrous thickening and fluid production, is historically the most common manifestation of radiation damage to the heart, but modern techniques have significantly reduced incidence [57]. One study of Hodgkin's disease survivors found thickened pericardium in 15% of patients after 5–10 years of follow-up [58]. No association was found between pericardial disease and gender, age, treatment parameters, or time after treatment. In another study, 7 of 16 esophageal cancer patients treated with radiation and 7 of 25 lung cancer patients developed cardiac complications, and the majority manifested as pericardial effusions. Prior histories of arrhythmias or heart failure were both predictive factors, likely because their hearts were more sensitive to radiation-induced changes in cardiac innervation [59].

Pericardial damage may present as acute, chronic, or intermittent disease, and as either effusive or restrictive [60]. Acute pericarditis occurs typically with a high dose of radiation, and symptoms usually resolve on their own [61]. Chronic disease manifests usually within 1 year of radiation treatment and is due to accumulation of fibrous adhesions and fluids with fibrous thickening of the pericardium [57].

32.3.2 Valvular Disease

Regurgitation or stenosis of the heart valves is increasingly being recognized as a major complication of radiation treatment for Hodgkin's disease. In one study, 5–10 years posttreatment 31% of patients had pathological regurgitation in either the aortic or mitral valve. Female gender was a predictor for valve disease, but no other demographic or treatment parameters, including anthracycline treatment, correlated [58, 62]. A follow-up to that study 12 years later found an even higher prevalence of regurgitation and aortic valve stenosis, as well as a progression to more severe disease in most patients [63]. These findings suggest that disease increases with time from treatment. Other studies confirm that valve thickening and regurgitation increase with length of follow-up, but are split as to whether the disease is clinically relevant in most patients [62, 64].

Several mechanisms of radiation-induced valve disease have been proposed. Endothelial dysfunction from chronic inflammation leading to fibrosis, direct radiation damage to the valves causing fibrous thickening, and reduced endothelial regenerative capacity have all been suggested as possible mechanisms of damage [63]. Valvular lesions may begin soon after radiation therapy as endocardial thickening, and then fibrosis builds up and, over time, the disease progresses from asymptomatic to physiologically important disease requiring surgical intervention. Damage usually occurs on the left side, to the mitral or aortic valves, likely due to higher pressure on those valves [65].

32.3.3 Accelerated Coronary Artery Disease

Accelerated coronary artery disease is a well-established complication of radiation. Young age at treatment and high radiation dose as well as traditional risk factors for coronary artery disease all increase risk. It is thus important to treat or control risk factors, such as smoking, hyperlipidaemia, and hypercholesterolaemia in cancer survivors with a history of radiation exposure [57].

Older studies showed a significant risk to patients with left-sided breast cancer over right-sided breast cancer [66], but some more recent studies have found no differences in risk [67, 68]. While one study found no greater incidence of myocardial infarction in breast cancer patients receiving radiation versus a general age-matched female population [68], most studies report that even the most modern techniques still cause a minor but significant increase (~10%) in cardiac morbidity and mortality with inclusion of radiation in the treatment plan [67, 69, 70].

Irradiation of the chest for other cancers also increases the risk of cardiac complications. Radiation for esophageal cancer causes a significantly higher prevalence of inferior wall ischemia even with modern techniques. Risk increases based on radiation dose and the volume of myocardium in the irradiation field [71]. Mediastinal radiation for non-Hodgkin's lymphoma increases risks of heart failure, myocardial infarction, and stroke in a dose-dependent manner. Doses higher than 40 Gy are particularly dangerous [72]. One study reported up to 18% of patients developed coronary artery disease 10 years after mantle field irradiation [65].

The mechanism of coronary artery disease pathogenesis in these patients is likely to be intimal and medial thickening of the vessels accompanying direct endothelial damage. Coronary lesions due to radiation have much less accumulation of lipids than typical atherosclerotic lesions [65]. Since the lesions are typically located in the proximal vessels due to typical anterior radiation fields, surgical treatment with coronary bypass is often possible [57, 65].

32.3.4 Cardiomyopathy

Symptomatic cardiomyopathy is a less common manifestation of radiation toxicity, and it is important to distinguish diagnostically the symptoms of heart failure due to cardiomyopathy versus constrictive pericarditis [57]. One study reported that preexisting hypertension increased the risks of heart failure and stroke, as did treatment at a younger age and treatment for relapsed cancer ("salvage treatment") [72]. Younger age at treatment most likely increases risk due to longer survival time, since it has also been shown that more disease appears with longer time from treatment. Another study conversely found that symptoms tended to appear in older patients, especially males [73]. Patients with known cardiac risk factors have a significantly increased risk of ischemic disease [64, 73].

Myocardial fibrosis and endocardial thickening are frequently observed in radiation-treated patients who develop cardiomyopathy without associated large-vessel coronary artery disease [74]. Ischemia caused by damage to the endothelial cells in the myocardial microvasculature leads to fibrosis, which then leads to decreased systolic and/or diastolic function. High-dose radiation alone typically leads to a restrictive cardiomyopathy, whereas radiation therapy plus anthracycline treatment tend to cause dilated cardiomyopathies [57].

32.3.5 Peripheral Vessel Stenosis

Radiation can also cause significant damage to the peripheral arteries. External cervical irradiation causes plaque-like thickening of the intima of the carotid artery, and strokes may also be increased in this patient population [75]. One study reported 4.8% of patients developed strokes following cervical irradiation for head and neck cancers. Risk was not correlated with hypertension, diabetes, surgical manipulation of the carotid arteries, or radiation dose [76]. Radiation damage in animal models produces lesions similar to those seen with typical atherosclerosis, including intimal proliferation, disruption of the internal elastic lamina, and necrosis [77].

A comparison of patients who developed carotid artery stenosis with or without prior radiation revealed that fewer cases of diabetes, ischemic heart disease, or other peripheral vascular disease were present in the radiation-treated group. Patients who were irradiated more commonly had bilateral disease or common carotid artery lesions [78]. These results suggest that radiation independently raises the risk of carotid artery disease significantly. Surgical repair of radiation-induced carotid occlusion or stenosis is more difficult due to scarring, risk of infection, more common restenosis, long lesion length, and increased risk of complications [77].

Peripheral vascular disease, including strokes, transient ischemic attack, carotid artery stenosis, and subclavian artery stenosis are also possible complications of radiation therapy for Hodgkin's disease. These effects are seen most frequently in two types of patients: older patients with preexisting atherosclerosis, who most often present with strokes or ischemia relatively shortly after treatment, and younger patients who present with carotid or subclavian stenosis after a longer interval [62]. Radiation for Hodgkin's disease or breast cancer can result in stenosis of multiple vessels coming off the aortic arch including subclavian, axillary, carotid, and vertebral arteries as well as stenosis of coronary arteries. Radiation-induced arterial disease presents at a much younger age than typically seen in the general population [74]. Most studies show that patients develop atherosclerosis in irradiated regions of the vasculature many years before developing age-related disease in the rest of the body [79].

The pathogenesis of radiation-induced peripheral vascular disease is similar to age-related hardening of the arteries. Radiation causes endothelial and fibroblast proliferation, collagen deposition, and fibrosis contributing to a phenotype of accelerated atherosclerosis. The media and adventitia of vessels with radiation-induced atherosclerosis look more diseased, with more medial degeneration and adventitial fibrosis than is typically seen [74].

32.3.6 Cardiac Baroreceptor Dysfunction

Another long-term complication of head and neck irradiation is cardiac baroreceptor dysfunction. Baroreceptors, located in the carotid arteries as well as in the aortic arch, heart, and pulmonary vessels, are responsible for regulating fluctuations in blood pressure. The baroreflex loop contains sympathetic and parasympathetic nerves that communicate changes in circulation and ventilation from the brain to the heart, and the carotid baroreceptors are a key component of that system [80]. Baroreflex syndrome occurs usually as a result of neck trauma, resection of bilateral carotid body tumors, carotid endartectomy, or radiation therapy to the neck region [81, 82]. The acute syndrome is characterized by volatile hypertension along with secondary symptoms of headache, palpitations, emotional instability, and diaphoresis [80, 81]. Cases of baroreflex failure usually develop after bilateral radiation or injury, as redundancy prevents symptoms from manifesting from only single-sided dysfunction [83]. Diagnosis of baroreceptor dysfunction should be considered in patients with volatile hypertension following neck irradiation, but pheochromocytoma, which has similar symptoms, should first be ruled out [80].

A study of 12 patients within 1–5 years of neck irradiation revealed that while none of the 12 had clinically significant baroreflex failure, all had lower baroreflex sensitivity than 15 controls [81]. In these patients, and in the cases reported of post-radiation baroreflex syndrome, exams showed decreased afferent input rather than decreased effector function to be the cause of barosystem failure [83–85]. Symptoms from radiation-induced baroreceptor dysfunction tend to develop gradually, in contrast to the immediate onset after endarterectomy or carotid tumor removal.

Treatment options should be focused on reducing the surges in blood pressure. Clonidine, a centrally acting alpha-adrenoreceptor agonist, has been shown to decrease the magnitude and frequency of hypertension [80, 84].

32.3.7 Conclusion

Even modern radiation techniques cannot shield all vulnerable vessels from doses sufficient to cause damage. Cardiac complications, particularly of mediastinal radiation therapy, but also from therapy for breast, lung, and esophageal cancers, are still a major source of morbidity and mortality for cancer survivors. Follow-up is recommended for all patients treated with radiation to the heart or major arteries, as extended time from treatment increases risk of complications. Aggressive medical management of traditional risk factors for coronary artery disease may be useful in preventing the cardiovascular complications of radiation therapy.

32.4 Conclusion

Clinicians treating patients with cancer should be aware of the possible complications of cancer and its therapies on the cardiovascular system. Cancer itself can occur in the heart or pericardium primarily, though tumors in this system are rare and mostly benign. More insidiously, metastases to the heart or pericardium can lead to devastating effects and signal a stage of disease that is very difficult to treat. Additionally, a number of cancers predispose patients to VTE, which can also often result from treatments or treatment methods. Early detection of cardiovascular complications prevents further damage to the system and may prevent death.

Patients who have undergone radiation therapy may be at risk for developing heart or vascular disease years or decades after undergoing the initial treatment, so lifelong monitoring may be beneficial to those treated with radiation in sensitive areas. Although modern radiation techniques have reduced some of the detrimental effects by lowering radiation dosage and narrowing the field of tissue exposed to radiation, cardiovascular complications can still occur. Radiation for cancers in the chest or mediastinum (including breast, lung, esophageal, and some lymphomas) can lead to a number of cardiac complications, including accelerated coronary artery disease, valve disease, and others. Cervical irradiation for head and neck cancers can cause cardiac baroreceptor dysfunction. Irradiation that includes any large blood vessels can also lead to vessel stenosis and an early atherosclerosis-like phenotype that occurs long before age-related disease in other vascular beds. Clinicians should be aware of the types of cardiovascular complications that can result from their patients' tumors or treatment regimens to better monitor and treat for these effects. In addition, research efforts directed towards developing strategies to prevent cardiovascular complications resulting from radiation therapy have the potential to substantially enhance the quality and quantity of life of cancer patients and cancer survivors.

References

1. Khakoo AY, Yeh ETH (2008) Therapy insight: management of cardiovascular disease in patients with cancer and cardiac complications of cancer therapy. Nat Clin Pract Oncol 5: 655–667
2. Yeh ETH (2006) Cardiotoxicity induced by chemotherapy and antibody therapy. Annu Rev Med 57:485–498
3. Yeh ETH, Tong AT, Lenihan DJ et al (2004) Cardiovascular complications of cancer therapy: diagnosis, pathogenesis, and management. Circulation 109:3122–3131
4. Grebenc ML, de Christenson ML Rosado, Burke AP, Green CE, Galvin JR (2000) Radiographics 20:1073–1103
5. Casey M, Vaughan CJ, He J et al (2000) Mutations in the protein kinase A R1alpha regulatory subunit cause familial cardiac myxomas and Carney complex. J Clin Invest 106: R31–R38
6. Reynen K (1995) Cardiac myxomas. N Engl J Med 333: 1610–1617
7. Mendoza CE, Rosado MF, Pacheco P (2001) Interleukin-6 production and recurrent cardiac myxoma. J Thorac Cardiovasc Surg 121:395–396
8. Bhan A, Mehrotra R, Choudhary SK et al (1998) Surgical experience with intracardiac myxomas: long-term follow-up. Ann Thorac Surg 66:810–813
9. Keeling IM, Oberwalder P, Anelli-Monti M et al (2002) Cardiac myxomas: 24 years of experience in 49 patients. Eur J Cardiothorac Surg 22:971–977
10. Jourdan M, Bataille R, Seguin J, Zhang XG, Chaptal PA, Klein B (1990) Constitutive production of interleukin-6 and immunologic features in cardiac myxomas. Arthritis Rheum 33:398–402

11. Saji T, Yanagawa E, Matsuura H et al (1991) Increased serum interleukin-6 in cardiac myxoma. Am Heart J 122: 579–580
12. Seino Y, Ikeda U, Shimada K (1993) Increased expression of interleukin 6 mRNA in cardiac myxomas. Br Heart J 69: 565–567
13. Yokomuro H, Yoshihara K, Watanabe Y, Shiono N, Koyama N, Takanashi Y (2007) The variations in the immunologic features and interleukin-6 levels for the surgical treatment of cardiac myxomas. Surg Today 37:750–753
14. Mendoza CE, Rosado MF, Bernal L (2001) The role of interleukin-6 in cases of cardiac myxoma. Clinical features, immunologic abnormalities, and a possible role in recurrence. Tex Heart Inst J 28:3–7
15. Munhoz Da Fontoura Tavares C, Araújo De Oliveira N, Miguel R, Atié J (2004) Recurrent ventricular fibrillation secondary to aortic valve tumor. Heart Rhythm 1:348–351
16. Gowda RM, Khan IA, Nair CK, Mehta NJ, Vasavada BC, Sacchi TJ (2003) Cardiac papillary fibroelastoma: a comprehensive analysis of 725 cases. Am Heart J 146:404–410
17. Khair T, Mazidi P, Laos LF (2010) Cardiac papillary fibroelastoma: case report and review of the literature. Int J Cardiol 139(1):102–104, Epub 2008 Aug 20
18. Kuwashiro T, Toyoda K, Otsubo R, Ishibashi-Ueda H, Tagusari O, Minematsu K (2009) Cardiac papillary fibroelastoma as a cause of embolic stroke: ultrasound and histopathological characteristics. Intern Med 48:77–80
19. Dereddy NR, Sett SS, Krishnan U (2008) Resection of ventricular rhabdomyomas in infants presenting with cardiac failure. Cardiol Young 18:635–637
20. D'Addario V, Pinto V, Di Naro E, Del Bianco A, Di Cagno L, Volpe P (2002) Prenatal diagnosis and postnatal outcome of cardiac rhabdomyomas. J Perinat Med 30:170–175
21. Farooki ZQ, Ross RD, Paridon SM, Humes RA, Karpawich PP, Pinsky WW (1991) Spontaneous regression of cardiac rhabdomyoma. Am J Cardiol 67:897
22. Krapp M, Baschat AA, Gembruch U, Gloeckner K, Schwinger E, Reusche E (1999) Tuberous sclerosis with intracardiac rhabdomyoma in a fetus with trisomy 21: case report and review of literature. Prenat Diagn 19:610–613
23. Kojima S, Sumiyoshi M, Suwa S et al (2003) Cardiac hemangioma: a report of two cases and review of the literature. Heart Vessels 18:153–156
24. Chiappini B, Gregorini R, Vecchio L et al (2009) Cardiac hemangioma of the left atrial appendag: a case report and discussion. J Card Surg 24:522–523
25. Antoniades L, Eftychiou C, Petrou PM, Bagatzounis A, Minas M (2009) Primary cardiac lymphoma: case report and brief review of the literature. Echocardiography 26: 214–219
26. Bagwan IN, Desai S, Wotherspoon A, Sheppard MN (2009) Unusual presentation of primary cardiac lymphoma. Interact Cardiovasc Thorac Surg 9:127–129
27. Piccioli A, Falanga A, Baccaglini U, Marchetti M, Prandoni P (2006) Cancer and venous thromboembolism. Semin Thromb Hemost 32:694–699
28. Lee A (2008) VTE in patients with cancer – diagnosis, prevention, and treatment. Thromb Res 123(Suppl 1):S50–S54
29. Kessler CM (2009) The link between cancer and venous thromboembolism: a review. Am J Clin Oncol 32:S3–S7
30. Lee AY, Levine MN (2003) Venous thromboembolism and cancer: risks and outcomes. Circulation 107:I17–I21
31. Deitcher SR (2003) Cancer-related deep venous thrombosis: clinical importance, treatment challenges, and management strategies. Semin Thromb Hemost 29:247–258
32. Gomes MP, Deitcher SR (2003) Diagnosis of venous thromboembolic disease in cancer patients. Oncology (Williston Park) 17:126–135, 139, discussion 39–44
33. Sohne M, Kruip MJ, Nijkeuter M et al (2006) Accuracy of clinical decision rule, D-dimer and spiral computed tomography in patients with malignancy, previous venous thromboembolism, COPD or heart failure and in older patients with suspected pulmonary embolism. J Thromb Haemost 4:1042–1046
34. Calvo-Romero JM, Perez-Miranda M, Bureo-Dacal P (2004) Syncope in acute pulmonary embolism. Eur J Emerg Med 11:208–209
35. Ullman E, Brady WJ, Perron AD, Chan T, Mattu A (2001) Electrocardiographic manifestations of pulmonary embolism. Am J Emerg Med 19:514–519
36. Sohne M, Ten Wolde M, Buller HR (2004) Biomarkers in pulmonary embolism. Curr Opin Cardiol 19:558–562
37. Agnelli G, Verso M (2006) Therapy insight: venous-catheter-related thrombosis in cancer patients. Nat Clin Pract Oncol 3:214–222
38. Knovich MA, Lesser GJ (2004) The management of thromboembolic disease in patients with central nervous system malignancies. Curr Treat Options Oncol 5:511–517
39. Hutten BA, Prins MH, Gent M, Ginsberg J, Tijssen JG, Buller HR (2000) Incidence of recurrent thromboembolic and bleeding complications among patients with venous thromboembolism in relation to both malignancy and achieved international normalized ratio: a retrospective analysis. J Clin Oncol 18:3078–3083
40. Lee AYY (2005) Management of thrombosis in cancer: primary prevention and secondary prophylaxis. Br J Haematol 128:291–302
41. Prandoni P (2005) How I treat venous thromboembolism in patients with cancer. Blood 106:4027–4033
42. Geerts WH, Pineo GF, Heit JA et al (2004) Prevention of venous thromboembolism: the Seventh ACCP Conference on Antithrombotic and Thrombolytic Therapy. Chest 126: 338S–400S
43. Thomason R, Schlegel W, Lucca M, Cummings S, Lee S (1994) Primary malignant mesothelioma of the pericardium. Case report and literature review. Tex Heart Inst J 21:170
44. Santos C, Montesinos J, Castañer E, Sole JM, Baga R (2008) Primary pericardial mesothelioma. Lung Cancer 60:291–293
45. Watanabe A, Sakata J, Kawamura H, Yamada O, Matsuyama T (2000) Primary pericardial mesothelioma presenting as constrictive pericarditis: a case report. Jpn Circ J 64: 385–388
46. Press OW, Livingston R (1987) Management of malignant pericardial effusion and tamponade. JAMA 257:1088–1092
47. Thomas CR, Edmondson EA (1991) Common emergencies in cancer medicine: cardiovascular and neurologic syndromes. J Natl Med Assoc 83:1001–1017
48. Crawford MH (2002) Current diagnosis and treatment in cardiology: diagnosis and treatment in cardiology. McGraw-Hill/Appleton & Lange, New York

49. Burstow DJ, Oh JK, Bailey KR, Seward JB, Tajik AJ (1989) Cardiac tamponade: characteristic Doppler observations. Mayo Clin Proc 64:312–324
50. Kronzon I, Glassman LR, Tunick PA (2003) Avoiding the left internal mammary artery during anterior pericardiocentesis. Echocardiography 20:533–534
51. Klein SV, Afridi H, Agarwal D, Coughlin BF, Schielke LH (2005) CT directed diagnostic and therapeutic pericardiocentesis: 8-year experience at a single institution. Emerg Radiol 11:353–363
52. Tsang TS, Oh JK, Seward JB (1999) Diagnosis and management of cardiac tamponade in the era of echocardiography. Clin Cardiol 22:446–452
53. Maher EA, Shepherd FA, Todd TJ (1996) Pericardial sclerosis as the primary management of malignant pericardial effusion and cardiac tamponade. J Thorac Cardiovasc Surg 112:637–643
54. Martinoni A, Cipolla CM, Cardinale D et al (2004) Long-term results of intrapericardial chemotherapeutic treatment of malignant pericardial effusions with thiotepa. Chest 126:1412–1416
55. Piehler JM, Pluth JR, Schaff HV, Danielson GK, Orszulak TA, Puga FJ (1985) Surgical management of effusive pericardial disease. Influence of extent of pericardial resection on clinical course. J Thorac Cardiovasc Surg 90:506–516
56. Gregory JR, McMurtrey MJ, Mountain CF (1985) A surgical approach to the treatment of pericardial effusion in cancer patients. Am J Clin Oncol 8:319–323
57. Heidenreich PA, Kapoor JR (2009) Radiation induced heart disease: systemic disorders in heart disease. Heart 95: 252–258
58. Lund MB, Ihlen H, Voss BM et al (1996) Increased risk of heart valve regurgitation after mediastinal radiation for Hodgkin's disease: an echocardiographic study. Heart 75:591–595
59. Gayed I, Gohar S, Liao Z, McAleer M, Bassett R, Yusuf SW (2009) The clinical implications of myocardial perfusion abnormalities in patients with esophageal or lung cancer after chemoradiation therapy. Int J Cardiovasc Imaging 25:487–495
60. Miller KD, Triano LR (2008) Medical issues in cancer survivors – a review. Cancer J 14:375–387
61. Schneider JS, Edwards JE (1979) Irradiation-induced pericarditis. Chest 75:560
62. Hull MC, Morris CG, Pepine CJ, Mendenhall NP (2003) Valvular dysfunction and carotid, subclavian, and coronary artery disease in survivors of hodgkin lymphoma treated with radiation therapy. JAMA 290:2831–2837
63. Wethal T, Lund M-B, Edvardsen T et al (2009) Valvular dysfunction and left ventricular changes in Hodgkin's lymphoma survivors. A longitudinal study. Br J Cancer 101: 575–581
64. Glanzmann C, Kaufmann P, Jenni R, Hess OM, Huguenin P (1998) Cardiac risk after mediastinal irradiation for Hodgkin's disease. Radiother Oncol 46:51–62
65. Carlson RG, Mayfield WR, Normann S, Alexander JA (1991) Radiation-associated valvular disease. Chest 99:538
66. Paszat LF, Mackillop WJ, Groome PA, Boyd C, Schulze K, Holowaty E (1998) Mortality from myocardial infarction after adjuvant radiotherapy for breast cancer in the surveillance, epidemiology, and end-results cancer registries. J Clin Oncol 16:2625–2631
67. Patt DA, Goodwin JS, Kuo Y-F et al (2005) Cardiac morbidity of adjuvant radiotherapy for breast cancer. J Clin Oncol 23:7475–7482
68. Vallis KA, Pintilie M, Chong N et al (2002) Assessment of coronary heart disease morbidity and mortality after radiation therapy for early breast cancer. J Clin Oncol 20:1036–1042
69. Pistevou-Gompaki K, Hatzitolios A, Eleftheriadis N et al (2008) Evaluation of cardiotoxicity five years after 2D planned, non-simulated, radiation therapy for left breast cancer. Ther Clin Risk Manag 4:1359–1362
70. Utehina O, Popovs S, Purina D et al (2009) Analysis of cardiac and pulmonary complication probabilites after radiation therapy for patients with early-stage breast cancer. Medicina (Kaunas) 45:276–285
71. Gayed IW, Liu HH, Yusuf SW et al (2006) The prevalence of myocardial ischemia after concurrent chemoradiation therapy as detected by gated myocardial perfusion imaging in patients with esophageal cancer. J Nucl Med 47:1756–1762
72. Moser EC, Noordijk EM, van Leeuwen FE et al (2006) Long-term risk of cardiovascular disease after treatment for aggressive non-Hodgkin lymphoma. Blood 107:2912–2919
73. Reinders JG, Heijmen BJ, Olofsen-van Acht MJ, van Putten WL, Levendag PC (1999) Ischemic heart disease after mantlefield irradiation for Hodgkin's disease in long-term follow-up. Radiother Oncol 51:35–42
74. Cavendish JJ, Berman BJ, Schnyder G et al (2004) Concomitant coronary and multiple arch vessel stenoses in patients treated with external beam radiation: pathophysiological basis and endovascular treatment. Catheter Cardiovasc Interv 62:385–390
75. Elerding SC, Fernandez RN, Grotta JC, Lindberg RD, Causay LC, McMurtrey MJ (1981) Carotid artery disease following external cervical irradiation. Ann Surg 194:609–615
76. Haynes JC, Machtay M, Weber RS, Weinstein GS, Chalian AA, Rosenthal DI (2002) Relative risk of stroke in head and neck carcinoma patients treated with external cervical irradiation. Laryngoscope 112(10):1883–1887
77. Harrod-Kim P, Kadkhodayan Y, Derdeyn CP, Cross DT, Moran CJ (2005) Outcomes of carotid angioplasty and stenting for radiation-associated stenosis. AJNR Am J Neuroradiol 26:1781–1788
78. Halak M, Fajer S, Ben-Meir H, Loberman Z, Weller B, Karmeli R (2002) Neck irradiation: a risk factor for occlusive carotid artery disease. Eur J Vasc Endovasc Surg 23:299–302
79. Farrugia M, Gowda KMS, Cheatle TR, Ashok TP (2006) Radiotherapy-related axillary artery occlusive disease: percutaneous transluminal angioplasty and stenting. Two case reports and review of the literature. Cardiovasc Interv Radiol 29:1144–1147
80. Timmers HJLM, Wieling W, Karemaker JM, Lenders JWM (2004) Baroreflex failure: a neglected type of secondary hypertension. Neth J Med 62:151–155
81. Timmers HJLM, Karemaker JM, Wieling W et al (2002) Arterial baroreflex and peripheral chemoreflex function after

radiotherapy for laryngeal or pharyngeal cancer. Int J Radiat Oncol Biol Phys 53:1203–1210
82. Timmers HJLM, Wieling W, Karemaker JM, Lenders JWM (2004) Cardiovascular responses to stress after carotid baroreceptor denervation in humans. Ann NY Acad Sci 1018:515–519
83. Hutchinson CD, Jardine DL, Hurrell M (2008) Vagolysis. Age Ageing 37:602–604
84. Park JW, Kim JH, Kim B-S, Park HK, Lee K, Park J-I (2007) Selective baroreflex failure complicated by unilateral neck irradiation. Int J Cardiol 115(1):117–119, The Netherlands
85. Sharabi Y, Dendi R, Holmes C, Goldstein DS (2003) Baroreflex failure as a late sequela of neck irradiation. Hypertension 42:110–116

Diffuse Alveolar Hemorrhage in Hematopoietic Stem Cell Transplant Recipients and Patients with Hematologic Malignancy

33

Bekele Afessa

Contents

B. Afessa
Division of Pulmonary and Critical Care Medicine, Mayo Clinic College of Medicine, 200 First St SW, Rochester, MN 55905, USA
e-mail: afessa.bekele@mayo.edu

33.1 Introduction

There are three major types of hematologic malignancies: leukemia, lymphoma, and plasma cell neoplasms [1]. More than 100,000 cases of hematologic malignancies were diagnosed in the United States in 2005, and over 53,000 people died from these cancers that same year [2]. Approximately 230,000 patients were estimated to have newly diagnosed hematologic malignancy in Europe in 2005 [1]. Blood and marrow transplantation (BMT) is used for the treatment of hematologic and solid tumors as well as various benign diseases worldwide. The Center for International Blood and Marrow Transplant Research (CIBMTR) reported 50,000–60,000 transplants to be performed annually worldwide [3, 4]. Among the 55,000 BMTs performed in 2006, 19,000 were allogeneic and 36,000 autologous.

Alveolar hemorrhage can be caused by infectious or noninfectious etiologies. It may involve the lungs diffusely or focally. In this chapter, we will focus on diffuse alveolar hemorrhage (DAH) of noninfectious etiology in patients with hematologic malignancy or BMT.

33.2 Diagnostic Criteria

DAH is a syndrome with nonspecific clinical and radiological features. Although pulmonary infections, cardiac insufficiency, thrombocytopenia, and coagulopathy may be associated with alveolar hemorrhage, we use the term DAH in this chapter to describe diffuse alveolar hemorrhage of noninfectious etiology, not related to cardiac pulmonary edema, and not

É. Azoulay (ed.), *Pulmonary Involvement in Patients with Hematological Malignancies*,
DOI: 10.1007/978-3-642-15742-4_33, © Springer-Verlag Berlin Heidelberg 2011

directly caused by thrombocytopenia or coagulopathy. The diagnostic criteria of DAH are [5–8]:

1. Evidence of widespread alveolar injury manifested by multilobar pulmonary infiltrates, symptoms and signs of pneumonia, and abnormal pulmonary physiology with increased alveolar to arterial oxygen gradient
2. Absence of infection compatible with the diagnosis
3. Bronchoalveolar lavage (BAL) showing progressively bloodier return from three separate subsegmental bronchi or the presence of ≥20% hemosiderin-laden macrophages or the presence of blood in at least 30% of the alveolar surfaces of lung tissue [7]

33.3 DAH in Patients with Hematologic Malignancy

As a result of their underlying diseases or the treatment, patients with hematologic malignancy are at risk for thrombocytopenia and angio-invasive fungal infections. Thrombocytopenia, coagulopathy, and angio-invasive fungal infections can lead to bleeding from any organ, including the lungs [9]. The incidence, clinical course, treatment, and prognosis of DAH in non-BMT recipients with hematologic malignancy have not been well described. In an autopsy study of patients with hematologic malignancy, DAH was reported in 23% of those with BMT compared to 5% without BMT [6].

Autopsy studies have shown pulmonary hemorrhage, mostly caused by infection, to be present in up to 74% of adult patients with leukemia [10]. In an autopsy study of 17 patients with adult T-cell leukemia, pulmonary hemorrhage was detected in 5 (29.4%) [11]. Although pulmonary hemorrhage had been known to be responsible for morbidity and mortality in patients with leukemia, it was rarely diagnosed during life. In 1975, Golde and colleagues reported five patients with pulmonary hemorrhage diagnosed by examining BAL fluid [12]. In a study of 98 patients with acute monocytic leukemia, 20 were admitted to the intensive care unit (ICU) for respiratory failure; 16 of these 20 had BAL, 7 of whom had hemorrhage [13]. Most of the publications addressing DAH in non-BMT patients with hematologic malignancy are limited to case reports [14–17]. Patients with hematologic malignancy and pulmonary hemorrhage are likely to have thrombocytopenia. However, platelet deficiency alone does not provide the entire explanation, since most patients with thrombocytopenia never experience pulmonary hemorrhage. Rituximab [18], all-trans retinoic acid [19, 20], and other chemotherapy agents [14, 21, 22] used to treat hematologic malignancies have been associated with DAH.

The pathogenesis of DAH in patients with hematologic malignancy has not been well studied. In a study of three patients with leukemia who died of massive pulmonary hemorrhage, the major finding at autopsy included diffuse alveolar damage with severe destruction of alveolar walls [23]. In a rat model of leukemia, accumulation of leukemic cells in capillaries increased simultaneously with the increase in the peripheral blood [24]. This was accompanied by increasing tachypnea, followed by aggregates consisting almost solely of leukemic cells in medium-sized blood vessels and then by complete obstruction of the lung vasculature, including the large arteries and veins, giving rise to extensive hemorrhages and edema. The histological and ultrastructural findings in this study suggest that beside the size and stiffness of individual leukemic cells, interactions not only between leukemic cells, but also between leukemic cells and the endothelium play a role in the pathogenesis of pulmonary leukostasis and DAH [24]. Alterations of cell adhesion associated with chemotherapy-induced blast lysis or cellular differentiation may also be contributing to DAH in hematologic malignancy [14].

The clinical presentation and radiologic findings in patients with hematologic malignancy do not differ from those described below for BMT recipients [25, 26]. BAL is often diagnostic by documenting the presence of alveolar hemorrhage and excluding infection [12].

Although correcting severe thrombocytopenia and coagulopathy is logical, there are no good studies to guide the treatment of DAH in patients with hematologic malignancy. Corticosteroids have been used to treat DAH in patients with leukemia [17]. Treatment with Sivelestat, a small molecule inhibitor of neutrophil elastase, has been reported to achieve rapid improvement in oxygenation and chest radiograph findings in a patient with DAH associated with all-trans retinoic acid [20].

33.4 DAH in BMT Recipients

33.4.1 Incidence

The frequency of DAH has varied among reported series because of differences in patient mix, diagnostic approaches, and diagnostic criteria [5]. The factors that influence the incidence of DAH have changed over time and varied among BMT centers. Although bronchoscopy and surgical lung biopsy have been used for decades, their application in BMT recipients with pulmonary infiltrates has not been well standardized. Since underlying conditions may prohibit invasive procedures, some clinicians prefer to initiate empiric antibiotics for suspected infection leading to underdiagnosis of DAH. Moreover, although BAL is widely used for the diagnosis of DAH, the diagnostic criteria have elements of subjectivity and are not uniformly applied.

Table 33.1 Frequency of DAH in BMT recipients

Reference number	Year	Total patients, *N*	Patients with DAH, *N* (%)
[30]	1986	130	2 (1.5)
[8]	1989	141	29 (20.6)
[44]	1991	288	39 (13.5)
[39]	1991	100	1 (1)
[67]	1991	77	4 (5.2)
[43]	1992	123	14 (11.4)
[42]	1992	178	2 (1.1)
[35]	1992	77	10 (13.0)
[38]	1994	603	65 (10.8)
[22]	1995	84	5 (6.0)
[47]	1998	1,380	29 (2.1)
[27]	1998	20	1 (5.0)
[41]	1999	74	4 (5.4)
[34]	1999	37	1 (2.7)
[36]	2000	990	28 (2.8)
[29]	2000	186	11 (5.9)
[32]	2001	339	24 (7.1)
[31]	2001	34	2 (5.9)
[45]	2002	1,215	48 (4.0)
[28]	2003	138	6 (4.4)
[37]	2006	1,919	45 (2.3)
[33]	2006	369	3 (0.8)
Total		8,502	373 (4.4)

BMT blood and marrow transplant, *DAH* diffuse alveolar hemorrhage

In 22 studies that included 8,502 BMT recipients, 373 cases of DAH were reported, for an overall frequency of 4.4%, with a range between 1% and 21% (Table 33.1) [8, 22, 27–45]. The reported frequency of DAH varies from 1% to 21% in autologous, and from 1% to 17% in allogeneic BMT recipients. DAH has been reported in 128 (4.0%) of 3,183 autologous [8, 29, 32, 35–39, 42, 46–48] compared to 139 (3.9%) of 3,607 allogeneic (28–34, 36–38, 41, 47) BMT recipients, with no statistically significant difference. The recent increase in the incidence of DAH has not been associated with the use of granulocyte colony-stimulating factor and peripheral blood stem cell source [36]. Limited DAH data are available in T-cell depleted allogeneic BMT recipients. In one study, 3 of 369 T-cell-depleted allogeneic BMT recipients (0.8%) developed DAH [33].

Among 1,261 BMT recipients who underwent bronchoscopy, DAH was reported in 161 (12.8%), with a range between 2% and 37% [45, 49–55]. In patients admitted to the intensive care unit for respiratory failure, the prevalence of DAH may exceed 40% [56, 57]. DAH has been reported in 23% (range 14–41%) of autopsies [6, 58–60].

33.4.2 Risk Factors

Several factors have been reported to predispose BMT recipients to DAH [5] (Table 33.2). Pre-transplant intensive chemotherapy, myeloablative conditioning regimen, total body irradiation, thoracic irradiation, and old age are associated with increased rates of DAH [8, 22, 35, 37, 39, 41, 60]. Despite few studies showing that solid tumors and breast cancer may be associated with the development of DAH in BMT recipients [8, 61], a review of several studies has not found such an association [5]. Although DAH occurs in both autologous and allogeneic BMT recipients, the initial studies included predominantly autologous recipients [8]. In data compiled from several studies, no significant difference was found in the incidence of DAH between

Table 33.2 Risk factors for DAH in BMT recipients

Pre-transplant
Age above 40 years
Indications for BMT
Thoracic radiation
Intensive chemotherapy
The presence of inflammatory cells in bronchial and BAL fluid
Peri-transplant
Conditioning regimen
Total body irradiation
Second transplants
Post-transplant
Fever
Mucositis
Leukocyte recovery
Elevated blood urea nitrogen
Elevated creatinine
Graft-versus-host disease

BAL bronchoalveolar lavage, *BMT* blood and marrow transplant, *DAH* diffuse alveolar hemorrhage

autologous and allogeneic BMT recipients: 123 of the 2,616 autologous recipients (5%) had DAH compared to 91 of the 1,748 allogeneic recipients (5%) [5]. In a more recent study, 38 of 1,318 allogeneic BMT recipients (2.9%) developed DAH compared to 7 of the 601 autologous recipients (1.2%), with no statistically significant difference [37].

Pre-transplant pulmonary function tests have shown that there is no association between the development of DAH and forced vital capacity (FVC), forced expiratory volume in 1 s (FEV1), total lung capacity (TLC), or diffusing capacity for carbon monoxide (DLCO) [8]. Pre-transplant bronchoscopy has shown a higher number of bronchial neutrophils and eosinophils in patients who develop DAH following BMT compared to those who do not develop DAH [43]. In the study by Sisson et al. in Hodgkin's disease patients, the pre-transplant presence of bronchial neutrophils >20% and eosinophils >0% was associated with the development of DAH [43]. White blood cell recovery and renal insufficiency, but not prolonged prothrombin or partial thromboplastin time or low platelets, are associated with the development of DAH [8, 35]. Although most patients with DAH have thrombocytopenia, the DAH is not corrected with platelet transfusion only [8].

33.4.3 Pathogenesis

Various conditions, including mitral valve disease, systemic vasculitides, collagen vascular diseases, drugs, anticoagulation, cocaine inhalation, and infections, have been implicated as causing alveolar hemorrhage in non-BMT recipients [5]. These conditions are associated with injury to the pulmonary arterioles, venules, and capillaries, disrupting the alveolar-capillary basement membrane. Penicillamine, abciximab, propythiouracil, amiodarone, nitrofurantoin, and cytotoxic medications are among drugs associated with alveolar hemorrhage. Drug-induced alveolar hemorrhage usually results from direct toxic effects, and indirect inflammatory or immunologic processes. Despite the recognition of the risk factors, the etiology and pathogenesis of DAH in the BMT recipient have not been clearly established. Lung tissue injury, inflammation, and cytokine release are implicated in the pathogenesis of both idiopathic pneumonia syndrome (IPS) and DAH. In a murine model of BMT, the critical early proinflammatory events associated with IPS have been found to be due to donor T cells [62].

33.4.3.1 Lung Injury

Pre-transplant high-dose chemotherapy, thoracic radiation, total body irradiation, and undocumented infections may be responsible for the initial injury to lung tissue leading to DAH in the BMT recipient. Vascular abnormalities, in the form of endothelial swelling and thrombi, are found in the autopsies of BMT recipients with acute hemorrhagic pulmonary edema [63]. The incidence of pulmonary hemorrhage is high in BMT recipients with graft-versus-host disease [37, 60]. In addition to the toxicity from therapy for graft-versus-host disease, antigen-specific injury to the endothelium may be a contributing factor to the development of DAH [64]. Mice receiving bone marrow cells with T lymphocytes have been shown to develop alveolitis, characterized by alveolar hemorrhage, increased alveolar leukocytes, platelet microthrombi, and damage to endothelial and epithelial cells during the acute phase of the graft-versus-host reaction [65].

Vasculopathy of small muscular arteries and thrombotic microangiopathy have been reported in BMT recipients with DAH [66]. The vasculopathy of small muscular arteries manifests as concentric intimal or medial hyperplasia with luminal narrowing, prominent myxoid change, extravasated red blood cells, and the presence of some foamy histiocytes with no evidence of thrombotic microangiopathy. Thrombotic microangiopathy has also been associated with DAH in the BMT recipient [66]. It is characterized by the presence of fragmented erythrocytes on peripheral smears, decreased hemoglobin and platelet count, refractoriness to platelet transfusions, and the absence of disseminated intravascular coagulation [66].

The use of dimethyl sulfoxide for cryopreservation of blood stem cells has been implicated in causing damage to the alveolar endothelial lining, thus leading to the development of DAH [67, 68].

33.4.3.2 Inflammation

Inflammatory cells are likely to play a role in the development of DAH. Animal studies have shown that alveolitis develops during the acute phase of the graft-versus-host reaction. This alveolitis is characterized by alveolar hemorrhage, increase in the alveolar leukocytes, platelet microthrombi, damage of alveolar endothelial and epithelial cells, increased turnover rate of alveolar cells, and increase in cell number and protein content of BAL fluid [65, 68]. Pre-transplant bronchoscopy has shown increased bronchial inflammatory cells in patients who develop DAH following BMT, suggesting that bronchial inflammation precedes alveolar inflammation [43, 68, 69]. The initial injury is compounded by damage related to the return of inflammatory cells to the lung coincident with marrow recovery [38]. Even in the presence of peripheral blood leukopenia, neutrophils and neutrophil products are seen in the lower respiratory tract of BMT recipients at the time of DAH [8, 38, 70, 71]. Hematopoietic growth factors, such as granulocyte colony-stimulating factor, may also play a role in worsening of the alveolar damage and capillary leakage by increasing neutrophil infiltration into the lungs [39, 72]. One study of 19 autologous BMT recipients has shown that about one-third of autologous BMT recipients with peri-engraftment respiratory distress syndrome have DAH [70]. Among the patients with peri-engraftment respiratory distress syndrome, those with DAH have higher absolute neutrophil counts than those without DAH [70].

33.4.3.3 Cytokine Release

Cytokine release may mediate the development of DAH. It is speculated that damage to alveolar capillary endothelial membranes begins during preparative chemotherapy or total body irradiation and results in release of inflammatory mediators [71]. In allogeneic transplants, donor T cells react to host alloantigens, become activated, proliferate, and secrete inflammatory mediators. This response may be amplified after the release of endotoxin into the circulation from the gut following injury from mucositis or graft-versus-host disease. It is suggested that the pathophysiology of acute graft-versus-host disease is a cytokine storm in which inflammatory cytokines mediate the response [73]. In autologous BMT recipients, the generation of cytokines is self-limited and resolves in 7–10 days [73]. Despite the more profound release of cytokines in allogeneic BMT recipients, the frequency of DAH is similar between allogeneic and autologous groups. This may be due to the immunosuppressive agents used for prophylaxis of graft-versus-host disease in the allogeneic group. The interleukin-12 level at the time of leukocyte recovery, tumor necrosis factor-α, and lipopolysaccharides have been associated with DAH in BMT recipients [65, 74].

33.4.4 Clinical Findings and Course

In the non-transplant patient population, the classic presentation of DAH consists of hemoptysis and dyspnea in the setting of iron deficiency anemia and a chest radiograph showing bilateral airspace consolidation with apical sparing. However, these features are variable and may be absent. In the BMT recipient, DAH is characterized by progressive dyspnea, hypoxia, cough, diffuse consolidation on chest radiograph, and characteristic BAL fluid findings developing within 1–7 days [5, 8]. DAH should be distinguished from localized pulmonary hemorrhage with diffuse aspiration of blood due to chronic bronchitis, bronchiectasis, tumors, or infections. BMT recipients with DAH often have dyspnea and dry cough [8, 45]. Although coexistent sepsis and mucositis may obscure the clinical picture, fever is a common finding [8, 35, 37, 41, 45, 67, 68]. Hemoptysis is uncommon [35, 45, 68]. None of the 29 BMT recipients with DAH had hemoptysis in the study by Robbins et al. [8]. Compared to patients without DAH, those with DAH have more severe mucositis [8].

The onset of DAH is usually within the first 30 (median 11–24) days following BMT [8, 35–37, 41, 45, 67]. However, reports of DAH with onset after the first month of transplant are not uncommon [37, 45, 60].

33.4.5 Laboratory and Radiographic Findings

BMT recipients with DAH are too ill to undergo pulmonary function testing. Arterial blood gas studies show hypoxemia [5]. BAL fluid shows a median leukocyte count of 130/μL and median red blood cell count 48,375/μL [36].

In BMT recipients with DAH, chest radiograph shows diffuse interstitial and alveolar infiltrates, primarily central, and involving predominantly the lower and middle lung zones [44]. The earliest radiographic manifestation is the presence of bilateral fine reticular opacities. Radiographic abnormalities present at a mean of 11 days after transplant (range 0–24) and 3 days before clinical diagnosis of DAH [44]. The radiographic findings deteriorate in the first 6 days. In a study of 39 BMT recipients with DAH, initial chest x-ray showed bilateral abnormality in 27, unilateral in 10, and normal in 2; interstitial in 27 and alveolar in 10 [44]. In the later phase of DAH, 70% of the patients develop an alveolar pattern, and the interstitial pattern persists in 30%. Pleural effusion is seen in 14% and cardiomegaly in 19%. Although computed tomography (CT) of the chest may be helpful in patients in whom a focal abnormality is suspected, CT and magnetic resonance imaging have a limited role in DAH. The most common CT finding is bilateral areas of ground-glass attenuation or consolidation [75].

BAL is the most commonly used diagnostic tool for confirming DAH [5]. The diagnosis of alveolar hemorrhage is made by progressively bloodier BAL return when hemorrhage is recent or by an increased number of hemosiderin-laden macrophages using Prussian blue staining (Fig. 33.1) [5, 7, 45]. The BAL appearance and the iron stain complement each other [45]. BAL may be progressively bloodier in early DAH, when hemosiderin-laden macrophages are absent. Iron staining adds an element of objectivity to the criteria used in the diagnosis of DAH. However, both false-positive and false-negative BAL have been reported [6, 53]. Because blood in the distal airways may give progressively bloodier BAL return regardless of the source, the appearance of BAL return is not reliable for the diagnosis of DAH. The mere presence of hemosiderin-laden macrophages is insufficient to diagnose DAH since normal individuals, particularly those who smoke cigarettes, may have hemosiderin-laden macrophages [76]. Following acute pulmonary hemorrhage, it may take 48–72 h for hemosiderin-laden macrophages to appear in respiratory secretions and 2–4 weeks for the hemosiderin-laden macrophages to clear from the lungs and airways [77]. Because of the delay in the appearance of hemosiderin-laden macrophages in BAL fluid and hemosiderin clearance after a few days, the absence of hemosiderin in alveolar macrophages does not exclude the possibility of recent (less than 48 h) or remote (greater than 12 days) alveolar bleeding [78]. To avoid BAL false-positive results, Golde et al. introduced ranking scores, the Golde score, based on the hemosiderin content of macrophages [12]. The Golde score

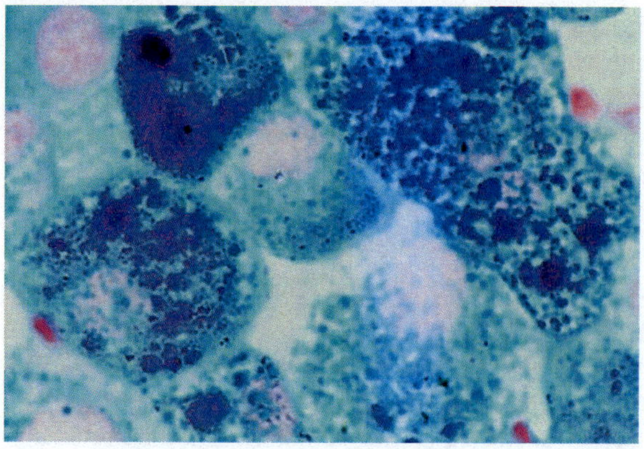

Fig. 33.1 Hemosiderin-laden macrophages in bronchoalveolar lavage fluid of a patient with diffuse alveolar hemorrhage (*Prussian blue stain*)

measures the hemosiderin content of pulmonary macrophages: 200–300 macrophages of BAL fluid are counted, each cell is graded for hemosiderin on a scale of 0–4, and a mean score for 100 cells is calculated. BAL hemosiderin-laden macrophages ≥20% correlate well with and are easier to measure than the Golde score for the diagnosis of alveolar hemorrhage [5, 7]. Early BAL is essential to exclude other pulmonary complications. Since hemosiderin-laden macrophages may not be present in BAL fluid early following acute alveolar hemorrhage, repeat bronchoscopy may be needed within 2–5 days of the first procedure [36]. Transbronchial lung biopsy is often contraindicated because of the bleeding risk due to coexisting thrombocytopenia. Lung tissues in DAH show histologic features consistent with diffuse alveolar damage [6, 8, 43, 45, 58, 59]. DAH at autopsy is defined by the presence of blood in at least 30% of the evaluated alveolar surfaces [6].

33.4.6 Differential Diagnosis

There are overlaps in the diagnostic criteria used to define DAH, idiopathic pneumonia syndrome (IPS), and peri-engraftment respiratory distress syndrome in BMT recipients [5, 70, 79]. DAH is a distinct subset of IPS. IPS is a heterogeneous entity characterized by evidence of widespread alveolar injury and absence of lower respiratory tract infection [79]. Despite similarities in the pathogenesis of DAH and IPS, DAH has its own peculiar characteristics.

IPS is characterized by diffuse interstitial pneumonitis and alveolitis leading to interstitial fibrosis. The early period following BMT is characterized by the presence of inflammatory cytokines whose net effect is to promote lymphocyte influx into lungs with minimal fibrosis [80]. During the later period, gradual changes in leukocyte influx and activation lead to dysregulated wound repair resulting from the shift in the balance of cytokines that promote fibrosis. DAH may be characterized by the prevalence of an antifibrotic cytokine milieu compared to a pro-fibrotic environment in IPS [5]. The onset of DAH mostly coincides with the stem cell engraftment period. The onset of IPS is not influenced by stem cell engraftment. Lung pathology in DAH is consistent with the proliferative phase of diffuse alveolar damage, without fibrosis. IPS is more common in allogeneic than autologous BMT recipients, whereas the incidence of DAH is similar between the two groups. The respiratory failure of most patients with DAH, unlike IPS, improves in response to corticosteroid therapy. More than 80% of the deaths in IPS are attributable to progressive respiratory failure compared to 15% in DAH [5].

Peri-engraftment respiratory distress syndrome is defined by the presence of fever, evidence of lung injury, absence of cardiac dysfunction, exclusion of infectious etiologies, and onset within 5 days of neutrophil engraftment [70]. It has been reported in both autologous and allogeneic BMT recipients. Despite the paucity of data, neutrophils are considered to play a major role in its development. One-third of BMT recipients with peri-engraftment respiratory distress syndrome also have DAH [70]. The absence of DAH in two-third of patients with peri-engraftment respiratory distress syndrome and the occurrence of DAH beyond the peri-engraftment period suggest differences between these two syndromes despite their overlap [5].

33.4.7 Treatment

Because the pathogenesis of DAH is considered to be an inflammatory response to various insults, and based on anecdotal experiences and retrospective studies, BMT recipients with DAH are treated with systemic corticosteroids [37, 38, 41, 45, 67, 71]. However, there are no prospective, randomized trials addressing the treatment of DAH in BMT recipients. In a retrospective study, Metcalf et al. compared three groups: those with no corticosteroids, daily methylprednisolone ≤30 mg, and daily methylprednisolone >30 mg [38]. The pretreatment arterial oxygen tension was lower in patients in the high-dose methylprednisolone group. However, the mortality rate was lower, and fewer patients required invasive mechanical ventilation in the high-dose methylprednisolone group. The methylprednisolone dose for the high-dose group was 125–250 mg every 6 h for the first 4–5 days and then tapered over 2–4 weeks. Low-dose methylprednisolone therapy was not better than no steroid therapy [38]. In another study of 15 BMT recipients with DAH treated with 250 mg–2 g/day of methylprednisolone, transient clinical improvement was seen in ten patients [36].

However, the overall mortality of 74% was not significantly different from previous reports of untreated patients. A more recent study showed no statistically significant difference in mortality between BMT recipients treated and not treated with corticosteroids for DAH [37]. Although many BMT recipients may subsequently die from other complications, the respiratory status of most patients with DAH improves in response to corticosteroid therapy [5]. The usually used corticosteroid is methylprednisolone at approximately 1 g daily in four divided doses for 5 days, followed by 1 mg/kg for 3 days, tapering off over 2–4 weeks [5].

Although immunosuppressive therapy, plasma exchange, and plasmapheresis have been tried to treat DAH in other patient populations, there is no evidence to justify their use in BMT recipients. There are case reports of allogeneic BMT recipients with DAH successfully treated with recombinant factor VIIa [81–83].

33.4.8 Prognosis

The overall mortality rate of DAH in BMT recipients is about 76%, ranging between 48% and 100% (Table 33.3) [8, 22, 28, 35–38, 43–45, 57]. Although the initial presentation of DAH in BMT recipients may be respiratory failure, the most common causes of death include multiple organ failure and sepsis [36, 38], in addition to respiratory failure [45].

The majority of BMT recipients with DAH require mechanical ventilator support for respiratory failure [32, 36, 37, 41, 43, 45, 57]. BMT recipients with DAH are at high risk for subsequent infectious complications [38]. Despite the high mortality rate, long-term survivors of BMT recipients with DAH may have normal respiratory function [36, 41]. However, one study had shown a more pronounced decline in FEV1 and FVC in BMT recipients who develop DAH compared to those who do not [8].

Table 33.3 Mortality rate of BMT recipients with DAH

Reference	Year	Patients, *N*	Dead, *N* (%)
[8]	1989	29	23 (79)
[44]	1991	39	30 (77)
[43]	1992	14	9 (64)
[35]	1992	10	10 (100)
[38]	1994	65	56 (86)
[22]	1995	5	4 (80)
[36]	2000	23	17 (74)
[57]	2000	26	21 (81)
[45]	2002	48	23 (48)
[28]	2003	6	5 (83)
[37]	2006	45	39 (87)
Total		310	237 (76)

BMT blood and marrow transplant, *DAH* diffuse alveolar hemorrhage

References

1. Rodriguez-Abreu D, Bordoni A, Zucca E (2007) Epidemiology of hematological malignancies. Ann Oncol 18(Suppl 1): i3–i8
2. US Cancer Statistics Working Group (2009). United States cancer statistics: 1999–2005 incidence and mortality web-based report. US department of health and human services, centers for disease control and prevention and national cancer institute. www.cdc.gov/uscs Accessed on 25 Nov 2010
3. Pasquini MC, Wang Z (2009) Current use and outcome of hematopoietic stem cell transplantation: part I – *CIBMTR Newsletter* [serial on line], 1:7–11. www.cibmtr.org/PUBLICATIONS/Newsletter Accessed on 16 Jan 2008
4. Pasquini MC, Wang Z (2007) Current use and outcome of hematopoietic stem cell transplantation: part II – CIBMTR summary slides, 2007. *CIBMTR Newsletter* [serial online] 2008;14:6–13. www.cibmtr.org/PUBLICATIONS/Newsletter Accessed on 16 Jan 2008
5. Afessa B, Tefferi A, Litzow MR et al (2002) Diffuse alveolar hemorrhage in hematopoietic stem cell transplant recipients. Am J Respir Crit Care Med 166:641–645
6. Agusti C, Ramirez J, Picado C et al (1995) Diffuse alveolar hemorrhage in allogeneic bone marrow transplantation. A postmortem study. Am J Respir Crit Care Med 151: 1006–1010
7. De Lassence A, Fleury-Feith J, Escudier E et al (1995) Alveolar hemorrhage. Diagnostic criteria and results in 194 immunocompromised hosts. Am J Respir Crit Care Med 151:157–163
8. Robbins RA, Linder J, Stahl MG et al (1989) Diffuse alveolar hemorrhage in autologous bone marrow transplant recipients. Am J Med 87:511–518
9. Panos RJ, Barr LF, Walsh TJ et al (1988) Factors associated with fatal hemoptysis in cancer patients. Chest 94:1008–1013
10. Maile CW, Moore AV, Ulreich S et al (1983) Chest radiographic-pathologic correlation in adult leukemia patients. Invest Radiol 18:495–499

11. Tashiro T (1992) Pulmonary complications in patients with adult T-cell leukemia. Nihon Kyobu Shikkan Gakkai Zasshi 30:756–762
12. Golde DW, Drew WL, Klein HZ et al (1975) Occult pulmonary haemorrhage in leukaemia. Br Med J 2:166–168
13. Azoulay E, Fieux F, Moreau D et al (2003) Acute monocytic leukemia presenting as acute respiratory failure. Am J Respir Crit Care Med 167:1329–1333
14. Wurthner JU, Kohler G, Behringer D et al (1999) Leukostasis followed by hemorrhage complicating the initiation of chemotherapy in patients with acute myeloid leukemia and hyperleukocytosis: a clinicopathologic report of four cases. Cancer 85:368–374
15. Saka H, Ito T, Ito M et al (1992) Diffuse pulmonary alveolar hemorrhage in acute promyelocytic leukemia. Intern Med 31:457–458
16. Russi E, Odermatt B, Joller-Jemelka HI et al (1993) Alveolar haemorrhage as a presenting feature of myeloma. Eur Respir J 6:267–270
17. Grigoriyan A, Rishi A, Molina J et al (2007) Diffuse alveolar damage and hemorrhage in acute myelogenous leukemia treated with corticosteroids. Conn Med 71:201–204
18. Alexandrescu DT, Dutcher JP, O'Boyle K et al (2004) Fatal intra-alveolar hemorrhage after rituximab in a patient with non-Hodgkin lymphoma. Leuk Lymphoma 45:2321–2325
19. Raanani P, Segal E, Levi I et al (2000) Diffuse alveolar hemorrhage in acute promyelocytic leukemia patients treated with ATRA–a manifestation of the basic disease or the treatment. Leuk Lymphoma 37:605–610
20. Kawasaki K, Akaike H, Miyauchi A et al (2006) Sivelestat relieves respiratory distress refractory to dexamethasone in all-trans retinoic acid syndrome: a report of two cases. Eur J Haematol 77:448–452
21. Wan TS, Yip SF, Yeung YM et al (2002) Fatal diffuse alveolar damage complicating acute myeloid leukemia with abnormal eosinophils and trisomy X. Ann Hematol 81: 167–169
22. Crilley P, Topolsky D, Styler MJ et al (1995) Extramedullary toxicity of a conditioning regimen containing busulphan, cyclophosphamide and etoposide in 84 patients undergoing autologous and allogenic bone marrow transplantation. Bone Marrow Transplant 15:361–365
23. Smith LJ, Katzenstein AL (1982) Pathogenesis of massive pulmonary hemorrhage in acute leukemia. Arch Intern Med 142:2149–2152
24. van Buchem MA, Hogendoorn PC, Levelt CN et al (1992) Development of pulmonary leukostasis in experimental myelocytic leukemia in the Brown-Norway rat. Leukemia 6:142–149
25. Tanaka N, Matsumoto T, Miura G et al (2002) CT findings of leukemic pulmonary infiltration with pathologic correlation. Eur Radiol 12:166–174
26. Lee WA, Hruban RH, Kuhlman JE et al (1992) High resolution computed tomography of inflation-fixed lungs: pathologic-radiologic correlation of pulmonary lesions in patients with leukemia, lymphoma, or other hematopoietic proliferative disorders. Clin Imaging 16:15–24
27. Baker WJ, Vukelja SJ, Burrell LM et al (1998) High-dose cyclophosphamide, etoposide and carboplatin with autologous bone marrow support for metastatic breast cancer: long-term results. Bone Marrow Transplant 21:775–778
28. Ben Abraham R, Paret G, Cohen R (2003) Diffuse alveolar hemorrhage following allogeneic bone marrow transplantation in children. Chest 124:660–664
29. Chao NJ, Snyder DS, Jain M et al (2000) Equivalence of two effective graft-versus-host disease prophylaxis regimens: results of a prospective double-blind randomized trial. Biol Blood Marrow Transplant 6:254–261
30. Cordonnier C, Bernaudin JF, Bierling P (1986) Pulmonary complications occurring after allogeneic bone marrow transplantation. A study of 130 consecutive transplanted patients. Cancer 58:1047–1054
31. Frankovich J, Donaldson SS, Lee Y et al (2001) High-dose therapy and autologous hematopoietic cell transplantation in children with primary refractory and relapsed Hodgkin's disease: atopy predicts idiopathic diffuse lung injury syndromes. Biol Blood Marrow Transplant 7: 49–57
32. Ho VT, Weller E, Lee SJ et al (2001) Prognostic factors for early severe pulmonary complications after hematopoietic stem cell transplantation. Biol Blood Marrow Transplant 7:223–229
33. Huisman C, van der Straaten HM, Canninga-van Dijk MR et al (2006) Pulmonary complications after T-cell-depleted allogeneic stem cell transplantation: low incidence and strong association with acute graft-versus-host disease. Bone Marrow Transplant 38:561–566
34. Jabro G, Koc Y, Boyle T et al (1999) Role of splenic irradiation in patients with chronic myeloid leukemia undergoing allogeneic bone marrow transplantation. Biol Blood Marrow Transplant 5:173–179
35. Jules-Elysee K, Stover DE, Yahalom J et al (1992) Pulmonary complications in lymphoma patients treated with high-dose therapy autologous bone marrow transplantation. Am Rev Respir Dis 146:485–491
36. Lewis ID, DeFor T, Weisdorf DJ (2000) Increasing incidence of diffuse alveolar hemorrhage following allogeneic bone marrow transplantation: cryptic etiology and uncertain therapy. Bone Marrow Transplant 26:539–543
37. Majhail NS, Parks K, DeFor TE et al (2006) Diffuse alveolar hemorrhage and infection-associated alveolar hemorrhage following hematopoietic stem cell transplantation: related and high-risk clinical syndromes. Biol Blood Marrow Transplant 12:1038–1046
38. Metcalf JP, Rennard SI, Reed EC (1994) Corticosteroids as adjunctive therapy for diffuse alveolar hemorrhage associated with bone marrow transplantation. University of Nebraska Medical Center Bone Marrow Transplant Group. Am J Med 96:327–334
39. Mulder PO, Meinesz AF, de Vries EG et al (1991) Diffuse alveolar hemorrhage in autologous bone marrow transplant recipients [letter; comment]. Am J Med 90:278–281
40. Nevo S, Enger C, Swan V et al (1999) Acute bleeding after allogeneic bone marrow transplantation: association with graft versus host disease and effect on survival. Transplantation 67:681–689
41. Raptis A, Mavroudis D, Suffredini A et al (1999) High-dose corticosteroid therapy for diffuse alveolar hemorrhage in allogeneic bone marrow stem cell transplant recipients. Bone Marrow Transplant 24:879–883
42. Seiden MV, Elias A, Ayash L et al (1992) Pulmonary toxicity associated with high dose chemotherapy in the treatment of

solid tumors with autologous marrow transplant: an analysis of four chemotherapy regimens. Bone Marrow Transplant 10:57–63

43. Sisson JH, Thompson AB, Anderson JR et al (1992) Airway inflammation predicts diffuse alveolar hemorrhage during bone marrow transplantation in patients with Hodgkin disease. Am Rev Respir Dis 146:439–443
44. Witte RJ, Gurney JW, Robbins RA et al (1991) Diffuse pulmonary alveolar hemorrhage after bone marrow transplantation: radiographic findings in 39 patients. AJR Am J Roentgenol 157:461–464
45. Afessa B, Tefferi A, Litzow MR et al (2002) Outcome of diffuse alveolar hemorrhage in hematopoietic stem cell transplant recipients. Am J Respir Crit Care Med 166: 1364–1368
46. Baker KS, Roncarolo MG, Peters C et al (1999) High spontaneous IL-10 production in unrelated bone marrow transplant recipients is associated with fewer transplant-related complications and early deaths. Bone Marrow Transplant 23:1123–1129
47. Nevo S, Swan V, Enger C et al (1998) Acute bleeding after bone marrow transplantation (BMT)—incidence and effect on survival. A quantitative analysis in 1,402 patients. Blood 91:1469–1477
48. Nevo S, Vogelsang GB (2001) Acute bleeding complications in patients after bone marrow transplantation. Curr Opin Hematol 8:319–325
49. Feinstein MB, Mokhtari M, Ferreiro R et al (2001) Fiberoptic bronchoscopy in allogeneic bone marrow transplantation: findings in the era of serum cytomegalovirus antigen surveillance. Chest 120:1094–1100
50. Glazer M, Breuer R, Berkman N et al (1998) Use of fiberoptic bronchoscopy in bone marrow transplant recipients. Acta Haematol 99:22–26
51. Gupta S, Jain A, Warneke CL et al (2007) Outcome of alveolar hemorrhage in hematopoietic stem cell transplant recipients. Bone Marrow Transplant 40:71–78
52. Hofmeister CC, Marinier DE, Czerlanis C et al (2007) Clinical utility of autopsy after hematopoietic stem cell transplantation. Biol Blood Marrow Transplant 13: 26–30
53. Huaringa AJ, Leyva FJ, Signes-Costa J et al (2000) Bronchoalveolar lavage in the diagnosis of pulmonary complications of bone marrow transplant patients. Bone Marrow Transplant 25:975–979
54. Kasow KA, King E, Rochester R et al (2007) Diagnostic yield of bronchoalveolar Llvage Ii low in allogeneic hematopoietic stem cell recipients receiving immunosuppressive therapy or with acute graft-versus-host disease: the St. Jude experience, 1990–2002. Biol Blood Marrow Transplant 13:831–837
55. Patel NR, Lee PS, Kim JH et al (2005) The influence of diagnostic bronchoscopy on clinical outcomes comparing adult autologous and allogeneic bone marrow transplant patients. Chest 127:1388–1396
56. Bojko T, Notterman DA, Greenwald BM et al (1995) Acute hypoxemic respiratory failure in children following bone marrow transplantation: an outcome and pathologic study. Crit Care Med 23:755–759
57. Huaringa AJ, Leyva FJ, Giralt SA et al (2000) Outcome of bone marrow transplantation patients requiring mechanical ventilation. Crit Care Med 28:1014–1017
58. Roychowdhury M, Pambuccian SE, Aslan DL et al (2005) Pulmonary complications after bone marrow transplantation: an autopsy study from a large transplantation center. Arch Pathol Lab Med 129:366–371
59. Sharma S, Nadrous HF, Peters SG et al (2005) Pulmonary complications in adult blood and marrow transplant recipients: autopsy findings. Chest 128:1385–1392
60. Wojno KJ, Vogelsang GB, Beschorner WE et al (1994) Pulmonary hemorrhage as a cause of death in allogeneic bone marrow recipients with severe acute graft-versus-host disease. Transplantation 57:88–92
61. Moreb JS, Kubilis PS, Mullins DL et al (1997) Increased frequency of autoaggression syndrome associated with autologous stem cell transplantation in breast cancer patients. Bone Marrow Transplant 19:101–106
62. Panoskaltsis-Mortari A, Taylor PA, Yaeger TM et al (1997) The critical early proinflammatory events associated with idiopathic pneumonia syndrome in irradiated murine allogeneic recipients are due to donor T cell infusion and potentiated by cyclophosphamide. J Clin Invest 100:1015–1027
63. Sloane JP, Depledge MH, Powles RL et al (1983) Histopathology of the lung after bone marrow transplantation. J Clin Pathol 36:546–554
64. Beschorner WE, Shinn CA, Hess AD et al (1989) Immune-related injury to endothelium associated with acute graft-versus-host disease in the rat. Transplant Proc 21:3025–3027
65. Piguet PF, Grau GE, Collart MA (1989) Pneumopathies of the graft-versus-host reaction. Alveolitis associated with an increased level of tumor necrosis factor mRNA and chronic interstitial pneumonitis. Lab Invest 61:37–45
66. Srivastava A, Gottlieb D, Bradstock KF (1995) Diffuse alveolar haemorrhage associated with microangiopathy after allogeneic bone marrow transplantation. Bone Marrow Transplant 15:863–867
67. Chao NJ, Duncan SR, Long GD et al (1991) Corticosteroid therapy for diffuse alveolar hemorrhage in autologous bone marrow transplant recipients. Ann Intern Med 114:145–146
68. Corso S, Vukelja SJ, Wiener D et al (1993) Diffuse alveolar hemorrhage following autologous bone marrow infusion. Bone Marrow Transplant 12:301–303
69. Vaughan WP, Linder J, Robbins R et al (1991) Pulmonary surveillance using bronchoscopy and bronchoalveolar lavage during high-dose antineoplastic therapy. Chest 99:105–111
70. Capizzi SA, Kumar S, Huneke NE et al (2001) Peri-engraftment respiratory distress syndrome during autologous hematopoietic stem cell transplantation. Bone Marrow Transplant 27:1299–1303
71. Haselton DJ, Klekamp JG, Christman BW et al (2000) Use of high-dose corticosteroids and high-frequency oscillatory ventilation for treatment of a child with diffuse alveolar hemorrhage after bone marrow transplantation: case report and review of the literature. Crit Care Med 28:245–248
72. Meng ZH, Dyer K, Billiar TR et al (2000) Distinct effects of systemic infusion of G-CSF vs. IL-6 on lung and liver inflammation and injury in hemorrhagic shock. Shock 14:41–48
73. Ferrara JL (1994) Cytokines other than growth factors in bone marrow transplantation. Curr Opin Oncol 6:127–134
74. Cooke KR, Kobzik L, Martin TRet al. (1996) An experimental model of idiopathic pneumonia syndrome after bone marrow transplantation: I. The roles of minor H antigens and endotoxin. Blood 88:3230–3239

75. Worthy SA, Flint JD, Muller NL (1997) Pulmonary complications after bone marrow transplantation: high-resolution CT and pathologic findings. Radiographics 17:1359–1371
76. Linder J, Robbins RA, Rennard SI (1988) Cytologic criteria for diffuse alveolar hemorrhage. Acta Cytol 32:763
77. Sherman JM, Winnie G, Thomassen MJ et al (1984) Time course of hemosiderin production and clearance by human pulmonary macrophages. Chest 86:409–411
78. Grebski E, Hess T, Hold G et al (1992) Diagnostic value of hemosiderin-containing macrophages in bronchoalveolar lavage. Chest 102:1794–1799
79. Clark JG, Hansen JA, Hertz MI et al (1993) NHLBI workshop summary. Idiopathic pneumonia syndrome after bone marrow transplantation. Am Rev Respir Dis 147:1601–1606
80. Shankar G, Cohen DA (2001) Idiopathic pneumonia syndrome after bone marrow transplantation: the role of pre-transplant radiation conditioning and local cytokine dysregulation in promoting lung inflammation and fibrosis. Int J Exp Pathol 82:101–113
81. Blatt J, Gold SH, Wiley JM et al (2001) Off-label use of recombinant factor VIIa in patients following bone marrow transplantation. Bone Marrow Transplant 28:405–407
82. Hicks K, Peng D, Gajewski JL (2002) Treatment of diffuse alveolar hemorrhage after allogeneic bone marrow transplant with recombinant factor VIIa. Bone Marrow Transplant 30:975–978
83. Pastores SM, Papadopoulos E, Voigt L et al (2003) Diffuse alveolar hemorrhage after allogeneic hematopoietic stem-cell transplantation: treatment with recombinant factor VIIa. Chest 124:2400–2403

Venous Thromboembolism in Patients with Hematologic Malignancies

34

Tarek Sousou and Alok A. Khorana

Contents

T. Sousou and A.A. Khorana (✉)
The Department of Medicine, James P. Wilmot Cancer Center, University of Rochester, 601 Elmwood Ave, P.O. Box 704, Rochester, NY 14642, USA
e-mail: alok_khorana@URMC.rochester.edu

34.1 Introduction

Venous thromboembolism (VTE) is an increasingly common complication of hematologic malignancies that can present as either a deep venous thrombosis (DVT) or a pulmonary embolism (PE) [1–3]. This illness has complications; in particular, analysis of a prospective observational study indicates that thrombosis is the second leading cause of death in cancer patients [1, 4]. In the past, cancer-associated VTE was primarily considered a complication of solid organ malignancies. However, emerging data indicate that the risk of VTE development is as great or greater in hematologic malignancies, including lymphoma, leukemia and multiple myeloma [5].

According to information from the Surveillance Epidemiology and End Results database in the United States, over 140,000 new cases of hematologic malignancies are expected to be diagnosed in 2009 with a prevalence of approximately 871,000 cases in the USA [6]. Hematologic cancer patients represent a population of cancer patients at highest risk for VTE (adjusted OR, 28.0; 95% CI, 4.0–199.7) for VTE development in some studies [5]. Despite the high incidence of malignancy-associated VTE, this diagnosis is underestimated according to autopsy-based studies [7]. With mounting evidence surrounding VTE incidence in hematologic malignancies, a greater emphasis has been placed on better identification of those at risk, prevention and appropriate treatment strategies to reduce recurrent VTE.

É. Azoulay (ed.), *Pulmonary Involvement in Patients with Hematological Malignancies*,
DOI: 10.1007/978-3-642-15742-4_34, © Springer-Verlag Berlin Heidelberg 2011

34.2 Risk Factors for VTE in Hematologic Malignancies

Several risk factors have been identified in cancer patients and can be categorized according to the type of malignancy, patient comorbidities and therapeutic interventions for cancer (Table 34.1).

34.2.1 Type of Malignancy

The type of malignancy is an important risk factor in VTE development. Historically, solid organ malignancies were associated with VTE. As discussed above, however, recent data from a large population-based case-controlled study, indicate the odds ratio for VTE development was highest in those with hematologic malignancies. Additional research demonstrates that amongst hematologic malignancies, lymphoma and multiple myeloma were associated with the highest rates of VTE in hospitalized hematologic cancer patients [1], and in some series, these diagnoses have accounted for more than a third of the total number of thrombotic events [8]. A retrospective analysis of 612 outpatients with plasma cell dyscrasia revealed a 9% incidence of VTE with a median time to VTE of 8.5 months following diagnosis [9]. The increased risk of VTE in myeloma patients varies according to the chemotherapy regimen employed as well as the disease status; for instance, patients with relapsed/refractory myeloma have lower rates of VTE compared to newly diagnosed patients [10, 11].

Table 34.1 Risk factors for VTE in hematologic cancer patients

Malignancy-associated risk factors
• Type of malignancy
– Myeloma
– Lymphoma
– Leukemia
• Initial period (3–6 months) after diagnosis
Comorbidities
• Older age
• Hospitalization
• Recent surgery
• Infection
• Obesity
• Renal disease
• Pulmonary disease
• Inherited prothrombotic mutations
– Factor V Leiden
– Prothrombin gene mutation
– Prior history of VTE
Therapy-associated risk factors
• Chemotherapy
• Stem cell transplantation
• Central venous catheters
• Erythropoiesis stimulating agents
• Anti-angiogenic agents
– Thalidomide
– Lenalidomide

34.2.2 Therapeutic Agents

Chemotherapy is associated with up to a sixfold increase in VTE risk as compared to the general population [2, 12, 13], with several studies demonstrating a direct link between the use of chemotherapy for hematologic malignancies and the incidence of thromboembolic events [14–17]. Specific therapeutic agents have been linked with VTE both in epidemiologic studies as well as in laboratory studies evaluating coagulation. For instance, asparaginase has been linked to reductions in antithrombin levels as well as elevations in factor VIII/von Willebrand levels [18]. Coupled with prednisone use, as is standard in acute lymphoblastic leukemia (ALL) treatment, a hypofibrinolytic state ensues due to a dose-dependent increase in plasminogen activator inhibitor-1 levels, thereby creating an environment suitable for VTE [18]. In some series, use of asparaginase, anthracyclines and prednisone was associated with a trend towards an increased risk of VTE with a 4.5% incidence [19, 20]. However, a meta-analysis of 17 prospective studies of pediatric ALL demonstrated asparaginase significantly increased VTE risk [21]. Larger adult ALL studies have supported this finding. A recent study from Italy, which included 379 hematologic cancer patients – of which 18% had ALL – revealed a significant 4.9-fold increase in VTE risk with asparaginase [22].

Doxorubicin, a key component of therapy for lymphoma, has been demonstrated in in vitro models to downregulate protein C activity, thereby promoting a prothrombotic state [23]. Novel therapeutics in the treatment of multiple myeloma, such as the anti-angiogenic class of agents, particularly thalidomide and lenalidomide, have also been associated with up to a sevenfold increase in the rate of DVT when given in combination with multiagent chemotherapy [17]. High rates of both venous and arterial events have been observed in clinical trials of other anti-angiogenic agents as well, suggesting this toxicity may be a class effect.

Not only is chemotherapy associated with a prothrombotic state, but also supportive care measures are linked to an increased risk of thrombotic events. The use of erythropoiesis-stimulating agents (ESAs) has been found to increase the risk of VTE as well, although it is unclear whether this accounts for the increased mortality associated with these agents in some studies [24, 25].

34.2.3 Initial Period After Diagnosis

The initial phase of treatment poses a risk for VTE development in hematologic cancer patients as well. VTE risk in cancer patients was found to be greatest within a 3-month period following the diagnosis of cancer and can remain elevated for up to 15 years [5]. A retrospective review of patients with diffuse large B-cell lymphoma (DLBCL) over an 11-year period revealed a VTE incidence of 12.8% with a greater number of events occurring in patients with advanced stage or high risk disease [26]. Over 80% of events occurred during the first three cycles of chemotherapy [26].

34.2.4 Stem Cell Transplantation

Stem cell transplantation also poses unique risks for VTE development given lengthy hospitalizations, prolonged risk for infection and use of chemotherapy. Furthermore, patients undergoing stem cell transplantation have decreased fibrinolysis, decreased antithrombin III levels, increased thrombin production and endothelial damage, all of which contribute to an increased risk for VTE [27–29]. A recent single-institution retrospective analysis of 589 patients undergoing hematopoietic stem cell transplantation revealed a 3.7% incidence of VTE 1-year post-transplant [30]. Risk factors for VTE in hematopoietic stem cell transplant patients have been identified in a cohort study of 1,514 cancer patients, which included 1,291 hematologic cancer patients. This study demonstrated that a prior history of VTE, the use of immunomodulators and the development of graft-versus-host disease was associated with up to an eightfold increase in risk of VTE development (OR: 8.36, 1.87 and 2.05, respectively) [31]. The universal use of central venous catheters for delivery of chemotherapy further increases this risk (HR = 3.4, CI: 1.8–6.5) [20].

34.2.5 Comorbid Conditions

Several patient comorbidities are associated with a higher incidence of VTE and include: older age, immobility, infection and obesity [13, 20]. Acquired prothrombotic states, such as a history of VTE, prothrombin gene mutation, protein C or S deficiency and factor V Leiden, may also increase the risk of VTE [13]. Hospitalization is well known to increase the risk of VTE in cancer patients [32, 33]. The average risk of VTE per hospitalization is 4.1%; however, this risk varies widely and is noted to be higher in certain hematologic malignancies [1]. The rate of VTE per hospitalization has increased by 47% in cancer patients receiving chemotherapy between 1995 and 2003, suggesting that newer chemotherapy regimens may be more thrombogenic [1].

34.3 Candidate Biomarkers of VTE

P-selectin is a cell adhesion molecule found in platelet granules and endothelial cells that has been implicated in tumor growth, leukocyte adhesion and most notably thrombosis. When activated, they are expressed on the cell surface and help mediate platelet adhesion in thrombosis with subsequent release of procoagulant microparticles [34]. A recent prospective cohort study of 687 patients revealed that P-selectin levels were significantly higher in cancer patients with VTE as compared to those without (HR 2.6, CI 1.4–4.9) [35]. Of note, there were no significant differences in P-selectin levels according to the type of malignancy [35]. However, only 91 patients (13% of the study population) had a hematologic malignancy.

D-dimer, a marker of hemostatic activation, has been found to be elevated in noncancer patients with VTE and is predictive of recurrent VTE [36]. A recent study of 821 cancer patients revealed D-dimer to be significantly higher in cancer patients with VTE with an HR of 1.8 for development of VTE [37]. This risk further increased with the simultaneous detection of elevated prothrombin fragments, products of thrombin generation. D-dimer and prothrombin fragment elevations were found to be as elevated if not higher in patients with hematologic malignancies as compared to solid organ malignancies [37].

Tissue factor (TF), a transmembrane glycoprotein that serves to initiate coagulation, also has a relationship to cancer progression and VTE. The majority of research in TF has been in solid organ malignancies; however, emerging data indicate that TF expression is increased in hematologic malignancies as well [38–40]. Furthermore, its expression levels correlate with angiogenesis in hematologic malignancies through its effect on several oncogenic proteins, such as vascular endothelial growth factor (VEGF) and extracellular-regulated kinase (ERK), among others [38, 41, 42]. Despite the known procoagulant properties of increased TF expression, any potential relationship between TF expression and clinical VTE in hematologic malignancies has not yet been described. More research into the potential use of TF assays in hematologic malignancies is needed before this can be used as a biomarker for VTE in this setting.

Research conducted in the ambulatory cancer population has identified novel candidate biomarkers that may be predictive of cancer-associated VTE as well. Data from the ANC Study Group Registry suggests that elevated pre-chemotherapy platelet counts are associated with VTE [2]. Over a 2.5-month period, the incidence of VTE was nearly 4% for patients with a pre-chemotherapy platelet count ≥350,000/mm^3 as compared to 1.25% for patients with a pre-chemotherapy platelet count of <200,000/mm^3 (p for trend = 0.0003). Further analysis of the ANC registry revealed a similar increase in risk of VTE with a pre-chemotherapy leukocyte count >11,000/mm^3 [43]. Although comprised primarily of solid tumor patients, this study targeted patients with lymphoma who comprised just over one-tenth of the study population.

Markers of hemostatic activation, such as C-reactive protein (CRP), have been observed to be elevated in cancer patients. Observational studies in cancer patients indicate that an increased CRP may be predictive of VTE [33, 44].

34.4 A Predictive Risk Assessment Score

Cancer-associated thrombosis is a multifactorial process that involves several risk factors. Identification of patients at risk for VTE requires a risk model that incorporates known risk factors and their relationships. Based upon data obtained from the ANC Study Group Registry, which included 512 (12.6%) patients with lymphoma, a validated risk model for chemotherapy-associated VTE has been developed [43].

Using a development cohort of 2,701 ambulatory cancer patients, five variables predictive for VTE were identified using a stage-adjusted multivariate model. These include: body mass index ≥35, site of cancer, pre-chemotherapy leukocyte count >11,000/mm^3, hemoglobin <10 g/dL and/or use of erythropoietin, and pre-chemotherapy platelet count ≥350,000/mm^3 [43]. Each variable was assigned a risk score using estimated regression coefficients, which was then validated in an independent cohort of 1,365 patients from the ANC registry. Rates of VTE in the high-risk patient subgroup approached 7%, similar to that seen in hospitalized patients [43]. Given thromboprophylaxis is safe and effective in hospitalized medical patients, similar assumptions can be made for cancer patients identified to be at high risk for VTE. A prospective study of thromboprophylaxis in ambulatory cancer patients deemed to be high risk based on this model is currently underway (NCT00876915).

34.5 VTE Thromboprophylaxis in Hematologic Malignancy

Several landmark studies have addressed thromboprophylaxis using unfractionated heparin (UFH), low molecular weight heparin (LMWH) or factor Xa inhibitors according to patient setting (Table 34.2).

Table 34.2 Trials evaluating thromboprophylaxis of hospitalized hematologic cancer patients

Study	Total patients	Cancer patients	Intervention	VTE
Samama 1999 *MEDENOX* [45]	1,102	157 (14)	Enoxaparin 40 mg Qday × 6–14 day vs placebo	5.5% vs 14.9%
Leizorovicz 2004 *PREVENT* [46]	3,706	190 (5)	Dalteparin 5,000 IU Qday × 14 days vs placebo	2.77% vs 4.96%
Cohen 2006 *ARTEMIS* [47]	849	131 (15)	Fondaparinux× 2.5 mg Qday × 6–14 days vs placebo	5.6% vs 10.5%

34.5.1 Hematologic Cancer Inpatients

Three large randomized controlled trials have examined the role of various anticoagulants in the prevention of VTE. Neither of these studies specifically focused on cancer patients, let alone patients with hematologic malignancies, with only 5–15% of the study populations of these studies comprising cancer patients.

The Comparison of Enoxaparin with Placebo for the Prevention of Venous Thromboembolism in Acutely Ill Medical Patients (MEDENOX) trial was a double-blinded, placebo-controlled study that randomly assigned patients to receive either enoxaparin or placebo for a total duration of up to 14 days. Patients older than 40 years of age who were not immobile for more than 3 days and had an estimated length of stay of at least 6 days were included. A total of 1,102 patients, 157 with cancer, were enrolled in this study and randomized to one of three arms: enoxaparin 40 mg daily ($N = 367$), enoxaparin 20 mg daily ($N = 364$) or placebo ($N = 371$). At day 14, 5.5% of participants randomized to the enoxaparin 40 mg arm developed VTE as compared to 14.9% within the placebo arm (RRR 0.63, $P < 0.001$) [45]. This difference among study arms was maintained during the 90-day follow-up phase [45]. However, there were no significant differences between the enoxaparin 20 mg arm and placebo. Adverse events were similar among all groups with the exception of injection site hematomas, which occurred at a greater frequency in the treatment arms [45].

The Prospective Evaluation of Dalteparin Efficacy for Prevention of VTE in Immobilized Patients (PREVENT) Trial is another study that sought to assess the efficacy of dalteparin in VTE prophylaxis. Patients over 40 years of age admitted for an acute medical illness with an estimated length of stay of at least 4 days were included [46]. A total of 3,706 patients, which included 190 cancer patients, were enrolled in this multicenter, placebo-controlled trial and were randomized to receive either dalteparin 5,000 U or placebo daily for 14 days. At day 21 of the study period, patients in the dalteparin study arm had a VTE incidence of 2.77% as compared to 4.96% in the placebo arm (RRR 0.45, $P = 0.0015$) [46]. There was a trend in the incidence of VTE favoring the dalteparin arm at day 90; however, this was not significant [46]. Adverse events were similar in both study arms.

The Arixtra for Thromboembolism Prevention in a Medical Indications (ARTEMIS) Study is a similar trial that evaluated the efficacy of the factor Xa inhibitor, fondaparinux, in VTE prophylaxis [47]. Patients older than 60 years of age, with congestive heart failure class III/IV and clinically diagnosed acute infections, were included in this study. A total of 849 patients, which included 131 cancer patients, were enrolled and randomized to receive either fondaparinux 2.5 mg daily or placebo for up to 14 days. Participants were assessed for VTE at day 15 of the study and were found to have a VTE incidence of 5.6% in the fondaparinux group as compared to 10.5% in the placebo group [47]. The adverse events using fondaparinux were not significantly different when compared to placebo, thus suggesting that fondaparinux is safe to use for thromboprophylaxis in hospitalized medical patients.

Alternatively, hospitalized cancer patients may be given UFH for thromboprophylaxis. Several trials have proven UFH to be a suitable means for thromboprophylaxis with a reduction in mortality for patients with extended lengths of stay as well as time to VTE development [48, 49]. A recent metaanalysis compared the use of LMWH to UFH in VTE incidence and found no significant difference in efficacy [50]. However, there was a 52% risk reduction in the incidence of major hemorrhage in the studies that used LMWH [50]. For patients who are at high risk of bleeding or actively bleeding, mechanical methods of thromboprophylaxis are an acceptable alternative. These include graduated compression stockings, intermittent pneumatic compression devices and a venous foot pump [51].

Cancer patients comprise a small percentage of the patient population evaluated in the majority of these studies, making it difficult to extrapolate the effects of prophylactic anticoagulation to this unique group of patients. Nonetheless, hospitalized hematologic cancer patients are at higher risk for VTE as compared to general medical patients. Given the safety and effectiveness of thromboprophylaxis in general medical patients, one could arguably assume similar results in hospitalized hematologic cancer patients. This has led various guidelines panels to recommend pharmacologic prophylaxis in hospitalized cancer patients without contraindications to prophylaxis, such as severe thrombocytopenia or active bleeding, where the risk of adverse bleeding events outweighs any potential benefit [52]. Current American Society of Clinical Oncology (ASCO) and National Comprehensive Cancer Network (NCCN) guidelines do not recommend thromboprophylaxis in cancer patients with a platelet count less than 50,000 [52, 53].

34.5.2 Hematologic Cancer Outpatients

Multiple myeloma patients receiving combination therapy using lenalidomide or thalidomide represent a unique subset of cancer patients at high risk for VTE. Initial studies utilizing thalidomide for treatment of myeloma were associated with a high rate of VTE [54–56]. Use of fixed low-dose warfarin for thromboprophylaxis in these patients produced conflicting results depending on the treatment regimen employed. VTE rates in patients treated with thalidomide and dexamethasone decreased by 50% with the use of fixed low-dose warfarin; however, this was not supported in a subsequent study [11, 57]. A study evaluating multiagent chemotherapy for treatment of MM revealed an inability of fixed low-dose warfarin to alter the rate of thrombotic complications; however, prophylactic LMWH was associated with a 50% reduction in VTE incidence [56]. In a related study of multiagent chemotherapy with or without thalidomide, use of LMWH did not alter VTE incidence, thus producing conflicting results [58].

Aspirin has also been evaluated in VTE prophylaxis with encouraging results. Data in abstract form from a large randomized trial of lenalidomide with either low- or high-dose dexamethasone revealed an 8% and 23% incidence of VTE, which decreased to 5% and 14%, respectively, with the use of aspirin [59]. Related trials utilizing lenalidomide in combination with dexamethasone and various chemotherapeutic agents have found similar results [60, 61]. Unfortunately, there are few trials evaluating the use of aspirin as prophylaxis. Moreover, there are no prospective randomized trials to date that address which anticoagulation regimen is best suited for MM patients. The choice of thromboprophylaxis should be tailored to any potential risk factor that predisposes one to VTE. The controversy surrounding thromboprophylaxis in MM patients is reflected in the published clinical guidelines. NCCN guidelines recommend the use of prophylactic anticoagulation, but do not specify which anticoagulant to use [62]. The ASCO guidelines recommend either LMWH or adjusted-dose warfarin but not aspirin for VTE prophylaxis [52]. A recent panel report of the Myeloma Working Group identified risk factors for thrombosis associated with thalidomide/lenalidomide-based therapy, including age, history of VTE, central venous catheter, comorbidities (infections, diabetes, cardiac disease), immobilization, surgery and inherited thrombophilia [63]. Myeloma-related risk factors included diagnosis and hyperviscosity. The panel recommended aspirin for patients with one or less risk factors for VTE. LMWH (equivalent to enoxaparin 40 mg/day) was recommended for those with two or more individual/myeloma-related risk factors. LMWH was also recommended for all patients receiving concurrent high-dose dexamethasone or doxorubicin. Full-dose warfarin targeting a therapeutic INR of 2–3 was suggested as an alternative to LMWH, although there are limited data in the literature with this strategy. It is important to emphasize that all of these guidelines and strategies are based on consensus rather than evidence, given the lack of randomized clinical trials data.

Despite the known association of VTE and cancer, it is not routine practice to place cancer patients on prophylactic anticoagulation. Data in abstract form from a recent meta-analysis of VTE prophylaxis in ambulatory cancer patients revealed a 36% relative risk reduction with the use of LMWH [64]. Unfortunately, the absolute risk reduction was 1.8%, and use of prophylactic anticoagulation was associated with a trend towards an increased risk for adverse bleeding events

[64]. Based upon these results, routine VTE prophylaxis in ambulatory cancer patients cannot be recommended at this time with the specific exception for patients with multiple myeloma as discussed above.

34.5.3 Central Venous Catheter Thromboprophylaxis

Cancer patients with central venous catheters (CVC) are at increased risk for VTE, prompting investigations into whether prophylactic LMWH or fixed low-dose warfarin can reduce its incidence. A recent systematic review evaluated nine prospective studies of thromboprophylaxis involving 1,932 cancer patients with CVC who received fixed low-dose warfarin, LMWH or UFH [65]. The result of this systematic review indicated no significant reduction in CVC-associated thrombosis in cancer patients [65]. The warfarin thromboprophylaxis in cancer patients with CVC catheters [66] trial sought to further address the role of warfarin in CVC-related thrombosis. This trial enrolled 1,590 cancer patients receiving active treatment via a CVC who were randomized to either fixed low-dose warfarin, dose-adjusted warfarin with a goal INR of 1.5–2.0 or placebo. The addition of either fixed low-dose warfarin or dose-adjusted warfarin did not significantly reduce the rate of CVC-associated VTE [66]. At this time, there is no role for prophylactic anticoagulation in patients with CVC.

34.6 Treatment of VTE in Cancer Patients

Historically, the standard treatment of VTE involved initial anticoagulation with either LMWH or UFH, which was overlapped with a vitamin K antagonist and discontinued when the prothrombin time is appropriately prolonged. Recent data have proven this model of anticoagulation to be suboptimal for cancer patients.

34.6.1 Initial Anticoagulation

Until the advent of LMWH, parenteral UFH was the sole mode of rapid onset initial anticoagulation. Unfortunately, this was at the expense of frequent monitoring, difficult dosage adjustments and at times wide fluctuations in the activated partial thromboplastin time (aPTT). With the discovery of LMWH, blood monitoring is no longer necessary, and consequently it allows for outpatient treatment, thereby simplifying the management of VTE. LMWHs have been proven to be as effective as UFH without any significant difference in the incidence of adverse outcomes [67–69]. Furthermore, there are data suggesting a statistically significant reduction in mortality with its use [67–70]. Based on these data, ASCO guidelines recommend LMWH as the preferred agent for initial anticoagulation in cancer patients [32]. Fondaparinux is an acceptable alternative to LMWH for initial anticoagulation [71].

34.6.2 Long-Term Anticoagulation

Warfarin has been the standard for long-term anticoagulation; however, it is fraught with difficulties in the cancer patient population. Long-term anticoagulation with warfarin has been associated with higher rates of adverse bleeding events in cancer patients as compared to those without cancer independent of INR levels [72, 73]. Warfarin has also been linked to an increased incidence of recurrent VTE in cancer patients as compared to noncancer patients (20.7% vs 6.8%, respectively) [73]. The outpatient management of anticoagulation with warfarin can be especially difficult due to the several dietary and drug-related interactions it has that can affect INR levels [74, 75]. Additionally, the process of reversal of anticoagulation followed by re-anticoagulation in the setting of an invasive procedure can be troublesome.

Given the inherent difficulties of long-term anticoagulation with warfarin, several studies have questioned if long-term anticoagulation with LMWH would be an acceptable alternative. The largest was the CLOT trial, wherein 672 cancer patients, 70 with hematologic malignancies, who had documented VTE, were randomized to receive either dalteparin ($N = 336$) or warfarin ($N = 336$) for a total of 6 months [76]. During the 6-month study period, 27 patients in the dalteparin group had recurrent VTE as compared to 53 patients receiving warfarin ($P = 0.002$) [76]. The use of LMWH was associated with a greater than 50% risk reduction in recurrent VTE. Coupled with an equivalent safety profile, LMWH was established as a superior agent for long-term anticoagulation in cancer patients. Similar results were obtained with tinzaparin in which 200 cancer patients, 23 with a hematologic malignancy, with documented VTE were randomized to receive either tinzaparin or warfarin for 3 months. At the end of 12 months, 7% of patients in the tinzaparin group had recurrent VTE as compared to 16% in the warfarin group ($P = 0.044$) [77]. The reported adverse events were similar across both study groups. Additional studies were performed using the LMWH enoxaparin, however were underpowered to show any statistically significant difference as compared to warfarin [78, 79].

The data supporting the efficacy for long-term anticoagulation using LMWH in cancer patients is mounting. A recent Cochrane database systematic review of LMWH for long-term anticoagulation conferred a statistically significant reduction in recurrent VTE (HR = 0.47, CI = 0.32–0.71) [80]. As per previous studies, there was no statistically significant difference in bleeding complications between LMWH and warfarin (RR = 0.91; CI = 0.64–1.31) [80]. As a result of the above-mentioned studies, the ASCO, NCCN and ACCP guidelines all recommend the use of LMWH for long-term anticoagulation of VTE in hematologic cancer patients [32, 81, 82].

The optimal duration of anticoagulation in cancer-associated thrombosis remains unknown. One can postulate that cancer patients should remain on anticoagulation indefinitely as long as the cancer is active, since this predisposes to an inherent prothrombotic state. Overall, the risk-benefit ratio should be weighed periodically, and an individualized decision regarding the duration of anticoagulation is recommended.

34.6.3 Use of Vena Caval Filters

Anticoagulation is the primary therapy for cancer patients with VTE. In situations where anticoagulation is contraindicated, an inferior vena cava (IVC) filter is a suitable alternative. A systematic review evaluating the benefit of IVC filters demonstrated a reduction in the incidence of pulmonary embolisms, but there has not been any documented survival benefit [83]. Data from long-term follow-up indicates that patients who received an IVC filter were at increased risk for DVT, but decreased risk for PE [84]. Unfortunately, none of these trials were exclusive to hematologic cancer patients or to a specific type of IVC filter. Therefore, the decision to use an IVC filter should be made on an individual basis when anticoagulation is contraindicated.

34.7 Summary and Future Directions

Cancer-associated thrombosis is a common complication of hematologic malignancies that is associated with an increased mortality and diminished quality of life. Risk factors for VTE have been identified related to the malignancy and its treatment. Emerging data have identified several potential candidate biomarkers predictive of VTE. Several studies have revealed LMWH, UFH and factor Xa inhibitors to be an effective means for thromboprophylaxis in hospitalized hematologic cancer patients. In select cases, thromboprophylaxis is also appropriate in the ambulatory setting. Using known risk factors for VTE, a validated risk model has been created to identify cancer patients at highest risk for VTE. Future application of this risk model in a prospective manner is currently ongoing and is important to assess the efficacy of thromboprophylaxis in high-risk hematologic malignancy patients.

Acknowledgment Dr. Khorana is supported by grants from the National Cancer Institute K23 CA120587, National Heart, Lung and Blood Institute 1R01HL095109-01 and the V Foundation.

References

1. Khorana AA, Francis CW, Culakova E, Kuderer NM, Lyman GH (2007) Frequency, risk factors, and trends for venous thromboembolism among hospitalized cancer patients. Cancer 110:2339–2346
2. Khorana AA, Francis CW, Culakova E, Lyman GH (2005) Risk factors for chemotherapy-associated venous thromboembolism in a prospective observational study. Cancer 104:2822–2829
3. Lee AY (2005) Deep vein thrombosis and cancer: survival, recurrence, and anticoagulant choices. Dis Mon 51: 150–157
4. Stein PD, Beemath A, Meyers FA, Kayali F, Skaf E, Olson RE (2006) Pulmonary embolism as a cause of death in patients who died with cancer. Am J Med 119:163–165

5. Blom JW, Doggen CJ, Osanto S, Rosendaal FR (2005) Malignancies, prothrombotic mutations, and the risk of venous thrombosis. JAMA 293:715–722
6. Horner MJ, Ries LAG, Krapcho M, Neyman N, Aminou R, Howlader N, Altekruse SF, Feuer EJ, Huang L, Mariotto A, Miller BA, Lewis DR, Eisner MP, Stinchcomb DG, Edwards BK (2009) SEER cancer statistics review, 1975–2006. http://seercancergov/csr/1975_2006/
7. Gomes MP, Deitcher SR (2003) Diagnosis of venous thromboembolic disease in cancer patients. Oncology (Huntingt) 17:126–135, 139, discussion 139–144
8. Khorana AA, Francis CW, Culakova E, Fisher RI, Kuderer NM, Lyman GH (2006) Thromboembolism in hospitalized neutropenic cancer patients. J Clin Oncol 24:484–490
9. Srkalovic G, Cameron MG, Rybicki L, Deitcher SR, Kattke-Marchant K, Hussein MA (2004) Monoclonal gammopathy of undetermined significance and multiple myeloma are associated with an increased incidence of venothromboembolic disease. Cancer 101:558–566
10. Barlogie B, Desikan R, Eddlemon P et al (2001) Extended survival in advanced and refractory multiple myeloma after single-agent thalidomide: identification of prognostic factors in a phase 2 study of 169 patients.[see comment]. Blood 98:492–494
11. Weber D, Rankin K, Gavino M, Delasalle K, Alexanian R (2003) Thalidomide alone or with dexamethasone for previously untreated multiple myeloma. J Clin Oncol 21: 16–19
12. Blom JW, Osanto S, Rosendaal FR (2006) High risk of venous thrombosis in patients with pancreatic cancer: a cohort study of 202 patients. Eur J Cancer 42:410–414
13. Heit JA, Silverstein MD, Mohr DN, Petterson TM, O'Fallon WM, Melton LJ 3rd (2000) Risk factors for deep vein thrombosis and pulmonary embolism: a population-based case-control study. Arch Intern Med 160:809–815
14. Gugliotta L, Mazzucconi MG, Leone G et al (1992) Incidence of thrombotic complications in adult patients with acute lymphoblastic leukaemia receiving L-asparaginase during induction therapy: a retrospective study. The GIMEMA Group. Eur J Haematol 49:63–66
15. Ottinger H, Belka C, Kozole G et al (1995) Deep venous thrombosis and pulmonary artery embolism in high-grade non Hodgkin's lymphoma: incidence, causes and prognostic relevance. Eur J Haematol 54:186–194
16. Seifter EJ, Young RC, Longo DL (1985) Deep venous thrombosis during therapy for Hodgkin's disease. Cancer Treat Rep 69:1011–1013
17. Zangari M, Anaissie E, Barlogie B et al (2001) Increased risk of deep-vein thrombosis in patients with multiple myeloma receiving thalidomide and chemotherapy. Blood 98:1614–1615
18. Athale UH, Chan AK (2003) Thrombosis in children with acute lymphoblastic leukemia. Part II. Pathogenesis of thrombosis in children with acute lymphoblastic leukemia: effects of the disease and therapy. Thromb Res 111:199–212
19. Caruso V, Iacoviello L, Di Castelnuovo A, Storti S, Donati MB (2007) Venous thrombotic complications in adults undergoing induction treatment for acute lymphoblastic leukemia: results from a meta-analysis. J Thromb Haemost 5:621–623
20. Ku GH, White RH, Chew HK, Harvey DJ, Zhou H, Wun T (2009) Venous thromboembolism in patients with acute leukemia: incidence, risk factors, and effect on survival. Blood 113:3911–3917
21. Caruso V, Iacoviello L, Di Castelnuovo A et al (2006) Thrombotic complications in childhood acute lymphoblastic leukemia: a meta-analysis of 17 prospective studies comprising 1752 pediatric patients. Blood 108:2216–2222
22. De Stefano V, Sora F, Rossi E et al (2005) The risk of thrombosis in patients with acute leukemia: occurrence of thrombosis at diagnosis and during treatment. J Thromb Haemost 3:1985–1992
23. Woodley-Cook J, Shin LY, Swystun L, Caruso S, Beaudin S, Liaw PC (2006) Effects of the chemotherapeutic agent doxorubicin on the protein C anticoagulant pathway. Mol Cancer Ther 5:3303–3311
24. Bennett CL, Silver SM, Djulbegovic B et al (2008) Venous thromboembolism and mortality associated with recombinant erythropoietin and darbepoetin administration for the treatment of cancer-associated anemia.[see comment]. JAMA 299:914–924
25. Bohlius J, Wilson J, Seidenfeld J et al (2006) Recombinant human erythropoietins and cancer patients: updated meta-analysis of 57 studies including 9353 patients. J Natl Cancer Inst 98:708–714
26. Komrokji RS, Uppal NP, Khorana AA et al (2006) Venous thromboembolism in patients with diffuse large B-cell lymphoma. Leuk Lymphoma 47:1029–1033
27. Kaufman PA, Jones RB, Greenberg CS, Peters WP (1990) Autologous bone marrow transplantation and factor XII, factor VII, and protein C deficiencies. Report of a new association and its possible relationship to endothelial cell injury. Cancer 66:515–521
28. Tsakiris DA, Marbet GA, Tichelli A, Gratwohl A, Speck B (1995) Activation of endothelium-dependent hemostatic factors following bone marrow transplantation. Schweiz Med Wochenschr J Suisse Med 125:416–419
29. Verheij M, Dewit LG, Boomgaard MN, Brinkman HJ, van Mourik JA (1994) Ionizing radiation enhances platelet adhesion to the extracellular matrix of human endothelial cells by an increase in the release of von Willebrand factor. Radiat Res 137:202–207
30. Gonsalves A, Carrier M, Wells PS, McDiarmid SA, Huebsch LB, Allan DS (2008) Incidence of symptomatic venous thromboembolism following hematopoietic stem cell transplantation. J Thromb Haemost 6:1468–1473
31. Gerber DE, Segal JB, Levy MY, Kane J, Jones RJ, Streiff MB (2008) The incidence of and risk factors for venous thromboembolism (VTE) and bleeding among 1514 patients undergoing hematopoietic stem cell transplantation: implications for VTE prevention. Blood 112: 504–510
32. Lyman GH, Khorana AA, Falanga A et al (2007) American society of clinical oncology guideline: recommendations for venous thromboembolism prophylaxis and treatment in patients with cancer. J Clin Oncol 25:5490–5505
33. Kroger K, Weiland D, Ose C et al (2006) Risk factors for venous thromboembolic events in cancer patients. Ann Oncol 17:297–303
34. Chen M, Geng JG (2006) P-selectin mediates adhesion of leukocytes, platelets, and cancer cells in inflammation,

thrombosis, and cancer growth and metastasis. Arch Immunol Ther Exp 54:75–84

35. Ay C, Simanek R, Vormittag R et al (2008) High plasma levels of soluble P-selectin are predictive of venous thromboembolism in cancer patients: results from the Vienna cancer and thrombosis study (CATS). [see comment]. Blood 112:2703–2708
36. Cushman M, Folsom AR, Wang L et al (2003) Fibrin fragment D-dimer and the risk of future venous thrombosis. [see comment]. Blood 101:1243–1248
37. Ay C, Vormittag R, Dunkler D et al (2009) D-dimer and prothrombin fragment 1 + 2 predict venous thromboembolism in patients with cancer: results from the Vienna cancer and thrombosis study. J Clin Oncol 27:4124–4129
38. Lopez-Pedrera C, Barbarroja N, Dorado G, Siendones E, Velasco F (2006) Tissue factor as an effector of angiogenesis and tumor progression in hematological malignancies. [see comment]. Leukemia 20:1331–1340
39. Sase T, Wada H, Yamaguchi M et al (2005) Haemostatic abnormalities and thrombotic disorders in malignant lymphoma. [see comment]. Thromb Haemost 93: 153–159
40. Wada H, Sase T, Yamaguchi M (2005) Hypercoagulant states in malignant lymphoma. Exp Oncol 27:179–185
41. Barbarroja N, Aristides-Torres L, Hernandez V et al (2007) Coordinated deregulation of cellular receptors, proangiogenic factors and intracellular pathways in acute myeloid leukaemia. Leuk Lymphoma 48:1187–1199
42. Versteeg HH, Spek CA, Peppelenbosch MP, Richel DJ (2004) Tissue factor and cancer metastasis: the role of intracellular and extracellular signaling pathways. Mol Med 10: 6–11
43. Khorana AA, Kuderer NM, Culakova E, Lyman GH, Francis CW (2008) Development and validation of a predictive model for chemotherapy-associated thrombosis. [see comment]. Blood 111:4902–4907
44. Cosmi B, Legnani C, Cini M, Guazzaloca G, Palareti G (2005) The role of D-dimer and residual venous obstruction in recurrence of venous thromboembolism after anticoagulation withdrawal in cancer patients. Haematologica 90: 713–715
45. Samama MM, Cohen AT, Darmon J-Y et al (1999) A comparison of enoxaparin with placebo for the prevention of venous thromboembolism in acutely ill medical patients. N Engl J Med 341(11):793–800
46. Leizorovicz A, Cohen AT, Turpie AG, Olsson CG, Vaitkus PT, Goldhaber SZ (2004) Randomized, placebo-controlled trial of dalteparin for the prevention of venous thromboembolism in acutely ill medical patients. Circulation 110: 874–879
47. Cohen AT, Davidson BL, Gallus AS et al (2006) Efficacy and safety of fondaparinux for the prevention of venous thromboembolism in older acute medical patients: randomised placebo controlled trial. Bmj 332:325–329
48. Gardlund B (1996) Randomised, controlled trial of low-dose heparin for prevention of fatal pulmonary embolism in patients with infectious diseases. The heparin prophylaxis study group. Lancet 347:1357–1361
49. Halkin H, Goldberg J, Modan M, Modan B (1982) Reduction of mortality in general medical in-patients by low-dose heparin prophylaxis. Ann Intern Med 96:561–565
50. Mismetti P, Laporte-Simitsidis S, Tardy B et al (2000) Prevention of venous thromboembolism in internal medicine with unfractionated or low-molecular-weight heparins: a meta-analysis of randomised clinical trials. Thromb Haemost 83:14–19
51. Geerts W, Pineo G, Heit J et al (2004) Prevention of venous thromboembolism. The seventh ACCP conference on antithrombotic and thrombolytic therapy. Am Coll Chest Phys 126:338–400
52. Khorana AA, Streiff MB, Farge D et al (2009) Venous thromboembolism prophylaxis and treatment in cancer: a consensus statement of major guidelines panels and call to action. J Clin Oncol 27:4919–4926
53. Rasmussen MS (2007) Prolonged thromboprophylaxis with low molecular weight heparin after major abdominal surgery. Curr Opin Pulm Med 13:389–392
54. Cavo M, Zamagni E, Cellini C et al (2002) Deep-vein thrombosis in patients with multiple myeloma receiving first-line thalidomide-dexamethasone therapy. Blood 100:2272–2273
55. Minnema MC, Breitkreutz I, Auwerda JJ et al (2004) Prevention of venous thromboembolism with low molecular-weight heparin in patients with multiple myeloma treated with thalidomide and chemotherapy. Leukemia 18: 2044–2046
56. Zangari M, Barlogie B, Anaissie E et al (2004) Deep vein thrombosis in patients with multiple myeloma treated with thalidomide and chemotherapy: effects of prophylactic and therapeutic anticoagulation. Br J Haematol 126:715–721
57. Cavo M, Zamagni E, Tosi P et al (2004) First-line therapy with thalidomide and dexamethasone in preparation for autologous stem cell transplantation for multiple myeloma. Haematologica 89:826–831
58. Barlogie B, Tricot G, Anaissie E et al (2006) Thalidomide and hematopoietic-cell transplantation for multiple myeloma. [see comment]. N Engl J Med 354:1021–1030
59. Rajkumar SV, Jacobus S, Callander N et al (2007) Phase III trial of lenalidomide plus high-dose dexamethasone versus lenalidomide plus low-dose dexamethasone in newly diagnosed multiple myeloma (E4A03): a trial coordinated by the Eastern Cooperative Oncology Group. J Clin Oncol (Meeting Abstracts). 25:LBA8025
60. Baz R, Walker E, Karam MA et al (2006) Lenalidomide and pegylated liposomal doxorubicin-based chemotherapy for relapsed or refractory multiple myeloma: safety and efficacy. Ann Oncol 17:1766–1771
61. Palumbo A, Falco P, Corradini P et al (2007) Melphalan, prednisone, and lenalidomide treatment for newly diagnosed myeloma: a report from the GIMEMA–Italian Multiple Myeloma Network. J Clin Oncol 25:4459–4465
62. NCCN clinical practice guidelines in oncology (2011) Multiple myeloma. http://wwwnccnorg/professionals/physician_gls/PDF/myelomapdf
63. Palumbo A, Rajkumar SV, Dimopoulos MA et al (2008) Prevention of thalidomide- and lenalidomide-associated thrombosis in myeloma. Leukemia 22:414–423
64. Kuderer NM, Khorana AA, Francis CW, Lyman GH, Falanga A, Ortel TL (2009) Low-molecular-weight heparin for venous thromboprophylaxis in ambulatory cancer patients: a meta-analysis. J Clin Oncol (Meeting Abstracts) 27:9537
65. Cunningham MS, White B, Hollywood D, O'Donnell J (2006) Primary thromboprophylaxis for cancer patients with

central venous catheters–a reappraisal of the evidence. Br J Cancer 94:189–194
66. Young AM, Billingham LJ, Begum G et al (2009) Warfarin thromboprophylaxis in cancer patients with central venous catheters (WARP): an open-label randomised trial. [see comment]. Lancet 373:567–574
67. Akl EA, Rohilla S, Barba M et al (2008) Anticoagulation for the initial treatment of venous thromboembolism in patients with cancer. Cochrane Database Syst Rev. Jan 23(1): CD006649
68. Dolovich LR, Ginsberg JS, Douketis JD, Holbrook AM, Cheah G (2000) A meta-analysis comparing low-molecular-weight heparins with unfractionated heparin in the treatment of venous thromboembolism: examining some unanswered questions regarding location of treatment, product type, and dosing frequency. Arch Intern Med 160:181–188
69. Gould MK, Dembitzer AD, Doyle RL, Hastie TJ, Garber AM (1999) Low-molecular-weight heparins compared with unfractionated heparin for treatment of acute deep venous thrombosis. A meta-analysis of randomized, controlled trials. Ann Intern Med 130:800–809
70. Kuenen BC, Levi M, Meijers JC et al (2003) Potential role of platelets in endothelial damage observed during treatment with cisplatin, gemcitabine, and the angiogenesis inhibitor SU5416. J Clin Oncol 21:2192–2198
71. Buller HR, Davidson BL, Decousus H et al (2003) Subcutaneous fondaparinux versus intravenous unfractionated heparin in the initial treatment of pulmonary embolism. N Engl J Med 349:1695–1702
72. Palareti G, Legnani C, Lee A et al (2000) A comparison of the safety and efficacy of oral anticoagulation for the treatment of venous thromboembolic disease in patients with or without malignancy. Thromb Haemost 84:805–810
73. Prandoni P, Lensing AWA, Piccioli A et al (2002) Recurrent venous thromboembolism and bleeding complications during anticoagulant treatment in patients with cancer and venous thrombosis. Blood 100:3484–3488
74. Ansell J, Hirsh J, Poller L, Bussey H, Jacobson A, Hylek E (2004) The pharmacology and management of the vitamin K antagonists: the Seventh ACCP Conference on Antithrombotic and Thrombolytic Therapy. Chest 126: 204S–233S
75. Wells PS, Holbrook AM, Crowther NR, Hirsh J (1994) Interactions of warfarin with drugs and food. Ann Intern Med 121:676–683
76. Lee AY, Levine MN, Baker RI et al (2003) Low-molecular-weight heparin versus a coumarin for the prevention of recurrent venous thromboembolism in patients with cancer. N Engl J Med 349:146–153
77. Hull RD, Pineo GF, Brant RF et al (2006) Long-term low-molecular-weight heparin versus usual care in proximal-vein thrombosis patients with cancer. Am J Med 119: 1062–1072
78. Deitcher SR, Kessler CM, Merli G, Rigas JR, Lyons RM, Fareed J (2006) Secondary prevention of venous thromboembolic events in patients with active cancer: enoxaparin alone versus initial enoxaparin followed by warfarin for a 180-day period. Clin Appl Thromb Hemost 12:389–396
79. Meyer G, Marjanovic Z, Valcke J et al (2002) Comparison of low-molecular-weight heparin and warfarin for the secondary prevention of venous thromboembolism in patients with cancer: a randomized controlled study. Arch Intern Med 162:1729–1735
80. Akl EA, Barba M, Rohilla S et al (2008) Low-Molecular-weight heparins are superior to vitamin K antagonists for the long term treatment of venous thromboembolism in patients with cancer: a Cochrane systematic review. J Exp Clin Cancer Res 27:21
81. Buller HR, Agnelli G, Hull RD, Hyers TM, Prins MH, Raskob GE (2004) Antithrombotic therapy for venous thromboembolic disease: the Seventh ACCP Conference on Antithrombotic and Thrombolytic Therapy.[see comment] [erratum appears in Chest. 2005 Jan;127(1):416]. Chest 126: 401S–428S
82. Wagman LD, Baird MF, Bennett CL et al (2006) Venous thromboembolic disease. Clinical practice guidelines in oncology. J Natl Compr Canc Netw 4:838–869
83. Girard P, Stern JB, Parent F (2002) Medical literature and vena cava filters: so far so weak. Chest 122:963–967
84. Group PS (2005) Eight-year follow-up of patients with permanent vena cava filters in the prevention of pulmonary embolism: the PREPIC (Prevention du Risque d'Embolie Pulmonaire par Interruption Cave) randomized study. [see comment]. Circulation 112:416–422

Transfusion-Related Acute Lung Injury in Children with Hematological Malignancies

35

Rachel S. Bercovitz, J. Bradley Ball, Marguerite R. Kelher, and Christopher C. Silliman

Contents

R.S. Bercovitz
Departments of Pediatrics,
School of Medicine,
University of Colorado Denver, Aurora,
CO, USA

J. Bradley Ball, and M.R. Kelher
Bonfils Blood Center, Denver, CO, USA and
Departments of Pediatrics and Surgery,
School of Medicine,
University of Colorado Denver, Aurora,
CO, USA

C.C. Silliman (✉)
Bonfils Blood Center, Denver, CO, USA and
Departments of Pediatrics and Surgery,
School of Medicine,
University of Colorado Denver, Aurora,
CO, USA and
Research Department, Bonfils Blood Center,
717 Yosemite Street, Denver, CO 80230, USA
e-mail: christopher.silliman@ucdenver.edu

35.1 Introduction

Acute lung injury (ALI) and its more severe form, acute respiratory distress syndrome (ARDS), are the rapid onset of severe pulmonary inflammation resulting in hypoxemia leading to respiratory failure [3, 6, 105]. A consensus definition was reached by the North American-European Consensus Conference (Table 35.1) to allow for proper research to better define the pathophysiology and to optimize clinical outcomes for affected patients [6]. ALI has been defined as the insidious onset of profound hypoxemia with $PaO_2/FiO_2 < 300$ mmHg (at sea level with lesser values at higher altitudes, e.g., 271 mmHg at 5,280 ft to 1,600 m) with bilateral infiltrates on x-ray without evidence of left atrial hypertension [6]. ARDS has the identical definition with PaO_2/FiO_2 ratios of <200 mmHg with similar altitude dependence [6]. These syndromes are characterized by massive leukocyte infiltration in the lungs with protein-rich exudates in the alveolar spaces [105].

The incidence of ARDS in children in the US is 12.8/100,000 person-years as calculated through a population-based, regional, prospective cohort study in contrast to previous studies from Australia-New Zealand and Germany, which demonstrated incidences of 2.95–3.4/100,000 person-years [9, 27, 109].

É. Azoulay (ed.), *Pulmonary Involvement in Patients with Hematological Malignancies*,
DOI: 10.1007/978-3-642-15742-4_35, © Springer-Verlag Berlin Heidelberg 2011

Table 35.1 Criteria for ALI [6] and TRALI [96]

The consensus definition of ALI
• Acute onset of respiratory symptoms
• No evidence of left atrial hypertension
– Pulmonary artery wedge pressure <18 mmHg[a]
• Hypoxemia
– $PaO_2/FIO_2 \leq 300$ mmHg
– Oxygen saturation ≤ 90% while on room air[b]
Additional criteria for TRALI
For patients without ALI risk factors (see Table 35.2)
– New ALI as outlined above
– Onset of symptoms during or within 6 h of the completion of a transfusion of one or more blood components
For patients with ALI risk factors[c]
– New or worsening ALI
– Onset of symptoms during or within 6 h of the completion of a transfusion of one or more blood components
Additional findings that can be associated with TRALI, but are not diagnostic
– Fever
– Hyper- or hypotension
– Transient leukopenia
– Leukocyte antibody–antigen match between donor and recipient

[a]If available. Catheter insertion is recommended only if clinically indicated

[b]Added by the NHLBI working group in 2005

[c]The clinician must evaluate the patient's course, hopefully with the assistance of the local blood bank to determine whether the patient's transfusion was causative or coincidental in the development of ALI

Table 35.2 Underlying diseases that can predispose patients to ALI and to TRALI [27, 88, 109]

Risk factors for ALI/ARDS
Direct
• Pneumonia (viral or bacterial or opportunistic)
• Bronchiolitis
• Aspiration
• Burns
• Near-drowning
Indirect
• Sepsis
• Trauma
• Pancreatitis
Risk factors for TRALI
• Patients with hematological malignancies
• Patients requiring cardiac surgery
• Recent major surgery (<24 h)
• Sepsis/acute active infection
• Massive transfusion
• Cytokine therapy
• HUS/TTP

In the past, mortality from ARDS was much higher (50–94%), but current data reported ARDS mortality between 18% and 35% with the largest single study of the syndrome at 22% [9, 27, 109]. As expected, the mortality from ALI is lower with current rates around 14–16% [27, 109]. Importantly, the largest number of children who die from ALI are immunocompromised hosts with hematopoietic stem cell transplants (HSCT) [109].

The risk factors associated with ALI/ARDS include bacterial pneumonia, sepsis, viral pneumonia, bronchiolitis, aspiration, non-pulmonary trauma, burns, near drowning, and pancreatitis (Table 35.2) [27, 109]. The largest prospective study of ALI in 328 children demonstrated that three risk factors were independently associated with mortality: (1) the initial severity of hypoxia, as documented by the PaO_2/FiO_2, (2) the presence of organ dysfunction excluding the lung and the central nervous system (CNS), and (3) CNS dysfunction [30]. For further information, the reader is encouraged to read the following articles to better understand the epidemiology, pathophysiology, risk factors for mortality and treatment [9, 27, 30, 73, 109].

Although it appears to be uncommon, ALI can be a serious complication in patients with cancer. These patients, because of the nature of their disease or its therapy, require immediate and special therapeutic interventions [10]. Unlike most of the patients who develop ALI, oncology patients have often received cytotoxic drugs, growth factors, and/or biologic response modifiers, radiation therapy, and transfusions of both packed red blood cells (PRBCs) and platelet concentrates (PCs). These treatment modalities may represent different risk factors for the development of ALI (Table 35.2). In addition to life-saving respiratory support with supplemental oxygen and proper mechanical ventilation, the patient with a hematological malignancy may require immediate cessation of the offending medication as well as the prompt administration of corticosteroids. Certainly patients with hematological malignancies are at risk for developing ALI secondary to the common risk factors, but their underlying disease, therapies, immunosuppression, and frequent need for transfusions make them a unique patient population. Lastly, transfusion-related acute lung injury (TRALI), a form of ALI that may also progress to ARDS, has been reported in a large number of patients with hematological malignancies, and TRALI may represent much of the ALI seen in the critically ill for its incidence is increasing and has been reported in 5–16.7% of critically ill patients requiring transfusion support [4, 5, 37].

35.2 Transfusion-Related Acute Lung Injury

35.2.1 Diagnosis and Treatment

In 2005, a working group from the National Heart Lung and Blood Institute expounded on the ALI criteria to define transfusion-related ALI (TRALI), which is new or worsening ALI that occurs during or within 6 h of transfusion of blood components with hypoxemia ($PaO_2/FiO_2 < 300$ mmHg) and a chest x-ray with bilateral infiltrates and a normal cardiac silhouette (Fig. 35.1). In patients who have clinical features that place them at risk for the development of ALI, the same criteria need to be met, but there is a chance that the onset of ALI in temporal relation to the transfusion is coincidental and not causative (Table 35.1) [96]. There are currently no laboratory tests or radiographic imaging that can distinguish TRALI from ALI due to other causes. Despite the definition of TRALI, it remains a diagnosis of exclusion, and all other potential causes of respiratory distress should be evaluated.

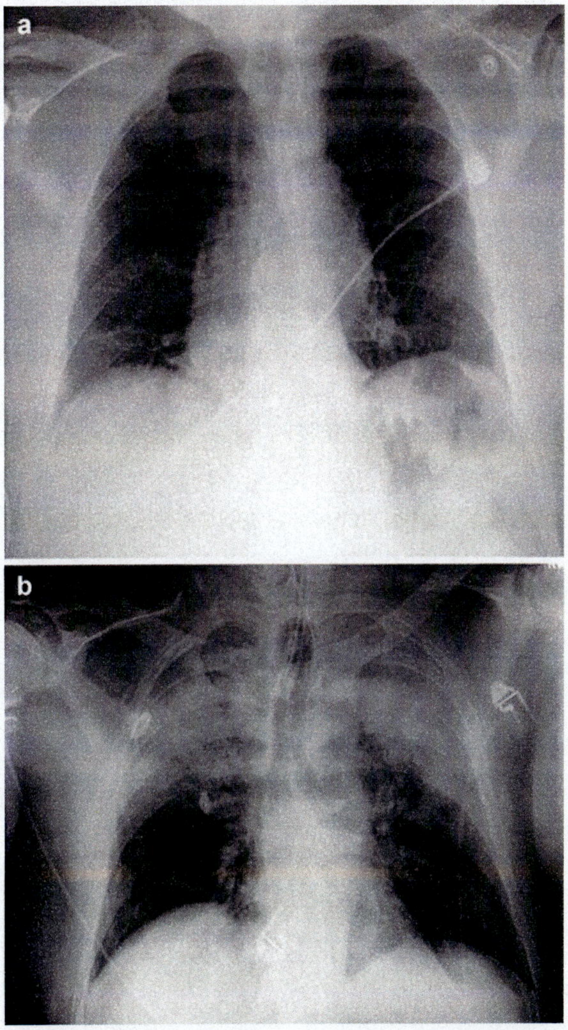

Fig. 35.1 A chest radiograph of a patient with fatal TRALI. (**a**) Radiograph taken prior to surgery. This X-ray shows normal cardiomediastinal silhouette, bilateral basilar atelectasis, and low lung volumes, but there is no evidence of pleural effusion, focal consolidation, or pneumothorax. (**b**) Radiograph taken at the time TRALI was identified. This X-ray demonstrates extensive bilateral areas of consolidation in the mid and upper lobes of the lung consistent with aspiration or edema with a normal cardiac silhouette, new since the previous examination earlier on the same day. Radiographs from N Leeborg and LK Boshkov, Deaprtment of Pathology, School of Medicine, Oregon Health Sciences University, Portland OR

That being said, there is likely underdiagnosis and underreporting of patients with clinical TRALI. The definition of TRALI also excludes patients who develop milder respiratory symptoms in the setting of a blood transfusion [19].

The etiology of TRALI has not been definitively elucidated. The pathogenesis of TRALI from both clinical studies and animal requires at least two distinct clinical events [90, 96]. The first event is the patient's underlying disease process, commonly an inflammatory process such as sepsis or newly diagnosed hematological malignancy. This inflammatory process leads to the adherence of neutrophils to the vascular endothelium and can lead to sequestration in the pulmonary vasculature. The second event is the passive transfer of antibodies or biologic response modifiers that activate the primed neutrophils causing their release of superoxide radicals. Such a model was initially proposed in the clinical "look back" studies by Van Buren, which was confirmed by the group in Denver and other "look back" studies [46, 50, 85, 90, 95, 100].

While the definition allows for symptoms to begin within 6 h of completing the transfusion, most patients become symptomatic during the transfusion or within 2 h of its completion [104]. The onset of symptoms may be as insidious as a cough, but can rapidly progress to severe dyspnea, tachypnea, hypoxia, and fatigue in the presence of a low-grade fever. The patient is usually severely hypoxemic with crackles upon auscultation of the lungs [10]. Chest radiograph demonstrates bilateral alveolar infiltrates indicative of edema, usually with a normal cardiac silhouette [10] (Fig. 35.1).

Treatment of TRALI is supportive in nature, and most patients recover within 72–96 h of the start of their symptoms. Severity can differ widely between patients; some patients may only require supplemental oxygen, while others may require either noninvasive pressure support or intubation and mechanical ventilation. There are reports of patients having sufficient respiratory failure to require extracorporeal membrane oxygenation (ECMO) [54, 57]. Steroids and diuretics are two additional therapies that have been used in patients with TRALI, but neither has been studied in a prospective trial. With regards to the use of steroids, there is no evidence that their use alters a patient's clinical course. Additional caution should be used in patients with lymphoblastic leukemia or lymphoma as corticosteroids play an important role in their therapy. A recent consensus conference has endorsed not using diuretics as they may be deleterious, presumably by decreasing the intravascular volume [88].

35.2.2 Epidemiology

TRALI has been described in patients of all ages, from infants to the elderly. While TRALI is most frequently associated with products containing more than 30 mL of plasma, all types of blood component therapy have been implicated in its development. Both patient and blood component factors contribute to the risk of developing TRALI. The patients with the highest risk of developing TRALI are those with hematological malignancies not yet in remission, patients undergoing cardiopulmonary bypass, critically ill patients, and patients with gastrointestinal (GI) bleeds [4, 37, 85]. Transfusion of blood products is an independent risk factor for the subsequent development of ALI in susceptible patients and acts in a dose-dependant manner [4].

Plasma-containing blood components are associated with the highest rates of TRALI morbidity and mortality [85]. Plasma obtained from multiparous females carries a higher risk of antibody-mediated TRALI [12, 47, 102]. In addition, studies reveal that biologic response modifiers associated with the priming of neutrophils (PMNs) accumulate in the storage of cellular blood products [48, 86, 87]. This is consistent with clinical studies associated higher rates of TRALI with older products [85].

Patients with hematological malignancies comprise a large portion of those patients who have TRALI. Silliman et al. (2003) reported on a case series of 46 patients who developed TRALI, looking at risk factors [85]. Their series included 15 pediatric patients and 31 adult patients. In the pediatric population, 12 out of the 15 patients had a hematological malignancy (leukemia or lymphoma) as their underlying disease process with 75% of those patients undergoing induction therapy at the time of their development of TRALI. Therefore, 60% of pediatric patients in this series who developed TRALI were patients with leukemia or lymphoma not in remission [85].

Of the 31 adult patients in this series, nine of them had underlying hematological malignancies (including three with myelodysplasia). The remaining six patients were undergoing induction therapy for either acute myelocytic leukemia (AML) or lymphoma. The most common underlying diagnosis in adult patients was cardiovascular disease in the setting of undergoing surgery with cardiopulmonary bypass [85]. The overall percent of patients in this series having an underlying oncologic diagnosis was 45% (21/46), and all patients had an absolute neutrophil count greater than 500/mm^3 [87], which is slightly higher than results from the Serious Hazards of Transfusion (SHOT) report published in 2009 reporting on 195 cases of TRALI, which showed 36% of patients having an underlying hematology/oncology diagnosis [12, 93]. The different incidences between these series may be due to the fact that in Silliman's series, 32% of the patients were under the age of 18, whereas in the SHOT report only 10% were pediatric patients.

The results of the Epidemiology and Survival of Transfusion Recipients (EASTR) survey recently reported on the indications for transfusion in the UK during a 12-month period in 2001–2002. Patients with benign and malignant hematological diseases made up 21% of the patients receiving PRBCs, 27% of patients receiving PCs, and 6% of patients receiving fresh frozen plasma (FFP) [106]. Comparing these results to the incidence in TRALI in a similar patient population reveals that patients with hematological malignancies are overrepresented in the population of patients who develop TRALI.

While it is more common for patients with hematological malignancies to develop TRALI during the early stages of treatment, either induction or consolidation [85], there are case reports of TRALI occurring in patients whose diseases are in remission [36]. Fung and colleagues describe two cases of pediatric patients who developed TRALI during therapy for acute myelocytic leukemia. One patient had just completed her sixth cycle of chemotherapy, while the second patient was treated with FFP prior to the initiation of any chemotherapy. In both patients, alternative diagnoses were considered including infection, fluid overload, pulmonary leukostasis, and pulmonary hemorrhage in addition to TRALI [36]. Given the frequency of blood component transfusions in oncology patients, it is important for the clinician to maintain a high level of suspicion for TRALI. Patients are not only at risk during their initial therapy; there are two case reports (one pediatric, one adult) describing patients who developed TRALI during the infusion of stem cells for treatment of acute leukemia [56, 98]. Additional case reports demonstrate patients are still at risk for TRALI following post-transplant engraftment [38, 56, 68].

35.2.3 The Role of the Neutrophil

The PMN has long been thought to be the effector cell in the pathogenesis of TRALI. Neutrophils are part of the innate immune system and emigrate to the tissues where they phagocytose invading microbes. The microbicidal arsenal of the PMNs includes both granule-based serine proteases and the NADPH oxidase, and PMNs kill bacterial or fungal pathogens by degranulation of proteases, and the formation and release of superoxide radicals into the phagolysosome or at areas of firm adherence (especially fungi). Neutrophils are not evenly distributed through the body: approximately 28% of an individual's neutrophils are located in the pulmonary pool [35]. This is a dynamic number and can increase in many clinical situations, especially in inflammation.

Neutrophils found in the body have three different stages: quiescent, primed, and activated [46]. Damaged or activated endothelium releases chemokines to recruit quiescent neutrophils, and surface selectins facilitate the tethering of PMNs to the endothelium (Fig. 35.2a). These firmly adherent PMNs are considered to be primed. Primed PMNs are firmly adherent to the vascular endothelium through β_2-integrins on the PMN and ligands, especially intercellular adhesion molecule-1 on the pulmonary microvascular endothelium (Fig. 35.2a). At this point the PMNs either diapedese through the capillary endothelial cells along a chemotactic gradient to the nidus of infection or they remain sequestered (Fig. 35.2). Importantly priming is a reversible phenomenon, and after minutes to hours these adherent PMNs regain their former malleable state of the quiescent cell and then traverse the pulmonary circulation to reenter the circulation.

With respect to PMN-mediated ALI, the adherent primed PMN is functionally hyperactive, such that agents that normally do not cause activation of the microbicidal arsenal of quiescent PMNs may activate a primed PMN [47] (Fig. 35.2b). Passive transfusion of antibodies or biologically active lipids can lead to the activation of these adherent/hyperactive PMNs, activating their microbicidal arsenal, causing release of oxidative (O_2^-) and nonoxidative (proteases) focused at the points of firm adhesion to the pulmonary vascular endothelium (Fig. 35.2b). This activation of the PMN

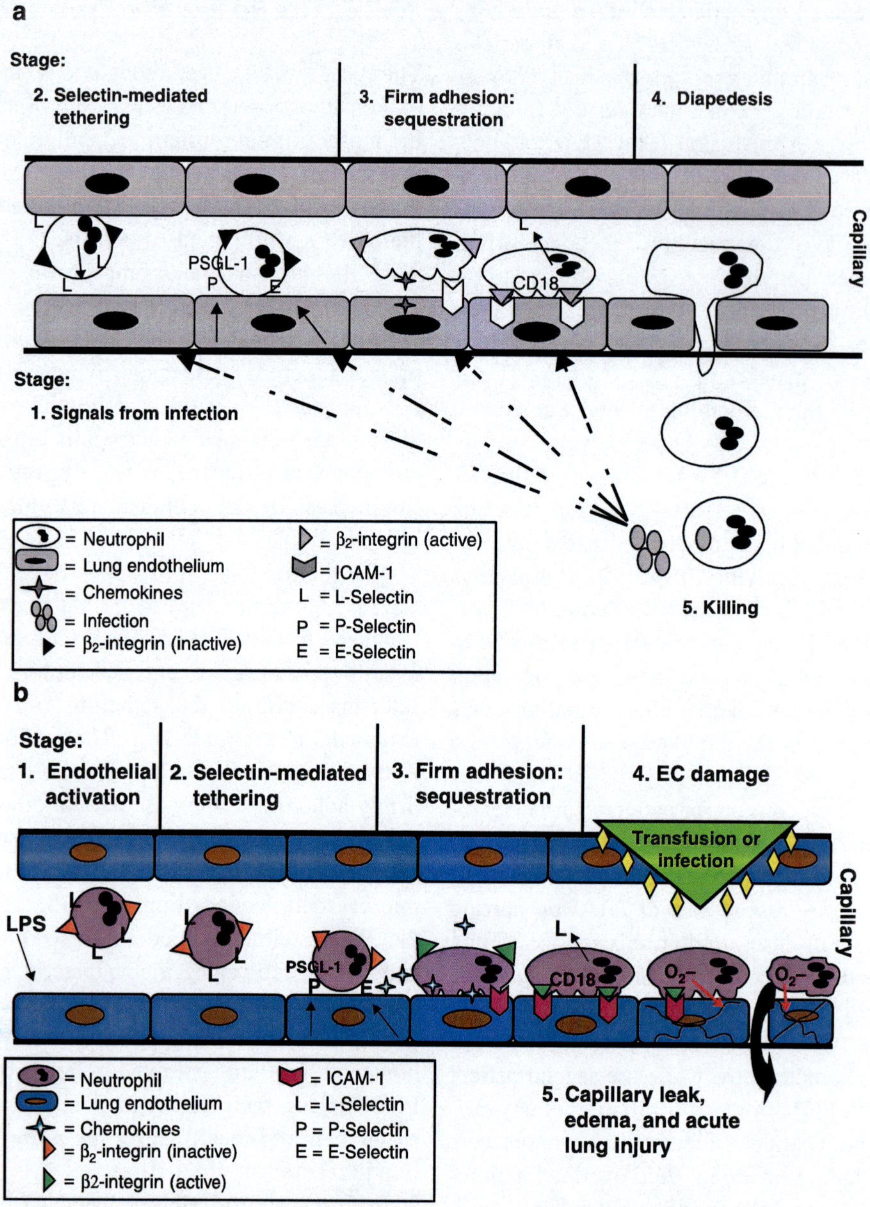

Fig. 35.2 (**a**) Normal PMN physiology. From an infection (*ovals*) in the tissues: (1) signals (*LPS*) are sent out (*arrows*) that activate ECs causing (2) chemokine release (*crosses*) and attraction, tethering, and (3) firm ICAM-1:CD11b/CD18 adherence. PMNs diapedese (4) and chemotax to the site of infection and kill the pathogens. (**b**) PMN-mediated ALI. In response to intravascular stimuli (LPS, cytokines, lipids), ECs become (1) activated and release chemokines (*crosses*), which cause PMN attraction, (2) tethering, and ICAM-1: CD11/CD18 firm adherence (3). A second intravascular stimulus including transfusion of specific antibodies against host PMN antigens or transfusion of BRMs activate these primed, adherent PMNs (4) causing EC damage, capillary leak, and TRALI (5). (This figure was published in Silliman CC et al. (2005) The role of endothelial activation in the pathogenesis of transfusion-related acute lung injury. Transfusion 45 (suppl) 109S–116s.)

microbicidal arsenal causes endothelial damage at the sites of sequestration, resulting in endothelial damage, capillary leak, and TRALI (Fig. 35.2b). Postmortem histological evaluation has confirmed that PMNs appear to be required for the lung injury in TRALI, and animal studies have demonstrated that TRALI can be inhibited by rendering the rodents neutropenic [45, 59] (Fig. 35.3).

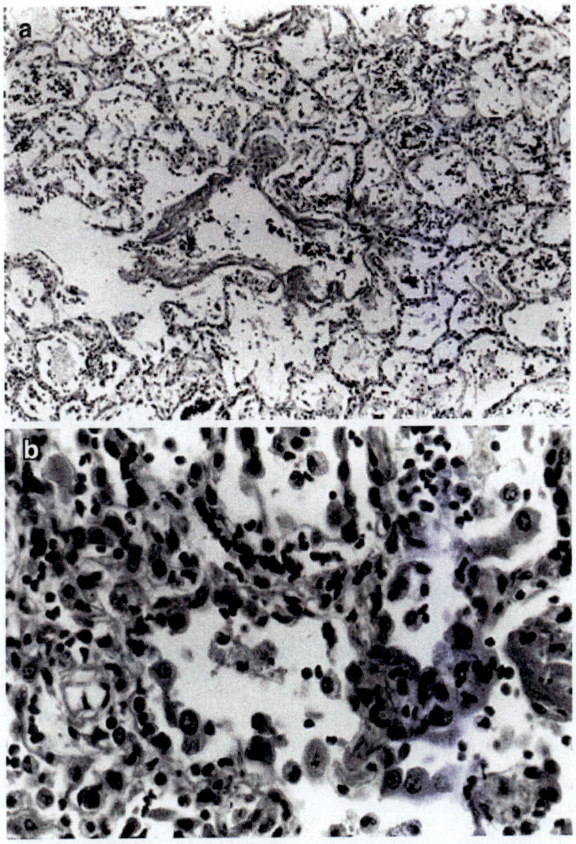

Fig. 35.3 Thin sections of fixed lung from a patient with fatal TRALI demonstrating acute diffuse alveolar infiltrate with intra-alveolar edema, hyaline membrane formation, and scant interstitial inflammation. There was not histological evidence of infection, and all cultures from the lung, bacterial, viral, and fungal, were negative, as were the patient's blood cultures. The magnification of the micrographs is 40× in image (**a**) and 440× in image (**b**). The images are taken from [89]

35.3 Etiology of TRALI: Antibody- and Nonantibody-Mediated TRALI

35.3.1 The Role of Human Leukocyte Antigen, Major Histocompatibility Complex Class I Antibodies

Anti-leukocyte antibodies are thought to be etiologic in most cases of TRALI, whether they are anti-human leukocyte antigen (HLA) or anti-human neutrophil antigen (HNA). Major histocompatibility complex (MHC) Class I antigens are expressed on all nucleated cells and present antigen fragments to cytotoxic T-cells alerting the immune system of a cell that is foreign, infected, or has become malignant. There is great variability in the portion of the MHC region responsible for antigen presentation. This variety stems from the over 2,500 possible Class I alleles and puts individuals at risk for developing HLA antibodies when exposed to blood products from either transfusion or childbirth.

Multiparous women are at the highest risk of having HLA antibodies, and the prevalence increases with each subsequent pregnancy [20,71]. Triulzi et al. (2009) demonstrated that 1.7% of nulliparous women and 1% of men have HLA antibodies, whereas nearly one third of women with four or more pregnancies have HLA antibodies [97]. This increase in HLA antibody prevalence increased incrementally with each pregnancy from 1.7% to 11.2%, 22.3%, 27.5% and 32.3% (1, 2, 3, and 4 pregnancies, respectively [97]. The difference in HLA antibody prevalence between male and multiparous female derived plasma has been well known and this difference prompted the British Transfusion Service to move to male-only plasma for transfusion in 2003. This switch has shown promise in decreasing rates of TRALI from a total of 59 cases in 2003–2004 to 34 cases in 2006–2007 [12, 97].

Early reports of TRALI showed the presence of anti-HLA or anti-granulocyte antibodies in almost 90% of units implicated in TRALI [71]. A meta-analysis of case reports and case series looking at the prevalence of HLA antibodies in TRALI confirmed this earlier observation and found HLA antibodies in 86% of TRALI cases compared to 28% of patients who did not develop TRALI [102]. These studies, while comprehensive, looked only for HLA antibodies in the donor and not for the cognate antigen in the recipient. Data from the Netherlands hemovigilance program suggest that not all patients who developed TRALI after being infused with donor HLA antibodies had the related antigen. They showed that in 49 patients with TRALI, while 73% (36/49) of donor samples had anti-leukocyte antibodies, only 58% (21/36) of those recipients had the cognate antigen [102]. Of the 21 donor samples with anti-HLA antibodies, 43% (9/21) were against HLA Class I. In another study of 44 patients with ALI after transfusion, 16% of cases had antibody–antigen matches despite 68% of the patients receiving products with HLA or anti-granulocyte antibodies [110].

The narrow focus of only looking for HLA antibodies in the donor without evaluating HLA antigens in the recipient can lead to an overestimation antibody-mediated TRALI. There is a report of a lung transplant patient developing TRALI in the transplanted lung, but not in her native lung [21]. Further laboratory investigation revealed that the donor blood contained anti-HLA-B44 antibodies. Only the donor lung had the cognate HLA-B44 antigen, whereas the patient only expressed HLA-B35 and HLA-B62 [21]. The marked difference in radiographic findings between the transplanted and native lung suggest that the presence of donor HLA antibodies is not sufficient to produce the second hit necessary for neutrophil priming. In addition, this case also represents one of immune complex deposition on the surface of the transplanted lung and provides clinical support for the animal model of Looney et al. [59]. There must be a specific antibody–antigen interaction to get the necessary immunologic response. One might conclude that the remaining 42% of patients in the Dutch study who did not have proven incompatibility with the donors HLA antibody, may have had nonimmune-mediated TRALI and that the finding of donor HLA-antibodies was coincidental, not causative.

The passive transfer of HLA antibodies to recipients who have the matching antigen is insufficient to cause TRALI in the absence of other risk factors. Two look-back studies have been performed to look at other patients receiving blood products from a donor implicated in a case of TRALI. Both of these studies demonstrate that despite having the cognate antigen to the donor's antibody (either HNA or HLA), the majority did not develop TRALI [50, 95, 108]. Kopko and associates looked at a donor with anti-HNA-3a antibodies and found that while only one recipient was diagnosed with clinical TRALI, 36% of the remaining studied recipients had some degree of respiratory distress in association with the transfusion, none of which was reported at possible TRALI a the time [50]. Their findings differ from those of both Win and Toy and their colleagues, who performed similar look-back studies, which did not show any other transfusion complications in patients with the matching HLA antigen to the donor's antibody [95, 108]. Given the under-reporting of TRALI and transfusion-associated respiratory symptoms [108], it is possible that some cases of TRALI were missed. These look-back studies suggest that TRALI is multi-factorial in nature: (1) requiring the transfusion of HLA or HNA antibodies into a patient with the cognate antigen and (2) an underlying condition that predisposes them to the development of TRALI.

Animal models have been developed to try to elucidate more information on the etiology of TRALI. Many of these models fail to recapitulate the exact process of TRALI and are not consistent with the clinical TRALI we see in patients [60, 82]. Lögdberg and colleagues published a summary of the available literature about current in vivo and ex vivo animal models [59]. Many of the models are based on the two-hit hypothesis and have used HNA antibodies, bioactive lipids, and HLA antibodies as the second insult [65, 82, 101]. Kelher and associates have developed a model in Sprague-Dawley rats that uses lipopolysaccharide (LPS) to produce underlying inflammation for the first hit and then infused the rats with MHC I antibodies [46]. They were able to demonstrate pulmonary capillary leak, which occurred over a similar time course as in clinical TRALI as well as a dose-dependent response to the antibodies. There was no evidence of pulmonary damage in the absence of either LPS or the MHC I antibodies [46]. This model not only confirms the two-hit hypothesis, but also the role that antibodies to MHC class I antigens play in the development of TRALI.

35.3.2 The Role of HLA MHC Class II Antibodies

Antibodies specific for HLA class II antigens have been implicated in a large number of patients with TRALI who express the cognate antigens [23, 37, 52, 103, 107]. Binding of specific HLA class II antibodies to their cognate antigens on monocytes in vitro resulted in intracellular synthesis of TNFα, IL-1β,and tissue factor over a 4-h time period as compared to identical monocytes incubated with control sera [51]. Moreover, incubation (20 h) of monocytes that express the cognate antigens with antibodies to these HLA class II antigens resulted in the production of both cytokines and chemokines (IL-8, GROα); the latter peptides could certainly activate neutrophils sequestered in the lung [79]. Recent in vitro studies demonstrated that co-cultures of human pulmonary microvascular endothelial cells (HMVECs) and monocytes stimulated with antibodies to HLA class II antigens expressed on the monocytes lead to the release of leukotriene B_4 (LTB_4) and TNFα into the supernatant with concomitant apoptosis of HMVECs [66, 67]. These experiments also identified the importance of monocytes and the HMVECs together because if alone, minimal LTB_4 was produced, and if an interfering anti-Dr antibody was introduced, HMVEC apoptosis and mediator release was inhibited [66, 67]. Lastly, because HLA class II antigens may be expressed on endothelial cells (EC), the infusion of class II antibodies into a recipient with the cognate antigen present on the pulmonary EC may manifest TRALI due to antibody-mediated EC activation, fenestration, and mild leak [51].

Although attractive, this model of TRALI raises two major issues: (1) while the synthesis of cytokines by circulating monocytes has the potential to cause TRALI, there is a significant time delay (4–20 h) for the synthesis of these cytokines and chemokines, and at 4 h these cytokines were never released extracellularly [51, 79]. By definition, TRALI occurs within 6 h of transfusion with most of the reactions occurring during or 1–2 h following transfusion; thus, the synthesis of chemokines and cytokines over a 20-h time period may have little to do with TRALI [40, 51, 79, 96]. In contrast, the production of LTB_4 and TNFα in the model of Nishimura et al. is temporally consistent with TRALI. However, this model requires further elucidation because the number of circulating monocytes in contact with the pulmonary EC must be relatively high as monocytes contain the LTA_4 hydrolase to synthesize LTB_4 from LTA_4. ECs alone can only synthesize the cysteinyl leukotrienes via activation of the LTA_4 synthetase and glutathione (LTC_4, LTD_4, and LTE_4) [40, 53, 70, 80, 83]. (2) Pathologic examination of lungs from a fatal TRALI reaction attributed to HLA class II antibodies documented that there were no HLA class II antigens on the pulmonary EC [39]. In addition, although prolonged (72 h) in vitro cytokine exposure has led to the surface expression of HLA class II molecules on neutrophils, HLA class II antigen expression on the neutrophil surface has only been demonstrated in patients treated with G-CSF or GM-CSF, and although such cytokine exposure may predispose these individuals to TRALI, this group of patients is largely neutropenic from chemotherapy and may not manifest neutrophil-mediated ALI [39, 58, 63, 74, 90, 92, 109]. These data are important because some interaction must occur between the pulmonary EC and the monocytes to produce clinically relevant amounts of LTB_4, and the expression of HLA class II molecules is one potential factor.

35.3.3 Laboratory Investigation of HLA Antibodies

The laboratory investigation of HLA class I and II antibodies will not be discussed in detail as the techniques are widely disseminated, and there are excellent, recent reviews available [32, 110]. It is important to note that many of the assays employed are highly sensitive techniques to detect the presence of any antibodies in donor or recipient sera that could be clinically relevant leading to graft rejection and/or graft versus host disease. Because HLA antibody screening is widely available, it is often the first step in many TRALI investigations when screening implicated donors; however, two reports revealed that a disproportionately small number of HLA class I antibodies actually induce TRALI [17, 95]. With this in mind, as well as the high sensitivity of current HLA techniques, one questions the clinical relevance of all of the HLA antibodies detected in TRALI because most of the current flow-based assays are so sensitive that a relatively high percentage of non-transfused males demonstrated antibodies [28, 97]. Similarly, current flow-based assays used to detect antibodies to HLA class II antigens in donors are designed to detect very small amounts of antibodies using a PRA luminex bead assay (One Lambda, Canoga Park, CA). These tests may overestimate the role of antibodies to HLA class II antigens in TRALI because: (1) no titers of antibody concentration are employed; (2) without sufficient modeling of HLA class II antibody-mediated TRALI, it is not known what concentration is applicable; (3) the role of the antibody has been thought to be neutrophil-dependent although neutrophils do not "naturally" express HLA class II antigens [32, 46, 71].

Recently, the current Leukocyte Antibody Prevalence Study (LAPS) determined the prevalence of HLA class I and II antibodies in large cohorts of non-transfused males, transfused males, nulliparous females, and parous females [97]. Separate analyses were generated for both antibodies to HLA class I and class II antigens and stratified by donor group, and the data were log transformed such that positives were defined as three standard deviations above the mean.

Samples were considered antibody positive with normalized background ratios of >10.8 for HLA class I antibodies and >6.9 for HLA class II antibodies. In the flow-based testing for HLA class II antibodies, which implicated them as etiologic for TRALI, percentage shifts as low as 8–10% in the mean fluorescence intensity were deemed positive, although these assays did not employ Luminex beads [39, 51, 72]. These very small flow shifts may be important for successful solid organ transplantation, but their relevance is not defined in TRALI.

Effective HLA antibody screening methods for blood donors from various testing sites reveal challenges in differentiating background noise and defining suitable cutoffs such that if this new normal range of cutoffs is employed, some antibodies implicated in TRALI never reach a positive titer [28, 44, 78, 97]. Furthermore, the clinical effects of transfused HLA antibodies may be attenuated due to absorption by lymphocytes or platelets, and neutralization by soluble HLA class I molecules, which comprise the majority of HLA class I antigens in the blood [45]. One notable exception is HLA-A2, which has been implicated in many TRALI cases and thus should be included in any first line TRALI investigation screen [41, 71,77].

35.3.4 Nonantibody TRALI: The Role of Biologic Response Modifiers

Many of the cases of TRALI can be linked to a donor-recipient antibody–antigen incompatibility. However, as the studies by van Stein and Zupanska show, there are some cases where no HLA or HNA antibodies are present in the blood component or the cognate antigen is not expressed by the recipient [102, 110]. These cases of nonimmune TRALI may be explained by the accumulation of agents in stored blood that have the ability to prime neutrophils, which then activate the respiratory burst of neutrophils sequestered in the pulmonary circulation. Such agents include proinflammatory lipids, lysophosphatidylcholines and neutral lipids, and CD40 ligand. Many of these agents have been shown to either damage human pulmonary microvascular endothelial cell monolayers or cause ALI in animal models, or both [46, 48].

Lipid accumulation during the routine storage of pRBCs is more prevalent in older products and is likely derived from the red blood cell membranes. Lysophosphatidylcholines and other neutral lipids accumulate during the storage interval such that their concentration is greatly increased during storage as compared to day 1 and have the ability to cause TRALI in animal models. These lipids augment the respiratory burst of fMLP-primed neutrophils and PMN cytotoxicity in vitro and in vivo.

Due to their underlying disease process, patients with hematological malignancies may have activated vascular endothelium, putting them at risk for pulmonary neutrophil sequestration. For patients who have undergone treatment for their disease, the therapy they have received, specifically total body irradiation (TBI) in preparation for HSCT, can activate the pulmonary endothelium [26]. This damage can serve as the first step of the neutrophil priming and activation cascade. With regards to traditional chemotherapies, their PMN priming activity has not been evaluated; however, a study of a novel priming agent designed to decrease bacterial infections during periods of neutropenia suggests that PMN activity can be enhanced after chemotherapy administration [34].

There is a report of ARDS occurring in neutropenic patients after bone marrow transplantation. These patients, at autopsy, had no findings consistent with neutrophil sequestration, but had typical findings of ALI, suggesting that the lung injury occurs by neutrophil-independent mechanisms [42]. ALI in neutropenic patients may be secondary to TRALI if the diagnostic criteria are met and can indicate that neutrophil-independent mechanisms may also play a role in the development of TRALI.

While there are a number of case reports of TRALI occurring in both cancer and HSCT patients, there are only a handful of cases that describe TRALI in the setting of neutropenia. Citak and colleagues report on an 18 month old who developed TRALI during late engraftment following an autologous HSCT for stage IV neuroblastoma [15]. The patient did not appear to show engraftment until day +67, when she had an absolute neutrophil count (ANC) of about 700/mL. On this day, she received a unit of PRBCs and developed respiratory distress consistent with TRALI. The following day, her ANC was significantly elevated at 4,000/mL, which puts her neutrophil count within the normal range, making this a case of TRALI that occurred concomitantly with engraftment. A more striking example was the case of a patient with

Burkitt's lymphoma who developed TRALI while at the neutropenic nadir. There was no identified antibody–antigen incompatibility; however, the implicated unit of PC was found to have very high levels of vascular endothelial growth factor (VEGF), a known capillary permeability agonist.

35.4 Treatment-Related Risk Factors for ALI in Patients with Hematologic Malignancies

Throughout this book, other clinical scenarios that may result in ALI in patients with hematological malignancies are reported. Because TRALI is a diagnosis of exclusion, it is particularly important to be aware of possible factors that may mimic ALI in this patient group.

35.5 TRALI Mitigation

Current mitigation strategies in the UK and by the American Red Cross have used male-only plasma transfusion regimens and have decreased the number of fatal TRALI reactions due to antibody-mediated TRALI [12, 22]. A number of blood centers use males plus nulliparous females to arrive at antibody-negative plasma transfusion regimes, including our center. Similar male-only platelet transfusion strategies are being implemented, and in some areas the replacement of plasma in PCs with additive solutions are being considered to decrease that amount of plasma transfused. Other investigators are developing rapid high-throughput assays to test for the presence of HLA antibodies in their donors. With regard to PRBCs, there are no mitigation strategies even in the planning stages, even though transfusion of PRBCs was responsible for 17% of the fatal TRALI cases [23]. Washing of cellular products eliminates all of the implicated HLA or HNA antibodies as well as the biologic response modifiers; however, it is time consuming, expensive, and may result in PCs that do not have the same hemostatic potential as unmodified PCs. Antibodies to HNAs present a particular problem, for they are not the result of maternal exposure to fetal leukocytes [97]. Their detection is cumbersome, and adequate testing for their presence is only performed in a few specialized laboratories worldwide.

35.6 Concluding Remarks

ALI and its more severe form, ARDS, are not common in children with hematological malignancies, but these patients do seem overrepresented among patients who develop TRALI. ALI, regardless of the etiology, presents a life-threatening complication that requires rapid intervention, including respiratory support and supportive care, cessation of the offending chemotherapy agent or biotherapeutic agent, and prompt intervention of corticosteroids if indicated. The therapy for TRALI is purely supportive, and generally patients have a resolution of their symptoms within 72–96 h. Supportive care for patients with hematological malignancies undergoing chemotherapy should be judicious, and it is important to note that certain modalities, especially the transfusion of plasma to children with ALI/ARDS correlated with increased mortality [14]. Patients with hematological malignancies have increased risk factors predisposing them to the development of TRALI: exposure to cytotoxic medications, frequent transfusion requirements, radiation therapy, but their frequent periods of neutropenia, which often coincide with their need for PRBC and platelet transfusions, may be protective against the development of TRALI, thought to be mediated by neutrophil priming and activation.

Acknowledgments This work was supported by Bonfils Blood Center, The Department of Pediatrics, School of Medicine, University of Colorado Denver, Aurora, CO, and grant GM49222 from NIGMS, NIH.

References

1. Arning M, Kliche KO, Schneider W (1991) GM-CSF therapy and capillary-leak syndrome. Ann Hematol 62:83
2. Asami K, Sasazaki Y, Utsumi J (1995) Successful treatment of retinoic acid syndrome with high-dose dexamethasone pulse therapy in a child with acute promyelocytic leukemia treated with ATRA. Acta Paediatr Jpn 37:384–387
3. Ashbaugh DG, Bigelow DB, Petty TL, Levine BE (1967) Acute respiratory distress in adults. Lancet 2:319–323
4. Benson AB, Moss M, Silliman CC (2009) Transfusion-related acute lung injury (TRALI): a clinical review with

emphasis on the critically ill. Br J Haematol 147(4): 431–443
5. Benson AG, Moss M, Silliman CC (2009) Transfusion-associated acute respiratory distress syndrome (ARDS) in patients with gastrointestinal bleeding: effect of end stage liver disease and the use of fresh frozen plasma. p A4639
6. Bernard GR, Artigas A, Brigham KL, Carlet J, Falke K, Hudson L, Lamy M, LeGall JR, Morris A, Spragg R (1994) Report of the American-European Consensus conference on acute respiratory distress syndrome: definitions, mechanisms, relevant outcomes, and clinical trial coordination. Consensus Committee. J Crit Care 9:72–81
7. Bernstein ML, Sobel DB, Wimmer RS (1982) Noncardiogenic pulmonary edema following injection of methotrexate into the cerebrospinal fluid. Cancer 50:866–868
8. Bilgrami S, Bona RD, Edwards RL, Li Z, Naqvi B, Shaikh A, Furlong F, Fox J, Clive J, Tutschka PJ (2001) Dexamethasone, paclitaxel, etoposide, cyclophosphamide (d-TEC) and G-CSF for stem cell mobilisation in multiple myeloma. Bone Marrow Transplant 28:137–143
9. Bindl L, Dresbach K, Lentze MJ (2005) Incidence of acute respiratory distress syndrome in German children and adolescents: a population-based study. Crit Care Med 33:209–312
10. Briasoulis E, Pavlidis N (2001) Noncardiogenic pulmonary edema: an unusual and serious complication of anticancer therapy. Oncologist 6:153–161
11. Buchali A, Feyer P, Groll J, Massenkeil G, Arnold R, Budach V (2000) Immediate toxicity during fractionated total body irradiation as conditioning for bone marrow transplantation. Radiother Oncol 54:157–162
12. Chapman CE, Stainsby D, Jones H, Love E, Massey E, Win N, Navarrete C, Lucas G, Soni N, Morgan C, Choo L, Cohen H, Williamson LM (2009) Ten years of hemovigilance reports of transfusion-related acute lung injury in the United Kingdom and the impact of preferential use of male donor plasma. Transfusion 49:440–452
13. Chen ZX, Xue YQ, Zhang R, Tao RF, Xia XM, Li C, Wang W, Zu WY, Yao XZ, Ling BJ (1991) A clinical and experimental study on all-trans retinoic acid-treated acute promyelocytic leukemia patients. Blood 78:1413–1419
14. Church GD, Matthay MA, Liu K, Milet M, Flori HR (2009) Blood product transfusions and clinical outcomes in pediatric patients with acute lung injury. Pediatr Crit Care Med 10:297–302
15. Citak EC, Kesik V, Atay AA, Sari E, Kismet E, Koseoglu V (2008) Transfusion-related acute lung injury in a child with neuroblastoma during a late engraftment period of autologous stem cell transplantation. Pediatr Transplant 12: 235–237
16. Cogliati AA, Conti G, Tritapepe L, Canneti A, Rosa G (2002) Noninvasive ventilation in the treatment of acute respiratory failure induced by all-trans retinoic acid (retinoic acid syndrome) in children with acute promyelocytic leukemia. Pediatr Crit Care Med 3:70–73
17. Cooling L (2002) Transfusion-related acute lung injury. JAMA 288:315–316
18. Cupitt JM (2000) A case for steroids in acute lung injury associated with the retinoic acid syndrome. Anaesth Intensive Care 28:202–204
19. Davis A, Mandal R, Johnson M, Makar R, Stowell C, Dzik S (2008) A touch of TRALI. Transfusion 48:541–545
20. Densmore TL, Goodnough LT, Ali S, Dynis M, Chaplin H (1999) Prevalence of HLA sensitization in female apheresis donors. Transfusion 39:103–106
21. Dykes A, Smallwood D, Kotsimbos T, Street A (2000) Transfusion-related acute lung injury (Trali) in a patient with a single lung transplant. Br J Haematol 109:674–676
22. Eder AF, Benjamin RJ (2009) TRALI risk reduction: donor and component management strategies. J Clin Apher 24: 122–129
23. Eder AF, Herron R, Strupp A, Dy B, Notari EP, Chambers LA, Dodd RY, Benjamin RJ (2007) Transfusion-related acute lung injury surveillance (2003–2005) and the potential impact of the selective use of plasma from male donors in the American Red Cross. Transfusion 47: 599–607
24. Eigen H, Wyszomierski D (1985) Bleomycin lung injury in children. Pathophysiology and guidelines for management. Am J Pediatr Hematol Oncol 7:71–78
25. Emminger W, Emminger-Schmidmeier W, Peters C, Susani M, Hawliczek R, Hocker P, Gadner H (1990) Capillary leak syndrome during low dose granulocyte-macrophage colony-stimulating factor (rh GM-CSF) treatment of a patient in a continuous febrile state. Blut 61:219–221
26. Epperly MW, Sikora CA, DeFilippi SJ, Gretton JE, Bar-Sagi D, Archer H, Carlos T, Guo H, Greenberger JS (2002) Pulmonary irradiation-induced expression of VCAM-I and ICAM-I is decreased by manganese superoxide dismutase-plasmid/liposome (MnSOD-PL) gene therapy. Biol Blood Marrow Transplant 8:175–187
27. Erickson S, Schibler A, Numa A, Nuthall G, Yung M, Pascoe E, Wilkins B (2007) Acute lung injury in pediatric intensive care in Australia and New Zealand: a prospective, multicenter, observational study. Pediatr Crit Care Med 8: 317–323
28. Fadeyi E, Adams S, Peterson B, Hackett J, Byrne P, Klein HG, Marincola FM, Leitman SF, Stroncek DF (2008) Analysis of a high-throughput HLA antibody screening assay for use with platelet donors. Transfusion 48: 1174–1179
29. Fauroux B, Meyer-Milsztain A, Boccon-Gibod L, Leverger G, Clement A, Biour M, Tournier G (1994) Cytotoxic drug-induced pulmonary disease in infants and children. Pediatr Pulmonol 18:347–355
30. Flori HR, Glidden DV, Rutherford GW, Matthay MA (2005) Pediatric acute lung injury: prospective evaluation of risk factors associated with mortality. Am J Respir Crit Care Med 171:995–1001
31. Frankel SR, Eardley A, Lauwers G, Weiss M, Warrell RP Jr (1992) The "retinoic acid syndrome" in acute promyelocytic leukemia. Ann Intern Med 117:292–296
32. Fuggle SV, Martin S (2008) Tools for human leukocyte antigen antibody detection and their application to transplanting sensitized patients. Transplantation 86:384–390
33. Fulkerson WJ, McLendon RE, Prosnitz LR (1986) Adult respiratory distress syndrome after limited thoracic radiotherapy. Cancer 57:1941–1946
34. Fung YL, Silliman CC (2009) The role of neutrophils in the pathogenesis of transfusion-related acute lung injury. Transfus Med Rev 23:266–283
35. Fung YL, Williams BA (2006) TRALI in 2 cases of leukemia. J Pediatr Hematol Oncol 28:391–394

36. Gajic O, Rana R, Winters JL, Yilmaz M, Mendez JL, Rickman OB, O'Byrne MM, Evenson LK, Malinchoc M, DeGoey SR, Afessa B, Hubmayr RD, Moore SB (2007) Transfusion-related acute lung injury in the critically ill: prospective nested case-control study. Am J Respir Crit Care Med 176:886–891
37. Ganguly S, Carrum G, Nizzi F, Heslop HE, Popat U (2004) Transfusion-related acute lung injury (TRALI) following allogeneic stem cell transplant for acute myeloid leukemia. Am J Hematol 75:48–51
38. Gosselin EJ, Wardwell K, Rigby WF, Guyre PM (1993) Induction of MHC class II on human polymorphonuclear neutrophils by granulocyte/macrophage colony-stimulating factor, IFN-gamma, and IL-3. J Immunol 151:1482–1490
39. Gronert K, Clish CB, Romano M, Serhan CN (1999) Transcellular regulation of eicosanoid biosynthesis. Methods Mol Biol 120:119–144
40. Hierholzer C, Harbrecht B, Menezes JM, Kane J, MacMicking J, Nathan CF, Peitzman AB, Billiar TR, Tweardy DJ (1998) Essential role of induced nitric oxide in the initiation of the inflammatory response after hemorrhagic shock. J Exp Med 187:917–928
41. Hirayama F (2009) Recent advances in laboratory assays for nonhemolytic transfusion reactions. Transfusion
42. Jules-Elysee K, White DA (1990) Bleomycin-induced pulmonary toxicity. Clin Chest Med 11:1–20
43. Kao GS, Wood IG, Dorfman DM, Milford EL, Benjamin RJ (2003) Investigations into the role of anti-HLA class II antibodies in TRALI. Transfusion 43:185–191
44. Kao KJ, Scornik JC, Riley WJ, McQueen CF (1988) Association between HLA phenotype and HLA concentration in plasma or platelets. Hum Immunol 21:115–124
45. Kelher MR, Masuno T, Moore EE, Damle S, Meng X, Song Y, Liang X, Niedzinski J, Geier SS, Khan SY, Gamboni-Robertson F, Silliman CC (2009) Plasma from stored packed red blood cells and MHC class I antibodies causes acute lung injury in a two-event in vivo rat model. Blood 113:2079–2087
46. Keller-Stanislawski B, Lohmann A, Gunay S, Heiden M, Funk MB (2009) The German Haemovigilance System-reports of serious adverse transfusion reactions between 1997 and 2007. Transfus Med 19(6):340–349
47. Khan SY, Kelher MR, Heal JM, Blumberg N, Boshkov LK, Phipps R, Gettings KF, McLaughlin NJ, Silliman CC (2006) Soluble CD40 ligand accumulates in stored blood components, primes neutrophils through CD40, and is a potential cofactor in the development of transfusion-related acute lung injury. Blood 108:2455–2462
48. Kopko PM, Holland PV (1999) Transfusion-related acute lung injury. Br J Haematol 105:322–329
49. Kopko PM, Marshall CS, MacKenzie MR, Holland PV, Popovsky MA (2002) Transfusion-related acute lung injury: report of a clinical look-back investigation. JAMA 287: 1968–1971
50. Kopko PM, Paglieroni TG, Popovsky MA, Muto KN, MacKenzie MR, Holland PV (2003) TRALI: correlation of antigen-antibody and monocyte activation in donor-recipient pairs. Transfusion 43:177–184
51. Kopko PM, Popovsky MA, MacKenzie MR, Paglieroni TG, Muto KN, Holland PV (2001) HLA class II antibodies in transfusion-related acute lung injury. Transfusion 41: 1244–1248
52. Krump E, Picard S, Mancini J, Borgeat P (1997) Suppression of leukotriene B4 biosynthesis by endogenous adenosine in ligand-activated human neutrophils. J Exp Med 186: 1401–1406
53. Kuroda H, Masuda Y, Imaizumi H, Kozuka Y, Asai Y, Namiki A (2009) Successful extracorporeal membranous oxygenation for a patient with life-threatening transfusion-related acute lung injury. J Anesth 23:424–426
54. Latini P, Aristei C, Aversa F, Checcaglini F, Maranzano E, Raymondi C, Panizza BM, Perrucci E, Martelli MF (1991) Lung damage following bone marrow transplantation after hyperfractionated total body irradiation. Radiother Oncol 22:127–132
55. Leach M, Vora AJ, Jones DA, Lucas G (1998) Transfusion-related acute lung injury (TRALI) following autologous stem cell transplant for relapsed acute myeloid leukaemia: a case report and review of the literature. Transfus Med 8:333–337
56. Lee AJ, Koyyalamudi PL, Martinez-Ruiz R (2008) Severe transfusion-related acute lung injury managed with extracorporeal membrane oxygenation (ECMO) in an obstetric patient. J Clin Anesth 20:549–552
57. Lei L, Altstaedt J, von der OM, Proft T, Gross U, Rink L (2001) Induction of interleukin-8 in human neutrophils after MHC class II cross-linking with superantigens. J Leukoc Biol 70:80–86
58. Logdberg LE, Vikulina T, Zimring JC, Hillyer CD (2009) Animal models of transfusion-related acute lung injury. Transfus Med Rev 23:13–24
59. Looney MR, Su X, Van Ziffle JA, Lowell CA, Matthay MA (2006) Neutrophils and their Fc gamma receptors are essential in a mouse model of transfusion-related acute lung injury. J Clin Invest 116:1615–1623
60. Loyd JE, Bolds JM, Wickersham N, Malcolm AW, Brigham KL (1988) Corticosteroids prevent acute lung dysfunction caused by thoracic irradiation in unanesthetized sheep. Am Rev Respir Dis 138:1227–1233
61. Marina NM, Greenwald CA, Fairclough DL, Thompson EI, Wilimas JA, Mackert PW, Hudson MM, Stokes DC, Bozeman PM (1995) Serial pulmonary function studies in children treated for newly diagnosed Hodgkin's disease with mantle radiotherapy plus cycles of cyclophosphamide, vincristine, and procarbazine alternating with cycles of doxorubicin, bleomycin, vinblastine, and dacarbazine. Cancer 75:1706–1711
62. Matsumoto S, Takei M, Moriyama M, Imanishi H (1987) Enhancement of Ia-like antigen expression by interferon-gamma in polymorphonuclear leukocytes. Chem Pharm Bull (Tokyo) 35:436–439
63. Matthews JH (1993) Pulmonary toxicity of ABVD chemotherapy and G-CSF in Hodgkin's disease: possible synergy. Lancet 342:988
64. Middelburg RA, Van SD, Briet E, van der Bom JG (2008) The role of donor antibodies in the pathogenesis of transfusion-related acute lung injury: a systematic review. Transfusion 48:2167–2176
65. Nishimura M, Hashimoto S, Satake M, Okazaki H, Tadokoro K (2007) Interference with TRALI-causing anti-HLA DR alloantibody induction of human pulmonary microvascular endothelial cell injury by purified soluble HLA DR. Vox Sang 93:78–82
66. Nishimura M, Takanashi M, Okazaki H, Satake M, Nakajima K (2006) Role of CD7 expressed in lung microvascular

endothelial cells as Fc receptor for immunoglobulin M. Endothelium 13:287–292
67. Noji H, Shichishima T, Ogawa K, Shikama Y, Ohto H, Maruyama Y (2004) Transfusion-related acute lung injury following allogeneic bone marrow transplantation in a patient with acute lymphoblastic leukemia. Intern Med 43:1068–1072
68. O'Driscoll BR, Hasleton PS, Taylor PM, Poulter LW, Gattameneni HR, Woodcock AA (1990) Active lung fibrosis up to 17 years after chemotherapy with carmustine (BCNU) in childhood. N Engl J Med 323:378–382
69. Palmantier R, Rocheleau H, Laviolette M, Mancini J, Borgeat P (1998) Characteristics of leukotriene biosynthesis by human granulocytes in presence of plasma. Biochim Biophys Acta 1389:187–196
70. Popovsky MA, Moore SB (1985) Diagnostic and pathogenetic considerations in transfusion-related acute lung injury. Transfusion 25:573–577
71. Powers A, Stowell CP, Dzik WH, Saidman SL, Lee H, Makar RS (2008) Testing only donors with a prior history of pregnancy or transfusion is a logical and cost-effective transfusion-related acute lung injury prevention strategy. Transfusion 48:2549–2558
72. Randolph AG (2009) Management of acute lung injury and acute respiratory distress syndrome in children. Crit Care Med 37:2448–2454
73. Reinisch W, Lichtenberger C, Steger G, Tillinger W, Scheiner O, Gangl A, Maurer D, Willheim M (2003) Donor dependent, interferon-gamma induced HLA-DR expression on human neutrophils in vivo. Clin Exp Immunol 133: 476–484
74. Ricardi U, Filippi AR, Biasin E, Ciammella P, Botticella A, Franco P, Corrias A, Vassallo E, Ragona R, Fagioli F (2009) Late toxicity in children undergoing hematopoietic stem cell transplantation with TBI-containing conditioning regimens for hematological malignancies. Strahlenther Onkol 185(Suppl 2):17–20
75. Ruiz-Arguelles GJ, Rizpe-Bravo D, Sanchez-Sosa S, Rojas-Ortega S, Moreno-Ford V, Ruiz-Arguelles A (1999) Fatal G-CSF-induced pulmonary toxicity. Am J Hematol 60: 82–83
76. Sachs UJ, Bux J (2003) TRALI after the transfusion of cross-match-positive granulocytes. Transfusion 43:1683–1686
77. Sachs UJ, Link E, Hofmann C, Wasel W, Bein G (2008) Screening of multiparous women to avoid transfusion-related acute lung injury: a single centre experience. Transfus Med 18:348–354
78. Sakagawa H, Miyazaki T, Fujihara M, Sato S, Yamaguchi M, Fukai K, Morioka M, Kato T, Azuma H, Ikeda H (2007) Generation of inflammatory cytokines and chemokines from peripheral blood mononuclear cells by HLA Class II antibody-containing plasma unit that was associated with severe nonhemolytic transfusion reactions. Transfusion 47:154–161
79. Sala A, Bolla M, Zarini S, Muller-Peddinghaus R, Folco G (1996) Release of leukotriene A4 versus leukotriene B4 from human polymorphonuclear leukocytes. J Biol Chem 271:17944–17948
80. Schilero GJ, Oropello J, Benjamin E (1995) Impairment in gas exchange after granulocyte colony stimulating factor (G-CSF) in a patient with the adult respiratory distress syndrome. Chest 107:276–278
81. Seeger W, Schneider U, Kreusler B, Von WE, Walmrath D, Grimminger F, Neppert J (1990) Reproduction of transfusion-related acute lung injury in an ex vivo lung model. Blood 76:1438–1444
82. Serhan CN (1993) Cell-cell interactions in the generation of eicosanoids: charting the routes and products of transcellular biosynthesis. J Lab Clin Med 121:372–374
83. Shearer P, Katz J, Bozeman P, Jenkins J, Laver J, Krance R, Hurwitz C, Mahmoud H, Mirro J (1994) Pulmonary insufficiency complicating therapy with high dose cytosine arabinoside in five pediatric patients with relapsed acute myelogenous leukemia. Cancer 74:1953–1958
84. Silliman CC, Boshkov LK, Mehdizadehkashi Z, Elzi DJ, Dickey WO, Podlosky L, Clarke G, Ambruso DR (2003) Transfusion-related acute lung injury: epidemiology and a prospective analysis of etiologic factors. Blood 101: 454–462
85. Silliman CC, Clay KL, Thurman GW, Johnson CA, Ambruso DR (1994) Partial characterization of lipids that develop during the routine storage of blood and prime the neutrophil NADPH oxidase. J Lab Clin Med 124:684–694
86. Silliman CC, Dickey WO, Paterson AJ, Thurman GW, Clay KL, Johnson CA, Ambruso DR (1996) Analysis of the priming activity of lipids generated during routine storage of platelet concentrates. Transfusion 36:133–139
87. Silliman CC, Fung YL, Bradley BJ, Khan SY (2009) Transfusion-related acute lung injury (TRALI): Current concepts and misconceptions. Blood Rev
88. Silliman CC, Kelher M (2005) The role of endothelial activation in the pathogenesis of transfusion-related acute lung injury. Transfusion 45:109S–116S
89. Silliman CC, Paterson AJ, Dickey WO, Stroneck DF, Popovsky MA, Caldwell SA, Ambruso DR (1997) The association of biologically active lipids with the development of transfusion-related acute lung injury: a retrospective study. Transfusion 37:719–726
90. SMITH JC (1964) Radiation pneumonitis. Case report of bilateral reaction after unilateral irradiation. Am Rev Respir Dis 89:264–269
91. Spagnoli GC, Juretic A, Rosso R, Van BJ, Harder F, Heberer M (1995) Expression of HLA-DR in granulocytes of polytraumatized patients treated with recombinant human granulocyte macrophage-colony-stimulating factor. Hum Immunol 43:45–50
92. Stainsby D, Jones H, Asher D, Atterbury C, Boncinelli A, Brant L, Chapman CE, Davison K, Gerrard R, Gray A, Knowles S, Love EM, Milkins C, McClelland DB, Norfolk DR, Soldan K, Taylor C, Revill J, Williamson LM, Cohen H (2006) Serious hazards of transfusion: a decade of hemovigilance in the UK 5. Transfus Med Rev 20: 273–282
93. Tallman MS, Andersen JW, Schiffer CA, Appelbaum FR, Feusner JH, Ogden A, Shepherd L, Willman C, Bloomfield CD, Rowe JM, Wiernik PH (1997) All-trans-retinoic acid in acute promyelocytic leukemia. N Engl J Med 337: 1021–1028
94. Toy P, Hollis-Perry KM, Jun J, Nakagawa M (2004) Recipients of blood from a donor with multiple HLA antibodies: a lookback study of transfusion-related acute lung injury. Transfusion 44:1683–1688

95. Toy P, Popovsky MA, Abraham E, Ambruso DR, Holness LG, Kopko PM, McFarland JG, Nathens AB, Silliman CC, Stroncek D (2005) Transfusion-related acute lung injury: definition and review. Crit Care Med 33:721–726
96. Triulzi DJ, Kleinman S, Kakaiya RM, Busch MP, Norris PJ, Steele WR, Glynn SA, Hillyer CD, Carey P, Gottschall JL, Murphy EL, Rios JA, Ness PM, Wright DJ, Carrick D, Schreiber GB (2009) The effect of previous pregnancy and transfusion on HLA alloimmunization in blood donors: implications for a transfusion-related acute lung injury risk reduction strategy. Transfusion 49(90):1825–1835
97. Urahama N, Tanosaki R, Masahiro K, Iijima K, Chizuka A, Kim SW, Hori A, Kojima R, Imataki O, Makimito A, Mineishi S, Takaue Y (2003) TRALI after the infusion of marrow cells in a patient with acute lymphoblastic leukemia. Transfusion 43:1553–1557
98. Valls A, Algara M, Marrugat J, Carreras E, Sierra J, Granena A (1993) Risk factors for early mortality in allogeneic bone marrow transplantation. A multivariate analysis on 174 leukaemia patients. Eur J Cancer 29A:1523–1528
99. Van Buren NL, Stroncek DF, Clay ME, McCullough J, Dalmasso AP (1990) Transfusion-related acute lung injury caused by an NB2 granulocyte-specific antibody in a patient with thrombotic thrombocytopenic purpura. Transfusion 30:42–45
100. Van SD, Beckers EA, Sintnicolaas K, Porcelijn L, Danovic F, Wollersheim JA, Brand A, Van Rhenen DJ (2010) Transfusion-related acute lung injury reports in the Netherlands: an observational study. Transfusion 50(1):213–220, Epub 2009 Aug 18
101. Varela M, Mas A, Nogues N, Escorsell A, Mazzara R, Lozano M (2002) TRALI associated with HLA class II antibodies. Transfusion 42:1102
102. Wallis JP (2007) Transfusion-related acute lung injury (TRALI): presentation, epidemiology and treatment. Intensive Care Med 33(Suppl 1):S12–S16
103. Ware LB, Matthay MA (2000) The acute respiratory distress syndrome. N Engl J Med 342:1334–1349
104. Wells AW, Llewelyn CA, Casbard A, Johnson AJ, Amin M, Ballard S, Buck J, Malfroy M, Murphy MF, Williamson LM (2009) The EASTR Study: indications for transfusion and estimates of transfusion recipient numbers in hospitals supplied by the National Blood Service. Transfus Med 19(6):315–328
105. Win N, Brown C, Navarrete C (2003) TRALI associated with HLA class II antibodies. Transfusion 43:545–546
106. Win N, Ranasinghe E, Lucas G (2002) Transfusion-related acute lung injury: a 5-year look-back study. Transfus Med 12:387–389
107. Zarco MA, Ribera JM, Villamor N, Balmes A, Urbano IA, Feliu E (1998) Phenotypic changes in neutrophil granulocytes after G-CSF administration in patients with acute lymphoblastic leukemia under chemotherapy. Haematologica 83:573–575
108. Zeevi A, Girnita A, Duquesnoy R (2006) HLA antibody analysis: sensitivity, specificity, and clinical significance in solid organ transplantation. Immunol Res 36:255–264
109. Zimmerman JJ, Akhtar SR, Caldwell E, Rubenfeld GD (2009) Incidence and outcomes of pediatric acute lung injury. Pediatrics 124:87–95
110. Zupanska B, Uhrynowska M, Michur H, Maslanka K, Zajko M (2007) Transfusion-related acute lung injury and leucocyte-reacting antibodies. Vox Sang 93:70–77

Acute Respiratory Distress Syndrome (ARDS) in Neutropenic Patients

36

Mokart Djamel, Textoris Julien, Ettori Florence, Bruno Chetaille, and Blache Jean-Louis

Contents

M. Djamel (✉)
Intensive Care Unit, Paoli-Calmette Institute, Marseille, France and
Department of Anesthesiology and Intensive Care Unit, Paoli-Calmette Institute, 232 bd Sainte Marguerite, 13273 Marseille Cedex 9, France
e-mail: mokartd@marseille.fnclcc.fr

T. Julien, E. Florence, B. Chetaille, and B. Jean-Louis
Intensive Care Unit, Paoli-Calmette Institute, Marseille, France

B. Chetaille
Division Département d'anatomopathologie, Paoli-Calmette Institute, Marseille, France

36.1 Introduction

Recent advances in the treatment of solid and hematological malignancies have significantly improved overall survival in cancer patients [1]. However, the new treatment strategies are not only more effective, but also more aggressive and therefore associated with a higher rate of neutropenia. An absolute circulating neutrophil count of 1,000–1,500/mm^3 defines mild neutropenia, 500–1,000/mm^3 moderate neutropenia, and less than 500/mm^3 severe neutropenia. Lung involvement is common in febrile neutropenic patients. Thus, among patients with severe neutropenia, 20% have lung infiltrates [2, 3]. Early radiologic lung infiltrates occur in two-thirds of severely neutropenic patients developing a fever [4] and are associated with high mortality rates [5]. Histopathological studies have identified many different causes of these infiltrates. The most frequently described causes include bacteria [6, 7], opportunist pathogens not covered by beta-lactam antibiotics (filamentous fungi, *Pneumocystis jiroveci,* and viruses), alveolar hemorrhage, infiltration by the underlying malignancy, organizing pneumonia, and lesions caused by chemotherapy or radiation [8–19]. Neutropenic patients with lung infiltrates may develop genuine acute respiratory distress syndrome (ARDS). Interestingly, although the role for neutrophils has been extensively studied in non-neutropenic patients with acute lung injury and ARDS [20–22], the pathophysiology of ARDS in patients with neutrophil depletion remains unclear. Animal studies produced conflicting results, with neutrophil depletion protecting against ARDS in some studies but not in others [23, 24]. Numerous studies [25–32] have documented the occurrence of authentic ARDS in patients with severe neutropenia.

É. Azoulay (ed.), *Pulmonary Involvement in Patients with Hematological Malignancies,*
DOI: 10.1007/978-3-642-15742-4_36, © Springer-Verlag Berlin Heidelberg 2011

This chapter reviews the most likely pathophysiological mechanisms involved in ARDS in neutropenic patients and highlights the points of ARDS management that are specific of neutropenic patients (Figs. 36.1–36.4).

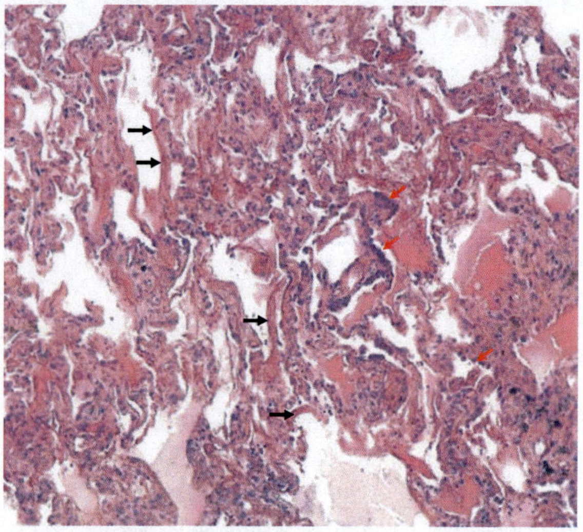

Fig. 36.1 ARDS in a neutropenic patient at the exudative phase of ARDS. Diffuse alveolar damage, early phase (hematoxylin and eosine, ×100). Alveolar septa are thickened by edema and scant mononuclear inflammation. Pneumocyte hyperplasia (*red arrows*) and hyaline membranes (*black arrows*) are seen

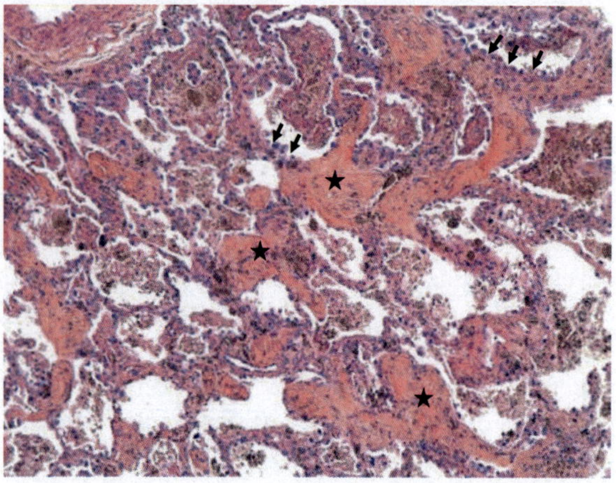

Fig. 36.2 ARDS in a neutropenic patient at the proliferative phase of ARDS, the patient was still neutropenic at this time. Diffuse alveolar damage, organizing phase (H&E, ×100). Alveolar septa are still thickened by congestion, mononuclear infiltrate, and scant interstitial fibrosis. Fibrosis is more prominent in the alveolar lumen (*black stars*). Note the alveolar pneumocyte hyperplasia (*black arrows*)

36.2 Epidemiology

In this chapter, acute respiratory failure (ARF) is defined clinically as tachypnea, recruitment of accessory respiratory muscles or respiratory muscle

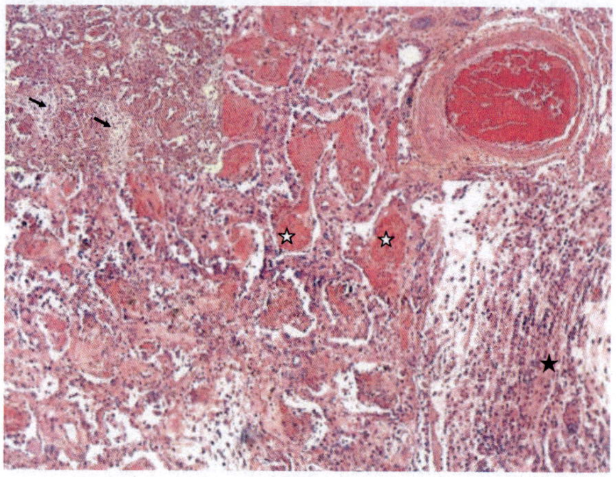

Fig. 36.3 ARDS occurring in a neutropenic patient; this patient presented a neutropenia recovery associated with an engraftment syndrome at the time of lung biopsy. Diffuse alveolar damage, acute phase. Prominent inflammation containing numerous neutrophils is seen within the alveolar septa, alveolar lumen, and bronchiolar lumen (*black star*). Some of the alveolar lumens contain a fibrinous material indicative of acute injury (*white stars*). Congestive endoluminal fibrosis (*top left corner, black arrows*) and recent organizing thrombus (*top right corner*) could also be seen (H&E ×100)

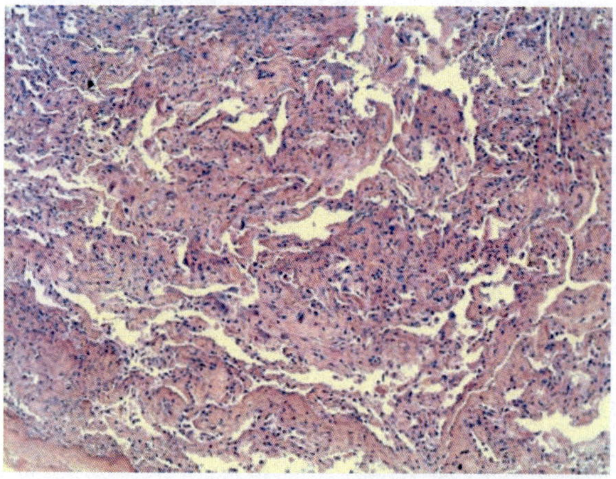

Fig. 36.4 ARDS occurring in a neutropenic patient; the lung biopsy was made at the fibrotic phase of ARDS and 12 days after the neutropenia recovery. Diffuse alveolar damage, late organizing phase, showing thickening of alveolar septa by extensive fibrosis and scant mononuclear inflammation (H&E, ×100). Despite the absence of neutropenia at this time, there is no obvious neutrophilic infiltration

exhaustion, arterial oxygen saturation lower than 90% on room air, pulmonary infiltrates, and a need for high-concentration facemask oxygen or for invasive or noninvasive mechanical ventilation. ARDS and acute lung injury (ALI) are defined as the abrupt onset (over less than 7 days) of clinically significant hypoxemia (PaO_2/FiO_2 <300 for ALI or 200 for ARDS) with diffuse bilateral pulmonary infiltrates (on the anterior–posterior radiograph, infiltrates consistent with pulmonary edema, which may be patchy and asymmetric; and possible presence of pleural effusions). The absence of left atrial hypertension (pulmonary-artery wedge pressure <18 mmHg if measured) is also required [33, 34]. ARF is a common reason for ICU admission in cancer patients. ARF occurs in 5% of patients with solid tumors, 50% of patients with hematological malignancies, and nearly 30% of patients with neutropenia [5, 35, 36]. In oncology and hematology patients requiring mechanical ventilation, mortality rates have ranged from 70% to 100% (in allogeneic BMT recipients) [5, 36, 37]. Among cancer patients with ARF, 70% require invasive mechanical ventilation. Among them, 83% develop authentic ARDS, which is associated with a hospital mortality rate of about 70%. Neutropenia is present in about 35% of cancer patients with ARF and, in this situation, the lack of neutrophils is not considered of adverse prognostic significance [5, 35, 36]. Few studies have addressed ARDS in neutropenic patients. Historical studies suggested a high mortality rate [25–32]. We showed recently [38] that hospital mortality in neutropenic ARDS patients was about 75% compared to 40% in the general population of ARDS patients [34]. The characteristics of the patients in our study are described in Tables 36.1–36.3.

Table 36.1 Causes of ARDS in 70 neutropenic cancer patients

Cause of ARDS ($n = 70$)	Number (%)
Gram-negative bacillus infection	17 (24.3%)
Gram-positive coccus infection	9 (12.9%)
Fungal infection	14 (20.0%)
Viral infection	5 (7.1%)
Other infection	2 (2.9%)
Noninfectious cause	4 (5.7%)
Unknown	19 (27.1%)
ARDS with direct pulmonary injury	30/51 (59%) (among the 51 patients with an identified cause)

Table 36.2 Characteristics and status of the malignancy in 70 neutropenic cancer patients with ARDS

Demographics	
Gender (male)	37 (53%)
Age (years)	55 (46–65)
Characteristics of Malignancy (n = 70)	*Number (%)*
Acute leukemia	39 (55.7%)
Lymphoma	19 (27.1%)
Myeloma	4 (5.7%)
Solid tumors	4 (5.7%)
Other cancers	4 (5.7%)
Autologous HSCT	10 (14.3%)
Allogeneic HSCT	5 (7.1%)
Radiotherapy	7 (10%)
Status of Malignancy	
First-line chemotherapy	41(58.6%)
Complete remission	5 (7%)
Relapse	20 (28.6%)
Secondary acute leukemia	4 (5.7%)

Table 36.3 Outcome of neutropenic cancer patients with ARDS during the ICU stay

Outcomes of patients ($n = 70$)	Number (%) or median (25th–75th percentile)
Noninvasive mechanical ventilation	39 (55.7%)
Invasive mechanical ventilation	66 (94.3%)
Use of vasopressors	60 (85.7%)
Dialysis	29 (41.4%)
Hospital mortality	52 (74.3%)
Day-90 mortality	52 (74.3%)

36.3 Pathophysiology

ALI and ARDS are characterized by acute diffuse damage to the lung parenchyma caused by a variety of local or systemic insults [39–41]. Increased alveolar capillary membrane permeability is the common end-organ injury and a central feature in all forms of ALI/ARDS. Investigations into the pathophysiology of lung injury make extensive use of three experimental ALI models in various species: the surfactant washout lavage model, the oleic acid intravenous injection model, and the endotoxin injection model [42]. These models, together with studies in human patients, have led to the identification of several mediators, cell types, and insults involved in the pathogenesis of ARDS. Circulating factors that are elevated in ARDS patients and ARDS models may contribute to lung injury. However, data on ARDS in neutropenic patients are still scarce.

36.3.1 Histological Features

In ARDS patients, histological studies show diffuse alveolar damage (DAD) that is not specific of the underlying cause. DAD progresses through three pathologic stages: the exudative phase, in which interstitial and alveolar edema and hemorrhage predominate; the proliferative phase, characterized by organization and repair; and the fibrotic phase, which represents end-stage disease [41]. In the mid-1980s, the first histological descriptions of ARDS in neutropenic patients were published [25, 26, 30–32]. The same three histological stages were found. The exudative phase was characterized by interstitial and alveolar edema, hyaline membranes, and hemorrhage; the proliferative phase by proliferation of alveolar-lining cells, alveolar macrophages, and fibroblasts; and the fibrotic phase by prominent interstitial fibrosis. In contrast to findings from non-neutropenic patients, neutrophil sequestration was not apparent at any of the disease stages in most of the neutropenic patients, nor was thromboembolism found.

36.3.2 Bronchoalveolar Lavage Fluid

In non-neutropenic patients with ARDS, bronchoalveolar lavage fluid (BALF) contains high concentrations of inflammatory mediators [40]. Activated complement components and pro-inflammatory cytokines are thought to mediate the host response to lung injury [43, 44]. Levels of interleukin (IL)-6 and IL-8 are elevated in BALF from non-neutropenic patients who have ARDS [40] or who are at risk for ARDS; [45] both cytokines may predict a complicated course of ARDS. Data regarding BALF and/or plasma cytokine concentrations in neutropenic cancer patients with ARDS are scarce. However, in neutropenic patients with pneumonia, BALF contains markedly higher levels of inflammatory mediators compared to neutropenic patients with fever of unknown origin [46]. BALF from febrile neutropenic patients may exhibit substantially elevated levels of IL-6, tumor necrosis factor alpha (TNFα), granulocyte/colony-stimulating factor (G-CSF), and activated complement components (C5a and C3a), even before the diagnosis of pneumonia [47]. These elevations may predict pneumonia and/or subsequent ARDS. In neutropenic patients with ARDS, the severity of lung injury measured based on BALF cytokine concentrations is a better predictor of the course of ARDS than plasma cytokine concentrations [48]. In fact, BALF concentrations of TNFα, IL-6, and IL-8 are significantly increased in patients who do not respond to ICU management, whereas plasma cytokine concentrations are not different compared to responders [48]. Neutropenic patients with pneumonia have low numbers of alveolar cells, particularly neutrophils and alveolar macrophages (AMs) [49]. In addition to reduced alveolar cellularity, profound neutropenia in patients with pneumonia may be associated with a distinctive alveolar cell profile characterized by predominance of AMs, low neutrophil counts, and lymphocyte counts similar to those seen in non-neutropenic patients. This cell profile has also been reported in neutropenic patients with ARDS [28], whereas BALF from non-neutropenic patients with ARDS contains large numbers of neutrophils [50]. Finally, the percentages of AMs, neutrophils, and lymphocytes in BALF from neutropenic ARDS patients are comparable to those of normal individuals [51], suggesting “alveolar anergy” in neutropenic patients. Thus, neither circulating nor lung neutrophils constitute the main source of lung inflammation and cytokine production. Other cells such as the endothelial cells, epithelial cells, or AMs may be alternative sources of cytokines in neutropenic patients [52, 53].

36.3.3 Neutropenia and Sequestered Neutrophils

Although neutrophils are considered pivotal in the pathophysiology of ARDS and ALI [54], their absence in neutropenic patients does not preclude the development of ARDS. The absence of neutrophils may indirectly modulate the inflammatory response in neutropenic patients [55]. In histological studies, most of the pulmonary specimens obtained during the early stages of neutropenic ARDS show diffuse alveolar damage (typical for ARDS) without neutrophil infiltrates, suggesting an alternative mechanism to neutrophil toxicity in the pathogenesis of ARDS (Table 36.4). BALF from neutropenic patients with ARDS or pneumonia contains few cells, with a very small number of neutrophils and a predominance of AMs. A study of experimental pneumonia [56] showed that the absence of neutrophils in the alveoli did not preclude neutrophil sequestration in the lung microvessels. Respiratory status deterioration during neutropenia may involve complex interactions between resident macrophages and migrated neutrophils sequestered in the lung interstitium, with upregulation of pro-inflammatory cytokines such as TNFα and IL-1β [8, 57]. In a rat model of endotoxemia, neutropenic rats had markedly lower plasma TNFα concentrations and higher plasma MIP-2 concentrations compared to non-neutropenic rats [55], and ALI was more severe in the neutropenic than in the non-neutropenic animals. Plasma MIP-2 elevation in endotoxemic neutropenic rats may

Table 36.4 Comparison of inflammatory responses during ARDS in neutropenic patients and in the general population

	ARDS in the general population	ARDS in neutropenic patients
Markers of lung injury	DAD, exudative phase (lung biopsy) [41]	DAD, exudative phase (lung biopsy) [25, 26, 30–32]
	Neutrophil influx (BALF or lung biopsy) [41, 50]	Absence of neutrophils (BALF or lung biopsy) [28, 30]
	High cellularity in BALF [50]	Low cellularity in BALF [28]
	Pro-inflammatory cytokines in BALF [40, 45]	Pro-inflammatory cytokines in BALF [48]
	Pro-inflammatory cytokines in blood [40]	Pro-inflammatory cytokines in blood [48]
	Platelets (lung biopsy) [41]	Absence of platelet and thromboembolic processes (lung biopsy) [30]
	Coagulation factors [40]	
	Alveolar macrophage activation [125]	Alveolar macrophage deactivation (BALF) [28]
		Monocyte deactivation (blood) [29]
Markers of lung repair	Normal or high cellularity in BALF [50]	Low cellularity in BALF [28]
	Predominance of alveolar macrophages (BALF) [50]	Predominance of alveolar macrophages (BALF) [28]
	Activated alveolar macrophages [40, 69, 73]	Alveolar macrophage deactivation [28]
	Anti-inflammatory cytokines in BALF [40, 73, 80]	Monocyte deactivation [28]
Immunosuppression	Anti-inflammatory cytokines in BALF [80]	Neutropenia
		Low cellularity in BALF [28]
		Alveolar neutropenia [28]
		Alveolar macrophage deactivation [28]
		Monocyte deactivation [28]
		Alveolar anergy?
		Use of G-CSF?

be secondary to the lack of a neutrophil response inhibiting the production or release of MIP-2. The role for neutrophils in TNFα production during inflammatory processes is controversial [58–60]. During experimental ALI, TNFα serum concentrations and pulmonary TNFα mRNA were not significantly different between neutropenic and non-neutropenic mice [54]. In contrast, other studies found no TNFα production and decreased TNFα mRNA levels in the lungs of neutropenic mice with ALI [55]. Plasma inflammatory cytokines may be increased in febrile neutropenic patients with or without sepsis or septic shock [61–64]. The production of inflammatory cytokines in neutropenic patients with sepsis or septic shock may be similar to that in non-neutropenic patients. During neutropenia, chemotherapy can decrease the ex-vivo production of pro-inflammatory cytokines in whole blood [65]. Interestingly, in neutropenic patients with hematological malignancies who did not receive chemotherapy, similar changes were found, suggesting a role for the neutropenia itself in cytokine production alterations [65]. The exact role for neutrophils in the pathogenesis of ARDS during neutropenia seems complex. It appears that ARDS can develop even when circulating and lung neutrophils are completely absent. However, conflicting experimental data suggest that neutropenia and/or sequestered neutrophils may modulate the lung inflammation in this situation. Although the number of neutrophils required to induce lung injury remains unknown, evidence suggests that neutrophil accumulation is not required for the onset of ALI and that other inflammatory cells may be involved.

36.3.4 Alveolar Macrophages and Circulating Monocytes

Few studies have investigated the importance of neutrophil-independent mechanisms in ARDS. In non-neutropenic patients, Steinberg et al. [50] compared the alveolar cell profile of BALF from patients with sepsis and ARDS and showed that high neutrophil counts were associated with greater severity of lung injury and poorer outcomes, whereas high AM counts were associated with better resolution and improved survival. There is convincing evidence that AMs play a key role in the resolution of inflammation, antibacterial defense, and the repair process following injury [40, 66]. However, studies have also shown that AMs and AM-derived products may contribute to lung injury [67]. Activated AMs can release a wide variety of mediators, most of which can damage the lung alveolar-capillary barrier [40, 68–70]. A study of ARDS patients [71] showed increased in vivo activation of the nuclear transcriptional regulatory factor nuclear factor κB in AMs, which may contribute to the increased expression of various cytokines. Consistent with a major role for macrophages in ARDS, primed AMs were used successfully to induce lung injury in a septic neutropenic guinea pig model of ARDS [24]. Thus, experimental studies suggest a critical role for AMs in the pathophysiology of ARDS in neutropenic patients. In contrast, in neutropenic patients with septic ARDS, we found not only evidence of local pulmonary immunosuppression related to AM deactivation [28], but also marked depression of the monocytic/macrophagic response [29]. In these patients, BALF contained few cells with a predominance of AMs. The human leukocyte antigen (HLA)-DR locus (HLA-DR) was down-regulated in AMs, and the LPS-induced macrophagic/monocytic cytokine responses were blunted, indicating severe hyporeactivity. This local macrophage hypoactivity was associated with severe "alveolar neutropenia," which contributed to local host immunosuppression. Indeed, systemic monocyte deactivation was also involved in the immunosuppression. Thus, these results do not support a direct role for monocytes/macrophages in lung injury induction during neutropenia. Interestingly, the monocyte/macrophage deactivation observed in these neutropenic patients extended to the anti-inflammatory cytokines, although all these patients received G-CSF therapy, which is also known to play a role in the upregulation of anti-inflammatory mediators [28, 72]. Therefore, this deactivation may hinder lung repair during ARDS [40, 73].

36.3.5 Possible Role for Platelets

Platelets may be involved in numerous inflammatory processes, including atherogenesis, ischemia-reperfusion injury, sepsis, and probably, lung injury [74, 75]. Importantly, neutrophil–platelet interactions promote mutual cell activation, and platelet–endothelial interactions facilitate the secondary capture not only of neutrophils, but also of other leukocytes. Platelets alone might be sufficient to mediate inflammatory lung disease, whereas platelet-derived mediators may contribute to the development of ARDS in neutropenic patients [76]. Platelet transfusions are frequently associated with the occurrence of ARDS [77]. Since neutropenic patients are more likely to receive platelet transfusions than the general population, the role for platelet transfusion in ARDS development in neutropenic patients should be evaluated.

36.3.6 Other Mechanisms and Other Mediators

Neither neutrophils nor monocytes/macrophages seem directly involved in lung injury during ARDS in neutropenic patients. Direct endothelial-cell injury by a host of soluble mediators may play a role [39–41]. Our experience suggests that indirect lung injury may be involved in about 40% of ARDS cases in neutropenic patients [38]. In this setting of indirect lung injury, a direct role for soluble mediators is plausible. Nevertheless, direct lung injury may be involved in the remaining 60% of cases and, in this situation, the cause of lung injury remains unknown. One interesting hypothesis involves the pulmonary endothelium. The pulmonary endothelium plays an active role in ALI development by mediating cell–cell adhesion, changing its barrier permeability, and releasing myriad soluble mediators, such as cytokines, serotonin, bradykinin, norepinephrine, nitric oxide, prostaglandins, and endothelins [40, 78]. Radiotherapy and a variety of chemotherapeutic antineoplastic agents induce pulmonary dysfunction and endothelial-cell lesions [79]. These treatments are commonly used in neutropenic patients and may constitute the first hit of a two-hit model, the second hit being pulmonary endothelium dysregulation [28–30].

36.4 Different Pathophysiological Pathways for Neutropenic and Non-neutropenic ARDS Patients: Clinical Implications

Contrary to non-neutropenic patients, neutropenic patients have a BALF profile characterized by low counts of alveolar cells, most notably neutrophils, predominance of AMs, and AM deactivation. In addition to neutropenia, deactivation of circulating monocytes may worsen the systemic immunosuppression. Systemic and lung inflammatory responses in neutropenic ARDS patients differ from those in non-neutropenic ARDS patients. In non-neutropenic ARDS patients, a predominant anti-inflammatory response combined with a limited pro-inflammatory response in the lungs is associated with better patient outcomes [80]. In neutropenic ARDS patients, in contrast, the deactivation of both AMs and circulating monocytes [28, 29] may contribute to the increased mortality. Despite these differences, neutropenic patients with sepsis or ARDS are treated according to standard guidelines developed for non-neutropenic patients [81]. These guidelines may be partly unsuitable for neutropenic patients. In addition, some of the recommendations for hematology patients need reappraisal [82, 83].

- First, routine growth factor therapy may be deleterious in neutropenic patients who have lung injury. The effects of G-CSF may influence the course of ALI. In a rat model of ALI during neutropenia, G-CSF therapy was associated with increased alveolar cell recruitment and pulmonary edema [57]. The results suggested that neutropenia recovery might worsen ALI and that G-CSF might further exacerbate ALI. Moreover, in a clinical study, G-CSF-induced neutropenia recovery was associated with respiratory status deterioration [84]. Furthermore, G-CSF may promote the development of infectious pneumonia-related ARDS in neutropenic patients [85] and may participate in macrophage deactivation during ARDS in neutropenic patients [28, 29]. These data suggest a need for evaluating the risk and benefits of G-CSF in neutropenic patients with lung injury. Other growth factors should also be evaluated [86].
- Second, clinical and experimental data have shown that ventilator-associated lung injury (VALI) involves ongoing lung inflammation resulting from lung overdistension and, perhaps, from excessively low lung volumes as well. In this situation, the decreased plasma levels of pro-inflammatory cytokines found in clinical studies are ascribable in part to lung-protective ventilation and are associated with better clinical outcomes [87]. Since neutropenic patients with ALI/ARDS appear to develop an atypical inflammatory response (Table 36.4), studies are needed to identify patient subgroups that are at high risk for VALI and therefore more likely to derive benefits from lung-protective ventilation.
- Third, corticosteroids have been investigated as a potential treatment for ARDS because of their

anti-inflammatory properties. However, whether corticosteroids decrease early mortality in patients with unresolving ARDS remains unclear [88]. Recent data suggest that corticosteroids may be effective on ALI/ARDS regardless of the occurrence of sepsis [89]. Furthermore, immunocompromised patients may develop acute noninfectious parenchymal lung damage that often meets ALI/ARDS criteria [90] and that usually responds to corticosteroids. Further studies are needed to evaluate the use of corticosteroids in immunocompromised patients (including neutropenic patients) with ALI/ARDS.

36.5 Therapeutic Management

The treatment of ARDS in neutropenic patients is not standardized. Importantly, neutropenia is not considered a prognostic factor in cancer patients with ARF. Data from neutropenic and non-neutropenic cancer patients show clearly that a prompt diagnosis, early appropriate antimicrobial therapy, adequate use of conventional and/or noninvasive mechanical ventilation, and early ICU admission are crucial to improving patient outcomes [4, 5, 36, 91]. In neutropenic patients with ARF/ARDS, sepsis should be considered the most likely cause, and the Surviving Sepsis Campaign guidelines [81] should be followed if possible. As mentioned above, neutropenia, autologous bone marrow transplantation, and the characteristics of the underlying malignancy [5] now seem to have little influence on ICU outcomes. The treatment initiated on the ward must not delay ICU admission [81]. Although criteria for ICU admission are not well established for these patients, delayed admission is associated with higher mortality rates [92].

Noninvasive mechanical ventilation (NIV) may improve survival in cancer patients requiring respiratory support [93]. However, prolonged NIV (>3 days) may lead to higher mortality rates [5], perhaps by delaying conventional mechanical ventilation (MV) and therefore optimal diagnostic procedures or treatment strategies [94–96]. Thus, in one clinical study, a longer time to conventional MV was associated with the highest mortality rate [5]. NIV may be appropriate for no more than 3 days, with a switch to conventional MV within the first 3 days of NIV initiation when the response is inadequate.

A tidal volume of 6 mL/kg (predicted) body weight and a plateau pressure <30 cm H_2O in a passively inflated patient are recommended [5, 34]. Identifying the cause of ARF is crucial; and early conventional MV, NIV, and antimicrobial therapy should be considered. Both invasive and noninvasive diagnostic strategies can be used to identify the cause of ARF in cancer patients [35]. The invasive strategy relies on fiberoptic bronchoscopy with bronchoalveolar lavage (FO-BAL) and the noninvasive strategy on imaging studies [97, 98] and on biological and microbiological tests on blood [99–102], urine [103, 104], sputa [105], and nasopharyngeal aspirates (Table 36.5) [16, 106]. Interestingly, the noninvasive strategy may be as effective as the FO-BAL strategy [36] and does not carry the risk of respiratory status deterioration associated with FO-BAL. In cancer patients with ARF, failure to identify the cause of ARF is associated with higher mortality. Therefore, the diagnostic strategy should be chosen and implemented early after ICU admission, before the onset of ARDS. However, the use of invasive techniques to identify the cause of lung infiltrates in febrile neutropenic patients has not clearly improved the outcomes [4, 17, 107, 108] despite enabling pathogen-directed antimicrobial treatment in up to 50% of patients [109].

36.5.1 Empirical Antimicrobial Therapy

Since febrile neutropenia in cancer patients is associated with high mortality, empirical antimicrobial therapy should be considered as soon as a fever develops. When the lungs are involved, the most common initial clinical picture on the ward is neutropenia, fever, pulmonary infiltrates, and ARF. At ICU admission, most patients are already on broad-spectrum antimicrobial agents for prophylactic, preemptive, or empirical treatment. Bacterial infections account for most cases of lung involvement in neutropenic patients [110–112]. The risk of bacterial infection is related both to neutropenia severity and to neutropenia duration [113]. In this situation, empirical antibiotic treatment must be prompt (<2 h after respiratory symptoms) and effective against the most common pathogens [81, 114, 115]. Gram-positive infections are common in neutropenic

Table 36.5 Interpretation of positive microbiological tests in neutropenic patients with lung infiltrates

	BAL or Sputum	Blood	Urine	Other
Treat immediately	*Pneumocystis jiroveci*, gram-negative aerobic pathogens,	Pneumococci, Alpha-hemolytic streptococci *Staphylococcus aureus*	Positive Legionella or pneumococcal antigen in urine	Any pathogens detected in biopsy material
	Pneumococci, Mycobacterium tuberculosis	Gram-negative aerobic pathogens (blood culture)		
	Aspergillus spp. Zygomycetes	Fungal pathogens (blood culture)		
	Positive rapid culture for CMV, detection of CMV "immediate early antigen" (in specific situations)	Positive Aspergillus galactomannan (blood samples)		
	Other pathogens such as toxoplasmosis, adenovirus or emerging viruses (allogeneic BMT recipients),			
Discuss before treating	Isolation of Enterococci from blood culture, smears, sputum, or BAL			
	Positive cytomegalovirus (CMV) PCR is not considered sufficient for the diagnosis of CMV pneumonia			
	Coagulase-negative staphylococci or *Corynebacterium* spp. obtained from any sample			
	Isolation of *Candida* spp. from swabs, saliva, sputum or tracheal aspirates			
	Findings from surveillance feces and urine cultures			
	Pneumocystis PCR in sputa or BAL in patients without risk for *Pneumocystis jirovecii* pneumonia			

patients, whereas gram-negative infections are associated with a higher mortality [116, 117]. Until now, empirical treatment with an anti-pseudomonal β-lactam in combination with an aminoglycoside in case of severe sepsis was the most widely used regimen [116]. Recent studies and recommendations for empirical treatment indicate that an antipseudomonal β-lactam alone is less toxic for the kidney and as effective as the combination with a β-lactam-aminoglycoside [118]. Therefore, initial combination therapy should be reserved for patients with severe sepsis, septic shock, or a high suspicion of resistant gram-negative microorganisms [118]. According to a recent report [119], 71% of experts used initial empirical monotherapy to manage febrile neutropenia; their antimicrobials of first choice were pipericillin/tazobactam (21%), meropenem (16%), imipenem (14.5%), cefepime (13.2%), and ceftazidime (7%). One-third of the experts added an aminoglycoside (preferably amikacin) for severe sepsis, suspected *Pseudomonas* infection, resistant gram-negative infections, secondary infections, or pneumonia. Even in patients with ARDS, glycopeptide antibiotics should be used in the event of severe sepsis, septic shock, a high suspicion of skin or soft-tissue infection (including catheter-tunnel infection), and a local bacterial ecology characterized by resistant gram-positive bacteria [120]. Combining an anti-pseudomonal β-lactam with a quinolone or macrolide may deserve discussion in patients with community-acquired pneumonia or a documented pathogen [115, 121]. The initial antibiotic regimen should be routinely reappraised to control the local bacterial ecology and to minimize the emergence of multiresistant bacteria [111, 116]. Antifungal agents should be introduced empirically in patients who remain neutropenic and febrile after 5 days or more despite the administration of broad-spectrum antibiotics as recommended [115, 119, 121]. Fungal infections should be more specifically considered in patients with severe or prolonged neutropenia, immunosuppressive therapy to control graft-versus-host disease, and, perhaps targeted therapies, such as rituximab [122]. To ensure early and effective action against filamentous fungi (predominantly *Aspergillus* spp.), the initial antifungal treatment should consist of voriconazole or liposomal amphotericin B [4]. Liposomal amphotericin B is preferred in patients recently treated with voriconazole or posaconazole [4]. After broad-spectrum azole prophylaxis, fungal infections with azole-resistant pathogens may develop. The place for echinocandins in this situation remains to be defined.

Empirical treatment with antiviral drugs in the absence of target pathogen isolation from clinically significant samples is not recommended [4, 121].

36.5.2 Directed Antimicrobial Therapy

Positive microbiological tests must be interpreted with discernment, and their clinical and/or etiological significance must be assessed. The identification of significant pathogens, particularly multiresistant bacteria, should lead to an immediate change in the initial antimicrobial treatment, as inadequate initial antimicrobial treatment is associated with a high risk of death [91].

In patients with neutropenia and pulmonary infiltrates, many pathogens may be etiologically significant.

Other findings such as community respiratory viruses, *Staphylococcus aureus*, *Legionella* spp. or atypical mycobacteria from respiratory secretions, or a positive CMV PCR (DNA) on BALF must be interpreted regarding their etiologic significance before starting specific antimicrobial treatment [4].

36.6 Prognosis and Prognostic Factors

To our knowledge, no data are available on the outcomes of patients who experience ARDS while neutropenic. Data from studies on outcomes of cancer patients admitted to the ICU are helpful, however. The survival rate in cancer patients with ARF has improved over time, to about 55%. When ventilatory assistance is required, the hospital mortality rate is about 75% [5, 36], except in allogeneic bone marrow or stem cell transplant recipients, who have even higher mortality rates [37]. The classic predictors of mortality have lost much of their significance [123]. In cancer patients with ARF [36], two malignancy-related factors independently predict hospital mortality, namely, malignancy remission and allogeneic bone marrow or stem cell transplantation. Interestingly, ICU admission during neutropenia recovery is protective, and neutropenia itself does not appear to increase the risk of death in this setting. The use of vasopressors or conventional MV is independently associated with death. Failure to identify the cause of ARF is an independent prognostic factor.

In a recent study of 70 neutropenic patients with ARDS, we found a hospital mortality rate of 75% [38]. At ICU admission, factors independently associated with hospital survival were first-line chemotherapy, lobar ARDS, neutropenia recovery, and initial broad-spectrum antibiotic treatment active on difficult-to-treat bacteria. During the ICU stay, all patients without neutropenia recovery in the ICU died, and 50% of patients with neutropenia recovery survived. Platelet transfusions were independently associated with the absence of neutropenia recovery. These data suggest several comments. First, ARDS in neutropenic patients should be considered an infectious emergency requiring immediate broad-spectrum antibiotic treatment appropriate for the local antibiotic resistance profiles. Second, transfusion strategies need to be evaluated in neutropenic patients. Third, achieving neutropenia recovery is a crucial objective. At the moment, ICU admission with full-code management followed by reappraisal on day 3–6 is recommended for cancer patients requiring mechanical ventilation [124]. Whether full-code management in neutropenic patients with ARDS should be continued until neutropenia recovery (even if achieved after more than 6 days) remains unclear, but may be particularly appropriate in patients receiving first-line chemotherapy. Neutropenia can be viewed as a transient and expected immune dysfunction. The first event is chemotherapy, which is usually associated with neutropenia severity, and the last event is neutropenia recovery. In real life, neutropenia duration, severity, and recovery depend on other factors including sepsis, lung injury, chemotherapy response, nature of the malignancy, and stage of the malignancy. Few published data on this issue are available. Neutropenic cancer patients constitute a highly heterogeneous population, and the differences across neutropenic subgroups should be considered. Thus, therapeutic decisions must take all the malignancy-related factors into consideration. For instance, the significance of neutropenia during first-line chemotherapy is very different from that during a relapse of the malignancy [110]. Further studies are needed to identify the factors predicting neutropenia recovery in cancer patients.

36.7 Conclusion

ARDS during neutropenia is a life-threatening condition. When ARDS occurs in a neutropenic patient with or without a fever, severe sepsis should be considered the cause unless documented otherwise. The physiopathology of lung injury during neutropenia remains to be elucidated. However, in neutropenic patients the local and systemic inflammatory responses are associated with profound immunosuppression. Therefore, the risks and benefits of immunomodulating treatments (corticosteroids, G-CSF, GM-CSF, blood transfusion, and platelet transfusion) should be carefully evaluated. Neutropenia recovery and prompt appropriate initial antimicrobial therapy are key determinants of survival. Further studies are needed to evaluate the prognostic factors and therapeutic management of these patients.

References

1. Brenner H, Gondos A, Arndt V (2007) Recent major progress in long-term cancer patient survival disclosed by modeled period analysis. J Clin Oncol 25:3274–3280
2. Link H, Maschmeyer G, Meyer P et al (1994) Interventional antimicrobial therapy in febrile neutropenic patients. Study Group of the Paul Ehrlich Society for Chemotherapy. Ann Hematol 69:231–243
3. Rossini F, Verga M, Pioltelli P et al (2000) Incidence and outcome of pneumonia in patients with acute leukemia receiving first induction therapy with anthracycline-containing regimens. Haematologica 85:1255–1260
4. Maschmeyer G, Link H, Hiddemann W et al (1994) Pulmonary infiltrations in febrile patients with neutropenia. Risk factors and outcome under empirical antimicrobial therapy in a randomized multicenter study. Cancer 73: 2296–2304
5. Azoulay E, Thiery G, Chevret S et al (2004) The prognosis of acute respiratory failure in critically ill cancer patients. Medicine (Baltimore) 83:360–370
6. Hachem RY, Chemaly RF, Ahmar CA et al (2007) Colistin is effective in treatment of infections caused by multidrug-resistant Pseudomonas aeruginosa in cancer patients. Antimicrob Agents Chemother 51:1905–1911
7. Safdar A, Rolston KV (2007) Stenotrophomonas maltophilia: changing spectrum of a serious bacterial pathogen in patients with cancer. Clin Infect Dis 45:1602–1609
8. Azoulay E, Darmon M, Delclaux C et al (2002) Deterioration of previous acute lung injury during neutropenia recovery. Crit Care Med 30:781–786
9. Bodey G, Bueltmann B, Duguid W et al (1992) Fungal infections in cancer patients: an international autopsy survey. Eur J Clin Microbiol Infect Dis 11:99–109
10. Canham EM, Kennedy TC, Merrick TA (1983) Unexplained pulmonary infiltrates in the compromised patient. An invasive investigation in a consecutive series. Cancer 52:325–329
11. Cazzadori A, Di PG, Todeschini G et al (1995) Transbronchial biopsy in the diagnosis of pulmonary infiltrates in immunocompromised patients. Chest 107:101–106
12. Cheson BD, Samlowski WE, Tang TT et al (1985) Value of open-lung biopsy in 87 immunocompromised patients with pulmonary infiltrates. Cancer 55:453–459
13. Commers JR, Robichaud KJ, Pizzo PA (1984) New pulmonary infiltrates in granulocytopenic cancer patients being treated with antibiotics. Pediatr Infect Dis 3:423–428
14. Danes C, Gonzalez-Martin J, Pumarola T et al (2002) Pulmonary infiltrates in immunosuppressed patients: analysis of a diagnostic protocol. J Clin Microbiol 40:2134–2140
15. Daniels CE, Myers JL, Utz JP et al (2007) Organizing pneumonia in patients with hematologic malignancies: a steroid-responsive lesion. Respir Med 101:162–168
16. Martino R, Ramila E, Rabella N et al (2003) Respiratory virus infections in adults with hematologic malignancies: a prospective study. Clin Infect Dis 36:1–8
17. Singer C, Armstrong D, Rosen PP et al (1979) Diffuse pulmonary infiltrates in immunosuppressed patients. Prospective study of 80 cases. Am J Med 66:110–120
18. Suzuki HI, Asai T, Tamaki Z et al (2008) Drug-induced hypersensitivity syndrome with rapid hematopoietic reconstitution during treatment for acute myeloid leukemia. Haematologica 93:469–470
19. Torres HA, Aguilera EA, Mattiuzzi GN et al (2007) Characteristics and outcome of respiratory syncytial virus infection in patients with leukemia. Haematologica 92: 1216–1223
20. Gougerot-Podicalo MA, Elbim C, Chollet-Martin S (1996) Modulation of the oxidative burst of human neutrophils by pro- and anti-inflammatory cytokines. Pathol Biol (Paris) 44:36–41
21. Nieman G, Searles B, Carney D et al (1999) Systemic inflammation induced by cardiopulmonary bypass: a review of pathogenesis and treatment. J Extra Corpor Technol 31: 202–210
22. Talbott GA, Sharar SR, Harlan JM et al (1994) Leukocyte-endothelial interactions and organ injury: the role of adhesion molecules. New Horiz 2:545–554
23. Heflin AC Jr, Brigham KL (1981) Prevention by granulocyte depletion of increased vascular permeability of sheep lung following endotoxemia. J Clin Invest 68:1253–1260
24. Tasaka S, Ishizaka A, Urano T et al (1995) BCG priming enhances endotoxin-induced acute lung injury independent of neutrophils. Am J Respir Crit Care Med 152:1041–1049
25. Braude S, Apperley J, Krausz T et al (1985) Adult respiratory distress syndrome after allogeneic bone-marrow transplantation: evidence for a neutrophil-independent mechanism. Lancet 1:1239–1242
26. Laufe MD, Simon RH, Flint A et al (1986) Adult respiratory distress syndrome in neutropenic patients. Am J Med 80:1022–1026
27. Maunder RJ, Hackman RC, Riff E et al (1986) Occurrence of the adult respiratory distress syndrome in neutropenic patients. Am Rev Respir Dis 133:313–316
28. Mokart D, Guery BP, Bouabdallah R et al (2003) Deactivation of alveolar macrophages in septic neutropenic ARDS. Chest 124:644–652

29. Mokart D, Kipnis E, Guerre-Berthelot P et al (2008) Monocyte deactivation in neutropenic acute respiratory distress syndrome patients treated with granulocyte colony-stimulating factor. Crit Care 12:R17
30. Ognibene FP, Martin SE, Parker MM et al (1986) Adult respiratory distress syndrome in patients with severe neutropenia. N Engl J Med 315:547–551
31. Sivan Y, Mor C, al-Jundi S et al (1990) Adult respiratory distress syndrome in severely neutropenic children. Pediatr Pulmonol 8:104–108
32. Vansteenkiste JF, Boogaerts MA (1989) Adult respiratory distress syndrome in neutropenic leukemia patients. Blut 58:287–290
33. Bernard GR, Artigas A, Brigham KL et al (1994) The American-European Consensus Conference on ARDS. Definitions, mechanisms, relevant outcomes, and clinical trial coordination. Am J Respir Crit Care Med 149:818–824
34. Wheeler AP, Bernard GR (2007) Acute lung injury and the acute respiratory distress syndrome: a clinical review. Lancet 369:1553–1564
35. Azoulay E, Schlemmer B (2006) Diagnostic strategy in cancer patients with acute respiratory failure. Intensive Care Med 32:808–822
36. Azoulay E, Mokart D, Rabbat A et al (2008) Diagnostic bronchoscopy in hematology and oncology patients with acute respiratory failure: prospective multicenter data. Crit Care Med 36:100–107
37. Pene F, Aubron C, Azoulay E et al (2006) Outcome of critically ill allogeneic hematopoietic stem-cell transplantation recipients: a reappraisal of indications for organ failure supports. J Clin Oncol 24:643–649
38. Mokart D, van Craenenbroeck T, Textoris J et al (2009) Early predictive factors of mortality in neutropenic patients with acute respiratory distress syndrome (submitted)
39. Hotchkiss RS, Karl IE (2003) The pathophysiology and treatment of sepsis. N Engl J Med 348:138–150
40. Pittet JF, Mackersie RC, Martin TR et al (1997) Biological markers of acute lung injury: prognostic and pathogenetic significance. Am J Respir Crit Care Med 155:1187–1205
41. Ware LB, Matthay MA (2000) The acute respiratory distress syndrome. N Engl J Med 342:1334–1349
42. Wang HM, Bodenstein M, Markstaller K (2008) Overview of the pathology of three widely used animal models of acute lung injury. Eur Surg Res 40:305–316
43. Chollet-Martin S, Montravers P, Gibert C et al (1994) Relationships between polymorphonuclear neutrophils and cytokines in patients with adult respiratory distress syndrome. Ann NY Acad Sci 725:354–366
44. Zilow G, Joka T, Obertacke U et al (1992) Generation of anaphylatoxin C3a in plasma and bronchoalveolar lavage fluid in trauma patients at risk for the adult respiratory distress syndrome. Crit Care Med 20:468–473
45. Donnelly SC, Strieter RM, Kunkel SL et al (1993) Interleukin-8 and development of adult respiratory distress syndrome in at-risk patient groups. Lancet 341:643–647
46. Kiehl M, Ostermann H, Birkfellner T et al (1996) Inflammatory mediators in the bronchoalveolar lavage fluid in leukocytopenic patients with fever. Am J Respir Crit Care Med 153:A616
47. Kiehl MG, Ostermann H, Thomas M et al (1997) Inflammatory mediators in BAL fluid as markers of evolving pneumonia in leukocytopenic patients. Chest 112:1214–1220
48. Kiehl MG, Ostermann H, Thomas M et al (1998) Inflammatory mediators in bronchoalveolar lavage fluid and plasma in leukocytopenic patients with septic shock-induced acute respiratory distress syndrome. Crit Care Med 26:1194–1199
49. Cordonnier C, Escudier E, Verra F et al (1994) Bronchoalveolar lavage during neutropenic episodes: diagnostic yield and cellular pattern. Eur Respir J 7:114–120
50. Steinberg KP, Milberg JA, Martin TR et al (1994) Evolution of bronchoalveolar cell populations in the adult respiratory distress syndrome. Am J Respir Crit Care Med 150: 113–122
51. Dakin J, Griffiths M (2002) The pulmonary physician in critical care 1: pulmonary investigations for acute respiratory failure. Thorax 57:79–85
52. Lamy M, by-Dupont G (1995) Is sepsis a mediator-inhibitor mismatch? Intensive Care Med 21(Suppl 2):S250–S257
53. Shelhamer JH, Levine SJ, Wu T et al (1995) NIH conference. Airway inflammation. Ann Intern Med 123:288–304
54. Abraham E (2003) Neutrophils and acute lung injury. Crit Care Med 31:S195–S199
55. Heidemann SM, Glibetic M (2007) Comparison of the systemic and pulmonary inflammatory response to endotoxin of neutropenic and non-neutropenic rats. J Inflamm (Lond) 4:7
56. Sato Y, van Eeden SF, English D et al (1998) Bacteremic pneumococcal pneumonia: bone marrow release and pulmonary sequestration of neutrophils. Crit Care Med 26:501–509
57. Azoulay E, Attalah H, Yang K et al (2003) Exacerbation with granulocyte colony-stimulating factor of prior acute lung injury during neutropenia recovery in rats. Crit Care Med 31:157–165
58. Abraham E, Kaneko DJ, Shenkar R (1999) Effects of endogenous and exogenous catecholamines on LPS-induced neutrophil trafficking and activation. Am J Physiol 276: L1–L8
59. Abraham E, Carmody A, Shenkar R et al (2000) Neutrophils as early immunologic effectors in hemorrhage- or endotoxemia-induced acute lung injury. Am J Physiol Lung Cell Mol Physiol 279:L1137–L1145
60. Pugin J, Ricou B, Steinberg KP et al (1996) Proinflammatory activity in bronchoalveolar lavage fluids from patients with ARDS, a prominent role for interleukin-1. Am J Respir Crit Care Med 153:1850–1856
61. Ostermann H, Rothenburger M, Mesters RM et al (1994) Cytokine response to infection in patients with acute myelogenous leukaemia following intensive chemotherapy. Br J Haematol 88:332–337
62. Schonbohn H, Schuler M, Kolbe K et al (1995) Plasma levels of IL-1, TNF alpha, IL-6, IL-8, G-CSF, and IL1-RA during febrile neutropenia: results of a prospective study in patients undergoing chemotherapy for acute myelogenous leukemia. Ann Hematol 71:161–168
63. Steinmetz HT, Herbertz A, Bertram M et al (1995) Increase in interleukin-6 serum level preceding fever in granulocytopenia and correlation with death from sepsis. J Infect Dis 171:225–228
64. Waage A, Steinshamn S (1993) Cytokine mediators of septic infections in the normal and granulocytopenic host. Eur J Haematol 50:243–249
65. Denecker NE, Kullberg BJ, Drenth JP et al (1997) Regulation of the production of pro-inflammatory cytokines and antagonists during chemotherapy-induced neutropenia in

patients with haematological malignancies. Cytokine 9: 702–710
66. Sibille Y, Reynolds HY (1990) Macrophages and polymorphonuclear neutrophils in lung defense and injury. Am Rev Respir Dis 141:471–501
67. Christner P, Fein A, Goldberg S et al (1985) Collagenase in the lower respiratory tract of patients with adult respiratory distress syndrome. Am Rev Respir Dis 131:690–695
68. Gibbs DF, Shanley TP, Warner RL et al (1999) Role of matrix metalloproteinases in models of macrophage-dependent acute lung injury. Evidence for alveolar macrophage as source of proteinases. Am J Respir Cell Mol Biol 20:1145–1154
69. Lohmann-Matthes ML, Steinmuller C, Franke-Ullmann G (1994) Pulmonary macrophages. Eur Respir J 7:1678–1689
70. Torii K, Iida K, Miyazaki Y et al (1997) Higher concentrations of matrix metalloproteinases in bronchoalveolar lavage fluid of patients with adult respiratory distress syndrome. Am J Respir Crit Care Med 155:43–46
71. Schwartz MD, Moore EE, Moore FA et al (1996) Nuclear factor-kappa B is activated in alveolar macrophages from patients with acute respiratory distress syndrome. Crit Care Med 24:1285–1292
72. Wiedermann FJ, Mayr AJ, Hobisch-Hagen P et al (2003) Association of endogenous G-CSF with anti-inflammatory mediators in patients with acute respiratory distress syndrome. J Interferon Cytokine Res 23:729–736
73. Dos Santos CC (2008) Advances in mechanisms of repair and remodelling in acute lung injury. Intensive Care Med 34:619–630
74. Zarbock A, Singbartl K, Ley K (2006) Complete reversal of acid-induced acute lung injury by blocking of platelet-neutrophil aggregation. J Clin Invest 116:3211–3219
75. Zarbock A, Polanowska-Grabowska RK, Ley K (2007) Platelet-neutrophil-interactions: linking hemostasis and inflammation. Blood Rev 21:99–111
76. Kuebler WM (2006) Selectins revisited: the emerging role of platelets in inflammatory lung disease. J Clin Invest 116: 3106–3108
77. Khan H, Belsher J, Yilmaz M et al (2007) Fresh-frozen plasma and platelet transfusions are associated with development of acute lung injury in critically ill medical patients. Chest 131:1308–1314
78. Lucas R, Verin AD, Black SM et al (2009) Regulators of endothelial and epithelial barrier integrity and function in acute lung injury. Biochem Pharmacol 77:1763–1772
79. Charpidou AG, Gkiozos I, Tsimpoukis S et al (2009) Therapy-induced toxicity of the lungs: an overview. Anticancer Res 29:631–639
80. Donnelly SC, Strieter RM, Reid PT et al (1996) The association between mortality rates and decreased concentrations of interleukin-10 and interleukin-1 receptor antagonist in the lung fluids of patients with the adult respiratory distress syndrome. Ann Intern Med 125:191–196
81. Dellinger RP, Levy MM, Carlet JM et al (2008) Surviving Sepsis Campaign: international guidelines for management of severe sepsis and septic shock: 2008. Intensive Care Med 34:17–60
82. Aapro MS, Cameron DA, Pettengell R et al (2006) EORTC guidelines for the use of granulocyte-colony stimulating factor to reduce the incidence of chemotherapy-induced febrile neutropenia in adult patients with lymphomas and solid tumours. Eur J Cancer 42:2433–2453
83. Kuderer NM, Dale DC, Crawford J et al (2007) Impact of primary prophylaxis with granulocyte colony-stimulating factor on febrile neutropenia and mortality in adult cancer patients receiving chemotherapy: a systematic review. J Clin Oncol 25:3158–3167
84. Karlin L, Darmon M, Thiery G et al (2005) Respiratory status deterioration during G-CSF-induced neutropenia recovery. Bone Marrow Transplant 36:245–250
85. Takahashi Y, Kobayashi Y, Chikayama S et al (1999) Effect of granulocyte/colony-stimulating factor on the onset of the adult respiratory distress syndrome. Acta Haematol 101:124–129
86. Meisel C, Schefold JC, Pschowski R et al (2009) Granulocyte-macrophage colony-stimulating factor to reverse sepsis-associated immunosuppression: a double-blind, randomized, placebo-controlled multicenter trial. Am J Respir Crit Care Med 180:640–648
87. Frank JA, Parsons PE, Matthay MA (2006) Pathogenetic significance of biological markers of ventilator-associated lung injury in experimental and clinical studies. Chest 130:1906–1914
88. Steinberg KP, Hudson LD, Goodman RB et al (2006) Efficacy and safety of corticosteroids for persistent acute respiratory distress syndrome. N Engl J Med 354:1671–1684
89. Tang BM, Craig JC, Eslick GD et al (2009) Use of corticosteroids in acute lung injury and acute respiratory distress syndrome: a systematic review and meta-analysis. Crit Care Med 37:1594–1603
90. Schwarz MI, Albert RK (2004) "Imitators" of the ARDS: implications for diagnosis and treatment. Chest 125:1530–1535
91. Hyle EP, Lipworth AD, Zaoutis TE et al (2005) Impact of inadequate initial antimicrobial therapy on mortality in infections due to extended-spectrum beta-lactamase-producing enterobacteriaceae: variability by site of infection. Arch Intern Med 165:1375–1380
92. Thiery G, Azoulay E, Darmon M et al (2005) Outcome of cancer patients considered for intensive care unit admission: a hospital-wide prospective study. J Clin Oncol 23: 4406–4413
93. Hilbert G, Gruson D, Vargas F et al (2001) Noninvasive ventilation in immunosuppressed patients with pulmonary infiltrates, fever, and acute respiratory failure. N Engl J Med 344:481–487
94. Delclaux C, L'Her E, Alberti C et al (2000) Treatment of acute hypoxemic nonhypercapnic respiratory insufficiency with continuous positive airway pressure delivered by a face mask: a randomized controlled trial. JAMA 284:2352–2360
95. Evans TW (2001) International Consensus Conferences in Intensive Care Medicine: non-invasive positive pressure ventilation in acute respiratory failure. Organised jointly by the American Thoracic Society, the European Respiratory Society, the European Society of Intensive Care Medicine, and the Societe de Reanimation de Langue Francaise, and approved by the ATS Board of Directors, December 2000. Intensive Care Med 27:166–178
96. Groeger JS, White P Jr, Nierman DM et al (1999) Outcome for cancer patients requiring mechanical ventilation. J Clin Oncol 17:991–997
97. Heussel CP, Kauczor HU, Heussel GE et al (1999) Pneumonia in febrile neutropenic patients and in bone marrow and blood stem-cell transplant recipients: use of high-resolution computed tomography. J Clin Oncol 17:796–805

98. Shorr AF, Susla GM, O'Grady NP (2004) Pulmonary infiltrates in the non-HIV-infected immunocompromised patient: etiologies, diagnostic strategies, and outcomes. Chest 125:260–271
99. Maertens J, Van EJ, Verhaegen J et al (2002) Use of circulating galactomannan screening for early diagnosis of invasive aspergillosis in allogeneic stem cell transplant recipients. J Infect Dis 186:1297–1306
100. Schvoerer E, Henriot S, Zachary P et al (2005) Monitoring low cytomegalovirus viremia in transplanted patients by a real-time PCR on plasma. J Med Virol 76:76–81
101. Templeton KE, Scheltinga SA, van den Eeden WC et al (2005) Improved diagnosis of the etiology of community-acquired pneumonia with real-time polymerase chain reaction. Clin Infect Dis 41:345–351
102. van Elden LJ, van Kraaij MG, Nijhuis M et al (2002) Polymerase chain reaction is more sensitive than viral culture and antigen testing for the detection of respiratory viruses in adults with hematological cancer and pneumonia. Clin Infect Dis 34:177–183
103. Mykietiuk A, Carratala J, Fernandez-Sabe N et al (2005) Clinical outcomes for hospitalized patients with Legionella pneumonia in the antigenuria era: the influence of levofloxacin therapy. Clin Infect Dis 40:794–799
104. Roson B, Fernandez-Sabe N, Carratala J et al (2004) Contribution of a urinary antigen assay (Binax NOW) to the early diagnosis of pneumococcal pneumonia. Clin Infect Dis 38:222–226
105. Rano A, Agusti C, Jimenez P et al (2001) Pulmonary infiltrates in non-HIV immunocompromised patients: a diagnostic approach using non-invasive and bronchoscopic procedures. Thorax 56:379–387
106. Chemaly RF, Ghosh S, Bodey GP et al (2006) Respiratory viral infections in adults with hematologic malignancies and human stem cell transplantation recipients: a retrospective study at a major cancer center. Medicine (Baltimore) 85:278–287
107. Ellis ME, Spence D, Bouchama A et al (1995) Open lung biopsy provides a higher and more specific diagnostic yield compared to broncho-alveolar lavage in immunocompromised patients. Fungal Study Group. Scand J Infect Dis 27:157–162
108. Rossiter SJ, Miller C, Churg AM et al (1979) Open lung biopsy in the immunosuppressed patient. Is it really beneficial? J Thorac Cardiovasc Surg 77:338–345
109. Peikert T, Rana S, Edell ES (2005) Safety, diagnostic yield, and therapeutic implications of flexible bronchoscopy in patients with febrile neutropenia and pulmonary infiltrates. Mayo Clin Proc 80:1414–1420
110. Azoulay E (2009) Pulmonary infiltrates in patients with malignancies: why and how neutropenia influences clinical reasoning. Eur Respir J 33:6–8
111. Maschmeyer G, Beinert T, Buchheidt D et al (2009) Diagnosis and antimicrobial therapy of lung infiltrates in febrile neutropenic patients: guidelines of the infectious diseases working party of the German Society of Haematology and Oncology. Eur J Cancer 45:2462–2472
112. Maschmeyer G, Haas A (2008) The epidemiology and treatment of infections in cancer patients. Int J Antimicrob Agents 31:193–197
113. Bodey GP, Buckley M, Sathe YS et al (1966) Quantitative relationships between circulating leukocytes and infection in patients with acute leukemia. Ann Intern Med 64: 328–340
114. Larche J, Azoulay E, Fieux F et al (2003) Improved survival of critically ill cancer patients with septic shock. Intensive Care Med 29:1688–1695
115. Mokart D, Sannini A, Brun JP et al (2008) Oncohematology patients with febrile neutropeniahospitalized in ICU: clinical practice guidelines. Réanimation 17:213–224
116. Bal AM, Gould IM (2007) Empirical antimicrobial treatment for chemotherapy-induced febrile neutropenia. Int J Antimicrob Agents 29:501–509
117. Wisplinghoff H, Seifert H, Wenzel RP et al (2003) Current trends in the epidemiology of nosocomial bloodstream infections in patients with hematological malignancies and solid neoplasms in hospitals in the United States. Clin Infect Dis 36:1103–1110
118. Drgona L, Paul M, Bucaneve G et al (2007) The need for aminoglycosides in combination with b-lactams for high-risk, febrile neutropaenic patients with leukaemia. Eur J Cancer supplement 5:13–22
119. Meunier F, Lukan C (2008) The First European Conference on Infections in Leukaemia – ECIL1: a current perspective. Eur J Cancer 44:2112–2117
120. Cometta A, Marchetti O, Calandra T (2007) Empirical use of anti-Gram-positive antibiotics in febrile neutropaenic cancer patients with acute leukaemia. Eur J Cancer supplements 5:23–31
121. Hughes WT, Armstrong D, Bodey GP et al (2002) 2002 guidelines for the use of antimicrobial agents in neutropenic patients with cancer. Clin Infect Dis 34:730–751
122. Gil L, Kozlowska-Skrzypczak M, Mol A et al (2009) Increased risk for invasive aspergillosis in patients with lymphoproliferative diseases after autologous hematopoietic SCT. Bone Marrow Transplant 43:121–126
123. Mayaud C (2002) Le SDRA de l'immunodéprimé: un pronostic amélioré ? Réanimation 11:5–8
124. Lecuyer L, Chevret S, Thiery G et al (2007) The ICU trial: a new admission policy for cancer patients requiring mechanical ventilation. Crit Care Med 35:808–814
125. Zhao M, Fernandez LG, Doctor A et al (2006) Alveolar macrophage activation is a key initiation signal for acute lung ischemia-reperfusion injury. Am J Physiol Lung Cell Mol Physiol 291:L1018–L1026

Pulmonary Venoocclusive Disease Following Hematopoietic Stem Cell Transplantation

37

Matthew C. Bunte and Linda J. Burns

Contents

M.C. Bunte
Department of Medicine, University of Minnesota, Minneapolis, MN 55455, USA

L.J. Burns (✉)
Department of Medicine, University of Minnesota, Minneapolis, MN 55455, USA and
Division of Hematology, Oncology and Transplantation, University of Minnesota, Mayo Mail Code 480,
420 Delaware St. SE, Minneapolis, MN 55455, USA
e-mail: burns019@umn.edu

37.1 Epidemiology

In 1984, Troussard reported on the first case of PVOD following HSCT [28] some 50 years after the disease was originally described [13].

In those 50 years, fewer than 70 cases of PVOD had been reported. Since that time, the number of reported cases has risen substantially, perhaps owing to greater recognition of the disease [1,11,18,21]. PVOD has been reported in association with a number of systemic inflammatory conditions, including infections, autoimmune disease, malignancy, toxic exposures and antineoplastic chemotherapy, and transplantation [19]. PVOD affects all ages, with cases reported in early infancy to 68 years, although the majority of cases affect those less than 50 years of age [11,19]. Nearly twice as many males are affected among those older than 18 years of age, a characteristic unique from PAH, which tends to favor females over males [11,18,21,29]. Children exhibit a more even male-to-female ratio. Familial forms linked to the pathway associated with bone-morphogenic protein receptor 2 (BMPR2), a member of the transforming growth factor-β family, have also been identified [4,21,30]. Of interest, the BMPR2 pathway has been linked in 60% of familial forms and 10–25% of sporadic cases of PAH [2]. An association of BMPR2 mutations in familial or sporadic cases of PVOD has not been well established.

This chapter's table summarizes reported cases of PVOD occurring in the post-HSCT population. Among HSCT recipients, most cases of PVOD have been described among those receiving myeloablative preparative regimens, although more recent reports also identify PVOD after reduced intensity, non-myeloablative regimens [1,8]. As seen in Table 37.1, among HSCT recipients PVOD tended to occur in those under age 25 years and predominantly among

É. Azoulay (ed.), *Pulmonary Involvement in Patients with Hematological Malignancies*,
DOI: 10.1007/978-3-642-15742-4_37, © Springer-Verlag Berlin Heidelberg 2011

Table 37.1 Case reports of pulmonary veno-occlusive disease (PVOD) after hematopoietic stem cell transplant

Case report (reference)	Age (years)/sex	Pre-HSCT diagnosis	Pre-transplant therapy	Transplant conditioning therapy	HSCT Type	GVHD prophylaxis	Onset of GVHD	Onset of PVOD post-HSCT	Presenting signs and symptoms	Treatment	Outcome
[35]	7/M	ALL	CY, AraC, vincristine, daunorubicin, mithramycin, pred	CY, TBI	allo-sib	MTX	Acute GVHD @ d+18	d+44	Interstitial pneumonitis	None	Deceased
[9]	4/F	ALL	Vincristine, pred, asparaginase, daunomycin, MTX (1st remission); CY, vincristine, pred, AraC, asparaginase, MTX (2nd remission)	CY, TBI, busulfan, MTX (transplant#1); CY, etoposide, BCNU (transplant#2)	allo-sib×2	NR	Acute - none; chronic - subclinical	d+46 (2nd HSCT)	Dyspnea	Steroids	Lived to d+106; deceased due to relapse of ALL
[9]	4/M	ALL	CY, TBI, MTX, Pred, AraC, vincristine, daunomycin, asparaginase, tenieposide, 6MP, etoposide, BCNU	CY, etoposide, BCNU	allo-sib	NR	Acute - none; chronic - none	d+60	Dyspnea, lethargy	Steroids	Alive at d+230[b]
[30]	39/M	NHL	CY, doxorubicin, vincristine, pred, AraC, etoposide, cisplatin	CY, etoposide, BCNU, dacarbazine	Auto	N/A	N/A	d+52	Dyspnea, cough, fever	Steroids	Deceased
[17]	19/F	ALL	NR	CY, TBI (transplant#1); mitoxantrone, AraC, busulfan, etoposide, melphalan (transplant#2)	Allo-sib×2	MTX, CSA (1st); none (2nd)	Acute - none; chronic - suspected clinically	d+342 (2nd HSCT)	Dyspnea	Steroids, PGE, heparin	Deceased

[41]	24/M	ALL	CY, doxorubicin, MTX, AraC, pred, CSA, dactinomycin, vincristine, BCNU, 6MP, asparaginase	NR	Allo	pred, CSA	None; skin biopsy neg	d+180	Dyspnea, cough	Steroids, heparin	Alive at d+360[b]
[29]	36/F	ALL	Daunorubicin	CY, TBI, TLI, melphalan, etoposide	Allo	None	None	d+6	Dyspnea	Oxygen, supportive care	Alive at d+27[b]
[32]	20/M	NHL	CY, doxorubicin, vincristine, pred, carboplatin, AraC, mitoxantrone	CY, TBI, AraC	Allo-sib	MTX, CSA	None	d+73	Dyspnea	Steroids	Deceased
[35]	1/M	Neuro-blastoma	CY, TBI, vincristine, doxorubicin, cisplatin, etoposide	Carboplatin, etoposide, Melphalan	Auto	N/A	N/A	d+13	Dyspnea	Steroids, heparin	Deceased
[26]	49/F	CML	Interferon-alpha	CY, TBI	Allo-sib	MTX, CSA	None	d+223	Dyspnea	Steroids	Deceased
[21]	48/M	Multiple myeloma	Vincristine, doxorubicin, pred	Melphalan	Auto	N/A	N/A	d+11	Dry cough, dyspnea	None	Alive at d+19[b]
Bunte (2007)[a] (unpublished data)	21/F	AML	Idarubicin, AraC	CY, TBI, fludarabine	Allo-DUCT	CSA, MMF	Acute - none; chronic - suspected clinically	d+138	Dyspnea, orthopnea, syncope	Prostacyclin, heparin	Alive at d+998[b]

those with hematologic malignancy as the indication for transplantation. Allogeneic transplant is represented more commonly than autologous transplant, which offers consideration for a possible immunologic role into development of this disease. Onset of PVOD typically occurred several weeks to months following HSCT, although it has been reported within days of transplant. The pathogenesis of PVOD is likely multifactorial, with transplantation providing a rich substrate of inflammation, endothelial injury, and opportunistic infections contributing to disease development.

37.2 Pathophysiology

Within recent years, larger case series of PVOD have provided improved recognition of this condition, enabling providers with enhanced characterization and understanding of the pathogenesis of this rare form of PAH [11,18,21]. Despite these important advances, many details of the development, progression, and resolution of PVOD are yet to be determined. On histological section, the hallmark of PVOD is patchy, diffuse intimal fibrosis among venules and small veins of the pulmonary bed [18,21]. Inter- and intralobular venular fibrosis commonly leads to intraluminal septae and vascular recanalization, eccentric intimal fibrosis, venular hypertrophy, and vascular obstruction (see Fig. 37.1) [18]. Capillary congestion proximal to these obstructions ensues, resulting in medial hypertrophy and intimal fibrosis of the pulmonary arterial circulation. Complex, plexiform lesions characteristic of PAH are not typically seen in PVOD. Severe PAH can subsequently develop nonetheless. Parenchymal evidence of PVOD may include interstitial edema and fibrosis, hemosiderosis, and diffuse alveolar damage. Lymphocytic infiltrates, lymphocytic venulitis, or leukocytoclastic vasculitis may be associated with this interstitial fibrosis as well [18,19]. Development of PVOD in the peri-transplant period has interesting similarities to other HSCT-associated complications that make this disease of interest to the transplant provider. Perhaps the most interesting feature of PVOD includes the histological and pathogenic similarities this disease has with other much more common complications of HSCT. Endothelial injury is a well-recognized feature of the complications affecting the HSCT recipient [3,34]. Many transplant-associated variables contribute to systemic inflammation and endothelial damage, including pretransplant malignancy, cytotoxic preparatory conditioning regimens, therapeutic radiation, opportunistic infections, and graft-versus-host disease. These pro-inflammatory factors contribute to a model of vascular injury that has been implicated in the pathogenesis of many common and clinically important HSCT complications including microangiopathic hemolytic anemia, hepatic venoocclusive disease (HVOD), acute lung injury, and multiple organ dysfunction syndrome, among others. Although these complications of HSCT certainly represent unique syndromes, transplant-associated endothelial injury provides a common pathophysiologic link of thrombosis, compromised vascular flow, and organ failure. Despite limited insight into the pathogenesis of PVOD due to its rare nature, endothelial injury may serve a critical role in the development of this disease. Among the HSCT-associated complications, HVOD represents a particularly important example of HSCT-related endothelial injury. Relative to PVOD, HVOD is a much more common and well-described complication of HSCT with an estimated incidence affecting 10–15% of transplant recipients [16,20]. While not specific to transplantation, HVOD has been linked to a number of transplant-associated variables including cytotoxic preparative regimens, radiation therapy, and allogeneic transplantation. HVOD is characterized by early loss of sinusoidal endothelial integrity, followed by hepatic sinusoidal and venular thrombosis, fibrosis,

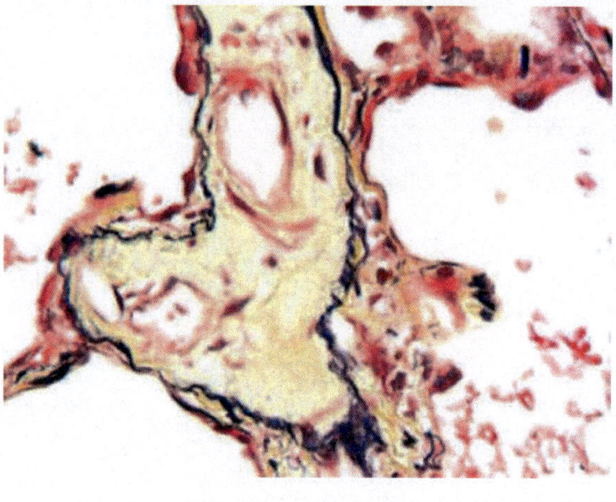

Fig. 37.1 Movat pentachrome stain shows collagen deposition in intima of a small venule, with the elastic layer (*black*) peripherally displaced. Recanalization within the collagen deposition is noted (40× objective) (Image courtesy of J. Gutman)

and eventual vascular obstruction [16]. A resultant triad of fluid retention, hyperbilirubinemia, and painful hepatomegaly produces a variable clinical syndrome ranging from mild disease to multiorgan failure and death. HVOD demonstrates distinct pathophysiologic and clinical similarities of early endothelial injury, thrombosis, and vascular remodeling that lead to venular obstruction and organ failure, which may serve as a useful conceptual model for the pathogenesis of PVOD. PVOD shares many common features with other forms of PAH, although important clinical and therapeutic differences exist that offer insight into the development of this disease. PVOD has been reported in a number of other inflammatory conditions, such as systemic sclerosis and myelodysplastic syndrome, among others. PAH is a common complication of systemic sclerosis; however, a higher rate of PAH non-responders is observed in this population. A weak, refractory, or paradoxical response to conventional vasodilator therapy among patients with systemic sclerosis presumed to have PAH may suggest an alternative diagnosis of PVOD [6,21]. A similar finding of unexplained pulmonary hypertension in chronic myeloproliferative disorders has also been described [5]. These findings not only suggest a unique association of PVOD with particular inflammatory conditions, but also illustrate that PVOD may be underdiagnosed and thereby represent a commonly misdiagnosed cause of PAH [9]. It is unclear if PVOD is represented in similar disproportion in the post-HSCT population. Nonetheless, accurate diagnosis of PVOD and the ability to distinguish it from other post-transplant pulmonary complications, including PAH, is critically important.

37.3 Clinical Manifestations and Diagnosis

Pulmonary complications following HSCT are common, clinically heterogeneous, and broadly represent a variety of pulmonary diseases [15,24,26,27]. In fact, retrospective reviews in the HSCT population suggest that the majority of pulmonary complications are not diagnosed antemortem, yet they remain the most common source of death among transplant recipients [24,26]. The diagnosis of PVOD is further challenged by a variable time course, heterogeneous clinical features, and need for invasive testing to confirm diagnosis. Nevertheless, recognition of PVOD as a complication of HSCT is critical, particularly as the disease must be distinguished from other forms of PAH given significant implications in treatment. Antemortem diagnosis of PVOD often proves difficult because of vague presenting symptoms, nonspecific radiographic findings, and atypical cardiopulmonary hemodynamics. A delay in diagnosis is common, with the mean duration of symptoms prior to diagnosis ranging from 12 to 49 months [18,21]. Milder and non-fatal forms with spontaneous resolution of pulmonary venular obstruction may be an under-recognized course of disease, contributing to an underestimation of the actual incidence of PVOD.

Although non-specific and similar to other forms of PAH, progressive dyspnea is the most consistent early complaint among those with subsequently diagnosed PVOD [18,19]. Consistent with this finding, dyspnea represented a consistent presenting symptom among HSCT recipients (see Table 37.1). Other symptoms of PVOD may include fatigue, chest pain, cough, clubbing, hemoptysis, orthopnea, paroxysmal nocturnal dyspnea, and syncope. As right ventricular function deteriorates, features of right heart failure, including lower extremity edema and hepatic congestion, may become more prominent. Physical examination findings of PVOD are typically nonspecific and consistent with that of PAH. Pulmonary crackles, elevated jugular venous pulse, cyanosis, congestive hepatomegaly, and lower extremity edema have been reported. Digital clubbing may be of value in considering the diagnosis of PVOD; commonly seen in interstitial lung disease, clubbing is not frequently reported among cases of PAH, including PVOD. Pleural effusions are frequently reported among cases of PVOD, yet are unusually seen in other forms of PAH.

Electrocardiography may reveal a rightward axis and reflect compensatory right ventricular enlargement from elevated pulmonary arterial pressures. Echocardiography may be of use in excluding other causes of right ventricular failure, including left ventricular failure and severe mitral valvular disease. Pulmonary function testing confirming a lower baseline partial pressure of oxygen at rest further reduced ambulatory arterial oxygen saturation, and reduced diffusion capacity of carbon monoxide may be more suggestive of PVOD than PAH [21].

Chest radiographic findings of PVOD include perihilar pulmonary vascular congestion and prominent septal lines; together, these findings are suggestive of post-arterial pulmonary capillary congestion and interstitial transudation of fluid [7]. Pleural effusions are commonly reported. Bilateral patchy parenchymal infiltrates appear similar to those of acute respiratory distress syndrome. Chest computed tomography (CT) of PVOD may demonstrate smooth interlobular septal thickening, poorly defined ground-glass opacification, and dilated central pulmonary arteries (see Fig. 37.2). Results of ventilation/perfusion (V/Q) scanning in PVOD may be variable from normal to diffuse irregularities or segmental V/Q mismatches. Pulmonary angiography may reveal enlarged pulmonary arteries and prolonged circulation time through the lungs, although flow through the pulmonary veins and left atrium is typically normal. Cardiac catheterization is a useful tool to confirm elevated pulmonary arterial, right ventricular, and right atrial pressures. A normal or paradoxically low pulmonary arterial wedge pressure (PAWP) is a classically described feature of PVOD. Despite the pulmonary venular occlusions associated with PVOD, the larger pulmonary veins are primarily responsible for determining resistance to blood flow beyond the wedged pulmonary artery catheter; these structures are hemodynamically normal in PVOD [32]. While an elevated PAWP does not exclude the diagnosis of PVOD, this finding may be more suggestive of another cause of elevated intrapulmonary pressures, including pulmonary vein stenosis, severe mitral stenosis, or left ventricular failure. Vasodilator challenge at the time of right heart catheterization, as is more routinely performed in PAH for predicting response to calcium channel blockers, may acutely worsen pulmonary congestion in PVOD. In addition, even if vasodilator challenge proves acutely helpful in PVOD, this test may not be useful in predicting long-term benefit from vasodilator therapy [21]. The triad of severe PAH, radiographic evidence of pulmonary edema, and normal PAWP is classically described clinical diagnostic criteria for PVOD [12,20]. Surgical lung biopsy remains the gold standard for diagnosis of PVOD. However, in many cases of PVOD, severely elevated pulmonary arterial pressures may make lung biopsy unfeasible. Therefore, clinical and radiographic findings may be reliable identifiers of PVOD and prove invaluable when surgical lung biopsy is not possible or not warranted due to clinical improvement.

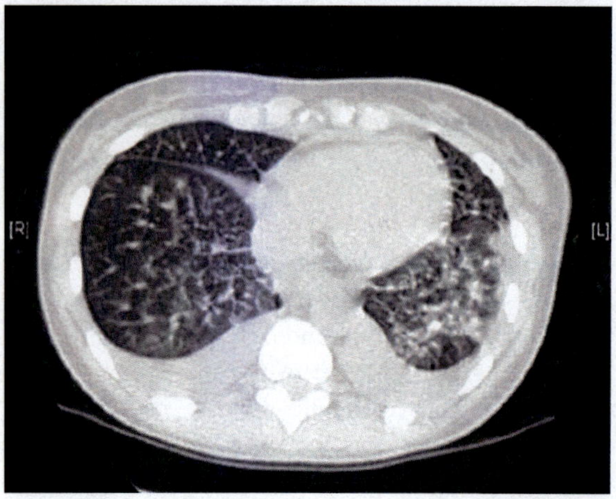

Fig. 37.2 Chest CT demonstrating septal thickening, small bilateral pleural effusions, scattered multifocal ground-glass opacities, and patchy left lower lobe airspace opacities (Image courtesy of J. Gutman)

37.4 Treatment

The rare nature of PVOD has offered little opportunity to evaluate preventative or treatment measures for this disease. Most accepted treatment options for PVOD have been extrapolated from the management of PAH and other complications associated with HSCT-induced microvascular injury. Overall, current treatment options for PVOD are quite limited. Vasodilators, such as nitrates, phosphodiesterase inhibitors, calcium channel blockers, prostacyclins, and endothelin antagonists, represent an important treatment class in the conventional management of PAH. Use of vasodilator therapy in PVOD has been reported with relatively mixed results and limited success. In fact, several reports demonstrate the dangerous potential of vasodilator treatment for PVOD, precipitating acute pulmonary edema, hypoxia, and even death. A limited or refractory response or paradoxical worsening of clinical status with vasodilator therapy in a presumed case of PAH may suggest PVOD [9]. Nevertheless, long-term improvement in respiratory symptoms associated with PVOD has been reported with the use of calcium-channel blockers and prostacyclins [17,23,25]. Despite these reports, no official recommendations have been made regarding the use of vasodilatory agents in the management of PVOD. Given the pathogenic hallmark of thrombotic occlusion of pulmonary venules, use of antithrombotic therapy in the management of PVOD has been reported. Use of antithrombotics/fibrinolytics has been extrapolated, in part, from trials of long-term anticoagulation in PAH, which has suggested a modest mortality benefit [14]. Use of antithrombotic therapy has been studied in HVOD, a more common post-transplant complication associated with endothelial dysfunction and thrombosis. When applied to HVOD, these therapies have been largely ineffective and associated with an excess of bleeding complications [16,31]. Defibrotide, a porcine-derived oligonucleotide with anti-thrombotic and endothelial reparative properties, has emerged as a novel treatment for HVOD [10]. Use of defibrotide for PVOD has been reported with favorable results [33], but requires further investigation. At present, it is unclear if defibrotide will have a role in the management of PVOD, although the pathophysiologic similarities between these conditions may suggest benefit in the pulmonary variant. Lung transplantation has traditionally been the only durable treatment option for severe, refractory PVOD. Epoprostenol may serve as a beneficial vasodilator "bridge" to lung transplantation [22]. However, with reports of recurrence of PVOD after lung transplantation, further study is needed to confirm the durability of this treatment option [13].

37.5 Complications and Prognosis

Classically, PVOD is associated with a dismal prognosis and high rate of death within 2 years of diagnosis [19]. More recently, cases of PVOD demonstrating partial recovery, improvement on vasodilator or antithrombotic therapy, or spontaneous resolution have been described. The typical clinical course for PVOD remains poorly defined. The clinical spectrum is likely variable, and the frequency of unrecognized or incorrectly diagnosed cases, including those that may resolve spontaneously, is unknown. Therefore, while prognosis of PVOD is traditionally poor, improved recognition and further study may demonstrate a broader spectrum of clinical disease. Further study in the pathogenesis of PVOD may subsequently result in more durable treatment options.

37.6 Conclusion

Although a rare condition, PVOD is likely underrecognized and misdiagnosed in many cases given its similar presentation to PAH and a number of other post-transplant pulmonary complications. The pathogenesis of PVOD is likely multifactorial, with a key role of endothelial dysfunction in the pathogenesis of this disease, as with other post-HSCT complications. Diagnosis of PVOD is challenged by vague presenting symptoms, non-specific clinical signs, and need for invasive testing to confirm the diagnosis. Accurate recognition of PVOD is warranted given the potentially devastating complications that may result from conventional PAH vasodilator therapy.

References

1. Bunte MC, Patnaik MM et al (2008) Pulmonary veno-occlusive disease following hematopoietic stem cell transplantation: a rare model of endothelial dysfunction. Bone Marrow Transplant 41(8):677–686
2. Chin KM, Rubin LJ (2008) Pulmonary arterial hypertension. J Am Coll Cardiol 51(16):1527–1538
3. Copelan EA (2006) Hematopoietic stem-cell transplantation. N Engl J Med 354(17):1813–1826
4. Davies P, Reid L (1982) Pulmonary veno-occlusive disease in siblings: case reports and morphometric study. Hum Pathol 13(10):911–915
5. Dingli D, Utz JP et al (2001) Unexplained pulmonary hypertension in chronic myeloproliferative disorders. Chest 120(3):801–808
6. Dorfmuller P, Humbert M et al (2007) Fibrous remodeling of the pulmonary venous system in pulmonary arterial hypertension associated with connective tissue diseases. Hum Pathol 38(6):893–902
7. Frazier AA, Franks TJ et al (2007) From the Archives of the AFIP: pulmonary venoocclusive disease and pulmonary capillary hemangiomatosis. Radiographics 27(3): 867–882
8. Gutman JA, Allen CT et al (2008) Pulmonary veno-occlusive disease following reduced intensity cord blood transplantation. Bone Marrow Transplant 42(8):559–561
9. Hackman RC, Madtes DK et al (1989) Pulmonary veno-occlusive disease following bone marrow transplantation. Transplantation 47(6):989–992
10. Harch S, Whitford H et al (2009) Failure of medical therapy in pulmonary arterial hypertension. Is there an alternative diagnosis? Chest 135(6):1462–1469
11. Ho VT, Revta C et al (2008) Hepatic veno-occlusive disease after hematopoietic stem cell transplantation: update on defibrotide and other current investigational therapies. Bone Marrow Transplant 41(3):229–237

12. Holcomb BW Jr, Loyd JE et al (2000) Pulmonary veno-occlusive disease: a case series and new observations. Chest 118(6):1671–1679
13. Hora J (1934) Zur histologie der klinischen 'primaren Pulmonalsklerose'. Frankf Z Pathol 47:100–118
14. Izbicki G, Shitrit D et al (2005) Recurrence of pulmonary veno-occlusive disease after heart-lung transplantation. J Heart Lung Transplant 24(5):635–637
15. Johnson SR, Granton JT et al (2006) Thrombotic arteriopathy and anticoagulation in pulmonary hypertension. Chest 130(2):545–552
16. Kotloff RM, Ahya VN et al (2004) Pulmonary complications of solid organ and hematopoietic stem cell transplantation. Am J Respir Crit Care Med 170(1):22–48
17. Kuga T, Kohda K et al (1996) Pulmonary veno-occlusive disease accompanied by microangiopathic hemolytic anemia 1 year after a second bone marrow transplantation for acute lymphoblastic leukemia. Int J Hematol 64(2):143–150
18. Kumar S, DeLeve LD et al (2003) Hepatic veno-occlusive disease (sinusoidal obstruction syndrome) after hematopoietic stem cell transplantation. Mayo Clin Proc 78(5): 589–598
19. Kuroda T, Hirota H et al (2006) Sildenafil as adjunct therapy to high-dose epoprostenol in a patient with pulmonary veno-occlusive disease. Heart Lung Circ 15(2):139–142
20. Lantuejoul S, Sheppard MN et al (2006) Pulmonary veno-occlusive disease and pulmonary capillary hemangiomatosis: a clinicopathologic study of 35 cases. Am J Surg Pathol 30(7):850–857
21. Malhotra P, Varma S et al (2005) Pulmonary veno–occlusive disease as a cause for reversible pulmonary hypertension in a patient with multiple myeloma undergoing peripheral blood stem cell transplantation. Am J Hematol 80(2):164–165
22. Mandel J, Mark EJ et al (2000) Pulmonary veno-occlusive disease. Am J Respir Crit Care Med 162(5):1964–1973, 16
23. McDonald GB, Hinds MS et al (1993) Veno-occlusive disease of the liver and multiorgan failure after bone marrow transplantation: a cohort study of 355 patients. Ann Intern Med 118(4):255–267
24. Montani D, Achouh L et al (2008) Pulmonary veno-occlusive disease: clinical, functional, radiologic, and hemodynamic characteristics and outcome of 24 cases confirmed by histology. Medicine (Baltimore) 87(4):220–233
25. Montani D, Jais X et al (2009) Cautious use of epoprostenol therapy is a safe bridge to lung transplantation in pulmonary veno-occlusive disease. Eur Respir J 34: 1204–1206
26. Mukai M, Kondo M et al (2003) Pulmonary veno-occlusive disease following allogeneic peripheral blood stem cell transplantation for chronic myeloid leukaemia. Br J Haematol 123(1):1
27. Okumura H, Nagaya N et al (2002) Effects of continuous IV prostacyclin in a patient with pulmonary veno-occlusive disease. Chest 122(3):1096–1098
28. Or R, Nagler A et al (1997) Noncardiogenic pulmonary congestion following bone marrow transplantation. Respiration 64:170–172
29. Roychowdhury M, Pambuccian SE et al (2005) Pulmonary complications after bone marrow transplantation: an autopsy study from a large transplantation center. Arch Pathol Lab Med 129(3):366–371
30. Salzman D, Adkins DR et al (1996) Malignancy-associated pulmonary veno-occlusive disease: report of a case following autologous bone marrow transplantation and review. Bone Marrow Transplant 18(4):755–760
31. Salzman GA, Rosa UW (1989) Prolonged survival in pulmonary veno-occlusive disease treated with nifedipine. Chest 95(5):1154–1156
32. Seguchi M, Hirabayashi N et al (2000) Pulmonary hypertension associated with pulmonary occlusive vasculopathy after allogeneic bone marrow transplantation. Transplantation 69(1):177–179
33. Sharma S, Nadrous HF et al (2005) Pulmonary complications in adult blood and marrow transplant recipients: autopsy findings. Chest 128(3):1385–1392
34. Soubani AO, Miller KB et al (1996) Pulmonary complications of bone marrow transplantation. Chest 109(4): 1066–1077
35. Trobaugh-Lotrario AD, Greffe B et al (2003) Pulmonary veno-occlusive disease after autologous bone marrow transplant in a child with stage IV neuroblastoma: case report and literature review. J Pediatr Hematol Oncol 25(5):405–409.
36. Troussard X, Bernaudin JF et al (1984) Pulmonary veno-occlusive disease after bone marrow transplantation. Thorax 39(12):956–957
37. Veeraraghavan S, Koss MN et al (1999) Pulmonary veno-occlusive disease. Curr Opin Pulm Med 5(5):310–313
38. Voordes CG, Kuipers JR et al (1977) Familial pulmonary veno-occlusive disease: a case report. Thorax 32(6): 763–766
39. Wadleigh M, Ho V et al (2003) Hepatic veno-occlusive disease: pathogenesis, diagnosis and treatment. Curr Opin Hematol 10(6):451–462
40. Weed HG (1991) Pulmonary "capillary" wedge pressure not the pressure in the pulmonary capillaries. Chest 100(4):1138–1140
41. Williams LM, Fussell S et al (1996) Pulmonary veno-occlusive disease in an adult following bone marrow transplantation. Case report and review of the literature. Chest 109(5):1388–1391
42. Willems E, Canivet JL et al (2009) Pulmonary veno-occlusive disease in myeloproliferative disorder. Eur Respir J 33(1):213–216
43. Woywodt A, Haubitz M et al (2004) Counting the cost: markers of endothelial damage in hematopoietic stem cell transplantation. Bone Marrow Transplant 34(12):1015–1023, 17

Radiation Pneumonitis

38

Miguel Gallego Díaz and Jordi Rello Condomines

Contents

Abbreviations

ACE	Angiotensin-converting enzyme
BMT	Bone marrow transplantation
COP	Criptogenic organizing pneumonia
COPD	Chronic obstructive lung disease
DLCO	Diffusing capacity of the lung for carbon monoxide
EGFR	Epidermal growth factor receptor
FEV1	Forced volume in the first second
Gy	Grays
HD	Hodgkin's disease
IL-6	Interleukin 6
PET	Positron emission tomography
PFT	Pulmonary function tests
RP	Radiation pneumonitis
TBI	Total body irradiation
TGF-β1	Transforming growth factor beta 1
TLC	Total lung volume
TNF-α	Tumor necrosis factor-alpha

38.1 Introduction

Radiotherapy has become the cornerstone of neoplasm treatment in recent decades. In neoplasms such as lung cancer, breast cancer, and lymphomas, radiotherapy is a powerful weapon and is used in most international protocols. Radiation pneumonitis (RP) is a diffuse interstitial disease that is the result of the normal lung response to radiotherapy and encompasses a wide range of clinical and radiological manifestations, from asymptomatic state to respiratory failure and death. Despite new advances in delivering radiation, such as conformal radiotherapy, intensity-modulated radiotherapy, and robotic stereotactic radiotherapy, acute and chronic

M.G. Díaz (✉)
Pulmonary Department, Corporació Sanitària Parc Taulí, CIBER Respiratorio, Sabadell, Barcelona, Spain
e-mail: mgallego@tauli.cat

J.R. Condomines
Critical Care Department, Hospital Universitari Joan XXIII, Universitat Rovira i Virgili, CIBER Respiratorio, Tarragona, Spain

É. Azoulay (ed.), *Pulmonary Involvement in Patients with Hematological Malignancies*,
DOI: 10.1007/978-3-642-15742-4_38, © Springer-Verlag Berlin Heidelberg 2011

toxicity still represents a major challenge, as does the risk of a second neoplasm.

Injury to the lung is common after therapeutic irradiation of intrathoracic and chest wall malignancies. In hematological diseases, the main indications for radiotherapy are lymphomas and conditioning myeloablative regimens to allow stem cell transplantation.

Radiologic manifestations of radiation-induced lung disease are well described in the literature. They include ground-glass opacities or consolidation in the acute phase, and traction bronchiectasis, volume loss, and consolidation in the late phase [7, 20]. In this chapter, we review the pathobiology of lung radiation injury and the associated risk factors, mainly in hematological diseases. We also discuss typical and atypical radiological manifestations and preventive approaches.

38.2 Incidence

Although estimates of the incidence of radiation pneumonitis depend heavily on the diagnostic criteria used, the condition is common in patients who undergo thoracic radiation, especially in lung cancer, breast cancer, and lymphomas. Its incidence in lung cancer is around 5–15% [25], and is somewhat lower in Hodgkin's disease (HD) and breast cancer patients. In a study of 590 patients with stage IA-IIIB Hodgkin's disease who received mantle radiation therapy alone, the incidence of radiation pneumonitis was 3%. The risk of radiation pneumonitis rose significantly to 11% when radiation therapy was combined with chemotherapy [36]. Patients with breast cancer who undergo breast radiation therapy as part of a breast-conserving approach have a less than 1% risk of radiation pneumonitis [13]. In fact, in a Danish cohort of more than 35,000 women, the accumulated incidence during follow-up was 14 cases per 100,000 person-years [8]. However, the concomitant use of chemotherapy increased the overall rate of pneumonitis from 1.4% to 3.9% [19]. Pulmonary complications occur frequently after bone marrow transplantation (BMT). In one study of 311 patients with hematologic malignancies who underwent autologous, allogeneic, or syngeneic BMT, the 2-year risk of interstitial pneumonitis was 26.8% and was as high as 34.1% in patients undergoing allogeneic BMT [11]. In that study, the median time from BMT to interstitial pneumonitis was 63.5 (7–720) days. Patients submitted to allogeneic BMT had a significantly higher risk of developing interstitial pneumonitis than patients receiving syngeneic or autologous BMT (34.1% vs 16.7% and 4.9%, respectively; $p = 0.0006$).

A lower incidence was reported in a recent retrospective study of 26 cohorts including 1,090 BMT patients, in which the incidence of interstitial pneumonitis was around 2.5% in patients with lung shielding and around 11% in patients without lung shielding [33].

38.3 Risk Factors

The factors that influence the degree of lung injury after irradiation of a thoracic malignancy may be related to the patient or to the irradiation techniques used [7]. The most important irradiation-related factors are the volume of irradiated lung, the total dose of delivered radiation, and the fractionation of the dose. The total dose of radiation delivered is important, as radiologic manifestations of radiation pneumonitis rarely appear at doses below 20 Gy, but are almost always present in patients receiving doses over 40 Gy [30]. In addition, chemotherapeutic agents such as actinomycin D, adriamycin, bleomycin, and busulfan can increase toxic effects of radiation [34]. Likewise, twice-daily doses in hyperfractionated treatment schedules are reported to cause less RP than single daily doses [17].

Among host factors, older age, female sex and prior respiratory disease have been identified as risk factors. In fact, chronic obstructive lung disease (COPD) is a very common underlying disease in lung cancer and has been identified as a risk factor for severe pneumonitis [28]. However, although this finding is controversial, tobacco seems to have a protective effect; the mechanism of this effect is not known, but it could be similar to the mitigating influence on the development of hypersensitivity pneumonitis. In a study of 606 patients with breast and esophageal carcinoma, the incidence of RP in smokers was 0.4% compared with 3.6% in non-smokers ($p = 0.022$) [16].

The abrupt withdrawal of steroid administration has been related to lung injury, since withdrawal can unmask latent radiation injury to the lung [6].

Animal studies and clinical observations have suggested the usefulness of plasma determination of some molecules as markers of the risk of pneumonitis [42]. Changes in the plasma concentrations of TGF-β1 and IL-6 during radiotherapy may identify patients at risk of RP, but unfortunately cytokines are also produced in tumors, and it is difficult to distinguish between the true effect of radiation and cytokine tumor production [32].

In the case of total body irradiation (TBI) as a part of a preconditioning regimen for BMT, the whole lung volume is included in the irradiation area. In patients who undergo allogeneic stem-cell transplantation, age over 20, a history of chronic myelogenous leukemia, alloimmunized donor, prior splenectomy, and graft-versus-host disease are risk factors for the development of interstitial pneumonitis [33].

The risk of pneumonitis depends not only on TBI, but also on the chemotherapeutic agent used. Thus, the most common combination (TBI plus cyclophosphamide) seems to produce less toxicity than regimens containing busulfan; likewise, fractionating doses and limiting the total dose to 12 Gy seem to decrease the risk of pneumonitis [33].

38.4 Pathobiology

The degree of radiosensitivity depends mainly on the tissue affected. Hematological tissue (especially bone marrow and peripheral lymphocytes) is the most radiosensitive, and in the thorax the most radiosensitive tissue is the lung (Table 38.1). Tissue damage will depend on absorbed doses that, in turn, are affected by the intensity of radiation. Radiation generates energy by accelerating electrons within the irradiated tissue; this release of energy produces free radicals that cause genetic damage and macromolecular injury. Genetic damage is more marked in cells with the highest mitotic rate. In the lung, the endothelial and epithelial cells are at risk of genetic damage, whereas macromolecular injury depends mainly on the direct effects of free radicals through lipid peroxidation and oxidation of protein sulfuryl groups [35]. Both genetic and macromolecular cellular injury triggers complex intracellular inflammatory pathways, inducing the production of cytokines and growth factors. Among the most prominent growth factor signaling cascades for which upregulation in (early responding) normal tissues after irradiation has been observed are the epidermal growth factor pathway (upregulation of the receptor EGFR) and the tumor necrosis factor-alpha (TNF-α) pathway (upregulation of the growth factor) [35]. The angiotensin system appears to be involved in the development of fibrosis, at least in the lung, presumably through interactions with TGF-β signaling [27]. In the kidney, angiotensin-converting enzyme (ACE) also contributes to the development of the radiation response. Therefore, ACE inhibitors, such as captopril and antagonists of the angiotensin II type 1 (AT1)- and type 2 (AT2) receptor, have been tested for their potential to mitigate or treat late radiation effects, particularly in kidney and lung.

From the histopathological point of view, the first changes occur within an hour of the initiation of radiation, when type II alveolar cells release surfactant. Subsequently, edema, increases in permeability, and alveolar filling drive the histological pattern of diffuse alveolar damage. In the next 2–9 months after irradiation, a repair process takes place with a reduction of the inflammatory response and an increase in collagen production. The last phase is pulmonary fibrosis due to sclerosis of the alveolar wall, endothelial damage, and alveolar fibrosis; although the airways usually remain unaffected, the interstitium is markedly thickened and the parenchyma distorted [9,12,25,38].

Table 38.1 Radiosensitivity of tissues

Highly radiosensitive	Moderately radiosensitive	Least radiosensitive
Lymphoid tissue	Skin	Central nervous system
Bone marrow	Vascular endothelium	Muscle
Gastrointestinal epithelium	Lung	Bone and cartilage
Gonads	Kidney	Connective tissue
Embryonic tissues	Liver	–

38.5 Diagnosis

38.5.1 Clinical Manifestations

The classic syndrome of acute radiation pneumonitis appears 4–6 weeks after irradiation. Only in 5–10% of cases does radiation pneumonitis become clinically significant [1]. Physical examination is unreliable: skin erythema may outline the radiation port, but these changes do not correlate well with the severity of pulmonary injury. Laboratory findings are also not specific. Acute radiation pneumonitis (RP), as a clinical syndrome, consists of non-productive mild cough, mild dyspnea, pleuritic chest pain, and low-grade fever. Fibrosis appears between 6 and 12 months after the end of radiation therapy and in general is irreversible; in these cases breathlessness is the most common complaint, and crackles may be heard. In some cases, respiratory failure is a terminal event, manifested as tachypnea and cyanosis.

38.5.2 Radiology

Chest X-ray and CT scan are the most common imaging techniques used to diagnose RP. Initial radiological manifestations of the acute phase of RP are ground-glass opacities and/or consolidation in the irradiated port. Occasionally, an ipsilateral moderate pleural effusion, often associated with atelectasis of the lung, develops at the time of radiation pneumonitis [18]. Because CT is more sensitive than chest radiography, homogeneous ground-glass attenuation representing early radiation pneumonitis can be seen a few weeks after the completion of radiation therapy, although the X-ray is normal [5,14,23].

Whereas classic pneumonitis occurs in the radiation port, sporadic radiation-induced lung injury develops in areas of untreated lung. In recent years, two different patterns have been described: (1) organizing pneumonia (COP), which occurs several months after irradiation and presents as migratory infiltrates outside the radiation portal, and (2) lymphocytic alveolitis, which occurs as bilateral lung injury 2–4 weeks after irradiation.

COP has been described only in females undergoing irradiation for breast cancer. COP usually appears 6 weeks to 10 months after radiation therapy, although longer periods have been reported (18 years) [26].

The most common images on CT scan are patchy, bilateral areas of consolidation or ground-glass infiltration characterized by a migratory pattern (Fig. 38.1).

Lymphocytic alveolitis has been observed in patients suffering from breast cancer; in a control study, the irradiated zones showed the same degree of alveolitis as non-irradiated areas. This finding was not predictive of radiological evidence of pneumonitis [24].

Eosinophilic pneumonia is a less frequently described complication that is thought to result from breast irradiation. In one study, five cases of females with chronic eosinophilic pneumonia following radiotherapy for breast cancer were reported. All patients had a history of asthma and/or atopic manifestation, and presented a marked peripheral blood and alveolar eosinophilia [10]. In this study, the median time interval between the end of radiation therapy and the onset of eosinophilic pneumonia was 3.5 (1–10) months.

Interactions between chemotherapy and radiotherapy are also a source of iatrogenic manifestations. The "radiation recall" syndrome may occur in a previously irradiated territory following chemotherapy. Radiation recall is an inflammatory skin reaction at a previously irradiated field subsequent to the administration of a

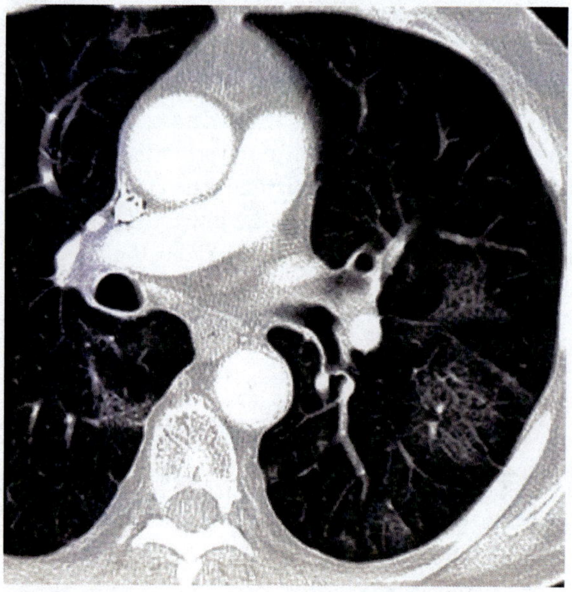

Fig. 38.1 Patient with breast cancer treated with RT. Patchy ground-glass opacities in both lungs

variety of pharmacologic agents. The skin is more frequently involved, but many organs can be affected, and pneumonitis has been described after gemcitabine, carmustine, paclitaxel, and anthracyclines [3].

Bronchial stump necrosis is an unusual manifestation described in irradiated lung cancer after pneumonectomy or lobectomy, causing a broncho-pleural fistula. This is a late complication, usually appearing between 1 and 7 years after radiation therapy [26].

In Hodgkin's disease, a mantle radiotherapy field that treats all lymph node areas above the diaphragm includes the lung apex and axilla bilaterally; in non-Hodgkin's lymphoma, smaller lung volumes are often treated. Follow-up chest radiographs show several abnormalities, such as apical and paramediastinal fibrosis and reduced lung volumes. Radiographic changes on CT scans are found in 30% of patients in whom the chest radiograph can be considered "normal" at 5 years follow-up [29]. Pulmonary necrosis can be seen, which is difficult to manage due to the possibility of lung infection (Fig. 38.2).

TBI is typically involved in the pathogenesis of idiopathic pneumonia syndrome; this syndrome can appear in the first 120 days after transplantation and is related not only to TBI, but also to the chemotherapy used, graft-versus-host disease, and older age. When suspected, clinicians should rule out other conditions before accepting a definitive diagnosis (Table 38.2).

Table 38.2 Diagnostic criteria for idiopathic pneumonia syndrome

1. Evidence of widespread alveolar injury, including:
Multilobar infiltrates on routine chest radiographs or CT scans
Symptoms and signs of pneumonia
Evidence of abnormal pulmonary physiology
Increased alveolar-to-arterial oxygen gradient
New or increased restrictive pulmonary function test abnormality
2. Absence of active lower respiratory tract infection. Appropriate evaluation includes:
Bronchoalveolar lavage negative for significant bacterial pathogens and/or lack of improvement with broad-spectrum antibiotics
Bronchoalveolar lavage negative for pathogenic nonbacterial microorganisms
Routine bacterial, viral, and fungal cultures
Shell-vial CMV culture
Cytology for CMV inclusions, fungi, and *Pneumocystis carinii*
Detection methods for respiratory syncytial virus, parainfluenza virus, other organisms

Radiographic findings are non-specific and include bilateral air-space opacification. CT scan shows progressive air-space consolidation with bibasilar prominence

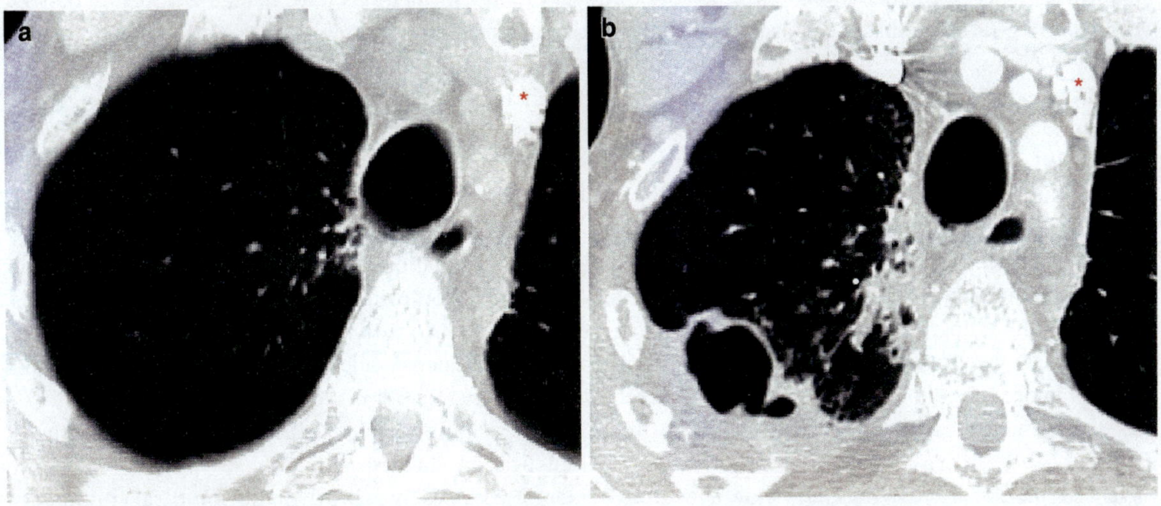

Fig. 38.2 (**a**) Subtle paramediastinal pneumonitis and calcified lymph nodes (*) after RT for Hodgkin's lymphoma. (**b**) Follow-up CT after 12 months shows increased pneumonitis and pulmonary necrosis in the apex of the right lung. No associated infection was identified

similar to non-cardiogenic pulmonary edema. Pleural effusions may be present [15].

In delayed-onset cases, the clinical course is more indolent and causes respiratory failure only on occasions [37].

38.5.3 Lung Functional Test

Pulmonary function tests (PFT) are the most objective way to evaluate the impact of irradiation on lung function. These tests have a variety of uses: (1) to evaluate the individual risk of RP, (2) to diagnose pulmonary fibrosis, and (3) to monitor the respiratory function closely. Although the forced volume in the first second (FEV1) is a useful and straightforward parameter for diagnosis of pulmonary fibrosis, it relies on a decrease of total lung volume (TLC) and diffusing capacity of the lung for carbon monoxide (DLCO). The DLCO test is the most sensitive indicator of interstitial disease; low DLCO levels are related to the loss of alveolar surface and thickening of intra-alveolar septa. Few long-term studies have assessed the impact of irradiation on lung function. It has only been determined in long-term survivors, mainly in lymphomas; follow-up studies in lymphomas show an initial reduction in TLC and DLCO at 3–6 months, and recovery rates of 50–60% by 18 months. Long-term (>10 years) follow-up reveals a moderate decrease in DLCO (up to 70–80% of predicted levels) and a minor reduction in TLC (to 90% of predicted levels) [4,21,29]. There were no long-term clinical sequelae, and exercise capacity was normal in 25 patients who underwent a graded stress test to assess the cardiac left ventricular ejection fraction in long-term follow-up for Hodgkin's disease [29].

In irradiated patients with breast cancer, significant changes in TLC have been reported. The maximal decrease was recorded 60 days after completion of radiotherapy and occurred without any apparent relationship with radiographic changes. These findings suggest that the reduction in pulmonary volume depends more on the diffuse lymphocytic alveolitis than on the extension of the localized lung damage [24].

In TBI, pulmonary functions tests show a restrictive pattern, with decreased TLC and DLCO.

38.6 Treatment

Corticosteroids are currently the most frequent treatment for RP. A dose of 1 mg/kg/day for 2–4 weeks, followed by gradual tapering over the next 6–12 months, is the most common approach. There are no trials for evaluating adequate dose or duration of treatment. It is recommended to start treatment as soon as toxicity is detected in order to avoid progression to fibrosis. Immunosuppressants used as steroid-sparing agents, like cyclosporine A and azathioprine, have proved useful, but only in case reports. There is also anecdotal evidence of the usefulness of inhaled corticosteroids [22].

In cases of pulmonary idiopathic pneumonia, the outcome is fatal in nearly 70% of cases despite the use of corticosteroids.

When fibrosis is established, only palliative therapy is possible. In these cases, only O_2 therapy relieves the sensation of dyspnea, apart from the use of morphine. The role of treatment with *N*-acetylcysteine (indicated in other types of fibrosis) remains uncertain because of the lack of studies in this area.

38.7 Prevention

38.7.1 Radiation Techniques

A number of methods have been developed to deliver an adequate or tumoricidal dose of radiation to tumors while limiting the amount of normal lung exposed, such as the use of limited radiation portals, tangential beams, conformal therapy, and intensity-modulated radiation therapy. The three-dimensional conformal irradiation technique, one of the most recent and sophisticated irradiation methods developed, uses multiple radiation beams to generate dose distributions that conform tightly to target volumes. This technique ensures that the entire target volume is adequately treated while minimizing doses to normal structures (Fig. 38.3).

Intensity-modulated radiation therapy delivers intensity-modulated radiation to irregularly shaped target volumes by using dynamic multileaf collimators in 3D conformal therapy. The use of new technologies,

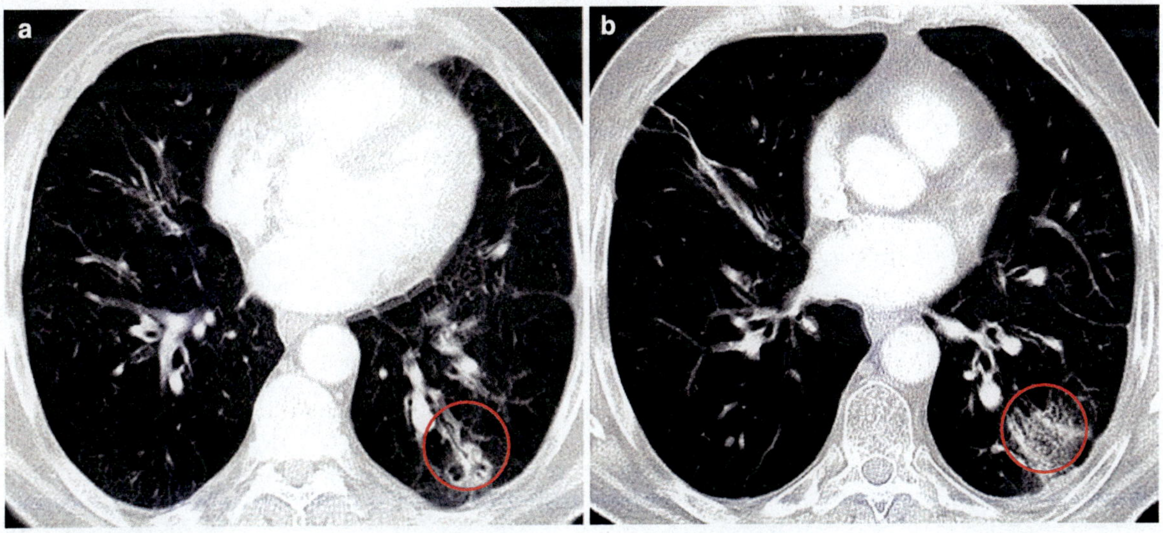

Fig. 38.3 (a) Patient with adenocarcinoma in LLL. (b) After 3D CRT, pneumonitis is limited to the area surrounding the tumor

such as 3D conformal radiotherapy or even newer developments such as stereotactic, allows the calculation of the exact area to be irradiated. In this way, planning with CT scan or positron emission tomography (PET) allows to define the exact area to be irradiated.

38.7.2 Drugs

Amifostine, an oxygen-free radical scavenger, has proven effectiveness in cytoprotection and reduces radiation pneumonitis in clinical trials. The administration of this drug has been associated with preventing the loss of DLCO when administered concurrently with chemoradiotherapy. Its administration before radiotherapy also reduced the macrophage levels and expression of lung tissue TGF-β1 [2,40].

Pentoxifylline is a xanthine derivate that inhibits platelet aggregation and enhances microvascular blood flow. A modest benefit was suggested in a trial with 40 patients treated for breast and lung cancer [31].

Captopril is an inhibitor of angiotensin-converting enzyme (ACE), which reduces radiation-induced lung fibrosis in rats, but no protective effect was found in a retrospective study in humans [41].

In TBI, to keep the dose to critical organs below their tolerance dose, the possibilities are: (1) fractionation, (2) lowering of the dose rate, (3) decreasing the dose locally by shielding of the organs concerned, or (4) a combination of the three. Fractionation is reported to lower the impact of the TBI on normal tissues, without modifying the effect on leukemia cells [39].

38.8 Conclusions

The development of radiation pneumonitis depends mainly on treatment-related factors, such as radiation dose, volume of lung irradiated, fraction schedule, use of concurrent chemotherapy and patient-related factors. Despite new advances in delivering radiation, reducing the incidence remains a challenge. Furthermore, the growing survival rates of patients with cancer make it essential to avoid toxicity in order to improve quality of life. Modern technologies, such as intensity-modulated radiation therapy or robotic stereotactic radiotherapy, may well help to achieve better outcomes in terms of survival and therapy-related morbidity. Research into drugs for preventing or treating toxicity is needed in the future.

References

1. Abratt RP, Onca FR, Morgan GW et al (2004) Pulmonary complications of radiation therapy. Clin Chest Med 25:167–177

2. Antonadou D, Petridis A, Synodinou M et al (2003) Amifostine reduces radiochemotherapy-induced toxicities in patients with locally advanced non-small cell lung cancer. Semin Oncol 30(Suppl):2–9
3. Azria D, Magne N, Zouhair A et al (2005) Radiation recall: a well recognized but neglected phenomenon. Cancer Treat Rev 31:555–570
4. Barrett A, Depledge MH, Powles RL (1983) Interstitial pneumonitis following bone marrow transplantation after low dose rate total body irradiation. Int J Radiat Oncol Biol Phys 9:1029–1033
5. Bell J, McGivern D, Bullimore J et al (1988) Diagnostic imaging of post-irradiation changes in the chest. Clin Radiol 39:109–119
6. Castellino RA, Glastein E, Turbow MM et al (1974) Latent radiation injury of lungs or heart activated by steroid withdrawal. Ann Intern Med 80:593–599
7. Choi YW, Munden RF, Erasmus JJ et al (2004) Effects of radiation therapy on the lung: radiologic appearances and differential diagnosis. Radiographics 24:985–998
8. Christensen S, Pedersen L, Grijota M et al (2008) Incidence of interstitial pneumonitis among breast cancer patients: a 10-year Danish population-based cohort study. Br J Cancer 98:1870–1875
9. Constine LS, Milano MT, Friedman D et al (2008) Late effects of cancer treatment on normal tissues. In: Perez CA, Brady L (eds) Principles and practice of radiation oncology, 5th edn. Lippincott, Williams & Wilkins, Philadelphia, PA
10. Cottin V, Frognier R, Monnot H et al (2004) Chronic eosinophilic pneumonia after radiation therapy for breast cancer. Eur Respir J 23:9–13
11. Granena A, Carreras E, Rozman C et al (1993) Interstitial pneumonitis after BMT: 15 years experience in a single institution. Bone Marrow Transplant 11:453–458
12. Gross NJ (1980) Experimental radiation pneumonitis. IV. Leakage of circulatory proteins onto the alveolar surface. J Lab Clin Med 95:19–31
13. Harris S (2001) Radiotherapy for early and advanced breast cancer. Int J Clin Pract 55:609–612
14. Ikezoe J, Takashima S, Morimoto S et al (1988) CT appearance of acute radiation-induced injury in the lung. AJR Am J Roentgenol 150:765–770
15. Jagannathan JP, Ramaiya N, Gill RR et al (2008) Imaging of complications of hematopoietic stem cell transplantation. Radiol Clin N Am 46:397–417
16. Johansson S, Bjermer L, Franzen L et al (1998) Effects of ongoing smoking on the development of radiation-induced pneumonitis in breast cancer and oesophagus cancer patients. Radiother Oncol 49:41–47
17. Libshitz HI (1993) Radiation changes in lung. Semin Roentgenol 28:303–320
18. Libshitz HI, Southard ME (1974) Complication of radiation therapy: the thorax. Semin Roentgenol 9:41–49
19. Lind PA, Marks LB, Hardenbergh PH et al (2002) Technical factors associated with radiation pneumonitis after local +/- regional radiation therapy for breast cancer. Int J Radiat Oncol Biol Phys 52:137–143
20. Logan PM (1998) Thoracic manifestations of external beam radiotherapy. AJR Am J Roentgenol 171:56
21. Lund MB, Kongerud J, Nome O et al (1995) Lung function impairment in long-term survivors of Hodgkin's disease. Ann Oncol 6:495–501
22. Magaña E, Crowell RE (2003) Radiation pneumonitis successfully treated with inhaled corticosteroids. South Med J 96:521–524
23. Mah K, Poon PY, Van Dyk J et al (1986) Assessment of acute radiation-induced pulmonary changes using computed tomography. J Comput Assist Tomogr 10:736–743
24. Martin C, Romero S, Sanchez-Paya J et al (1999) Bilateral lymphocytic alveolitis: a common reaction after unilateral thoracic irradiation. Eur Respir J 13:727–732
25. McDonald S, Rubin P, Phillips TL et al (1995) Injury to the lung from cancer therapy: clinical syndromes, measurable endpoints, and potential scoring systems. Int J Radiat Oncol Biol Phys 31:1187–1203
26. Mesurolle B, Qanadli SD, Merad M et al (2000) Unusual radiologic findings in the thorax alter radiation. Radiographics 20:67–81
27. Molteni A, Moulder JE, Cohen EF et al (2000) Control of radiation-induced pneumopathy and lung fibrosis by angiotensin-converting enzyme inhibitors and an angiotensin II type 1 receptor blocker. Int J Radiat Biol 76:523–532
28. Moreno M, Aristu J, Ramos L et al (2007) Predictive factors for radiation-induced pulmonary toxicity after-three-dimensional conformal chemoradiation in locally advanced non-small-cell lung cancer. Clin Transl Oncol 9:596–602
29. Morgan GW, Freeman AP, McLean RG et al (1985) Late cardiac, thyroid and pulmonary sequelae of mantle radiotherapy for Hodgkin's disease. Int J Radiat Oncol Biol Phys 11:1925–1931
30. Movsas B, Raffin TA, Epstein AH et al (1997) Pulmonary radiation injury. Chest 111:1061–1076
31. Ozturk B, Egehan I, Atavci S et al (2004) Pentoxifilline in prevention of radiation-induced lung toxicity in patients with breast and lung cancer: a double-blind randomized trial. Int J Radiat Oncol Biol Phys 58:213
32. Rübe CE, Palm J, Erren M et al (2008) Cytokine plasma levels: reliable predictors for radiation pneumonitis? PLoS ONE 3(8):e2898. doi:10.1371/journal.pone.0002898
33. Sampath S, Schultheiss TE, Wong J (2005) Dose response and factors related to interstitial pneumonitis after bone marrow transplant. Int J Radiat Oncol Biol Phys 63:876–884
34. Sostman HD, Putnam CE, Gamsu G (1981) Diagnosis of chemotherapy lung. AJR Am J Roentgenol 136:33–40
35. Stewart FA, Dörr W (2009) Milestones in normal tissue radiation biology over the past 50 years: from clonogenic cell survival to cytokine networks and back to stem cell recovery. Int J Radiat Biol 85:574–586
36. Tarbell NJ, Thompson L, Mauch P (1990) Thoracic irradiation in Hodgkin's disease: disease control and long-term complications. Int J Radiat Oncol Biol Phys 18:275–281
37. Tichelli A, Rovó A, Gratwohl A (2008) Late pulmonary, cardiovascular, and renal complications after hematopoietic stem cell transplantation and recommended screening practices. Hematology 1:125–133
38. Tsouttsou PG, Koukourakis MI (2006) Radiation pneumonitis and fibrosis: mechanisms underlying its pathogenesis and implications for future research. Int J Radiat Oncol Biol Phys 66:1281–1293

39. Vriesendorp HM (1990) Prediction of effects of therapeutic total body irradiation in man. Radiother Oncol 1(Suppl): 37–50
40. Vujaskovic Z, Feng QF, Rabbani ZN et al (2002) Assessment of the protective effect of amifostine on radiation-induced pulmonary toxicity. Exp Lung Res 157:577–590
41. Wang LW, Fu XL, Clough R et al (2000) Can angiotensin-converting enzyme inhibitors protect against symptomatic radiation pneumonitis? Radiat Res 153:405
42. Zhao L, Sheldon K, Chen M et al (2008) The predictive role of plasma TGF-beta1 during therapy for radiation-induced lung toxicity deserves further study in patients with non-small cell lung cancer. Lung Cancer 59:232

Leukostasis, Infiltration and Pulmonary Lysis Syndrome Are the Three Patterns of Leukemic Pulmonary Infiltrates

39

François Vincent

Contents

F. Vincent
Medico-Surgical Intensive Care Unit,
Avicenne Teaching Hospital, 125, rue de Stalingrad,
93009 Bobigny Cedex, France
e-mail: francois.vincent@avc.aphp.fr

39.1 Introduction

Noninfectious causes of pulmonary involvement in patients with early or relapsing hyperleukocytic leukemia include pulmonary leukostasis, leukemic lung infiltration, and acute lysis pneumopathy [1, 2]. Pulmonary leukostasis associated with nonlymphocytic or lymphocytic leukemia usually occurs when the leukocyte count is greater than 100,000/mm^3 or increases rapidly [3–5]. Acute lysis pneumopathy can develop at chemotherapy initiation in these patients [2, 6–13]. In contrast, symptomatic leukemic infiltration of the lungs has been reported in acute leukemia with or without hyperleukocytosis, suggesting that the type of blasts and their affinity for the pulmonary endothelium may be involved in the development of acute respiratory distress syndrome [14]. Clinically significant leukemic pulmonary infiltrates are recognized antemortem in fewer than 7% of leukemic patients [1]. The incidence of leukemic lung infiltration found at autopsy is much greater, ranging from 25% to 46% of patients. Histology shows leukemic blasts occupying most or all of the vascular lumens, with or without the presence of fibrin [15]. Distinguishing among leukostasis, leukemic infiltration, and acute lysis pneumopathy may be difficult, particularly as these conditions may occur concomitantly [10].

39.2 Pulmonary Leukostasis

Pulmonary leukostasis is one of the manifestations of hyperleukocytic syndrome, which also causes other clinical and laboratory abnormalities (Table 39.1). Pulmonary leukostasis is best defined as a pathological

É. Azoulay (ed.), *Pulmonary Involvement in Patients with Hematological Malignancies*,
DOI: 10.1007/978-3-642-15742-4_39, © Springer-Verlag Berlin Heidelberg 2011

Table 39.1 Clinical manifestations of leukostasis

Central nervous system circulation
Headache, confusion, somnolence, dizziness, slurred speech, impaired hearing, tinnitus, diplopia, delirium, stupor, coma
Retinal vein distension, retinal hemorrhage, papilledema
Intracranial hemorrhage
Penile circulation
Priapism
Cardiovascular system
Acute myocardial infarction
Right ventricular overload
Acral lividosis
Acute limb ischemia, bowel infarction, renal vein thrombosis
Laboratory findings
Real or spurious decreases in PaO_2 and/or $PaCO_2$
Decreased plasma glucose
Spurious hyperkalemia
Real or spurious hypophosphatemia and hypokaliema
Increases in red-blood-cell count, hemoglobin, and hematocrit

entity that is usually, but not invariably, associated with very high counts of circulating leukemic cells [14]. Pulmonary leukostasis occurs mainly in acute myeloid leukemia (AML) and in advanced chronic myelogenous leukemia (CML) at the blast-crisis stage. In early autopsy studies, the incidence of pulmonary leukostasis was as high as 29/82 patients with AML and 14/47 patients with CML [15]. Pulmonary leukostasis was found in all patients with leukocyte counts greater than 200 G·10^9/L and half of those with leukocyte counts between 50 and 200 G·10^9/L. In half the patients, pulmonary leukostasis was thought to be a major cause of death. Pulmonary leukostasis is rare in patients with chronic lymphocytic leukemia (CLL), as well as in those with acute lymphocytic leukemia (ALL) and leukocyte counts lower than 250 G·10^9/L [4]. For example, of 636 patients with CLL followed over 8 years, only 5 (0.78%) required admission for pulmonary leukostasis [16]. Among AML patients, 5–29% of adults and a slightly higher percentage of children had leukocyte counts greater than 50 G·10^9/L [17]. AML subsets associated with hyperleukocytosis and pulmonary leukostasis include myelomonocytic (M4) or monocytic (M5) AML and the microgranular variant of acute promyelocytic leukemia (M3) (Fig. 39.1) with inv16 (p13;q22), 11q23 rearrangements, and duplications of the activating mutations in the Fms-like tyrosine-3 (*FLT3*) gene [17–19]. Hyperleukocytosis with or without pulmonary leukostasis was the single worst prognostic factor in patients with AML in some studies, but not in the most recent reports [5, 20, 21]. Pathogenic mechanisms that may contribute to pulmonary leukostasis include increased blood viscosity in the microcirculation [22, 23], leukocyte aggregation, leukocytic microthrombi, changes in vascular impedance [23], release of toxic products from leukemic cells, endothelial cell damage and activation [24], complement activation [25], oxygen steal and hypoxia, and microvascular invasion [23, 26, 27].

Table 39.1 lists the most common symptoms of leukostasis. Because none of these symptoms is specific, leukostasis is difficult to prove, and no universally accepted diagnostic criteria exist [28]. Table 39.2 shows the four-point clinical score developed to assist in the diagnosis of leukostasis; 0 indicates no leukostasis; 1, possible leukostasis; 2, probable leukostasis; and 3, highly probable leukostasis [29]. This score was developed based on 95 patients (59 males and 36 females with a median age of 52 years) with leukocyte counts greater than 50 G·10^9/L including 48 with AML, 31 with CML, 13 with ALL, and 3 with chronic myelomonocytic leukemia (CMML). The score rests on criteria that are simple and fast to evaluate: overall symptom severity (slight, marked, or severe limitation), presence of pulmonary symptoms (from no limitation to dyspnea at rest), and presence of neurological symptoms (tinnitus, visual disturbances, confusion, and/or somnolence). It was validated in a different group of 31 patients (27 with AML and 4 with ALL) whose median leukocyte count was 219 G·10^9/L [30]. Of these 31 patients, 6 (18.2%) died early on, mainly of pulmonary failure; all six patients had AML, which was of monocytic lineage in three patients [85–87].

In patients with severe hyperleukocytosis, tissue oxygenation is difficult to evaluate. Pulse oximetry is unreliable because of increased methemoglobinemia, and blood gas analysis can be affected by excessive oxygen consumption by the leukocytes [23, 31–33]. Interestingly, blasts consume more oxygen than do normal leukocytes due to an increase in Na^+-K^+ ATPase activity [34]. Although many methods for

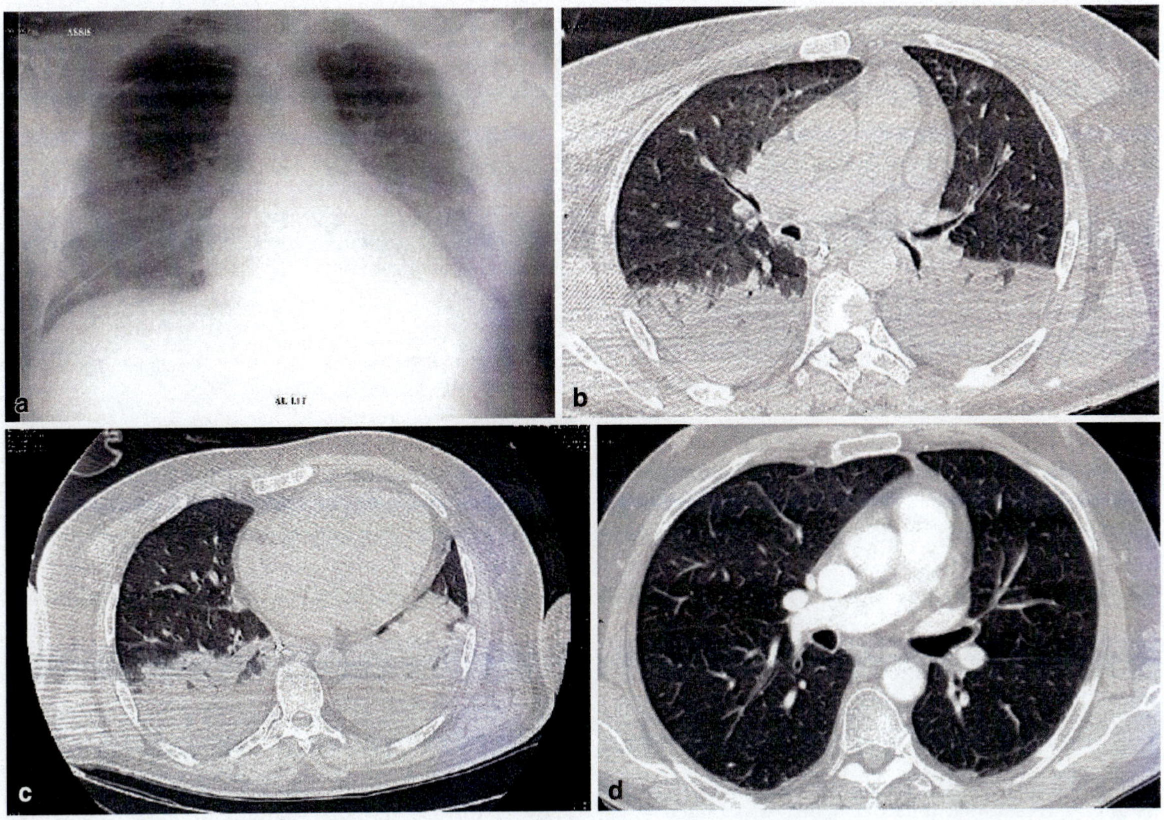

Fig. 39.1 A 28-year-old man with hyperleukocytic AML type 3 (15–17 translocation). (**a**) High-resolution computed tomography of the chest on day 1 (leukocyte count, 108.8 G·10^9/L; LDH, 9·N). (**b**) High-resolution computed tomography of the chest on day 3 (treatment with idarubicin, aracytine, ATRA, and dexamethasone; leukocyte count, 59.9 G·10^9/L; LDH, 10·N). (**c**) High-resolution computed tomography of the chest on day 4 (treatment with idarubicin, aracytine, ATRA, and dexamethasone; leukocyte count, 10.9 G·10^9/L; LDH, 11·N; admission to the intensive care unit for acute respiratory failure; invasive mechanical ventilation; bronchoalveolar lavage fluid, no pathogens, siderophages, or blast cells). (**d**) High-resolution computed tomography of the chest on day 16 (leukocyte count, 0.9 G·10^9/L; LDH, normal; invasive mechanical ventilation discontinued 5 days earlier). (**e**) High-resolution computed tomography of the chest 2 months after the first remission

performing blood gas analysis in patients with severe hyperleukocytosis have been tested (ice versus no ice, immediate versus delayed analysis), they remain controversial [35]. Laboratory tests often show metabolic disturbances such as hypokalemia and hypophosphatemia in patients with extreme hyperleukocytosis [36]. These findings may reflect in vivo abnormalities or the metabolic activity of leukocytes in vitro. Appropriate sampling techniques and immediate analysis are therefore crucial. Pseudohyperkalemia due to in vitro potassium release by leukocytes undergoing lysis during the clotting process has been reported [37].

No radiological findings have been clearly associated with pulmonary leukostasis. The chest radiograph may be normal or show an atypical bilateral reticular pattern with septal lines or bilateral airspace consolidation (Fig. 39.2) [38]. Perfusion lung scanning for the diagnosis (diffuse vascular occlusive pattern) and monitoring of pulmonary leukostasis remains controversial [39, 40]. Pulmonary leukostasis may mimic pulmonary embolism or suggest tuberculosis in endemic areas [41, 42].

39.3 Pulmonary Leukemic Infiltration

Symptomatic leukemic infiltration of the lung is the least common cause of pulmonary infiltrates in patients with leukemia, although the incidence at autopsy may be as high as 64% [43–46]. Pulmonary infiltrates are

Table 39.2 Clinical score to identify patients with leukostasis

Group	Probability of leukostasis syndrome	Severity of symptoms	Pulmonary symptoms	Neurological symptoms	Other organ systems
0	Not present	No limitation	No symptom and no limitation in ordinary activities	No neurological symptoms	No symptom
1	Possible	Slight limitation	Mild symptoms and slight limitation during ordinary activity, comfortable at rest	Mild tinnitus, headache, dizziness	Moderate fatigue
2	Probable	Marked limitation	Marked limitation in activity because of symptoms, even during less than ordinary activity, comfortable only at rest	Slight visual disturbances,[a] severe tinnitus, headache, dizziness	Severe fatigue
3	Highly probable	Severe limitation	Dyspnea at rest, oxygen or ventilation required	Severe visual disturbances[a] (acute inability to read), confusion, delirium, somnolence, intracranial hemorrhage	Myocardial infarction, priapism, ischemic necrosis

Adapted from [29]

[a]Blurred vision, diplopia, hemianopsia

usually microscopic and frequently associated with hyperleukocytosis, although they have been reported in non-hyperleukocytic AML patients [46–49]. The diagnosis is based on histological or cytological studies and on negative findings from a comprehensive investigation for more common causes. The infiltrates typically follow the lymphatic routes along the bronchovascular bundles, interlobular septa, and pleural interstitial tissue. Nodules are uncommon [50].

Pulmonary leukemic infiltration is frequently found at autopsy but rarely documented in clinical practice because of the lack of specific clinical and radiological signs, unless hyperleukocytosis is present [51]. It seems more common in AML than in ALL [4, 52]. Most of the cases reported in patients with AML had M4 or M5 disease [46–49]. Pulmonary leukemic infiltration seems especially rare during the course of CLL, with only two of 636 hospital admissions [16]. Clinical symptoms of leukemic pulmonary infiltration are nonspecific, such as cough, pyrexia, and dyspnea. Lung biopsy or bronchoalveolar lavage may be required to confirm the diagnosis, but are often contraindicated because of hypoxia or thrombocytopenia. Studies have sought to define the radiological pattern of pulmonary leukemic infiltration. Radiographs may show a diffuse reticular pattern or, less frequently, pulmonary nodules or focal homogeneous opacities [53–55]. Three studies report the findings from high-resolution computed tomography (HRCT). In a study of ten patients with leukemic infiltrates diagnosed by transbronchial biopsy and BAL ($n=8$), open lung biopsy ($n=1$), or autopsy ($n=1$) [56], four patients had T-cell leukemia (ATL), two had CML, two had CLL, and two had AML (subtype not specified). The main findings were thickening of the interlobular septa and bronchovascular bundles, and presence of parenchymal nodules smaller than 10 mm. Subsequently, similar findings were obtained in 11 patients (six with AML, three with ATL, one with chronic myelomonocytic leukemia, and one with plasma cell leukemia) [57]. HRCT findings in these 11 patients with leukemic pulmonary infiltration were compared with those of 22 leukemic patients who had other lung diseases. HRCT histopathology correlations were assessed in seven patients with leukemic infiltration, from whom specimens were obtained by autopsy ($n=6$) or transbronchial lung biopsy ($n=1$). Frequent parenchymal HRCT findings were thickening of bronchovascular bundles (81.8%), prominence of peripheral pulmonary arteries (81.8%), and non-lobular non-segmental

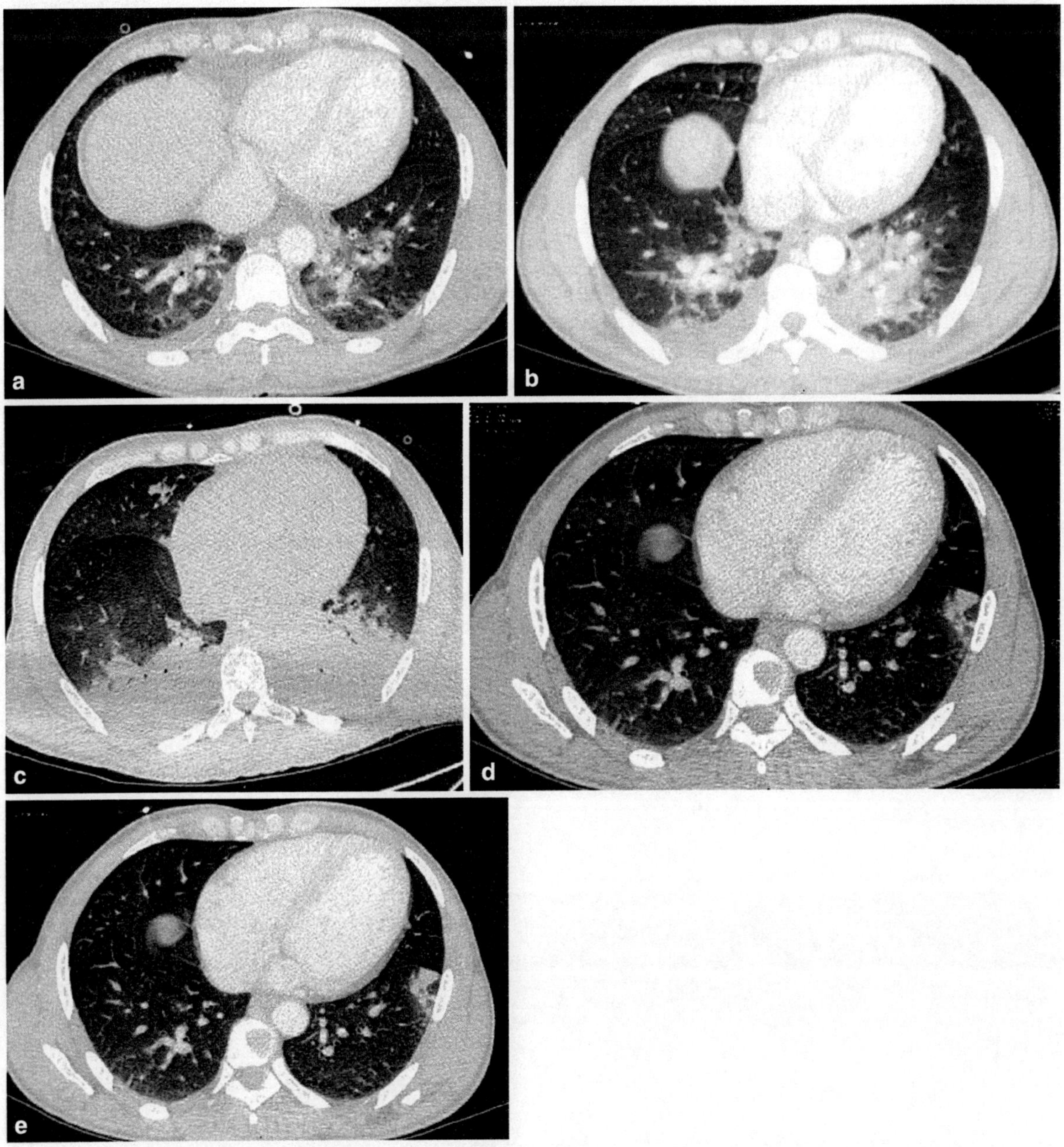

Fig. 39.2 A 52-year-old man with type 1 AML (no cytogenetic abnormality, 10% monoblasts) admitted to the intensive care unit for acute respiratory failure. (**a**) Chest X-ray on day 1 (leukocyte count, 447 G·10^9/L). (**b**) High-resolution computed tomography of the chest on day 2 (leukocyte count, 46 G·10^9/L, treatment with hydroxyurea and dexamethasone, no antiinfectious agents. (**c**) High-resolution computed tomography of the chest on day 14 (leukocyte count, 0.1 G·10^9/L), treatment with idarubicin from day 7 to day 10 and aracytine from day 7 to day 12, broad-spectrum antibiotics (ceftazidime, amikacin, and vancomycin) despite negative findings from microbiological studies. (**d** and **e**) High-resolution computed tomography of the chest 2 months after the first remission

ground-glass opacities (90.9%). The first two findings were significantly more common in the group with leukemic infiltration than in the control group; had good interobserver agreement; and corresponded to leukemic cell infiltration around the pulmonary arteries, bronchi, or bronchioles. The third study was done in four patients with AML, low leukocyte counts, and respiratory symptoms. HRCT showed pulmonary infiltrates with alveolar, interstitial, mixed, and peribronchial/perivascular patterns in all patients, including one with normal standard radiographic findings [51]. Infectious agents were excluded. Histology of the lung specimens (autopsy, $n=2$; open lung biopsy, $n=1$; and transbronchial lung biopsy, $n=1$) demonstrated leukemic infiltrates. These findings suggest that pulmonary leukemic infiltration may produce pulmonary infiltrates even in AML patients with low blast counts.

39.4 Acute Lysis Pneumopathy

Infections are the most common cause of respiratory failure in acute leukemia patients during induction therapy [58] (Table 39.3). However, the potential of AML treatment to precipitate acute respiratory failure (ARF) in hyperleukocytic patients has long been recognized. The term "leukemic cell lysis pneumopathy" was first used in 1982 [6] in a report about five patients with de novo AML (subtype not specified). All five patients had high circulating blast cell counts initially (range, 192–245 G·10^9/L) and had recently received chemotherapy. Within 4 days of the leukocyte count nadir, patchy and often multilobar pneumonitis developed. Cultures for bacteria, fungi, and viruses were negative, and broad-spectrum antibiotics produced no clinical response. Lung biopsies from all five patients (open lung biopsy, $n=4$; or transbronchial biopsies, $n=1$) showed diffuse alveolar damage (DAD) at the proliferative phase with degenerating blast cells within the interstitium and organizing alveolar exudates. No potentially pathogenic organisms were seen. In all five patients, the pulmonary infiltrate resolved without specific therapy. It was postulated that lysis of leukemic cells with release of their enzyme contents led to the histological DAD. This clinical picture was later called "lysis pneumopathy" [8]. Two patients with hyperleukocytic myelomonocytic leukemia (M4) and abnormal marrow eosinophils developed ARF within 1–3 days after starting high-dose induction chemotherapy [8]. Arguments for pulmonary injury due to resident

Table 39.3 Acute lysis pneumopathy

First author	Reference	Population	Cases (leukemia type, FAB subtype)	Onset of symptoms/ beginning of chemotherapy	Chemotherapy
Tryka et al. (1982)	[6]	Adults	5 (3 AML, type unprecised, 2 CML)	16±5 days	Aracytine in all patients + diverse chemotherapeutic agents
Myers et al. (1983)	[7]	Adults	4 (AML, type unprecised)	10–48 h	Aracytine/6-thioguanine
Dombret et al. (1992)	[8]	Adults	2 (M4 eosino)	7–12 h	Daunorubicin (in both patients)/ aracytine (in one)
Würthner et al. (1999)	[10]	Adults	2 (1 M4, 1 M2)	7–36 h[a]	Aracytine
Lester et al. (2000)	[9]	Adults	2 (M4 eosino)	16–24 h	Daunorubicin/ aracytine/ATRA
Wan et al. (2002)	[11]	Adult	1 (M4 with abnormal eosinophils)	72 h	Daunorubicin/ aracytine
Hijiya et al. (2005)	[2]	Children	5 (3 M4 eosino, 2 M5)	1–2 days	Daunorubicin/ aracytine

ATRA All-trans-retinoic acid

[a]One patient had intracerebral bleeding, myocardial and kidney infarction, and peripheral arterial thrombi

leukemic cell lysis included the presence of moderate pulmonary leukostasis (leukocyte counts, 200 G·10^9/L and 257 G·10^9/L, respectively), simultaneous occurrence of acute tumor lysis syndrome, lack of evidence of other causes of ARF, improvement in respiratory symptoms in correlation with declining leukocyte counts, and regression of acute tumor lysis syndrome. A single patient had not yet been treated with aracytine, a drug known to induce myeloid maturation of immature leukemic blasts and to cause ARF [59–64]. More recently, leukostasis followed by histologically proven hemorrhagic pulmonary infarctions with blast accumulation in the vessels was reported in a patient with AML type 2 and hyperleukocytosis who had just started chemotherapy [10]. Similar findings, combined with DAD, were described in a patient with AML-M2, abnormal eosinophils, and trisomy X who developed fatal ARF 3 days after starting induction chemotherapy [11]. In the absence of hyperleukocytosis, DAD may be related to chemotherapy-induced cell lysis with the release of eosinophil constituents such as enzymes or reactive oxygen species on [8, 11]. Among 155 children with de novo AML followed up for 11 years, five (three with AML-M4eo with inv16 and two with AML-M5) experienced severe ARF attributed to tumor lysis, associated in four patients with circulatory failure requiring vasopressor support [2]. This complication was significantly more common in AML-M4 and -M5 than in the other subtypes ($P=0.010$) and was significantly more common in AML-M4eo than in AML-M4/M5 ($P=0.008$). Interestingly, four of these five patients required invasive mechanical ventilation and were successfully extubated 2–13 days after chemotherapy initiation. No specific clinical or radiological signs have been identified to date, as the number of reported cases remains small. The most suggestive symptoms seem to be hemoptyis and extensive bilateral airspace consolidations [1]. Pulmonary lysis syndrome must be considered in patients with ARF within the first few hours or days after chemotherapy initiation, especially in patients who have AML with monocytic and eosinophilic components.

39.5 Management

The clinical management of the pulmonary manifestations of hyperleukocytosis in patients with leukemia remains unsatisfactory. No specific treatment is available. Importantly, patients with pulmonary leukostasis or other manifestations of hyperleukocytic syndrome who survive the first few days of treatment, especially those with AML, have the same complete remission rates and median disease-free survival times as patients with lower leukocyte counts [20, 65]. Every effort must be made to diminish early mortality in these patients, including ICU admission and invasive or noninvasive mechanical ventilation [47, 66, 67]. Interventions that increase blood viscosity should to avoided, especially red-blood-cell transfusions that are not absolutely required by the clinical condition of the patient (Fig. 39.3) [68]. All patients must receive hyperhydration to induce hemodilution (isotonic saline, 3 L/m^2/day without inducing alkalinization) and rasburicase to prevent acute tumor lysis syndrome and acute kidney injury from uratic nephropathy, which worsen the prognosis [69–72]. Even initially asymptomatic patients may deteriorate clinically within a few hours, and, consequently, immediate leukapheresis holds theoretical appeal as a means of diminishing the leukemic cellular burden faster than can be achieved by chemotherapy. However, no published randomized trials or evidence-based guidelines on leukapheresis are available. Leukapheresis should not be used in patients with hyperleukocytic AML-M3, in whom it might worsen the coagulation disorders [73]. Table 39.4 lists the main results of the four largest studies of leukapheresis. Controversial data have been obtained, most notably in patients with AML-M4 or -M5 [65]. Leukapheresis is generally performed as an emergency procedure in acutely ill patients with severe thrombocytopenia and coagulopathy. Although leukapheresis may be feasible through a large peripheral vein, it often needs the placement of a large-bore central venous access, which may result in complications, especially sepsis and bleeding [17]. Symptomatic hypocalcemia induced by citrate is the most often reported side effect [17]. In a recent study, severe procedural complications occurred in 18 (85.7%) of 21 children (femoral vein thrombosis, $n=5$; coagulopathy, $n=6$; sinus bradycardia, $n=4$; hypotension, $n=4$; hypertension, $n=3$; hypokalemia, $n=4$; and hypomagnesemia, $n=1$) [74]. Cytoreduction may be obtained with conventional chemotherapy. However, hydroxyurea at a dosage of 3–6 g/m^2 has been used for more than 30 years as a means of rapidly diminishing the leukocyte count without causing metabolic disturbances [75, 76]. The most recent case series,

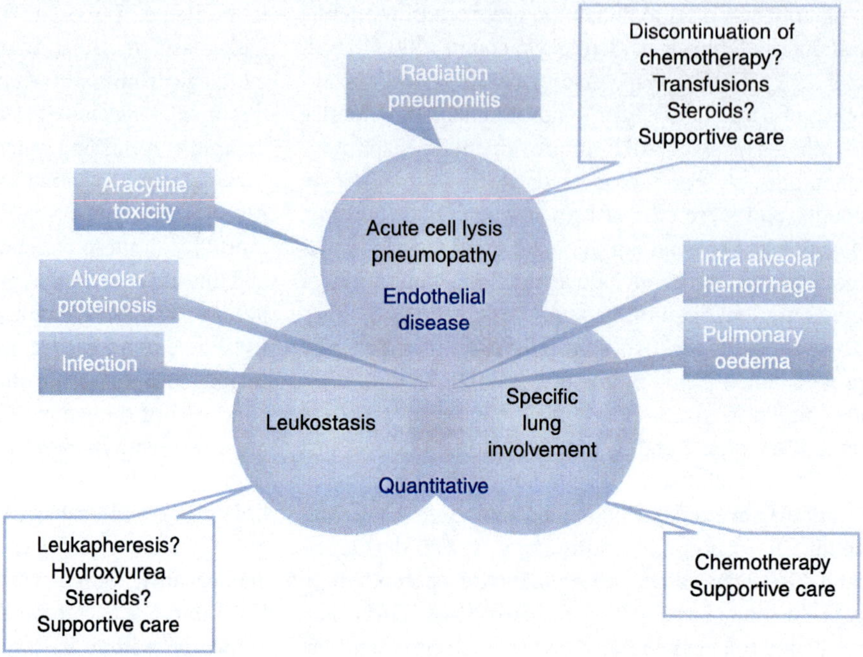

Fig. 39.3 Possible interventions

Table 39.4 Leukapheresis in patients with hyperleukocytic leukemia

Author	Reference	Population	Leukemia	Responders	Early deaths	Remission
Cuttner et al. (1983)	[88]	22 (19 adults, 3 children) WBC >100 G·10^9/L	22 AML (13M4, 6M5, 3M2)	17/22 (77.3%)[a]	–	15/17 responders vs
Porcu et al. (1997)	[89]	48 (not specified) WBC >100 G·10^9/L	AML and CML (not specified)	31/48 (64.6%)[b]	14/48 (29.2%)[c]	–
Giles et al. (2001)	[90]	71 (not specified) WBC >50 G·10^9/L	AML (not specified)	–	17/71 (24%)[d]	44/71 (62%)[e]
Inaba et al. (2008)	[21]	20 children WBC >100 G·10^9/L	AML (50% M4 or M5)	–	2/20[f]	–

[a]Greater than 30% decrease in the leukocyte count
[b]Greater than 50% decrease in the leukocyte count
[c]Death within 1 week
[d]Death within 6 weeks; $P=0.58$ vs 28% in patients treated without leukapheresis
[e]$P=0.81$ vs 59% in patients treated without leukapheresis
[f]Death within 2 weeks; $P=0.1$ vs 22.8% in patients treated without leukapheresis; both died of pulmonary hemorrhage and acute renal failure

including 87 pediatric and adult patients with hyperleukocytic AML, supports the use of oral hydroxyurea (50 mg/kg/day for 4 days), which produced cytoreduction in 62 (71.3%) patients [77]. Interestingly, only four (4.6%) patients developed acute tumor lysis syndrome. Preliminary results of a randomized study of early AML management with leukapheresis versus hydroxyurea (median cumulative dose, 18 g within the first 4 days) showed no benefits from leukapheresis [78]. These data have been incorporated into the most recent recommendations about managing hyperleukocytic AML, which suggest hydroxyurea treatment in dosages of up to 50–60 mg/kg/day until the leukocyte count falls below 10–20 G·10^9/L [79]. The existence of interactions between adhesion receptors expressed by blast cells and endothelial cells (e.g., selectins, integrins, VCAM-1, and ICAM-1) supports the use of corticosteroids [80, 81]. At our institution, we currently use dexamethasone 10 mg/12 h until resolution of the pulmonary symptoms. A recent report suggests the use of the multikinase and FLT3 inhibitor sorafenib in patients with AML FLT3, as this drug seems able to decrease the leukocyte count without inducing tumor lysis syndrome, thereby facilitating induction therapy [82]. Several patients with CML in myeloid blast crisis who presented with pulmonary leukostasis were treated with imatinib mesylate, with or without hydroxyurea, and experienced rapid leukocyte count decreases and marked improvements in their respiratory status [42, 83, 84].

There is no clear recommendation for managing acute lysis pneumopathy. Interruption of chemotherapy has been suggested to improve the clinical manifestations [2]. The roles for corticosteroids, anti-inflammatory agents, or inhibitors of cytokines or leukotrienes have not been well defined [2]. Supportive care, including mechanical ventilation, seems to be the most important therapeutic intervention. Given the presence of alveolar hemorrhage, we recommend an aggressive blood transfusion strategy (hemoglobin level above 10 g/L and platelet count above 50 G·10^9/L), especially if invasive mechanical ventilation is required [10].

References

1. Koh TT, Colby TV, Muller NL (2005) Myeloid leukemias and lung involvement. Semin Respir Crit Care Med 26(5):514–519
2. Hijiya N, Metzger ML, Pounds S, Schmidt JE, Razzouk BI, Rubnitz JE, Howard SC, Nunez CA, Pui CH, Ribeiro RC (2005) Severe cardiopulmonary complications consistent with systemic inflammatory response syndrome caused by leukemia cell lysis in childhood acute myelomonocytic or monocytic leukemia. Pediatr Blood Cancer 44(1):63–69
3. Dutcher JP, Schiffer CA, Wiernik PH (1987) Hyperleukocytosis in adult acute nonlymphocytic leukemia: impact on remission rate and duration, and survival. J Clin Oncol 5(9):1364–1372
4. Bunin NJ, Pui CH (1985) Differing complications of hyperleukocytosis in children with acute lymphoblastic or acute nonlymphoblastic leukemia. J Clin Oncol 3(12): 1590–1595
5. Lester TJ, Johnson JW, Cuttner J (1985) Pulmonary leukostasis as the single worst prognostic factor in patients with acute myelocytic leukemia and hyperleukocytosis. Am J Med 79(1):43–48
6. Tryka AF, Godleski JJ, Fanta CH (1982) Leukemic cell lysis pneumonopathy. A complication of treated myeloblastic leukemia. Cancer 50(12):2763–2770
7. Myers TJ, Cole SR, Klatsky AU, Hild DH (1983) Respiratory failure due to pulmonary leukostasis following chemotherapy of acute nonlymphocytic leukemia. Cancer 51(10):1808–1813
8. Dombret H, Hunault M, Faucher C, Dombret MC, Degos L (1992) Acute lysis pneumopathy after chemotherapy for acute myelomonocytic leukemia with abnormal marrow eosinophils. Cancer 69(6):1356–1361
9. Lester WA, Hull DR, Fegan CD, Morris TC (2000) Respiratory failure during induction chemotherapy for acute myelomonocytic leukaemia (FAB M4Eo) with ara-C and all-trans retinoic acid. Br J Haematol 109(4):847–850
10. Wurthner JU, Kohler G, Behringer D, Lindemann A, Mertelsmann R, Lubbert M (1999) Leukostasis followed by hemorrhage complicating the initiation of chemotherapy in patients with acute myeloid leukemia and hyperleukocytosis: a clinicopathologic report of four cases. Cancer 85(2):368–374
11. Wan TS, Yip SF, Yeung YM, Chan LC, Ma SK (2002) Fatal diffuse alveolar damage complicating acute myeloid leukemia with abnormal eosinophils and trisomy X. Ann Hematol 81(3):167–169
12. Perez-Zincer F, Juturi JV, Hsi ED, Hoeltge GA, Rybicki LA, Kalaycio ME (2003) A pulmonary syndrome in patients with acute myelomonocytic leukemia and inversion of chromosome 16. Leuk Lymphoma 44(1):103–109
13. Ventura GJ, Hester JP, Smith TL, Keating MJ (1988) Acute myeloblastic leukemia with hyperleukocytosis: risk factors for early mortality in induction. Am J Hematol 27(1):34–37
14. Soares FA, Landell GA, Cardoso MC (1992) Pulmonary leukostasis without hyperleukocytosis: a clinicopathologic study of 16 cases. Am J Hematol 40(1):28–32
15. McKee LC Jr, Collins RD (1974) Intravascular leukocyte thrombi and aggregates as a cause of morbidity and mortality in leukemia. Medicine (Baltimore) 53(6):463–478
16. Ahmed S, Siddiqui AK, Rossoff L, Sison CP, Rai KR (2003) Pulmonary complications in chronic lymphocytic leukemia. Cancer 98(9):1912–1917
17. Blum W, Porcu P (2007) Therapeutic apheresis in hyperleukocytosis and hyperviscosity syndrome. Semin Thromb Hemost 33(4):350–354
18. Frohling S, Schlenk RF, Breitruck J, Benner A, Kreitmeier S, Tobis K, Dohner H, Dohner K (2002) Prognostic significance of activating FLT3 mutations in younger adults (16 to 60 years) with acute myeloid leukemia and normal cytogenetics: a study of the AML Study Group Ulm. Blood 100(13):4372–4380
19. Thornton KA, Levis M (2007) FLT3 mutation and acute myelogenous leukemia with leukostasis. N Engl J Med 357(16):1639
20. Marbello L, Ricci F, Nosari AM, Turrini M, Nador G, Nichelatti M, Tedeschi A, Vismara E, Morra E (2008)

Outcome of hyperleukocytic adult acute myeloid leukaemia: a single-center retrospective study and review of literature. Leuk Res 32(8):1221–1227
21. Inaba H, Fan Y, Pounds S, Geiger TL, Rubnitz JE, Ribeiro RC, Pui CH, Razzouk BI (2008) Clinical and biologic features and treatment outcome of children with newly diagnosed acute myeloid leukemia and hyperleukocytosis. Cancer 113(3):522–529
22. Lichtman MA, Rowe JM (1982) Hyperleukocytic leukemias: rheological, clinical, and therapeutic considerations. Blood 60(2):279–283
23. Lichtman MA, Heal J, Rowe JM (1987) Hyperleukocytic leukaemia: rheological and clinical features and management. Baillières Clin Haematol 1(3):725–746
24. Stucki A, Rivier AS, Gikic M, Monai N, Schapira M, Spertini O (2001) Endothelial cell activation by myeloblasts: molecular mechanisms of leukostasis and leukemic cell dissemination. Blood 97(7):2121–2129
25. van Buchem MA, Levelt CN, Hogendoorn PC, Colly LP, Kluin PM, Willemze R, Daha MR (1993) Involvement of the complement system in the pathogenesis of pulmonary leukostasis in experimental myelocytic leukemia. Leukemia 7(10):1608–1614
26. van Buchem MA, Colly LP, Hogendoorn PC, Kluin PM, Willemze R (1991) Experimental myelocytic leukemia in the Brown-Norway rat as a model for pulmonary leukostasis. Am J Pathol 138(3):777–780
27. van Buchem MA, Hogendoorn PC, Bruijn JA, Kluin PM (1993) Endothelial activation antigens in pulmonary leukostasis in leukemia. Acta Haematol 90(1):29–33
28. Porcu P, Farag S, Marcucci G, Cataland SR, Kennedy MS, Bissell M (2002) Leukocytoreduction for acute leukemia. Ther Apher 6(1):15–23
29. Novotny JR, Muller-Beissenhirtz H, Herget-Rosenthal S, Kribben A, Duhrsen U (2005) Grading of symptoms in hyperleukocytic leukaemia: a clinical model for the role of different blast types and promyelocytes in the development of leukostasis syndrome. Eur J Haematol 74(6): 501–510
30. Piccirillo N, Laurenti L, Chiusolo P, Sora F, Bianchi M, De Matteis S, Pagano L, Zini G, D'Onofrio G, Leone G et al (2009) Reliability of leukostasis grading score to identify patients with high-risk hyperleukocytosis. Am J Hematol 84(6):381–382
31. Chillar RK, Belman MJ, Farbstein M (1980) Explanation for apparent hypoxemia associated with extreme leukocytosis: leukocytic oxygen consumption. Blood 55(6):922–924
32. Gartrell K, Rosenstrauch W (1993) Hypoxaemia in patients with hyperleukocytosis: true or spurious, and clinical implications. Leuk Res 17(11):915–919
33. Lele AV, Mirski MA, Stevens RD (2005) Spurious hypoxemia. Crit Care Med 33(8):1854–1856
34. Gorski TF, Ajemian M, Hussain E, Talhouk A, Ruskin G, Hanna A, Jacobs M (1999) Correlation of pseudohypoxemia and leukocytosis in chronic lymphocytic leukemia. South Med J 92(8):817–819
35. Vincent F, Levy V, Bensousan T, Escudier B, Leclercq B (1994) Blood gas analysis in patients with hyperleucocytosis: validity of repeated measures on same sampling without ice? Leuk Res 18(7):553–554
36. Polak R, Huisman A, Sikma MA, Kersting S (2010) Spurious hypokalaemia and hypophosphataemia due to extreme hyperleukocytosis in a patient with a haematological malignancy. Ann Clin Biochem. Mar;47(Pt 2):179–81
37. Sevastos N, Theodossiades G, Savvas SP, Tsilidis K, Efstathiou S, Archimandritis AJ (2006) Pseudohyperkalemia in patients with increased cellular components of blood. Am J Med Sci 331(1):17–21
38. Van Buchem MA, Wondergem JH, Kool LJ, Te Velde J, Kluin PM, Bode PJ, Busscher DL (1987) Pulmonary leukostasis: radiologic-pathologic study. Radiology 165(3): 739–741
39. Nagler A, Brenner B, Zuckerman E, Hazani A, Israel O (1988) Acute respiratory failure in hyperleukocytotic acute myeloid leukemia: the role of perfusion lung scintigraphy. Am J Hematol 27(1):65–66
40. Szyper-Kravitz M, Strahilevitz J, Oren V, Lahav M (2001) Pulmonary leukostasis: role of perfusion lung scan in diagnosis and follow up. Am J Hematol 67(2):136–138
41. Kaminsky DA, Hurwitz CG, Olmstead JI (2000) Pulmonary leukostasis mimicking pulmonary embolism. Leuk Res 24(2):175–178
42. Pinheiro RF, Santiago SP, Lopes A, Araujo VN, Magalhaes SM (2010) Pulmonary leukostasis mimicking tuberculosis in endemic area. Leuk Res 34(5):e128–e129
43. Tenholder MF, Hooper RG (1980) Pulmonary infiltrates in leukemia. Chest 78(3):468–473
44. Hildebrand FL Jr, Rosenow EC III, Habermann TM, Tazelaar HD (1990) Pulmonary complications of leukemia. Chest 98(5):1233–1239
45. Poletti V, Salvucci M, Zanchini R, Molinari AL, Zuffa E, Poletti G, Zaccaria A (2000) The lung as a target organ in patients with hematologic disorders. Haematologica 85(8):855–864
46. Valentino DJ III, Gelfand MC, Nava VE, Garvin DF, Roberts AH II (2005) Hypoxemic respiratory failure in a 57-year-old woman with acute monocytic leukemia. Chest 128(5): 3629–3633
47. Prakash UB, Divertie MB, Banks PM (1979) Aggressive therapy in acute respiratory failure from leukemic pulmonary infiltrates. Chest 75(3):345–350
48. Rossi GA, Balbi B, Risso M, Repetto M, Ravazzoni C (1985) Acute myelomonocytic leukemia. Demonstration of pulmonary involvement by bronchoalveolar lavage. Chest 87(2): 259–260
49. Azoulay E, Fieux F, Moreau D, Thiery G, Rousselot P, Parrot A, Le Gall J-R, Dombret H, Schlemmer B (2003) Acute monocytic leukemia presenting as acute respiratory failure. Am J Respir Crit Care Med 167(10):1329–1333
50. Callahan M, Wall S, Askin F, Delaney D, Koller C, Orringer EP (1987) Granulocytic sarcoma presenting as pulmonary nodules and lymphadenopathy. Cancer 60(8):1902–1904
51. Potenza L, Luppi M, Morselli M, Tonelli S, D'Apollo N, Facchini L, Torricelli P, Tazzioli G, Saviola A, Bresciani P et al (2003) Leukaemic pulmonary infiltrates in adult acute myeloid leukaemia: a high-resolution computerized tomography study. Br J Haematol 120(6):1058–1061
52. Bodey GP, Powell RD Jr, Hersh EM, Yeterian A, Freireich EJ (1966) Pulmonary complications of acute leukemia. Cancer 19(6):781–793
53. Kovalski R, Hansen-Flaschen J, Lodato RF, Pietra GG (1990) Localized leukemic pulmonary infiltrates. Diagnosis by bronchoscopy and resolution with therapy. Chest 97(3):674–678

54. Okura T, Tanaka R, Shibata H, Kukita H (1992) Adult T-cell leukemia with a solitary lung mass. Chest 101(5): 1471–1472
55. Sueyoshi E, Uetani M, Hayashi K, Tawara M (1996) Adult T-cell leukemia with multiple pulmonary nodules due to leukemic cell infiltration. AJR Am J Roentgenol 167(2): 540–541
56. Heyneman LE, Johkoh T, Ward S, Honda O, Yoshida S, Muller NL (2000) Pulmonary leukemic infiltrates: high-resolution CT findings in 10 patients. AJR Am J Roentgenol 174(2):517–521
57. Tanaka N, Matsumoto T, Miura G, Emoto T, Matsunaga N, Satoh Y, Oka Y (2002) CT findings of leukemic pulmonary infiltration with pathologic correlation. Eur Radiol 12(1): 166–174
58. Specchia G, Pastore D, Carluccio P, Mele G, Montagna MT, Liso A, Rizzi R, Ianora AS, Liso V (2003) Pneumonia in acute leukemia patients during induction therapy: experience in a single institution. Leuk Lymphoma 44(1): 97–101
59. Fabian I, Shur I, Bleiberg I, Rudi A, Kashman Y, Lishner M (1995) Growth modulation and differentiation of acute myeloid leukemia cells by jaspamide. Exp Hematol 23(7): 583–587
60. Lubbert M, Koeffler HP (1988) Myeloid cell lines: tools for studying differentiation of normal and abnormal hematopoietic cells. Blood Rev 2(2):121–133
61. Andersson BS, Luna MA, Yee C, Hui KK, Keating MJ, McCredie KB (1990) Fatal pulmonary failure complicating high-dose cytosine arabinoside therapy in acute leukemia. Cancer 65(5):1079–1084
62. Jehn U, Goldel N, Rienmuller R, Wilmanns W (1988) Noncardiogenic pulmonary edema complicating intermediate and high-dose Ara C treatment for relapsed acute leukemia. Med Oncol Tumor Pharmacother 5(1):41–47
63. Forghieri F, Luppi M, Morselli M, Potenza L (2007) Cytarabine-related lung infiltrates on high resolution computerized tomography: a possible complication with benign outcome in leukemic patients. Haematologica 92(9):e85–e90
64. Chagnon K, Boissel N, Raffoux E, Dombret H, Tazi A, Bergeron A (2009) A new pattern of cytosine-arabinoside-induced lung toxicity. Br J Haematol 147(5):771–774
65. Hiroto I, Ying F, Stanley P, Terrence LG, Jeffrey ER, Raul CR, Ching-Hon P, Bassem IR (2008) Clinical and biologic features and treatment outcome of children with newly diagnosed acute myeloid leukemia and hyperleukocytosis. Cancer 113(3):522–529
66. Vernant JP, Brun B, Mannoni P, Dreyfus B (1979) Respiratory distress of hyperleukocytic granulocytic leukemias. Cancer 44(1):264–268
67. Darmon M, Azoulay E (2005) Prognosis of acute monocytic leukemia (French-American-British classification M5). J Clin Oncol 23(6):1327, author reply 1327–1328
68. Harris AL (1978) Leukostasis associated with blood transfusion in acute myeloid leukaemia. Br Med J 1(6121): 1169–1171
69. Coiffier B, Altman A, Pui CH, Younes A, Cairo MS (2008) Guidelines for the management of pediatric and adult tumor lysis syndrome: an evidence-based review. J Clin Oncol 26(16):2767–2778
70. Tosi P, Barosi G, Lazzaro C, Liso V, Marchetti M, Morra E, Pession A, Rosti G, Santoro A, Zinzani PL et al (2008) Consensus conference on the management of tumor lysis syndrome. Haematologica 93(12):1877–1885
71. Darmon M, Guichard I, Vincent F, Schlemmer B, Azoulay E (2010) Prognostic significance of acute renal injury in acute tumor lysis syndrome. Leuk Lymphoma 51(2): 221–227
72. Ricci Z, Ronco C (2010) Pulmonary/renal interaction. Curr Opin Crit Care 16(1):13–18
73. Vahdat L, Maslak P, Miller WH Jr, Eardley A, Heller G, Scheinberg DA, Warrell RP Jr (1994) Early mortality and the retinoic acid syndrome in acute promyelocytic leukemia: impact of leukocytosis, low-dose chemotherapy, PMN/RAR-alpha isoform, and CD13 expression in patients treated with all-trans retinoic acid. Blood 84(11): 3843–3849
74. Abla O, Khanani MF, Hitzler JK, Sung L, Geary D, Abdelhaleem M, Weitzman S, Naqvi A (2004) Complications of hyperleukocytosis and leukapheresis in pediatric acute leukemias. ASH Ann Meet Abstr 104(11):1963
75. Grund FM, Armitage JO, Burns P (1977) Hydroxyurea in the prevention of the effects of leukostasis in acute leukemia. Arch Intern Med 137(9):1246–1247
76. Berg J, Vincent PC, Gunz FW (1979) Extreme leucocytosis and prognosis of newly diagnosed patients with acute non-lymphocytic leukaemia. Med J Aust 1(11):480–482
77. Quessar AM, Khoubila NR, Ribeiro RCU, Rachid MA, Zafad SD, Harif MM, Madani AL, Hda NZ, Howard S, Benchekroun SI (2007) Hydroxyurea in the early management of acute myeloid leukemia and hyperleukocytosis. ASH Ann Meet Abstr 110(11):4368
78. Kuo KHM, Callum J, Brandwein J, Crump M, Curtis JE, Gupta V, Lipton JH, Pantalony D, Schimmer A, Schuh A et al (2006) Management of hyperleukocytosis in acute myelogenous leukemia using hydroxyurea rather than leukopheresis. ASH Ann Meet Abstr 108(11):2007
79. Dohner H, Estey EH, Amadori S, Appelbaum FR, Buchner T, Burnett AK, Dombret H, Fenaux P, Grimwade D, Larson RA et al (2010) Diagnosis and management of acute myeloid leukemia in adults: recommendations from an international expert panel, on behalf of the European LeukemiaNet. Blood 115(3):453–474
80. Rowe JM, Lichtman MA (1984) Hyperleukocytosis and leukostasis: common features of childhood chronic myelogenous leukemia. Blood 63(5):1230–1234
81. Ozdemir MA, Karakukcu M, Patiroglu T, Torun YA, Kose M (2009) Management of hyperleukocytosis and prevention of tumor lysis syndrome with low-dose prednisone continuous infusion in children with acute lymphoblastic leukemia. Acta Haematol 121(1):56–62
82. Schroeder T, Saure C, Bruns I, Zohren F, Czibere AG, Safaian NN, Fenk R, Haas R, Kobbe G (2009) Clinical efficacy of sorafenib in patients with acute myeloid leukemia (AML) and activating FLT3-mutations. ASH Ann Meet Abstr 114(22):2057
83. Leis JF, Primack SL, Schubach SE, Curtin PT, Druker BJ, Maziarz RT (2004) Management of life-threatening pulmonary leukostasis with single agent imatinib mesylate during CML myeloid blast crisis. Haematologica 89(9):ECR30
84. Ramanujam D, McNicholl F, Furby D, Richardson D, Cuthbert RJG, McMullin MF (2009) Dramatic resolution of respiratory symptoms with imatinib mesylate in patients with chronic myeloid leukemia presenting with lower airway

symptoms resembling asthma. Leuk Lymphoma 50(10): 1721–1722

85. Frankel DH, Larson RA, Lorincz AL (1987) Acral lividosis – a sign of myeloproliferative diseases. Hyperleukocytosis syndrome in chronic myelogenous leukemia. Arch Dermatol 123(7):921–924
86. Mataix R, Gomez-Casares MT, Campo C, Jimenez S, Malcorra JJ (1996) Acute leg ischaemia as a presentation of hyperleukocytosis syndrome in acute myeloid leukaemia. Am J Hematol 51(3):250
87. Cohen Y, Amir G, Da'as N, Gillis S, Rund D, Polliack A (2002) Acute myocardial infarction as the presenting symptom of acute myeloblastic leukemia with extreme hyperleukocytosis. Am J Hematol 71(1):47–49
88. Cuttner J, Holland JF, Norton L, Ambinder E, Button G, Meyer RJ (1983) Therapeutic leukapheresis for hyperleukocytosis in acute myelocytic leukemia. Med Pediatr Oncol 11(2):76–78
89. Porcu P, Danielson CF, Orazi A, Heerema NA, Gabig TG, McCarthy LJ (1997) Therapeutic leukapheresis in hyperleucocytic leukaemias: lack of correlation between degree of cytoreduction and early mortality rate. Br J Haematol 98(2):433–436
90. Giles FJ, Shen Y, Kantarjian HM, Korbling MJ, O'Brien S, Anderlini P, Donato M, Pierce S, Keating MJ, Freireich EJ et al (2001) Leukapheresis reduces early mortality in patients with acute myeloid leukemia with high white cell counts but does not improve long- term survival. Leuk Lymphoma 42(1–2):67–73

Pulmonary MALT Lymphoma: Clinical, Molecular and Therapeutic Aspects

40

Marie Wislez, Raphael Borie, Catherine Thieblemont, Marie-France Carette, Martine Antoine, and Jacques Cadranel

Contents

M. Wislez (✉) and J. Cadranel
Service de Pneumologie et Réanimation, Centre de Compétence des Maladies Rares pulmonaires, Hôpital Tenon, AP-HP Université Paris 6, 4 Rue de la Chine, 75020 Paris, France
e-mail: marie.wislez@tnn.aphp.fr

R. Borie
Service de Pneumologie, Hôpital Bichat, AP-HP, Paris, France

C. Thieblemont
Service d'Hémato-oncologie, Hôpital Saint-Louis, AP-HP – Université Paris Diderot VII – INSERM U 728 – Institut Universitaire d'hématologie, Paris, France

M.-F. Carette
Service de Radiologie, Hôpital Tenon, AP-HP, Paris, France

M. Antoine
Service d'Anatomie Pathologique, Hôpital Tenon, AP-HP, Paris, France

Primary pulmonary lymphoma (PPL) is defined as clonal lymphoid proliferation affecting one or both lungs (parenchyma and/or bronchi) in a patient with no detectable extrapulmonary involvement at diagnosis or during the subsequent 3 months [1, 2]. When the lung is the principal tumor site, the other sites of involvement may be diverse: [1] multifocal inside lung; [2] pulmonary with satellite nodes (hilar or mediastinal) and [3] pulmonary with multi-organ involvement. These different clinical presentations are associated to the distinct histological subtypes, respectively [2, 3]: (a) the extranodal marginal zone lymphoma (MZL) of mucosa-associated lymphoid tissue (MALT lymphoma), (b) diffuse large B cell lymphoma (DBCL), and (c) lymphomatoid granulomatosis (LG), which is much rarer. T-cell lymphoma may occur in lung, either as a primitive site or as a secondary site after dissemination from extrapulmonary T-cell lymphoma. This general review aims to clarify the pathophysiological, diagnostic, prognostic, and therapeutic features of pulmonary MALT lymphoma.

40.1 Terminology

Extranodal MZL of mucosa-associated lymphoid tissue (MALT lymphoma) is the most common indolent *B-PPL* [4]. The cell of origin is thought to be identical to the other subtypes of MZL, i.e., nodal and splenic

É. Azoulay (ed.), *Pulmonary Involvement in Patients with Hematological Malignancies*,
DOI: 10.1007/978-3-642-15742-4_40, © Springer-Verlag Berlin Heidelberg 2011

subtypes [4]. However, clinical presentation and cytogenetic characteristics are different [5–9]. These lymphomas represent 8% of diagnosed cases of NHL [10], making them the third most common histological sub-type after diffuse large-cell B lymphomas and follicular lymphomas [6].

40.2 MALT Lymphoma

40.2.1 Marginal Zone and Bronchial Mucosa-Associated Lymphoid Tissue

In terms of anatomy, the marginal zone (MZ) was first described in the spleen [11] and was recognized as MZ-like in organs, such as Peyer patch, nodes, or MALT. Functionaly B-lymphocytes of MZ are memory B cells, involved in T-dependent or T-independent immune responses.

MALT is a lymphoid tissue that is specialized in defending the mucosa [2]. It was first described in the digestive tract (GALT) in animal models, and later in the ileum in humans. It consists of Peyer's patches, the lamina propria, and intraepithelial lymphocytes. Peyer's patches are mucosal nodules of lymphoid tissue, the structure of which is similar to that of lymph node lymphoid follicles, though the B cell MZ is more fully developed. The lamina propria contains T lymphocytes and plasma cells that secrete IgA. Intraepithelial lymphocytes are of T and CD8+ phenotype. The stomach is the organ that is most frequently affected by MALT-type lymphomatous disease, and the stomach model can be extrapolated to other locations of MALT-type MZL, such as the lungs.

Lymphomas of the MZ generally appear to be associated with chronic antigen stimulation, frequently from microbial origin [12]. This is an unusual model of lymphoproliferation, in which the infectious agent does not infect lymphoid cells and does not directly transform them, unlike lymphomas associated with the EBV, HHV8, or HTLV1 viruses. In MZLs, the infectious agent increases the risk of lymphomatous transformation via chronic stimulation of antigen-specific B lymphocyte proliferation. Under normal circumstances there is no MALT in the stomach. In cases of chronic antigen stimulation, for example, in *Helicobacter pylori* infection, MALT develops, which can later undergo lymphomatous transformation starting in the B lymphocytes in the MZ. The malignant B cell clone requires the presence of *H. pylori* antigen in order to multiply. For this reason, *H. pylori* is present in the majority of gastric biopsies from patients with gastric MALT lymphoma. The incidence of gastric lymphoma is higher in regions in which *H. pylori* is endemic, and the seroprevalence of *H. pylori* is greater in patients with gastric lymphoma than in control patients who do not have lymphoma. Finally, eradication of *H. pylori* leads to complete and prolonged disease remission in 80% of early-stage gastric lymphoma cases [13]. Other infectious agents have been suggested as possible candidates for causes of MALT lymphoma in other sites, such as *Borrelia burgdorferi* (the agent that causes Lyme disease) for skin lymphoma [12, 14], *Chlamydia psittaci* for orbital lymphoma, and *Campylobacter jejuni* for small-intestine lymphoma, formerly known as alpha-chain disease or Mediterranean lymphoma [15]. Chronic antigen stimulation may be of autoimmune origin. MALT lymphomas in the salivary glands and thyroid are observed more frequently in patients with Sjögren's syndrome or Hashimoto's thyroiditis. A recent meta-analysis looked at the link between autoimmune diseases and lymphoma, examining the data from 29,423 patients involved in 12 case control studies [16]. This meta-analysis confirms that patients with Sjögren's syndrome or lupus have an increased risk of MZ lymphoma. Primary or secondary Sjögren's syndrome was associated with a 6.5-fold increased risk of lymphoma in general, a 1,000-fold increased risk of parotid gland MZ lymphoma, and a fivefold increased risk of lymphoma in other extranodal sites. Lupus was associated with a 2.7-fold increased risk of lymphoma in general and a 12.9-fold increased risk in extranodal lymphoma (after deduction of cases of secondary Sjögren's syndrome).

No antigen was identified in the lungs. A recent study examined detection of *C. pneumoniae*, *trachomatis* and *psittacci* DNA, and the DNA of *Mycoplasma pneumoniae*, using PCR on tissue from patients with pulmonary MALT lymphoma ($n=69$), using other pulmonary lymphoproliferative disorders (LPD) ($n=30$) and tissue free from LPD ($n=44$) as control specimens [17]. *Chlamydiae* sp. DNA was detected more frequently in MALT tissue than in non-LPD tissue, but the difference was not statistically significant. *M. pneumoniae* DNA was not detected.

Finally, conditions in which there is chronic antigen stimulation, such as systemic lupus erythematosus, multiple sclerosis, Hashimoto's thyroiditis, and, in particular, Sjögren's syndrome, are also recognized as factors that can lead to development of MALT-type pulmonary lymphoma.

40.2.2 Molecular Basis

The cytogenetic abnormalities that characterize MALT lymphomas have been known for several years (Table 40.1). Their frequency and type vary depending on the lymphoma site, and possibly depending on the patient's geographical location. These are trisomy 3 and 18, as well as various translocations. Translocation t(11;18)(q21;q21) is the most common abnormality and is specific to MZLs of the MALT type. It is found in 42% of pulmonary cases, 22% of gastric cases, and 15% of intestinal cases [18]. It is in most cases absent if disease is in the thyroid, salivary glands, or liver. This translocation is associated with a risk of greater dissemination, resistance to antibiotic treatment for *H. pylori*, and less risk to histological progression. It corresponds to a fusion of the API2 gene (apoptosis inhibitor 2), which is situated on chromosome 11, and of the MALT1 gene (MALT lymphoma-associated translocation), which is situated on chromosome 18. The t(1;14)(p22;q32)/IGH-BCL10, t(14;18)(q32;q21)/IGH-MALT1 and t(3;14)/IGH-FOXP1 translocations are rarer and are particularly found when disease is located in the gastrointestinal tract or lungs [18]. The most recently described translocation, t(3;14)(p14.1;q32), is more frequent when disease is located in the thyroid. All these translocations, except the last one, activate the NF-kB pathway, which suggests that this pathway plays a role in causing MALT-type MZ lymphomas. These translocations are mutually exclusive and can be studied with morphological techniques (interphase in situ hybridization to visualize the translocation in tumor cells), using paraffin-embedded tissue or with RT-PCR (fusion transcript), most often using frozen specimens but also involving paraffin-embedded tissue.

Table 40.1 Main cytogenetic abnormalities involved in marginal zone lymphomas (From [14])

Cytogenetic abnormality	Site (frequency)
t(11;18)(q21;q21)	Lung (30–50%)
API2-MALT1	Intestine (~40%)
	Stomach (5–30%)
	Ocular adnexa (0–5%)
t(14;18)(q32;q21)	Ocular adnexa, skin, salivary glands, liver (frequent)
IgH-MALT1	Lung (10%)
	Stomach (rare)
t(1;14)(p22;q32)	Stomach (5%)
BCL10-IgH	Lung (rare)
t(3;14)(p14.1;q32)	All sites (10%)
FOXP1-IgH	Thyroid (50%)
	Ocular adnexa (20%)
	Skin (10%)
Trisomy 3, 12, 18	Intestine
	Salivary glands
	Ocular adnexa
	Other

40.2.3 Epidemiology

PPL is rare, representing 0.5–1% of lung neoplasias. MALT-type lymphomas represent more than half of PPL and are the most common type of pulmonary lymphoma [19–21]. Age of onset is around 50–60 years and very occasionally those under 30 are affected [22, 23]. The rate of smoking (37%) is no higher among these patients than in the general population [21]. Women are affected as often as men. The presence of immune system disorder is a predisposing factor for development of MALT-type PPL. In a recent study, 16% of patients had an autoimmune disease at the time of diagnosis [21].

40.3 Clinical and Radiological Signs of Pulmonary MALT Lymphoma

In nearly half of the cases, patients are asymptomatic, and investigations are initiated because of an abnormal lung finding on X-ray. If symptoms are present, they are non-specific (cough, minimal dyspnea, chest pain, and sometimes hemoptysis). On pulmonary auscultation, there are crackles in less than 20% of cases. General signs (fever or weight loss) are observed in less than a quarter of patients, particularly in aggressive forms [22, 23]. The usual radiological appearance is alveolar opacity, which is localized, less than 5 cm in diameter, and associated in nearly 50% of cases with air bronchogram [24–29]. CT scanning (see Fig. 40.1), which is more sensitive than standard X-ray, has shown that lesions are most often bilateral (60–70% of cases) and multiple (70–77% of cases) [30, 31] and that there is almost always a clear patch within each lesion, corresponding to the intact bronchial lumen. Presence of distended bronchi within the lesions is suggestive of diagnosis [31]. In less than 10% of cases, there are diffuse reticulonodular opacities in both lungs, atelectasis or pleural effusion [24–27, 29]. Hilar or mediastinal lymphadenopathy may be present on CT scanning [24, 26]. The mean time between initial clinical or radiological findings and diagnosis is 9 months, ranging between 15 days and several years (8 years) [21, 24–28, 32].

40.4 Diagnostic Approach

The diagnostic approach to a patient who has pulmonary lesions that are suspicious for involvement could require different modalities to provide sufficient tissue to diagnose lymphoma and classify the lymphoma and to exclude other inflammatory conditions and malignancies. Tissue biopsy is the gold standard for diagnosis. Samples will be analyzed for histology assessment, paraffin section immunohistochemistry, and molecular genetic analysis (PCR for immunoglobulin gene rearrangements). These modalities could also provide cells for cytological examination and flow cytometry. Diagnostic approaches are going from the minimally invasive technique such as bronchoscopy to the highly invasive thoracotomy with surgical biopsies.

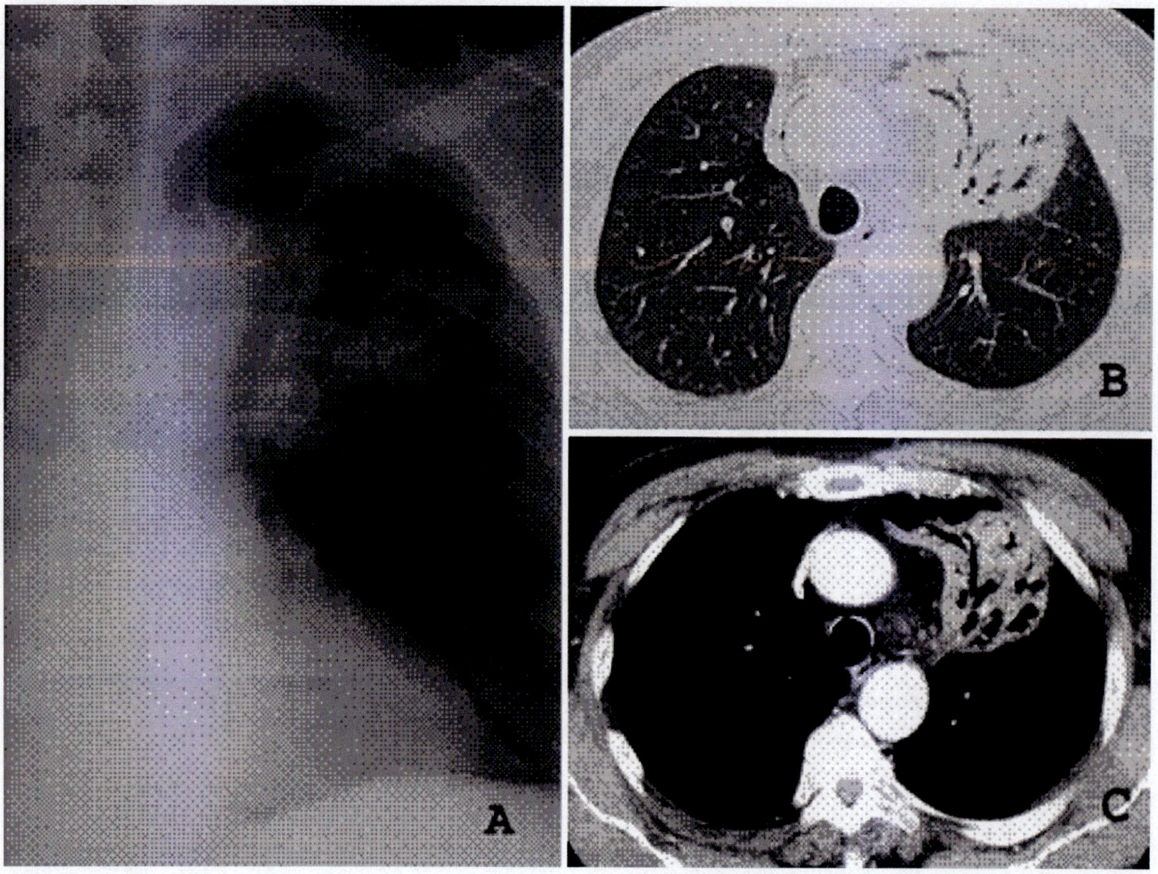

Fig. 40.1 MALT-type pulmonary lymphoma. Chronic alveolar opacity of the left upper lobe with air bronchogram. Chest X-ray (*panel A*) and CT scan (*B and C*)

40.4.1 Contribution of Bronchoscopy

Macroscopic findings of bronchoscopy are usually normal [24]. Abnormalities, from inflammatory mucosa to bronchial stenosis, may be observed [24, 29]. Bronchial biopsies are more fruitful when they are carried out on endobronchial lesions. Transbronchial biopsies must be guided by the topography of abnormalities seen on CT scanning [24]. In a recent series, the sensitivity of bronchial and transbronchial biopsy was 31% and 88%, respectively [21]. Bronchioloalveolar lavage may play a major role in the differential diagnosis of chronic alveolar opacity, showing the absence of tumor cells that could be seen in other malignancies, such as bronchoalveolar carcinoma or of pathogens seen in chronic infections. Presence of lymphocytic alveolitis could also suggest the diagnosis of PPL [33]. This lymphocytosis, which is most often of T phenotype, does not appear to have specific characteristics unless more than 10% B-lymphocytes are present [24, 29, 34, 35]. Morphological analysis of lymphocytes from lavage could sometimes reveal monocytoid or plasmacytoid cells. The diagnostic value of this B-lymphocyte alveolitis is greater if the clonality can be demonstrated by clonal rearrangement of immunoglobulin genes using molecular biology techniques [36–40]. However, a negative result does not exclude the diagnosis. In a recent study, involving 35 patients with MALT-type PPL, 84% of patients had more than 15% lymphocytic alveolitis. B-lymphocytes were more than 10% of total alveolar lymphocytes in cases for which phenotyping was available. Clonality analysis identified a B-cell clone in 71% of them [21].

40.4.2 Contribution of Other Diagnostic Alternatives

If there is no specific lesion seen on such specimens, CT-guided aspiration and biopsy must be considered, especially for peripheral nodules or masses. Sensitivity of this test was 80% in series [21]. Diagnostic surgery may be carried out as last resort. It is an invasive procedure that requires significant effort, expense, and post-biopsy recovery time for the patient. However, surgery provides larger biopsy samples than the less invasive procedures. In certain situations, lymphomas are morphologically and immunophenotypically complex, and are associated with reactive elements (non-neoplastic reacting T cells, granulomas, amyloid, fibrosis, etc.) such that they are not diagnosable in small sample size biopsies. Lastly, surgical biopsy in case of a localized lesion will allow radical treatment at the same time.

40.4.3 Diagnostic Criteria

Diagnosis of MALT-type PPL is made on the basis of histology and is based on analysis of tumor tissue.

40.4.3.1 Results of Conventional Histology Analysis

The macroscopic appearance is of a whitish mass, which is soft and poorly delimited. The microscopic appearance of MALT-type PPL is defined using the following criteria, which do not always appear in association [20, 25, 32, 41–43]: (1) a proliferation of neoplastic cells made up of small to medium-sized lymphocytic cells, similar to MZ cells of Peyer's patch follicles or of the spleen, in the form of centrocyte-like cells or monocytoid or plasmacytoid cells; (2) presence of a lymphoepithelial lesion with migration of the lymphoid cells of the MZ into the bronchiolar epithelium; (3) reactive follicular hyperplasia, sometimes with the appearance of follicular colonization; and (4) in rare cases, blast cells. The neoplastic cell population is located interstitially, in the alveolar and bronchiolar walls [44] (see Fig. 40.2). Because of the density of the lesions, they tend to collapse the residual alveoli rather than invading the lumen, and they destroy the pulmonary architecture. Some more distinctive appearances should be recognized, such as forms with amyloid or granulomatous deposits, presence of lymphatic invasion [43–47], and, finally, fibrosis of varying degrees [44], but these features are not key diagnostic element.

40.4.3.2 Contribution of Immunohistochemistry

Immunohistochemistry analysis on paraffin-embedded tissue contributes to a positive and differential diagnosis of MALT-type PPL. It identifies a CD20 B-cell phenotype [20, 25, 27, 28, 32, 42–44, 48]

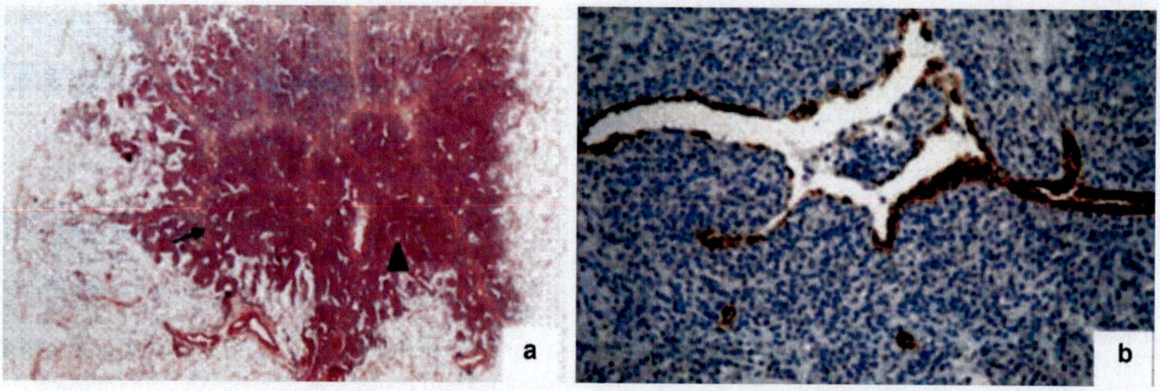

Fig. 40.2 MALT-type pulmonary lymphoma. *Panel A*: Proliferation in peribronchovascular interstitium (*arrowhead*: *septa; arrow*: *vascular lumen*). *Panel B*: Lymphoepithelial lesion, with bronchiolar epithelium masked or partially destroyed by lymphoid infiltrate. Residual epithelial cells shown using anticytokeratin antibody

(see Fig. 40.2) with coexpression of CD43 and determines clonality by showing immunoglobulin light chain monotype [49, 50] in the lymphocytic infiltrate, which invades follicular structures and damages the bronchial/bronchiolar epithelium (see Fig. 40.2). These B lymphocytes also express CD79 (particularly if there is plasmacytic differentiation) and bcl-2 [43]. This technique also reveals, by showing whether there are persistent dendritic cells (CD21, CD35) [32, 42, 44], whether follicles have been destroyed within the tumor proliferation and whether there are usually small reactive T-lymphocytes (CD3) within the parietal alveolar infiltrate and around the peribronchiolar nodules [42, 44]. In particular, it can be used to rule out indolent lymph node lymphoma (follicular NHL-B, mantle NHL-B, and CLL-type lymphoma) if there is a negative result for the expression of surface antigens CD5, CD10, and CD23 [42, 44, 51, 52], cyclin D1, and bcl-6.

40.4.3.3 Contribution of Molecular Biology

Current molecular biology techniques involve PCR on frozen tissue or cells or paraffin-embedded tissue (sometimes with prior microdissection). These help to determine clonality by showing how the immunoglobulin repertoire is restricted.

Each normal mature B cell has rearranged immunoglobulin heavy and light chain genes. Since all of the neoplastic cells in B cell lymphoma are thought to derive from a single cell that undergoes neoplastic transformation and then proliferates, all of the cells would have identical immunoglobulin gene rearrangements. This is the property of B cell populations that is assessed by PCR analysis of immunoglobulin heavy and light chain gene rearrangements. PCR can also be used to detect the fusion genes that result from chromosomal translocations in MALT lymphoma. FISH (fluorescence in situ hybridization) techniques can recognize the involved genes in the chromosomal translocations and can detect extra copies of chromosomes 3, 8, and 18 that are common in MALT lymphomas. Lastly, FISH relies on the use of probes on immunoglobulin kappa and lambda light chain mRNA to determine if the B cell and plasma cell populations of interest express both kappa and lambda light chain mRNA (polyclonal) or show light chain mRNA restriction (clonal).

40.5 Differential Diagnosis: Clinical and Pathological

In clinical terms, the problem is how to identify a diagnosis of MALT-type PPL from a radiological finding of chronic diffuse or localized alveolar opacity, which can correspond to one of many etiologies (Tables 40.2 and 40.3).

In terms of histology, particularly with a small specimen, the difficulty is to distinguish MALT-type NHL from diffuse lymphoid hyperplasia or lymphocytic interstitial pneumonia (LIP) on transbronchial

Table 40.2 Main etiologies to be considered in cases of chronic single or multiple alveolar opacities

Frequent causes
Bacterial or viral pneumonia, slow to resolve
Organizing pneumonia
Tuberculosis
Pulmonary infarction
Pulmonary contusion
Localized pulmonary edema
Less frequent causes
Bronchioloalveolar carcinoma
Pseudo-alveolar sarcoidosis
Hypersensitivity lung disease
Lymphoma
Alveolar proteinosis
Radiation-induced lung disease
Eosinophilic lung disease
Alveolar hemorrhage
Bacterial pneumonia involving slow-growing organisms (nocardiosis, actinomycosis)

The diagnoses in italics are those that are most often evoked, because of their subacute clinical onset

Table 40.3 Main etiologies to be considered in cases of multiple nodular opacities, which may be excavated

Frequent causes
Metastasis (ENT cancer, cervical or testicular cancer, choriocarcinoma)
Septic metastases (endocarditis)
Tuberculosis
Post-embolism pulmonary infarction
Less frequent causes
Wegener's granulomatosis
Sarcoidosis, which may be necrotizing
Rheumatoid arthritis
Benign granulomatous and lymphocytic vasculitis
Lymphomatoid granulomatosis, lymphoma
Bacterial pneumonia involving slow-growing organisms (nocardiosis, actinomycosis)
Invasive or semi-invasive aspergillosis, other mycoses: cryptococcosis, American histoplasmosis
Multiple chondromatous hamartomas
Multiple hydatid cysts
Amyloidosis
Pneumoconiosis

The diagnoses in italics are those that are most often evoked in the context of extrapulmonary signs and excavation visible on X-ray

biopsy, follicular bronchitis (FB) or chronic aspecific inflammatory reaction on bronchial biopsy, or lymphoid nodular hyperplasia on transthoracic biopsy [43, 53]. A finding of intraepithelial lymphocytic infiltrate with dual CD20/CD43-positive phenotype is a significant argument in favor of MALT lymphoma [43]. This discussion may seem artificial to clinicians, however, as the X-ray and clinical presentation of these conditions differs from that of MALT-type PPL [54].

40.6 Pretreatment Staging

Lymph node lymphoma with secondary dissemination to the lungs can be ruled out using CT scan of the chest, abdomen, and pelvis with contrast injection. Bone marrow biopsy is essential and will show whether there are any signs of bone marrow involvement, which was present in 13–30% of patients in a MALT lymphoma series [8, 21, 55–57]. Similarly, concomitant disease in other mucosa-associated lymphoid sites is present in 25–35% of cases [56–58] and is more frequent in non-digestive MALT lymphomas. In a recent study of 63 MALT-type PPLs, extrapulmonary involvement was found in around half of the cases, with stomach involvement in one third of cases and bone marrow involvement in 14% of cases [21]. Assessment of other mucosa sites should include ophthalmological and ENT examination (MRI or ultrasound of the salivary and lacrimal glands if in doubt), gastroscopy, and colonoscopy (and in some cases, small bowel transit study).

Positron emission tomography using 18-fluorodeoxyglucose (PET-FDG) has not been studied in detail. Sensitivity and specificity do not seem to be as high as for staging of aggressive lymphomas. In addition, the sensitivity and specificity of PET-FDG vary depending on the organ that is being considered. Assessment of the stomach appears to be associated with excessive false negatives, and sensitivity of PET-FDG is between 50% and 89% [59–61]. Assessment of pulmonary disease produces better results, with sensitivity of between 80% and 100% [62, 63]. PET-FDG does not seem to assess bone marrow involvement well; neither of the two patients with bone marrow involvement in the recent series of 63 MALT-type PPL patients had pathological hyperfixation [21]. Plasmacytic differentiation seems to be associated with better sensitivity [60].

The only laboratory tests that are useful in pretreatment screening are LDH and serum electrophoresis and immunoelectrophoresis. Monoclonal gammopathy, in eight in ten cases of IgM type, is found in 20–60% of cases, particularly if there is plasmacytic differentiation [24, 26–28] and seems to be detected more frequently in cases of extrapulmonary disease [21]. Increased β_2 microglobulin seems to be an independent poor prognostic factor [57].

40.7 Progression, Prognosis, and Treatment

40.7.1 Progression and Prognostic Factors

In general, the *prognosis* for patients with *MALT lymphomas* is *good*, with overall 5-year survival rates that are greater than 80% and median survival of >10 years [20, 24–28, 32, 46, 56–58, 64]. It has been demonstrated that overall survival is longer for MALT-type PPL than for nodal and spleen MZ lymphomas [8]. Conversely, however, it has not been demonstrated that survival of patients with MALT-type PPL is equivalent to that of the general population [19, 46]. Median survival of MALT-type PPL of the digestive tract does not differ from disease in other sites, but progression-free survival seems to be shorter for disease in other sites, particularly in the lungs [55]. A long period of monitoring is required, because it is common for disease to recur at a late stage (almost 50% of cases experience disease recurrence after more than 2 years), either in the same location or outside the thoracic region, following surgical resection [24, 28, 32, 46, 48].

Prognostic factors for MALT-type lymphomas have not been clearly demonstrated. In a multivariate analysis, studying disease in all sites, the following were found to influence prognosis: in one study, elevated β_2 microglobulin [57] and stage IV in the Ann Arbor classification in another [65]. In a series of 63 patients with pulmonary MALT lymphoma, poor prognostic factors for overall survival were age and performance status, and for progression-free survival the prognostic factors were cyclophosphamide or anthracycline-based chemotherapy in comparison to chlorambucil [21]. In another retrospective series, this time involving 48 patients, no prognostic factors were demonstrated [66]. Time to diagnosis, disease presentation, whether the lesions were bilateral or not, postoperative classification, surgery, and extrapulmonary involvement were not found to be prognostic factors [19, 21]. In terms of histology, amyloid deposits within the tumor seem to signal poor prognosis, while lymphoepithelial lesions indicate a good prognosis [19].

Transformation of MALT-type PPL into large B-cell lymphoma [67] is suggested by the fact that the *two* histological subtypes may be observed on sequential biopsies in one single patient, with identical rearrangements of the Ig genes and accumulation of genetic abnormalities [18, 20, 26, 28, 42, 44, 68]. Of note, the t(11;18) translocation has only been observed primarily in MALT-type PPLs [18, 69] and not in transformed forms [18].

40.7.2 Principles Underlying Treatment

There are no current written treatment guidelines. As no microorganism has been identified that plays the role that *H. pylori* does in gastric lymphoma, we are unable to use effective antibiotic treatment for cases of MALT-type pulmonary lymphoma. Treatments currently used are surgery, chemotherapy, and radiotherapy [22, 23]. It is not possible to analyze the respective levels of effectiveness of these treatments, because of the lack of comparative groups; non-treatment can even be considered [32]. Nevertheless, surgical resection is commonly carried out if the lesion is localized [24–29, 32, 48]. Use of chemotherapy alone is permitted in cases of bilateral or extrapulmonary disease, or of disease recurrence or progression; multiple-agent chemotherapy treatment such as CHOP has not been shown to be superior to single-agent chemotherapy treatment using chloraminophene, cyclophosphamide, azathioprine, or corticosteroid [24, 26, 27, 32]. A recent study showed that progression-free survival was greater in the group treated with chlorambucil compared with those treated with cyclophosphamide or anthracyclin-based chemotherapy [21]. Anti-CD20 monoclonal antibodies (Rituximab) are effective and have a 70% response rate in MALT in all sites [70], but have a high disease recurrence rate (36%). Consolidation studies involving anti-CD20 and combinations of anti-CD20 and other first-line chemotherapy agents such as chloraminophene are currently ongoing. MALT-type PPLs are also sensitive to fludarabine, a purine analog [71], and to bortezomib, a drug that targets the NFB [72] pathway, though indications for these treatments still need to be defined. Finally, radiotherapy is little used to treat pulmonary forms of this disease [20, 26–28].

40.8 Conclusion

Significant progress has been made in identifying the pathophysiology of primary pulmonary lymphomas. No infectious agent has been isolated that plays a role in the development of MALT-type pulmonary lymphomas, as has been demonstrated for *H. pylori* in gastric MALT lymphomas. Diagnosis of clonal LPD has also greatly benefited from immunohistochemistry and molecular biology; these techniques should be more widely evaluated, in particular using small endoscopic specimens, in order to spare patients thoracotomy procedures that are sometimes performed purely for diagnostic purposes. In the absence of randomized trials involving pulmonary lymphoma specifically, treatment is the same as that offered for lymphomas of similar histology, whether MALT-type or large B-cell. In the absence of disseminated disease and respiratory contraindications, surgery or radiotherapy should be considered. Otherwise, chlorambucil, given as a single-agent chemotherapy, remains the gold-standard treatment. On a case-by-case basis, consideration can be given to simply monitoring the patient.

References

1. Freeman C, Berg JW, Cutler SJ (1972) Occurrence and prognosis of extranodal lymphomas. Cancer 29(1):252–260
2. Isaacson PG, Norton AJ (1994) Extranodal lymphomas. Churchill Livingstone, New York
3. Jaffe ES, Travis WD (1991) Lymphomatoïd granulomatosis and lymphoproliferative disorders of the lung. Lippincott company, Philadelphia
4. IARC (2008) WHO classification of tumours of heamatopoietic and lymphoid tissues, 4th edn. IARC press, Lyon
5. Harris NL, Jaffe ES, Stein H, Banks PM, Chan JK, Cleary ML et al (1994) A revised European-American classification of lymphoid neoplasms: a proposal from the International Lymphoma Study Group. Blood 84(5):1361–1392
6. Jaffe ES, Harris NL, Stein H, Vardiman JW (2001) Pathology and genetics of tumours of haematopoietic and lymphoid tissues. World Health Organization Classification of Tumours. IARC Press, Lyon
7. Campo E, Miquel R, Krenacs L, Sorbara L, Raffeld M, Jaffe ES (1999) Primary nodal marginal zone lymphomas of splenic and MALT type. Am J Surg Pathol 23(1):59–68
8. Nathwani BN, Anderson JR, Armitage JO, Cavalli F, Diebold J, Drachenberg MR et al (1999) Marginal zone B-cell lymphoma: a clinical comparison of nodal and mucosa-associated lymphoid tissue types Non-Hodgkin's Lymphoma Classification Project. J Clin Oncol 17(8):2486–2492
9. Remstein ED, James CD, Kurtin PJ (2000) Incidence and subtype specificity of API2-MALT1 fusion translocations in extranodal, nodal, and splenic marginal zone lymphomas. Am J Pathol 156(4):1183–1188
10. A clinical evaluation of the International Lymphoma Study Group classification of non-Hodgkin's lymphoma (1997) The non-Hodgkin's Lymphoma Classification Project. Blood 89(11):3909–3918, 1 Jun 1997
11. Mebius RE, Kraal G (2005 Aug) Structure and function of the spleen. Nat Rev Immunol 5(8):606–616
12. Suarez F, Lortholary O, Hermine O, Lecuit M (2006) Infection-associated lymphomas derived from marginal zone B cells: a model of antigen-driven lymphoproliferation. Blood 107(8):3034–3044, 15 Apr 2006
13. Isaacson PG (1999) Mucosa-associated lymphoid tissue lymphoma. Semin Hematol 36(2):139–147
14. Ferry JA (2008 Apr) Extranodal lymphoma. Arch Pathol Lab Med 132(4):565–578
15. Bertoni F, Zucca E (2005) State-of-the-art therapeutics: marginal-zone lymphoma. J Clin Oncol 23(26):6415–6420, 10 Sept 2005
16. Ekstrom Smedby K, Vajdic CM, Falster M, Engels EA, Martinez-Maza O, Turner J et al (2008) Autoimmune disorders and risk of non-Hodgkin lymphoma subtypes: a pooled analysis within the InterLymph Consortium. Blood 111(8):4029–4038, 15 Apr 2008
17. Chanudet E, Adam P, Nicholson AG, Wotherspoon AC, Ranaldi R, Goteri G et al (2007) Chlamydiae and Mycoplasma infections in pulmonary MALT lymphoma. Br J Cancer 97(7):949–951, 8 Oct 2007
18. Farinha P, Gascoyne RD (2005) Molecular pathogenesis of mucosa-associated lymphoid tissue lymphoma. J Clin Oncol 23(26):6370–6378, 10 Sept 2005

19. Kurtin PJ, Myers JL, Adlakha H, Strickler JG, Lohse C, Pankratz VS et al (2001 Aug) Pathologic and clinical features of primary pulmonary extranodal marginal zone B-cell lymphoma of MALT type. Am J Surg Pathol 25(8): 997–1008
20. Li G, Hansmann ML, Zwingers T, Lennert K (1990) Primary lymphomas of the lung: morphological, immunohistochemical and clinical features. Histopathology 16(6):519–531
21. Borie R, Wislez M, Thabut G, Antoine M, Rabbat A, Couderc LJ et al (2009 Dec) Clinical characteristics and prognostic factors of pulmonary MALT lymphoma. Eur Respir J 34(6):1408–1416
22. Cadranel J, Wislez M, Antoine M (2002) Primary pulmonary lymphoma. Eur Respir J 20(3):750–762
23. Wislez M, Cadranel J (2002) Lymphomes pulmonaires primitifs. Encycl Méd Chir 6-002-H-5, 9 p
24. Cordier JF, Chailleux E, Lauque D, Reynaud-Gaubert M, Dietemann-Molard A, Dalphin JC et al (1993) Primary pulmonary lymphomas. A clinical study of 70 cases in nonimmunocompromised patients. Chest 103(1): 201–208
25. Herbert A, Wright DH, Isaacson PG, Smith JL (1984) Primary malignant lymphoma of the lung: histopathologic and immunologic evaluation of nine cases. Hum Pathol 15(5):415–422
26. Kennedy JL, Nathwani BN, Burke JS, Hill LR, Rappaport H (1985) Pulmonary lymphomas and other pulmonary lymphoid lesions. A clinicopathologic and immunologic study of 64 patients. Cancer 56(3):539–552
27. Le Tourneau A, Audouin J, Garbe L, Capron F, Servais B, Monges G et al (1983) Primary pulmonary malignant lymphoma, clinical and pathological findings, immunocytochemical and ultrastructural studies in 15 cases. Hematol Oncol 1(1):49–60
28. L'Hoste RJ Jr, Filippa DA, Lieberman PH, Bretsky S (1984) Primary pulmonary lymphomas. A clinicopathologic analysis of 36 cases. Cancer 54(7):1397–1406
29. Muller C, Grivaux M, Schwartz F, Blanchon F (1990) Primary pulmonary lymphoma. Current data. Apropos of 9 cases. Rev Pneumol Clin 46(4):166–171
30. Lee DK, Im JG, Lee KS, Lee JS, Seo JB, Goo JM et al (2000) B-cell lymphoma of bronchus-associated lymphoid tissue (BALT): CT features in 10 patients. J Comput Assist Tomogr 24(1):30–34
31. Wislez M, Cadranel J, Antoine M, Milleron B, Bazot M, Mayaud C et al (1999) Lymphoma of pulmonary mucosa-associated lymphoid tissue: CT scan findings and pathological correlations. Eur Respir J 14(2):423–429
32. Addis BJ, Hyjek E, Isaacson PG (1988) Primary pulmonary lymphoma: a re-appraisal of its histogenesis and its relationship to pseudolymphoma and lymphoid interstitial pneumonia. Histopathology 13(1):1–17
33. Drent M, Wagenaar SS, Mulder PH, van Velzen-Blad H, Diamant M, van den Bosch JM (1994) Bronchoalveolar lavage fluid profiles in sarcoidosis, tuberculosis, and non-Hodgkin's and Hodgkin's disease. An evaluation of differences. Chest 105(2):514–519
34. Costabel U, Bross KJ, Matthys H (1985) Diagnosis by bronchoalveolar lavage of cause of pulmonary infiltrates in haematological malignancies. Br Med J (Clin Res Ed) 290 (6474):1041
35. Kobayashi H, Ii K, Hizawa K, Maeda T (1985) Two cases of pulmonary Waldenstrom's macroglobulinemia. Chest 88(2):297–299
36. Pisani RJ, Witzig TE, Li CY, Morris MA, Thibodeau SN (1990) Confirmation of lymphomatous pulmonary involvement by immunophenotypic and gene rearrangement analysis of bronchoalveolar lavage fluid. Mayo Clin Proc 65(5):651–656
37. Schwaiger A, Prior C, Weyrer K, Umlauft F, Gattringer C, Grunewald K et al (1991) Non-Hodgkin's lymphoma of the lung diagnosed by gene rearrangement from bronchoalveolar lavage fluid: a fast and noninvasive method. Blood 77(11):2538–2539
38. Shiota T, Chiba W, Ikeda S, Ikei N (1993) Gene analysis of pulmonary pseudolymphoma. Chest 103(2):335–338
39. Subramanian D, Albrecht S, Gonzalez JM, Cagle PT (1993) Primary pulmonary lymphoma. Diagnosis by immunoglobulin gene rearrangement study using a novel polymerase chain reaction technique. Am Rev Respir Dis 148(1):222–226
40. Zompi S, Couderc LJ, Cadranel J, Antoine M, Epardeau B, Fleury-Feith J et al (2004) Clonality analysis of alveolar B lymphocytes contributes to the diagnostic strategy in clinical suspicion of pulmonary lymphoma. Blood 103(8):3208–3215, 15 Apr 2004
41. Isaacson PG (1991) B cell lymphomas of mucosa associated lymphoid tissue (MALT). Bull Cancer 78(2):203–205
42. Nicholson AG, Wotherspoon AC, Diss TC, Butcher DN, Sheppard MN, Isaacson PG et al (1995) Pulmonary B-cell non-Hodgkin's lymphomas. The value of immunohistochemistry and gene analysis in diagnosis. Histopathology 26(5):395–403
43. Begueret H, Vergier B, Parrens M, Lehours P, Laurent F, Vernejoux JM et al (2002 Jan) Primary lung small B-cell lymphoma versus lymphoid hyperplasia: evaluation of diagnostic criteria in 26 cases. Am J Surg Pathol 26(1):76–81
44. Fiche M, Caprons F, Berger F, Galateau F, Cordier JF, Loire R et al (1995) Primary pulmonary non-Hodgkin's lymphomas. Histopathology 26(6):529–537
45. Foulet A, Petrella T, Viard H, Jeannin L, Drouot F, Arnould L et al (1994) Lympho-epithelial lesions induced by plasma cells in a pulmonary MALT lymphoma. Ann Pathol 14(1): 36–40
46. Koss MN, Hochholzer L, Nichols PW, Wehunt WD, Lazarus AA (1983) Primary non-Hodgkin's lymphoma and pseudolymphoma of lung: a study of 161 patients. Hum Pathol 14(12):1024–1038
47. Turner RR, Colby TV, Doggett RS (1984) Well-differentiated lymphocytic lymphoma. A study of 47 patients with primary manifestation in the lung. Cancer 54(10):2088–2096
48. Peterson H, Snider HL, Yam LT, Bowlds CF, Arnn EH, Li CY (1985) Primary pulmonary lymphoma. A clinical and immunohistochemical study of six cases. Cancer 56(4): 805–813
49. Davis WB, Gadek JE (1987) Detection of pulmonary lymphoma by bronchoalveolar lavage. Chest 91(5):787–790
50. Dee PM, Arora NS, Innes DJ Jr (1982) The pulmonary manifestations of lymphomatoid granulomatosis. Radiology 143(3):613–618
51. Dorfman DM, Pinkus GS (1995) Utility of immunophenotypic studies in the diagnosis of low-grade lymphoma of

mucosa-associated lymphoid tissue (MALT) and other low-grade non Hodgkin's lymphomas of extra-nodal sites. Appl Immunohistochem 3:160–167
52. Harris NL, Isaacson PG (1999) What are the criteria for distinguishing MALT from non-MALT lymphoma at extranodal sites? Am J Clin Pathol 111(1 Suppl 1):S126–S132
53. Abbondanzo SL, Rush W, Bijwaard KE, Koss MN (2000 Apr) Nodular lymphoid hyperplasia of the lung: a clinicopathologic study of 14 cases. Am J Surg Pathol 24(4): 587–597
54. Yousem SA, Colby TV (1991) Pulmonary lymphomas and lymphomatoid hyperplasias. In: Knowles DM (ed) Neoplastic hematology. Williams & Wilkins, Baltimore, pp 979–1007
55. Thieblemont C, Bastion Y, Berger F, Rieux C, Salles G, Dumontet C et al (1997) Mucosa-associated lymphoid tissue gastrointestinal and nongastrointestinal lymphoma behavior: analysis of 108 patients. J Clin Oncol 15(4):1624–1630
56. Zinzani PL, Magagnoli M, Galieni P, Martelli M, Poletti V, Zaja F et al (1999) Nongastrointestinal low-grade mucosa-associated lymphoid tissue lymphoma: analysis of 75 patients. J Clin Oncol 17(4):1254
57. Thieblemont C, Berger F, Dumontet C, Moullet I, Bouafia F, Felman P et al (2000) Mucosa-associated lymphoid tissue lymphoma is a disseminated disease in one third of 158 patients analyzed. Blood 95(3):802–806
58. Raderer M, Vorbeck F, Formanek M, Osterreicher C, Valencak J, Penz M et al (2000) Importance of extensive staging in patients with mucosa-associated lymphoid tissue (MALT)-type lymphoma. Br J Cancer 83(4):454–457
59. Enomoto K, Hamada K, Inohara H, Higuchi I, Tomita Y, Kubo T et al (2008 May) Mucosa-associated lymphoid tissue lymphoma studied with FDG-PET: a comparison with CT and endoscopic findings. Ann Nucl Med 22(4):261–267
60. Hoffmann M, Wohrer S, Becherer A, Chott A, Streubel B, Kletter K et al (2006 Dec) 18F-Fluoro-deoxy-glucose positron emission tomography in lymphoma of mucosa-associated lymphoid tissue: histology makes the difference. Ann Oncol 17(12):1761–1765
61. Radan L, Fischer D, Bar-Shalom R, Dann EJ, Epelbaum R, Haim N et al (2008 Aug) FDG avidity and PET/CT patterns in primary gastric lymphoma. Eur J Nucl Med Mol Imaging 35(8):1424–1430
62. Beal KP, Yeung HW, Yahalom J (2005 Mar) FDG-PET scanning for detection and staging of extranodal marginal zone lymphomas of the MALT type: a report of 42 cases. Ann Oncol 16(3):473–480
63. Bae YA, Lee KS, Han J, Ko YH, Kim BT, Chung MJ et al (2008 Feb) Marginal zone B-cell lymphoma of bronchus-associated lymphoid tissue: imaging findings in 21 patients. Chest 133(2):433–440
64. Stefanovic A, Morgensztern D, Fong T, Lossos IS (2008) Pulmonary marginal zone lymphoma: a single centre experience and review of the SEER database. Leuk Lymphoma 49(7):1311–1320
65. Zucca E, Conconi A, Pedrinis E, Cortelazzo S, Motta T, Gospodarowicz MK et al (2003) Nongastric marginal zone B-cell lymphoma of mucosa-associated lymphoid tissue. Blood 101(7):2489–2495, 1 Apr 2003
66. Ferraro P, Trastek VF, Adlakha H, Deschamps C, Allen MS, Pairolero PC (2000) Primary non-Hodgkin's lymphoma of the lung. Ann Thorac Surg 69(4):993–997
67. Harris NL, Jaffe ES, Diebold J, Flandrin G, Muller-Hermelink HK, Vardiman J (2000) Lymphoma classification–from controversy to consensus: the R.E.A.L. and WHO Classification of lymphoid neoplasms. Ann Oncol 11 (Suppl 1):3–10
68. Chan JK, Ng CS, Isaacson PG (1990 May) Relationship between high-grade lymphoma and low-grade B-cell mucosa-associated lymphoid tissue lymphoma (MALToma) of the stomach. Am J Pathol 136(5):1153–1164
69. Morgner A, Miehlke S, Fischbach W, Schmitt W, Muller-Hermelink H, Greiner A et al (2001) Complete remission of primary high-grade B-cell gastric lymphoma after cure of Helicobacter pylori infection. J Clin Oncol 19(7): 2041–2048
70. Conconi A, Martinelli G, Thieblemont C, Ferreri AJ, Devizzi L, Peccatori F et al (2003) Clinical activity of rituximab in extranodal marginal zone B-cell lymphoma of MALT type. Blood 102(8):2741–2745, 15 Oct 2003
71. Salar A, Domingo-Domenech E, Estany C, Canales MA, Gallardo F, Servitje O et al (2009) Combination therapy with rituximab and intravenous or oral fludarabine in the first-line, systemic treatment of patients with extranodal marginal zone B-cell lymphoma of the mucosa-associated lymphoid tissue type. Cancer 115(22):5210–5217, Aug 11
72. Troch M, Jonak C, Mullauer L, Puspok A, Formanek M, Hauff W et al (2009 May) A phase II study of bortezomib in patients with MALT lymphoma. Haematologica 94(5): 738–742

ARDS During Neutropenia Recovery

41

Élie Azoulay, Eric Ezingeard, Choupi-Salomon Berckowski, and Michael Darmon

Contents

É. Azoulay (✉) and C.-S. Berckowski
Service de Réanimation Médicale, Hôpital Saint-Louis, 1 avenue Claude Vellefaux, 75010, Paris, France and Medical Intensive Care Units, Saint-Louis Hospital, Paris 7 University, Paris, France
e-mail: elie.azoulay@sls.aphp.fr

E. Ezingeard
Medical ICU, Saint-Etienne University Hospital, Saint-Etienne, France

M. Darmon
Medical ICU, Saint-Etienne University Hospital, Saint-Etienne, France and
Saint-Etienne School of Medicine, Saint-Etienne, France

41.1 Introduction

Acute respiratory failure (ARF) is a major cause of morbidity in cancer patients. At least one respiratory complication occurs in about 20% of patients with solid tumors or hematological malignancies and in nearly half the patients with neutropenia or bone marrow transplantation [1, 2]. ARF, together with shock, is the most common organ failure leading to ICU admission in neutropenic patients. In these patients, ARF often stems from a combination of factors that may be closely intertwined, such as infection and cardiogenic edema or alveolar hemorrhage.

Neutropenia recovery may be associated with an increased risk of deteriorating oxygenation and of exacerbation of prior acute lung injury resulting from infectious or noninfectious causes. Overall, 104 cases of respiratory failure during neutropenia recovery have been reported. Recent studies have more clearly evaluated the prevalence, risk factors, and outcomes associated with respiratory failure at the onset of neutropenia recovery.

Here, we review the evidence suggesting that neutropenia recovery may be associated with exacerbation of ARF, and we will discuss the factors suspected to be associated with respiratory failure during neutropenia recovery.

41.2 Clinical Presentation and Risk Factors

Neutropenia recovery is clinically silent in the vast majority of patients. However, respiratory failure has been reported during neutropenia recovery [3, 4], that

É. Azoulay (ed.), *Pulmonary Involvement in Patients with Hematological Malignancies*,
DOI: 10.1007/978-3-642-15742-4_41, © Springer-Verlag Berlin Heidelberg 2011

is, during the 2–3 days preceding and following, the neutrophil count increases to 500/mm^3 or leukocyte count increases to 1,000/mm^3 (Fig. 41.1) [4, 5]. Both clinical and experimental findings suggest that granulocyte colony-stimulating factor (G-CSF) may exacerbate the clinical consequences of neutropenia recovery [5, 6]. The development of lung infiltrates during the neutropenic period is a risk factor for acute lung injury/acute respiratory distress syndrome (ALI/ARDS) during neutropenia recovery (Table 41.1) [4–6]. Other suggested risk factors include delayed or prolonged neutropenia [4], a fast rate of neutrophil recovery [7], and invasive pulmonary aspergillosis [7]. Overall, the prevalence of respiratory failure during neutropenia recovery may be as high as 50% in high-risk patients [8].

Respiratory failure during neutropenia recovery usually presents as ARDS [4]. Radiographic changes are always present at the onset of ARF and usually consist in bilateral alveolar infiltrates (two thirds of the patients) [4, 5]. Interstitial pneumonia, pleural effusion, or nodules may occur less frequently [4, 5]. Finally, patients with invasive aspergillosis may experience hemoptysis or pneumothorax [7].

Among patients with ARF during neutropenia recovery, 75–90% require invasive or noninvasive mechanical ventilation [4, 5, 8]. When bronchoalveolar lavage is performed, alveolar macrophages are always the predominant cell type [4]. The rates of neutrophil counts above 10% and alveolar hemorrhage are lower than 20% [4].

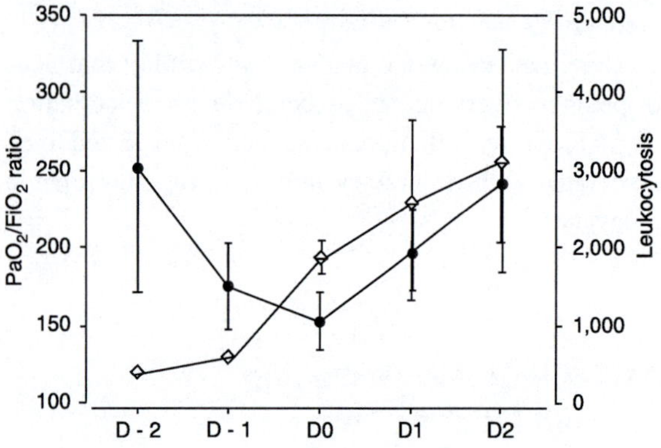

Fig. 41.1 Time course of the PaO_2/FiO_2 ratio (*closed circles*) and total leukocyte count (*diamonds*) during the 5-day period centered on the day of neutropenia recovery (*D0*) (From [5]. With permission)

Table 41.1 Risk factors for respiratory failure during neutropenia recovery

Delayed neutropenia (time from cancer chemotherapy to neutropenia >10 days) [4]
Prolonged neutropenia (neutropenia duration >10 days) [4]
Fast neutrophil recovery [7]
Clinically or microbiologically documented infection [4–6]
Aspergillosis [7]
G-CSF use [5, 6]

In the three largest cohorts reported in the literature, ARF at the onset of neutropenia recovery carried a poor outcome, with a 66% ICU mortality rate (51 of 79 patients) [4, 5, 8]. In addition, ARF at neutropenia recovery onset was an independent risk factor for death [8].

41.3 Evidence Supporting a Risk of Respiratory Failure During Neutropenia Recovery

Although several studies described cases of ARF during neutropenia recovery, none demonstrated a causal relationship between neutropenia recovery and ARF. In addition, no large-scale prospective study has evaluated the prevalence of ARF during neutropenia recovery. Five strong arguments support the existence of an increased risk of ARDS during neutropenia recovery: a large proportion of patients who experience pneumonia during the neutropenic period exhibit substantial respiratory deterioration during neutropenia recovery; the ALI/ARDS rate in neutropenic patients with pneumonia is far higher during than before or after neutropenia recovery; several groups in different parts of the world have described cases of ALI/ARDS during neutropenia recovery; experimental studies in neutropenic rats have replicated the occurrence of ALI/ARDS during neutropenia recovery and suggested reasonable pathophysiological hypotheses; the occurrence of ALI/ARDS is clinically plausible, as neutropenic cancer patients have a well-established predisposition to lung disease and infections [9] that is related to lung toxicity from cancer chemotherapy agents and G-CSF and, in some patients, to lung involvement by the malignancy. Nevertheless, although these arguments support the existence of a risk of respiratory failure following neutropenia recovery, we need large prospective studies to demonstrate that an association exists between these two events.

41.4 Pathophysiology

Cancer chemotherapy is administered every day to numerous patients, many of whom experience neutropenia as one of the expected adverse events [10]. In patients with neutropenia, the risk of bacterial sepsis is of grave concern [11, 12]. The main sites of bacterial infection are the lungs, gastrointestinal tract, and bloodstream [12–15]. Prolonged neutropenia, for instance, in patients with acute leukemia or recipients of stem cell or bone marrow transplants, promotes the occurrence of non-bacterial infections [16, 17]. Although neutrophils are believed to play a pivotal role in the pathophysiology of ALI and ARDS, convincing evidence has accumulated since the 1980s that ALI/ARDS can occur in patients with severe neutropenia [18–21]. Hypotheses put forward to explain the occurrence of apparently neutrophil-independent ALI/ARDS involve deactivation of macrophages [22] or monocytes [23] caused by the malignancy, cancer chemotherapy, and sepsis. Neutropenia recovery and G-CSF treatment have been suspected to exacerbate previous lung injury, possibly via accumulation of neutrophils in the lungs [24, 25]. However, during respiratory failure following neutropenia recovery, macrophages, but not neutrophils, were recovered from bronchoalveolar lavage fluid, suggesting that ALI during neutropenia recovery may be nosologically similar to ARDS during neutropenia [18, 20]. In a lamb model of experimental lung injury, G-CSF enhanced alveolar neutrophil functions, increasing both cytokine production and the oxidative burst [26, 27]. G-CSF upregulates the production of cytokines that increase alveolar permeability or neutrophil influx, such as tumor necrosis factor-α, interleukin-1β, and IL-8 [28, 29]. In vitro studies also found enhanced secretion of pro-inflammatory cytokines by isolated alveolar macrophages obtained during neutropenia recovery from rats that received G-CSF, compared with rats that did not receive G-CSF, providing a possible explanation for lung injury exacerbation during G-CSF-induced neutropenia recovery [6].

41.5 Conclusions

Early recognition of patients at high risk for ALI/ARDS during neutropenia recovery may help to improve outcomes. Risk factors in each individual patient should be assessed routinely, as the first ARDS symptoms may antedate the increase in leukocyte counts. A high degree of suspicion for this complication should be maintained in patients with clinically or microbiologically documented pneumonia complicating neutropenia who are at higher risk for respiratory failure during neutropenia recovery. Since G-CSF may increase the risk of respiratory failure in these patients, the risk/benefit ratio of G-CSF should be carefully evaluated [30]. When G-CSF is used, we believe that it is imperative that G-CSF be discontinued as soon as bone marrow function improves (neutrophils >500/mm^3).

Despite recent studies, several questions remain unanswered. First, all of the recent studies were performed in critically ill patients. Therefore, risk factors for respiratory failure at the onset of neutropenia recovery have not been evaluated in the overall population of oncology and hematology patients, nor has the incidence of respiratory failure at the onset of neutropenia recovery been evaluated in an unselected population of cancer patients. Information regarding this event is therefore scarce and mainly related to a specific subgroup of critically ill patients. Last, although a previous study suggested a high risk of respiratory failure during neutropenia recovery in patients with invasive aspergillosis [7], this finding was not confirmed by more recent studies. Further studies are therefore required to clarify the incidence of respiratory failure at the onset of neutropenia recovery in the general population of cancer patients, to describe risk factors, and to further explore the impact of invasive aspergillosis on this event.

References

1. Azoulay E, Thiery G, Chevret S et al (2004) The prognosis of acute respiratory failure in critically ill cancer patients. Medicine (Baltimore) 83:360–370
2. Kress JP, Christenson J, Pohlman AS et al (1999) Outcomes of critically ill cancer patients in a university hospital setting. Am J Respir Crit Care Med 160:1957–1961
3. Rinaldo JE, Borovetz H (1985) Deterioration of oxygenation and abnormal lung microvascular permeability during

resolution of leukopenia in patients with diffuse lung injury. Am Rev Respir Dis 131:579–583
4. Azoulay E, Darmon M, Delclaux C et al (2002) Deterioration of previous acute lung injury during neutropenia recovery. Crit Care Med 30:781–786
5. Karlin L, Darmon M, Thiery G et al (2005) Respiratory status deterioration during G-CSF-induced neutropenia recovery. Bone Marrow Transplant 6:1–6
6. Azoulay E, Attalah H, Yang K et al (2003) Exacerbation with granulocyte colony-stimulating factor of prior acute lung injury during neutropenia recovery in rats. Crit Care Med 31:157–165
7. Todeschini G, Murari C, Bonesi R et al (1999) Invasive aspergillosis in neutropenic patients: rapid neutrophil recovery is a risk factor for severe pulmonary complications. Eur J Clin Invest 29:453–457
8. Rhee CK, Kang JY, Kim YH et al (2009) Risk factors for acute respiratory distress syndrome during neutropenia recovery in patients with hematologic malignancies. Crit Care 13:R173
9. Lehrnbecher T, Koehl U, Wittekindt B et al (2008) Changes in host defence induced by malignancies and antineoplastic treatment: implication for immunotherapeutic strategies. Lancet Oncol 9:269–278
10. Bodey GP (1986) Infection in cancer patients. A continuing association. Am J Med 81:11–26
11. Bodey GP, Rodriguez V, Chang HY et al (1978) Fever and infection in leukemic patients: a study of 494 consecutive patients. Cancer 41:1610–1622
12. Cartoni C, Dragoni F, Micozzi A et al (2001) Neutropenic enterocolitis in patients with acute leukemia: prognostic significance of bowel wall thickening detected by ultrasonography. J Clin Oncol 19:756–761
13. Maschmeyer G (2001) Pneumonia in febrile neutropenic patients: radiologic diagnosis. Curr Opin Oncol 13:229–235
14. Puig N, De La Rubia J, Jarque I et al (2007) Characteristics of and risk factors for pneumonia in patients with hematological malignancies developing fever after autologous blood stem cell transplantation. Leuk Lymphoma 48: 2367–2374
15. Meyer E, Beyersmann J, Bertz H et al (2007) Risk factor analysis of blood stream infection and pneumonia in neutropenic patients after peripheral blood stem-cell transplantation. Bone Marrow Transplant 39:173–178
16. Darmon M, Azoulay E, Alberti C et al (2002) Impact of neutropenia duration on short-term mortality in neutropenic critically ill cancer patients. Intensive Care Med 28: 1775–1780
17. Hughes WT, Armstrong D, Bodey GP et al (2002) 2002 guidelines for the use of antimicrobial agents in neutropenic patients with cancer. Clin Infect Dis 34:730–751
18. Ognibene FP, Martin SE, Parker MM et al (1986) Adult respiratory distress syndrome in patients with severe neutropenia. N Engl J Med 315:547–551
19. Braude S, Apperley J, Krausz T et al (1985) Adult respiratory distress syndrome after allogeneic bone-marrow transplantation: evidence for a neutrophil-independent mechanism. Lancet 1:1239–1242
20. Maunder RJ, Hackman RC, Riff E et al (1986) Occurrence of the adult respiratory distress syndrome in neutropenic patients. Am Rev Respir Dis 133:313–316
21. Laufe MD, Simon RH, Flint A et al (1986) Adult respiratory distress syndrome in neutropenic patients. Am J Med 80:1022–1026
22. Mokart D, Guery BP, Bouabdallah R et al (2003) Deactivation of alveolar macrophages in septic neutropenic ARDS. Chest 124:644–652
23. Mokart D, Kipnis E, Guerre-Berthelot P et al (2008) Monocyte deactivation in neutropenic acute respiratory distress syndrome patients treated with granulocyte colony-stimulating factor. Crit Care 12:R17
24. Glauser FL, Fairman RP (1985) The uncertain role of the neutrophil increased permeability pulmonary edema. Chest 88:601–607
25. Tate RM, Repine JE (1983) Neutrophils and the adult respiratory distress syndrome. Am Rev Respir Dis 128:552–559
26. King J, Deboisblanc BP, Mason CM et al (1995) Effect of granulocyte colony-stimulating factor on acute lung injury in the rat. Am J Respir Crit Care Med 151:302
27. Azoulay E, Herigault S, Levame M et al (2003) Effect of granulocyte colony-stimulating factor on bleomycin-induced acute lung injury and pulmonary fibrosis. Crit Care Med 31:1442–1448
28. Aggarwal A, Baker CS, Evans TW et al (2000) G-CSF and IL-8 but not GM-CSF correlate with severity of pulmonary neutrophilia in acute respiratory distress syndrome. Eur Respir J 15:895–901
29. Wiedermann FJ, Mayr AJ, Hobisch-Hagen P et al (2003) Association of endogenous G-CSF with anti-inflammatory mediators in patients with acute respiratory distress syndrome. J Interferon Cytokine Res 23:729–736
30. Azoulay E, Attalah H, Harf A et al (2001) Granulocyte colony-stimulating factor or neutrophil-induced pulmonary toxicity: myth or reality? Systematic review of clinical case reports and experimental data. Chest 120:1695–1701

Fibrosing Alveolitis in Hematologic Malignancy Patients Undergoing Hematopoietic Cell Transplantation

42

Huda Salman, Kenneth R. Cooke, and Hillard M. Lazarus

Contents

H. Salman (✉) and H.M. Lazarus
Divisions of Hematology-Oncology, Departments of Medicine, Blood and Marrow Transplant Program, University Hospitals Case Medical Center, Case Comprehensive Cancer Center, Case Western Reserve School of Medicine, Cleveland, OH 44106, USA
e-mail: huda.salman@case.edu

K.R. Cooke
Divisions of Hematology-Oncology, Departments of Pediatrics, Blood and Marrow Transplant Program, University Hospitals Case Medical Center, Case Comprehensive Cancer Center, Case Western Reserve School of Medicine, Cleveland, OH 44106, USA

Case Presentation

A 20-year-old man patient with *de novo* acute myelogenous leukemia (AML) was induced into complete remission with chemotherapy consisting of idarubicin and cytarabine. After consolidation with high-dose cytarabine, he later received conditioning with cyclophosphamide 60 mg/kg/day intravenously for 2 days and fractionated total body irradiation (TBI) 1,200 cGy followed by allogeneic hematopoietic cell transplant (HSCT) using a HLA-identical sibling donor. Graft-versus-host disease (GVHD) prophylaxis consisted of tacrolimus and short-course methotrexate. His clinical course was uncomplicated, but after withdrawal of immunosuppression he developed extensive chronic GVHD involving skin and liver. This complication was controlled with the re-institution of tacrolimus.

Surveillance pulmonary function testing completed 180 days after HSCT showed evidence of mild reductions in forced expiratory volume in 1 s (FEV_1) with preservation of forced vital capacity (FVC). Follow-up study revealed significant and rapid worsening of obstructive lung disease (OLD) despite resolution of hepatic and skin GVHD and continued prophylaxis against viral, fungal and *Pneumocystis* infections using acyclovir, fluconazole and trimethoprim-sulfamethoxazole, respectively. Reductions in pulmonary function ultimately were associated with shortness of breath and dyspnea with exertion. Subsequent workup revealed ground-glass opacities with air trapping on chest computed tomography (CT) scan and evidence of progressive AFO on pulmonary function testing based on reduction of FEV_1 (50% of predicted normal), a ratio of FEV_1 to FVC of 0.64 and a residual volume of 1.52 L (157% of predicted normal). Bronchoalveolar lavage was negative for infection. Video-assisted thoracoscopic biopsy of the lungs

É. Azoulay (ed.), *Pulmonary Involvement in Patients with Hematological Malignancies*,
DOI: 10.1007/978-3-642-15742-4_42, © Springer-Verlag Berlin Heidelberg 2011

revealed changes consistent with bronchiolitis obliterans with early fibrosis. The patient continued to receive tacrolimus, and ultimately a course of oral prednisone (2 mg/kg/day) and etanercept 50 mg subcutaneous once weekly was initiated. Clinical symptoms resolved and pulmonary function improved. He remains in complete remission regarding the AML.

42.1 Introduction

Fibrosing alveolitis (FA) is a progressive and often fatal disorder characterized by sequential acute lung injury with subsequent scarring and end-stage lung disease. Historically, idiopathic pulmonary fibrosis (IPF) encompassed a heterogeneous group of histologic and clinical entities arising in an idiopathic setting [1]. Patients with hematologic malignancies treated with chemotherapy, radiation or HSCT, such as the patient described above, commonly develop a wide variety of late and chronic pulmonary dysfunction states [2]. These complications share many of the clinical and pathologic features described in typical idiopathic FA.

This spectrum of pulmonary toxicity observed during FA can be simplified by considering the time of diagnosis in relation to institution of therapy, whether the radiographic abnormalities are focal or diffuse, and by underlying histopathology. In addition, there are individual patient factors that should be considered when formulating a differential diagnosis. These include:

- Radiotherapy delivered to the chest wall or as part of total body irradiation (TBI)
- Exposure to pulmonary- or cardio-toxic chemotherapeutic agents
- Current or prior immunosuppressant therapy
- History of high-dose chemotherapy exposure prior to autologous or allogeneic HSCT
- History of opportunistic pulmonary infection (fungal or otherwise)

In the case described herein, the patient was exposed to radiation therapy in preparation for HSCT and received an allogeneic graft from his HLA-matched sibling. While his early posttransplant course was uncomplicated, he developed chronic GVHD of the skin and liver lung after immunosuppression was tapered. The widespread and appropriate use of prophylactic antibiotics has shifted the spectrum of pulmonary dysfunction in HSCT recipients from infectious to noninfectious etiologies. This chapter will address the chronic lung complications that lead to pulmonary fibrosis and persistent organ dysfunction in each context with specific focus on hematologic malignancy patients treated using HSCT.

42.2 Fibrosing Alveolitis Secondary to Pulmonary Infections

In patients with hematologic malignancies, severe lung infections frequently lead to the development of acute respiratory distress syndrome (ARDS). Bacterial infections predominate (see Table 42.1) and arise because of severe immune suppression inherent to these disorders and their treatments. The pathology of ARDS involves severe alveolar epithelial cell damage, hyaline membrane formation, and festinate myofibroblast proliferation and fibrosis in the intra-alveolar spaces. Affected HSCT recipients who deteriorate and require intubation and mechanical ventilation for ARDS experience a high mortality. In one series, overall intensive care unit (ICU) mortality was 74% [3]. In recent years, advancements in supportive care have resulted in significant improvement in survival [4]. However, long-term survivors continue to have residual lung dysfunction that may progress over time. In one series, autopsy evaluation revealed pulmonary fibrosis in 55% of such patients, underscoring the importance of dysregulated reparative mechanisms in the lung after an acute insult [5]. Factors influencing progression to the fibro-proliferative phase of ARDS versus resolution and reconstitution of the normal parenchymal architecture are poorly understood. Abnormal repair and remodeling may be profoundly affected by both environmental and genetic factors. In this context, mechanical ventilation may affect the macromolecules that constitute the extracellular matrix (collagen, elastin, fibronectin, laminin, proteoglycan and glycosaminoglycans) and impact the biomechanical balance within the lung parenchyma.

Fungal infections also may follow a chronic course of prolonged inflammation with focal or diffuse

Table 42.1 Timing of likely infections among allogeneic hematopoietic cell transplant (HCT) recipients receiving antimicrobial prophylaxis

	Pre-engraftment: <3 weeks after HCT	Immediate post-HCT: 3 weeks-3 months after HCT	Late post-HCT: >3 months after HCT
Risk factors	Mucositis	Acute GVHD and its therapy	Chronic GVHD and its therapy
	Organ dysfunction		
	Neutropenia and other immune defects	Mucocutaneous damage	Mucocutaneous damage
		Cellular immune dysfunction	Cellular and humoral immune dysfunction
		Immune modulating viruses	Hyposplenism and decreased opsonization
			Decrease in reticuloendothelial function
Infecting			
Bacterial species	Many gram-positive spp. including coagulase-negative staphylococci, Staphylococcus aureus, viridans streptococci	Listeria monocytogenes	Encapsulated organisms, e.g., Streptococcus pneumoniae, Haemophilus influenzae, Neisseria meningitides
		Legionella pneumophila	
	Many gram-negative spp. including Legionella spp, Pseudomonas aeruginosa, Enterobacteriaceae, Stenotrophomonas maltophilia		
Fungal species	*Candida* sp.	*Candida* sp.	*Aspergillus* sp
		Aspergillus sp.	*Pneumocystis jiroveci*
		Pneumocystis jiroveci	
Viral species	Herpes simplex	Respiratory viruses, CMV, HHV6, HHV7	CMV, HHV6, HHV7, VZV, Bk adenovirus, JC virus, EBV
Parasitic species		Toxoplasmosis	

HCT hematopoietic cell transplant, *GVHD* graft-versus-host disease, *HHV6 and HHV7* human herpes virus 6 and 7, *CMV* cytomegalovirus, *JC virus* John Cunningham virus

scarring ultimately resulting in significant pulmonary dysfunction. Invasive aspergillosis (IA) occurs frequently in hematologic malignancy patients, particularly after an allogeneic HSCT, presenting classically as angio-invasive or airway-invasive disease. Angio-invasive IA is characterized histologically by invasion and occlusion of small to medium-sized pulmonary arteries by fungal hyphae. This effect leads to the formation of necrotic hemorrhagic nodules or pleural-based, wedge-shaped hemorrhagic infarcts. The "halo sign" (nodules surrounded by areas of ground-glass attenuation) on chest CT scan strongly suggests a diagnosis of IA [6].

Airway-invasive aspergillosis is characterized by the presence of organisms in the basement membrane of the bronchioles and within the airway lumen. Positive yield from respiratory samples such as sputa examination or broncho-alveolar lavage (BAL) is more likely in this subtype of IA than in the angio-invasive variety. Clinical manifestations of acute airway-invasive aspergillosis include: acute tracheobronchitis, exudative bronchiolitis and bronchopneumonia. Using high-resolution CT, the associated bronchiolitis is characterized by the presence of peri-bronchial consolidation, centri-lobular micro-nodules, and branching linear or nodular areas of ground-glass attenuation having a "tree-in-bud" appearance [7]. This form of airway-invasive aspergillosis can be associated with pseudo-membranous necrotizing tracheal involvement that can cause pneumo-mediastinum and has a high mortality [8]. Airway-invasive aspergillosis can also follow a chronic course known as chronic necrotizing aspergillosis. This condition is characterized by an indolent, granulomatous cavitary infection that may mimic reactivation of tuberculosis radiographically [9]. Mortality is lower compared with the other forms of IA and often is related to the underlying disease of the patient.

42.3 Fibrosing Alveolitis Secondary to Noninfectious Etiologies

Hematologic malignancy patients treated with chemotherapy or chest wall radiation therapy, or those who proceed to receive a HSCT may develop a wide variety inflammatory noninfectious lung disorders that ultimately may lead to pulmonary fibrosis.

42.3.1 *Radiation Therapy*

Radiation-induced lung injury first was described in 1898, soon after the development of roentgenograms [10]. In 1925 the distinction between two separate types of radiation-induced lung injury, radiation pneumonitis and radiation fibrosis, was made [11]. An entire chapter from Drs. Gallego and Rello in this book is dedicated to radiation-related lung injury. Radiation-induced lung injury results from the combination of direct cytotoxicity upon normal lung tissue and, perhaps more importantly, the development of fibrosis triggered by radiation-induced cellular signal transduction. The cytotoxic effect is largely a consequence of DNA damage and death in normal lung epithelial cells. The development of fibrosis that can compromise lung function is mediated by a number of different cytokines. Clinically, the most extensively studied radiation-induced cytokine is transforming growth factor beta 1 (TGF-β), which can induce fibroblast collagen deposition. A normal plasma TGF-β concentration at the conclusion of a clinical course of radiotherapy has been observed to be a predictor for the risk of pneumonitis [12]. Other proinflammatory cytokines, including, but not limited to, interleukin IL-6, tumor necrosis factor-alpha TNFα and IL-1, are upregulated immediately after irradiation. Increased IL-6 plasma concentrations correlate with an increased risk of radiation-induced lung injury [13, 14]. Platelet-derived growth factor (PDGF) and basic fibroblast growth factor (βFGF) are upregulated in animal models of lung irradiation injury and antedate the development of fibrosis [15]. Factors affecting the development of radiation-induced lung disease are numerous and are included in Table 42.2 [16–19]; all have been reported to raise the risk of radiation pneumonitis.

Radiographic and bronchoscopic findings are nonspecific, and the diffusion capacity for carbon monoxide (DL) typically is depressed in patients with radiation-induced lung damage. Long-term glucocorticoids may be effective in the treatment of radiation-associated lung injury in which COP is the leading pulmonary involvement; however, symptoms and radiographic abnormalities, as well as immunologically mediated lymphocytic alveolitis frequently recur with discontinuation of therapy [20, 21]. Early studies suggested that pentoxifylline may have a role

Table 42.2 Factors affecting the development of radiation-induced lung disease [16–19]

- Method of irradiation such as conformal radiation therapy or specialized techniques including intensity-modulated radiation therapy and stereotactic body radiation therapy
- Volume of lung tissue irradiated
- Radiation dosage and time-dose factor administered
- Use of concurrent chemotherapy
- Prior thoracic irradiation
- Volume loss due to lung collapse
- Younger patient age
- Smoking history
- Poor pretreatment clinical performance status
- Reduced pretreatment lung function
- Chronic obstructive pulmonary disease
- Female gender
- Endocrine therapy for breast cancer
- Glucocorticoid withdrawal during radiotherapy

in the treatment of radiation-induced fibrosis involving the skin and subcutaneous tissues as this agent also inhibits experimental bleomycin-induced pulmonary fibrosis in rats, likely via its anti-TNFα effects [22]. Pentoxifylline showed a significant protective effect for both early and late lung radiotoxicity. Amifostine is a pro-drug that is de-phosphorylated by alkaline phosphatase in tissues to a pharmacologically active free thiol metabolite. This drug can reduce the toxic effects of chemotherapy by acting as a scavenger of free radicals generated in tissues exposed to radiation. Early evidence suggests that amifostine may decrease radiation-induced pulmonary injury without diminishing the therapeutic effect [23, 24]. Captopril and other ACE inhibitors also have been shown to reduce radiation-induced lung fibrosis in rats [25], but there are no published data in humans.

Improvements in the perfusion and ventilation of radiation-injured lung tissue may be expected from 3 to 18 months after radiation therapy. Beyond 18 months, however, further significant improvement appears unusual [26, 27].

42.3.2 Chemotherapy

Patients with hematologic diseases are exposed to a host of traditional and newer chemotherapeutic agents that can cause lung injury at an incidence that ranges from less than 5% to as high as 60% [28, 29]. The increased complexity of multi-modality treatments and high-dose protocols designed to augment antineoplastic efficacy, particularly in the context of HSCT, has increased the incidence of pulmonary complications. The diagnosis of drug-induced respiratory disease often is complex because: (1)1 patients may be exposed to several pneumo-toxic drugs concurrently or in sequence due to earlier treatment failure; (2)2 time to onset of pulmonary toxicity may be delayed, making it difficult to ascertain which agent is responsible for the pulmonary reaction; (3)3 the combination of drugs to treat malignant hematologic conditions may lead to unexpected drug interactions, producing enhanced toxicity compared with the toxicity of each agent considered separately; and (4)4 radiation therapy to the chest or TBI. Other factors that play a role in the development of pulmonary toxicity include advanced age, current smoking, abrupt withdrawal of corticosteroids and the use of HSCT (allogeneic vs autologous). Changes in blood neutrophil counts, thrombocytopenia, coagulation deficits, volume overload or left ventricular dysfunction also can influence the spectrum and severity of pulmonary drug toxicity. In addition to overt pulmonary toxicity, subclinical drug-induced lung dysfunction often occurs in the form of reduced DLCO and lung volumes or changes in cell populations in BAL fluid. Upon cessation of exposure to the agent, most of these changes reverse slowly in a few weeks or months.

Drug-induced lung injury can manifest in several patterns (Table 42.3). Nonspecific interstitial pneumonia (NSIP) is a common pattern of pulmonary injury to

Table 42.3 Lung toxicities associated with chemotherapeutic agents

Pattern of toxicity	Drug
Nonspecific interstitial pneumonia	Methotrexate, azathioprine, chlorambucil, cyclophosphamide, procarbazine, and rarely, vinca alkaloids
Pulmonary infiltrates and eosinophilia	Fludarabine, rarely: interferons, inhaled or parenteral pentamidine and radiographic contrast media
Organizing pneumonia	Bleomycin
Diffuse alveolar damage (DAD)	BCNU, lomustine, CCNU, bleomycin, busulfan, chlorambucil, cyclophosphamide, melphalan, procarbazine, vinblastine
Diffuse pulmonary fibrosis	BCNU, lomustine, CCNU, bleomycin, busulfan, chlorambucil, cyclophosphamide, melphalan, vinca alkaloids, radiation therapy
Granulomatosis	Bleomycin
Pulmonary nodules	Bleomycin, cyclophosphamide, vinblastine, rarely fludarabine

chemotherapeutic agents. Drugs causing the syndrome include methotrexate (accounting for the majority of cases), azathioprine, chlorambucil, cyclophosphamide, procarbazine and, rarely, vinca alkaloids. The onset of this condition is unpredictable; symptoms may develop a few days to years after exposure. The clinical picture includes increasing dyspnea, dry cough, high fevers and rash. The severity of illness can vary from mild to progressive respiratory failure, and associated radiographic findings may range from bilateral (usually symmetrical) interstitial or alveolar opacities to extensive consolidation with air bronchograms and volume loss [30–32]. Pleural effusions and mediastinal lymph node enlargement have been reported in patients with methotrexate-induced lung injury [33, 34]. BAL fluid usually shows lymphocyte predominance. A low ratio of CD4 to CD8 lymphocytes is suggestive, but not specific, for drug-induced lung disease. Other BAL findings include neutrophilia or a combined pattern of lymphocytosis with neutrophilia or eosinophilia [35]. Appropriate stains, cultures and molecular techniques in BAL fluid should be performed to exclude opportunistic infections. A lung biopsy may be required in selected cases. Histopathologic features include interstitial inflammation and pulmonary granulomas. Fibrosis can be present, but is generally not the dominant histopathologic feature. Alveolar edema or hemorrhage may be found as a manifestation of severe methotrexate pneumonitis [34]. High-dose corticosteroids may be indicated with more advanced disease, as drug-induced NSIP can lead to mortality if it is not treated promptly, but in milder cases, symptoms can subside after simple drug withdrawal [36]. Although rechallenge with the drug may be safe, it is not generally recommended [37].

Eosinophilic pneumonia (EP) is an unusual and unpredictable pattern of response to chemotherapeutic agents as opposed to that described following the use of some antibiotics. EP in patients with hematologic malignancies can result from treatment with fludarabine and, rarely, interferons, inhaled or parenteral pentamidine, and radiographic contrast media [33]. Although methotrexate and procarbazine pneumonitis can often be associated with peripheral eosinophilia, BAL and histopathologic features are not those of EPs. Typically, the syndrome of EP develops during or shortly after termination of treatment. A history of an allergic disorder, or repeated courses of treatment with the specific drug, may predict for a higher risk. The diseases could manifest as acute pneumonia and progress to respiratory failure [38, 39]. Radiograghic findings of EP include alveolar infiltrates and the classic pattern of "photographic negative" pulmonary edema [40]. It also could cause faint ground-glass opacities, or Kerley's "B" lines (dense and diffuse). EP is diagnosed by the presence of increased percentages or numbers of eosinophils in blood, BAL, or lung tissue. A lung biopsy is rarely required, but discontinuance of the offending drug is essential. Corticosteroid drug therapy is suggested in cases with severe involvement. The prognosis for this condition usually is good.

Chemotherapy-induced organizing pneumonia (OP) may manifest with chest pain, dyspnea and diffuse radiographic abnormalities with [41] or without acute respiratory failure [42], or may be discovered incidentally on chest imaging [36]. Nodular OP typically is seen in patients exposed to chemotherapy who develop round-shaped foci that localize mainly in lung bases, may abut the pleura and simulate metastatic nodules [43–45]. Nonspecific findings are retrieved from BAL, such as increases in the percentage of lymphocytes, neutrophils or eosinophils. Open lung biopsy guided by the results of CT scan is the procedure of choice. The nodules correspond to sterile aggregates of mononuclear cells. Histology reveals interstitial inflammation, superimposed on the dominant background of alveolar and ductal fibrosis. Lung nodules with the histopathologic features of cryptogenic organizing pneumonia or of localized fibrosis can be observed after treatment with bleomycin, cyclophosphamide, vinblastine and, rarely, fludarabine [46–49]. Drug discontinuation and, if required, corticosteroid therapy usually are followed by improvement in most cases. Organizing pneumonia (formerly BOOP) can be seen following HSCT and is described in detail later in the chapter.

Diffuse alveolar damage (DAD) is a serious form of pulmonary pathology that may develop in the context of drug-related lung injury. Single chemotherapeutic agents (e.g., BCNU or other nitrosoureas, bleomycin, busulfan, chlorambucil, cyclophosphamide, melphalan, procarbazine, vinblastine) or multiagent cytostatic chemotherapy have been reported to cause this lung toxicity [50]. Some regimens may be associated with a greater likelihood of DAD than others even if they differ in one agent only. For instance, in patients with de novo-treated Hodgkin's lymphoma, the substitution of gemcitabine for dacarbazine, e.g., ABVG rather than ABVD (doxorubicin, bleomycin, vinblastine and gemcitabine instead of dacarbazine), was associated with a 42% incidence rate of pulmonary toxicity [51]. Likewise, the substitution of gemcitabine for etoposide in the dose-escalated BEACOPP regimen (bleomycin, doxorubicin, cyclophosphamide, vincristine, procarbazine, prednisone and gemcitabine rather than etoposide) significantly escalated the likelihood of pulmonary toxicity [52–54]. Concurrent administration of radiation therapy to the chest or use of TBI, supplemental oxygen and possibly colony-stimulating factors (CSFs) may increase the risk of DAD.

Time to onset of DAD can vary from shortly after the first administration of the offending drug to much later into the treatment course [55]. Restrictive lung function patterns and hypoxemia are typical. DLCO abnormalities often precede clinical symptoms. The clinical evolution of drug-induced DAD varies from an isolated decrease in DLCO [56, 57] or evidence of fibrosis in trans-bronchial or pulmonary biopsies [58, 59] as the only manifestation of toxicity to bilateral, interstitial and alveolar infiltrates [57, 60]. Severe cases progress to an ARDS picture and death [61].

High-resolution CT scanning may show ground-glass opacities and intra-lobular septal thickening, and the extent of changes correlates with clinical severity [62]. Dysplastic pneumocytes may be retrieved by BAL [63, 64]. A lung biopsy is reserved for patients with an atypical presentation or for those who do not improve with empirical antibiotic and corticosteroid treatment [65]. The main histopathologic feature of DAD is consistent with hyaline membranes and fibrin deposits lining the alveolar border, dysplasia of type II cells, free alveolar fibrin, cells and debris in alveolar spaces and various stages of interstitial edema, inflammation and organization [66]. DAD may be reversible after discontinuation of drugs or after the addition of corticosteroids, or both [67]. The usual doses of oral corticosteroids may not prevent the condition from developing, but higher doses are reported to reduce the incidence [68].

The high incidence, severity and unpredictability of DAD associated with chemotherapy suggest that it is reasonable to discontinue such treatment once the DLCO has decreased 50% compared with pre-therapy values. Although smaller decrements in DLCO do not equate to toxicity and should not lead to withdrawal of chemotherapy, a precipitous decrease in the DLCO indicates impending toxicity [69]. When radiation therapy is planned after the administration of chemotherapeutic agents, it is advisable to wait for any chemotherapy-induced decrease in the DLCO to stabilize or show a trend toward improvement before starting radiation.

Finally, drug-induced pulmonary fibrosis may develop in patients receiving cytotoxic agents, such as bleomycin, busulfan, BCNU, lomustine, CCNU chlorambucil, cyclophosphamide, melphalan, vinca alkaloids, radiation therapy and TBI [70]. This entity more often is diagnosed months or years after termination of treatment. Early signs of this disease are basilar or diffuse streaky opacities and volume loss. This condition can progress to honeycombing and fibrotic changes; reversal of this toxicity and the response to corticosteroids are unpredictable and often unsatisfying. Histologic exam can demonstrate the characteristic dysplasia of type II pneumocytes that reflects exposure to alkylating agents and radiation therapy. In a few patients, especially children treated for hematologic malignancies, pleural or pulmonary fibrosis may develop [71]. This process results in thoracic deformity, encasement of the lungs and severely restricts lung physiology. An accelerated variant of pulmonary fibrosis, acute interstitial pneumonia (formerly termed the Hamman and Rich syndrome), has been described after treatment with chlorambucil and methotrexate [72–74]. The prognosis of this condition is poor despite drug withdrawal and institution of high-dose corticosteroids.

42.3.3 Chronic Pulmonary Dysfunction After Hematopoietic Cell Transplantation

As seen in the patient description at the start of this chapter, a decline in lung function long has been identified as a significant complication in the months to years that follow allogeneic HSCT. A clinical pearl from Dr. Bergeron in this book also very nicely describes this type of pulmonary involvement. Noninfectious conditions now represent the major pulmonary causes of morbidity and mortality after HSCT. Idiopathic pneumonia syndrome (IPS), discussed in another chapter in this book, remains one of the more common and serious pulmonary complications occurring within months after HSCT. Although graft-versus-host reactions may play an etiologic role, the major contributing factor is conditioning-related toxicity. Among lung conditions that are more closely associated with GVHD, both bronchiolitis obliterans (BrOb) (onset months to years after HSCT) and bronchiolitis obliterans with organizing pneumonia (COP) may lead to FA. The term COP should not be used interchangeably with bronchiolitis obliterans (BO) to describe a patient with chronic lung dysfunction after HSCT, although such usage unfortunately is widespread. The two disorders differ with respect to histopathology, pulmonary function characteristics and, most importantly, response to therapy. BrOb is an inexorably progressive condition, whereas COP behaves similarly to idiopathic COP seen in other populations. COP after HSCT usually is quite responsive to corticosteroids and in other settings may resolve spontaneously, whereas BrOb is not [75, 76]. Organizing pneumonia also is associated with restrictive (rather than obstructive) changes on pulmonary function testing (Table 42.4).

In allogeneic HSCT recipients, the disparity in match between the donor graft and the recipient for the human leukocyte antigens (HLAs) mediate both GVHD and graft rejection (host-versus-graft reaction). The presence of alloreactive injury to the lung attributed to GVHD is poorly defined and remains debated. In the skin, liver and intestine, GVHD produces a characteristic T-lymphocyte-mediated epithelial destruction. There are few data to support such a defined lesion with the exception of lymphocytic pneumonitis [77]. A variety of pulmonary complications have been described as manifestations of GVHD, but these associations are based primarily on the simultaneous occurrence of pulmonary abnormalities, the absence of an infectious agent and nonspecific histopathologic lesions in the setting of established GVHD in other organs. Nevertheless, both acute and late-onset lung injury syndromes have shown a clinical association with GVHD, including IPS, engraftment syndrome, diffuses alveolar hemorrhage, BrOb and COP [78]. Several murine models also demonstrate pathologic lung changes in the setting of GVHD, thus supporting a mechanistic relationship between GVHD and lung injury.

OLD and chronic AFO are the most common noninfectious late pulmonary complications of allogeneic HSCT. These entities are manifested on pulmonary function testing by a diminished FEV1 or FEV1/FVC. The incidence of these syndromes ranges from 6% to 32%, depending upon the definition of AFO applied in each study [79, 80]. Typically, the presentation occurs beyond the third month after HSCT [81]. Among patients who develop chronic GVHD, new-onset AFO may develop in up to one third of the patients. In a study of 11 cases the underlying process accounting for AFO was BrOb in 70% [82]. Histologically, this process demonstrates fibrous obliteration of the lumen

Table 42.4 Clinical factors present in obstructive versus restrictive lung disease

Clinical Factor	Obstructive lung disease	Restrictive lung disease
Onset	Late (3–12 months after HCT)	Early (within 3 months after HSCT)
Symptoms	Dyspnea, nonproductive cough	Dyspnea, nonproductive cough
Physical exam	Wheezing	Crackles
PFTs	Obstructive physiology	Restrictive physiology
FEV_1/FVC	Decreased	Normal
TLC	Normal	Decreased
DLco	Decreased	Decreased
CT scan findings	Air trapping Bronchial wall thickening Centrilobular nodules	Patchy consolidation Organizing pneumonia Ground-glass opacities
Chronic GVHD	Strong association	Variable, association with organizing pneumonia

PFTs pulmonary function tests, *FEV1/FVC* forced expiratory volume in 1 s/forced vital capacity, *TLC* total lung capacity, *DLco* diffusion capacity for carbon monoxide of respiratory and membranous bronchioles. In the absence of histopathologic evidence, new onset AFO after allogeneic HSCT often is referred to as "bronchiolitis obliterans syndrome" (BOS). In addition to chronic GVHD, risk factors for the development of AFO include increasing recipient age, pre-transplant reduction in the ratio FEV1/FVC, low serum immunoglobulin levels, use of methotrexate and a history of respiratory viral infection within the first 100 days [79]. The onset typically is insidious with presenting symptoms including dry cough (60–100%), dyspnea (50–70%) and wheezing (40%), but fever is uncommon [79, 82, 83]. The chest radiograph is usually normal, but high-resolution CT scans often demonstrate evidence of expiratory air trapping, hypo-attenuation and bronchial dilation [80, 84–86]. Demonstrating persistent AFO using pulmonary function testing and exclusion of other causes of AFO such as asthma, tobacco-related emphysema, and viral or bacterial respiratory infection establish the diagnosis. Except for its utility in excluding an infectious etiology, BAL is usually nonspecific [87], and transbronchial biopsies typically are nondiagnostic due to the patchy nature of this small airway process and the limited size of samples obtained. Surgical lung biopsy is rarely indicated.

The etiology of new onset AFO after HSCT is unknown. Those recognized causes in otherwise normal hosts rarely include recurrent aspiration, viral infection (influenza, adenovirus, measles) and bacterial infection (*Mycoplasma* sp.) [88]. Immunologic mechanisms inducing bronchial epithelial injury are suggested by the strong association between chronic GVHD and new onset AFO. Indeed, the lung epithelium may be the target of immune-mediated injury induced by donor cytotoxic T cells in chronic GVHD [89]. Thus, BrOb after HSCT may represent a manifestation of GVHD in the lung.

Disease progression is variable; however, the syndrome is associated with significantly increased mortality rates, and improvement in lung function is uncommon. Many patients develop a progressive decline in lung function resulting in respiratory failure [79, 80]. There are no prospective studies of the treatment of new onset AFO after HSCT. OLD in the presence of chronic GVHD is managed primarily by controlling GVHD. Various immunosuppressive agents have been reported to result in stabilization of lung function in 30–50%, but improvement in only 8–30% [37, 51]. In the hope that early recognition and treatment may improve outcome, routine spirometry among patients with chronic GVHD is encouraged to detect the insidious onset of this process.

Restrictive lung disease (RLD) is defined by reductions in FVC, total lung capacity (TLC) and DLCO as measured by standard pulmonary function tests (PFTs). In RLD, the ratio FEV_1/FVC is maintained near 100% [90, 91]. RLD is common after HSCT. Significant decreases in FVC or TLC have been reported in as many as 25–45% of allogeneic HSCT recipients by day 100. A decline in TLC or FVC after HSCT (even if the absolute values for each measurement remained within the normal range) has been associated with an increase in nonrelapse mortality. TBI-containing conditioning regimens and the presence of acute GVHD have been associated with RLD, in addition to obstructive lung disease [92–94]; however, the impact of age on the development of RLD is less clear. Early reports suggested that the incidence of RLD is lower in children compared to adults and that the incidence increases with advancing recipient age [95]. More recent studies have revealed significant RLD in children receiving HSCT [96]. Organizing pneumonia after HSCT falls under the RLD pattern on liver function tests and recently was shown to be associated with prior acute and chronic GVHD. Organizing pneumonia has been described in case reports as occurring after both allogeneic and syngeneic HSCT; these data suggest an association of the lung lesion with chronic GVHD and intestinal ulcerations. In addition, corticosteroid therapy appeared beneficial in the resolution of the lesion. In a recent case control study, Freudenberger et al. reviewed 49 cases of histologic COP [97]. The clinical features of COP in this population were similar to idiopathic and other etiologies with an association between acute and chronic GVHD and the subsequent development of COP. Affected patients were more likely to have skin involvement with acute GVHD and chronic GVHD affecting the gut and oral mucosa. The causes of COP following HSCT remain enigmatic, but possible etiologies include direct allo-immunologic reactions, atypical infection or atypical manifestations of IPS. Regardless, the clinical presentations and responses of COP are similar to other cases of idiopathic COP.

The published literature contains a paucity of therapeutic trials for chronic lung injury after HSCT. A study by Payne and colleagues showed that the use of cyclosporine and methotrexate as GVHD prophylaxis prevented the development of OLD when compared to historic controls receiving prednisone and methotrexate [98], but results of prospective, randomized trials in this setting are not available. Three recently published case series have exploited the antiinflammatory effects of azithromycin to treat OLD in both allogeneic HSCT and lung allograft recipients. Each study suggested a beneficial effect of this drug on pulmonary function when administered for 12 or more weeks [99–101]. The potential role for TNFα in the pathogenesis of both OLD and RLD suggests that agents such as etanercept may have promise, and several studies have demonstrated a potential benefit of this drug in some HSCT patients with chronic lung injury [102, 103].

The immunologic mechanisms responsible for chronic, fibrotic pulmonary dysfunction after HSCT remain poorly defined, in large part because of the lack of correlative data obtained from afflicted HSCT recipients and the paucity of suitable SCT animal models for either RLD or OLD. Chronic pulmonary disease following allogeneic HSCT likely involves an initial insult to lung parenchyma followed by an ongoing inflammatory process involving the interplay between recruited donor-derived immune cells and the resident cells of the pulmonary vascular endothelium and interstitium. Mechanistic insights into OLD following HSCT have been derived from studies of lung allograft rejection. Data generated from both humans and mice support the hypothesis that the development of BrOb in this scenario involves the secretion of inflammatory cytokines and chemokines, along with interactions between APCs and activated lymphocytes [104, 105]

A tri-phasic model of chronic noninfectious lung injury after HSCT has been proposed [106]. In phase I, an acute pneumonitis develops as a consequence of an allogeneic immune response, resulting in the sequential influx of lymphocytes, macrophages and neutrophils into an inflamed pulmonary parenchyma. In phase II, a persistent inflammatory signal, in the setting of dysregulated repair mechanisms, promotes the transition from acute to chronic injury. If the inciting injurious stimulus predominantly involves bronchiolar epithelial cells, phase II is associated with the concentric infiltration of lymphocytes and collagen deposition in the peri-bronchiolar areas resulting in the development of chronic bronchiolitis. If, however, the alveolar epithelium is the primary target, leukocyte recruitment and matrix deposition are confined primarily to the interstitial space. As chronic inflammation proceeds to phase III, lung fibroblasts increase dramatically in number and contribute to the enhanced deposition of collagen and granulation tissue in and around bronchial structures, ultimately resulting in complete obliteration of small airways and fixed OLD. By contrast, fibroblast proliferation and intra-septal collagen deposition during phase III ultimately result in interstitial thickening, septal fibrosis, significant volume loss and severe RLD.

Clinical and experimental data suggest that the progression to a chronic, pro-fibrotic form of pulmonary toxicity involves the secretion of cytokines and chemokines [107–109], and in this context, TNFα may be a central factor in the proposed tri-phasic model of disease. Evidence for a role of TNFα in the transition from acute to chronic lung injury comes from studies using targeted over-expression of TNFα in the lungs of rodents [110]. In these models, early lung histopathology includes a lymphocytic infiltrate similar to that seen in experimental IPS models [111, 112], whereas the histologic changes associated with more prolonged exposure to TNFα show both interstitial and peribronchial inflammation that closely resemble changes seen at later time points after HSCT [107, 113].

42.4 Conclusion

FA is characterized by sequential acute lung injury that can culminate in scarring and end-stage lung disease. Despite the high success rate in treating hematologic malignancies with or without using HSCT, this sequence of events continues to be a significant contributor to nonrelapse morbidity and mortality in patients with hematologic malignancies because of either the disease itself or as a result of treatment modalities employed. The pathophysiologic mechanisms contributing to the initiation and progression of disease remain poorly defined. To this end, current treatment options remain suboptimal and primarily limited to supportive care measures and antiinflammatory agents, such as corticosteroids or other immunosuppressant therapy. Further research is necessary (in the form of clinical trials and pre-clinical models) to improve our understanding of fibrosing alveolits and related disorders and to ultimately design and implement targeted therapeutic strategies.

References

1. Fellrath JM, du Bois RM (2003) Idiopathic pulmonary fibrosis/cryptogenic fibrosing alveolitis. Clin Exp Med 3:65–83
2. Sharma S, Nadrous HF, Peters SG, Tefferi A, Litzow MR, Aubry MC, Afessa B (2005 Sept) Pulmonary complications in adult blood and marrow transplant recipients: autopsy findings. Chest 128(3):1385–1392
3. Soares M, Silva UV, Teles JM, Silva E, Caruso P, Lobo SM, Dal Pizzol F, Azevedo LP, de Carvalho FB, Salluh JI (2010 Jul) Validation of four prognostic scores in patients with cancer admitted to Brazilian intensive care units: results from a prospective multicenter study. Intensive Care Med 36(7):1188–1195
4. Vandijck DM, Benoit DD, Depuydt PO et al (2008) Impact of recent intravenous chemotherapy on outcome in severe sepsis and septic shock patients with hematological malignancies. Intensive Care Med 34:847–855
5. Vourlekis JS, Brown KK, Schwarz MI (2001) Acute interstitial pneumonitis: current understanding regarding diagnosis, pathogenesis, and natural history. Semin Respir Crit Care Med 22:399–408
6. Pinto PS (2004) The CT halo sign. Radiology 230:109–110
7. Okada F, Ando Y, Yoshitake S et al (2007) Clinical/pathologic correlations in 553 patients with primary centrilobular findings on high-resolution CT scan of the thorax. Chest 132:1939–1948
8. Kradin RL, Mark EJ (2008) The pathology of pulmonary disorders due to Aspergillus spp. Arch Pathol Lab Med 132:606–614
9. Gefter WB, Weingrad TR, Epstein DM, Ochs RH, Miller WT (1981) "Semi-invasive" pulmonary aspergillosis: a new look at the spectrum of aspergillus infections of the lung. Radiology 140:313–321
10. Bergonie J, Teissier J (1898) Rapport sur l'action des rayons X sur la tuberculose. Arch Electr Med 6:334
11. Evans WA, Leucutia T (1925) Intrathoracic changes induced by heavy irradiation. AJR Am J Roentgenol 13:203
12. Anscher MS, Kong FM, Andrews K et al (1998) Plasma transforming growth factor beta1 as a predictor of radiation pneumonitis. Int J Radiat Oncol Biol Phys 41:1029–1035
13. Chen Y, Williams J, Ding I et al (2002) Radiation pneumonitis and early circulatory cytokine markers. Semin Radiat Oncol 12(1 Suppl 1):26–33
14. Chen Y, Rubin P, Williams J, Hernady E, Smudzin T, Okunieff P (2001) Circulating IL-6 as a predictor of radiation pneumonitis. Int J Radiat Oncol Biol Phys 49: 641–648
15. Rubin P, Johnston CJ, Williams JP, McDonald S, Finkelstein JN (1995) A perpetual cascade of cytokines postirradiation leads to pulmonary fibrosis. Int J Radiat Oncol Biol Phys 33:99–109
16. McDonald S, Rubin P, Phillips TL, Marks LB (1995) Injury to the lung from cancer therapy: clinical syndromes, measurable endpoints, and potential scoring systems. Int J Radiat Oncol Biol Phys 31:1187–1203
17. Rancati T, Ceresoli GL, Gagliardi G, Schipani S, Cattaneo GM (2003) Factors predicting radiation pneumonitis in lung cancer patients: a retrospective study. Radiother Oncol 67:275–283
18. Robnett TJ, Machtay M, Vines EF, McKenna MG, Algazy KM, McKenna WG (2000) Factors predicting severe radiation pneumonitis in patients receiving definitive chemoradiation for lung cancer. Int J Radiat Oncol Biol Phys 48: 89–94
19. Monson JM, Stark P, Reilly JJ et al (1998) Clinical radiation pneumonitis and radiographic changes after thoracic radiation therapy for lung carcinoma. Cancer 82:842–850
20. Katayama N, Sato S, Katsui K et al (2009) Analysis of factors associated with radiation-induced bronchiolitis obliterans organizing pneumonia syndrome after breast-conserving therapy. Int J Radiat Oncol Biol Phys 73:1049–1054
21. Arbetter KR, Prakash UB, Tazelaar HD, Douglas WW (1999) Radiation-induced pneumonitis in the "nonirradiated" lung. Mayo Clin Proc 74:27–36
22. Ozturk B, Egehan I, Atavci S, Kitapci M (2004) Pentoxifylline in prevention of radiation-induced lung toxicity in patients with breast and lung cancer: a double-blind randomized trial. Int J Radiat Oncol Biol Phys 58:213–219
23. Antonadou D (2002) Radiotherapy or chemotherapy followed by radiotherapy with or without amifostine in locally advanced lung cancer. Semin Radiat Oncol 12(1 Suppl 1): 50–58
24. Antonadou D, Coliarakis N, Synodinou M et al (2001) Randomized phase III trial of radiation treatment +/– amifostine in patients with advanced-stage lung cancer. Int J Radiat Oncol Biol Phys 51:915–922
25. Ward WF, Molteni A, Ts'ao CH (1989) Radiation-induced endothelial dysfunction and fibrosis in rat lung: modification by the angiotensin converting enzyme inhibitor CL242817. Radiat Res 117:342–350
26. Borst GR, De Jaeger K, Belderbos JS, Burgers SA, Lebesque JV (2005) Pulmonary function changes after radiotherapy in non-small-cell lung cancer patients with long-term disease-free survival. Int J Radiat Oncol Biol Phys 62: 639–644
27. Theuws JC, Seppenwoolde Y, Kwa SL et al (2000) Changes in local pulmonary injury up to 48 months after irradiation for lymphoma and breast cancer. Int J Radiat Oncol Biol Phys 47:1201–1208
28. Fryer CJ, Hutchinson RJ, Krailo M et al (1990) Efficacy and toxicity of 12 courses of ABVD chemotherapy followed by low-dose regional radiation in advanced Hodgkin's disease in children: a report from the Children's Cancer Study Group. J Clin Oncol 8:1971–1980
29. Rossi HA, Becker PS, Emmons RV et al (2003) High-dose cyclophosphamide, BCNU, and VP-16 (CBV) conditioning before allogeneic stem cell transplantation for patients with non-Hodgkin's lymphoma. Bone Marrow Transplant 31: 441–446
30. Erasmus JJ, McAdams HP, Rossi SE (2002) Drug-induced lung injury. Semin Roentgenol 37:72–81
31. Erasmus JJ, McAdams HP, Rossi SE (2002) High-resolution CT of drug-induced lung disease. Radiol Clin North Am 40:61–72
32. Rossi SE, Erasmus JJ, McAdams P, Sporn TA, Goodman PC (2000) Pulmonary drug toxicity: radiologic and pathologic manifestations. Radiographics 20:1245–1259
33. Zisman DA, McCune WJ, Tino G, Lynch JP 3rd (2001) Drug-induced pneumonitis: the role of methotrexate. Sarcoidosis Vasc Diffuse Lung Dis 18:243–252

34. Imokawa S, Colby TV, Leslie KO, Helmers RA (2000) Methotrexate pneumonitis: review of the literature and histopathological findings in nine patients. Eur Respir J 15:373–381
35. Fuhrman C, Parrot A, Wislez M et al (2001) Spectrum of CD4 to CD8 T-cell ratios in lymphocytic alveolitis associated with methotrexate-induced pneumonitis. Am J Respir Crit Care Med 164:1186–1191
36. Berkani K, Bayle JY, Perol M, Bejui-Thivolet F, Perrot D, Guerin JC (2003) "Spontaneous" resolution of two severe methotrexate-induced pneumonias. Rev Pneumol Clin 59:301–305
37. Fehr T, Jacky E, Bächli EB (2003) Successful reintroduction of methotrexate after acute pneumonitis in a patient with acute lymphoblastic leukemia. Ann Hematol 82:193–196
38. Oddo M, Liaudet L, Lepori M, Broccard AF, Schaller MD (2003) Relapsing acute respiratory failure induced by minocycline. Chest 123:2146–2148
39. Baptista JP, Casanova PC, Sousa JP et al (2004) Acute eosinophilic pneumonia associated with acute respiratory distress syndrome: case report. Rev Port Pneumol 10: 355–364
40. Jeong YJ, Kim KI, Seo IJ, Lee CH, Lee KN, Kim KN, Kim JS, Kwon WJ (2007 May–Jun) Eosinophilic lung diseases: a clinical, radiologic, and pathologic overview. Radiographics 27(3):617–637, discussion 637–9
41. Egerer G, Witzens M, Spaeth A et al (2001) Successful treatment of bronchiolitis obliterans organizing pneumonia with low-dose methotrexate in a patient with Hodgkin's disease. Oncology 61:23–27
42. Kalambokis G, Stefanou D, Arkoumani E, Kitsanou M, Bourantas K, Tsianos EV (2004) Fulminant bronchiolitis obliterans organizing pneumonia following 2 d of treatment with hydroxyurea, interferon-alpha and oral cytarabine ocfosfate for chronic myelogenous leukemia (case report). Eur J Haematol 73:67–70
43. Ferriby D, Stojkovic T (2001) Bronchiolitis obliterans with organizing pneumonia during interferon b-1a treatment. Lancet 357:751
44. Santrach PJ, Askin FB, Wells RJ, Azizkhan RG, Merten DF (1989) Nodular form of bleomycin-related pulmonary injury in patients with osteogenic sarcoma. Cancer 64: 806–811
45. Gehl HB, Hauptmann S, Sohn M, Bohndorf K (1992) Late pulmonary changes following bleomycin administration in computed tomography. Nodular fibrosis mimicking a seminoma metastasis. Radiologe 32:80–82
46. Glasier CM, Siegel MJ (1981) Multiple pulmonary nodules: unusual manifestation of bleomycin toxicity. AJR Am J Roentgenol 137:155–156
47. Franchi F, Seminara P, Gualdi GF (1984) Lung pseudometastases due to vinblastine toxicity. Klin Wochenschr 62:1047–1048
48. Scharstein R, Johnson JF, Cook BA, Stephenson SR (1987) Bleomycin nodules mimicking metastatic osteogenic sarcoma. Am J Pediatr Hematol Oncol 9:219–221
49. Garg S, Garg MS, Basmaji N (2002) Multiple pulmonary nodules: an unusual presentation of fludarabine pulmonary toxicity: case report and review of literature. Am J Hematol 70:241–245
50. Kreisman H, Wolkove N (1992) Pulmonary toxicity of antineoplastic therapy. Semin Oncol 19:508–520
51. Friedberg JW, Neuberg D, Kim H et al (2003) Gemcitabine added to doxorubicin, bleomycin, and vinblastine for the treatment of de novo Hodgkin disease: unacceptable acute pulmonary toxicity. Cancer 98:978–982
52. Stuart MJ, Chao NS, Horning SJ et al (2001) Efficacy and toxicity of a CCNU-containing high-dose chemotherapy regimen followed by autologous hematopoietic cell transplantation in relapsed or refractory Hodgkin's disease. Biol Blood Marrow Transplant 7:552–560
53. Bredenfeld H, Franklin J, Nogova L et al (2004) Severe pulmonary toxicity in patients with advanced-stage Hodgkin's disease treated with a modified bleomycin, doxorubicin, cyclophosphamide, vincristine, procarbazine, prednisone, and gemcitabine (BEACOPP) regimen is probably related to the combination of gemcitabine and bleomycin: a report of the German Hodgkin's lymphoma Study Group. J Clin Oncol 22:2424–2429
54. Quigley M, Brada M, Heron C, Horwich A (1988) Severe lung toxicity with a weekly low dose chemotherapy regimen in patients with non-Hodgkin's lymphoma. Hematol Oncol 6:319–324
55. Todd NW, Peters WP, Ost AH, Roggli VL, Piantadosi AC (1993) Pulmonary drug toxicity in patients with primary breast cancer treated with high-dose combination chemotherapy and autologous bone marrow transplantation. Am Rev Respir Dis 147:1264–1270
56. Brice P, Tredaniel J, Monsuez JJ et al (1991) Cardiopulmonary toxicity after three courses of ABVD and mediastinal irradiation in favorable Hodgkin's disease. Ann Oncol 2(Suppl 2):73–76
57. Kalaycioglu M, Kavuru M, Tuason L, Bolwell B (1995) Empiric prednisone therapy for pulmonary toxic reaction after high-dose chemotherapy containing carmustine (BCNU). Chest 107:482–487
58. Maher J, Daly PA (1993) Severe bleomycin lung toxicity: reversal with high dose corticosteroids. Thorax 48:92–94
59. Segura A, Yuste A, Cercos A et al (2001) Pulmonary fibrosis induced by cyclophosphamide. Ann Pharmacother 35: 894–897
60. Maher J, Daly PA (1993) Severe bleomycin lung toxicity: reversal with high dose corticosteroids. Thorax 48:92–94
61. Rubio C, Hill ME, Milan S, O'Brien MER, Cunningham D (1997) Idiopathic pneumonia syndrome after high dose chemotherapy for relapsed Hodgkin's disease. Br J Cancer 75:1044–1048
62. Cleverley JR, Screaton NJ, Hiorns MP, Flint JD, Müller NL (2002) Drug-induced lung disease: high-resolution CT and histological findings. Clin Radiol 57:292–299
63. Huang MS, Colby TV, Goellner JR, Martin WJ (1989) Utility of bronchoalveolar lavage in the diagnosis of drug induced pulmonary toxicity. Acta Cytol 33:533–538
64. Du EZ, Yung GL, Le DT, Masliah E, Yi ES, Friedman PJ (2001) Severe alveolar proteinosis following chemotherapy for acute myeloid leukemia in a lung allograft recipient. J Thorac Imaging 16:307–309
65. Dai MS, Lee SC, Ho CL, Chen YC, Kao WY, Chao TY (2001) Impact of open lung biopsy for undiagnosed pulmonary infiltrates in patients with hematological malignancies. Am J Hematol 68:87–90
66. Colby TV (2000) Surgical pathology of non-neoplastic lung disease. Mod Pathol 13:343–358

67. Maher J, Daly PA (1993) Severe bleomycin lung toxicity: reversal with high dose corticosteroids (case report). Thorax 48:92–94
68. Wadhwa PD, Fu P, Koc ON et al (2005) High-dose carmustine, etoposide and cisplatinum for autologous stem cell transplantation with or without involved-field radiation for relapsed/refractory lymphoma: an effective regimen with low morbidity and mortality. Biol Blood Marrow Transplant 11:13–22
69. Bell MR, Meredith DJ, Gill PG (1985) Role of carbon monoxide diffusing capacity in the early detection of major bleomycin induced pulmonary toxicity. Aust N Z J Med 15:235–240
70. Tucker AS, Newman AJ, Alvorado C (1977) Pulmonary, pleural and thoracic changes complicating chemotherapy. Radiology 125:805–809
71. Malik SW, Myers JL, DeRemee RA, Specks U (1996) Lung toxicity associated with cyclophosphamide use: two distinct patterns. Am J Respir Crit Care Med 154:1851–1856
72. No authors listed (1975) The Hamman-Rich syndrome following treatment of lymphoma with chlorambucil. J La State Med Soc 127:311–315
73. Bedrossian CWM, Miller WC, Luna MA (1979) Methotrexate induced diffuse interstitial pulmonary fibrosis. South Med J 72:313–318
74. Attar EC, Ervin T, Janicek M, Deykin A, Godleski J (2000) Acute interstitial pneumonitis related to gemcitabine. J Clin Oncol 18:697–698
75. Williams KM, Chien JW, Gladwin MT (2009) Pavletic SZ Bronchiolitis obliterans after allogeneic hematopoietic stem cell transplantation. JAMA 302:306–314
76. Afessa B, Litzow MR, Tefferi A (2001) Bronchiolitis obliterans and other late onset noninfectious pulmonary complications in hematopoietic stem cell transplantation. Bone Marrow Transplant 28:425–434
77. Stein R, Hummel D, Bohn D, Levison H, Roifman CM (1991) Lymphocytic pneumonitis following bone marrow transplantation in severe combined immunodeficiency. Am Rev Respir Dis 143:1406–1408
78. Yousem SA (1995) The histological spectrum of pulmonary graft-versus-host disease in bone marrow transplant recipients. Hum Pathol 26:668–675
79. Chien JW, Martin PJ, Gooley TA et al (2003) Airflow obstruction after myeloablative allogeneic hematopoietic stem cell transplantation. Am J Respir Crit Care Med 168:208–214
80. Clark JG, Crawford SW, Madtes DK, Sullivan KM (1989) Obstructive lung disease after allogeneic marrow transplantation: clinical presentation and course. Ann Intern Med 111:368–376
81. Paz HL, Crilley P, Patchefsky A, Schiffman RL, Brodsky I (1992) Bronchiolitis obliterans after autologous bone marrow transplantation. Chest 101:775–778
82. Chan CK, Hyland RH, Hutcheon MA et al (1987) Small-airways disease in recipients of allogeneic bone marrow transplants: an analysis of 11 cases and a review of the literature. Medicine (Baltimore) 66:327–340
83. Ralph DD, Springmeyer SC, Sullivan KM, Hackman RC, Storb R, Thomas ED (1984) Rapidly progressive air-flow obstruction in marrow transplant recipients: possible association between obliterative bronchiolitis and chronic graft-versushost disease. Am Rev Respir Dis 129:641–644
84. Schultz KR, Green GJ, Wensley D et al (1994) Obstructive lung disease in children after allogeneic bone marrow transplantation. Blood 84:3212–3220
85. Philit F, Wiesendanger T, Archimbaud E, Mornex JF, Brune J, Cordier JF (1995) Post-transplant obstructive lung disease ("bronchiolitis obliterans"): a clinical comparative study of bone marrow and lung transplant patients. Eur Respir J 8:551–558
86. Palmas A, Tefferi A, Myers JL et al (1998) Late-onset non-infectious pulmonary complications after allogeneic bone marrow transplantation. Br J Haematol 100:680–687
87. St John RC, Gadek JE, Tutschka PJ, Kapoor N, Dorinsky PM (1990) Analysis of airflow obstruction by bronchoalveolar lavage following bone marrow transplantation: implications for pathogenesis and treatment. Chest 98:600–607
88. Clark JG, Schwartz DA, Flournoy N, Sullivan KM, Crawford SW, Thomas ED (1987) Risk factors for airflow obstruction in recipients of bone marrow transplants. Ann Intern Med 107:648–656
89. Holland HK, Wingard JR, Beschorner WE, Saral R, Santos GW (1988) Bronchiolitis obliterans in bone marrow transplantation and its relationship to chronic graft-v-host disease and low serum IgG. Blood 72:621–627
90. Freudenberger TD, Madtes DK, Curtis JR et al (2003) Association between acute and chronic graft-versus-host disease and bronchiolitis obliterans organizing pneumonia in recipients of hematopoietic stem cell transplants. Blood 102:3822–3828
91. Afessa B, Litzow MR, Tefferi A (2001) Bronchiolitis obliterans and other late onset non-infectious pulmonary complications in hematopoietic stem cell transplantation. Bone Marrow Transplant 28:425–434
92. Clark JG, Schwartz DA, Flournoy N, Sullivan KM, Crawford SW, Thomas ED (1987) Risk factors for air-flow obstruction in recipients of bone marrow transplants. Ann Intern Med 107:648–656
93. Crawford SW, Pepe M, Lin D, Benedetti F, Deeg HJ (1995) Abnormalities of pulmonary function tests after marrow transplantation predict nonrelapse mortality. Am J Respir Crit Care Med 152:690–695
94. Badier M, Guillot C, Delpierre S, Vanuxem P, Blaise D, Maraninchi D (1993) Pulmonary function changes 100 days and one year after bone marrow transplantation. Bone Marrow Transplant 12:457–461
95. Cerveri I, Zoia MC, Fulgoni P et al (1999) Late pulmonary sequelae after childhood bone marrow transplantation. Thorax 54:131–135
96. Quigley PM, Yeager AM, Loughlin GM (1994) The effects of bone marrow transplantation on pulmonary function in children. Pediatr Pulmonol 18:361–367
97. Freudenberger TD, Madtes DK, Curtis JR et al (2003) Association between acute and chronic graft-versus-host disease and bronchiolitis obliterans organizing pneumonia in recipients of hematopoietic stem cell transplants. Blood 102:3822–3828
98. Payne L, Chan CK, Fyles G et al (1993) Cyclosporine as possible prophylaxis for obstructive airways disease after allogeneic bone marrow transplantation. Chest 104:114–118
99. Verleden GM, Dupont LJ (2004) Azithromycin therapy for patients with bronchiolitis obliterans syndrome after lung transplantation. Transplantation 77:1465–1467

100. Gerhardt SG, McDyer JF, Girgis RE et al (2003) Maintenance azithromycin therapy for bronchiolitis obliterans syndrome: results of a pilot study. Am J Respir Crit Care Med 168:121–125
101. Khalid M, Al Saghir A, Saleemi S et al (2005) Azithromycin in bronchiolitis obliterans complicating bone marrow transplantation: a preliminary study. Eur Respir J 25: 490–493
102. Chiang KY, Abhyankar S, Bridges K et al (2002) Recombinant human tumor necrosis factor receptor fusion protein as complementary treatment for chronic graft-versus-host disease. Transplantation 73:665–667
103. Yanik G, Uberti J, Ferrara JLM et al (2003) Etanercept for sub-acute lung injury following allogeneic stem cell transplantation (abstract). Blood 102:471a
104. Belperio JA, DiGiovine B, Keane MP et al (2002) Interleukin-1 receptor antagonist as a biomarker for bronchiolitis obliterans syndrome in lung transplant recipients. Transplantation 73:591–599
105. Elssner A, Jaumann F, Dobmann S et al (2000) Elevated levels of interleukin-8 and transforming growth factor-beta in bronchoalveolar lavage fluid from patients with bronchiolitis obliterans syndrome: proinflammatory role of bronchial epithelial cells. Munich Lung Transplant Group. Transplantation 70:362–367
106. Cooke KR, Yanik G (2009) Lung injury following hematopoietic stem cell transplantation. In: Appelbaum FR, Forman SJ, Negrin RS, Blume KG (eds) Thomas' hematopoietic cell transplantation, 4th edn. Wiley-Blackwell, Oxford
107. Shankar G, Cohen DA (2001) Idiopathic pneumonia syndrome after bone marrow transplantation: the role of pre-transplant radiation conditioning and local cytokine dysregulation in promoting lung inflammation and fibrosis. Int J Exp Pathol 82:101–113
108. Coker RK, Laurent GJ (1998) Pulmonary fibrosis: cytokines in the balance. Eur Respir J 11:1218–1221
109. Sime PJ, Marr RA, Gauldie D et al (1998) Transfer of tumor necrosis factor-a to rat lung induces severe pulmonary inflammation and patchy interstitial fibrogenesis with induction of transforming growth factor-b1 and myofibroblasts. Am J Pathol 153:825–832
110. Miyazaki Y, Araki K, Vesin C, Garcia I, Kapanci Y, Whitsett JA et al (1995) Expression of a tumor necrosis factor-alpha transgene in murine lung causes lymphocytic and fibrosing alveolitis. A mouse model of progressive pulmonary fibrosis. J Clin Invest 96:250–259
111. Cooke KR, Kobzik L, Martin TR, Brewer J, Delmonte J, Crawford JM et al (1996) An experimental model of idiopathic pneumonia syndrome after bone marrow transplantation. I. The roles of minor H antigens and endotoxin. Blood 88:3230–3239
112. Piguet PF, Grau GE, Collart MA, Vassalli P, Kapanci Y (1989) Pneumopathies of the graft-versus-host reaction. Alveolitis associated with an increased level of tumor necrosis factor MRNA and chronic interstitial pneumonitis. Lab Invest 61:37–45
113. Yousem SA (1995) The histological spectrum of pulmonary graft-versus-host disease in bone marrow transplant recipients. Hum Pathol 26:668–675

Part VI

Treatment and Difficult Decisions in Patients with HM and ARF

Antibiotic Therapy in Neutropenic Patients 43

Matthieu Legrand, Adeline Max, and Bertrand Gachot

Contents

M. Legrand
Department of Anesthesiology and Critical Care, Lariboisière Hospital, Assistance Publique – Hopitaux de Paris, University of Paris 7 Denis Diderot, 2 rue Ambroise-Paré, 75475 Paris Cedex 10, France and
Medical Intensive Care Unit, AP-HP, Saint-Louis Hospital, Assistance Publique – Hopitaux de Paris, University of Paris 7 Denis Diderot, 1 rue Claude Vellefaux, 75010 Paris, France

A. Max
Medical Intensive Care Unit, AP-HP, Saint-Louis Hospital, Assistance Publique – Hopitaux de Paris, University of Paris 7 Denis Diderot, 1 rue Claude Vellefaux, 75010 Paris, France

B. Gachot (✉)
Department of Intensive Care and Infectious Diseases, Institut Gustave Roussy, 39, rue Camille Desmoulins, 94805 Villejuif cedex, France
e-mail: gachot@igr.fr

43.1 Introduction

Infection remains a major cause of hospital mortality in cancer patients [1, 2]. Infections often require a decrease in the chemotherapy dosage, which may adversely affect the prognosis of the malignancy. Neutropenia is defined as a neutrophil count ≤500/mm^3, or ≤1,000/mm^3 with a predicted decrease to ≤500/mm^3 [3].

Fever, defined as a single oral temperature of ≥38.3°C or as a temperature of ≥38.0°C for at least 1 h, is common in neutropenic patients. A fever develops in 10–50% of patients after chemotherapy for solid tumors and in more than 80% of patients with hematological malignancies [4]. Fever of unknown origin (FUO), defined as new-onset fever with no clear cause detected clinically or microbiologically, accounts for 30–65% of febrile episodes in neutropenic patients compared to 10–30% for clinically documented infections defined as fever and unambiguous diagnostic signs of localized infection (e.g., pneumonia or skin/soft tissue inflammation) and 10–40% for microbiologically documented infections [4].

The occurrence of a fever in a neutropenic patient poses several challenges. The first-line antibiotics should cover the pathogens deemed to be most likely based on the patient's characteristics, neutropenia, and local epidemiology. However, the changing epidemiology of infections, global increase in resistant strains, and need to contain health care costs require careful selection of antibiotics.

The aim of this review is to provide an up-to-date guide that will assist physicians in choosing the optimal antibiotic regimen in neutropenic patients based on the above-mentioned considerations and on the most recent international guidelines and literature.

É. Azoulay (ed.), *Pulmonary Involvement in Patients with Hematological Malignancies*,
DOI: 10.1007/978-3-642-15742-4_43,

43.2 Bacterial Epidemiology in Neutropenic Patients

In the 1990s, gram-positive bacteria emerged as the leading agents responsible for infections in neutropenic patients worldwide. In adults with bloodstream infections and malignancies in the United States, the proportion of gram-positive organisms increased from 62% in 1995 to 76% in 2000, whereas the proportion of gram-negative infections decreased from 22% to 15% [5]. Factors that may increase the risk of gram-positive sepsis in neutropenic patients include the widespread use of central venous catheters, introduction of prophylactic quinolone therapy, increased use of proton pump inhibitors, and rising prevalence of chemotherapy-induced mucositis [6]. Importantly, gram-negative bacteria seem to have been causing an increasing number of infections in neutropenic patients since the early 2000s [7] (Table 43.1). The selection of empirical antimicrobials depends in part on an assessment of which pathogens are most likely to be involved [16]. Table 43.2 shows a non-exhaustive list of pathogens with their possible sites of development in neutropenic patients. While gram-negative bacteria are usually associated with severe infections that carry high mortality rates [17], coagulase-negative staphylococci (CNS), which are recognized as the most common causes of nosocomial bacteremia, are often associated with more indolent forms of infections and have been more prevalent among low-risk than among high-risk patients [18]. However, in the setting of sustained bacteremia, CNS is an emerging cause of nosocomial endocarditis, usually occurring as a complication of catheter-related infection [19]. Viridans group streptococcal bacteremia may be associated with fulminant infection and is particularly common in patients with hematological malignancies and profound neutropenia [5].

A major concern is the emergence of multidrug-resistant bacteria [20, 21]. Among gram-negative rods, *Pseudomonas aeruginosa*, *Escherichia coli*, *Citrobacter freundii*, *Acinetobacter* species, and *Stenotrophomonas maltophilia* are increasingly found to exhibit multidrug resistance (i.e., resistance to three or more classes of antimicrobials), extensive drug resistance (i.e., resistance to all but one or two classes); or pandrug-resistance (i.e., resistance to all available classes) [22]. Antibiotic selection pressure promotes the induction of extended-spectrum chromosomal β-lactamases (ESBL) after the use of β-lactams [23, 24] and the selection of enterobacteria with decreased porin production after the use of carbapenems [20]. ESBL-producing *Enterobacteriaceae* are now commonly isolated in the community (Fig. 43.1) [16, 25]. Furthermore, Enterobacteriaceae that produce *Klebsiella pneumoniae* carbapenemases (KPCs) are now reported worldwide, and KPCs have become the leading class A carbapenemases. KPC β-lactamases confer decreased susceptibility or resistance to virtually all β-lactams [26]. Similarly, fluoroquinolone exposure is associated with the emergence of methicillin-resistant *Staphylococcus aureus* (MRSA) and penicillin-resistant streptococci [27–29]. Widespread use of vancomycin has been described to cause outbreaks of bacteremia due to nosocomial vancomycin-resistant enterococci associated with high mortality rates [5, 30]. Finally, other gram-positive organisms with limited susceptibility or with resistance to β-lactams have been increasingly isolated in cancer patients with febrile neutropenia; examples include *Corynebacterium jeikeium*, *Lactobacillus*, *Bacillus* species, and *Rhodococcus* species [22, 31]. Antibiotic resistance rates vary widely across countries. For instance, the proportion of *P. aeruginosa* strains exhibiting carbapenem resistance is below 10% in Denmark, The Netherlands, Switzerland, Sweden, and Finland; greater than 25% in Croatia, Turkey, Germany, Italy, and the Czech Republic; and as high as 45% in Greece [32].

43.3 Strategies for Empirical Antibiotic Therapy

43.3.1 Principles Underlying First-Line Antibiotic Therapy

Antibiotic therapy must be initiated immediately in febrile patients with neutropenia [33]. The antibiotics used for first-line therapy must be active against the most likely pathogens, as estimated based on the suspected source of infection, the patient's medical history, careful clinical examination, bacteriological findings, and X-ray results [16]. Signs and symptoms of inflammation are frequently minimal or absent in

Table 43.1 Bloodstream bacterial isolates in clinical trials enrolling neutropenic adults between 1998 and 2009

	Carratala et al. [8]	Gruson et al. [9]	Feld et al. [10]	Regazzoni et al. [11]	Harter et al. [12]	Klastersky et al. [13]	Metallidis et al. [14]	De La Rubia et al. [15]
Number of patients	39	38	411	62	161	2142	75	428
Number of organisms	43	5	93	16	96	556	13	125
Gram-positive organisms	18 (41.9)	4 (80)	41 (44.1)	7 (43.7)	70 (72.9)	353 (63.5)	6 (46.1)	81 (64.8)
Staphylococcus spp.	3 (7)	3 (60)	13 (14)	2 (12.5)	52 (54.5)	187 (33.6)	6 (46.1)	56 (44.8)
Streptococcus spp.	15 (34.9)	1 (20)	27 (29)	4 (25)	15 (15.6)	114 (20.5)	–	10 (8)
Other	–	–	1 (1.1)	1 (6.2)	3 (3.1)	52 (9.4)	–	15 (12)
Gram-negative organisms	25 (58.1)	1 (20)	52 (55.9)	9 (56.3)	26 (27.1)	203 (36.5)	7 (53.9)	44 (35.2)
Enterobacteriaceae	6 (14)	–	42 (45.2)	6 (37.5)	22 (23)	123 (22.1)	4 (76.9)	–
Pseudomonas aeruginosa	17 (39.5)	1 (20)	6 (6.5)	2 (12.5)	3 (3.1)	49 (8.8)	2 (15.3)	–
Other	2 (4.6)	–	4 (4.3)	1 (6.3)	1 (1)	31 (5.6)	1 (7.7)	–

Table 43.2 Non-exhaustive list of bacteria that cause disease in febrile neutropenic patients, with their possible sites of development

Gram-positive bacteria		*Site of infection*
	Coagulase-negative staphylococci	Bloodstream infections, catheter-associated sepsis
	Viridans group streptococci	Bloodstream infections, endocarditis
	Enterococcus faecium	Bloodstream infections, endocarditis
	E. faecalis	
	Stomatococcus mucilaginosus	Bloodstream infections, catheter-associated sepsis
	Pediococcus spp.	Urine and bloodstream infections
	Corynebacterium jeikeium	Endocarditis, catheter-related bacteremia, cutaneous lesions, and nodular pulmonary infiltrates
	Lactobacillus spp.	Bloodstream infections endocarditis, meningitis, intraabdominal abscesses, and pneumonia
	Rhodococcus equi	Suppurative pneumonia with pulmonary abscesses and empyema
	Clostridium septicum	Metastatic myonecrosis, typhlitis
Gram-negative bacteria		
	Pseudomonas aeruginosa	Pneumonia, bloodstream infections
	Escherichia coli, Klebsiella species, Enterobacter	Bloodstream infections, catheter-associated sepsis, and pneumonia
	Stenotrophomonas maltophilia	Pneumonia
	Alcaligenes xylosoxidans and *Burkholderia cepacia*	Catheter-associated sepsis
	Capnocytophaga species	Bloodstream infections in bone marrow transplant recipients
Anaerobes		
	Fusobacterium nucleatum	Bloodstream infections, ulcerative pharyngitis, and nodular pulmonary infiltrates due to septic emboli
	Leptotrichia buccalis	Bloodstream infections with extensive mucosal involvement in severely immunosuppressed patients
Mycobacteria		
	Mycobacterium chelonae	Pneumonia, disseminated infections
	M. fortuitum	

patients with neutropenia [31]. The initial assessment of patients with febrile neutropenia should include a careful physical examination for subtle signs and symptoms of infection, with special attention to the sinuses and oropharynx, skin and skin folds, intravenous lines, genital organs, and anal area [34]. Obtaining bacterial samples is crucial to ensure the detection and susceptibility testing of the causative pathogen. Most pathogens are isolated from blood cultures, which must be drawn both from the catheter and from a peripheral vein. Cultures of stool, urine, cerebrospinal fluid, and/or skin lesions should be performed as indicated by the clinical picture. Previous microbiological results should be considered, as carriage of multiresistant

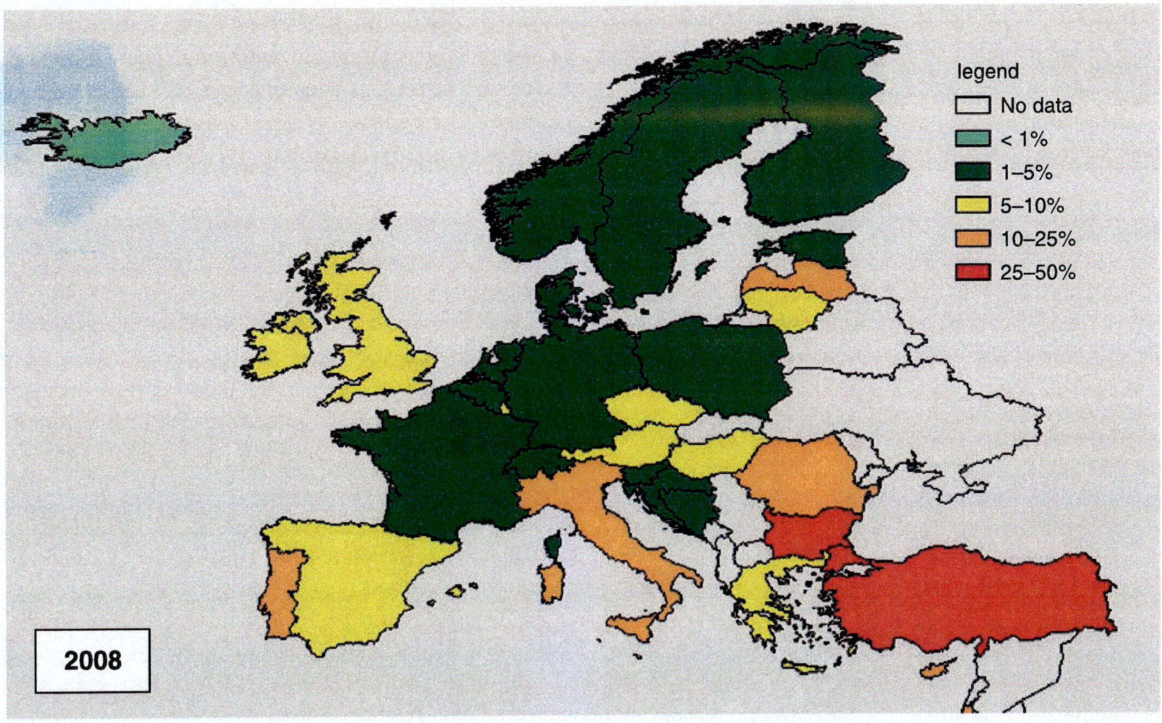

Fig. 43.1 Map showing the proportion of *Escherichia coli* strains resistant to third-generation cephalosporins in European countries participating in the European Antimicrobial Resistance Surveillance System database in 2008

strains may last several weeks or months. A chest radiograph should be obtained, and high-resolution computed tomography of the chest may be indicated if the patient has pulmonary symptoms with an uninformative chest radiograph or if an invasive mold infection is suspected. Finally, the choice of antibiotics should take into account the risk of complications of the underlying malignancy; nature of the treatment; degree, duration, and type of immunosuppression; and clinical presentation [31].

43.3.2 Choice of the First-Line Antibiotic Regimen

43.3.2.1 Site of Care and Route of Empirical Antibiotic Therapy

Oral antibiotic administration and home care may benefit selected patients by avoiding the risks associated with prolonged hospitalization (i.e., hospital-acquired infections and intravenous line-associated complications), while being cost-effective [35, 36]. However, this strategy is reserved for carefully selected patients at low risk for complications [18, 37]. Scores have been developed for identifying low-risk patients who may be eligible for oral treatment and either early discharge after initial stabilization in the hospital or outpatient care [10]. This strategy is widely used by hematologists and oncologists in the United States [38] and is supported by several large randomized studies and meta-analyses [38–43]. However, in-hospital intravenous antibiotic therapy is required in patients with factors that predict complications, such as hemodynamic instability, abdominal pain, nausea, and/or vomiting, diarrhea, neurological or mental changes, catheter-related infection, new pulmonary infiltrates, renal failure, or liver failure [31, 34, 44]. The Multinational Association for Supportive Care in Cancer (MASCC) predictive score, developed and validated prospectively in cancer patients, seems simple to use [10]. The score can range from 3 to 26 depending on age, outpatient status, acute clinical status, history, and disease severity. A score greater than 20 predicts a risk of severe complications lower than 10% (Table 43.3). Patients with a low risk of complications are eligible for

Table 43.3 The Multinational Association for Supportive Care in Cancer (MASCC) risk prediction model score. The points are added to obtain the total score. A total score >20 predicts a low risk (<10%) of serious medical complications during the course of febrile neutropenia

Characteristic	No. of points
Age <60 years	2
Outpatient at fever onset	3
No dehydration	3
Solid tumor or (in hematology patients) no previous fungal infection	4
No chronic obstructive pulmonary disease	4
No hypotension	5
Burden of underlying illness	
No symptoms	5
Mild symptoms	5
Moderate symptoms	3

home-based therapy and oral medication provided they can return immediately to the hospital in the event of a clinical deterioration, an inability to tolerate oral medications, or inadequate enteral absorption [37]. The best oral regimen recommended to date is the combination of a quinolone (e.g., ciprofloxacin) with amoxicillin/clavulanic acid [3]. Oral moxifloxacin seems promising [45], and oral cefixime has been proven effective in low-risk children with cancer [3].

43.3.2.2 Antibiotic Combinations

The advantages of combination therapy include coverage of a broad spectrum of pathogens and, theoretically, synergistic activity with a decrease in the emergence of resistant strains. The main downsides are ototoxicity and nephrotoxicity, most notably with aminoglycosides, and increased cost. It should be pointed out that nephrotoxicity may occur even with very short courses of aminoglycosides, particularly with multiple-dose regimens and in patients receiving or having received other toxic substances (e.g., cisplatin, ciclosporin, amphotericin B, colistin, acyclovir, or contrast media) [46, 47].

So far, no randomized study or metaanalysis has proven that adding an aminoglycoside or quinolone to a β-lactam is superior to using a broad-spectrum β-lactam alone. Given that *P. aeruginosa* is common and associated with high mortality rates in neutropenic patients [8], the empirical antibiotic regimen should cover this pathogen. Monotherapy with ceftazidime, cefepime, imipenem, or piperacillin/tazobactam was as effective as β-lactam/aminoglycoside combinations, even in the subset of bacteremic patients [48–50]. There are no studies of β-lactam/aminoglycoside combinations in critically ill patients. According to the recent guidelines issued by the European Conference on Infections in Leukemia, β-lactam-aminoglycoside combinations may be justified in patients with severe sepsis or septic shock and in those with suspected resistant gram-negative infections [51]. Fluoroquinolones are associated with the emergence of antibiotic-resistant pathogens, and their use in initial empirical regimens should therefore be discouraged, particularly in patients with a history of quinolone-based prophylaxis.

In febrile neutropenic patients, efficacy seems equivalent with β-lactam monotherapy, cefepime, piperacillin/tazobactam, and carbapenems [12, 45, 49, 52–57] (Table 43.4). Ceftazidime monotherapy may be an effective strategy [38, 58]. However, the limited activity of ceftazidime against gram-positive bacteria [59] is of concern in high-risk neutropenic patients, as streptococcal bacteremia is associated with high complication rates [60]. In a randomized study of 219 patients with acute leukemia or autologous peripheral-blood stem-cell transplantation, ceftazidime monotherapy was less effective than carbapenems (i.e., imipenem and meropenem) [10, 61], but as effective as piperacillin/tazobactam [12]. Although most broad-spectrum β-lactams (cefepime, piperacillin/tazobactam, and carbapenems) provide coverage against most gram-positive bacteria, some gram-positive organisms, such as *S. mitis*, methicillin-resistant *S. aureus*, *Enterococcus faecium*, and *Corynebacterium* species, may be resistant to β-lactams and susceptible only to glycopeptides (i.e., vancomycin and teicoplanin), quinupristin-dalfopristin, or linezolid. The appropriateness of adding vancomycin to a β-lactam has long been a matter of debate [62, 63]. Given the risk of emergence of resistant pathogens due to widespread vancomycin use [30] and the often relatively indolent course of infections due to the most commonly isolated resistant gram-positive organisms (i.e., CNS), routinely adding vancomycin to the first-line regimen is now strongly discouraged [3, 64]. In contrast, the vancomycin/β-lactam combination remains recommended for the first-line treatment

Table 43.4 Suggested dosages for empirical antibiotic therapy in high-risk adult neutropenic patients with normal renal function. The local bacterial ecology and patient's bacterial history must be considered when selecting empirical antibiotics

	Dosage	Targets for serum concentrations	
Cefepime	2 g iv every 8–12 h	Max. T>MIC (at least 70% of the dosing interval)	
Piperacillin–tazobactam[a]	4 g/500 mg iv every 6–8 h	Max. T>MIC (at least 70% of the dosing interval)	
Ceftazidime[a]	1–2 g every 8 h or 2 g loading dose followed by 6 g continuous iv infusion every 24 h	Max. T>MIC (at least 70% of the dosing interval)	
Imipenem[a]	500 mg every 6 h to 1 g iv every 6–8 h up to 50 mg/kg/day	Max. T>MIC (at least 70% of the dosing interval)	
Meropenem[a]	0.5–1 g iv infusion every 8 h	Max. T>MIC (at least 70% of the dosing interval)	
Amikacin[b]	15–20 mg/kg once daily for seriously ill patients: 25–30 mg/kg once daily	Peak/MIC ratio >8–10	Peak: 64–80 μg/mL Trough <2.5 μg/mL
Gentamicin[b] tobramycin[b]	3–5 mg/kg iv once daily for seriously ill patients: 7–8 mg/kg iv once daily	Peak/MIC ratio >8–10	Peak: 32–40 μg/mL Trough <0.5 μg/mL
Vancomycin[b]	15–20 mg/kg ¤ given every 8–12 h for seriously ill patients: loading dose of 25–30 mg/kg or loading dose of 15 mg/kg iv followed by 30–60 mg/kg continuous iv infusion every 24 h	Optimal 24 h AUC/MIC ratio >400	Trough: >15–20 mg/L, 25–35 mg/L if severe infection Always >10 mg/L to avoid the development of resistance
Teicoplanin[b]	6–12 mg/kg every 12 h iv from day 1 to 4 followed by 6–12 mg/kg every 24 h	Optimal 24 h AUC/MIC ratio >400	Trough: 20–30 mg/L
Ciprofloxacin[a]	400 mg every 8–12 h	Optimal 24 h AUC/MIC ratio ~125 for gram-negative bacteria. Optimal 24 h AUC/MIC ratio ~40 for gram-positive bacteria	
Colimycin	75,000 to 150,000 IU/kg (2.5–5 mg/kg colistin base) every 24 h in 3 divided doses		

[a]Note that the highest suggested dosage is active against *Pseudomonas aeruginosa*

[b]Routine determination of trough serum levels is required. For aminoglycosides, renal impairment may occur after a few days of treatment; therefore, treatment duration should be limited to 48–72 h and should not exceed 5 days. Multiple daily doses of aminoglycosides are discouraged, since this regimen does not reduce toxicity and cannot provide sufficient peak serum concentrations; peak concentration should be determined 30 min after the end of the infusion and trough concentration just before the next infusion. For vancomycin, trough serum concentrations should be obtained just before the fourth dose. There is no evidence that continuous infusion regimens improve patient outcomes. The recommended infusion rate is 0.5–1 g/h. Monitoring of trough serum vancomycin concentrations is recommended in patients receiving aggressive dose targeting, in patients with unstable renal function and in patients receiving concurrent treatment with nephrotoxic agents; ¤should be calculated based on actual body weight; *iv*, intravenous

of patients with severe sepsis or septic shock and of patients at high risk for infection by antibiotic-resistant gram-positive cocci [3] (Table 43.4). In a randomized controlled study of neutropenic patients with cancer, linezolid and vancomycin produced similar outcomes [65]. Quinupristin-dalfopristin and daptomycin have not been specifically assessed in patients with neutropenia. The limited data on linezolid and the bacteriostatic activity of this drug are of concern when treating neutropenic patients.

In all likelihood, no guidelines of universal relevance can be developed. Instead, the global epidemiology of bacterial infections should be considered in conjunction with local rates of pathogen isolation and resistance. The patient's own ecology should be considered also. Valuable information can be garnered from a review of previous anterior nasal and rectal swabs, which may have shown colonization by antibiotic-resistant bacteria (e.g. methicillin-resistant *S. aureus*, *P. aeruginosa*, multidrug-resistant gram-negative bacilli, and vancomycin-resistant enterococci). A history of infection should raise the possibility of a recurrence and should prompt the use of antibiotics active against the pathogen involved. Finally, renal and hepatic function and the risk of allergies may influence the choice of the first-line antibiotics.

43.3.3 Adapting the Antibiotics: Treatment Duration

Failure to respond to empirical therapy is defined as persistent fever and the development of serious medical complications. The median time to defervescence in hospitalized patients with cancer is 5–7 days, although low-risk patients often respond within 2 days or less [3]. International guidelines recommend a reassessment of the initial antibiotic regimen after 3–5 days if the fever persists [3]. Persistence of fever with clinical deterioration or infectious disease progression should be distinguished from persistence of fever in a clinically stable patient. Patients whose clinical status deteriorates require a complete reassessment, including a careful physical examination and the collection of new culture specimens to look for a second infection. Ultrasonography and high-resolution computed tomography should be performed as indicated by the clinical data, and the indwelling catheter should be removed if a catheter-related infection is proven or strongly suspected. If a resistant pathogen is isolated or suspected to be responsible for the deterioration (i.e., if present in a recent stool culture) and is not covered by initial empirical regimen, the treatment should be modified promptly. Empirical addition of a glycopeptide, if not used initially, may be warranted, and switching to a carbapenem as second-line therapy should be considered (Fig. 43.2). Finally, empirical addition of antifungal agents deserves consideration in patients who have risk factors for fungal infection [3, 64, 66]. The management of antifungal therapy is beyond the scope of this chapter, but readers can refer to specific reviews on this topic [67–69]. For clinically stable patients with persistent fever, there is no published evidence supporting a change in the antibiotic regimen. Moreover, the widespread emergence of multiresistant and panresistant bacterial strains should discourage "escalating" strategies, such as switching from piperacillin-tazobactam or cefepime to a carbapenem or adding vancomycin [63]. When a causative pathogen is identified, the antibiotic regimen should be adapted based on the antibiotic susceptibility test results. The dwindling number of drugs in the pharmaceutical pipeline and the increased incidence of multidrug-resistant bacteria have led to the increasing use of old antibiotics such as colistin. Colistin exhibits rapid and concentration-dependent bactericidal activity with relatively low rates of resistance. Good rates of clinical responses have been reported in patients infected with multidrug-resistant bacteria and treated with intravenous colistin as salvage therapy. Colistin may act synergistically with rifampin or carbapenems against metallo-β-lactamase-producing (MBL) *K. pneumoniae* or *A. baumannii* strains. However, these data on colistin come chiefly from nonrandomized studies in small numbers of patients. Although the manufacturer recommends not exceeding six million units per day, a growing number of clinicians now routinely use daily dosages of up to nine million IU in two to four divided doses (12,500 IU of colistin is equivalent to 1 mg of the prodrug colistin methanesulfonate). Inhalational colistin therapy has long been used in patients with cystic fibrosis and is now given to critically ill patients with ventilator-associated pneumonia. However, we have very little information on colistin pharmacokinetics and pharmacodynamics, especially in critically ill patients. Nephrotoxicity associated with the use of colistin remains a matter of concern. In vitro studies have shown that the toxic effects of colistin on mammalian cells are concentration-dependent and time-dependent. Colistin nephrotoxicity seems rare in young patients with normal renal function

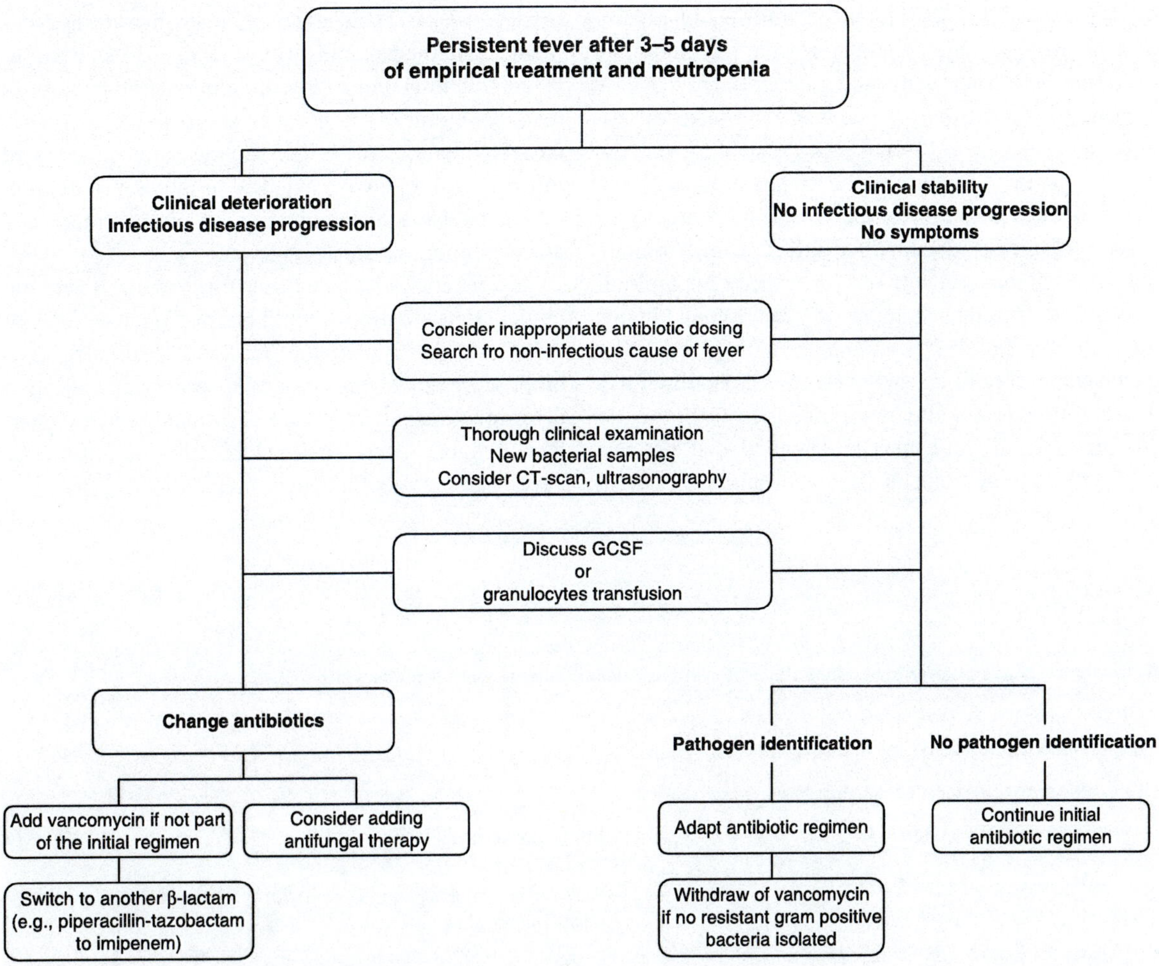

Fig. 43.2 Suggested adjustments to the empirical antibiotic regimen in patients with persistent fever after 3–5 days of treatment

and common in patients with underlying renal insufficiency. The risk may depend on the cumulative dose. Colistin nephrotoxicity is usually mild and almost always reversible within a few weeks or months after treatment discontinuation.

When no antibiotic-resistant gram-positive bacteria are isolated, withdrawal of glycopeptides is warranted and may limit the emergence of vancomycin-resistant enterococci and the risk of nephrotoxicity [20, 39]. Similarly, de-escalation (e.g., switching from carbapenem to cefepime or piperacillin-tazobactam) should be encouraged when no microorganism resistant to the first-line regimen is isolated.

In patients with sustained bacteremia and/or persistent fever and clinical deterioration, a portal of entry requiring specific treatment should be sought. Necrotizing cellulitis or peritonitis requires surgery. One of the most common problems is deciding whether to remove the indwelling central venous catheter in bacteremic patients. The decision rests on the clinical presentation (septic shock, local tunnel, or port infection), pathogen, presence of intestinal colonization, and differential time to blood culture positivity of samples drawn simultaneously by phlebotomy and through the catheter. In patients with bacteremia due to *Enterobacteriaceae*, enterococci or *Pseudomonas*, with no local signs of catheter infection or septic shock, the conjunction of intestinal colonization and microbial growth in peripheral blood before or within 2 h after growth in a sample obtained simultaneously from the catheter hub often indicates bacterial translocation from the intestine [70, 71]. Further information regarding the management of catheter-related infections can be found in recently published guidelines [72].

Current guidelines recommend continued intravenous administration of antibiotics after 48 h of apyrexia for at least 2 days after neutropenia resolution or for 4–5 days if the fever persists [3]. Clinically or microbiologically documented infection may require longer treatment, but with narrower spectrum antibiotics (i.e., a neutropenic patient who has bacteremia due to multisusceptible *E. coli* treated with piperacillin-tazobactam should be switched to amoxicillin for a few additional days after neutrophil recovery).

International guidelines recommend that patients with persistent neutropenia be kept on antibiotics for at least 2 weeks. Then, if no infection has been documented and the patient is free of significant symptoms, discontinuation under close monitoring can be considered. This time frame may be shortened to 7 days in closely monitored low-risk patients with no signs of infection, who may be switched to the oral route after 48–72 h, using a combination of ciprofloxacin and amoxicillin-clavulanic acid.

All patients with persistent fever, with or without clinical deterioration, should be investigated for noninfectious causes of fever (Table 43.5). Finally, antibiotic dose adjustment based on serum concentration determination may be required, as changes in the pharmacodynamics and pharmacokinetics of antibiotics have been reported in neutropenic patients [73–75].

Table 43.5 Causes of fever persistence after initial empirical antibiotic in neutropenic patients

Infectious causes of persistent fever	
Inappropriate antibiotic dosing and concentration	
Clostridium difficile-induced diarrhea	
Antibiotic-resistant pathogen	Multidrug-resistant bacteria Mycobacteria Fastidious pathogens (e.g., *Legionella, Mycoplasma, Chlamydia pneumoniae, Bartonella*)
Fungal infection	Molds: *Aspergillus* and Mucormycosis Yeasts: *Candida* and *Cryptococcus*
Parasitic infection	For example, *Toxoplasma gondii*
Viral infection	For example, herpesviruses (cytomegalovirus, Epstein–Barr virus, human herpesvirus 6, varicella-zoster virus, herpes simplex virus) parainfluenza virus, respiratory syncytial virus, influenza viruses
Persistent focus of infection (e.g., catheter)	
Uncontrolled infection (e.g., endocarditis or peritonitis)	
Noninfectious causes of persistent fever	
Transfusion-related fever	
Hemophagocytic lymphohistiocytosis	
Venous thrombosis	
Drug- or transfusion-induced fever	
Graft-versus-host disease	
Underlying malignancy	
Pancreatitis	

43.4 Pharmacodynamic and Pharmacokinetic Considerations

The pharmacokinetics and pharmacodynamics of many antibiotics are modified in neutropenic [73] and/or critically ill patients [76]. The volumes of distribution and clearance are increased, and therefore the half-life and plasma concentrations may be lower than in control patients.

Many animal studies found decreases in the bactericidal activity of β-lactams in neutropenic animals. Given that the activity of β-lactams and glycopeptides depends on the time spent with serum drug concentrations greater than the minimum inhibitory concentration of the organism, decreasing the interval between doses or using a continuous infusion may be the best strategy for administering β-lactams and glycopeptides to neutropenic patients. In any case, therapeutic drug monitoring is valuable for guiding dosage adjustments and ensuring that therapeutic concentrations are achieved in order to increase the chances of eradicating the organism and to minimize the risk of selecting antibiotic-resistant bacteria [73, 75, 77]. Serum vancomycin and teicoplanin levels should be monitored routinely [74]. In neutropenic patients receiving the recommended 2 g/day dose of imipenem, many may have serum concentrations below the therapeutic range [77]. When using carbapenems in neutropenic patients, 50–60% of the dosing interval must be spent above the minimum inhibitory concentration to achieve bactericidal activity, and success rates improve when 75–100% of the dosing interval is spent above the minimum inhibitory concentration [77–79]. Plasma carbapenem levels can be measured using high-performance liquid chromatography in patients with persistent fever to ensure that the plasma concentrations are within the therapeutic range.

Aminoglycosides, in contrast, have a concentration-dependent bactericidal activity. Elimination of aminoglycosides is highly dependent on renal clearance, and accumulation is likely to occur in patients with renal failure. Once-daily administration of aminoglycosides is often preferred over multiple daily dosing to reduce the risk of nephrotoxicity and is recommended in the few neutropenic patients who require an aminoglycoside in combination with a wide-spectrum β-lactam [64]. When using aminoglycosides, therapeutic drug monitoring is important to minimize the risk of renal and cochlear/vestibular toxicity [75]. A recently published review is available for readers who wish to have further information on antibiotic pharmacokinetics and pharmacodynamics in neutropenic patients [73].

43.5 Prophylactic Antibiotics

Two recent large randomized double-blind placebo-controlled trials and one meta-analysis found that prophylactic antibiotics given to cancer patients diminished the numbers of febrile episodes and bacterial infections, the use of empirical antibiotics and possibly mortality rates [80–82]. Based on these studies and others, the guidelines issued by the European Conference on Infections in Leukemia recommend prophylactic ciprofloxacin or levofloxacin therapy in neutropenic patients with acute leukaemia or in recipients of haematopoietic stem cell transplantation. [64]. However, many centers still do not give quinolone prophylaxis to patients with afebrile neutropenia because of concerns about the emergence of antibiotic resistance in the long run [28, 83]. The selection of resistant organisms by quinolones is a serious hazard, as reemphasized recently [84]. The emergence of resistant strains should therefore be monitored in centers where quinolone-based prophylaxis is used [20, 85].

43.6 Conclusion

Antibiotic therapy must be initiated promptly in febrile neutropenic patients. Oral antibiotics can be used in carefully selected low-risk patients. In high-risk patients, initial empirical treatment with a single antibiotic is recommended. The antibiotic should be selected based on the initial clinical assessment, bacterial ecology in the hospital, and bacterial history of the patient. The use of vancomycin should be reserved for patients with suspected methicillin-resistant gram-positive infections and/or signs of severe sepsis or septic shock. There is no evidence to support adding an aminoglycoside to most of the extended-spectrum β-lactams in non-critically ill patients. Persistent fever requires adaptation of the initial antibiotic regimen if the clinical condition deteriorates or if a resistant pathogen is isolated. Addition of an antifungal agent must be considered. Giving the growing emergence of multidrug-resistant bacteria, the implementation of antibiotic stewardship programs is now mandatory.

References

1. Pene F, Percheron S, Lemiale V, Viallon V, Claessens YE, Marque S, Charpentier J, Angus DC, Cariou A, Chiche JD, Mira JP (2008) Temporal changes in management and outcome of septic shock in patients with malignancies in the intensive care unit. Crit Care Med 36:690–696
2. Thiery G, Azoulay E, Darmon M, Ciroldi M, De Miranda S, Levy V, Fieux F, Moreau D, Le Gall JR, Schlemmer B (2005) Outcome of cancer patients considered for intensive care unit admission: a hospital-wide prospective study. J Clin Oncol 23:4406–4413
3. Hughes WT, Armstrong D, Bodey GP, Bow EJ, Brown AE, Calandra T, Feld R, Pizzo PA, Rolston KV, Shenep JL, Young LS (2002) 2002 guidelines for the use of antimicrobial agents in neutropenic patients with cancer. Clin Infect Dis 34:730–751
4. Buchheidt D, Bohme A, Cornely OA, Fatkenheuer G, Fuhr HG, Heussel G, Junghanss C, Karthaus M, Kellner O, Kern WV, Schiel X, Sezer O, Sudhoff T, Szelenyi H (2003) Diagnosis and treatment of documented infections in neutropenic patients – recommendations of the Infectious Diseases Working Party (AGIHO) of the German Society of Hematology and Oncology (DGHO). Ann Hematol 82 (Suppl 2):S127–S132
5. Wisplinghoff H, Bischoff T, Tallent SM, Seifert H, Wenzel RP, Edmond MB (2004) Nosocomial bloodstream infections in US hospitals: analysis of 24, 179 cases from a prospective nationwide surveillance study. Clin Infect Dis 39:309–317
6. Zinner SH (1999) Changing epidemiology of infections in patients with neutropenia and cancer: emphasis on gram-positive and resistant bacteria. Clin Infect Dis 29:490–494
7. Du B, Long Y, Liu H, Chen D, Liu D, Xu Y, Xie X (2002) Extended-spectrum beta-lactamase-producing Escherichia coli and Klebsiella pneumoniae bloodstream infection: risk factors and clinical outcome. Intensive Care Med 28: 1718–1723
8. Carratala J, Roson B, Fernandez-Sevilla A, Alcaide F, Gudiol F (1998) Bacteremic pneumonia in neutropenic patients with cancer: causes, empirical antibiotic therapy, and outcome. Arch Intern Med 158:868–872
9. Gruson D, Hilbert G, Portel L, Boiron JM, Bebear CM, Vargas F, Bebear C, Reiffers J, Gbikpi-Benissan G, Cardinaud JP (1999) Severe respiratory failure requiring ICU admission in bone marrow transplant recipients. Eur Respir J 13:883–887
10. Klastersky J, Paesmans M, Rubenstein EB, Boyer M, Elting L, Feld R, Gallagher J, Herrstedt J, Rapoport B, Rolston K, Talcott J (2000) The Multinational Association for Supportive Care in Cancer risk index: A multinational scoring system for identifying low-risk febrile neutropenic cancer patients. J Clin Oncol 18:3038–3051
11. Regazzoni CJ, Khoury M, Irrazabal C, Myburg C, Galvalisi NR, O'Flaherty M, Sarquis SG, Poderoso JJ (2003) Neutropenia and the development of the systemic inflammatory response syndrome. Intensive Care Med 29:135–138
12. Harter C, Schulze B, Goldschmidt H, Benner A, Geiss HK, Hoppe-Tichy T, Ho AD, Egerer G (2006) Piperacillin/tazobactam vs ceftazidime in the treatment of neutropenic fever in patients with acute leukemia or following autologous peripheral blood stem cell transplantation: a prospective randomized trial. Bone Marrow Transplant 37: 373–379
13. Klastersky J, Ameye L, Maertens J, Georgala A, Muanza F, Aoun M, Ferrant A, Rapoport B, Rolston K, Paesmans M (2007) Bacteraemia in febrile neutropenic cancer patients. Int J Antimicrob Agents 30(Suppl 1):S51–S59
14. Metallidis S, Kollaras P, Giannakakis T, Seitanidis B, Kordosis T, Nikolaidis J, Hatzitolios A, Nikolaidis P (2008) A prospective, controlled, randomized, non-blind, comparative study of the efficacy and safety of a once daily high dose of ceftriaxone plus ciprofloxacin versus thrice daily ceftazidime plus amikacin in empirical therapy for febrile neutropenic patients. Eur J Intern Med 19:619–624
15. de la Rubia J, Montesinos P, Martino R, Jarque I, Rovira M, Vazquez L, Lopez J, Batlle M, de la Camara R, Julia A, Lahuerta JJ, Deben G, Diaz J, Garcia R, Sanz MA (2009) Imipenem/cilastatin with or without glycopeptide as initial antibiotic therapy for recipients of autologous stem cell transplantation: results of a Spanish multicenter study. Biol Blood Marrow Transplant 15:512–516
16. Rolston KV (2005) Challenges in the treatment of infections caused by gram-positive and gram-negative bacteria in patients with cancer and neutropenia. Clin Infect Dis 40(Suppl 4):S246–S252
17. Ramzi J, Mohamed Z, Yosr B, Karima K, Raihane B, Lamia A, Hela BA, Zaher B, Balkis M (2007) Predictive factors of septic shock and mortality in neutropenic patients. Hematology 12:543–548
18. Kamana M, Escalante C, Mullen CA, Frisbee-Hume S, Rolston KV (2005) Bacterial infections in low-risk, febrile neutropenic patients. Cancer 104:422–426
19. Chu VH, Woods CW, Miro JM, Hoen B, Cabell CH, Pappas PA, Federspiel J, Athan E, Stryjewski ME, Nacinovich F, Marco F, Levine DP, Elliott TS, Fortes CQ, Tornos P, Gordon DL, Utili R, Delahaye F, Corey GR, Fowler VG Jr (2008) Emergence of coagulase-negative staphylococci as a cause of native valve endocarditis. Clin Infect Dis 46: 232–242
20. Ramphal R (2004) Changes in the etiology of bacteremia in febrile neutropenic patients and the susceptibilities of the currently isolated pathogens. Clin Infect Dis 39(Suppl 1): S25–S31
21. Irfan S, Idrees F, Mehraj V, Habib F, Adil S, Hasan R (2008) Emergence of carbapenem resistant gram negative and vancomycin resistant gram positive organisms in bacteremic isolates of febrile neutropenic patients: a descriptive study. BMC Infect Dis 8:80
22. Kanamaru A, Tatsumi Y (2004) Microbiological data for patients with febrile neutropenia. Clin Infect Dis 39(Suppl 1):S7–S10

23. Tumbarello M, Sanguinetti M, Montuori E, Trecarichi EM, Posteraro B, Fiori B, Citton R, D'Inzeo T, Fadda G, Cauda R, Spanu T (2007) Predictors of mortality in patients with bloodstream infections caused by extended-spectrum-beta-lactamase-producing Enterobacteriaceae: importance of inadequate initial antimicrobial treatment. Antimicrob Agents Chemother 51:1987–1994
24. Moland ES, Black JA, Ourada J, Reisbig MD, Hanson ND, Thomson KS (2002) Occurrence of newer beta-lactamases in *Klebsiella pneumoniae* isolates from 24 US hospitals. Antimicrob Agents Chemother 46:3837–3842
25. Rodriguez-Bano J, Picon E, Gijon P, Hernandez JR, Ruiz M, Pena C, Almela M, Almirante B, Grill F, Colomina J, Gimenez M, Oliver A, Horcajada JP, Navarro G, Coloma A, Pascual A (2010) Community-onset bacteremia due to extended-spectrum beta-lactamase-producing *Escherichia coli*: risk factors and prognosis. Clin Infect Dis 50:40–48
26. Cuzon G, Naas T, Nordmann P (2010) KPC carbapenemases: what issue in clinical microbiology? Pathol Biol (Paris) 58:39–45
27. Kern WV, Steib-Bauert M, de With K, Reuter S, Bertz H, Frank U, von Baum H (2005) Fluoroquinolone consumption and resistance in haematology–oncology patients: ecological analysis in two university hospitals 1999–2002. J Antimicrob Chemother 55:57–60
28. Cattaneo C, Quaresmini G, Casari S, Capucci MA, Micheletti M, Borlenghi E, Signorini L, Re A, Carosi G, Rossi G (2008) Recent changes in bacterial epidemiology and the emergence of fluoroquinolone-resistant *Escherichia coli* among patients with haematological malignancies: results of a prospective study on 823 patients at a single institution. J Antimicrob Chemother 61:721–728
29. Razonable RR, Litzow MR, Khaliq Y, Piper KE, Rouse MS, Patel R (2002) Bacteremia due to viridans group Streptococci with diminished susceptibility to Levofloxacin among neutropenic patients receiving levofloxacin prophylaxis. Clin Infect Dis 34:1469–1474
30. DiazGranados CA, Jernigan JA (2005) Impact of vancomycin resistance on mortality among patients with neutropenia and enterococcal bloodstream infection. J Infect Dis 191: 588–595
31. Klastersky J (2004) Management of fever in neutropenic patients with different risks of complications. Clin Infect Dis 39(Suppl 1):S32–S37
32. European Antimicrobial Resistance surveillance System (2008) http://www.rivm.nl/earss/database/
33. Mebis J, Goossens H, Berneman ZN (2010) Antibiotic management of febrile neutropenia: current developments and future directions. J Chemother 22:5–12.
34. Kern WV (2001) Risk assessment and risk-based therapeutic strategies in febrile neutropenia. Curr Opin Infect Dis 14:415–422
35. Innes H, Lim SL, Hall A, Chan SY, Bhalla N, Marshall E (2008) Management of febrile neutropenia in solid tumours and lymphomas using the Multinational Association for Supportive Care in Cancer (MASCC) risk index: feasibility and safety in routine clinical practice. Support Care Cancer 16:485–491
36. Klastersky J, Paesmans M, Georgala A, Muanza F, Plehiers B, Dubreucq L, Lalami Y, Aoun M, Barette M (2006) Outpatient oral antibiotics for febrile neutropenic cancer patients using a score predictive for complications. J Clin Oncol 24:4129–4134
37. Kern WV (2006) Risk assessment and treatment of low-risk patients with febrile neutropenia. Clin Infect Dis 42: 533–540
38. Freifeld A, Marchigiani D, Walsh T, Chanock S, Lewis L, Hiemenz J, Hiemenz S, Hicks JE, Gill V, Steinberg SM, Pizzo PA (1999) A double-blind comparison of empirical oral and intravenous antibiotic therapy for low-risk febrile patients with neutropenia during cancer chemotherapy. N Engl J Med 341:305–311
39. Paul M, Borok S, Fraser A, Vidal L, Cohen M, Leibovici L (2005) Additional anti-gram-positive antibiotic treatment for febrile neutropenic cancer patients. Cochrane Database Syst Rev CD003914
40. Minotti V, Gentile G, Bucaneve G, Iori AP, Micozzi A, Cavicchi F, Barbabietola G, Landonio G, Menichetti F, Martino P, Del Favero A (1999) Domiciliary treatment of febrile episodes in cancer patients: a prospective randomized trial comparing oral versus parenteral empirical antibiotic treatment. Support Care Cancer 7:134–139
41. Hidalgo M, Hornedo J, Lumbreras C, Trigo JM, Colomer R, Perea S, Gomez C, Ruiz A, Garcia-Carbonero R, Cortes-Funes H (1999) Outpatient therapy with oral ofloxacin for patients with low risk neutropenia and fever: a prospective, randomized clinical trial. Cancer 85:213–219
42. Gupta A, Swaroop C, Agarwala S, Pandey RM, Bakhshi S (2009) Randomized controlled trial comparing oral amoxicillin-clavulanate and ofloxacin with intravenous ceftriaxone and amikacin as outpatient therapy in pediatric low-risk febrile neutropenia. J Pediatr Hematol Oncol 31:635–641
43. Malik IA, Abbas Z, Karim M (1992) Randomised comparison of oral ofloxacin alone with combination of parenteral antibiotics in neutropenic febrile patients. Lancet 339: 1092–1096
44. Sipsas NV, Bodey GP, Kontoyiannis DP (2005) Perspectives for the management of febrile neutropenic patients with cancer in the 21st century. Cancer 103:1103–1113
45. Sebban C, Dussart S, Fuhrmann C, Ghesquieres H, Rodrigues I, Geoffrois L, Devaux Y, Lancry L, Chvetzoff G, Bachelot T, Chelghoum M, Biron P (2008) Oral moxifloxacin or intravenous ceftriaxone for the treatment of low-risk neutropenic fever in cancer patients suitable for early hospital discharge. Support Care Cancer 16:1017–1023
46. Cosgrove SE, Vigliani GA, Fowler VG Jr, Abrutyn E, Corey GR, Levine DP, Rupp ME, Chambers HF, Karchmer AW, Boucher HW (2009) Initial low-dose gentamicin for *Staphylococcus aureus* bacteremia and endocarditis is nephrotoxic. Clin Infect Dis 48:713–721
47. Bayer AS, Murray BE (2009) Initial low-dose aminoglycosides in *Staphylococcus aureus* bacteremia: good science, urban legend, or just plain toxic? Clin Infect Dis 48: 722–724
48. Cometta A, Calandra T, Gaya H, Zinner SH, de Bock R, Del Favero A, Bucaneve G, Crokaert F, Kern WV, Klastersky J, Langenaeken I, Micozzi A, Padmos A, Paesmans M, Viscoli C, Glauser MP, The International Antimicrobial Therapy Cooperative Group of the European Organization for Research and Treatment of Cancer, The Gruppo Italiano Malattie Ematologiche Maligne dell'Adulto Infection Program (1996) Monotherapy with meropenem versus com-

bination therapy with ceftazidime plus amikacin as empiric therapy for fever in granulocytopenic patients with cancer. Antimicrob Agents Chemother 40:1108–1115

49. De Pauw BE, Deresinski SC, Feld R, Lane-Allman EF, Donnelly JP, The Intercontinental Antimicrobial Study Group (1994) Ceftazidime compared with piperacillin and tobramycin for the empiric treatment of fever in neutropenic patients with cancer. A multicenter randomized trial. Ann Intern Med 120:834–844
50. Del Favero A, Menichetti F, Martino P, Bucaneve G, Micozzi A, Gentile G, Furno P, Russo D, D'Antonio D, Ricci P, Martino B, Mandelli F (2001) A multicenter, double-blind, placebo-controlled trial comparing piperacillin-tazobactam with and without amikacin as empiric therapy for febrile neutropenia. Clin Infect Dis 33:1295–1301
51. Cordonnier C, Thiebaut A, Ribaud P, Gachot B, Herbrecht R (2008) Résumé des premières et seconde conférences de l'ECIL (*European Conference on Infections in Leukemia*) à propos de la prise en charge des infections bactériennes et fongiques chez les patients leucémiques. Hématologie14:406–19.
52. Bow EJ, Rotstein C, Noskin GA, Laverdiere M, Schwarer AP, Segal BH, Seymour JF, Szer J, Sanche S (2006) A randomized, open-label, multicenter comparative study of the efficacy and safety of piperacillin-tazobactam and cefepime for the empirical treatment of febrile neutropenic episodes in patients with hematologic malignancies. Clin Infect Dis 43:447–459
53. Cometta A, Zinner S, de Bock R, Calandra T, Gaya H, Klastersky J, Langenaeken J, Paesmans M, Viscoli C, The International Antimicrobial Therapy Cooperative Group of the European Organization for Research and Treatment of Cancer (1995) Glauser MP: piperacillin-tazobactam plus amikacin versus ceftazidime plus amikacin as empiric therapy for fever in granulocytopenic patients with cancer. Antimicrob Agents Chemother 39:445–452
54. Viscoli C, Cometta A, Kern WV, Bock R, Paesmans M, Crokaert F, Glauser MP, Calandra T (2006) Piperacillin-tazobactam monotherapy in high-risk febrile and neutropenic cancer patients. Clin Microbiol Infect 12:212–216
55. Paul M, Yahav D, Fraser A, Leibovici L (2006) Empirical antibiotic monotherapy for febrile neutropenia: systematic review and meta-analysis of randomized controlled trials. J Antimicrob Chemother 57:176–189
56. Shah PM, Heller A, Fuhr HG, Walther F, Halir S, Schaumann R, Bohme A, Jung B, Kohler A, Lips-Schulte C, Stille W (1996) Empirical monotherapy with meropenem versus imipenem/cilastatin for febrile episodes in neutropenic patients. Infection 24:480–484
57. Gorschluter M, Hahn C, Fixson A, Mey U, Ziske C, Molitor E, Horre R, Sauerbruch T, Marklein G, Schmidt-Wolf IG, Glasmacher A (2003) Piperacillin-tazobactam is more effective than ceftriaxone plus gentamicin in febrile neutropenic patients with hematological malignancies: a randomized comparison. Support Care Cancer 11:362–370
58. Vandercam B, Gerain J, Humblet Y, Ferrant A, Wauters G, Moreau M, Longueville J, Symann M, Straetmans N (2000) Meropenem versus ceftazidime as empirical monotherapy for febrile neutropenic cancer patients. Ann Hematol 79:152–157
59. Diekema DJ, Coffman SL, Marshall SA, Beach ML, Rolston KV, Jones RN (1999) Comparison of activities of broad-spectrum beta-lactam compounds against 1, 128 gram-positive cocci recently isolated in cancer treatment centers. Antimicrob Agents Chemother 43:940–943
60. Han XY, Kamana M, Rolston KV (2006) Viridans streptococci isolated by culture from blood of cancer patients: clinical and microbiologic analysis of 50 cases. J Clin Microbiol 44:160–165
61. Liang R, Yung R, Chiu E, Chau PY, Chan TK, Lam WK, Todd D (1990) Ceftazidime versus imipenem-cilastatin as initial monotherapy for febrile neutropenic patients. Antimicrob Agents Chemother 34:1336–1341
62. Raad II, Escalante C, Hachem RY, Hanna HA, Husni R, Afif C, Boktour MR, Whimbey EE, Kontoyiannis D, Jacobson K, Kantarjian H, Levett LM, Rolston KV (2003) Treatment of febrile neutropenic patients with cancer who require hospitalization: a prospective randomized study comparing imipenem and cefepime. Cancer 98:1039–1047
63. Cometta A, Kern WV, De Bock R, Paesmans M, Vandenbergh M, Crokaert F, Engelhard D, Marchetti O, Akan H, Skoutelis A, Korten V, Vandercam M, Gaya H, Padmos A, Klastersky J, Zinner S, Glauser MP, Calandra T, Viscoli C (2003) Vancomycin versus placebo for treating persistent fever in patients with neutropenic cancer receiving piperacillin-tazobactam monotherapy. Clin Infect Dis 37:382–389
64. Meunier F, Lukan C (2008) The first european conference on infections in leukaemia – ECIL1: a current perspective. Eur J Cancer 44:2112–2117
65. Jaksic B, Martinelli G, Perez-Oteyza J, Hartman CS, Leonard LB, Tack KJ (2006) Efficacy and safety of linezolid compared with vancomycin in a randomized, double-blind study of febrile neutropenic patients with cancer. Clin Infect Dis 42:597–607
66. Maertens J, Marchetti O, Herbrecht R, Cornely OA, Flückiger U, Frêre P, Gachot B, Heinz WJ, Lass-Flörl C, Ribaud P, Thiebaut A, Cordonnier C (2010) European guidelines for antifungal management in leukemia and hematopoietic stem cell transplant recipients: summary of the ECIL 3-2009 Update. Bone Marrow Transplant (in press).
67. Almyroudis NG, Segal BH (2009) Prevention and treatment of invasive fungal diseases in neutropenic patients. Curr Opin Infect Dis 22:385–393
68. Ruping MJ, Vehreschild JJ, Cornely OA (2008) Patients at high risk of invasive fungal infections: when and how to treat. Drugs 68:1941–1962
69. Spanakis EK, Aperis G, Mylonakis E (2006) New agents for the treatment of fungal infections: clinical efficacy and gaps in coverage. Clin Infect Dis 43:1060–1068
70. Raad I, Hanna H, Maki D (2007) Intravascular catheter-related infections: advances in diagnosis, prevention, and management. Lancet Infect Dis 7:645–657
71. Blot F, Nitenberg G, Chachaty E, Raynard B, Germann N, Antoun S, Laplanche A, Brun-Buisson C, Tancrede C (1999) Diagnosis of catheter-related bacteraemia: a prospective comparison of the time to positivity of hub-blood versus peripheral-blood cultures. Lancet 354:1071–1077
72. Mermel LA, Allon M, Bouza E, Craven DE, Flynn P, O'Grady NP, Raad II, Rijnders BJ, Sherertz RJ, Warren DK (2009) Clinical practice guidelines for the diagnosis and management of intravascular catheter-related infection: 2009 Update by the Infectious Diseases Society of America. Clin Infect Dis 49:1–45

73. Lortholary O, Lefort A, Tod M, Chomat AM, Darras-Joly C, Cordonnier C (2008) Pharmacodynamics and pharmacokinetics of antibacterial drugs in the management of febrile neutropenia. Lancet Infect Dis 8:612–620
74. Rybak MJ, Lomaestro BM, Rotscahfer JC, Moellering RC, Craig WA, Billeter M, Dalovisio JR, Levine DP (2009) Vancomycin therapeutic guidelines: a summary of consensus recommendations from the infectious diseases Society of America, the American Society of Health-System Pharmacists, and the Society of Infectious Diseases Pharmacists. Clin Infect Dis 49:325–327
75. Bartal C, Danon A, Schlaeffer F, Reisenberg K, Alkan M, Smoliakov R, Sidi A, Almog Y (2003) Pharmacokinetic dosing of aminoglycosides: a controlled trial. Am J Med 114:194–198
76. Roberts JA, Lipman J (2009) Pharmacokinetic issues for antibiotics in the critically ill patient. Crit Care Med 37:840–851, quiz 859
77. Lamoth F, Buclin T, Pascual A, Calandra T, Marchetti O (2009) Imipenem underdosing as a cause of persistent neutropenic fever? J Antimicrob Chemother 64:665–667
78. Ariano RE, Nyhlen A, Donnelly JP, Sitar DS, Harding GK, Zelenitsky SA (2005) Pharmacokinetics and pharmacodynamics of meropenem in febrile neutropenic patients with bacteremia. Ann Pharmacother 39:32–38
79. Mouton JW, Touzw DJ, Horrevorts AM, Vinks AA (2000) Comparative pharmacokinetics of the carbapenems: clinical implications. Clin Pharmacokinet 39:185–201
80. Gafter-Gvili A, Fraser A, Paul M, Leibovici L (2005) Meta-analysis: antibiotic prophylaxis reduces mortality in neutropenic patients. Ann Intern Med 142:979–995
81. Bucaneve G, Micozzi A, Menichetti F, Martino P, Dionisi MS, Martinelli G, Allione B, D'Antonio D, Buelli M, Nosari AM, Cilloni D, Zuffa E, Cantaffa R, Specchia G, Amadori S, Fabbiano F, Deliliers GL, Lauria F, Foa R, Del Favero A (2005) Levofloxacin to prevent bacterial infection in patients with cancer and neutropenia. N Engl J Med 353:977–987
82. Cullen M, Steven N, Billingham L, Gaunt C, Hastings M, Simmonds P, Stuart N, Rea D, Bower M, Fernando I, Huddart R, Gollins S, Stanley A (2005) Antibacterial prophylaxis after chemotherapy for solid tumors and lymphomas. N Engl J Med 353:988–998
83. Oliveira AL, de Souza M, Carvalho-Dias VM, Ruiz MA, Silla L, Tanaka PY, Simoes BP, Trabasso P, Seber A, Lotfi CJ, Zanichelli MA, Araujo VR, Godoy C, Maiolino A, Urakawa P, Cunha CA, de Souza CA, Pasquini R, Nucci M (2007) Epidemiology of bacteremia and factors associated with multi-drug-resistant gram-negative bacteremia in hematopoietic stem cell transplant recipients. Bone Marrow Transplant 39:775–781
84. Reuter S, Kern WV, Sigge A, Dohner H, Marre R, Kern P, von Baum H (2005) Impact of fluoroquinolone prophylaxis on reduced infection-related mortality among patients with neutropenia and hematologic malignancies. Clin Infect Dis 40:1087–1093
85. Rangaraj G, Granwehr BP, Jiang Y, Hachem R, Raad I (2010) Perils of quinolone exposure in cancer patients: breakthrough bacteremia with multidrug-resistant organisms. Cancer 116(4):967–973

Antifungal Therapy in Patients with Hematological Malignancies

44

Raoul Herbrecht and Yasmine Nivoix

Contents

R. Herbrecht (✉) and Y. Nivoix
Department of Hematology and Oncology, Hôpital de Hautepierre, 67098 Strasbourg, France
e-mail: raoul.herbrecht@chru-strasbourg.fr

44.1 Introduction

Improvement during the last 2 decades in the outcome in invasive aspergillosis and invasive candidiasis, the two most frequent invasive fungal diseases, is the result of the availability of more effective and better tolerated agents in our antifungal armamentarium together with improved diagnostic tools and new strategies promoting earlier onset of effective therapy. Several antifungal agents are now available for the treatment of invasive fungal diseases. Echinocandins, triazoles, and polyenes are the three dominant classes of antifungal agents used in hematological patients. Beside these agents, flucytosine has a restricted use, and terbinafine is only used in very rare cases of invasive fungal disease in hematological patients; these indications are still controversial. Recommendations for use in hematological patients have been provided by the ECIL (European Conference on Infections in Leukemia) [57, 74, 78]. They are summarized in Tables 44.1 and 44.2.

44.2 Polyenes

Amphotericin B is a macrocyclic polyene characterized by a broad spectrum covering most of the fungal pathogens involved in human disease [8, 38, 91, 98]. However some species, including *Candida lusitaniae*, *Trichosporon* sp, *Geotrichum* sp, *Scedosporium apiospermum*, and the causative agents of dermatomycoses, are resistant or poorly sensitive to amphotericin B [1, 124]. Nystatin, another polyene, is only used as a topical agent due to its toxicity by a systemic route. Nystatin has been encapsulated in liposomes, and the

É. Azoulay (ed.), *Pulmonary Involvement in Patients with Hematological Malignancies*,
DOI: 10.1007/978-3-642-15742-4_44, © Springer-Verlag Berlin Heidelberg 2011

Table 44.1 Recommendations for prevention of fungal diseases and for empiric therapy of persistent febrile neutropenia in leukemic patients and hematopoietic stem cell transplant recipients (adapted from European Conference on Infections in Leukemia guidelines [74, 78] updated at 3rd conference held in September 2009)

	First choice[1]	Alternative[2]	Comments
Prophylaxis of fungal infections			
Allogeneic stem cell transplantation			
• Before engraftment	Fluconazole (400 mg qd, oral/iv) Voriconazole (200 mg bid, oral)	Itraconazole (200 mg iv followed by 200 mg bid oral solution) Aerosolized liposomal amphotericin B (10 mg twice weekly) + fluconazole	Fluconazole only in centers with low incidence of aspergillosis, with HEPA filtered-air rooms and with a mould-directed diagnostic approach
• With graft versus host disease	Posaconazole (200 mg tid, oral) Voriconazole (200 mg bid, oral)	Itraconazole (200 mg iv followed by 200 mg bid oral solution)	
Induction chemotherapy in leukemia or myelodysplastic syndromes	Posaconazole (200 mg tid, oral)	Aerosolized liposomal amphotericin B (10 mg twice weekly) + fluconazole	
Empiric therapy of persistent febrile neutropenia	Liposomal amphotericin B (3 mg/kg, iv) Caspofungin (70 mg on day 1 then 50 mg, iv)	Amphotericin B colloidal dispersion (4 mg/kg, iv) Amphotericin B lipid complex (5 mg/kg, iv) Itraconazole (200mg, iv) Voriconazole (3 mg/kg bid, iv) Micafungin (100 mg, iv) Amphotericin B deoxycholate (0.5–1.0 mg/kg, iv)	Amphotericin B deoxycholate not recommended if renal impairment, nephrotoxic co-medication or history of previous nephrotoxicity

[1]First choice refers to drugs graded A (good evidence to support a recommendation for use / strongly recommended)

[2]Alternative refers to drugs graded B (moderate evidence to support a recommendation for use /generally recommended)

drug has been assessed in invasive aspergillosis in a pilot trial but was not further developed [84].

Amphotericin B has strong affinity for ergosterol, the principal sterol of fungal membranes, while it shows less affinity for cholesterol, the principal sterol of mammalian cell membranes [14]. Amphotericin B and ergosterol form micelles that combine to form transmembrane channels leading to leakage of ions and other cellular components [117]. Other mechanisms of action include proton pump inhibition and induction of membrane lipid peroxidation [106].

Amphotericin B deoxycholate use is limited by a significant toxicity, with both infusion-related effects (fever, chills, hypotension, dyspnea) and nephrotoxicity. Because of its strong lipophilic properties, encapsulation of the drug in liposomes or binding to lipid complexes has led to the development of lipid formulations of amphotericin B in an attempt to increase the efficacy and the safety profile. Three lipid formulations of amphotericin B are currently commercially available: a liposomal preparation, a lipid complex, and a colloidal dispersion.

44.2.1 Amphotericin B Deoxycholate

Amphotericin B deoxycholate has been on the market for nearly 50 years and was extensively used before the lipid formulation of amphotericin B, the broad-spectrum azoles, and the echinocandins were developed. Its poor safety profile compared to these more recent agents now represents a major limitation to its use.

44.2.1.1 Pharmacokinetics

Amphotericin B is very weakly absorbed by the oral route. After intravenous injection, it is strongly bound to plasma protein (91–95%). The distribution

Table 44.2 Recommendations for the treatment of invasive aspergillosis and mucormycosis in leukemic patients and hematopoietic stem cell transplant recipients (adapted from European Conference on Infections in Leukemia guidelines [57] updated at 3rd conference held in September 2009)

	First choice[1]	Alternative[2]	Comments
Invasive pulmonary aspergillosis	Voriconazole (6 mg/kg bid on day 1 then 4 mg/kg bid, iv, followed by 200 mg bid, oral)	Liposomal amphotericin B (3–5 mg/kg, iv) Amphotericin B lipid complex (5 mg/kg, iv) Caspofungin (70 mg on day 1 then 50 mg, iv) Posaconazole (800 mg/day divided in two or four doses, oral) Voriconazole (6 mg/kg bid on day 1 then 4 mg/kg bid, iv) if not given as primary therapy Combination therapy for second line: • Caspofungin + voriconazole • Caspofungin + liposomal amphotericin B • Caspofungin + amphotericin B lipid complex	Initiation with iv voriconazole is preferred Caspofungin 70 mg if weight ≥80 kg Primary combination therapy is not routinely recommended but is an alternative for second line therapy Surgery may be indicated in: • Sinus disease • Pulmonary lesion close to a large vessel • Endocarditis • Single extra-pulmonary lesion Monitoring of azole serum level is recommended especially in case of failure or of suspicion of toxicity
Mucormycosis	Liposomal amphotericin B for primary therapy (3–5 mg/kg) Amphotericin B lipid complex for primary therapy (5 mg/kg) Control of underlying condition: • Control of diabetes • Hematopoietic growth factor if neutropenia • Discontinuation/tapering of steroids • Reduction in immunosuppressive therapy Surgery for rhino-orbito-cerebral and soft tissue localisations	Posaconazole (800 mg/day divided in 2 or 4 doses, oral) for second line and for maintenance therapy Combination of a lipid amphotericin B and caspofungin for second line therapy	Posaconazole may be used as an alternative for primary therapy when amphotericin B is absolutely contra-indicated Surgery for pulmonary and for disseminated disease should be considered on a case by case basis Insufficient data to recommend use of a combination of posaconazole and a lipid amphotericin B or a combination including deferasirox

[1]First choice for aspergillosis refers to drugs graded A (good evidence to support a recommendation for use/strongly recommended); for mucormycosis no drug was graded A because of insufficient data

[2]Alternative for aspergillosis refers to drugs graded B (moderate evidence to support a recommendation for use/generally recommended)

corresponds to a three-phase model [6]. The plasma half-life is 24–48 h, but the elimination half-life is approximately 15 days [26]. High concentrations are found in the liver, kidneys, and lungs [20, 53, 133]. The metabolic pathways followed by amphotericin B in humans are not known, and biliary and renal excretions are both weak. Because of the complex pharmacokinetics, the concentrations of amphotericin B in the blood do not accurately reflect the concentrations in the tissue, and measuring them is therefore of little value [67]. Amphotericin B is not significantly cleared by dialysis.

44.2.1.2 Clinical Efficacy

Despite mediocre tolerability, amphotericin B was the standard treatment for most deep-seated fungal diseases. Amphotericin B was usually administered by slow i.v. infusion at a daily dosage varying from 0.5 to 1.0 mg/kg depending on the severity of the disease, the nature of the pathogen, renal function, and drug tolerance. In general, response rates were low, and over 40% of the patients with invasive candidiasis or invasive aspergillosis treated with amphotericin B died [56, 73, 119].

44.2.1.3 Tolerability

Infusion-related adverse events occur in 70–90% of patients, and include nausea, vomiting, fever, chills, pain at the injection site, gastrointestinal disorders, thrombophlebitis, bronchospasm, hypotension, and cardiac arrhythmia [41, 47, 72]. An infusion duration of at least 6 h is recommended and helps to reduce the severity of the infusion-related events.

The limiting factor is nephrotoxicity, which is cumulative and can cause renal impairment, hypokalemia, hypomagnesemia, and acidosis [41]. Renal toxicity occurs in 24–80% of treatments [21, 41, 92, 95]. It is worsened by combination with other nephrotoxic drugs, such as ciclosporin, vancomycin, aminoglycosides, and cisplatin. Regular biological monitoring is required during therapy and also sometimes after treatment cessation because of prolonged renal potassium leakage. Sodium loading (up to 150 mmol in the absence of contraindications) before amphotericin B infusion may reduce the renal toxicity [52].

44.2.2 *Amphotericin B Colloidal Dispersion*

Amphotericin B colloidal dispersion (ABCD) has market access limited only to some countries. ABCD is composed of cholesteryl sulfate bilayers in which the amphotericin B molecule inserts itself at an equimolar ratio. The particles have a disk-like structure, and are 120–140 nm in diameter and 4 nm thick.

44.2.2.1 Pharmacokinetics

ABCD is rapidly taken up by the reticuloendothelial system, explaining why the maximal plasma concentration is low and the volume of distribution high, and also why tissue concentrations are high in the liver, spleen, and bone marrow [37]. The elimination half-life increases with the dose, from 86 h at 0.25 mg/kg to 238 h at 1 mg/kg [101].

44.2.2.2 Clinical Efficacy

The therapeutic potential of ABCD has been assessed in open-label studies demonstrating activity in various invasive fungal diseases, including candidiasis, aspergillosis, and mucormycosis (zygomycosis) [58, 59]. A randomized trial comparing ABCD (6 mg/kg/day) and amphotericin B deoxycholate (1–1.5 mg/kg/day) in invasive aspergillosis showed low response rates with no differences in both arms [17]. Similar response rates between ABCD and amphotericin B deoxycholate have also been shown in the treatment of persistent febrile neutropenia [130].

44.2.2.3 Tolerability

The infusion-related effects are equivalent to or even more frequent than those of amphotericin B [17, 58, 130]. Daily doses over 4 mg/kg are associated with more adverse effects. Pre-treatment medication (acetaminophen or diphenhydramine) and lowering of the infusion rate to no more than 1 mg kg^{-1} h^{-1} reduce the frequency and severity of infusion-related events. Renal tolerability is improved compared to amphotericin B deoxycholate.

44.2.3 *Amphotericin B Lipid Complex*

Amphotericin B lipid complex (ABLC) is a suspension of amphotericin B complexed to dimyristoylphosphatidylcholine and dimyristoyl phosphatidylglycerol. The particles are ribbon-shaped and 1,600–6,000 nm long [63].

44.2.3.1 Pharmacokinetics

After injection, ABLC is taken up by the macrophagic and monocytic cells of the reticuloendothelial system in complex form, explaining why ABLC concentrates mainly in the liver, spleen and lungs, and bone marrow [108, 133]. The lipid complexes are disorganized by the action of fungal or host cell-derived phospholipases, thus releasing amphotericin B [107].

44.2.3.2 Clinical Efficacy

Clinical data supporting the activity of ABLC are mostly derived from open non-comparative trials and from a registry [19, 62, 89, 123]. They showed significant response rates of invasive candidiasis, aspergillosis, fusariosis, and mucormycosis. There is still a lack of well-designed randomized trials to fix the exact role of ABLC in clinical practice.

44.2.3.3 Tolerability

The adverse effects of ABLC are similar in nature to those of amphotericin B deoxycholate, but their frequency is far lower. In randomized comparison to liposomal amphotericin, patients treated with ABLC experienced more acute infusion-related events, including dyspnea, and more nephrotoxicity [132].

44.2.4 Liposomal Amphotericin B

Liposomal amphotericin B is a formulation of amphotericin B encapsulated in unilamellar liposomes. The liposomes are composed of hydrogenated soya phosphatidylcholine, cholesterol, and distearoyl phosphatidylglycerol at a ratio of 10:5:4 [108]. They have a diameter of approximately 80 nm.

44.2.4.1 Pharmacokinetics

The pharmacokinetic behavior of liposomal amphotericin B is very different from that of amphotericin B deoxycholate and the other lipid formulations. The high plasma concentrations achieved with liposomal amphotericin B are explained by the fact that the small rigid liposomes are taken up less rapidly by the reticuloendothelial system [108]. The strongest concentrations are found in liver and spleen, while pulmonary concentrations are variable. Studies have suggested that liposomal amphotericin B delivers amphotericin B to fungal cells by liposome fusion with the cell membrane, leading to the death of the fungal cell [2].

44.2.4.2 Clinical Efficacy

Several randomized trials have confirmed the efficacy of liposomal amphotericin B for the treatment of persistent febrile neutropenia and for invasive aspergillosis. In this latter study, a standard dose (3 mg/kg/day) of liposomal amphotericin B was compared to a high-dose regimen (10 mg/kg/day for 10 days followed by standard dose). Efficacy was similar in both arms, but tolerance was better with the standard dose. Most prophylaxis studies failed to demonstrate a decrease in the incidence of pulmonary aspergillosis, with the exception of a randomized trial comparing aerosolized liposomal amphotericin B to a placebo [97].

44.2.4.3 Tolerability

The studies of empirical treatment of patients with febrile neutropenia serve as a good basis for appreciating tolerability [92, 122]. Patients treated with liposomal amphotericin B (3 mg/kg/day) had fewer infusion-related events and less nephrotoxicity than patients treated with amphotericin B deoxycholate. Liposomal amphotericin B was also better tolerated than ABLC in a double-blind trial [132]. However, in studies comparing liposomal amphotericin B to caspofungin or to micafungin, the echinocandins arm showed better tolerability [70, 127].

44.3 Azoles

Imidazoles are mostly used as topical agents, whereas triazoles have a greater affinity for fungal than mammalian CYP450 enzymes and are therefore safer for systemic use compared to the imidazoles. Triazoles used in hematological patients include fluconazole, itraconazole, voriconazole, and posaconazole. Among the azoles under development, isavuconazole seems to be the most promising.

Azole antifungal agents act by inhibiting ergosterol synthesis. Ergosterol is the predominant cell membrane sterol of most fungi, in contrast to mammalian cells where the membrane is mainly composed of cholesterol. Azole antifungals inhibit the fungal cytochrome P450-dependent enzyme lanosterol 14α-demethylase. This inhibition results in an interruption of ergosterol synthesis and the accumulation of toxic 14-methylsterol intermediates. Both events cause an alteration of the fungal cell membrane. Antifungal azoles agents are mostly fungistatic rather than fungicidal. As azole antifungals can also inhibit many mammalian cytochrome P450-dependent isoenzymes involved in hormone synthesis or drug metabolism, there is potential for toxicity or drug-to-drug interactions.

Various factors interfere with the pharmacokinetics and metabolism of antifungal azoles, especially for itraconazole, voriconazole, or posaconazole. These conditions include the formulation of the antifungal agent, variation in gastric pH, digestive tract dysfunction, genetic polymorphism of CYP450 isoenzymes, saturation of intestinal absorption or of metabolism, potential liver disease, and potential for interactions with food or with other drugs. The large variations seen with these agents in serum levels may be associated with decreased efficacy, increased toxicity, or occurrence of breakthrough infections, and monitoring of the serum levels may be useful [46, 87, 109, 110].

44.3.1 Fluconazole

Fluconazole has a spectrum restricted to yeasts. *Candida krusei* is resistant to fluconazole, and *Candida glabrata* has limited susceptibility. Fluconazole is water-soluble and has been available as oral and intravenous formulations since the late 1980s.

44.3.1.1 Pharmacokinetics

Oral formulations of fluconazole have a bioavailability exceeding 90%, and the plasma concentration–dose relationship is linear. Absorption is not influenced by gastric pH or by food intake. Maximum serum levels are achieved between 0.5 and 1.5 h when taken in a fasting state. A loading double dose is recommended for the treatment of invasive diseases.

Protein binding is low (11%), and tissue diffusion is excellent with levels ranging from 0.8 to 3 times the serum levels, allowing the treatment of a variety of systemic fungal diseases [28]. Fluconazole undergoes minimal CYP450-mediated metabolism and is mainly eliminated unchanged in the urine; the average elimination half-life is approximately 30 h. A dosage adjustment is required for patients with reduced creatinine clearance (<50 mL/min).

44.3.1.2 Clinical Efficacy

Several studies have shown a beneficial role of fluconazole (400 mg/day) for prophylaxis of yeast infections in allogeneic stem cell transplant patients with a significant reduction of the incidence of invasive fungal diseases and of overall mortality [45, 103]. Despite some controversial results in clinical studies, meta-analyses also demonstrated a benefit of fluconazole prophylaxis in patients undergoing intensive chemotherapy for acute leukemia: the incidence of proven invasive fungal diseases and fungal-related mortality is decreased, but the overall mortality and incidence of aspergillosis are not [16, 65]. Benefit is highest in centers with incidences of invasive fungal diseases >15% and for leukemia patients receiving doses of fluconazole >200 mg/day.

The role of fluconazole in the empiric therapy of febrile neutropenia is limited by its lack of activity against molds and against some *Candida* spp. Therefore, its use as empiric therapy should be restricted to patients at lowest risk of aspergillosis, excluding allogeneic stem transplant recipients, patients with prolonged severe neutropenia, and patients with a prior exposition to an azole who are more likely infected with a fluconazole-resistant *Candida* sp.

Epidemiology of invasive *Candida* infection has changed over the last 2 decades, and now more than half of the strains isolated in candidemia are non-*albicans Candida*. Among these *C. glabrata* and *C. krusei* have reduced susceptibility to fluconazole and are associated with a high mortality rate. Fluconazole is therefore only considered as an option before species identification in invasive *Candida* disease. In this setting, a lipid formulation of amphotericin B or an echinocandin is preferred. Fluconazole can be proposed for deep-seated infections, including lung infections, when activity has been confirmed in vitro, especially when a long duration of therapy is required, as it is well tolerated and available as an oral formulation.

Fluconazole is active in vitro against *Cryptococcus* spp. While combination of amphotericin B deoxycholate (0.7–1.0 mg/kg/day) and flucytosine (100 mg/kg/day) given for 6 weeks has been the standard for treatment of CNS cryptococcosis in HIV positive and negative patients, a switch to maintenance therapy with fluconazole (400 mg/g) after 2 weeks of combination therapy is also accepted in guidelines [90]. Immunocompromised patients with severe pulmonary cryptococcal infections or with cryptococcal fungemia should be treated in the same fashion as patients with CNS disease. Upfront fluconazole is a reasonable approach for patients with mild to moderate pulmonary infection.

44.3.1.3 Tolerability

Fluconazole is well tolerated. The most frequent adverse events are gastrointestinal. However, these events were not more frequent in fluconazole-treated patients than in patients receiving placebo in prophylaxis studies. Transaminase elevations are common, but usually do not need discontinuation of the therapy. Very high doses, far higher than those recommended for clinical use, have been associated with neurological intolerance [5]. As fluconazole is less lipohilic than the other triazoles, it interacts less with cytochrome P450 isoenzymes and is therefore less subject to drug-to-drug interactions.

A shift toward *C. glabrata* and *C. krusei* infections in patients receiving fluconazole has been reported.

44.3.2 Itraconazole

Itraconazole was introduced in 1987 when amphotericin B was the only anti-*Aspergillus* active agent available for systemic use [43]. Itraconazole was initially available as capsules and later as a solution in hydroxypropyl-β-cyclodextrin for oral and intravenous use. The spectrum of itraconazole includes *Candida* spp. (with high resistance rates in *C. glabrata* and *C. krusei*), *Cryptococcus neoformans*, *Aspergillus* spp., dimorphic fungi, and agents of dermatomycosis.

44.3.2.1 Pharmacokinetics

Itraconazole is highly lipophilic. Absorption from the capsules is limited, is enhanced by food and an acidic beverage, and is decreased by concomitant antacid drugs. In contrast to the capsules, itraconazole in oral solution has a 30–40% higher bioavailability than that of the capsule formulation [9, 131]. Absorption of itraconazole oral solution is highest in the fasted state [10].

Itraconazole is extensively metabolized in the liver into many metabolites by CYP3A4. The main metabolite, hydroxyitraconazole, has antifungal activity [61]. Itraconazole and hydroxyitraconazole are both inhibitors of CYP3A4.

Itraconazole's pharmacokinetics are not affected by renal function [13]. However, the intravenous formulation is contraindicated in patients with a creatinine clearance below 30 mL/min due to the accumulation of the solubilizing agent, hydroxypropyl-β-cyclodextrin. In patients with minor or moderate degrees of hepatic insufficiency, initial dosing of itraconazole does not need to be changed. Monitoring of serum levels is recommended to adjust further dosage targeting through concentrations of 500–2,000 ng/mL.

44.3.2.2 Clinical Efficacy

A small randomized study showed no difference in efficacy in a comparison of itraconazole (capsules at a dosage of 400 mg/day) versus a low dose of amphotericin B deoxycholate plus flucytosine for the treatment of suspected fungal infections in neutropenic patients [114]. An open trial was conducted in 76 patients with invasive aspergillosis. Itraconazole capsules were given at a dose of 600 mg/day for 4 days followed by 400 mg/day [30]. An overall favorable response rate was 39%, suggesting at this time that itraconazole could be an alternative to amphotericin B deoxycholate for invasive aspergillosis and that a controlled trial should be performed. This trial has never been performed because of the development of more promising agents such as the lipid formulations of amphotericin B and voriconazole, and also because of the erratic absorption of itraconazole capsules.

In the 1990s, itraconazole capsules were mainly used with some satisfactory results as oral follow-up therapy in patients with invasive aspergillosis who responded to amphotericin B deoxycholate, and also in patients with chronic necrotizing aspergillosis, aspergilloma, and allergic bronchopulmonary aspergillosis who required a long duration of therapy [27, 29, 31, 128]. The further development of an oral and an intravenous solution led to the assessment of itraconazole in empiric and in prophylactic therapy of invasive fungal diseases in high-risk hematological patients and solid organ recipients. Several studies suggested a superiority of itraconazole over fluconazole in the prevention of fungal disease in leukemic patients, including a reduction in the incidence of aspergillosis [74]. Patients with a chronic granulomatous disease may also benefit from prophylaxis with itraconazole as shown in a randomized placebo controlled trial in 39 patients [40]. Currently, the role of itraconazole is mostly restricted to prophylaxis (preferably with the i.v. formulation followed by the oral solution) and to maintenance therapy of invasive aspergillosis in case of contraindications to voriconazole and posaconazole.

44.3.2.3 Tolerability

Itraconazole capsules are generally well tolerated. Itraconazole oral solution is associated with digestive tract intolerance, mainly nausea, vomiting, diarrhea, and abdominal pain, which can lead to a very high rate of discontinuation (up to 36%) [42]. These events are more likely to be due to the vehicle, hydroxypropyl-β-cyclodextrin, than to the antifungal agent itself. Itraconazole has also been associated with mild hepatic toxicity [15, 44].

Severe hepatic events have been reported in allogeneic hematopoietic stem cell transplant recipients receiving itraconazole prophylaxis concomitantly to cyclophosphamide [80, 81]. Analysis demonstrated higher exposure to toxic cyclophosphamide metabolites among recipients of itraconazole compared with fluconazole, explaining the conditioning-related liver toxicities.

Fifty-eight cases suggestive of congestive heart failure in association with the use of itraconazole have been summarized in a publication [3]. The labeling of itraconazole has been changed to alert physicians to this finding, and itraconazole is now contraindicated for the treatment of superficial fungal infections in patients with signs of congestive heart failure or other ventricular dysfunction.

As with other azoles, neurotoxicity, sometimes severe, has been observed when itraconazole is concomitantly administered with vincristine [18]. The proposed mechanism cans most likely be attributed to either the inhibition by the azole of CYP3A4 enzymes that are involved in vincristine metabolism or the blockade of P-glycoprotein pumps that participate in the cellular efflux of vinca alkaloids [18, 82]. This interaction with vincristine is likely to occur with other vinca alkaloids as they share similar metabolic pathways. Rare cases of neuropathy have also been reported in the absence of concomitant vincristine administration.

Itraconazole serum levels should be monitored in all patients treated with itraconazole capsules for a prolonged period for invasive fungal diseases such as aspergillosis or histoplasmosis [46]. A trough serum level of 500 ng/mL of itraconazole, measured by HPLC, has been considered as adequate for prophylaxis [44]. A trough concentration of itraconazole around 1,000 ng/mL should be considered as a target concentration for activity against invasive aspergillosis [43]. The additional concentration of the active first-pass metabolite of itraconazole, hydroxyitraconazole, more than doubles the total serum concentration.

44.3.3 Voriconazole

Voriconazole is available for oral administration as tablets, as an oral suspension, and as an intravenous formulation using sulphobutyl ether β-cyclodextrin sodium as the solubilizing agent. Voriconazole has broad-spectrum activity against most pathogenic yeasts, dimorphic fungi, and *Aspergillus* spp. and opportunistic molds, excluding Zygomycetes [35, 50, 118].

44.3.3.1 Pharmacokinetics

Voriconazole is absorbed rapidly after oral administration, reaching maximum serum concentrations within 1–2 h [71]. Administering voriconazole with food delays the time to reach maximum plasma levels to approximately 2.5 h, and fat decreases the bioavailability of voriconazole, with reductions of approximately 30% in the area under the curve and peak plasma concentration. Bioavailability >90% has been reported in healthy volunteers. Absorption is not affected by antacid agents.

Interpatient variability in peak serum concentration and area under the curve values have been observed after multiple doses; therefore, a wide range of plasma drug concentrations can be expected in patients treated with the same dose of voriconazole. Steady-state trough plasma concentrations are reached after 5 days of oral or intravenous administration, but can be achieved after 3 days if a loading dose is given.

Voriconazole exhibits non-linear pharmacokinetics in adult patients due to saturable first-pass metabolism and systemic clearance; thus, peak plasma concentrations and the area under the curve increase disproportionately with increasing dose [71]. It is estimated that, on average, increasing the oral dose in healthy subjects from 200 to 300 mg leads to a 2.5-fold increase in exposure (area under the curve), while increasing the intravenous dose from 3 to 4 mg/kg produces a 2.3-fold increase in exposure. The mean elimination half-life of orally administered voriconazole is 6–12 h, although this is also dose-dependent. Voriconazole binds moderately to plasma proteins (58–65%). The drug penetrates well into body fluids, including the CSF.

Extensive metabolism of voriconazole takes place in the liver via the hepatic cytochrome P450 isoenzymes CYP3A4, CYP2C19, and CYP2C9. Metabolites have minimal antifungal activity. The major enzyme involved in the metabolism of voriconazole is CYP2C19, which exhibits genetic polymorphism. Between 15% and 20% of Asians are expected to be poor metabolizers of voriconazole and have a consequent fourfold higher exposure to voriconazole. Conversely, only 3–5% of Caucasians and Blacks are expected to show genetic polymorphism.

Patients with mild to moderate hepatic impairment have an area under the curve threefold higher than that of normal patients. High accumulation of voriconazole has been shown in a patient with liver cirrhosis [129]. It is recommended that the standard loading dose regimens should be used, but the maintenance dose halved in patients with mild to moderate hepatic cirrhosis receiving voriconazole. The drug is contraindicated in patients with severe hepatic dysfunctions.

Patients with renal disease had similar voriconazole pharmacokinetics to healthy volunteers. Renal impairment was found to decrease the clearance of sulphobutyl ether β-cyclodextrin sodium used as the solubilizing agent in the intravenous preparation. This i.v. formulation is thus contraindicated in patients with a creatinine clearance <30 mL/min.

44.3.3.2 Clinical Efficacy

Voriconazole has a major role in the treatment of invasive aspergillosis, in addition to its activity in oropharyngeal and esophageal candidiasis, candidemia, and in some of the more unusual fungal diseases, such as fusariosis and scedosporiosis, where treatment options are limited [56, 64].

Voriconazole has been compared to amphotericin B deoxycholate for primary therapy in 277 patients with invasive aspergillosis [56]. Patients given voriconazole had a higher successful outcome rate with a 53% (complete 21%, partial 32%) response compared to a 32% response of those given amphotericin B (complete 17%, partial 15%). Twelve-week survival was higher in the voriconazole group (71%) compared with only 58% in the amphotericin B group. Voriconazole was more effective than amphotericin B regardless of the underlying condition, the site of infection, the presence or absence of neutropenia, or the degree of certainty of the diagnosis of aspergillosis.

Voriconazole has been compared to liposomal amphotericin B for the empiric treatment of invasive fungal disease in neutropenic patients with persistent fever [125]. The non-inferiority of voriconazole could not be demonstrated, but a difference was reported in favor of voriconazole in the number of patients who developed a breakthrough fungal infection during the treatment. Voriconazole was better tolerated than liposomal amphotericin B. Voriconazole has not been approved for this indication, but is nevertheless recommended by the Infectious Diseases Society of America guidelines, similarly to liposomal amphotericin B and caspofungin, for empiric therapy in persistent febrile neutropenia [121].

44.3.3.3 Tolerability

Voriconazole has a good safety profile. The most frequent adverse reactions reported after administration of oral or intravenous voriconazole are visual disturbances, hepatic abnormalities, and skin reactions. Visual disturbances (enhanced light perception, blurred vision, photophobia, or altered color discrimination) are usually mild to moderate in severity, occur shortly after dosing, and usually last up to 30 min. Visual disturbances have been reported in approximately 30–45% of patients receiving voriconazole in clinical studies and are most common during the first days of therapy [55]. The retina has been shown to be the site of these side effects with decreased amplitude of electroretinogram waveforms in dogs and humans. However, no long-term visual sequelae have been reported.

Elevations in hepatic enzymes occur in 4–27% of patients receiving voriconazole and are generally associated with high plasma levels and/or doses of the drug

[55, 64]. The usual pattern is increased in aspartate aminotransferase and alanine aminotransferase, but an increase in alkaline phosphatase and bilirubin levels have also been reported. Rare cases of severe hepatic reactions have been reported during clinical trials, including clinical hepatitis, cholestasis, and fulminant hepatic failure with resulting fatalities. Patients should be warned about the possible visual disturbances associated with voriconazole. Patients with mild-to-moderate hepatic cirrhosis should receive the normal loading dose of voriconazole, but the maintenance dose should be reduced by half. Data are insufficient for patients with severe hepatic cirrhosis, and voriconazole is therefore contraindicated. Patients with renal insufficiency and reduced creatinine clearance (<50 mL/min) should take oral voriconazole and should not be given the intravenous preparation to prevent accumulation of the solubilizing agent, sulphobutyl ether β-cyclodextrin sodium, unless the benefit/risk to the patient justifies the use of intravenous form.

Skin reactions, mostly rashes, have been reported in 1–19% of patients receiving voriconazole [55, 64]. Photosensitivity can occur, and patients taking voriconazole should be advised to avoid strong, direct sunlight during the course of their treatment. Other adverse reactions reported with voriconazole include nausea, vomiting, diarrhea, headaches, and visual hallucinations or confusion. Similar to itraconazole, concomitant administration of voriconazole and vinca alkaloids should be avoided.

Voriconazole therapy has been identified as a risk factor for developing mucormycosis [68, 110]. In most cases voriconazole has been administered for primary or secondary prophylaxis in hematopoietic stem cell transplant recipients, and most patients also had several of the previously established risk factors for mucormycosis. In a multivariate analysis, voriconazole therapy as well as diabetes mellitus and malnutrition were independently associated with the occurrence of mucormycosis [68]. It has also been suggested that an increased rate of mucormycosis might more likely be related to recent improved diagnostic procedures of this disease rather than a selection of the agents of mucormycosis by voriconazole.

Large variability of voriconazole serum levels has been documented in patients [87, 109, 110]. Underexposure to voriconazole (serum level ≤1,000 ng/mL) can result in failure to cure the infection and in increased risk of breakthrough infection. Overexposure also needs to be documented in patients with unexpected toxicity: a correlation has been found between high serum levels (>5,500 ng/mL) and occurrence of encephalopathy. As under- and overexposure lead to adverse events or to failures to respond, monitoring of voriconazole through the serum level is recommended to optimize the safety and efficacy [121].

44.3.4 Posaconazole

Posaconazole is an extended-spectrum triazole that is currently only available as an oral suspension. An intravenous formulation is under development. Like other triazoles, posaconazole inhibits fungal ergosterol synthesis. Posaconazole is active against *Candida* spp., including *C. krusei* and *C. glabrata, C. neoformans*, dimorphic fungi such as *Coccidioides immitis* and *Histoplasma*, *Aspergillus* spp., *Fusarium* spp., and some other filamentous fungi involved in human disease. Importantly, the spectrum of activity includes also Zygomycetes, and clinical trials have shown the efficacy of posaconazole in invasive mucormycosis [4, 48, 112].

44.3.4.1 Pharmacokinetics

Posaconazole exhibits dose-proportional pharmacokinetics up to 800 mg/day [24, 36]. No increase in area under the curve is observed when the posaconazole dose is further increased. Posaconazole exposure is enhanced two to four times by administration with food, with peak plasma concentrations attained at ~5–6 h post dose [25]. Similarly, administration of posaconazole with a nutritional supplement increases approximately threefold the maximum plasma concentration and the area under the curve. To optimize absorption, each dose of posaconazole should be administered with a full meal or a liquid nutritional supplement. Alternative antifungal therapy must be considered in patients not able to take food or oral nutritional supplement.

Posaconazole has extensive tissue distribution and a long half-life. Steady-state concentrations are achieved within 7–10 days. Posaconazole is primarily metabolized in the liver, where it undergoes glucuronidation and transformation into other biologically inactive metabolites [69]. Approximately 14% of an administered dose is excreted as multiple glucuronidated derivatives in the urine; an additional 77% is eliminated as unchanged drug in the feces. Minor amounts are excreted in the urine.

Posaconazole is not primarily metabolized by CYP enzymes [54]. Thus, coadministering drugs that interact with the CYP enzyme system is unlikely to alter posaconazole plasma concentrations. An evaluation of the effects of posaconazole on the various CYP enzymes demonstrated an inhibitory effect on CYP3A4 activity, but no influence on the activity of the other isoenzymes (CYP1A2, CYP2C8/9, CYP2D6, or CYP2E1). Posaconazole may have the potential for fewer drug interactions compared with other azole antifungal agents.

Posaconazole pharmacokinetics are not significantly influenced by age, ethnicity, or renal or hepatic function [54]. No dose adjustment is necessary to accommodate for differences in these patient factors.

44.3.4.2 Clinical Efficacy

Two large randomized studies demonstrated the efficacy of posaconazole given for prophylaxis of invasive fungal diseases in high-risk patients [23, 111]. The first study compared oral posaconazole (200 mg three times a day) to oral fluconazole in allogeneic stem cell transplant recipients with graft-versus-host disease who received immunosuppressive therapy [111]. Posaconazole was as effective as fluconazole in preventing all invasive fungal diseases and was superior to fluconazole in preventing proven or probable invasive aspergillosis. Posaconazole significantly reduced the fungal-related mortality, but overall mortality was similar in both arms. The second study compared posaconazole (200 mg three times a day) to either fluconazole or itraconazole in patients with prolonged neutropenia following intensive chemotherapy for acute myeloblastic leukemia or myelodysplastic syndrome [23]. Fewer patients receiving posaconazole had a probable or proven invasive fungal disease, and fewer patients had aspergillosis. The overall survival rate was significantly higher in patients treated with posaconazole.

The efficacy and safety of posaconazole oral suspension (200 mg/day four times a day or 400 twice a day) have been investigated in an open-label study in patients with invasive aspergillosis who were refractory to or intolerant of conventional antifungal therapy [126]. Posaconazole conferred a response and survival benefit as compared to an external control group. Interestingly, a dose response analysis showed a 75% response rate in the quartile of patients with the highest posaconazole serum levels and only a 24% response rate in the quartile of patients with the lowest serum levels.

Posaconazole has also shown efficacy as salvage therapy of mucormycosis [48, 112]. A 60% favorable response rate has been obtained. Outcome may differ according to the genus and species of the Mucorales. While response rates were high in *Absidia* spp., *Cunninghamella* spp., and *Mucor* spp., they were lower in *Rhizopus* spp. and *Rhizomucor* spp. infections. So far, posaconazole cannot be recommended for first-line therapy of mucormycosis except in case of contraindication to amphotericin B formulations. Its role in salvage and in maintenance therapy has been recognized.

44.3.4.3 Tolerability

Posaconazole oral solution is usually well accepted by the patients. Posaconazole has a safety profile similar to fluconazole [23, 111]. Most frequent adverse events are gastrointestinal events, such as nausea, vomiting, diarrhea, anorexia, and abdominal pain. Hepatic toxicity is low and rarely requires discontinuation of the treatment [126]. Skin rashes have been reported in 4% of the patients. As for other azoles, posaconazole may increase the neurotoxicity of vinca alkaloids [77].

Little information is available regarding the use of posaconazole drug monitoring. Monitoring serum levels in a clinical trial showed a variability in through serum levels of more than a 1–10 ratio [126]. The highest serum levels were associated with the highest response rates. Conversely, 25% of the patients had very low serum levels, and only 24% of them responded to therapy. Early identification of these patients allows switching to another therapy to increase the probability of efficacy of the antifungal treatment.

44.3.5 Isavuconazole

Isavuconazole is a new broad-spectrum oral and intravenous azole currently in phase III clinical trials. In vitro, isavuconazole is active against *Candida* spp., including fluconazole-resistant strains, and against *Aspergillus* species most frequently involved in human infections, including *Aspergillus terreus* [50]. Isavuconazole has also activity against dermatophytes and some Zygomycetes.

The drug is being developed as a water-soluble prodrug (BAL8557) suitable for oral and intravenous administration. The prodrug is rapidly and almost totally (>99%) converted by esterases into BAL8728 (prodrug cleavage product) and to the active drug (isavuconazole, BAL4815). The drug is characterized by a long elimination half life (56–77 h after oral administration and 76–104 h after intravenous administration) [88]. The most frequent adverse events reported in phase two studies were headache, nasopharyngitis, and rhinitis. Phase III studies are ongoing in invasive aspergillosis (compared to voriconazole) and in invasive candidiasis (compared to caspofungin followed by oral voriconazole).

44.4 Echinocandins

The echinocandins are semisynthetic lipopeptides produced via chemical modification of natural products of fungi [34]. Echinocandins block the synthesis of β (1,3)-D-glucan, an essential carbohydrate component of the cell wall of numerous fungal species, by non-competitive inhibition of the enzyme β (1,3)-D-glucan synthase. Inhibition of the synthesis of β (1,3)-D-glucan produces a double effect – fungistatic and fungicidal. The fungistatic effect results from blockade of the cell wall synthesis, reducing fungal growth. The fungicidal effect results from a change in the integrity of the wall, which loses its properties of mechanical resistance and becomes unable to resist the intracellular osmotic pressure, leading ultimately to destruction of the fungal cell. Mammalian cells do not contain β (1,3)-D-glucan, thus avoiding direct human cell toxicity of the echinocandins.

Three echinocandins are approved: caspofungin, micafungin, and anidulafungin. They are active against *Candida* spp., including azole-resistant *Candida* spp., and *Aspergillus* spp., but lack activity against *Cryptococcus* spp., *Trichosporon* spp., *Fusarium* spp., and Zygomycetes.

44.4.1 Caspofungin

Caspofungin was the first echinocandin on the market in the USA and Europe. It has been assessed in candidiasis, aspergillosis, and empiric therapy of persistent febrile neutropenia.

44.4.1.1 Pharmacokinetics

The oral bioavailability of caspofungin is very low, requiring parenteral administration. Pharmacokinetics are linear in humans after single doses ranging from 5 to 100 mg [105]. The β-phase half-life is long (9–11 h), leading to moderate accumulation after administration of multiple doses. Caspofungin is mainly eliminated in the urine and the feces as metabolites [7]. Very little caspofungin is excreted in urine.

Metabolism of caspofungin is thought to be independent of the cytochrome system, and caspofungin does not inhibit the cytochrome P450 isoenzymes. Nevertheless, interaction studies suggest that caspofungin concentrations are reduced during concomitant administration of cytochrome inducers. Caspofungin does not cause any significant change in the pharmacokinetics of amphotericin B, itraconazole, cyclosporine, or mycophenolate [66]. However, concentrations of tacrolimus are reduced by around 20% during administration of caspofungin, necessitating closer monitoring of serum tacrolimus concentrations. In contrast, cyclosporine increases the area under the curve of caspofungin by about 35%, but these alterations are not sufficient to suggest any dosage modification.

There is no need to reduce the dosage in elderly subjects, nor in cases of moderate renal insufficiency or mild hepatic insufficiency. In patients with moderate hepatic insufficiency, it is recommended to reduce the dosage to 35 mg/day after a loading dose of 70 mg on day 1. Insufficient data are available in patients with severe hepatic failure. Caspofungin is not dialysable.

44.4.1.2 Clinical Efficacy

Large studies have convincingly shown excellent efficacy and safety in invasive candidiasis [83, 86]. Response rates were also satisfactory with caspofungin given as monotherapy or in combination for salvage therapy of invasive aspergillosis [75, 76]. Data are however less convincing for primary therapy of invasive aspergillosis with a low response rate and survival in leukemic patients, but higher rates in allogeneic stem cell transplant recipients [60, 120]. Of note, all these patients had a mycologically documented infection, which was not the case in studies with voriconazole or liposomal amphotericin B [22, 56]. Caspofungin has also been successfully assessed for empiric therapy of persistent febrile neutropenia [127].

44.4.1.3 Tolerability

Caspofungin is a well-tolerated antifungal drug [12, 83, 86, 127]. Serious drug-related adverse effects and discontinuation of therapy because of drug-related adverse events were uncommon in clinical trials. The most commonly encountered drug-related adverse effects are fever, phlebitis at the infusion site, headache, and nausea. Renal tolerability is excellent, even on prolonged treatment. Transient mild to moderate elevations in alanine aminotransferase levels can be seen.

44.4.2 *Micafungin*

Micafungin is a semisynthetic, water-soluble, lipopeptide, antifungal agent of the echinocandin class with fungicidal activity toward *Candida* spp. and fungistatic activity toward *Aspergillus* spp.

44.4.2.1 Pharmacokinetics

Similarly to the other echinocandins, micafungin has a low oral bioavailability requiring parenteral administration. It exhibits a linear relationship between systemic exposure and dosage. The mean elimination half-life is 14.6 h, which is compatible with a once-daily dosing strategy. Steady state is achieved by day 4. Seventy to ninety percent of a dose is excreted as unchanged drug or metabolites in feces through the biliary route [51, 100]. Micafungin is not metabolized by hepatic cytochrome P450 (CYP450) isoenzymes. Hepatic biotransformation of micafungin is primarily mediated by arylsulfatase followed by catechol-*O*-methyltransferase. Moderate hepatic impairment conferred no clinically significant difference on micafungin pharmacokinetic parameters. Renal excretion of the parent drug is negligible, and severe renal impairment has no effect on micafungin disposition.

44.4.2.2 Clinical Efficacy

Most clinical trials have investigated the efficacy and safety of micafungin in the treatment of invasive candidiasis and its prophylactic capacity in neutropenic patients undergoing hematopoietic stem cell transplantation [70, 86, 113].

Micafungin was as effective as and better tolerated than liposomal amphotericin B in patients with invasive candidiasis [70]. In a second study, micafungin was not inferior to caspofungin [86]. Micafungin (50 mg/day) proved to be as effective as fluconazole for prophylaxis of invasive fungal disease in patient undergoing autologous or allogeneic hematopoietic stem cell transplantation [113]. Fewer episodes of aspergillosis occurred in the micafungin group; the difference was close to statistical significance.

Clinical data regarding the use of micafungin in the management of invasive aspergillosis are so far insufficient to allow any recommendation.

44.4.2.3 Tolerability

The most frequently reported treatment-related adverse events are nausea, vomiting, phlebitis, hypokalemia, fever, and diarrhea, as well as increases in alkaline phosphatase, aspartate aminotransferase, and alanine aminotransferase. Micafungin was as well tolerated as caspofungin in a double-blind comparative study [86].

44.4.3 Anidulafungin

Anidulafungin is the third approved echinocandin, with a spectrum and activity similar to caspofungin and micafungin. Anidulafungin is a semi-synthetic derived from a fermentation product of *Aspergillus nidulans* [99]. As for the other echinocandins, oral bioavailability is low, and i.v. administration is required. Anidulafungin has been successfully assessed in *Candida* infections [39, 93, 115].

44.4.3.1 Pharmacokinetics

Anidulafungin is distinct among the echinocandins in that it undergoes slow degradation from a ring form into a linear peptide by non-specific chemical peptidases in human plasma with no evidence of hepatic-mediated metabolism [99]. Anidulafungin is eliminated predominantly as degradation products in the feces. As a consequence, impairments in renal or hepatic function do not substantially alter its pharmacokinetics [32]. The primary degradation product does not retain antifungal activity. The terminal half-life is longer (approximately 1 day) than for micafungin and caspofungin.

Anidulafungin has not demonstrated any drug–drug interactions because it is not a substrate, inhibitor, or inducer of the cytochrome P450 enzyme system.

44.4.3.2 Clinical Efficacy

A large phase III study compared anidulafungin and fluconazole in invasive candidiasis in adult patients [93]. The response rate was higher in the group of patients receiving anidulafungin. The frequency and types of adverse events were similar in the two groups. A combination of anidulafungin plus liposomal amphotericin B has been assessed in invasive aspergillosis in a very low number of patients. Safety analysis did not demonstrate any unexpected toxicity. Efficacy analysis has not yet been published.

44.4.3.3 Tolerability

Anidulafungin is well tolerated in adults and pediatric patients, with few reported adverse drug events.

44.5 Flucytosine

Flucytosine (5-fluorocytosine) acts as an antimetabolite. It is activated by deamination within the fungal cells to 5-fluorouracil, resulting in an inhibition of fungal DNA and proteins synthesis. Flucytosine is available in an oral form and as an i.v. preparation.

Its spectrum is restricted to *Candida* species and *C. neoformans* with evidence of primary and acquired resistance in some strains. Flucytosine is also active against some of the dematiaceous fungi [116].

Flucytosine should not be used as monotherapy with the exception of the treatment of urinary tract infections due to non-*albicans Candida* species [85]. Resistance may develop rapidly during therapy. Flucytosine has been recommended by expert panels for severe *Candida* infections in combination with amphotericin B. It is also the partner of amphotericin B in the standard of care for the initial therapy of *C. neoformans* neuromeningeal and disseminated infections, especially in AIDS patients [90]. In this latter indication, flucytosine is given at a daily dose of 100 mg/kg/day concomitantly with amphotericin B deoxycholate (0.7–1.0 mg/kg/day) for 2 weeks.

Most common toxicities are hematopoietic, occurring mainly in patients with renal impairment and liver toxicity [116].

44.6 Combination Antifungal Therapy

Combination of two antifungal agents has been proposed to improve further the outcome of the most severe of these infections. Combination therapy could confer antimicrobial synergy (resulting from inhibition of different stages of the same pathway, increased intracellular penetration of an agent by the action of another agent on the cell wall or membrane, transport interaction, or action on different molecular targets), complementary pharmacokinetics, a broader spectrum for empiric or pre-emptive therapy, or reduced acquired resistance. Expected clinical results are: increased response rate and survival, accelerated response to therapy allowing shorter treatment duration, and reduction in length of hospitalization. However, a combination of antifungal agents may also lead to antagonism or to increased toxicity, and will considerably increase antifungal drug acquisition costs. Substantial amounts of in vitro and experimental data support the use of antifungal combination. Unfortunately, clinical data are only limited and somewhat controversial.

The best example of the beneficial effect of combination therapy was shown in cryptococcosis more than 2 decades ago and is still recommended for treatment of neuromeningeal cryptococcosis and of severe non-neuromeningeal infections [90]. The combination of amphotericin B and flucytosine provided a higher response rate and a lower relapse rate in patients with neuromeningeal cryptococcosis [11]. These results were later confirmed in HIV positive patients, and combination therapy is now recommended for first-line therapy of neuromeningeal and severe pulmonary cryptococcosis.

Data are less convincing in invasive candidiasis. Combination of amphotericin B and flucytosine has also been recommended in guidelines for the most severe forms of invasive candidiasis, but this recommendation was based on expert opinions and not on data [33]. Later a large clinical trial compared fluconazole alone and a combination of amphotericin B plus fluconazole in candidemia, showing a higher response rate and less failure to clear the cultures, but also a higher rate of nephrotoxicity and no difference in survival [33, 96]. Currently, the recommendation is to treat invasive candidiasis using monotherapy except for in cases of endocarditis, endophtalmitis, or central nervous system infections where combination therapy seems, according to expert opinions, to be a better approach [85].

Combinations including echinocandins look most promising in invasive aspergillosis. In vitro and experimental results suggest potential synergy with amphotericin B plus echinocandin or with triazoles plus echinocandins against *Aspergillus*. Successful outcomes after failure of a previous line of antifungal therapy have been presented in invasive aspergillosis in single case reports, short series, or comparison to a historical control group [79, 102]. In the absence of results from a randomized trial and according to international guidelines, combination therapy cannot yet be recommended for the primary treatment of patients with invasive aspergillosis [57, 121]. Combination therapy remains, however, an alternative to salvage therapy after failure of primary monotherapy.

Echinocandins alone are not active in vitro against Mucorales, but synergy with amphotericin B has been shown in experimental models. Preliminary clinical data suggest these experimental results could translate into a major benefit in clinical practice [94]. Two preclinical studies assessed the effect of combining posaconazole and amphotericin B [104]. In the first study an increase in survival was observed in neutropenic mice; in the second study there was no benefit from combination therapy. In vitro, data also suggest the synergistic effect of the combination of caspofungin and posaconazole [49]. No clinical data are available. Deferasirox, an iron chelator, inhibits growth of some of the Mucorales species. Interestingly, animal models show major synergy of deferasirox and amphotericin B, resulting in major expectations for clinical use. So far, combination therapy is not recommended for the primary treatment of mucormycosis, but is an alternative for second line therapy.

References

1. Abi-Said D, Anassie EJ (1995) New emerging fungal pathogens. Baillieres Clin Infect Dis 2:71–87
2. Adler-Moore J (1994) AmBisome targeting to fungal infections. Bone Marrow Transplant 14(Suppl 5):S3–S7
3. Ahmad SR, Singer SJ, Leissa BG (2001) Congestive heart failure associated with itraconazole. Lancet 357:1766–1767
4. Almyroudis NG, Sutton DA, Fothergill AW, Rinaldi MG, Kusne S (2007) In vitro susceptibilities of 217 clinical isolates of zygomycetes to conventional and new antifungal agents. Antimicrob Agents Chemother 51:2587–2590
5. Anaissie EJ, Kontoyiannis DP, Huls C, Vartivarian SE, Karl C, Prince RA, Bosso J, Bodey GP (1995) Safety, plasma concentrations, and efficacy of high-dose fluconazole in invasive mold infections. J Infect Dis 172:599–602
6. Atkinson AJ Jr, Bennett JE (1978) Amphotericin B pharmacokinetics in humans. Antimicrob Agents Chemother 13: 271–276
7. Balani SK, Xu X, Arison BH, Silva MV, Gries A, DeLuna FA, Cui D, Kari PH, Ly T, Hop CE, Singh R, Wallace MA, Dean DC, Lin JH, Pearson PG, Baillie TA (2000) Metabolites of caspofungin acetate, a potent antifungal agent, in human plasma and urine. Drug Metab Dispos 28:1274–1278
8. Barchiesi F, Colombo AL, McGough DA, Rinaldi MG (1994) Comparative study of broth macrodilution and microdilution techniques for in vitro antifungal susceptibility testing of yeasts by using the National Committee for Clinical Laboratory Standards' proposed standard. J Clin Microbiol 32:2494–2500
9. Barone JA, Moskovitz BL, Guarnieri J, Hassell AE, Colaizzi JL, Bierman RH, Jessen L (1998) Enhanced bioavailability of itraconazole in hydroxypropyl-beta-cyclodextrin solution versus capsules in healthy volunteers. Antimicrob Agents Chemother 42:1862–1865

10. Barone JA, Moskovitz BL, Guarnieri J, Hassell AE, Colaizzi JL, Bierman RH, Jessen L (1998) Food interaction and steady-state pharmacokinetics of itraconazole oral solution in healthy volunteers. Pharmacotherapy 18: 295–301
11. Bennett JE, Dismukes WE, Duma RJ, Medoff G, Sande MA, Gallis H, Leonard J, Fields BT, Bradshaw M, Haywood H, McGee ZA, Cate TR, Cobbs CG, Warner JF, Alling DW (1979) A comparison of amphotericin B alone and combined with flucytosine in the treatment of cryptoccal meningitis. N Engl J Med 301:126–131
12. Betts RF, Nucci M, Talwar D, Gareca M, Queiroz-Telles F, Bedimo RJ, Herbrecht R, Ruiz-Palacios G, Young JA, Baddley JW, Strohmaier KM, Tucker KA, Taylor AF, Kartsonis NA (2009) A Multicenter, double-blind trial of a high-dose caspofungin treatment regimen versus a standard caspofungin treatment regimen for adult patients with invasive candidiasis. Clin Infect Dis 48:1676–1684
13. Boelaert J, Schurgers M, Matthys E, Daneels R, van Peer A, de Beule K, Woestenborghs R, Heykants J (1988) Itraconazole pharmacokinetics in patients with renal dysfunction. Antimicrob Agents Chemother 32:1595–1597
14. Bolard J (1986) Interaction of polyene antibiotics with membrane lipids: physicochemical studies of the molecular basis of selectivity. Drugs Exp Clin Res 12:613–618
15. Boogaerts M, Winston DJ, Bow EJ, Garber G, Reboli AC, Schwarer AP, Novitzky N, Boehme A, Chwetzoff E, de Beule K (2001) Intravenous and oral itraconazole versus intravenous amphotericin B deoxycholate as empirical antifungal therapy for persistent fever in neutropenic patients with cancer who are receiving broad-spectrum antibacterial therapy. A randomized, controlled trial. Ann Intern Med 135:412–422
16. Bow EJ, Laverdiere M, Lussier N, Rotstein C, Cheang MS, Ioannou S (2002) Antifungal prophylaxis for severely neutropenic chemotherapy recipients: a meta analysis of randomized-controlled clinical trials. Cancer 94:3230–3246
17. Bowden R, Chandrasekar P, White MH, Li X, Pietrelli L, Gurwith M, van Burik JA, Laverdiere M, Safrin S, Wingard JR (2002) A double-blind, randomized, controlled trial of amphotericin B colloidal dispersion versus amphotericin B for treatment of invasive aspergillosis in immunocompromised patients. Clin Infect Dis 35:359–366
18. Chan JD (1998) Pharmacokinetic drug interactions of vinca alkaloids: summary of case reports. Pharmacotherapy 18:1304–1307
19. Chandrasekar PH, Ito JI (2005) Amphotericin B lipid complex in the management of invasive aspergillosis in immunocompromised patients. Clin Infect Dis 40(Suppl 6): S392–S400
20. Christiansen KJ, Bernard EM, Gold JW, Armstrong D (1985) Distribution and activity of amphotericin B in humans. J Infect Dis 152:1037–1043
21. Clements JS Jr, Peacock JE Jr (1990) Amphotericin B revisited: reassessment of toxicity. Am J Med 88:22N–27N
22. Cornely OA, Maertens J, Bresnik M, Ebrahimi R, Ullmann AJ, Bouza E, Heussel CP, Lortholary O, Rieger C, Boehme A, Aoun M, Horst HA, Thiebaut A, Ruhnke M, Reichert D, Vianelli N, Krause SW, Olavarria E, Herbrecht R (2007) Liposomal amphotericin B as initial therapy for invasive mold infection: a randomized trial comparing a high-loading dose regimen with standard dosing (AmBiLoad trial). Clin Infect Dis 44:1289–1297
23. Cornely OA, Maertens J, Winston DJ, Perfect J, Ullmann AJ, Walsh TJ, Helfgott D, Holowiecki J, Stockelberg D, Goh YT, Petrini M, Hardalo C, Suresh R, Angulo-Gonzalez D (2007) Posaconazole vs. fluconazole or itraconazole prophylaxis in patients with neutropenia. N Engl J Med 356: 348–359
24. Courtney R, Pai S, Laughlin M, Lim J, Batra V (2003) Pharmacokinetics, safety, and tolerability of oral posaconazole administered in single and multiple doses in healthy adults. Antimicrob Agents Chemother 47:2788–2795
25. Courtney R, Wexler D, Radwanski E, Lim J, Laughlin M (2004) Effect of food on the relative bioavailability of two oral formulations of posaconazole in healthy adults. Br J Clin Pharmacol 57:218–222
26. Daneshmend TK, Warnock DW (1983) Clinical pharmacokinetics of systemic antifungal drugs. Clin Pharmacokinet 8:17–42
27. de Almeida MB, Bussamra MH, Rodrigues JC (2006) Allergic bronchopulmonary aspergillosis in paediatric cystic fibrosis patients. Paediatr Respir Rev 7:67–72
28. Debruyne D, Ryckelynck JP (1993) Clinical pharmacokinetics of fluconazole. Clin Pharmacokinet 24:10–27
29. Denning DW (1996) Therapeutic outcome in invasive aspergillosis. Clin Infect Dis 23:608–615
30. Denning DW, Lee JY, Hostetler JS, Pappas P, Kauffman CA, Dewsnup DH, Galgiani JN, Graybill JR, Sugar AM, Catanzaro A (1994) NIAID mycoses study group multicenter Trial of oral itraconazole therapy for invasive aspergillosis. Am J Med 97:135–144
31. Denning DW, Van Wye JE, Lewiston NJ, Stevens DA (1991) Adjunctive therapy of allergic bronchopulmonary aspergillosis with itraconazole. Chest 100:813–819
32. Dowell JA, Knebel W, Ludden T, Stogniew M, Krause D, Henkel T (2004) Population pharmacokinetic analysis of anidulafungin, an echinocandin antifungal. J Clin Pharmacol 44:590–598
33. Edwards JE Jr, Bodey GP, Bowden RA, Buchner T, De Pauw BE, Filler SG, Ghannoum MA, Glauser M, Herbrecht R, Kauffman CA, Kohno S, Martino P, Meunier F, Mori T, Pfaller MA, Rex JH, Rogers TR, Rubin RH, Solomkin J, Viscoli C, Walsh TJ, White M (1997) International conference for the development of a consensus on the management and prevention of severe candidal infections. Clin Infect Dis 25:43–59
34. Eschenauer G, Depestel DD, Carver PL (2007) Comparison of echinocandin antifungals. Ther Clin Risk Manag 3: 71–97
35. Espinel-Ingroff A (1998) In vitro activity of the new triazole voriconazole (UK-109, 496) against opportunistic filamentous and dimorphic fungi and common and emerging yeast pathogens. J Clin Microbiol 36:198–202
36. Ezzet F, Wexler D, Courtney R, Krishna G, Lim J, Laughlin M (2005) Oral bioavailability of posaconazole in fasted healthy subjects: comparison between three regimens and basis for clinical dosage recommendations. Clin Pharmacokinet 44: 211–220
37. Fielding RM, Singer AW, Wang LH, Babbar S, Guo LS (1992) Relationship of pharmacokinetics and drug distribution in tissue to increased safety of amphotericin B colloidal

dispersion in dogs. Antimicrob Agents Chemother 36: 299–307
38. Franzot SP, Hamdan JS (1996) In vitro susceptibilities of clinical and environmental isolates of Cryptococcus neoformans to five antifungal drugs. Antimicrob Agents Chemother 40:822–824
39. Gafter-Gvili A, Vidal L, Goldberg E, Leibovici L, Paul M (2008) Treatment of invasive candidal infections: systematic review and meta-analysis. Mayo Clin Proc 83:1011–1021
40. Gallin JI, Alling DW, Malech HL, Wesley R, Koziol D, Marciano B, Eisenstein EM, Turner ML, DeCarlo ES, Starling JM, Holland SM (2003) Itraconazole to prevent fungal infections in chronic granulomatous disease. N Engl J Med 348:2416–2422
41. Gallis HA, Drew RH, Pickard W (1990) Amphotericin B: 30 years of clinical experience. Rev Infect Dis 12:308–329
42. Glasmacher A, Cornely O, Ullmann AJ, Wedding U, Bodenstein H, Wandt H, Boewer C, Pasold R, Wolf HH, Hanel M, Dolken G, Junghanss C, Andreesen R, Bertz H (2006) An open-label randomized trial comparing itraconazole oral solution with fluconazole oral solution for primary prophylaxis of fungal infections in patients with haematological malignancy and profound neutropenia. J Antimicrob Chemother 57:317–325
43. Glasmacher A, Prentice A (2006) Current experience with itraconazole in neutropenic patients: a concise overview of pharmacological properties and use in prophylactic and empirical antifungal therapy. Clin Microbiol Infect 12(Suppl 7):84–90
44. Glasmacher A, Prentice A, Gorschluter M, Engelhart S, Hahn C, Djulbegovic B, Schmidt-Wolf IG (2003) Itraconazole prevents invasive fungal infections in neutropenic patients treated for hematologic malignancies: evidence from a meta-analysis of 3, 597 patients. J Clin Oncol 21:4615–4626
45. Goodman JL, Winston DJ, Greenfield RA, Chandrasekar PH, Fox B, Kaizer H, Shadduck RK, Shea TC, Stiff P, Friedman DJ (1992) A controlled trial of fluconazole to prevent fungal infections in patients undergoing bone marrow transplantation. N Engl J Med 326:845–851
46. Goodwin ML, Drew RH (2008) Antifungal serum concentration monitoring: an update. J Antimicrob Chemother 61:17–25
47. Goodwin SD, Cleary JD, Walawander CA, Taylor JW, Grasela TH Jr (1995) Pretreatment regimens for adverse events related to infusion of amphotericin B. Clin Infect Dis 20:755–761
48. Greenberg RN, Mullane K, van Burik JA, Raad I, Abzug MJ, Anstead G, Herbrecht R, Langston A, Marr KA, Schiller G, Schuster M, Wingard JR, Gonzalez CE, Revankar SG, Corcoran G, Kryscio RJ, Hare R (2006) Posaconazole as salvage therapy for zygomycosis. Antimicrob Agents Chemother 50:126–133
49. Guembe M, Guinea J, Pelaez T, Torres-Narbona M, Bouza E (2007) Synergistic effect of posaconazole and caspofungin against clinical zygomycetes. Antimicrob Agents Chemother 51:3457–3458
50. Guinea J, Pelaez T, Recio S, Torres-Narbona M, Bouza E (2008) In Vitro antifungal activity of isavuconazole (BAL4815), voriconazole, and fluconazole against 1, 007 isolates of Zygomycetes, Candida, Aspergillus, Fusarium, and Scedosporium species. Antimicrob Agents Chemother 52:1396–4000
51. Hebert MF, Smith HE, Marbury TC, Swan SK, Smith WB, Townsend RW, Buell D, Keirns J, Bekersky I (2005) Pharmacokinetics of micafungin in healthy volunteers, volunteers with moderate liver disease, and volunteers with renal dysfunction. J Clin Pharmacol 45:1145–1152
52. Heidemann HT, Gerkens JF, Spickard WA, Jackson EK, Branch RA (1983) Amphotericin B nephrotoxicity in humans decreased by salt repletion. Am J Med 75:476–481
53. Heinemann V, Bosse D, Jehn U, Kahny B, Wachholz K, Debus A, Scholz P, Kolb HJ, Wilmanns W (1997) Pharmacokinetics of liposomal amphotericin B (Ambisome) in critically ill patients. Antimicrob Agents Chemother 41:1275–1280
54. Herbrecht R (2004) Posaconazole: a potent, extended-spectrum triazole anti-fungal for the treatment of serious fungal infections. Int J Clin Pract 58:612–624
55. Herbrecht R (2004) Voriconazole: therapeutic review of a new azole antifungal. Expert Rev Anti Infect Ther 2:485–497
56. Herbrecht R, Denning DW, Patterson TF, Bennett JE, Greene RE, Oestmann JW, Kern WV, Marr KA, Ribaud P, Lortholary O, Sylvester R, Rubin RH, Wingard JR, Stark P, Durand C, Caillot D, Thiel E, Chandrasekar PH, Hodges MR, Schlamm HT, Troke PF, de Pauw B (2002) Voriconazole versus amphotericin B for primary therapy of invasive aspergillosis. N Engl J Med 347:408–415
57. Herbrecht R, Flueckiger U, Gachot B, Ribaud P, Thiebaut A, Cordonnier C (2007) Treatment of invasive Candida and invasive Aspergillus infections in adult haematological patients. Eur J Cancer 5(Suppl 2):49–59
58. Herbrecht R, Letscher V, Andres E, Cavalier A (1999) Safety and efficacy of amphotericin B colloidal dispersion. An overview. Chemotherapy 45:67–76
59. Herbrecht R, Letscher-Bru V, Bowden RA, Kusne S, Anaissie EJ, Graybill JR, Noskin GA, Oppenheim AE, Pietrelli LA (2001) Treatment of 21 cases of invasive mucormycosis with amphotericin B colloidal dispersion. Eur J Clin Microbiol Infect Dis 20:460–466
60. Herbrecht R, Maertens J, Baila L, Aoun M, Heinz W, Martino R, Schwartz S, Ullmann AJ, Meert L, Paesmans M, Marchetti O, Akan H, Ameye L, Shivaprakash M, Viscoli C (2010) Caspofungin first-line therapy for invasive aspergillosis in allogeneic hematopoietic stem cell transplant patients: an EORTC study. Bone Marrow Transplant 45(7): 1227–1233
61. Heykants J, van Peer A, Van dV V, Van Rooy P, Meuldermans W, Lavrijsen K, Woestenborghs R, Van Cutsem J, Cauwenbergh G (1989) The clinical pharmacokinetics of itraconazole: an overview. Mycoses 32(Suppl 1):67–87
62. Ito JI, Hooshmand-Rad R (2005) Treatment of Candida infections with amphotericin B lipid complex. Clin Infect Dis 40(Suppl 6):S384–S391
63. Janoff AS, Boni LT, Popescu MC, Minchey SR, Cullis PR, Madden TD, Taraschi T, Gruner SM, Shyamsunder E, Tate MW (1988) Unusual lipid structures selectively reduce the toxicity of amphotericin B. Proc Natl Acad Sci USA 85:6122–6126
64. Johnson LB, Kauffman CA (2003) Voriconazole: a new triazole antifungal agent. Clin Infect Dis 36:630–637

65. Kanda Y, Yamamoto R, Chizuka A, Hamaki T, Suguro M, Arai C, Matsuyama T, Takezako N, Miwa A, Kern W, Kami M, Akiyama H, Hirai H, Togawa A (2000) Prophylactic action of oral fluconazole against fungal infection in neutropenic patients. A meta-analysis of 16 randomized, controlled trials. Cancer 89:1611–1625
66. Keating GM, Jarvis B (2001) Caspofungin. Drugs 61: 1121–1129
67. Khoo SH, Bond J, Denning DW (1994) Administering amphotericin B-a practical approach. J Antimicrob Chemother 33:203–213
68. Kontoyiannis DP, Lionakis MS, Lewis RE, Chamilos G, Healy M, Perego C, Safdar A, Kantarjian H, Champlin R, Walsh TJ, Raad II (2005) Zygomycosis in a tertiary-care cancer center in the era of Aspergillus-active antifungal therapy: a case-control observational study of 27 recent cases. J Infect Dis 191:1350–1360
69. Krieter P, Flannery B, Musick T, Gohdes M, Martinho M, Courtney R (2004) Disposition of posaconazole following single-dose oral administration in healthy subjects. Antimicrob Agents Chemother 48:3543–3551
70. Kuse ER, Chetchotisakd P, da Cunha CA, Ruhnke M, Barrios C, Raghunadharao D, Sekhon JS, Freire A, Ramasubramanian V, Demeyer I, Nucci M, Leelarasamee A, Jacobs F, Decruyenaere J, Pittet D, Ullmann AJ, Ostrosky-Zeichner L, Lortholary O, Koblinger S, Diekmann-Berndt H, Cornely OA (2007) Micafungin versus liposomal amphotericin B for candidaemia and invasive candidosis: a phase III randomised double-blind trial. Lancet 369:1519–1527
71. Leveque D, Nivoix Y, Jehl F, Herbrecht R (2006) Clinical pharmacokinetics of voriconazole. Int J Antimicrob Agents 27:274–284
72. Levy M, Domaratzki J, Koren G (1995) Amphotericin-induced heart-rate decrease in children. Clin Pediatr 34:358–364
73. Lin SJ, Schranz J, Teutsch SM (2001) Aspergillosis case-fatality rate: systematic review of the literature. Clin Infect Dis 32:358–366
74. Maertens J, Frère P, Lass-Floerl C, Heinz W, Cornely OA (2007) Primary antifungal prophylaxis in leukaemia patients. Eur J Cancer 5(suppl 2):43–48
75. Maertens J, Glasmacher A, Herbrecht R, Thiebaut A, Cordonnier C, Segal BH, Killar J, Taylor A, Kartsonis N, Patterson TF, Aoun M, Caillot D, Sable C (2006) Multicenter, noncomparative study of caspofungin in combination with other antifungals as salvage therapy in adults with invasive aspergillosis. Cancer 107:2888–2897
76. Maertens J, Raad I, Petrikkos G, Boogaerts M, Selleslag D, Petersen FB, Sable CA, Kartsonis NA, Ngai A, Taylor A, Patterson TF, Denning DW, Walsh TJ (2004) Efficacy and safety of caspofungin for treatment of invasive aspergillosis in patients refractory to or intolerant of conventional antifungal therapy. Clin Infect Dis 39: 1563–1571
77. Mantadakis E, Amoiridis G, Kondi A, Kalmanti M (2007) Possible increase of the neurotoxicity of vincristine by the concurrent use of posaconazole in a young adult with leukemia. J Pediatr Hematol Oncol 29:130
78. Marchetti O, Cordonnier C, Calandra T (2007) Empirical antifungal therapy in neutropenic cancer patients with persistent fever. Eur J Cancer 5(Suppl 2):32–42
79. Marr KA, Boeckh M, Carter RA, Kim HW, Corey L (2004) Combination antifungal therapy for invasive aspergillosis. Clin Infect Dis 39:797–802
80. Marr KA, Crippa F, Leisenring W, Hoyle M, Boeckh M, Balajee SA, Nichols WG, Musher B, Corey L (2004) Itraconazole versus fluconazole for prevention of fungal infections in patients receiving allogeneic stem cell transplants. Blood 103:1527–1533
81. Marr KA, Leisenring W, Crippa F, Slattery JT, Corey L, Boeckh M, McDonald GB (2004) Cyclophosphamide metabolism is affected by azole antifungals. Blood 103:1557–1559
82. Miyama T, Takanaga H, Matsuo H, Yamano K, Yamamoto K, Iga T, Naito M, Tsuruo T, Ishizuka H, Kawahara Y, Sawada Y (1998) P-glycoprotein-mediated transport of itraconazole across the blood-brain barrier. Antimicrob Agents Chemother 42:1738–1744
83. Mora-Duarte J, Betts R, Rotstein C, Colombo AL, Thompson-Moya L, Smietana J, Lupinacci R, Sable C, Kartsonis N, Perfect J (2002) Comparison of caspofungin and amphotericin B for invasive candidiasis. N Engl J Med 347:2020–2029
84. Offner F, Krcmery V, Boogaerts M, Doyen C, Engelhard D, Ribaud P, Cordonnier C, de Pauw B, Durrant S, Marie JP, Moreau P, Guiot H, Samonis G, Sylvester R, Herbrecht R (2004) Liposomal nystatin in patients with invasive aspergillosis refractory to or intolerant of amphotericin B. Antimicrob Agents Chemother 48:4808–4812
85. Pappas PG, Kauffman CA, Andes D, Benjamin DK Jr, Calandra TF, Edwards JE Jr, Filler SG, Fisher JF, Kullberg BJ, Ostrosky-Zeichner L, Reboli AC, Rex JH, Walsh TJ, Sobel JD (2009) Clinical practice guidelines for the management of candidiasis: 2009 update by the Infectious Diseases Society of America. Clin Infect Dis 48:503–535
86. Pappas PG, Rotstein CM, Betts RF, Nucci M, Talwar D, De Waele JJ, Vazquez JA, Dupont BF, Horn DL, Ostrosky-Zeichner L, Reboli AC, Suh B, Digumarti R, Wu C, Kovanda LL, Arnold LJ, Buell DN (2007) Micafungin versus caspofungin for treatment of candidemia and other forms of invasive candidiasis. Clin Infect Dis 45:883–893
87. Pascual A, Calandra T, Bolay S, Buclin T, Bille J, Marchetti O (2008) Voriconazole therapeutic drug monitoring in patients with invasive mycoses improves efficacy and safety outcomes. Clin Infect Dis 46:201–211
88. Pasqualotto AC, Denning DW (2008) New and emerging treatments for fungal infections. J Antimicrob Chemother 61(Suppl 1):i19–i30
89. Perfect JR (2005) Treatment of non-Aspergillus moulds in immunocompromised patients, with amphotericin B lipid complex. Clin Infect Dis 40(Suppl 6):S401–S408
90. Perfect JR, Dismukes WE, Dromer F, Goldman DL, Graybill JR, Hamill RJ, Harrison TS, Larsen RA, Lortholary O, Nguyen MH, Pappas PG, Powderly WG, Singh N, Sobel JD, Sorrell TC (2010) Clinical Practice Guidelines for the Management of Cryptococcal Disease: 2010 Update by the Infectious Diseases Society of America. Clin Infect Dis 50(3):291–322
91. Pfaller MA, Messer S, Jones RN (1997) Activity of a new triazole, Sch 56592, compared with those of four other antifungal agents tested against clinical isolates of Candida spp. and Saccharomyces cerevisiae. Antimicrob Agents Chemother 41:233–235

92. Prentice HG, Hann IM, Herbrecht R, Aoun M, Kvaloy S, Catovsky D, Pinkerton CR, Schey SA, Jacobs F, Oakhill A, Stevens RF, Darbyshire PJ, Gibson BE (1997) A randomized comparison of liposomal versus conventional amphotericin B for the treatment of pyrexia of unknown origin in neutropenic patients. Br J Haematol 98: 711–718
93. Reboli AC, Rotstein C, Pappas PG, Chapman SW, Kett DH, Kumar D, Betts R, Wible M, Goldstein BP, Schranz J, Krause DS, Walsh TJ (2007) Anidulafungin versus fluconazole for invasive candidiasis. N Engl J Med 356:2 472–2482
94. Reed C, Bryant R, Ibrahim AS, Edwards J Jr, Filler SG, Goldberg R, Spellberg B (2008) Combination polyene-caspofungin treatment of rhino-orbital-cerebral mucormycosis. Clin Infect Dis 47:364–371
95. Rex JH, Bennett JE, Sugar AM, Pappas PG, van der Horst CM, Edwards JE, Washburn RG, Scheld WM, Karchmer AW, Dine AP, Levenstein MJ, Webb CD, Candidemia Study Group and the National Institute of Allergy and Infectious Diseases Mycosis Study Group (1994) A randomized trial comparing fluconazole with amphotericin B for the treatment of candidemia in patients without neutropenia. N Engl J Med 331:1325–1330
96. Rex JH, Pappas PG, Karchmer AW, Sobel J, Edwards JE, Hadley S, Brass C, Vazquez JA, Chapman SW, Horowitz HW, Zervos M, McKinsey D, Lee J, Babinchak T, Bradsher RW, Cleary JD, Cohen DM, Danziger L, Goldman M, Goodman J, Hilton E, Hyslop NE, Kett DH, Lutz J, Rubin RH, Scheld WM, Schuster M, Simmons B, Stein DK, Washburn RG, Mautner L, Chu TC, Panzer H, Rosenstein RB, Booth J (2003) A randomized and blinded multicenter trial of high-dose fluconazole plus placebo versus fluconazole plus amphotericin B as therapy for candidemia and its consequences in nonneutropenic subjects. Clin Infect Dis 36:1221–1228
97. Rijnders BJ, Cornelissen JJ, Slobbe L, Becker MJ, Doorduijn JK, Hop WC, Ruijgrok EJ, Lowenberg B, Vulto A, Lugtenburg PJ, de Marie S (2008) Aerosolized liposomal amphotericin B for the prevention of invasive pulmonary aspergillosis during prolonged neutropenia: a randomized, placebo-controlled trial. Clin Infect Dis 46:1401–1408
98. Rotowa NA, Shadomy HJ, Shadomy S (1990) In vitro activities of polyene and imidazole antifungal agents against unusual opportunistic fungal pathogens. Mycoses 33: 203–211
99. Sabol K, Gumbo T (2008) Anidulafungin in the treatment of invasive fungal infections. Ther Clin Risk Manag 4:71–78
100. Sakaeda T, Iwaki K, Kakumoto M, Nishikawa M, Niwa T, Jin JS, Nakamura T, Nishiguchi K, Okamura N, Okumura K (2005) Effect of micafungin on cytochrome P450 3A4 and multidrug resistance protein 1 activities, and its comparison with azole antifungal drugs. J Pharm Pharmacol 57:759–764
101. Sanders SW, Buchi KN, Goddard MS, Lang JK, Tolman KG (1991) Single-dose pharmacokinetics and tolerance of a cholesteryl sulfate complex of amphotericin B administered to healthy volunteers. Antimicrob Agents Chemother 35:1029–1034
102. Singh N, Limaye AP, Forrest G, Safdar N, Munoz P, Pursell K, Houston S, Rosso F, Montoya JG, Patton P, Del Busto R, Aguado JM, Fisher RA, Klintmalm GB, Miller R, Wagener MM, Lewis RE, Kontoyiannis DP, Husain S (2006) Combination of voriconazole and caspofungin as primary therapy for invasive aspergillosis in solid organ transplant recipients: a prospective, multicenter, observational study. Transplantation 81:320–326
103. Slavin MA, Osborne B, Adams R, Levenstein MJ, Schoch HG, Feldman AR, Meyers JD, Bowden RA (1995) Efficacy and safety of fluconazole prophylaxis for fungal infections after marrow transplantation–a prospective, randomized, double-blind study. J Infect Dis 171:1545–1552
104. Spellberg B, Walsh TJ, Kontoyiannis DP, Edwards J Jr, Ibrahim AS (2009) Recent advances in the management of mucormycosis: from bench to bedside. Clin Infect Dis 48:1743–1751
105. Stone JA, Holland SD, Wickersham PJ, Sterrett A, Schwartz M, Bonfiglio C, Hesney M, Winchell GA, Deutsch PJ, Greenberg H, Hunt TL, Waldman SA (2002) Single- and multiple-dose pharmacokinetics of caspofungin in healthy men. Antimicrob Agents Chemother 46: 739–745
106. Surarit R, Shepherd MG (1987) The effects of azole and polyene antifungals on the plasma membrane enzymes of Candida albicans. J Med Vet Mycol 25:403–413
107. Swenson CE, Perkins WR, Roberts P, Ahmad I, Stevens R, Stevens DA, Janoff AS (1998) In vitro and in vivo antifungal activity of amphotericin B lipid complex: are phospholipases important? Antimicrob Agents Chemother 42: 767–771
108. Tiphine M, Letscher-Bru V, Herbrecht R (1999) Amphotericin B and its new formulations: pharmacologic characteristics, clinical efficacy, and tolerability. Transpl Infect Dis 1:273–283
109. Trifilio S, Pennick G, Pi J, Zook J, Golf M, Kaniecki K, Singhal S, Williams S, Winter J, Tallman M, Gordon L, Frankfurt O, Evens A, Mehta J (2007) Monitoring plasma voriconazole levels may be necessary to avoid subtherapeutic levels in hematopoietic stem cell transplant recipients. Cancer 109:1532–1535
110. Trifilio S, Singhal S, Williams S, Frankfurt O, Gordon L, Evens A, Winter J, Tallman M, Pi J, Mehta J (2007) Breakthrough fungal infections after allogeneic hematopoietic stem cell transplantation in patients on prophylactic voriconazole. Bone Marrow Transplant 40:451–456
111. Ullmann AJ, Lipton JH, Vesole DH, Chandrasekar P, Langston A, Tarantolo SR, Greinix H, Morais DA, Reddy V, Boparai N, Pedicone L, Patino H, Durrant S (2007) Posaconazole or fluconazole for prophylaxis in severe graft-versus-host disease. N Engl J Med 356:335–347
112. van Burik JA, Hare RS, Solomon HF, Corrado ML, Kontoyiannis DP (2006) Posaconazole is effective as salvage therapy in zygomycosis: a retrospective summary of 91 cases. Clin Infect Dis 42:e61–e65
113. van Burik JA, Ratanatharathorn V, Stepan DE, Miller CB, Lipton JH, Vesole DH, Bunin N, Wall DA, Hiemenz JW, Satoi Y, Lee JM, Walsh TJ (2004) Micafungin versus fluconazole for prophylaxis against invasive fungal infections during neutropenia in patients undergoing hematopoietic stem cell transplantation. Clin Infect Dis 39:1407–1416

114. van't Wout JW, Novakova I, Verhagen CA, Fibbe WE, De Pauw BE, van der Meer JW (1991) The efficacy of itraconazole against systemic fungal infections in neutropenic patients: a randomised comparative study with amphotericin B. J Infect 22:45–52
115. Vazquez JA, Schranz JA, Clark K, Goldstein BP, Reboli A, Fichtenbaum C (2008) A phase 2, open-label study of the safety and efficacy of intravenous anidulafungin as a treatment for azole-refractory mucosal candidiasis. J Acquir Immune Defic Syndr 48:304–309
116. Vermes A, Guchelaar HJ, Dankert J (2000) Flucytosine: a review of its pharmacology, clinical indications, pharmacokinetics, toxicity and drug interactions. J Antimicrob Chemother 46:171–179
117. Vertut-Croquin A, Bolard J, Gary-Bobo CM (1985) Transfer of amphotericin B from gel state vesicles to mycoplasma cells: biphasic action on potassium transport and permeability. Antimicrob Agents Chemother 28:167–171
118. Verweij PE, te Dorsthorst DT, Rijs AJ, Vries-Hospers HG, Meis JF (2002) Nationwide survey of in vitro activities of itraconazole and voriconazole against clinical Aspergillus fumigatus isolates cultured between 1945 and 1998. J Clin Microbiol 40:2648–2650
119. Viscoli C, Girmenia C, Marinus A, Collette L, Martino P, Vandercam B, Doyen C, Lebeau B, Spence D, Krcmery V, de Pauw B, Meunier F (1999) Candidemia in cancer patients: a prospective, multicenter surveillance study by the Invasive Fungal Infection Group (IFIG) of the European Organization for Research and Treatment of Cancer (EORTC). Clin Infect Dis 28:1071–1079
120. Viscoli C, Herbrecht R, Akan H, Baila L, Sonet A, Gallamini A, Giagounidis A, Marchetti O, Martino R, Meert L, Paesmans M, Ameye L, Shivaprakash M, Ullmann AJ, Maertens J (2009) An EORTC Phase II study of caspofungin as first-line therapy of invasive aspergillosis in haematological patients. J Antimicrob Chemother 64: 1274–1281
121. Walsh TJ, Anaissie EJ, Denning DW, Herbrecht R, Kontoyiannis DP, Marr KA, Morrison VA, Segal BH, Steinbach WJ, Stevens DA, van Burik JA, Wingard JR, Patterson TF (2008) Treatment of aspergillosis: clinical practice guidelines of the Infectious Diseases Society of America. Clin Infect Dis 46:327–360
122. Walsh TJ, Finberg RW, Arndt C, Hiemenz J, Schwartz C, Bodensteiner D, Pappas P, Seibel N, Greenberg RN, Dummer S, Schuster M, Holcenberg JS (1999) Liposomal amphotericin B for empirical therapy in patients with persistent fever and neutropenia. National Institute of Allergy and Infectious Diseases Mycoses Study Group. N Engl J Med 340:764–771
123. Walsh TJ, Hiemenz JW, Seibel NL, Perfect JR, Horwith G, Lee L, Silber JL, DiNubile MJ, Reboli A, Bow E, Lister J, Anaissie EJ (1998) Amphotericin B lipid complex for invasive fungal infections: analysis of safety and efficacy in 556 cases. Clin Infect Dis 26:1383–1396
124. Walsh TJ, Melcher GP, Rinaldi MG, Lecciones J, McGough DA, Kelly P, Lee J, Callender D, Rubin M, Pizzo PA (1990) Trichosporon beigelii, an emerging pathogen resistant to amphotericin B. J Clin Microbiol 28:1616–1622
125. Walsh TJ, Raad I, Patterson TF, Chandrasekar P, Donowitz GR, Graybill R, Greene RE, Hachem R, Hadley S, Herbrecht R, Langston A, Louie A, Ribaud P, Segal BH, Stevens DA, van Burik JA, White CS, Corcoran G, Gogate J, Krishna G, Pedicone L, Hardalo C, Perfect JR (2007) Treatment of invasive aspergillosis with posaconazole in patients who are refractory to or intolerant of conventional therapy: an externally controlled trial. Clin Infect Dis 44:2–12
126. Walsh TJ, Raad I, Patterson TF, Chandrasekar P, Donowitz GR, Graybill R, Greene RE, Hachem R, Hadley S, Herbrecht R, Langston A, Louie A, Ribaud P, Segal BH, Stevens DA, van Burik JA, White CS, Corcoran G, Gogate J, Krishna G, Pedicone L, Hardalo C, Perfect JR (2007) Treatment of invasive aspergillosis with posaconazole in patients who are refractory to or intolerant of conventional therapy: an externally controlled trial. Clin Infect Dis 44:2–12
127. Walsh TJ, Teppler H, Donowitz GR, Maertens JA, Baden LR, Dmoszynska A, Cornely OA, Bourque MR, Lupinacci RJ, Sable CA, de Pauw BE (2004) Caspofungin versus liposomal amphotericin B for empirical antifungal therapy in patients with persistent fever and neutropenia. N Engl J Med 351:1391–1402
128. Wark PA, Gibson PG, Wilson AJ (2004) Azoles for allergic bronchopulmonary aspergillosis associated with asthma. Cochrane Database Syst Rev CD001108
129. Weiler S, Zoller H, Graziadei I, Vogel W, Bellmann-Weiler R, Joannidis M, Bellmann R (2007) Altered pharmacokinetics of voriconazole in a patient with liver cirrhosis. Antimicrob Agents Chemother 51: 3459–3460
130. White MH, Bowden RA, Sandler ES, Graham ML, Noskin GA, Wingard JR, Goldman M, van Burik JA, McCabe A, Lin JS, Gurwith M, Miller CB (1998) Randomized, double-blind clinical trial of amphotericin B colloidal dispersion vs. amphotericin B in the empirical treatment of fever and neutropenia. Clin Infect Dis 27:296–302
131. Willems L, van Der GR, de Beule K (2001) Itraconazole oral solution and intravenous formulations: a review of pharmacokinetics and pharmacodynamics. J Clin Pharm Ther 26:159–169
132. Wingard JR, White MH, Anaissie E, Raffalli J, Goodman J, Arrieta A (2000) A randomized, double-blind comparative trial evaluating the safety of liposomal amphotericin B versus amphotericin B lipid complex in the empirical treatment of febrile neutropenia. L Amph/ABLC Collaborative Study Group. Clin Infect Dis 31:1155–1163
133. Wong-Beringer A, Jacobs RA, Guglielmo BJ (1998) Lipid formulations of amphotericin B: clinical efficacy and toxicities. Clin Infect Dis 27:603–618

Antiviral Agents in Patients with Hematological Malignancies and Acute Respiratory Failure

45

Michael Sandherr

Contents

M. Sandherr
Gemeinschaftspraxis für Hämatologie und Onkologie,
Röntgenstr. 4, 82362 Weilheim, Germany
e-mail: michael.sandherr@web.de

45.1 Introduction

Despite substantial advances in antiviral therapy, opportunistic viral infections with HSV, VZV and CMV have a major impact on morbidity and mortality in immunocompromised patients, such as patients with hematological malignancies or after hematopoietic stem cell transplantation (HSCT). Since reactivation of latent viruses is the predominant mechanism of clinically relevant infection, antiviral prophylaxis is an attractive approach for patients expecting immunosuppression [1]. Beside prevention of viral transmission, the use of antiviral agents is the key element in treatment and prophylaxis of viral infection in immunocompromised hosts.

Currently, a variety of antiviral agents is approved for clinical use, as well as for prophylaxis or for treatment of an established infection [2]. The purpose of this review is to discuss antiviral agents used for the treatment of herpes viruses (HSV, VZV, and CMV) and respiratory viruses.

This review will not discuss or support the use of immunoglobulins in prophylaxis or treatment of viral infection because its efficacy has not been demonstrated in randomized trials so far.

45.2 Herpes Viruses

45.2.1 Acyclovir and Valacyclovir

Acyclovir is a nucleoside analog with in vitro antiviral activity against HSV, VZV and CMV [3]. Valacyclovir is a prodrug of acyclovir and shares the same mechanism of action with similar adverse effects [4].

É. Azoulay (ed.), *Pulmonary Involvement in Patients with Hematological Malignancies*,
DOI: 10.1007/978-3-642-15742-4_45, © Springer-Verlag Berlin Heidelberg 2011

Intravenous acyclovir is the treatment of choice for systemic and severe HSV disease. It acts as a competitive inhibitor of viral polymerase and HSV thymidine kinase and host cellular enzymes to become active as acyclovir triphosphate. Since CMV does not encode thymidine kinase, it is less susceptible to acyclovir than HSV and VZV. Both acyclovir and valacyclovir are commonly used as prophylaxis against HSV reactivation in patients who are treated with agents resulting in profound T-cell suppression as purine analogs, alemtuzumab or after autologous or allogeneic stem cell transplantation (Table 45.1).

The oral absorption of acyclovir results in a bioavailability of 15–30%. It should be administered intravenously to reach high serum levels in the treatment of less susceptible herpes viruses as VZV. Valacyclovir is the L-valyl ester prodrug of acyclovir and is rapidly hydrolyzed to acyclovir by the liver and the gastrointestinal tract. This results in three to five times higher plasma levels than achieved with oral acyclovir. The bioavailability of valacyclovir was found to be 54.2% after an oral dose of 1,000 mg.

Both drugs have excellent safety profiles. Common adverse events are rash, headache, nausea and diarrhea. Confusion, renal failure and severe thrombocytopenic syndromes have been reported after treatment with high doses of intravenous acyclovir. Since acyclovir is primarily eliminated by the kidney through glomerular

Table 45.1 Antiviral Agents

Agent	Indication	Treatment		
Acyclovir	HSV, VZV, CMV	PROPHYLAXIS		
		HSV	2–3 × 400 mg/day	
		VZV	2 × 800 mg/day	allo SCT
			2 × 400 mg/day	Bortezomib
		CMV	4 × 800 mg/day	allo SCT
		TREATMENT		
		HSV	5 mg/kg iv every 8 h for 7–10 day	
		VZV	5 mg/kg iv every 8 h for 7–10 day	
			5 × 800 mg/day	
		Diss. infection	10 mg/kg iv every 8 h	
Valacyclovir	HSV, VZV	PROPHYLAXIS		
		HSV/VZV	2–3 × 500 mg/day	
		CMV	4 × 2 g/day	allo SCT
		TREATMENT		
		HSV/VZV	3 × 1 g/day	
Ganciclovir	CMV	PROPHYLAXIS	5–6 mg/kg iv/day for 5 day/week	
		PREEMPTIVE THERAPY	5 mg/kg iv/day every 12 h for 2 weeks	
		TREATMENT	5 mg/kg iv/day every 12 h for 2 weeks	
		Followed by	6 mg/kg iv/d on 5 day/week for 2 weeks	
Valganciclovir	CMV	PROPHYLAXIS	900 mg/day	
		PREEMPTIVE THERAPY	2 × 900 mg/day for 2 weeks	
		Followed by	900 mg/day for 7 days	

filtration and tubular secretion, dosages of both drugs must be adjusted in renal malfunction.

Acyclovir and valacyclovir are indicated for prophylaxis and treatment of HSV and VZV reactivation and infection. For prophylaxis according to guidelines, acyclovir is given 400 mg three to four times daily or 800 mg twice daily [1]. In the case of intravenous prophylaxis, acyclovir is dosed at 5 mg/kg bodyweight every 12 h. Oral valacyclovir 500 mg two to three times daily is equivalent to acyclovir in the prevention of HSV reactivation [5]. For treatment of systemic infection of HSV with organ involvement, the dose of intravenous acyclovir should be 5 mg/kg bodyweight every 8 h.

Higher doses and plasma concentrations are needed to treat VZV infections. For herpes zoster reactivation, intravenous acyclovir should be given 10 mg/kg every 8 h and oral valacyclovir 1,000 mg three times daily for 10–14 days. For prophylaxis against VZV reactivation, the same doses as given for HSV prophylaxis appear to be safe in the treatment of patients with hematological malignancies or aplastic anemia. VZV prophylaxis is an important issue after allogeneic stem cell transplantation and treatment with purine analogs, alemtuzumab or bortezomib.

Penciclovir is a competitive and selective inhibitor of viral DNA polymerase, while famciclovir is an oral prodrug of penciclovir with improved oral bioavailability [6]. It is active against HSV, VZV, hepatitis B virus (HBV) and EBV. Famciclovir is indicated for the treatment of HSV and VZV infections. A dose of 500 mg twice daily appears to be equivalent to a treatment of HSV reactivation with acyclovir 400 mg five times daily. In patients after stem cell or solid organ transplantation, famciclovir 500 mg three times daily has proven the same efficacy as acyclovir 800 mg five times daily in the treatment of herpes zoster [7]. Famciclovir was well tolerated with adverse events similar to acyclovir.

Resistance to acyclovir or famciclovir has been rarely reported. The primary mechanism of resistance is associated with mutations in the thymidine kinase gene. Since most acyclovir-resistant HSV and VZV isolates show cross-resistance to penciclovir, treatment with famciclovir in acyclovir-resistant viruses is not recommended.

Efficacy of acyclovir or valacyclovir in the prevention or treatment of CMV reactivation or CMV disease is different. In patients after stem cell transplantation, the risk of CMV infection and CMV disease can be reduced by prophylactic treatment with high-dose acyclovir with a daily dose of 500 mg/m^2 three times daily [8]. In a large randomized study, high-dose valacyclovir with 2 g four times daily reduced the incidence of CMV infection from 40% to 28% in comparison to high-dose acyclovir [9]. There was, however, no difference in CMV disease or survival.

45.2.2 Ganciclovir and Valganciclovir

Ganciclovir is an acyclic nucleoside analog of 2′-deoxyguanosine that interferes with the replication of herpes viruses [10]. It is the standard agent used in prophylaxis, preemptive therapy and treatment of CMV infection and disease [11]. Since it has a poor bioavailability, a prodrug, valganciclovir, was developed and approved for the treatment of CMV retinitis in AIDS patients and for CMV prophylaxis in patients with solid organ transplants. Valganciclovir is the L-valyl ester of ganciclovir with a bioavailability of 60%. After 900 mg oral valganciclovir, the systemic exposure is similar to a dose of 5 mg/kg bodyweight intravenous ganciclovir. Elimination of both drugs is by renal excretion through glomerular filtration and tubular secretion. The adverse effects are similar. Myelosuppression, especially neutropenia, is the dose-limiting toxicity. Other adverse events are nausea and vomiting, diarrhea, pyrexia and, clinically most important, renal failure.

Induction dosing for intravenous ganciclovir is 5 mg/kg every 12 h followed by maintenance therapy with 5 mg/kg daily. For valganciclovir, the induction dose is 900 mg twice daily orally with food followed by maintenance with 900 mg daily. Dose adjustment is mandatory in patients with reduced creatinine clearance.

Prophylaxis with ganciclovir in patients after hematopoietic cell transplantation shows a reduction in CMV disease but no improved survival [12, 13]. Its use at engraftment results in prolonged neutropenia with a higher incidence of invasive bacterial and fungal infections. In addition, a substantial number of patients not at risk for the disease will unnecessarily receive a potentially marrow-toxic drug. Thus, this strategy is not established as standard procedure for prophylaxis of CMV disease in patients after stem cell transplantation [14]. Since no valid data exist for valganciclovir used as prophylaxis, it cannot be recommended. All prophylaxis strategies will result in the unnecessary treatment of patients who will not develop CMV infection or disease.

Preemptive antiviral therapy has evolved as the standard of care in the prevention of CMV disease [14]. It is initiated at the detection of CMV reactivation in the blood by diagnostic techniques, such as the pp65 antigenemia assay or DNA detection methods. Weekly monitoring of CMV replication by PCR or pp65 antigen detection is recommended to trigger antiviral therapy, as this approach lowers the rate of CMV infections and mortality.

Initiation of preemptive ganciclovir therapy is recommended after a single positive pp65 antigen test or after two consecutive positive CMV PCR assays. Weekly monitoring should continue for at least 100 days after HSCT.

In view of an increased risk of delayed CMV reactivations, prolonged monitoring for up to 1 year after transplantation should be conducted in patients with chronic GvHD, prolonged immunosuppression and after T-cell depletion [15]. The same procedure applies to patients having received antiviral treatment for a number of weeks, to recipients of transplantation with reduced conditioning and to those with GvHD.

CMV gastrointestinal disease and pneumonia are the most common manifestations of CMV disease [16]. The incidence in the first year after hematopoietic cell transplantation is 8–10% in seropositive patients. CMV pneumonia is the most feared complication. Standard of care is the treatment with ganciclovir in combination with intravenous immunoglobulin. There does not appear to be a specific advantage of CMV-specific immune globulin compared with pooled immunoglobulin.

45.2.3 Foscarnet

Foscarnet has activity against HSV, VZV and CMV [17]. It is clinically important due to its efficacy in acyclovir-resistant HSV and VZV and ganciclovir-resistant CMV. Foscarnet inhibits viral DNA polymerase by binding to the pyrophosphate binding site and blocking the cleavage of pyrophosphate from the terminal nucleoside triphosphate. The effect of foscarnet on human DNA polymerase appears to be negligible. It has poor bioavailability and should be given intravenously. Renal elimination occurs by glomerular filtration as well as tubular secretion. Dose adjustment in patients with renal insufficiency is therefore mandatory. The main adverse effects of foscarnet include nephrotoxicity, symptomatic hypocalcemia, hypomagnesemia, hyperphosphatemia, hypokalemia and CNS effects. Dose-limiting toxicity is renal failure. Adequate hydration, avoidance of other nephrotoxic agents, and close monitoring of renal function and electrolytes is mandatory during treatment with foscarnet.

Foscarnet is indicated as the second-line treatment in patients with CMV infections [18]. It is standard of care in patients with ganciclovir-associated cytopenias or ganciclovir-resistant CMV. In a randomized trial for prevention of CMV disease after HSCT, foscarnet has been proven to be as efficacious as ganciclovir with a reduction of mortality within 180 days after HSCT [19].

45.2.4 Cidofovir

Cidofovir is an acyclic nucleoside phosphonate analogue of deoxynucleoside monophosphate and has broad antiviral activity against herpes viruses and other DNA viruses [20]. It has a low bioavailability of less than 5% and must be given as intravenous infusion. Renal elimination is the primary route of metabolism, and the simultaneous administration of oral probenecid to reduce nephrotoxicity is mandatory. Renal insufficiency is the dose-limiting toxicity, which may be caused by its accumulation in the renal cortex. The most serious side effects of cidofovir are proteinuria and neutropenia.

Cidofovir is indicated as the second-line treatment for CMV infection. In allogeneic HSCT patients it has been used as salvage treatment of CMV infection and disease not responding to ganciclovir or foscarnet [21]. Induction therapy starts with 5 mg/kg once weekly for 2 weeks followed by maintenance doses of 5 mg/kg intravenously every 2 weeks. In addition to probenecid, patients receive at least 1000 mL of 0.9% saline infusion over a 1–2-h period immediately before the cidofovir infusion.

Cidofovir has also been studied for the prevention and treatment of adenovirus infections in patients after stem cell or solid organ transplantation [22]. There are still limited published data on its efficacy in this setting. Patients with refractory GvHD, umbilical cord transplantation, haploidentical cell transplantation or substantial T-cell depletion have a high risk for adenoviral disease and should be monitored weekly for active adenovirus infection by PCR. The available data suggest that cidofovir could be used as preemptive antiviral therapy of adenoviral disease in selected high-risk patients. The duration of this treatment depends on treatment tolerance and viral load.

Cidofovir has not shown efficacy in the preemptive treatment of asymptomatic patients after HSCT who develop viruria or viremia with polyomaviruses BK or JC.

45.2.5 Maribavir

Maribavir is an oral riboside analogue that of inhibits viral DNA synthesis of CMV and EBV but not other herpes viruses. In patients after allogeneic HSCT, maribavir was effective in the prophylaxis of CMV infection and reduced the incidence of initiation of CMV-directed therapy [23]. Treatment with maribavir was well tolerated, and it did not appear to cause any myelosuppression based on neutrophil and platelet counts. To date, it is not standard of care, but is currently being tested for CMV prevention in several randomized phase III trials.

45.3 Respiratory Viruses

Respiratory viral infections are an important cause of morbidity and mortality in hematopoietic cell transplant recipients and immunosuppressed patients with hematological malignancies [24]. Respiratory syncytial virus (RSV), parainfluenza viruses (PIVs) and influenza viruses are a common cause of upper and lower respiratory tract infection. The epidemiology of these viruses is similar to their occurrence in the community.

Patients with hematological malignancies and after HSCT are at increased risk for infection with influenza virus [25]. Progression to the lower respiratory tract may be a devastating complication with pneumonia, lung injury and death. It occurs after a median of 1 week after the onset of symptoms, and presents radiographically and clinically as viral pneumonia. Upper respiratory tract infection with RSV may progress to fatal pneumonia as well and is associated with the highest attributable mortality of all respiratory viruses [26]. Winter season, male gender and the use of bone marrow as stem cell source were identified as risk factors for infection with RSV during stem cell transplantation.

Parainfluenza virus (PIV) type 3 is the most detected type in HSCT with an incidence of 7%. The only identified risk factor for infection with PIV is transplantation of an unrelated donor. The most important risk factors for the progression from upper respiratory tract infection to pneumonia are the use of systemic corticosteroids and lymphopenia. PIV pneumonia has a high incidence of infection with copathogens such as *Aspergillus fumigatus*.

Recommendations for prophylaxis and treatment of infection with respiratory viruses are limited since controlled or even randomized data are missing. It should be taken into account that viral pneumonia may often be complicated by bacterial and fungal pathogens. Specific management guidelines are difficult to define. An aggressive diagnostic workup is recommended [27].

45.3.1 Neuraminidase Inhibitors

45.3.1.1 Oseltamivir

Oseltamivir is an ethyl ester prodrug of its active metabolite and oseltamivir carboxylate inhibiting influenza neuraminidase, which is responsible for cleaving the cellular-receptor sialic acid residues responsible for the release of progeny influenza virus from infected host cells that can then infect new cells [29]. Neuraminidase inhibitors should be given early in the course of the disease since influenza virus replication in the respiratory tract reaches its peak 1–2 days after the onset of symptoms. Oseltamivir is administered orally as oseltamivir phosphate and converted to its active metabolite oseltamivir carboxylate. It is eliminated mainly by renal excretion.

Oseltamivir has been studied at doses of 75 or 150 mg daily in immunocompetent patients. An advantage of the higher dose could not be demonstrated. The relevance of these studies for highly immunosuppressed patients remains unclear to date. There are minimal data concerning treatment of patients with hematological malignancies with respect to longer duration of symptoms or treatment. It is reasonable to believe that the course of disease is much different in immunocompromised patients due to longer ongoing viral replication, only mild symptoms at disease onset or progression to the lower respiratory tract even later than 1 week of ongoing infection [28].

Oseltamivir is a well-tolerated drug with most common side effects including upper gastrointestinal symptoms such as nausea and vomiting. Allergic skin reactions and rash are rare. Oseltamivir is indicated for the treatment or prophylaxis of influenza viruses type A and B as well as the treatment of avian influenza and infection with seasonal H1N1 influenza viruses. Since a high prevalence of resistance in the latter influenza type occurs, an empiric combination treatment with rimantidine is recommended. Few data exist on the duration of treatment in patients with hematological malignancies and after HSCT. While healthy immunocompetent patients should be treated 5 days, longer treatment should be considered during immunosuppression. The median time from diagnosis of upper respiratory infection to lower tract disease is 7 days in patients after HSCT. Thus, a 5-day course may be too short to prevent cases of late progression.

45.3.1.2 Zanamivir

Zanamivir is a potent inhibitor of influenza types A and B neuraminidase [29]. In influenza enzymatic assays, the antiviral activity of zanamivir is similar to that of oseltamivir carboxylate. Zanamivir has a low bioavailability of approximately 2% and is dispensed as a dry powder for oral inhalation. Drug tolerance is quite good with an incidence of adverse events of less than 4%. The most common side effects in patients with chronic disease or with immunosuppression were sinubronchial distress symptoms and diarrhea. The recommended adult dose of zanamivir for the treatment of influenza type A and B is two oral inhalations twice daily for 5 days. Treatment should start not later than after 48 h of flu-like symptoms. It is also indicated for prophylaxis of influenza infection during periods of increased influenza activity.

45.3.2 Amantadine and Rimantadine

Amantadine and rimantadine are M2 ion channel-blocking antiviral agents that interfere with viral uncoating intracellularly. They are active against influenza A but have no activity against influenza B [30]. The adamantanes are associated with rapid emergence of resistance, and influenza A may be shed for extended periods in immunocompromised patients under amantadine treatment. Thus, adamantanes should not be used until the susceptibility of circulating influenza A strains is established. Amantadine has a high bioavailability after oral administration. The normal daily dose is 200 mg for influenza A prophylaxis given either as a single dose or 100 mg twice daily. Rimantadine is well absorbed after oral administration, and the recommended dose is 200 mg daily.

The main toxicity is CNS-related with dizziness, headache, insomnia and confusion. Patients with a history of seizures should be monitored closely.

45.3.3 Ribavirin

Ribavirin is approved for the treatment of patients with RSV infections. It is a structural analogue of guanosine and inhibits the enzyme IMP dehydrogenase, and has shown in-vitro activity against a variety of respiratory viruses. Ribavirin is administered as a small-particle aerosol using a mask or mechanical ventilator for 12–18 h daily.

Data supporting the use of ribavirin in immunocompromised patients are limited and exist only in the form of nonrandomized studies. It is the treatment of choice in patients with established RSV pneumonia after HSCT and may be used as prophylaxis for progression to pneumonia in patients with RSV upper respiratory tract infection [14]. Systemic ribavirin is not effective for the treatment of pneumonia, but seems to be more effective at the upper respiratory tract infection stage.

45.3.4 Palivizumab

Palivizumab is a RSV-specific humanized monoclonal antibody that is approved for the treatment of RSV disease in high-risk pediatric patients. There are limited data on its efficacy in immunocompromised patients. To date, there are no sufficient data to support its use in combination with ribavirin for treatment of documented pneumonia with RSV in severely immunocompromised children and adults [31].

References

1. Sandherr M, Einsele H, Hebart H et al (2006) Antiviral prophylaxis in patients with haematological malignancies and solid tumors: guidelines of the Infectious Diseases Working Party (AGIHO) of German Society for Hematology and Oncology (DGHO). Ann Oncol 17(7):1051–1059
2. Jancel T, Penzak SR (2009) Antiviral therapy in patients with hematologic malignancies, transplantation and aplastic anemia. Semin Hematol 46(3):230–247
3. Wagstaff AJ, Faulds D, Goa KL (1994) Aciclovir. A reappraisal of its antiviral activity, pharmacokinetic properties and therapeutic efficacy. Drugs 47:153–205
4. Beutner K (1995) Valacyclovir: a review of its antiviral activity, pharmacokinetic properties, and clinical efficacy. Antiviral Res 28:281–290
5. Eisen D, Essell J, Broun ER et al (2003) Clinical utility of oral Valacyclovir compared with oral acyclovir for the prevention of herpes simplex virus Mucositis following autologous bone marrow transplantation or stem cell rescue therapy. Bone Marrow Transplant 31:51–55
6. Bacon TH, Howard BA, Spender LC et al (1996) Activity of penciclovir in antiviral assays against herpes simplex virus. J Antimicrob Chemother 37:303–313
7. Tyring S, Belanger R, Bezwoda W et al (2001) A randomized, double-blind trial of famciclovir versus acyclovir for the treatment of localized dermatomal herpes zoster in immunocompromised patients. Cancer Invest 19: 13–22
8. Meyers JD, Reed EC, Shepp DH et al (1988) Acyclovir for prevention of cytomegalievirus infection and disease after allogeneic marrow transplantation. N Engl J Med 318: 70–75
9. Ljungman P, De la Camara R, Milpied N et al (2002) Randomized study of Valacyclovir as prophylaxis against cytomegalovirus reactivation in recipients of allogeneic bone marrow transplants. Blood 99:3050–3056
10. Curran M, Noble S (2001) Valganciclovir. Drugs 61: 1145–1150
11. Boeckh M, Ljungman P (2009) How I treat cytomegalovirus in haematopoietic cell transplant recipients. Blood 113: 5711–5719
12. Winston DJ, Yeager AM, Chandrasekar PH et al (2003) Randomized comparison of oral valacyclovir and intravenous ganciclovir for prevention of cytomegalovirus disease after allogeneic bone marrow transplantation. Clin Infect Dis 36:749–758
13. Goodrich JM, Bowden RA, Fisher L et al (1993) Ganciclovir prophylaxis to prevent cytomegalovirus disease after allogeneic bone marrow transplant. Ann Intern Med 118:173–178
14. Zaia J, Baden L, Boeckh MJ et al (2009) Viral diease prevention after hematopoietic cell transplantation. Bone Marrow Transplant 44:471–482
15. Boeckh M, Nichols W, Chemaly R et al (2008) Prevention of late CMV disease after HCT: a randomized double-blind multicenter trail of valganciclovir prophylaxis versus PCR-guided GCV/VGCV preemptive therapy. Biol Blood Marrow Transplant 14:30, abstract 75
16. Ljungman P, Griffiths P, Paya C (2002) Definitions of cytomegalovirus infection and disease in transplant recipients. Clin Infect Dis 34:1094–1097
17. Crumpacker CS (1992) Mechanism of action in foscarnet against viral polymerases. Am J Med 92:3S–7S
18. Razonable RR, Emery VC (2004) Management of CMV infection and disease in transplant patients. Herpes 11:77–86
19. Reusser P, Einsele H, Lee J et al (2002) Randomized multicenter trial of foscarnet versus ganciclovir for preemptive therapy of cytomegalovirus infection after allogeneic stem cell transplantation. Blood 99:1159–1164
20. De Clercq E, Holy A (2005) Acyclic nucleoside phosphonates: a key class of antiviral drugs. Nat Rev Drug Discov 4:928–940
21. Ljungman P, Deliliers GL, Platzbecker U et al (2001) Cidofovir for cytomegalovirus infection and disease in allogeneic stem cell transplant recipients. Blood 97: 388–392
22. Ison MG (2006) Adenovirus infections in transplant recipients. Clin Infect Dis 43:331–339
23. Winston D, Young J, Pullarkat V et al (2008) Maribavir prophylaxis for prevention of cytomegalovirus infection in allogeneic stem cell transplant recipients: a multicenter randomized, double-blind, placebo-controlled, dose-ranging study. Blood 111:5403–5410
24. Englund JA (2001) Diagnosis and epidemiology of community-acquired respiratory virus infections in the immunocompromised host. Biol Blood Marrow Transplant 7(Suppl):2S–4S
25. Boeckh M (2008) The challenge of respiratory virus infections in hematopoietic cell transplant recipients. Br J Haematol 143:455–467
26. Anaissie E, Mahfouz TH, Aslan T et al (2004) The natural history of respiratory syncytial virus infection in cancer and transplant patients: implications for management. Blood 103:1611–1617
27. Nichols WG, Campbell AJ, Boeckh M (2008) Respiratory viruses other than Influenza virus: impact and therapeutic advances. Clin Microbiol Rev 21(2):274–290
28. Casper C, Englung J, Boeckh M (2010) How we treat influenza in patients with hematologic malignancies. Blood 115(7):1331–1342
29. Moscona A (2005) Neuraminidase inhibitors for influenza. N Engl J Med 353:1363–1373
30. Jefferson T, Demicheli V, Rivetti D et al (2006) Antivirals for influenza in healthy adults: systematic review. Lancet 367:303–313
31. de Fontbrune FS, Robin M, Porcher R, Scieux C, de Latour RP, Ferry C, Rocha V, Boudjedir K, Devergie A, Bergeron A, Gluckman E, Azoulay E, Lapalu J, Socié G, Ribaud P (2007) Palivizumab treatment of respiratory syncytial virus infection after allogeneic hematopoietic stem cell transplantation. Clin Infect Dis 45(8):1019–1024, 15 Oct 2007

Mechanical Ventilation in Patients with Hematological Malignancies

46

Márcio Soares, Jorge I.F. Salluh, and Pieter O. Depuydt

Contents

Acute respiratory failure (ARF) requiring mechanical ventilation (MV) is a severe and frequent complication in patients with hematological malignancies (HMs). For many years, ARF developing in these patients was considered a consequence of refractory pulmonary diseases invariably associated with dismal outcomes, and, as a result, physicians felt that admission to the intensive care unit (ICU) was inappropriate. However, the situation has changed. Now, there is no scientific reason to deny ICU admission to patients with HMs and ARF. In recent years, several specialized centers have reported improved survival rates. In addition to advances in hematological and critical care, this improvement has been ascribed to better patient selection for ICU admission and to the use of MV.

However, patient selection is complex, as it depends on multiple factors, and disagreements are still common among hematologists and intensivists. In addition to ICU admission guidelines, clinicians should take into consideration patient-related characteristics, expectations regarding post-ICU outcomes, published evidence, personal experience, and each patient's wishes and values. These multiple factors can only be analyzed on a case-by-case basis.

This chapter addresses the epidemiology and outcomes of HM patients and bone marrow transplant (BMT) recipients who require invasive positive-pressure ventilation (IPPV). Also discussed are the criteria used to identify patients likely to benefit from IPPV instead of noninvasive positive-pressure ventilation (NIPPV) as the initial ventilatory strategy. However, aspects

M. Soares (✉)
Intensive Care Unit, Instituto Nacional de Câncer; Centro de Tratamento Intensivo, Pça. Cruz Vermelha, 23 – 10° Andar, Rio de Janeiro – RJ, Brazil, CEP: 20230-130
e-mail: marciosoaresms@yahoo.com.br

J.I.F. Salluh
Intensive Care Unit, Instituto Nacional de Câncer, Praça Cruz Vermelha, 23–10° andar, 20230-120 Rio de Janeiro – RJ, Brazil
e-mail: jorgesalluh@yahoo.com.br

P.O. Depuydt
Department of Intensive Care Medicine, Ghent University Hospital, De Pintelaan 185, 9000 Ghent, Belgium
e-mail: pieter.depuydt@ugent.be

Conflicts of interest: none.

Financial support: Dr. Soares is supported in part by an individual research grant from CNPq – Conselho Nacional de Desenvolvimento Científico e Tecnológico (Brazil).

É. Azoulay (ed.), *Pulmonary Involvement in Patients with Hematological Malignancies*,
DOI: 10.1007/978-3-642-15742-4_46, © Springer-Verlag Berlin Heidelberg 2011

related to patients supported with NIPPV are discussed in greater detail in chapters from Drs. Antonelli, Hilbert, and Nava of this book.

46.1 Epidemiology

Up to 50% of HM patients develop ARF requiring MV during the course of their disease [1–9]. ARF is a major reason for ICU admission, and 43–88% of patients require mechanical ventilation during the ICU stay [10–18]. In general, patients with acute leukemia and allogeneic BMT recipients are at highest risk for this severe complication [1, 19, 20]. In two large multicenter studies of patients with HM admitted to both specialized and general ICUs, MV was provided to 55% and 71% of patients, respectively [18, 21].

46.2 Outcome Evaluation and Prognostic Factors

ARF requiring MV is usually associated with high mortality and morbidity in patients with HMs. Until the 1990s, the outcome for these patients was considered very poor, as the hospital mortality rates were consistently greater than 80% [22–30] overall and 90–95% in BMT recipients. Mortality was highest after HLA-mismatched BMT and in patients who both required MV and had cardiovascular, renal, or hepatic dysfunction [6, 7, 25, 31–34]. In a large study of outcomes in 782 cancer patients (including 61% with HMs) treated with IPPV in the ICUs of five academic tertiary care hospitals, hospital mortality was 76% overall, 85% in HM patients, and 87% in BMT recipients [30]. By multivariate analysis, leukemia and allogeneic BMT were independently associated with higher mortality [30]. These data led to the recommendation that a restrictive ICU admission policy be used in HM patients and BMT recipients requiring MV [7, 35].

Fortunately, studies done over the last few years have documented improved survival rates in critically ill patients with HMs, including those requiring MV [1, 11, 20, 36–38]. Nonetheless, the need for invasive MV remains a major outcome predictor in these patients and is still associated with relatively high mortality rates [1, 12, 14, 17, 18, 39]. In the following section, aspects related to the outcomes of HM patients requiring IPPV are discussed based on data published over the last decade.

46.2.1 Short- and Long-Term Outcomes

46.2.1.1 Specific Diagnoses and Characteristics Related to the Malignancy

Until recently, HM patients were considered at higher risk for mortality than patients with solid tumors. However, studies done over the last decade have documented equivalent mortality rates for hematology and oncology patients requiring MV [11–15, 30, 38–42]. Mortality in these patients varies according to multidimensional variables, including patient-related characteristics, in terms of underlying diagnosis and comorbidities, severity of acute illness, level of ICU support, and ICU policies (e.g., criteria used to implement end-of-life care and to admit and discharge patients from the ICU). Table 46.1 reports the results of the main studies published over the last decade and done in HM patients requiring IPPV. Overall hospital mortality rates ranged from 62% to 80%, with an average of 71% [1, 5, 11–15, 17, 18, 21, 34, 41, 43–46]. Most of the studies were single-centered and carried out in specialized institutions. However, there is still limited information on medium- and long-term outcomes. In one study, only 21 (25%) of 84 HM patients (including 57% who were mechanically ventilated) were alive after 6 months [15], and in another, done in 100 patients with HMs (including 81 mechanically ventilated), the 2-year survival rate was 15% [14].

Nevertheless, the term HM encompasses myriad diseases with diverse clinical and biological behaviors. In general, after adjustment on other prognostic indicators, the type or group of HM per se is not associated with short-term outcomes of patients requiring IPPV [11, 15, 41], although worse outcomes have been reported in patients with acute leukemia [39] or lymphoma [21]. On the other hand, higher survival rates were observed in patients with multiple myeloma [37]. In addition, short-term mortality is significantly worse in patients with disease recurrence or progression compared to those with newly diagnosed disease or disease remission (partial or complete) [15]. However, studies evaluating specific groups of patients are still scarce.

Table 46.1 Mortality rates and prognostic indicators in studies published over the last decade (2000–2009) and conducted in patients with hematological malignancies requiring mechanical ventilation in the intensive care unit

Author, year	Study design	Patients	IPPV patients		Independent prognostic factors
			n (%)	Hospital mortality (%)	
Azoulay et al. 2001 [41]	Cohort, retrospective, single center	203	169 (71%)	71[a]	SAPS II score was associated with mortality; NIPPV use was protective.
Evison et al. 2001 [13]	Cohort, retrospective, single center	78	42 (53%)	62	Number of organ failures
Krochinsky et al. 2002 [12]	Cohort, retrospective, single center	104	54 (52%)	74	Mechanical ventilation, SAPS II score
Massion et al. 2002 [15]	Cohort, retrospective, single center	84	48 (57%)	75	Number of organ failures, fungal infection, BMT, disease progression
Benoit et al. 2003 [11]	Cohort, retrospective, single center	124	58 (47%)	69	Leukopenia, vasopressor use, and kidney injury were associated with mortality. Bacteremia was protective
Azoulay et al. 2004 [1]	Cohort, prospective, single center	203	148 (73%)	62	Invasive aspergillosis, lack of definite diagnosis of cause of ARF, vasopressor use, NIPPV failure (especially after 2 days on NIPPV), and need for first-line IPPV were associated with mortality; congestive heart failure and successful use of NIPPV were protective
Depuydt et al. 2004 [39]	Cohort, retrospective, single center	166	140 (84%)	72	SAPS II score and diagnosis of AML were associated with mortality; female gender, endotracheal intubation <24 h of ICU admission, and bacteremia were protective
Rabbat et al. 2005 [17]	Cohort, prospective, single center	83	47 (57%)	72	SAPS II score and need for mechanical ventilation
Owczuk et al. 2005 [44]	Cohort, prospective, single center	40	40 (100%)	65[b]	SAPS II score
Lim et al. 2006 [5]	Cohort, prospective, single center	55	40 (73%)	74	Multivariate analysis not performed
Lamia et al. 2006 [43]	Cohort, retrospective, single center	92	58 (63%)	79	Septic shock, BMT, severity of illness, and organ dysfunction scores

(continued)

Table 46.1 (continued)

Author, year	Study design	Patients	IPPV patients		Independent prognostic factors
			n (%)	Hospital mortality (%)	
Ferrá et al. 2007 [14]	Cohort, single center	100	81 (81%)	70[b]	Hemodynamic instability and need for IPPV.
Lecuyer et al. 2008 [18]	Cohort, retrospective, multicenter, secondary analysis	1753	967 (55%)	67	SAPS II score, need for IPPV, renal replacement therapy and vasopressors, ARDS, shock, and coma were associated with ICU mortality
Azoulay et al., 2008 [46]	Cohort, prospective, multicenter	148	110 (74%)	69	History of BMT, vasopressor use or dialysis, and intubation during the ICU stay were associated with mortality
Hampshire et al. 2009 [21]	Cohort, prospective, Multicenter, secondary analysis	7,689	4,244 (55%)	70	Severe sepsis, older age, longer time from hospital to ICU admission, BMT, lymphoma, and several variables related to organ dysfunctions and acute illness severity (including hematocrit, systolic blood pressure, respiratory rate, heart rate, Glasgow coma scale, sedation, PaO_2, arterial pH, urine output, serum sodium, and serum urea)
Depuydt et al. 2009 [45]	Cohort, retrospective, single center	137	104 (76%)	80	SOFA and cancer-specific scores were associated with mortality; bacterial infection was protective
Combined	–	1,1059	6490 (59%)	71	–

HM hematological malignancies, *IPPV* invasive positive-pressure ventilation, *NIPPV* non-invasive positive-pressure ventilation, *BMT* bone marrow transplant, *AML* acute myeloid leukemia, *ARDS* acute respiratory distress syndrome, *SAPS* Simplified Acute Physiology Score, *SOFA* Sequential Organ Dysfunction Score, *ICU* intensive care unit

[a]30-day mortality; hospital mortality was not reported

[b]ICU mortality; hospital mortality was not reported

Finally, in recent studies neither the presence of neutropenia nor recent exposure to chemotherapy was associated with an increased risk of death [40, 46, 47].

Although improvements in survival have been achieved, outcomes of BMT patients requiring IPPV remain relatively poor. In recent studies, short-term mortality rates ranged from 74% to 86%, with an average of 82% (Table 46.2) [8, 9, 48–52]. Mortality remains extremely high in allogeneic BMT recipients with severe graft-versus-host disease or concomitant hepatic, renal, or cardiovascular dysfunction [29, 30, 32, 46, 48, 50–52]. In contrast, autologous BMT recipients have survival rates that are closer to those seen in non-transplanted patients [9, 20, 30, 37, 48, 50]. For example, in a cohort of 78 autologous peripheral BMT patients who received MV, 26% of the patients were discharged alive from the hospital, and 60% were alive after 6 months [20]. In a population-based cohort study, Scales et al. reported a 13% 1-year survival rate in BMT patients who required MV in subsequent hospitalizations [53].

46.2.1.2 Main Prognostic Factors

As expected, the severity of acute physiologic disturbances and organ dysfunctions correlates directly with short-term mortality [30, 39–41, 46, 49]. Although severity of illness scores are inaccurate for predicting outcomes in HM patients [54], they have been used as surrogate markers for acute disease severity and correlate strongly with mortality [12, 17, 18, 39, 41, 44, 50]. Moreover, HM patients frequently require MV in the context of multiple organ failure, and mortality increases with the number of additional failing organs [1, 13, 14, 16, 18, 21, 30, 39–42, 44, 55]. Both baseline values and subsequent changes in organ dysfunction scores over the first few days of ICU stay (such as the Sequential Organ Failure Assessment [SOFA] and Logistic Organ Dysfunction (LOD) scores) correlate strongly with mortality [43]. In addition, the need for additional life-sustaining therapies, such as renal replacement therapy or vasopressors, after a few days on MV suggests that the patient's clinical condition may be unresponsive to intensive care and therefore indicates a high risk of death [55].

Outcomes vary largely across conditions requiring MV. For instance, survival is higher in patients with respiratory failure secondary to cardiogenic pulmonary edema than in patients with pulmonary infiltration by the malignancy or invasive fungal infections [1, 3, 28]. Additionally, failure to identify the cause of ARF is independently associated with mortality [1, 2, 46]. Although ARF due to bacterial infections remains associated with high mortality rates, the prognosis is better than in patients with opportunistic infections, severe sepsis, and ARF [1, 2, 11, 29, 39, 45, 56, 57].

In HM patients, the severity of comorbid conditions and functional impairments (as evaluated by the performance status) has a major impact on outcomes, and self-sufficiency is routinely evaluated by the performance status [40, 58, 59]. Older age per se does not seem to be a major risk factor for short-term mortality [1, 30, 38, 39, 41, 42, 45, 46]. However, aging is associated with a decrease in physiologic capacity and a higher prevalence of chronic diseases, including cancer. Therefore, in elderly patients with HM and ARF, selection for ICU admission may need to be somewhat restrictive.

46.3 When to Reach for the Tube Instead of the Mask

Although the final outcome of ARF depends upon the reversibility of its cause, gas exchange disorders must be corrected to ensure patient survival when this cause is identified and treated. MV is often necessary to reverse severe hypoxemia or hypercapnic acidosis, and the clinician must choose between invasive and noninvasive modalities [60, 61]. IPPV (i.e., ventilation delivered through endotracheal intubation) couples a secure airway with full control of alveolar ventilation superseding the patient's respiratory efforts and permits aggressive alveolar recruitment by high intra-alveolar pressures, thus rapidly reversing profound hypoxemia and respiratory acidosis. As intubation is fraught with major complications, such as airway trauma and ventilator-associated pneumonia, the use of NIPPV has generated increasing interest since suitable facial and nasal masks became available in the 1980s. By avoiding airway intubation, NIPPV preserves the integrity of the upper airway functions and defense mechanisms, allowing for swallowing, coughing, and vocalization, and decreases the need for sedation. As a consequence, the incidence of ventilator-associated pneumonia is lower with NIPPV than with IPPV. Over

Table 46.2 Mortality rates and prognostic indicators in various studies published over the last decade (2000–2009) and conducted in bone marrow transplant patients requiring mechanical ventilation in the intensive care unit

Author, year	Study design	Patients	Type of BMT (auto/allo)	IPPV patients		Independent prognostic factors
				n (%)	Hospital mortality (%)	
Huaringa et al. 2000 [48]	Cohort, prospective, single center	60	26/34	60 (100%)	49 (82%)[a]	Multivariate analysis not performed
Bach et al. 2001 [49]	Cohort, prospective, multicenter	226	66/160	226 (100%)	194 (86%)	Hepatic and kidney dysfunctions, IPPV longer than 4 days
Khassawneh et al., 2002 [20]	Cohort, retrospective, single center	78	78/0	78 (100%)	58 (74%)	Multivariate analysis not performed
Afessa et al. 2003 [50]	Cohort, retrospective, single center	112	62/50	62 (55%)	46 (74%)	APACHE III score and allogeneic BMT
Soubani et al. 2004 [9]	Cohort, retrospective, single center	85	40/45	51 (60%)	41 (80%)	Lactic acidosis, multiple organ failure, need for IPPV
Naeem et al. 2006 [51]	Cohort, single center	44	0/44	12 (27%)	10 (83%)[a]	Multivariate analysis not performed
Pene et al. 2006 [52]	Cohort, retrospective, multicenter	209	0/209	122 (58%)	103 (84%)	Corticosteroid treatment for GVHD, vasopressor use, and bilirubin level were associated with mortality; time interval from BMT to ICU admission <30 days was protective
Yang et al. 2007 [8]	Cohort, retrospective, single center	41	6/35	41 (100%)	34 (83%)	Multivariate analysis not performed
Combined	–	855	278/577	652 (76%)	535 (82%)	–

IPPV invasive positive-pressure ventilation, *BMT* bone marrow transplant, *APACHE* Acute Physiology and Chronic Health Evaluation, *GVHD* graft-versus-host disease, *ICU* intensive care unit

[a]ICU mortality; hospital mortality was not reported

the last decade, NIPPV has been increasingly used in various patient groups with ARF. Among patient subsets in which NIPPV has been proven to decrease complications and to improve survival are immunocompromised patients with hypoxemic ARF [60, 62, 63] (see also Chap. 47)]. It should be kept in mind that the absence of airway intubation in NIPPV, while clearly beneficial in selected patients with ARF, precludes the use of NIPPV in patients who require stringent control of gas exchange (such as hemodynamically unstable patients or patients with profound hypoxemia), patients in whom airway patency is compromised (e.g., by excessive sputum, hemoptysis, or vomiting), and uncooperative patients (e.g., patients with coma or agitation). The British Thoracic Society guidelines [64] and the recent German S3 guidelines [65] list a number of absolute and relative contraindications to the use of NIPPV in patients with ARF (Table 46.3). Clearly, HM patients with ARF and one or more of these general contraindications should immediately receive endotracheal MV without a previous NIPPV trial. As argued above, outcomes in invasively ventilated HM patients have improved sufficiently over the last decade to classify intubation among potential first-line lifesaving techniques rather than among treatments of last resort or harbingers of a fatal outcome [66].

Table 46.3 Contraindications for non-invasive positive-pressure ventilation [61, 64, 65]

Absolute
Impending respiratory arrest
Inability to protect airway or airway obstruction
Gastrointestinal bleeding
Bowel obstruction, ileus, vomiting
Relative
Coma
Agitation, lack of cooperation
Excessive respiratory secretions
Severe hypoxemia or acidosis (pH < 7.1)
Hemodynamic instability
Not able to fit interface (anatomical or functional incompatibility)
Recent facial, upper gastrointestinal, or airway surgery
Untreated pneumothorax

Evidently, this set of contraindications restricts the use of NIPPV to the subset of HM patients with hypoxemic or hypercapnic ARF who are hemodynamically stable, awake, cooperative, and free of evidence of impending respiratory arrest. In both randomized trials of NIPPV in immunocompromised patients with hypoxemic ARF, the standard-care group received supplemental oxygen, and, therefore, the included patients were likely to be identified early on and referred to the ICU while still having a good physiological reserve [62, 63]. In observational studies of patients with HMs or other malignancies and hypoxemic ARF, NIPPV was used in only 4–39% of patients [1, 39–41, 45]. Nevertheless, failure was common, with roughly half the patients requiring subsequent intubation. More worryingly, some studies found high mortality rates in patients who failed NIPPV [1, 39, 67]. Thus, in one study the in-hospital mortality rate in patients switched from NIPPV to invasive ventilation was 91% [39], and in another, mortality in patients intubated after 48 h of NIPPV was 92% [1]. In contrast, mortality in patients who received first-line invasive ventilation was 72% [39] and 78% [1] in these two studies. In addition, switching from IPPV to NIPPV was an independent predictor of mortality [1, 67]. Although this effect on mortality may be due to the poor prognosis associated with non-reversible ARF (where NIPPV is more likely to fail than in rapidly reversible ARF), it may also point to a causal relationship between adverse outcomes and the inappropriate use of NIPPV. The potential of NIPPV to cause harm by delaying instead of avoiding intubation has been demonstrated in an interventional trial in patients with postextubation hypoxemic ARF, who were randomly allocated to NIPPV or standard therapy (supplemental oxygen) to avoid reintubation [68]. ICU mortality was significantly higher in patients who were reintubated after a trial of NIPPV than in patients who were reintubated after standard care (38% vs 22%,), and the interval between respiratory failure onset and reintubation was higher in the NIPPV group than in the standard-care group.

In addition to the set of well-known contraindications to NIPPV in ARF, other factors play a more subtle role in the success or failure of a trial of NIPPV. Identifying predictors for NIPPV failure in patients with HMs is therefore important to improve patient selection. Knowledge of the baseline determinants of NIPPV success or failure may help to identify patients who are likely to respond to NIPPV (and may avoid futile and possibly deleterious NIPPV exposure in other patients). Furthermore, the identification of early predictors of NIPPV failure during NIPPV therapy may allow earlier substitution of IPPV for NIPPV, thus avoiding the deleterious outcomes of late NIPPV failure [39]. Predictors of NIPPV failure in non-cancer patients with hypoxemic ARF include acute lung injury (ALI) or acute respiratory distress syndrome (ARDS); pneumonia; high severity-of-illness scores; and the presence of metabolic acidosis, shock, and profound hypoxemia, especially after 1 h of NIPPV (Table 46.4) [60]. Observational data on NIPPV in cancer patients have led to the identification of factors associated with NIPPV failure in this specific patient subset. In one study, NIPPV failure was associated with a newly diagnosed malignancy, short symptom duration at ARF onset, steroid treatment, increasing NIPPV duration, ARDS, vasopressor therapy, and failure to identify the cause of ARF [1]. In another study, where the NIPPV failure rate was as high as 75%, the patients had high SAPS II scores (mean, 52 ± 15) and low PaO_2/FiO_2 ratios (mean, 95 ± 42) [39]. Finally, in 99 cancer patients managed with NIPPV, factors significantly associated with NIPPV failure were a delay in NIPPV initiation, a diagnosis of ARDS at NIPPV initiation, and presence of extrapulmonary organ failures (need for vasopressors and renal replacement therapy) [67]. In addition, an increasing respiratory rate under NIPPV predicted NIPPV failure. While organ failure at admission (as assessed by LOD score) was not significantly different between patients who responded and those who failed NIPPV, the LOD score was significantly higher in patients failing NIPPV on days 2 and 3.

Table 46.4 Predictors of NIPPV failure [1, 39, 60, 67, 69]

In general patients [1]
High severity-of-illness scores (APACHE II ≥29, SAPS II ≥35)
Pneumonia
ARDS
pH <7.25
Respiratory rate ≥35 breaths per minute
PaO_2/FIO_2 ≤146 (≤175 for ARDS) after 1 h of NIPPV
Excessive air leak, lack of tolerance, agitation during NIPPV
In patients with hematological malignancies [9, 11, 13]
High severity-of-illness scores
Need for vasopressor therapy
Need for renal replacement therapy
ARDS
Absence of etiologic diagnosis
Higher respiratory rate under NIPPV
Longer duration of NIPPV dependency

NIPPV noninvasive positive-pressure ventilation, *APACHE* Acute Physiology and Chronic Health Evaluation, *SAPS* Simplified Acute Physiology Score, *ARDS* acute respiratory distress syndrome

In summary, NIPPV should be used with discernment in HM patients with ARF, and the clinician should always consider whether intubation might be the better choice. After ruling out the formal contraindications for NIPPV, the likelihood that NIPPV will be successful should be estimated based on the presenting symptoms, degree of hypoxemia, presence of extrapulmonary organ failures, and likelihood that the underlying disease process can be reversed quickly. If the odds for NIPPV success are low, the safest approach is immediate intubation. In patients with an acceptable chance of success, NIPPV should be applied with caution. The response to NIPPV (in terms of hypoxemia reversal and respiratory rate decline) should be assessed after 1 or 2 h, and the patient should remain under close monitoring for early signs of NIPPV failure. If increasing organ failure or persistent ARF is observed over the next few days, switching to IPPV should be strongly considered [69].

References

1. Azoulay E, Thiéry G, Chevret S et al (2004) The prognosis of acute respiratory failure in critically ill cancer patients. Medicine (Baltimore) 83:360–370
2. Azoulay E, Schlemmer B (2006) Diagnostic strategy in cancer patients with acute respiratory failure. Intensive Care Med 32:808–822
3. Azoulay E, Fieux F, Moreau D et al (2003) Acute monocytic leukemia presenting as acute respiratory failure. Am J Respir Crit Care Med 167:1329–1333
4. Chaoui D, Legrand O, Roche N et al (2004) Incidence and prognostic value of respiratory events in acute leukemia. Leukemia 18:670–675
5. Lim Z, Pagliuca A, Simpson S et al (2007) Outcomes of patients with haematological malignancies admitted to intensive care unit. A comparative review of allogeneic

haematopoietic stem cell transplantation data. Br J Haematol 136:448–450
6. Rubenfeld GD, Crawford SW (1996) Withdrawing life support from mechanically ventilated recipients of bone marrow transplants: a case for evidence-based guidelines. Ann Intern Med 125:625–633
7. Faber-Langendoen K, Caplan AL, McGlave PB (1993) Survival of adult bone marrow transplant patients receiving mechanical ventilation: a case for restricted use. Bone Marrow Transplant 12:501–507
8. Yang TM, Wang PN, Kao KC, Huang CC, Tsai YH, Hsieh MJ et al (2007) Outcome of hematopoietic stem cell recipients who were mechanically ventilated and admitted to intensive care units. J Formos Med Assoc 106:295–301
9. Soubani AO, Kseibi E, Bander JJ et al (2004) Outcome and prognostic factors of hematopoietic stem cell transplantation recipients admitted to a medical ICU. Chest 126: 1604–1611
10. Taccone FS, Artigas AA, WSprung CL et al (2009) Characteristics and outcomes of cancer patients in European ICUs. Crit Care 13:R15
11. Benoit DD, Vandewoude KH, Decruyenaere JM et al (2003) Outcome and early prognostic indicators in patients with a hematologic malignancy admitted to the intensive care unit for a life-threatening complication. Crit Care Med 31: 104–112
12. Kroschinsky F, Weise M, Illmer T et al (2002) Outcome and prognostic features of intensive care unit treatment in patients with hematological malignancies. Intensive Care Med 28:1294–1300
13. Evison J, Rickenbacher P, Ritz R et al (2001) Intensive care unit admission in patients with haematological disease: incidence, outcome and prognostic factors. Swiss Med Wkly 131:681–686
14. Ferrà C, Marcos P, Misis M et al (2007) Outcome and prognostic factors in patients with hematologic malignancies admitted to the intensive care unit: a single-center experience. Int J Hematol 85:195–202
15. Massion PB, Dive AM, Doyen C et al (2002) Prognosis of hematologic malignancies does not predict intensive care unit mortality. Crit Care Med 30:2260–2270
16. Silfvast T, Pettilä V, Ihalainen A et al (2003) Multiple organ failure and outcome of critically ill patients with haematological malignancy. Acta Anaesthesiol Scand 47:301–306
17. Rabbat A, Chaoui D, Montani D et al (2005) Prognosis of patients with acute myeloid leukaemia admitted to intensive care. Br J Haematol 129:350–357
18. Lecuyer L, Chevret S, Guidet B et al (2008) Case volume and mortality in haematological patients with acute respiratory failure. Eur Respir J 32:748–754
19. Shorr AF, Moores LK, Edenfield WJ et al (1999) Mechanical ventilation in hematopoietic stem cell transplantation: can We effectively predict outcomes? Chest 116:1012–1018
20. Khassawneh BY, White P Jr, Anaissie EJ et al (2002) Outcome from mechanical ventilation after autologous peripheral blood stem cell transplantation. Chest 121: 185–188
21. Hampshire PA, Welch CA, McCrossan LA et al (2009) Admission factors associated with hospital mortality in patients with haematological malignancy admitted to UK adult, general critical care units: a secondary analysis of the ICNARC Case Mix Programme Database. Crit Care 13:R137
22. Peters SG, Meadows JA 3rd, Gracey DR (1988) Outcome of respiratory failure in hematologic malignancy. Chest 94:99–102
23. Lloyd-Thomas AR, Wright I, Lister TA et al (1988) Prognosis of patients receiving intensive care for life-threatening medical complications of haematological malignancy. Br Med J (Clin Res Ed) 296:1025–1029
24. Schuster DP, Marion JM (1983) Precedents for meaningful recovery during treatment in a medical intensive care unit. Outcome in patients with hematologic malignancy. Am J Med 75:402–408
25. Epner DE, White P, Krasnoff M et al (1996) Outcome of mechanical ventilation for adults with hematologic malignancy. J Investig Med 44:254–260
26. Hauser MJ, Tabak J, Baier H (1982) Survival of patients with cancer in a medical critical care unit. Arch Intern Med 142:527–529
27. Snow RM, Miller WC, Rice DL et al (1979) Respiratory failure in cancer patients. JAMA 241:2039–2042
28. Ewig S, Torres A, Riquelme R et al (1998) Pulmonary complications in patients with haematological malignancies treated at a respiratory ICU. Eur Respir J 12:116–122
29. Gruson D, Hilbert G, Portel L et al (1999) Severe respiratory failure requiring ICU admission in bone marrow transplant recipients. Eur Respir J 13:883–887
30. Groeger JS, White P Jr, Nierman DM et al (1999) Outcome for cancer patients requiring mechanical ventilation. J Clin Oncol 17:991–997
31. Paz HL, Garland A, Weinar M et al (1998) Effect of clinical outcomes data on intensive care unit utilization by bone marrow transplant patients. Crit Care Med 26:66–70
32. Price KJ, Thall PF, Kish SK et al (1998) Prognostic indicators for blood and marrow transplant patients admitted to an intensive care unit. Am J Respir Crit Care Med 158: 876–884
33. Afessa B, Tefferi A, Hoagland HC et al (1992) Outcome of recipients of bone marrow transplants who require intensive-care unit support. Mayo Clin Proc 67:117–122
34. Crawford SW, Petersen FB (1992) Long-term survival from respiratory failure after marrow transplantation for malignancy. Am Rev Respir Dis 145:510–514
35. Carlon GC (1989) Just say no. Crit Care Med 17:106–107
36. Azoulay E, Recher C, Alberti C et al (1999) Changing use of intensive care for hematological patients: the example of multiple myeloma. Intensive Care Med 25:1395–1401
37. Peigne V, Rusinová K, Karlin L et al (2009) Continued survival gains in recent years among critically ill myeloma patients. Intensive Care Med 35:512–518
38. Kress JP, Christenson J, Pohlman AS et al (1999) Outcomes of critically ill cancer patients in a university hospital setting. Am J Respir Crit Care Med 160:1957–1961
39. Depuydt PO, Benoit DD, Vandewoude KH et al (2004) Outcome in noninvasively and invasively ventilated hematologic patients with acute respiratory failure. Chest 126:1299–1306
40. Soares M, Salluh JI, Spector N et al (2005) Characteristics and outcomes of cancer patients requiring mechanical ventilatory support for >24 hrs. Crit Care Med 33:520–526

41. Azoulay E, Alberti C, Bornstain C et al (2001) Improved survival in cancer patients requiring mechanical ventilatory support: impact of noninvasive mechanical ventilatory support. Crit Care Med 29:519–525
42. Vallot F, Paesmans M, Berghmans T et al (2003) Leucopenia is an independent predictor in cancer patients requiring invasive mechanical ventilation: a prognostic factor analysis in a series of 168 patients. Support Care Cancer 11:236–241
43. Lamia B, Hellot MF, Girault C et al (2006) Changes in severity and organ failure scores as prognostic factors in onco-hematological malignancy patients admitted to the ICU. Intensive Care Med 32:1560–1568
44. Owczuk R, Wujtewicz MA, Sawicka W et al (2005) Patients with haematological malignancies requiring invasive mechanical ventilation: differences between survivors and non-survivors in intensive care unit. Support Care Cancer 13:332–338
45. Depuydt PO, Benoit DD, Roosens CD et al (2009) The impact of the initial ventilatory strategy on survival in hematological patients with acute hypoxemic respiratory failure. J Crit Care. doi:10.1016/j.jcrc.2009.02.016
46. Azoulay E, Mokart D, Rabbat A et al (2008) Diagnostic bronchoscopy in hematology and oncology patients with acute respiratory failure: prospective multicenter data. Crit Care Med 36:100–107
47. Vandijck DM, Benoit DD, Depuydt PO et al (2008) Impact of recent intravenous chemotherapy on outcome in severe sepsis and septic shock patients with hematological malignancies. Intensive Care Med 34:847–855
48. Huaringa AJ, Leyva FJ, Giralt SA et al (2000) Outcome of bone marrow transplantation patients requiring mechanical ventilation. Crit Care Med 28:1014–1017
49. Bach PB, Schrag D, Nierman DM et al (2001) Identification of poor prognostic features among patients requiring mechanical ventilation after hematopoietic stem cell transplantation. Blood 98:3234–3240
50. Afessa B, Tefferi A, Dunn WF et al (2003) Intensive care unit support and Acute Physiology and Chronic Health Evaluation III performance in hematopoietic stem cell transplant recipients. Crit Care Med 31:1715–1721
51. Naeem N, Eyzaguirre A, Kern JA et al (2006) Outcome of adult umbilical cord blood transplant patients admitted to a medical intensive care unit. Bone Marrow Transplant 38: 733–738
52. Pène F, Aubron C, Azoulay E et al (2006) Outcome of critically ill allogeneic hematopoietic stem-cell transplantation recipients: a reappraisal of indications for organ failure supports. J Clin Oncol 24:643–649
53. Scales DC, Thiruchelvam D, Kiss A et al (2009) Intensive care outcomes in bone marrow transplant recipients: a population-based cohort analysis. Crit Care 12:R77
54. den Boer S, de Keizer NF, de Jonge E (2005) Performance of prognostic models in critically ill cancer patients - a review. Crit Care 9:R458–R463
55. Lecuyer L, Chevret S, Thiery G et al (2007) The ICU trial: a new admission policy for cancer patients requiring mechanical ventilation. Crit Care Med 35:808–814
56. Salluh JI, Bozza FA, Pinto TS et al (2005) Cutaneous periumbilical purpura in disseminated strongyloidiasis in cancer patients: a pathognomonic feature of potentially lethal disease? Braz J Infect Dis 9:419–424
57. Benoit DD, Depuydt PO, Peleman RA et al (2005) Documented and clinically suspected bacterial infection precipitating intensive care unit admission in patients with hematological malignancies: impact on outcome. Intensive Care Med 31:934–942
58. Groeger JS, Lemeshow S, Price K et al (1998) Multicenter outcome study of cancer patients admitted to the intensive care unit: a probability of mortality model. J Clin Oncol 16:761–770
59. Soares M, Salluh JI, Ferreira CG et al (2005) Impact of two different comorbidity measures on the 6-month mortality of critically ill cancer patients. Intensive Care Med 31: 408–415
60. Mehta S, Hill NS (2001) Noninvasive ventilation: State of the art. Am J Respir Crit Care Med 163:540–577
61. Hill NS, Brennan J, Garpestad E et al (2007) Noninvasive ventilation in acute respiratory failure. Crit Care Med 35:2402–2407
62. Hilbert G, Gruson D, Vargas D et al (2001) Noninvasive ventilation in immunosuppressed patients with pulmonary infiltrates, fever, and acute respiratory failure. N Engl J Med 344:481–487
63. Antonelli M, Conti G, Bufi M et al (2000) Noninvasive ventilation for treatment of acute respiratory failure in patients undergoing solid organ transplantation: a randomized trial. JAMA 283:235–241
64. British Thoracic Society Standards of Care Committee (2002) Non-invasive ventilation in acute respiratory failure. Thorax 57:192–211
65. Schönhofer B, Kuhlen R, Neumann P et al (2008) Nichtinvasive Beatmung als Therapie der akuten respiratorische Insuffizienz: das wichtigste der neuen S3-Leitlinie. Der Anaesthestist 57:1091–1102
66. Azoulay E, Afessa B (2006) The intensive care support of the patient with malignancy: do everything that can be done. Intensive Care Med 32:3–5
67. Adda M, Coquet I, Darmon M et al (2008) Predictors of noninvasive ventilation failure in patients with hematologic malignancy and acute respiratory failure. Crit Care Med 36:2766–2772
68. Esteban A, Frutos-Vivar F, Ferguson N et al (2004) Noninvasive positive-pressure ventilation for respiratory failure after extubation. N Engl J Med 350:2452–2460
69. Soares M, Salluh JIF, Azoulay E (2009) Noninvasive ventilation in patients with malignancies and hypoxemic acute respiratory failure: a still pending question. J Crit Care. doi:10.1016/j.jcrc.2009.04.001

Optimizing Noninvasive Ventilation in Hematological Patients with Acute Respiratory Failure

47

Gilles Hilbert

Contents

G. Hilbert
The Division of Medical Intensive Care, University Hospital, Bordeaux, France and
Service de Réanimation Médicale, Hôpital Pellegrin, F 33076 Bordeaux Cedex, France
e-mail: gilles.hilbert@chu-bordeaux.fr

47.1 Introduction/Rationale for Optimizing Noninvasive ventilation

Pulmonary complications are an important cause of illness in immunocompromised patients and contribute to a large extent to the mortality associated with various types of immunosuppression [1, 2]. With the increasing use of these treatment modalities and the growing potency of immunosuppressive regimens, physicians will more frequently be asked to evaluate and to care for these individuals.

Strategies for management include both a specific approach, in terms of the diagnostic tools and treatment regimens used, and a symptomatic approach, in terms essentially of treatment of acute respiratory failure (ARF). Classically, these recipients required frequent intubation and mechanical ventilatory assistance. Too often, this intervention has been followed by further, ultimately fatal complications, including sepsis. Although invasive mechanical ventilation is highly effective and reliable in supporting alveolar ventilation, endotracheal intubation is associated with numerous complication risks [3]. Furthermore, in hematological patients with ARF, mechanical ventilation is associated with a significant risk of death [4–7]. The outcome predictors that consistently predicted poor outcome of hematopoietic stem cell transplantation recipients admitted to the ICU were the need for mechanical ventilation and the presence of multiple organ system failure [8].

Even if over the last years overall survival rates of hematological patients admitted to the ICU have been improving, due, in part, to the benefits of noninvasive ventilation (NIV) in selected patients, which has led some experts to defend the concept of "doing

É. Azoulay (ed.), *Pulmonary Involvement in Patients with Hematological Malignancies*,
DOI: 10.1007/978-3-642-15742-4_47,

everything that can be done," the negative impact of intubation and mechanical ventilation has been confirmed in several recent studies. In a study published in 2001 in patients with hematological malignancy, the overall mortality in the ICU was 44%: only 12% in patients without mechanical ventilation, but 74% among those under mechanical ventilation ($p<0.001$); multivariate analysis revealed mechanical ventilation and SAPS II as independent prognostic factors of both ICU mortality and long-term survival [7]. In their literature review, Soubani et al. showed clearly that the lower the percentage of patients receiving mechanical ventilation was, the higher the survival rate [8]. Thus, above all, the key driving force behind the increasing use of NIV has been the desire to avoid the complications of invasive ventilation.

Among the 64 neutropenic patients with febrile acute hypoxemic normocapnic respiratory failure treated by CPAP in addition to standard therapy in the study by Hilbert at al., CPAP was efficient in only 25% of cases [9]. The enrolled patients were critically ill, with a PaO_2/FiO_2 ratio of 128 ± 32, and with a high SAPS II score and more than two organ dysfunctions, explaining, in part, the poor results obtained. Nevertheless, all the responders and only four nonresponders survived their ICU stay. More recently, a case control study on 34 patients was performed to evaluate the effectiveness of early administration of CPAP through a helmet in hematological malignancy patients with ARF [10]. Each patient was treated by CPAP outside an ICU, directly in the hematological ward. The authors described a success rate as high as possible in patients ventilated with the helmet, while eight NIV failures were registered in the group ventilated with a facemask because of intolerance of this interface.

Several noncontrolled studies have reported encouraging results with NIV in hematological patients with ARF when a technique of spontaneous ventilation with pressure support (PS) and positive end expiratory pressure (PEEP) was used [11–13]. Azoulay et al. retrospectively studied a cohort of patients with solid or hematologic cancer admitted to the ICU for ARF [13]. The first group of 132 patients was admitted between 1990 and 1995, while the second group, composed of 105 patients, was admitted between 1996 and 1998. The survival rate in the 1996–1998 period was significantly higher than that in the previous period. In a matched-pair analysis of cancer patients requiring MV support, the mortality among NIV patients was significantly lower than in conventionally ventilated patients (43.7% vs 70.8%, $p=0.008$) [13]. In a multivariate analysis two variables were found to predict ICU outcome: higher SAPS II at admission was associated with an increased mortality rate, whereas the use of NIV during the 1996–1998 period was associated with a marked improvement in survival. Another study compared NIV with invasive intubation and ventilation for this patient group [14]. In this retrospective study, 27 patients who received NIV were matched for SAPS II with 52 patients who required immediate intubation on a 1:2 basis. In contrast to several earlier reports, the authors could not demonstrate the presence of a survival benefit for the use of NIV. Indeed, treatment with NIV successfully averted the need for intubation in eight patients (31%), five of whom (62.5%) survived their hospital stay; this last rate was similar to that recorded in patients who required immediate intubation. Nevertheless, these results must be evaluated cautiously because hypoxemic ARF was dramatically most severe in the NIV group compared to the invasive ventilation group (median PaO_2/FiO_2 ratio 71 vs 141, respectively, $p<0.001$).

We hypothesized that the intermittent use of NIV at an early stage of hypoxemic ARF would reduce the need for endotracheal intubation and the incidence of complications [15]. In a prospective, randomized, controlled study, we compared the efficacy of NIV delivered intermittently through a mask with that of standard medical treatment with supplemental oxygen and no ventilatory support in patients with immunosuppression of various causes in whom hypoxemic ARF had been precipitated by pulmonary infiltrates and fever. It is important to underline that randomization was done at an early stage of respiratory failure, well before the patients were even headed for intubation. The immunosuppression could have been caused by neutropenia after chemotherapy or bone marrow transplantation in patients with hematological cancers, drug-induced immunosuppression in organ-transplant recipients, or as a result of corticosteroid or cytotoxic therapy for a nonmalignant disease or AIDS. In the NIV group, as compared with standard therapy, fewer patients required endotracheal intubation (12 vs 20, $p=0.03$), and there were fewer complications (13 vs 21, $p=0.02$). Overall, with NIV, there were improvements in mortality in the ICU (10 vs 18, $p=0.03$) and in total in-hospital mortality (13 vs 21, $p=0.02$). Neutropenia in patients with hematological malignancies was the most frequent type of immunosuppression in patients included in this last study [15]. Although NIV enabled avoiding intubation in only 47% of neutropenic patients, this rate was still significantly higher than in the standard treatment group (7%, $p=0.02$).

ARF in immunocompromised patients is a recognized indication of NIV, and according to recent international recommendations (of level I), NIV should be used whenever possible in this indication to reduce the risk of nosocomial pneumonia [16]. Above all, NIV makes it possible to reduce the mortality of oncohematology patients of with ARF.

47.2 Optimizing Noninvasive Ventilation

47.2.1 *Taking into Consideration the Mechanisms of Improvement with NIV*

As recalled by M. Tobin, the objectives of mechanical ventilation are primarily to decrease the work of breathing and reverse life-threatening hypoxemia or acute progressive respiratory acidosis [17].

In patients with hypoxemic ARF, intrapulmonary shunt and ventilation-perfusion imbalances may cause life-threatening hypoxemia. Moreover, hard work of breathing because of increased alveolar dead space and reduced respiratory system compliance may cause ventilatory failure with hypercapnia and respiratory acidosis. When employed during episodes of hypoxemic ARF, the goal of NIV is to ensure an adequate PaO_2 level until the underlying problem can be reversed.

NIV can improve the pathophysiology of hypoxemic respiratory failure. Mechanisms of improvement can include the beneficial effects of PEEP on the distribution of extravascular lung water, on alveolar recruitment of under-ventilated alveoli by increasing lung volume at end expiration and in early treatment of atelectasis. In addition, improvements in ventilation/perfusion ratios or even shunt undoubtedly occur in patients with acute respiratory distress syndrome (ARDS) in whom the application of expiratory pressure should have an effect similar to that of PEEP in invasively ventilated patients. By lowering left ventricular transmural pressure, CPAP may reduce afterload and increase cardiac output, making it an attractive modality for therapy of acute pulmonary edema. Even if CPAP alone is able to improve lung mechanics in patients with ARF and decrease work of breathing compared with unsupported ventilation [18], the addition of PS has a positive effect in reducing work of breathing and maintaining a tidal volume compatible with adequate alveolar ventilation.

Numerous case series and reports have shown that CPAP and NIV improve oxygenation, reduce the respiratory rate and lessen dyspnea in patients with hypoxemic ARF. Confalonieri et al. compared NIV to invasive mechanical ventilation in AIDS patients with *Pneumocystis jirovecii* pneumonia [19]. Changes in arterial blood gas and respiratory rate were comparable in the two groups of patients during the first 72 h of the study.

Several prospective controlled studies, comparing CPAP or NIV with standard medical treatment, have shown that use of these methods of ventilation in hypoxemic ARF was associated with prompt improvement in pulmonary gas exchange as determined by arterial blood gases obtained within the first few hours [15, 20–22]. Antonelli et al. conducted a prospective, randomized trial of NIV as compared with endotracheal intubation with conventional mechanical ventilation in 64 patients with hypoxemic ARF who required mechanical ventilation [20]. Seven (22%) of 32 patients randomized to NIV had ARDS of varied etiology. The patients in the two groups had a similar initial change in the PaO_2/FiO_2 ratio: Within the first hour of ventilation, 20 patients (62%) in the NIV group and 15 (47%) in the conventional ventilation group had an improvement in the PaO_2/FiO_2 ratio. Their PaO_2/FiO_2 ratios increased significantly from 116 ± 24 to 230 ± 76 mmHg with NIV and from 124 ± 25 to 211 ± 68 mmHg with conventional ventilation. In a study comparing NIV with standard treatment using supplemental oxygen administration in recipients of solid organ transplantation with hypoxemic ARF, 7 (22%) of 32 patients randomized to NIV had ARDS of varied etiology [21]. Within the first hour of treatment, 14 patients (70%) in the NIV group and only 5 patients (25%) in the standard treatment group improved their PaO_2/FiO_2 ratio. In another randomized controlled trial, the physiologic effects of CPAP versus standard oxygen therapy were compared in 123 patients with hypoxemic ARF and $PaO_2/FiO_2\leq300$ due to bilateral pulmonary edema,

102 of them with acute lung injury [22]. After 1 h of treatment, the median PaO_2/FiO_2 ratio was greater with CPAP (203 vs 151, $p = 0.02$). In a prospective, randomized trial of NIV, as compared with standard medical treatment with supplemental oxygen in immunosuppressed patients with hypoxemic ARF, initial improvement in the PaO_2/FiO_2 ratio was observed in 46% in the NIV group and in 15% in the standard group ($p = 0.02$) [15]. Even if NIV was used intermittently in a sequential mode, the protocol of NIV used in this study achieved significantly higher rates of improvement in gas exchange abnormalities than in patients with standard treatment. Reducing the work of breathing during NIV sessions may also allow respiratory muscles to be more efficient during nonassisted breaths.

47.2.2 Optimizing the Selection of Patients

Before starting NIV we should always consider the possible contraindications to its use [23]. In a randomized, controlled trial, the patients were selected, and exclusion criteria were a requirement for emergent intubation for cardiopulmonary resuscitation, respiratory arrest, or a rapid deterioration in neurological status with a Glasgow Coma Scale score ≤8; hemodynamic instability or electrocardiogram instability; chronic obstructive pulmonary disease; a cardiac origin of the respiratory failure, which was established by physical signs, chest X-ray and echocardiogram; a partial pressure of arterial carbon dioxide ($PaCO_2$) more than 55 mmHg, with acidosis (pH < 7.35); failure of more than two new organs; uncorrected bleeding diathesis; and tracheotomy, a facial deformity or recent oral, esophageal or gastric surgery [15].

It is essential to know the arterial blood gas tensions before making a decision on whether NIV is indicated. The patient should first be established on appropriate oxygen therapy and the arterial blood gases interpreted in the light of the FiO_2.

Conti et al. have evaluated treatment with NIV as an alternative to endotracheal intubation and conventional mechanical ventilation in 16 patients with hematological malignancies complicated by ARF and having intubation criteria (at inclusion, $PaO_2/FiO_2 = 87 \pm 22$) [12]. NIV was delivered via nasal mask by means of a BiPAP mode. Five patients died in the ICU following complications independent of the respiratory failure, while 11 were discharged from the ICU in stable condition after a mean stay of 4.3 ± 2.4 days and were discharged from the hospital. Thus, NIV proved to be feasible for the treatment of respiratory failure in hematological patients who were at high risk of intubation-related complications.

However, in immunocompromised patients with "lung failure," NIV is more indicated at an earlier stage of ARF when the PaO_2/FiO_2 ratio is below 200 or when oxygen saturation does not reach 90% despite high-flow oxygen therapy [15, 21]. Indeed, in those randomized, controlled studies, NIV helped avert the need for endotracheal intubation and improved the outcomes in selected immunocompromised patients with hypoxemic ARF [15, 21]. The early involvement of intensivists in hematological patients care and the better definitions of patients who require ICU admission will probably play a major role in the future.

47.2.3 Optimizing Equipment and Techniques

The time suitable to appreciate improvement or, contrarily, NIV failure may depend on many factors. The lack of ARF resolving at 1–2 h makes it possible to select the patients for whom efforts to try improving adaptation and outcome will be most important. Thus, it is important to consider if it could be possible to ameliorate several factors to improve adaptation of the patient to NIV and the outcome of the technique. This reasoning is helpful within the first few hours of NIV when the patient needs to adapt and also later when prolonged ventilation is required.

Many factors can be improved. Some of them are well known and similar to those we consider when PS with PEEP is used in intubated patients. Several others are more specific to NIV.

47.2.3.1 Interface

NIV uses a tight-fitting facemask as an alternative interface between the patient and the ventilator to avoid the complications of invasive ventilation. In contrast to invasive ventilation, NIV leaves the upper airway intact, preserves airway defense mechanisms, and allows patients to eat, drink, verbalize and expectorate secretions. The development of improved masks and ventilator technology has made this mode of ventilation acceptable.

NIV can be administered to immunocompromised patients with different types of interfaces. The patient interface most commonly employed is a full face or nasal mask secured firmly, but not tightly, with a head strap [23]. The full facemask delivers higher ventilation pressures with fewer leaks, requires less patient cooperation and permits mouth breathing. However, it is less comfortable, increases the dead space, impedes communication and limits oral intake. The nasal mask needs patent nasal passages and requires mouth closure to minimize air leaks. The leaks through the mouth decrease alveolar ventilation and may decrease the efficacy of NIV to reduce the work of breathing. Furthermore, high flows of gas passing through the nose in case of mouth leaks can markedly increase nasal resistance and thus further reduce the efficacy of nasal NIV [24]. In order to improve success rates in awake and cooperative patients, it is essential to gently hold the device on the patient's face before tightening it in order to improve patient comfort. It is also recommended that physicians do not tighten the device excessively or weakly, since excessive pressure can cause skin breakdown and reduce patient tolerance, while weak sealing may facilitate air leakage and patient–ventilator asynchronies. It is also beneficial to reassure the patient and explain the technique in detail.

Patients may develop complications related to the use of NIV such as skin necrosis, gastric distention or evidence of barotrauma (pneumothorax, pneumomediastinum, pneumoperitoneum or pulmonary interstitial emphysema). Data from the literature and observations from our practice suggest the highest incidence of facial-skin breakdown and/or intolerance of the interface in the subgroup of patients with hypoxemic ARF and hematological malignancies. The incidence of pressure necrosis of the skin over the nasal bridge reached 31% in an uncontrolled study [12]. Hilbert et al. excluded three patients from the study because they refused to keep the facial mask during the first CPAP session [9]. The reason was acute stress in one case and major painful mucositis in two cases. A bad tolerance of CPAP was reported in five other patients enrolled in this study who were intubated. Mask intolerance because of pain, discomfort or claustrophobia may require discontinuation of NIV and endotracheal intubation.

Various modifications are available to minimize this complication, such as use of forehead spacers or the addition of a thin plastic flap that permits air sealing with less mask pressure on the nose. Straps that hold the mask in place are also important for patient comfort, and many types of strap assemblies are available. Most manufacturers provide straps that are designed for use with a particular mask. More points of attachment add to stability, and strap systems with Velcro fasteners are useful.

There is no evidence to support the use of particular patient interface devices in patients with hypoxemic ARF [23]. Nevertheless, clinical experience suggests that full facemasks improve efficacy by reducing leaks and are more appropriate for use in the setting of severe hypoxemic ARF. In addition, a facial mask was used preferentially in studies examining the efficacy of NIV in immunocompromised patients with hypoxemic ARF.

The fact that most NIV failures are due to technical problems justifies the studies that have evaluated new interface devices. Attempting to improve tolerability of patients, Antonelli et al. adopted a transparent helmet made from latex-free polyvinyl chloride that allows patients to see, read and speak as an interface during NIV. They conducted a prospective trial with a matched control group in order to investigate the efficacy of NIV using the helmet to treat patients with hypoxemic ARF [25]. Six patients (18%) in the helmet group and nine patients (13%) in the facial mask group had ARDS. Eight patients (24%) in the helmet group and 21 patients (32%) in the facial mask group failed NIV and were intubated. No patients failed NIV because of intolerance of the technique in the helmet group in comparison with eight patients (38%) in the mask group ($p=0.047$). Complications related to the technique (skin necrosis, gastric distension and eye irritation) were fewer in the helmet group compared with the standard mask group (no patients vs 14 patients [21%], $p=0.002$). The helmet allowed the continuous application of NIV for a longer period of time ($p=0.05$). The authors concluded that NIV by helmet successfully treated hypoxemic ARF with better tolerance and fewer complications than facial mask NIV. The helmet is very popular in Italy, and excellent results have been reported with the administration of CPAP through a helmet in hematological malignancy patients with ARF [10]. Better tolerance of the helmet compared to a conventional interface was also found in a case control study [26]. However, this interface can be responsible for increased work of breathing and for dyspnea [27, 28], as well as a potential risk of rebreathing CO_2, which have to be carefully weighed against the major benefits achieved respecting the integrity of the face. In practice, in many units, including ours, the helmet is used in the second or even third line as an alternative to facemasks in case of skin lesions responsible for intolerance with a risk of failure of the method.

47.2.3.2 Ventilators and Ventilatory Modes

NIV can be performed with either modern ICU ventilators or chronic long-term home ventilators. The choice of ventilator type to deliver NIV should depend on both the patient's conditions and the technical characteristics of the machine, such as quality of monitoring (detection of asynchronies and quantification of air leaks); mechanisms of compensation for leaks; and performance. Indeed, these aspects have a clinical impact in terms of work of breathing and represent a key factor to improve the tolerability of the technique, as well as the patient–ventilator interaction during NIV. The use of ICU ventilators is generally preferable in the acute setting, since they are more powerful and have more adjustable features compared with home ventilators. Additionally, circuits with dual tubes reduce the risk of rebreathing CO_2 in patients with ARF. A recent survey conducted to evaluate the application of NIV in ICUs showed that an ICU ventilator was used in 79% of cases, a ventilator dedicated to NIV in 12% and a home device in 5% [29].

One of the main differences between management of COPD patients and of patients with hypoxemic ARF is the place of CPAP in the therapeutic armamentarium of physicians treating patients with hypoxemic ARF. CPAP represents the application of a constant level of positive pressure at the airway opening during spontaneous breathing. CPAP results in a higher mean intrathoracic pressure than unassisted spontaneous breathing, but a lower pressure than positive pressure mechanical ventilation and PEEP. Mean airway pressure increases, with possible beneficial effects on atelectasis and improvement in oxygenation; lung compliance can increase, reducing the work of breathing, and the presence of intrinsic PEEP can be counterbalanced with a partial reduction of the inspiratory effort. An advantage of CPAP over modes of mechanical ventilatory assistance is that CPAP does not require patient–ventilator synchronization. Pressures commonly used to deliver CPAP to patients with hypoxemic ARF range from 5 to 15 cmH_2O. Such pressures can be applied using a wide variety of devices, including CPAP valves connected to a compressed gas source, small portable units used for home therapy of obstructive sleep apnea and ventilators designed for use in the ICU. Depending on the critical care ventilator selected, CPAP may be administered using "demand," "flow-by" or "continuous flow" techniques, with imposed work differing slightly between them. CPAP is widely used in the belief that it may reduce the need for intubation and mechanical ventilation in patients with acute hypoxemic respiratory insufficiency. Nevertheless, to our knowledge, although several studies have shown the ability of the method to improve hypoxemia, only one randomized study has demonstrated that the use of CPAP reduces the need for endotracheal intubation in patients with severe hypercapnic cardiogenic pulmonary edema [30]. A recent study showed that, as compared with standard oxygen therapy, CPAP neither reduced the need for intubation nor improved outcomes in patients with hypoxemic ARF [22].

On the contrary, positive results have been reported in randomized controlled studies where PS + PEEP was used [15, 21]. During PS ventilation, the ventilator is triggered by the patient, delivers a set pressure for each breath, and cycles to expiration either when it senses a fall in inspiratory flow rate below a threshold value or at a preset time. Noninvasive PS ventilation offers the potential of excellent patient–ventilator synchrony, reduced diaphragmatic work and improved patient comfort.

The choice of NIV with PS and PEEP, rather than CPAP, a technique previously systematically used for hypoxemic ARF in our ICU [9], has undoubtedly contributed to the good results recently reported in immunosuppressed patients [15]. In our practice, after the mask has been secured, the level of PS is progressively increased and adjusted for each patient to obtain an expired tidal volume of 7–9 mL/kg of body weight and a respiratory rate of fewer than 25 breaths/min. PEEP is repeatedly increased by 2 cmH_2O, up to a level of 10 cmH_2O, until the FiO_2 requirement is 70% or less.

The FiO_2 level is adjusted to maintain SaO_2 above 90%. Ventilator settings are adjusted on the basis of continuous monitoring of SpO_2, clinical data and measurements of arterial blood gases. Studies comparing the impact on clinical outcome of CPAP and PS + PEEP in patients with hypoxemic ARF will be useful. For the moment, and looking forward to the results of further studies, PS ventilation + PEEP could be the ventilatory mode recommended for treatment with NIV of hypoxemic ARF.

Many factors must be considered when PS + PEEP is used. Some of them are well known (for instance, inspiratory trigger sensitivity, inspiratory flow) and close to those we consider when this ventilatory mode is used in intubated patients.

Flow triggering has been shown to slightly reduce the effort needed to trigger the ventilator compared with pressure triggering. Moreover, a less sensitive trigger could be associated with a higher incidence of ineffective triggering events. These data indicate that a sensitive flow trigger should be used to take full advantage of patient's efforts without inducing auto-triggering. Auto-triggering is a frequent asynchrony during NIV, and a flow triggering set around 3 L/min (when possible settings range 0.5–10 L/min, for instance) could represent an optimal adjustment, being sensitive enough and avoiding auto-triggering. Some ventilators self-adjust trigger sensitivity as a function of leaks.

Several other factors are more specific to NIV, for instance, the negative impact of leaks on work of breathing with a risk of patient–ventilator asynchrony [31]. Gas leaks around the mask or from the mouth limit the efficacy of the device, make monitoring of tidal volume difficult; it may prevent adequate ventilatory assistance in patients who require high inspiratory airway pressures and represents an important cause of failure. Leaks may also indicate low compliance or ventilation close to total lung capacity. Thus, particular attention should be given to leaks during application of NIV in patients with hypoxic ARF. When large leaks occur during inspiration, the ventilator continues to insufflate because the delivered flow remains above the cycling criterion so that cycling off does not occur. In this situation, the patient attempts to expire and can fight against the ventilator because the expiratory valve remains closed, generating ineffective efforts during persistent insufflation. Several adjustments can eliminate prolonged inspiration by reducing either the leaks or the ventilator insufflation time. First, the mask position should be adjusted to minimize leaks around the mask. Secondly, limiting the total inspiratory pressure should be considered, reducing the PS and/or PEEP level. Persistent leaks indicate a need for limiting the ventilator insufflation time. In a study on six patients with acute lung injury due to AIDS-related opportunistic pneumonia, a time-cycled expiratory trigger provided a better patient–machine interaction than a flow-cycled expiratory trigger in the presence of air leaks during NIV [31]. Another possibility is to increase the threshold of flow cutoff. Most of the new-generation ICU ventilators and many NIV-dedicated ventilators allow adjustment of the expiratory trigger or maximal inspiratory time.

We believe the first hours of delivering NIV, with careful attention to mask fit, patient comfort and patient–ventilator synchrony, represent a critical opportunity to improve outcome.

47.2.3.3 Chosing a Continuous or Discontinuous Approach

In immunocompromised patients with "lung failure," NIV is indicated at an earlier stage of ARF when the PaO_2/FiO_2 ratio is below 200 or when oxygen saturation does not reach 90% despite high-flow oxygen therapy [15, 21]. Treating with NIV at an early stage of ARF allows a discontinuous approach.

In two trials dealing with immunocompromised recipients, NIV was used intermittently, since the onset of management [15] or after the first 24 h of treatment [21] at a less advanced stage of hypoxemic ARF than in other studies that assessed the value of NIV in patients who met the criteria for intubation [12, 20]. On the basis of our previous experience, we use NIV in a sequential mode [9, 32, 33]. This mode is a discontinuous mode, with some specificity, i.e., the predetermination of the duration of the ventilation sessions and of the time between the NIV sessions. One of the potential advantages of the sequential approach is a harmonious distribution of NIV sessions, a better acceptance and tolerance by the patients, and a better management by nursing staff. The protocol of sequential ventilation is appreciated by our staff and has contributed to the standardization of techniques of NIV in our ICU. It has not been necessary to modify the organization of our unit since the introduction of these new techniques.

In practice, NIV is delivered through a facemask in a discontinuous mode with a protocol close to that previously described for COPD patients [32, 33], i.e., periods of NIV lasting at least 45 min and alternating every 3 h with periods of spontaneous breathing. Between periods of ventilation, patients breathe oxygen spontaneously while SpO_2 is continuously monitored. NIV is automatically resumed when the arterial oxygen saturation is less than 85% or when dyspnea worsens, as evidenced by a respiratory rate of more than 30 breaths/min.

In the randomized controlled trial, NIV was administered for a mean of 9 ± 3 h during the first 24 h [15]. Subsequently, the mean duration of NIV was 7 ± 3 h/day; the mean duration of NIV was 4 ± 2 days.

47.2.3.4 Predictive Factors of NIV Outcome

In the randomized study by Hilbert et al., the effect on outcomes of the presence and the absence of a final diagnosis of the cause of pneumonitis with respiratory failure was studied [25]. In the NIV group, the patients with a final diagnosis had significantly lower rates of intubation ($p = 0.03$), and death in the ICU ($p = 0.04$) or in the hospital ($p = 0.006$). Thus, a positive diagnosis and a well-adapted treatment could be the main determinants of improved outcome of immunosuppressed patients managed with NIV. It is important to establish the specific causes of a hematological patient's pulmonary disease so that specific therapy can be instituted. Furthermore, a positive diagnosis and a well-adapted treatment could be the main determinants in the improved outcome of immunosuppressed patients managed with NIV [15]. Consequently, fiberoptic bronchoscopy and bronchoalveolar lavage are major tools for diagnosing the diffuse infiltrates that often occur in association with fever and new onset of respiratory symptoms in immunosuppressed patients [15, 34–36]. In a recent prospective randomized trial on 26 patients, NIV was shown superior to conventional oxygen supplementation in preventing gas exchange deterioration and provided better hemodynamic tolerance during fiberoptic bronchoscopy in patients with less severe forms of hypoxemia ($PaO_2/FiO_2 < 200$) [37]. In this study, PS was 15–17 cmH_2O, PEEP was set at 5 cmH_2O and FiO_2 at 0.9; the session of NIV was started 10 min before the fiberoptic bronchoscopy and continued at least 30 min after the procedure. We currently have the same approach.

In a prospective study, variables predictive of NIV failure were investigated in 354 patients with hypoxemic ARF, 37 of them with immunosuppression [38]. Multivariate analysis identified age >40 years (OR 1.72, 95% CI 0.92–3.23), a higher SAPS II ≥ 35 (OR 1.81, 95% CI 1.07–3.06), the presence of ARDS or community-acquired pneumonia (OR 3.75, 95% CI 2.25–6.24) and a $PaO_2/FiO_2 \leq 146$ after 1 h of NIV (OR 2.51, 95% CI 1.45–4.35) as factors independently associated with failure of NIV. In a retrospective, monocentric study dealing with patients with hematologic malignancy, factors independently associated with NIV failure by multivariate analysis were respiratory rate under NIV, longer delay between admission and NIV first use, need for vasopressors or renal replacement therapy, and ARDS [39].

Nevertheless, in practice, it can be difficult to predict an individual outcome and decide promptly to withdraw noninvasive ventilatory support, keeping in mind the poor prognosis of intubation in numerous patients. However, it is crucial, in my opinion, to do all that can be done to try to optimize the technical aspects, which are crucial for a successful application of NIV.

While learning NIV techniques is described as simple in some studies, it is essential and must be continuous, allowing for better indications of the technique, optimizing the technical aspects and monitoring, which are the sole guarantors of avoiding too much delay of intubation when the method fails. Indeed, the use of NIV with a delay in reintubation can lead to excess mortality, and we should not delay the moment of reintubation if this becomes necessary. The success of NIV is also strictly dependent upon local factors. The best venue depends on the training and experience of the staff, available resources (beds, staff, equipment) and monitoring capacity.

Undoubtedly, ARF in hematological patients is one of the indications for NIV that requires experience and good mastery of the technique; in my opinion, this justifies practicing NIV in the ICU for this indication.

47.3 Conclusions

A reduction in the incidence of nosocomial infection is a consistent and important advantage of NIV compared with invasive ventilation and is probably one of the most important advantages of avoiding endotracheal intubation using NIV. ARF in immunocompromised patients is a recognized indication for NIV, and according to recent international recommendations (level I), NIV should be used whenever possible for this indication to reduce the risk of nosocomial pneumonia [16]. Above all, NIV makes it possible to reduce the mortality of onco-hematology patients with ARF.

Given the risks of serious complications and death associated with intubation, the relative safety of appropriately applied NIV should change our approach to ventilation in hematological patients with respiratory failure; patients in whom respiratory distress develops should be treated conventionally with oxygen and other indicated therapies and should be monitored closely; if moderate to severe respiratory distress develops with tachypnea and hypoxemia, NIV should be initiated unless there are contraindications [40].

Patients for whom ARF does not resolve in 1–2 h are most in need of efforts to try to improve their adaptation and outcome. Clinical experience suggests that full facemasks are more appropriate for use in the setting of severe hypoxemic ARF. Many factors must be considered when PS + PEEP is used, and particular attention should be paid to the leaks responsible for ineffective efforts during persistent insufflations; several adjustments can eliminate prolonged inspiration by reducing either the leaks or the ventilator insufflation time.

The experiences gradually acquired by the different units, the regular training of the personnel, further technological advances and future research will position NIV more accurately in the therapeutic armamentarium of physicians dealing with hematological patients with ARF and are likely to improve the conditions for performing NIV in the future.

References

1. Masur H, Shelhamer J, Parrillo JE (1985) The management of pneumonias in immunocompromised patients. JAMA 253(12):1769–1773, Mar 22–29
2. Estopa R, Torres-Marti A, Kastanos N et al (1984) Acute respiratory failure in severe hematologic disorders. Crit Care Med 12:26–28
3. Stauffer JL (1994) Complications of translaryngeal intubation. In: Tobin MJ (ed) Principles and practice of mechanical ventilation. Marcel Dekker, New York, pp 711–747
4. Ewig S, Torres A, Riquelme R et al (1998) Pulmonary complications in patients with haematological malignancies treated at a respiratory intensive care unit. Eur Respir J 12:116–122
5. Gruson D, Hilbert G, Portel L et al (1999) Severe respiratory failure requiring ICU admission in bone marrow transplant recipients. Eur Respir J 13:883–887
6. Bach PB, Schrag D, Nierman DM et al (2001) Identification of poor prognostic features among patients requiring mechanical ventilation after hematopoietic stem cell transplantation. Blood 98:3234–3240
7. Kroschinsky F, Weise M, Illmer T et al (2002) Outcome and prognostic features of ICU treatment in patients with hematological malignancies. Intensive Care Med 28:1294–1300
8. Soubani AO, Kseibi E, Bander JJ et al (2004) Outcome and prognostic factors of hematopoietic stem cell transplantation recipients admitted to a medical ICU. Chest 126:1604–1611
9. Hilbert G, Gruson D, Vargas F et al (2000) Non-invasive continuous positive airway pressure in neutropenic patients with acute respiratory failure requiring intensive care unit admission. Crit Care Med 28:3185–3190
10. Principi T, Pantanetti S, Catani F et al (2004) Noninvasive continuous positive airway pressure delivered by helmet in hematological malignancy patients with hypoxemic acute respiratory failure. Intensive Care Med 30:147–150
11. Tognet E, Mercatello A, Polo P et al (1994) Treatment of acute respiratory failure with non-invasive intermittent positive pressure ventilation in haematological patients. Clin Intensive Care 5:282–288
12. Conti G, Marino P, Cogliati A et al (1998) Noninvasive ventilation for the treatment of acute respiratory failure in patients with hematologic malignancies: a pilot study. Intensive Care Med 24:1283–1288
13. Azoulay E, Alberti C, Bornstain C et al (2001) Improved survival in cancer patients requiring mechanical ventilatory support: impact of noninvasive mechanical ventilatory support. Crit Care Med 29:519–525
14. Depuydt PO, Benoit DD, Vandewoude KH, Decruyenaere JM, Colardyn FA (2004) Outcome in noninvasively and invasively ventilated hematologic patients with acute respiratory failure. Chest 126:1299–1306
15. Hilbert G, Gruson D, Vargas F et al (2001) Noninvasive ventilation for treatment of acute respiratory failure in immunosuppressed patients with pulmonary infiltrates and fever, a randomized trial. N Engl J Med 344:481–487
16. American Thoracic Society; Infectious Diseases Society of America (2005) Guidelines for the management of adults with hospital-acquired, ventilator-associated, and healthcare-associated pneumonia. Am J Respir Crit Care Med 171:388–416
17. Tobin MJ (2001) Advances in mechanical ventilation. N Engl J Med 344:1986–1996
18. Katz JA, Marks JD (1985) Inspiratory work with and without continuous positive airway pressure in patients with acute respiratory failure. Anesthesiology 63:598–607
19. Confalonieri M, Calderini E, Terraciano S et al (2002) Noninvasive ventilation for treating acute respiratory failure in AIDS patients with Pneumocystis carinii pneumonia. Intensive Care Med 28:1233–1238
20. Antonelli M, Conti G, Rocco M et al (1998) A comparison of noninvasive positive pressure ventilation and conventional

mechanical ventilation in patients with acute respiratory failure. N Engl J Med 339:429–435
21. Antonelli M, Conti G, Bufi M et al (2000) Noninvasive ventilation for treatment of acute respiratory failure in patients undergoing solid organ transplantation. A randomized trial. JAMA 283:235–241
22. Delclaux C, L'Her E, Alberti C et al (2000) Treatment of acute hypoxemic nonhypercapnic respiratory insufficiency with continuous positive airway pressure delivered by a face mask: a randomized controlled trial. JAMA 284:2352–2360
23. International Consensus Conferences in Intensive Care Medicine (2001) Noninvasive positive pressure ventilation in acute respiratory failure. Am J Respir Crit Care Med 163:283–291
24. Richards GN, Cistulli PA, Ungar RG et al (1996) Mouth leak with nasal continuous positive airway pressure increases nasal airway resistance. Am J Respir Crit Care Med 154:182–186
25. Antonelli M, Conti G, Pelosi P et al (2002) New treatment of acute hypoxemic respiratory failure: noninvasive pressure support ventilation delivered by helmet – a pilot controlled trial. Crit Care Med 30:602–608
26. Rocco M, Dell'Utri D, Morelli A et al (2004) Noninvasive ventilation by helmet or facemask in immunocompromised patients: a case-control study. Chest 126:1508–1515
27. Racca F, Appendini L, Gregoretti C et al (2005) Effectiveness of mask and helmet interfaces to deliver noninvasive ventilation in a human model of resistive breathing. J Appl Physiol 99:1262–1271
28. Vargas F, Thille A, Lyazidi A et al (2009) Helmet with specific settings versus facemask for noninvasive ventilation. Crit Care Med 37:1921–1928
29. Demoule A, Girou E, Richard JC, Taille S, Brochard L (2006) Increased use of noninvasive ventilation in French intensive care units. Intensive Care Med 32:1747–1755
30. Bersten AD, Holt AW, Vedig AE et al (1991) Treatment of severe cardiogenic pulmonary edema with continuous positive airway pressure delivered by face mask. N Engl J Med 325:1825–1830
31. Calderini E, Confalonieri M, Puccio PG et al (1999) Patient–ventilator asynchrony during noninvasive ventilation: the role of expiratory trigger. Intensive Care Med 25:662–667
32. Hilbert G, Gruson D, Gbikpi-Benissan G et al (1997) Sequential use of noninvasive pressure support ventilation for acute exacerbations of COPD. Intensive Care Med 23: 955–961
33. Hilbert G, Gruson D, Portel L et al (1998) Non-invasive pressure support ventilation in COPD patients with postextubation hypercapnic respiratory insufficiency. Eur Respir J 11:1349–1353
34. Stover DE, Zaman NB, Hadjou SI et al (1984) Bronchoalveolar lavage in the diagnosis of diffuse pulmonary infiltrates in the immunosuppressed host. Ann Intern Med 101:1–7
35. Gruson D, Hilbert G, Valentino R et al (2000) Utility of fiber-optic bronchoscopy in neutropenic patients admitted to intensive care unit with pulmonary infiltrates. Crit Care Med 28:2224–2230
36. Hilbert G, Gruson D, Vargas F et al (2001) Bronchoscopy with bronchoalveolar lavage via the laryngeal mask airway in high-risk hypoxemic immunosuppressed patients. Crit Care Med 29:249–255
37. Antonelli M, Conti G, Rocco M et al (2002) Noninvasive positive-pressure ventilation vs. conventional oxygen supplementation in hypoxemic patients undergoing diagnostic bronchoscopy. Chest 121:1149–1154
38. Antonelli M, Conti G, Moro ML et al (2001) Predictors of failure of noninvasive positive pressure ventilation in patients with acute hypoxemic respiratory failure: a multi-center study. Intensive Care Med 27:1718–1728
39. Adda M, Coquet I, Darmon M et al (2008) Predictors of noninvasive ventilation failure in patients with hematologic malignancy and acute respiratory failure. Crit Care Med 36: 2766–2772
40. Hill NS (2001) Noninvasive ventilation for immunocompromised patients. N Engl J Med 344:522–524

Noninvasive Ventilation to Ensure the Safety of Fiberoptic Bronchoscopy

48

Massimo Antonelli, Giuseppe Bello, and Riccardo Maviglia

Contents

M. Antonelli (✉), G. Bello, and R. Maviglia
Istituto di Anestesiologia e Rianimazione,
Policlinico Universitario A. Gemelli, Università Cattolica del Sacro Cuore, Largo A. Gemelli 8, 00168 Rome, Italy
e-mail: m.antonelli@rm.unicatt.it

Abbreviations

BAL	Bronchoalveolar lavage
COPD	Chronic obstructive pulmonary disease
CPAP	Noninvasive constant continuous positive airway pressure
ETI	Endotracheal intubation
FB	Fiberoptic bronchoscopy
FiO_2	Inspired oxygen fraction
NIV	Noninvasive ventilation
NPPV	Noninvasive intermittent positive pressure ventilation
$PaCO_2$	Arterial carbon dioxide tension
PaO_2	Arterial oxygen partial pressure
PEEP	Positive end-expiratory pressure
SpO_2	Arterial oxygen saturation of hemoglobin measured by pulse oximetry

48.1 Introduction

Noninvasive ventilation (NIV) is the provision of ventilatory assistance using techniques that do not bypass the upper airway. The theoretical advantages of NIV include avoiding the complications associated with conventional mechanical ventilation [11, 28], improving patient comfort, and preserving the airway defense mechanism.

Over the last 2 decades, the encouraging results obtained in the treatment of acute respiratory failure by using NIV [3, 4, 9, 13, 24] have stimulated investigations of various applications of NIV in the acute care setting. In hypoxemic patients needing fiberoptic bronchoscopy (FB) with bronchoalveolar lavage (BAL), NIV has been employed to prevent gas-exchange

É. Azoulay (ed.), *Pulmonary Involvement in Patients with Hematological Malignancies*,
DOI: 10.1007/978-3-642-15742-4_48, © Springer-Verlag Berlin Heidelberg 2011

deterioration accompanying FB and compensate for the increase in work of breathing occurring during FB, thus avoiding endotracheal intubation (ETI) and its complications [2, 5, 6, 12, 22]. This application of NIV to improve the safety of FB has been found of particular interest in the diagnosis of pneumonia in immunocompromised patients, such as those with hematological malignancies. The prognosis of these patients may worsen under invasive ventilation [14, 15, 27], despite the improved outcome achieved in the last few years also when ETI is required [7].

The treatment of patients with hematological malignancies is frequently associated with infectious pulmonary complications [10, 30]. The diagnosis of pneumonia in these patients constitutes a major challenge to the clinician, since the classical presentation is variable, and other causes of fever and chest infiltrates may occur in hematological malignancies. FB with BAL is widely recognized as a valuable diagnostic tool for detection of the respiratory pathogens in patients with pulmonary infiltrates. The prompt identification of the responsible microorganisms is crucial to start an appropriate antimicrobial therapy and to avoid the empirical administration of unnecessary and often toxic antibiotics. Non-intubated, spontaneously breathing patients with hypoxemia [defined as the inability to maintain an arterial oxygen partial pressure (PaO_2) <75 mmHg or an oxygen saturation >90% despite oxygen supplementation] should not undergo FB because of their high risk of developing respiratory failure or serious cardiac arrhythmias [16]. Until a few years ago, the available options for hypoxemic patients with a suspicion of pneumonia were to avoid FB and to administer empirical treatment, or to perform ETI and to start mechanical ventilation for ensuring adequate gas exchange during FB. The following sections review the rationale for using NIV to assist patients undergoing FB, the available literature supporting this method, and some procedural considerations.

In this chapter, the term CPAP is referred to as noninvasive continuous positive airway pressure delivered to spontaneously breathing patients, whereas NPPV is referred to as noninvasive intermittent positive pressure ventilation with or without positive end-expiratory pressure (PEEP). NIV is considered to include either CPAP or NPPV.

48.2 Rationale for Using NIV During FB

In critically ill patients, even a standard FB is associated with transient alterations in pulmonary mechanics and gas exchange [21, 23]. PaO_2 may fall significantly below its baseline value during FB and remain decreased for a few minutes to several hours after removing the bronchoscope [21, 23]. In a group of 107 mechanically ventilated patients undergoing FB, an average decline in PaO_2 of 26% was observed at the end of the procedure compared to the baseline value [29]. Hypoxemia may be more marked when BAL is performed because of ventilation and perfusion abnormalities induced by the saline solution instillation [19].

In a non-intubated adult male, a 5.7-mm outside diameter flexible bronchoscope occupies about 10% of the tracheal cross-sectional area and about 15% of the cross-sectional area at the cricoid ring [21]. Positioning the bronchoscope into the major airways decreases the area available for airway flow and, consequently, increases airway resistance [21]. The high exhalation resistance rapidly results in an increase in functional residual capacity and, therefore, in the development of an intrinsic PEEP mechanism [23]. This finally leads to increased work of breathing and risk of barotraumas.

Besides the physical presence of the bronchoscope in the airway, a frequent suction through the instrument working channel may be another cause of the alterations in pulmonary mechanics and gas exchange during FB. Removal of tracheobronchial gas by excessive use of suction evacuates respiratory gas from the airways, decreasing functional residual capacity, or causing de-recruitment under positive pressure ventilation with consequent hypoxemia [20, 21].

By improving oxygenation and reducing the work of breathing [18], NIV has been demonstrated to be a useful method to avoid ETI in hypoxemic patients undergoing FB. The application of NIV during FB has been described both in at-risk patients who were initially breathing spontaneously and who started NIV to assist FB, and in patients who were already receiving NIV and who were scheduled to undergo FB during NIV.

48.3 Review of the Literature

In an early study on the use of NIV in patients requiring diagnostic FB, Antonelli et al. [2] described the application of facemask NPPV during FB in eight immunocompromised hypoxemic (i.e., PaO_2 to inspired oxygen fraction [FiO_2] ratio, <100) patients with suspected pneumonia. NPPV was associated with a significant improvement in PaO_2/FiO_2 during FB. The technique was well tolerated, and no patient required ETI.

Favorable results were also obtained using NPPV during FB in patients with chronic obstructive pulmonary disease (COPD). Da Conceiçao et al. [12] investigated ten consecutive COPD patients with pneumonia who were admitted to the intensive care unit with hypercapnia (i.e., arterial carbon dioxide tension [$PaCO_2$], 67 ± 11 mmHg) and hypoxemia (i.e., PaO_2, 53 ± 13 mmHg). During FB with NPPV, arterial oxygen saturation of hemoglobin measured by pulse oximetry (SpO_2) increased from 91 ± 4.7% at baseline to 97 ± 1.7%. There were no changes in $PaCO_2$ and PaO_2 during the hour following the end of the procedure, and no patients were intubated within 24 h.

Maitre et al. [19] conducted a randomized double-blind study of 30 patients with PaO_2/FiO_2 <300 to compare facemask CPAP to oxygen administration in maintaining oxygenation during FB. CPAP allowed minimal alterations in gas exchange and prevented subsequent respiratory failure. During FB and 30 min thereafter, SpO2 was significantly higher in the CPAP group than the oxygen group. Arterial blood gas measurements 15 min after termination of FB showed that the PaO_2 had increased by 10.5 ± 16.9% in the CPAP group and decreased by 15 ± 16.6% in the oxygen group ($p = 0.01$). Five patients in the oxygen group, but none in the CPAP group, developed respiratory failure and required ETI in the 6 h following the FB procedure.

In a subsequent trial, Antonelli et al. [5] randomized 26 hypoxemic (i.e., PaO_2/FiO_2, <200) patients needing diagnostic FB to receive a FiO_2 of 0.9 via facemask, or NPPV via oronasal mask with pressure support ventilation of 15–17 cmH_2O, expiratory pressure of 5 cmH_2O and FiO_2 of 0.9. PaO_2/FiO_2 was substantially higher both during FB (261 vs 139 mmHg) and 1 h after FB (176 vs 140 mmHg), although both groups started at essentially the same PaO_2/FiO_2 at baseline (143 vs 155 mmHg). One hour after FB, the NPPV group had a lower mean heart rate (91 vs 108 beats/min; $p = 0.02$), and no reduction in mean arterial pressure in comparison to a 15% decrease from the baseline in the control group. Three patients required non-emergent ETI after undergoing FB, one patient in the NPPV group (7 h after the procedure) and two patients in the control group (9 and 5 h after the procedure). In all three cases, the ETI was not apparently related to FB.

In a more recent study [6] of patients with hypoxemic acute respiratory failure receiving NPPV through the helmet, FB with BAL was shown to be a safe and feasible technique, capable of avoiding ETI and discontinuation of assisted ventilation.

48.4 Contraindications

The risks associated with either the bronchoscopic examination or NIV application should be weighed against the potential benefits of the procedure. The criteria for excluding patients from NIV treatment include severe central neurological disturbances, inability to protect the airway, unstable hemodynamic conditions, vomiting, facial deformities, and recent oral, esophageal, or gastric surgery. The following situations are considered contraindications to FB: (1) absence of consent from the patient; (2) lack of trained personnel; (3) refractory hypoxemia even during NIV; (4) inability to normalize platelet count and coagulation if biopsy or brushing are anticipated; (5) unstable cardiac disease; and (6) uncontrolled bronchospasm [8]. In COPD patients, oxygen supplementation as well as intravenous sedation should be avoided or given with extreme caution during the procedure to prevent dangerous increases in $PaCO_2$ [26].

48.5 Practical Considerations

Technical aspects of the procedure are slightly different depending on the type of interface that is adopted to deliver NIV. When NIV is given through a facial mask, a T-adapter is attached to the mask for insertion

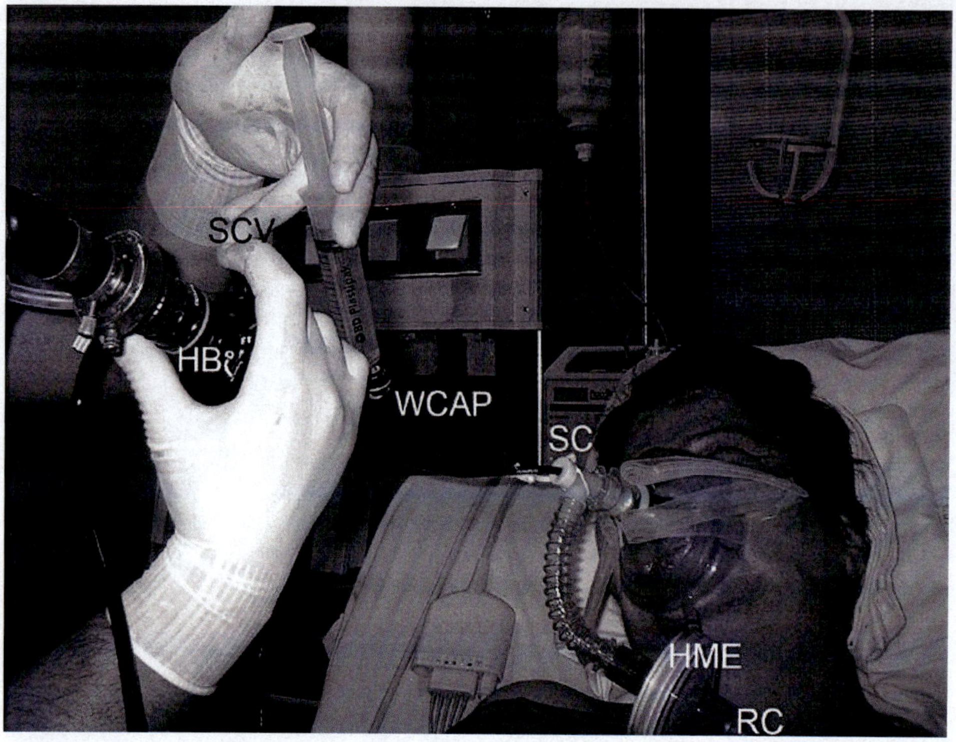

Fig. 48.1 Fiberoptic bronchoscopy with bronchoalveolar lavage performed during noninvasive ventilation delivered through an oronasal mask. *HB* handle of the bronchoscope, *HME* heat and moisture exchanger, *RC* respiratory circuit, *SC* seal connection, *SCV* suction control valve, *WCAP* working channel access port (Photograph printed with the permission of the patient)

of the bronchoscope through the nose or the mouth (Fig. 48.1). Differently, when a helmet is used, the bronchoscope is passed through the specific seal connector placed in the plastic ring of the helmet (Fig. 48.2). This connector is also used to spray local anaesthetics into the nostrils and pharynx of the patient. The internal adjustable diaphragm of the seal connection can prevent loss of the respiratory gases, maintaining ventilation throughout FB [6].

Prior to FB, NIV is delivered (if not yet started) for at least 15 min in order to obtain an adequate patient-ventilator interaction. NIV is maintained during FB and for at least 30 min after completion of the procedure, after which it is discontinued if the patient is not showing respiratory difficulties or significant gas exchange deterioration. The FiO_2 is kept at 0.9–1 while the patient adjusts to the ventilator and during the examination. PEEP should be decreased or discontinued during the FB procedure. For the first 30 min after termination of FB, the applied FiO_2 is gradually reduced to the pre-FB requirements as long as the patient is able to maintain SpO_2 at >92%.

Topical anesthesia of the nose and pharynx can be performed by spraying a 10% lidocaine solution. Topical anesthesia of the larynx and vocal cords can be obtained by injecting 2% lidocaine through the working channel of the bronchoscope. When FB is used to obtain samples from the lower respiratory tract for the diagnosis of pneumonia, the sampling area is selected by localizing new or progressive infiltrates on chest radiograph or the segment visualized during FB as having purulent secretions [25]. There are no clear recommendations regarding the sampling site in patients with diffuse lung infiltrates. In the supine patient, the BAL fluid recovery is best from the right middle lobe or lingula. When BAL is performed, the tip of the bronchoscope is wedged as far as possible into a distal airway, generally fourth to fifth order bronchi, and sterile saline solution is instilled through the bronchoscope and then aspirated into a sterile trap. Additional aliquots of 20–60 mL are injected and aspirated back after each instillation. The total amount of fluid used to obtain BAL ranges from 100 to 240 mL [16, 17, 25]. Bacterial pneumonia is diagnosed when a positive quantitative

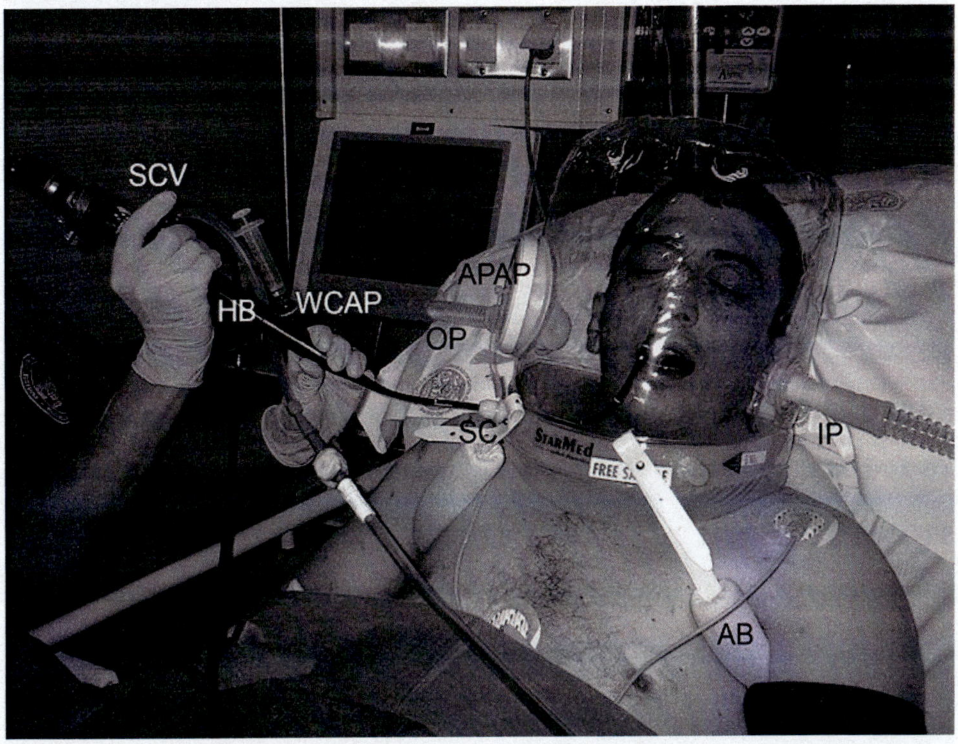

Fig. 48.2 Fiberoptic bronchoscopy performed during noninvasive ventilation delivered through a helmet. *AB* armpit braces, *APAP* airtight patient access port, *HB* handle of the bronchoscope, *IP* inlet port, *OP* outlet port, *SC* seal connection, *SCV* suction control valve, *WCAP* working channel access port (Photograph printed with the permission of the patient)

culture at 10^4 colony-forming units or more per milliliter of bacteria are measured in the BAL fluid [1].

The patient should have no oral feeding (or enteral nutrition) for 4 h and no clear oral fluids for 2 h before FB [8]. Subjects with a history of asthma should be premedicated with a bronchodilator before FB.

Cardiorespiratory monitoring during the procedure should include continuous electrocardiogram and SpO_2, continuous intra-arterial blood pressure or intermittent cuff blood pressure measurement at least every 5 min, tidal volume, minute ventilation, and airway pressure.

Finally, the feasibility of the technique may be affected by the type of NIV interface. When NIV is delivered through a helmet, performing FB could be difficult if there is a large distance between the plastic ring of the helmet and the patient's nose or mouth. One possibility to help the procedure might be removing the screw cap of the patient access port of the helmet [Fig. 48.2] for a few seconds to allow the operator to insert one hand into the helmet, helping the introduction of the bronchoscope into the patient's nose or mouth. Once the bronchoscope is paced in the upper airway, the patient access port is closed and NIV is resumed.

The technique using a facial mask is in general easier. If a facial mask is used, transnasal FB may involve some difficulties when the seal connector of the catheter mount, which joints the mask to the ventilator circuit, is not positioned over the patient's nose axis. When it occurs, it may be difficult either to introduce the bronchoscope into the nose or to maneuver the instrument through the airways. Replacing the facemask with another model can overcome this problem.

48.6 Conclusion

The use of NIV during FB appears to be a safe and valuable alternative to ETI for maintaining gas exchange in hypoxemic high-risk patients, especially those with hematological malignancies, allowing a prompt diagnosis and avoiding unnecessary empirical therapy.

References

1. American Thoracic Society; Infectious Diseases Society of America (2005) Guidelines for the management of adults with hospital-acquired, ventilator-associated, and health-care-associated pneumonia. Am J Respir Crit Care Med 171:388–416
2. Antonelli M, Conti G, Riccioni L et al (1996) Noninvasive positive-pressure ventilation via face mask during bronchoscopy with BAL in high-risk hypoxemic patients. Chest 110:724–728
3. Antonelli M, Conti G, Rocco M et al (1998) A comparison of noninvasive positive-pressure ventilation and conventional mechanical ventilation in patients with acute respiratory failure. N Engl J Med 339:429–435
4. Antonelli M, Conti C, Bufi M et al (2000) Noninvasive ventilation for treatment of acute respiratory failure in patients undergoing solid organ transplantation. JAMA 283: 235–241
5. Antonelli M, Conti G, Rocco M et al (2002) Noninvasive positive-pressure ventilation vs. conventional oxygen supplementation in hypoxemic patients undergoing diagnostic bronchoscopy. Chest 121:1149–1154
6. Antonelli M, Pennisi MA, Conti G et al (2003) Fiberoptic bronchoscopy during noninvasive positive pressure ventilation delivered by helmet. Intensive Care Med 29:126–129
7. Azoulay E, Afessa B (2006) The intensive care support of patients with malignancy: do everything that can be done. Intensive Care Med 32:3–5
8. British Thoracic Society Bronchoscopy Guidelines Committee, a Subcommittee of Standards of Care Committee of British Thoracic Society (2001) British Thoracic Society guidelines on diagnostic flexible bronchoscopy. Thorax 56(Suppl 1):i1–i21
9. Brochard L, Isabey D, Piquet J et al (1990) Reversal of acute exacerbations of chronic obstructive lung disease by inspiratory assistance with a face mask. N Engl J Med 323: 1523–1530
10. Campbell JH, Blessing N, Burnett AK et al (1993) Investigation and management of pulmonary infiltrates following bone marrow transplantation: an eight year review. Thorax 48:1248–1251
11. Craven DE, Kunches LM, Kilinsky V et al (1986) Risk factors for pneumonia and fatality in patients receiving continuous mechanical ventilation. Am Rev Respir Dis 113: 792–796
12. Da Conceiçao M, Genco G, Favier JC et al (2000) Fiberoptic bronchoscopy during noninvasive positive-pressure ventilation in patients with chronic obstructive lung disease with hypoxemia and hypercapnia. Ann Fr Anesth Rèanim 19:231–236
13. Elliott MW, Steven MH, Phillips GD et al (1990) Noninvasive mechanical ventilation for acute respiratory failure. BMJ 300:358–360
14. Estopa R, Torres Marti A, Kastanos N et al (1984) Acute respiratory failure in severe hematologic disorders. Crit Care Med 12:26–28
15. Ewig S, Torres A, Riquelme R et al (1998) Pulmonary complications in patients with haematological malignancies treated at a respiratory ICU. Eur Respir J 12:116–122
16. Goldstein RA, Rohatgi PK, Bergofsky EH et al (1990) Clinical role of bronchoalveolar lavage in adults with pulmonary disease. Am Rev Respir Dis 142:481–486
17. Klech H, Pohl W (1989) Technical recommendations and guidelines for bronchoalveolar lavage (BAL). Report of the European Society of Pneumology Task Group. Eur Respir J 2:561–585
18. L'Her E, Deye N, Lellouche F et al (2005) Physiologic effects of noninvasive ventilation during acute lung injury. Am J Respir Crit Care Med 172:1112–1118
19. Lin CC, Wu JL, Huang WC (1988) Pulmonary function in normal subjects after bronchoalveolar lavage. Chest 93: 1049–1053
20. Lindgren S, Odenstedt H, Erlandsson K et al (2008) Bronchoscopic suctioning may cause lung collapse: a lung model and clinical evaluation. Acta Anaesthesiol Scand 52:209–218
21. Lindholm CE, Ollman B, Snyder JV et al (1978) Cardiorespiratory effects of flexible fiberoptic bronchoscopy in critically ill patients. Chest 74:362–368
22. Maitre B, Jaber S, Maggiore SM et al (2000) Continuous positive airway pressure during fiberoptic bronchoscopy in hypoxemic patients: a randomized double-blind study using a new device. Am J Respir Crit Care Med 162: 1063–1067
23. Matsushima Y, Jones RL, King EG et al (1984) Alterations in pulmonary mechanics and gas exchange during routine fiberoptic bronchoscopy. Chest 86:184–188
24. Meduri GU, Conoscenti CC, Menashe P et al (1989) Noninvasive face mask ventilation in patients with acute respiratory failure. Chest 95:865–870
25. Meduri GU, Chastre J (1992) The standardization of bronchoscopic techniques for ventilator-associated pneumonia. Chest 102:557S–564S
26. Peacock MD, Johnson JE, Blanton HM (1994) Complications of flexible bronchoscopy in patients with severe obstructive pulmonary disease. J Bronchol 1:181–186
27. Peters SG, Meadows JA 3rd, Gracey DR (1988) Outcome of respiratory failure in hematologic malignancy. Chest 94: 99–102
28. Pingleton SK (1988) Complications of acute respiratory failure. Am Rev Respir Dis 137:1463–1493
29. Trouillet JL, Guiguet M, Gibert C et al (1990) Fiberoptic bronchoscopy in ventilated patients: evaluation of cardiopulmonary risk under midazolam sedation. Chest 97: 927–933
30. Wardman AG, Milligan DW, Child JA et al (1984) Pulmonary infiltrates and adult acute leukaemia: empirical treatment and survival related to the extent of pulmonary radiological disease. Thorax 39:568–571

NIV Outside the ICU

49

Stefano Nava and Sebastiano Mercadante

Contents

S. Nava (✉)
Respiratory and Critical Care Ospedale, S. Orsola-Malpighi, Via Albertom n. 15, Bologna, Italy
e-mail: stefanava@gmail.com

S. Mercadante
Anesthesia & Intensive Care Unit and Pain Relief & Palliative Care Unit, La Maddalena Cancer Center, Palermo, Italy

49.1 Introduction

It is known that with the technological innovations both in the diagnosis and in multidisciplinary treatment, the mortality rate at least for selected types of hematological malignancies has decreased. However, patients with hematological malignancies may often develop respiratory complications related to the underlying disorder and/or the aggressive treatment strategy. This may aversely affect their outcome, even if intensive care measures are adopted [1].

Prolonging survival, however, is not always a desirable goal to achieve for both the physician and the patient according to patient-centered management of diseases [2]. Conversely, palliation of symptoms and shared end of life decisions are the main targets of the care in order to maintain human dignity in the transition to the death [3]. With the introduction of non-invasive ventilation (NIV) to treat acute respiratory failure (ARF) of different etiologies about 2 decades ago, classical outcome measures – such as hospital mortality, need for endotracheal intubation, complications of invasive ventilation, and length of hospital stay – have been drastically improved [4]. In parallel, mechanical ventilation is no longer associated with death in more than 80% of the cases. The feasibility and usefulness of NIV both in the treatment of ARF in patients with hematological malignancies and its use a palliative tool in the same group of patients near the end of their lives are still under debate [5, 6]. In this chapter, the rationale for using NIV outside the ICU and the little available literature will be discussed.

É. Azoulay (ed.), *Pulmonary Involvement in Patients with Hematological Malignancies*,
DOI: 10.1007/978-3-642-15742-4_49, © Springer-Verlag Berlin Heidelberg 2011

49.2 When to Start NIV Outside the ICU

We need to keep in mind that the application of NIV outside a "protected" environment like the intensive care unit (ICU) or a respiratory intensive or high dependency unit (RICU or HDU) in the large majority of cases results in avoiding intubation and/or providing relief of dyspnea rather than being a real alternative to invasive mechanical ventilation. An ICU bed may not be available, and NIV can be initiated in the hematological wards. Reasons for this include monitoring systems and the patient/nurse ratio; also, the physician's training in performing cardiorespiratory maneuvers, including intubation, may be profoundly different in the ICU compared to a "classical" medical ward.

On one hand, the early application of NIV is recommended outside the ICU in patients with acute respiratory failure due hematological malignancies to avoid the complications of invasive ventilation, but on the other hand, the clinicians should be aware of not going "too far" if NIV is not rapidly effective in order not to unduly delay the time of intubation. Therefore, the time to start and the time to eventually stop NIV are critical in a non-protected environment [7].

The "early" use of NIV is recommended because the opportunity to initiate NIV successfully may be lost if initiation is delayed and the patient's underlying disease progresses too far. However, NIV can be started too early when the patient's condition is so mild that no ventilatory assistance is needed and the patient is more likely to be intolerant than to be helped [8].

In our practice, it is essential to know the arterial blood gas tensions before making a decision about whether NIV is indicated. The patient should first be established on appropriate oxygen therapy and the arterial blood gases interpreted in the light of the inspired fraction of oxygen (FiO_2). It is important to note that a relatively small proportion of patients who fulfill arterial blood gas criteria for NIV at the time of admission to hospital do in fact improve rapidly with initial medical treatment and an appropriate FiO_2. Measurement of arterial blood gas tensions should be considered in all individuals with breathlessness of sufficient severity. Oximetry alone may provide false reassurance in patients on supplemental oxygen in whom oxygenation is well maintained despite dangerous hypercapnia [9].

In patients affected by "pump" failure, there is agreement that NIV in the medical ward should be started when the pH is below 7.35 and the $PaCO_2$ is above 45–50 mmHg [4]. In patients with "lung" failure, NIV is indicated when the PaO_2/FiO_2 ratio is below 250 or when oxygen saturation does not reach 90% despite high-flow oxygen therapy [4]. Although a "magic" threshold does not exist, it is strongly recommended that in the case of a pH <7.28–7.30 and a PaO_2/FiO_2 <180–200, the patients should be transferred to an ICU or RICU, unless there is a "do-not-intubate" (DNI) order or the patient is in a terminal and irreversible phase of the disease.

The institution of NIV also depends on other factors such as the severity of the patient's clinical condition. NIV is not indicated if consciousness is altered [10, 11], or if there is hemodynamic stability or association with other organ dysfunction [12]. For example, a patient with organ failure other than acute respiratory failure (i.e., coma or shock, etc.) is not a candidate for NIV, but rather for prompt intubation, even if the arterial blood gases are still not severely compromised. Making the decision about when to start NIV is above all clinical and not only based on arterial blood gases. Most practitioners seek evidence of increased dyspnea as well as work of breathing (tachypnea or increased accessory muscle use) [13].

It must also be said that the inability to recognize those patients in whom NIV will fail early on can lead to delayed intubation, clinical deterioration and increased morbidity and mortality. Therefore, recognition of those clinical and instrumental features that can help the physician to predict NIV failure early in the course of the disease is of great importance in order to avoid undue delay in the transfer of these patients to the ICU or RICU. Failure of gas exchange, pH, respiratory rate, or dyspnea to improve after 1–3 h or deterioration in hemodynamic or mental status should prompt referral to the ICU service for intubation [10, 11]. This is true for the "classical" NIV indications and for the specific group with hematological malignancy [14].

Overall, the delivery of NIV does not appear to increase the workload of nursing staff or respiratory therapists [15, 16], but this may be only true in specific environments where the experience and the training of the whole team may explain these conclusions. In particular, we have shown that staff training is a key factor in determining the outcome of the patient undergoing a NIV trial [17]. Indeed, with few exceptions, all the studies dealing with the use of NIV were performed in units where the patient-to-nurse ratio was in the worst case 1:5 or 1:6.

Figure 49.1 shows a possible flow chart for the use of NIV outside the ICU in most of the Italian hospitals with an NIV service.

49.3 The Rationale for Using NIV in Hematological Patients with Acute Respiratory Failure

The use of NIV to treat an episode of respiratory failure in acutely ill hematological cancer patients is a relatively new field of application that is expanding

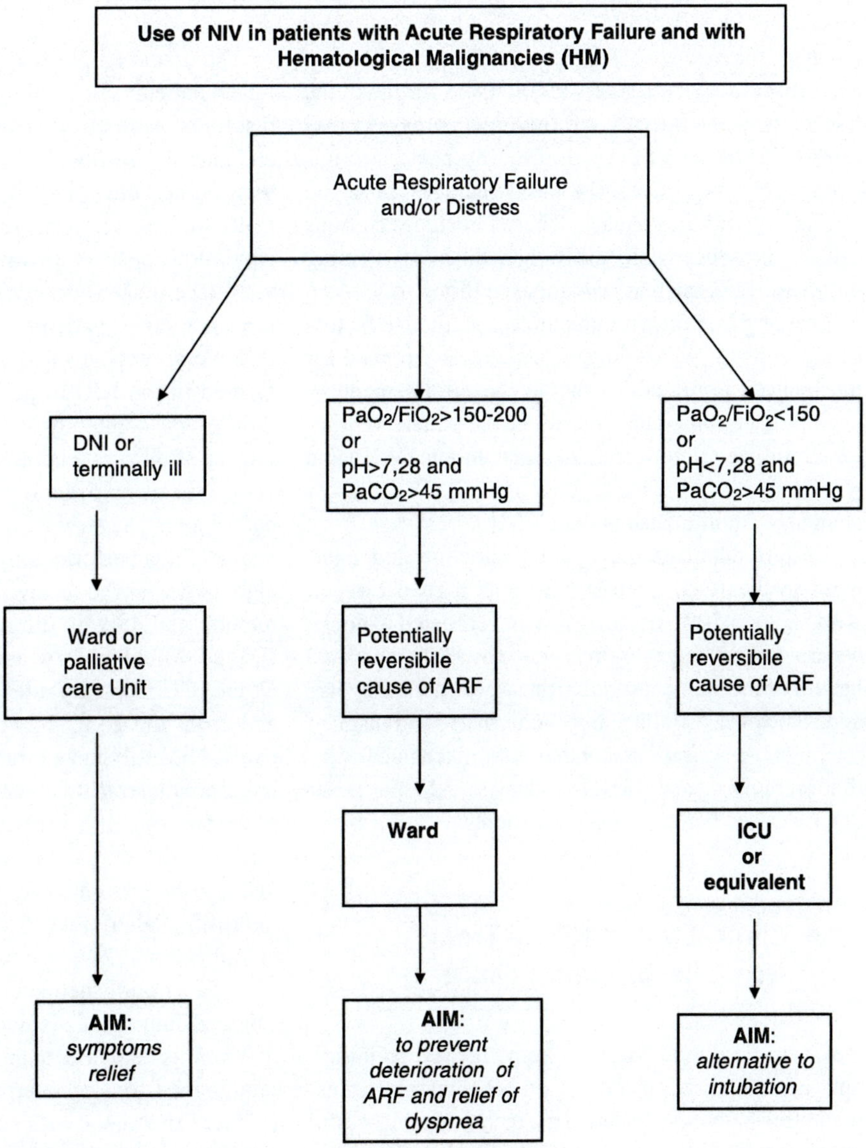

Fig. 49.1 Possible flow chart for the use of NIV outside the ICU in most of the Italian hospitals with an NIV service

very quickly given the very promising results obtained. Up to 30–40% of the patients with neutropenia may develop severe pulmonary infections. Other patients may also be prone to develop other respiratory complications, such as alveolar hemorrhage, capillary leak syndrome, radiation toxicity, or drug-related toxicity [18–20].

Endotracheal intubation increases the mortality risk because it concerns the sickest patients who cannot survive without being ventilated. Intubated patients have a greater possibility of developing new or superimposed infections, such as sinusitis and ventilator-associated pneumonia [21]. The endotracheal tube bypasses the mechanical defenses of the upper airways and causes local damage. In addition, the portion of the trachea between the cuff and the vocal cords becomes a reservoir of secretions colonized by bacteria originating from the sinuses, the nasal passages, pharynx, oral cavity, and the stomach. These infected secretions can be introduced into the lung with every nursing maneuver [22], such as bronchoaspiration.

One of the strongest independent predictive factors of mortality in hematological patients is the need for mechanical ventilation. Despite the efforts made to prevent bacterial contamination of the patient/ventilator circuit, ventilator-associated pneumonia (VAP) and worsening of a pre-existing infection are still the major challenges in intubated patients [23].

Despite adequate diagnostic evaluation and treatment in the ICU, mortality remains high. However, with an up to 50% mortality rate in ventilated patients, we are now no longer asking questions about the actual benefit of mechanical ventilation, as was done 20 years ago. However, in allogeneic bone marrow transplant recipients, outcomes associated with mechanical ventilation remain poor [24]. Nevertheless, NIV has never demonstrated benefits in BMT patients.

49.4 Clinical Use of NIV to Treat Acute Respiratory Failure

New types and modalities of chemotherapy, radiotherapy, hematopoietic stem cell or bone marrow transplantation have contributed to the increase in successful treatment of hematological malignancies. However, these regimens may predispose patients to various life-threatening complications. The lung has been recognized as the target organ most frequently involved in these complications. The implementation of NIV services outside a protected environment may be theoretically useful to avoid ICU bed congestion and to treat not only the respiratory distress directly caused by the hematological disease, but also the acute exacerbations of an underlying respiratory or cardiac disease, which are often present in patients with blood malignancies and mainly due to the tobacco abuse.

In this book, Antonelli and colleagues provide a contribution on the use of NIV to ensure the safety of bronchoscopy and BAL in hematological patients. Also, a review on palliative NIV is provided by Meert and colleagues.

The first attempts to apply NIV in immunocompromised patients, although not those with hematological disorders, were made in the early 1990s by Gregg [25] and later by Gachot [26] in patients with acute respiratory failure due to *Pneumocystis jiroveci* infection. Both studies, although uncontrolled, concluded that continuous positive airway pressure (CPAP) delivered via a facemask was an effective supportive therapy in these acutely ill patients.

Several uncontrolled or pilot studies were performed in the ICU in patients with acute respiratory failure and hematological malignancy. To define the impact of NIV vs. endotracheal intubation on the survival of cancer patients (mainly with hematological pathologies), a pairwise, matched, exposed-unexposed analysis was performed by Azoulay et al. [27]. Forty-eight patients who received NIV as the first ventilation method and 48 who did not were matched for SAPS II, type of malignancy, and period of ICU admission. Crude ICU mortality rates from those exposed to NIV and from the controls were 44% and 71%, respectively. NIV still had a protective effect against mortality after adjustment for matching variables. According to the risk of death attributable to mechanical ventilation, about four patients had to receive NIV for one death to be prevented. NIV seems therefore to be an interesting alternative because of the lower risk of complications [28].

A paper published later by Hilbert [29] in the New England Journal of Medicine gave scientific dignity to NIV in this field. The authors conducted a prospective, randomized trial of intermittent NIV compared with standard treatment with supplemental oxygen and no ventilatory support in 52 immunocompromised patients with pulmonary infiltrates, fever, and an early stage of hypoxemic acute respiratory failure (PaO_2/FiO_2 ratio <200). Half the patients had a hematological malignancy and neutropenia. Periods of NIV delivered through a facemask were alternated every 3 h with periods of spontaneous breathing with supplemental oxygen. The decision to intubate was made according to standard, predetermined criteria. The main results of the study were that fewer patients in the NIV group than in the standard treatment group required endotracheal intubation, had serious complications, or died in the ICU or in the hospital.

Although the study was performed in the ICU, some important conclusions may be drawn for the use of NIV outside this protected environment. The authors stressed the "early" use of NIV as a major factor of success. One of the enrollment criteria was a PaO_2/FiO_2 of <200 that corresponds to a PaO_2 of 60 mmHg at an FiO_2 of 30%; very often these patients in the "real world" are not always admitted to the ICU, especially if medical therapy and oxygen have not yet been started. The study indicates on one hand that NIV is superior to oxygen alone, but on the other hand that at this stage of severity NIV may also be initiated outside the ICU provided a prompt transfer to an ICU or RICU is possible. Indeed, although in the ICU so-called "isolated" or "negative pressure" rooms are not frequently available, most of the hematological wards probably have these facilities, so that these patients could be treated early with NIV, without exposing them to a high risk of infection.

Several other studies [14, 27, 29–37], illustrated in Table 49.1, follow along the line of Hilbert's study, but they were performed mainly in the ICU, with the exception of a couple of studies.

Table 49.1 No. of patients and locations of published studies using NIV in hematological patients

Author	References	No. of patients	Location
Conti et al.	[30]	16	ICU
Hilbert et al.	[29]	26	ICU
Tognet et al.	[31]	18	ICU
Azoulay et al.	[27]	42	ICU
Depuydt et al.	[32]	166	ICU
Rabitsh et al.	[33]	35	Bone marrow transplant unit
Hilbert et al.	[34]	64	ICU
Principi et al.	[35]	17	Oncology ward
Rocco et al.	[36]	8	ICU
Marin et al.	[37]	1	Hematological ward

In 1998 the first report of the use of NIV outside the ICU in a patient with respiratory failure after hematopoietic progenitor transplantation was published [37]. Also, Principi et al. [35] described the use of NIV directly in the hematological unit of a university hospital in a prospective clinical study with historical matched controls. They compared the efficacy of early administration of noninvasive CPAP delivered by the helmet vs. facemask to treat hematological malignancy patients with fever, pulmonary infiltrates, and hypoxemic acute respiratory failure (PaO_2/FiO_2 <200). A total of 34 patients were enrolled with a mean oxygenation ratio of about 140. Oxygenation improved in all patients after nCPAP. No patient failed helmet nCPAP because of intolerance, while eight patients in the mask group did so. nCPAP could be applied continuously for a longer period of time in the helmet group, so that the authors concluded that early nCPAP with a helmet improves oxygenation in selected immunocompromised patients with hypoxemic acute respiratory failure even outside the ICU. Indeed the tolerance of helmet nCPAP seems better than that of nCPAP delivered by a mask.

There are several new pieces of information from the Principi's study. First, they assessed the safety and feasibility of NIV outside the ICU in hematologic patients with severe acute respiratory failure. Second, they applied a particular interface, the helmet, which is probably the most simple and easiest way to apply CPAP outside a protected unit, since it does not require any electrical power and/or need a ventilator. The helmet should however be used with caution, especially in hypercapnic patients, when applying pressure support ventilation with a commonly used ventilator because of the possibility of rebreathing CO_2 and of poor patient/ventilator interaction. Third, this study indirectly highlighted that interdisciplinary collaboration between hematologists and intensivists appears crucial for achieving an early implementation of noninvasive mechanical ventilation and improving the quality of care. One year later, Rabitsh et al. [33] retrospectively analyzed the efficacy of NIV in 35 patients with acute hypoxemic respiratory failure after autologous or allogeneic stem cell transplantation directly ventilated in the bone marrow transplant unit. NIV was delivered by a standard facemask or helmet. Of the 82 patients who developed respiratory failure, 47 patients were initially intubated and mechanically ventilated. None of these patients survived. Thirty-five patients initially underwent NIV. Seven of these patients survived and were discharged from the hospital (20%). Eleven of the 35 (31%) patients improved within the first 4 h of NIV with respect to oxygenation and were regarded as responders. In all survivors, the partial pressure of arterial oxygen (PaO_2) improved after the initiation of NIV, whereas in non-survivors, PaO_2 improved in only 4/28 patients (17%) ($P<0.0001$). The authors concluded that in patients with acute respiratory failure after stem cell transplantation, NIV could improve prognosis when compared to a group of patients who constantly die if they receive mechanical ventilation.

49.5 Conclusions

Using early NIV in an environment less prone to infectious contamination (i.e., sterile rooms in the hematological ward) may be interesting for hematological patients. The choice to perform NIV outside a protected environment should be made carefully in order to balance the severity of acute respiratory failure and the intensity of care needed together with the optimization of the limited economic resources of national health systems. The number and the experience of the team (medical doctors, respiratory therapists, nurses) have to be adequate and adapted to the severity of the acute illness. The more expert the team is in NIV, the greater the severity of the ARF that can be managed [17], provided that switching from NIV to invasive ventilation can be done very quickly. Sometimes NIV use may only delay the time to more aggressive treatment. Clinical evaluation when NIV is implemented and then regularly is warranted. Last but not least, ethical and palliative issues should be taken in account when implementing NIV [3, 5].

References

1. Adam AK, Soubani AO (2008) Outcome and prognostic factors of lung cancer patients admitted to the medical intensive care unit. Eur Respir J 31:47–53
2. Claessens MT, Lynn J, Zhong Z, Desbiens NA, Phillips RS, Wu AW, Harrell FE Jr, Connors AF Jr (2000) Dying with lung cancer or chronic obstructive pulmonary disease: insights from SUPPORT. Study to Understand Prognoses and Preferences for Outcomes and Risks of Treatments. J Am Geriatr Soc 48(5 Suppl):S146–S153
3. Curtis JR, Cook DJ, Sinuff T, White DB, Hill N, Keenan SP, Benditt JO, Kacmarek R, Kirchhoff KT, Levy MM (2007) Society of Critical Care Medicine Palliative Noninvasive Positive Ventilation Task Force. Noninvasive positive pressure ventilation in critical and palliative care settings: understanding the goals of therapy. Crit Care Med 35:932–939
4. Nava S, Hill N (2009) Non-invasive ventilation in acute respiratory failure. Lancet 374:250–259
5. Sinuff T, Cook DJ, Keenan SP, Burns KE, Adhikari NK, Rocker GM, Mehta S, Kacmarek R, Eva K, Hill NS (2008) Noninvasive ventilation for acute respiratory failure near the end of life. Crit Care Med 36:789–794
6. Truog RD, Campbell ML, Curtis JR, Haas CE, Luce JM, Rubenfeld GD, Rushton CH, Kaufman DC (2008) Recommendations for end-of-life care in the intensive care unit: A consensus statement by the American Academy of Critical Care Medicine. Crit Care Med 36:953–963
7. Nava S, Navalesi P, Conti G (2006) Time of noninvasive ventilation. Intensive Care Med 32:361–370
8. Barbè F, Togores B, Rubi M et al (1996) Noninvasive ventilatory support does not facilitate recovery from acute respiratory failure in chronic obstructive pulmonary disease. Eur Respr J 9:1240–1245
9. Jubran A, Tobin MJ (1996) Monitoring during mechanical ventilation. Clin Chest Med 17:453–473
10. Anton A, Guell R, Gomez J et al (2000 Mar) Predicting the result of noninvasive ventilation in severe acute exacerbations of patients with chronic airflow limitation. Chest 117: 828–833
11. Ambrosino N, Foglio K, Rubini F, Clini E, Nava S, Vitacca M (1995) Non-invasive mechanical ventilation in acute respiratory failure due to chronic obstructive pulmonary disease: correlates for success. Thorax 50:755–757
12. Moretti M, Cilione C, Tampieri A, Fracchia C, Marchioni A, Nava S (2000) Incidence and causes of non-invasive mechanical ventilation failure after an initial (>48 h) successful attempt. Thorax 55:819–825
13. Keenan SP, Powers CE, McCormack DG (2005) Noninvasive positive-pressure ventilation in patients with milder chronic obstructive pulmonary disease exacerbations: a randomized controlled trial. Respir Care 50:610–616
14. Adda M, Coquet I, Darmon M et al (2008) Predictors of noninvasive ventilation failure in patients with hematologic malignancy and acute respiratory failure. Crit Care Med 36:2766–2772
15. Kramer N, Meyer TJ, Meharg J, Cece RD, Hill NS (1995) Randomized, prospective trial of noninvasive positive pressure ventilation in acute respiratory failure. Am J Respir Crit Care Med 151:1799–1806
16. Nava S, Evangelisti I, Rampulla C, Fracchia C, Rubini F (1997) Human and financial costs of non-invasive mechanical ventilation in patients affected by chronic obstructive pulmonary disease and acute respiratory failure. Chest 111:1631–1638
17. Carlucci A, Delmastro M, Rubini F, Fracchia C, Nava S (2003) Changes in the practice of non-invasive ventilation in treating COPD patients over 8 years. Intensive Care Med 29:419–425
18. Ewing S, Torres A, Riquelme R et al (1988) Pulmonary complications in patients with haematological malignancies treated at a respiratory ICU. Eur Respir J 12:116–122

19. Kress JP, Christenson J, Pohlman AS, Linkin DR, Hall JB (1999) Outcomes of critically ill cancer patients in a university hospital setting. Am J Respir Crit Care Med 160: 1957–1961
20. Chaflin DB, Carlon GC (1990) Age and utilization of ICU resources of critically ill cancer patients. Crit Care Med 18: 694–698
21. Fagon JY, Chastre J, Domart Y et al (1989) Nosocomial pneumonia in patients receiving continuous mechanical ventilation. Prospective analysis of 52 episodes with use of protected specimen brush and quantitative culture techniques. Am Rev Respir Dis 139:877–884
22. Elpern EH, Scott MG, Petro L, Ries MH (1994) Pulmonary aspiration in mechanically ventilated patients with tracheostomies. Chest 105:563–566
23. American Thoracic Society; Infectious Diseases Society of America (2005) Guidelines for the management of adults with hospital-acquired, ventilator-associated, and healthcare-associated pneumonia. Am J Respir Crit Care Med 171: 388–416
24. Rubenfeld GD, Crawford SW (1996) Withdrawing life support from mechanically ventilated recipients of bone marrow transplant: a case for evidence-based guidelines. Ann Intern Med 125:625–633
25. Gregg RW, Friedman BC, Williams JF, McGrath BJ, Zimmerman JE (1990) Continuous positive airway pressure by face mask in Pneumocystis carinii pneumonia. Crit Care Med 18:21–24
26. Gachot B, Clair B, Wolff M, Reigner B, Vachon F (1992) Continuous positive airway pressure administered by face mask or mechanical ventilation in patients with immunodeficiency virus infection and severe Pneumocystis carinii pneumonia. Intens Care Med 18:155–159
27. Azoulay E, Alberti C, Bornstain C, Leleu G, Moreau D, Recher C, Cevret S, Le Gall JR, Brochard L, Schlemmer B (2001) Improved survival in cancer patients requiring mechanical ventilator support: impact of noninvasive mechanical ventilator support. Crit Care Med 29:519–524
28. Hess DR (2004) The evidence for noninvasive positive-pressure ventilation in the care of patients in acute respiratory failure: a systematic review of the literature. Respir Care 49: 810–829
29. Hilbert G, Gruson D, Vargas F, Valentino R, Gbikpi-Benissan G, Dupon M, Reiffers J, Cardinaud JP (2001) Noninvasive ventilation in immunodepressed patients with pulmonary infiltrates, fever and acute respiratory failure. N Engl J Med 344:481–487
30. Conti G, Marino P, Cogliati A, Dell'Utri D, Lappa A, Rosa G, Gasparetto A (1998) Noninvasive ventilation for treatment of acute respiratory failure in patients with haematological malignancies: a pilot study. Intensive Care Med 24: 1283–1288
31. Tognet E, Mercatello A, Polo P, Coronel B, Bret M, Archimbaud E, Moskovtchenko JF (1994) Treatment of acute respiratory failure with non-invasive intermittent positive pressure ventilation in haematological patients. Clin Intensive Care 5:282–288
32. Depuydt PO, Benoit DD, Wandewoude KH et al (2004) Outcome in noninvasively and invasively ventilated hematologic patients with acute respiratory failure. Chest 126: 1299–06
33. Rabitsch W, Staudinger T, Locker GJ et al (2005) Respiratory failure after stem cell transplantation: improved outcome with non-invasive ventilation. Leuk Lymphoma 46: 1151–1157
34. Hilbert G, Gruson D, Vargas F, Valentino R, Chene G, Boiron JM, Pigneux A, Reiffers J, Gbikpi-Benissan G, Cardinaud JP (2000) Noninvasive continuous positive airway pressure in neutropenic patients with acute respiratory failure requiring ICU admission. Crit Care Med 28: 3185–3190
35. Principi T, Pantanetti S, Catani F, Elisei D, Gabbanelli V, Pelaia P, Leoni P (2004) Noninvasive continuous positive airway pressure delivered by helmet in hematological malignancy patients with hypoxemic acute respiratory failure. Intensive Care Med 30:147–150
36. Rocco M, Dell'Utri D, Morelli A et al (2004) Noninvasive ventilation by helmet or face mask in immunocompromised patients. Chest 126:1508–1515
37. Marin D, Gonzales-Barca E, Domingo E et al (1998) Noninvasive mechanical ventilation in a patient with respiratory failure after hematopoietic progenitor transplantation. Bone Marrow Transpl 22:1123–1124

Palliative Noninvasive Mechanical Ventilation in Patients with Hematological Malignancies

50

Anne-Pascale Meert, Thierry Berghmans, and Jean-Paul Sculier

Contents

Noninvasive mechanical ventilation (NIV) can be used in two categories of palliative care patients with hematological malignancies: patients with do-not-intubate (DNI) orders and patients very near the end of life who receive comfort measures only.

The role for NIV in patients with DNI orders has been assessed in a few studies (Table 50.1). In a study published in 1992 [1], nasal-mask ventilation was used as the treatment of last resort in 30 elderly noncancer patients in whom endotracheal intubation was deemed inappropriate. Of the 30 patients, 18 were successfully weaned off NIV and 12 failed to improve; in this last group, eight died and four received endotracheal mechanical ventilation. The first study that included cancer patients was done in 11 terminally ill patients who refused endotracheal intubation, including three patients with cancer [2]. Facial mask NIV used to treat hypercapnic or hypoxemic acute respiratory failure was effective in 7 of the 11 patients, all of whom survived and were discharged from the ICU, and five of whom were discharged alive from the hospital. The four patients who died in the ICU had hypercapnic respiratory failure. In another study [3], the same team evaluated 26 patients with advanced disease (three with lung cancer and the others with end-stage chronic obstructive pulmonary disease (COPD), liver disease, or AIDS) and who refused intubation. Nine patients died during the ICU stay, including five in whom NIV was not effective and was discontinued at the patient's or family's request. Thus, NIV is feasible and effective in terminally ill patients.

These results prompted several larger studies. Levy et al. [4] reported a study of 114 patients (including 14 with malignancies) with DNI orders who were treated with NIV. Among them, 43% were discharged alive from the hospital. In patients with COPD, the results of palliative NIV seem good. A study assessed the role

A.-P. Meert (✉), T. Berghmans, and J.-P. Sculier
Department of Intensive Care and Thoracic Oncology, Institut Jules Bordet, Université Libre de Bruxelles (ULB), 1 rue Héger Bordet, B-1000, Brussels, Belgium
e-mail: ap.meert@bordet.be

É. Azoulay (ed.), *Pulmonary Involvement in Patients with Hematological Malignancies*,
DOI: 10.1007/978-3-642-15742-4_50, © Springer-Verlag Berlin Heidelberg 2011

Table 50.1 Studies assessing noninvasive ventilation in patients with do-not-intubate orders

Author	No. patients	No. cancer patients	Patients	Overall hospital discharge rate	Hospital discharge rate in cancer patients
Meduri [2]	11	3	Terminally ill patients	45%	
Meduri [3]	26	3	COPD, liver disease, AIDS, lung cancer	64%[a]	
Benhamou [1]	17	0	Elderly	47%	
Farha [17]	14	0	COPD, pulmonary edema, obesity hypoventilation, neuromuscular disease	50%	
Chu [5]	37	0	COPD	179 days[b]	
Scarpazza [6]	62	0	COPD	87%	
Levy [4]	114	14	COPD, pneumonia, other (one lymphoma and one chronic myelogenous leukemia)	43%	
Schettino [8]	131	40	COPD, pulmonary edema, non-COPD hypercapnic failure, postextubation respiratory failure, hypoxemic respiratory failure	35%	15%
Fernandez [7]	36	6	COPD, non-COPD	26%	
Meert [9]	18	18	17 solid tumors and one leukemia	55%	55%
Cuomo [10]	23	23	Solid tumors	56%	56%

AIDS acquired immune deficiency syndrome, *COPD* chronic obstructive pulmonary disease
[a]ICU discharge
[b]Median survival

for NIV in 37 COPD patients who had DNI orders and who developed acute respiratory failure [5]. Median survival was 179 days with a 1-year survival rate of about 30%. Most of the survivors experienced another life-threatening event within the next year. In a more recent study, NIV was successful in 54 of 62 hypercapnic COPD patients with DNI orders [6]. In a retrospective study of 233 ICU patients managed with NIV in 2002–2004, 36 patients (including six with cancer) had DNI orders [7]. Hospital survival in these 36 patients was only 26%, compared to 74% in the other 199 patients [7]. A prospective study of patients with DNI orders who received NIV showed that this modality was effective in reversing acute respiratory failure and preventing hospital mortality in patients with COPD or cardiogenic pulmonary edema, but not in those with postextubation failure, hypoxemic respiratory failure, or end-stage cancer ($n=40$) [8]. A score combining the SAPS II value and the serum albumin level predicted survival in NIV-treated patients with DNI orders [8].

Only two studies focused specifically on cancer patients. We evaluated the role for NIV in 18 cancer patients with treatment-limitation decisions (including DNI orders). Among them, 12 had lung cancer, two head and neck cancer, two bladder carcinoma, one prostate cancer, and one acute myeloblastic leukemia [9]. The reasons for NIV were hypoxemic respiratory failure in 11 patients and hypercapnic respiratory failure in 7. NIV was well tolerated. Total median NIV duration was 29 h (over a median of 2.5 days). Total median ICU stay duration was 7 days. Only four patients failed to respond to NIV. Fourteen patients were discharged alive from the ICU and ten from the hospital. Overall median survival was 50 days, and 1-year survival was 10%. Among the 12 lung-cancer patients, nine (75%) survived to hospital discharge, compared to only 16% of the six other patients. These results suggested a role for NIV in cancer patients with treatment-limitation decisions, although the long-term survival rate was low, in large part because of cancer progression. A single patient, aged 76 years, had a hematological malignancy (leukemia); this patient was managed successfully with NIV for acute cardiogenic pulmonary edema. The other study in cancer patients included 23 palliative-care patients with solid tumors and acute respiratory failure [10]. Among them, 13 were managed successfully with NIV and discharged alive, two failed NIV and accepted endotracheal mechanical ventilation, and eight died after a period of NIV. Higher SAPS II and lower PaO_2/FiO_2 were associated with a lower survival rate. The 1-year survival rate was 13% [10].

Thus, in patients with advanced cancer and treatment-limitation decisions, NIV seems useful. That over 50% of these cancer patients are discharged alive from the hospital after an acute illness managed using NIV is encouraging. However, about 90% of these patients die within the next year, usually from progression of the cancer, which recovers its independent influence on survival after resolution of the acute complication [11]. Our group has reported that the characteristics of the cancer do not predict hospital or ICU survival, but do predict survival after discharge [11]. Furthermore, the response to life-supporting treatments (cardiorespiratory resuscitation [12], endotracheal mechanical ventilation [13], NIV [14], and continuous veno-venous hemodialfiltration [15]) are independent from cancer characteristics. In patients with DNI orders, NIV is well tolerated and can prolong life, allowing further anti-cancer therapy or giving the patient time to complete life-closure tasks. NIV may be offered to cancer patients with reversible causes of acute respiratory failure for whom potentially life-extending treatments are available. For example, many cancer patients are smokers or former smokers who experience COPD exacerbations or episodes of cardiogenic pulmonary edema that may respond promptly to NIV.

However, when rapid death is unavoidable, care should be taken to avoid prolonging the dying process. No study has fully assessed the effectiveness and safety of NIV in patients who are very near the end of life and who receive comfort measures only. NIV may alleviate dyspnea due to acute respiratory failure complicating COPD [2] or cancer [10]. In a few patients, the relief from dyspnea and improved level of consciousness provided by NIV might improve communication at the end of life. However, further research is needed to determine whether these patients benefit from NIV. Importantly, many dying patients may find NIV undesirable because they feel the potential for dyspnea relief does not outweigh the discomfort caused by the tight-fitting facemask. Furthermore, the technical aspect of NIV might cause stress, and the facemask impedes communication. No studies have compared NIV in this setting with pharmacological treatments, such as morphine.

The palliative use of NIV is controversial. It has been argued that the decision to use NIV is up to the patient and family once they are fully informed about the risks and potential benefits [16]. The ethical and economic costs of using NIV to delay death have been described as unacceptably high. Informed consent is one of the main challenges raised by using NIV for palliative care. Patients do not always discuss end-of-life issues with their physicians, and many physicians are reluctant to discuss advance directives with their patients. Importantly, the patient must be informed of the risks and benefits of NIV and must consent to NIV. Then, the patient must be able to decide at any time to continue or to stop NIV. If the patient wants only comfort care without life-sustaining measures, NIV may be inappropriate, whereas NIV might deserve consideration in patients who are willing to use life-prolonging techniques but do not want to be intubated. In all cases, if NIV induces more discomfort than relief, the patient can simply choose to discontinue NIV, and comfort is then achieved using pharmacological treatments. Continued NIV despite patient discomfort may lead to painful facial skin irritation or necrosis, dryness of the nose and throat, distension of the esophagus and stomach, ocular irritation, and inadequate rest and sleep due to the noise caused by the ventilator. Intensivists must be careful not to give unreasonable expectations to the patient and family, and not to merely prolong the dying process. Often, a private room where the loved ones can remain at the bedside is the best means of providing comfort and a dignified death. With this in mind, we have developed an algorithm for decisions about

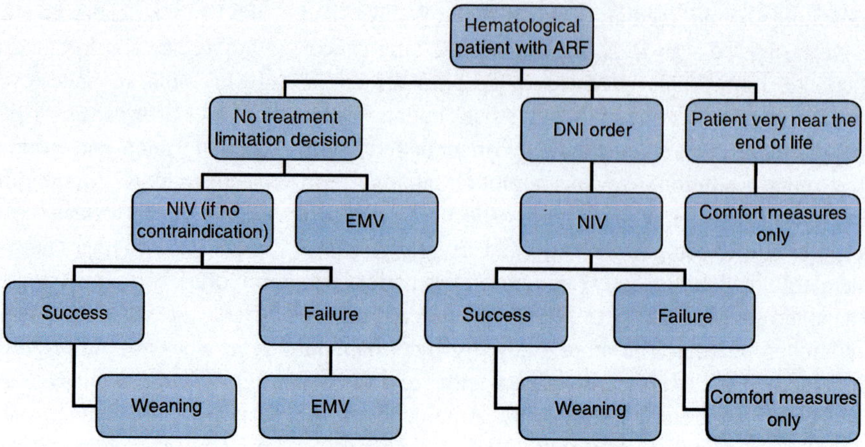

Fig. 50.1 Algorithm for deciding when to use mechanical ventilation applied in our institution. *ARF* acute respiratory failure, *DNI* do not intubate, *NIV* noninvasive ventilation, *EMV* endotracheal mechanical ventilation

using mechanical ventilation in our institution (Fig. 50.1).

The success of NIV depends on two factors: early use and delivery by experienced personnel. NIV improves patient outcomes only when used early. NIV used for palliative care in patients close to the end of life may be feasible on the wards, provided the staff is well trained and patient monitoring is adequate. In a study of 14 patients (COPD, neuromuscular disease, pulmonary edema, pneumonia, and pulmonary fibrosis) who had DNI orders and who received NIV on the hospital ward, survival was 50%, that is, similar to the rate seen when NIV is used in the ICU.

In conclusion, very few data are available on the role for NIV in palliative care patients with hematological malignancies. Experience acquired in patients with solid tumors indicates that NIV is feasible and effective provided the cause of acute respiratory failure is reversible and life-extending cancer treatment is available. For patients who are very near the end of life and who are receiving comfort measures only, NIV may alleviate dyspnea, although there is no evidence that NIV is better than pharmacological treatments such as morphine. In all cases, the patient must be fully informed and asked to provide or deny consent. Further studies are clearly needed to identify the subsets of palliative care patients with hematological malignancies who are most likely to benefit from NIV.

References

1. Benhamou D, Girault C, Faure C, Portier F, Muir JF (1992) Nasal mask ventilation in acute respiratory failure. Experience in elderly patients. Chest 102(3):912–917
2. Meduri GU, Fox RC, bou-Shala N, Leeper KV, Wunderink RG (1994) Noninvasive mechanical ventilation via face mask in patients with acute respiratory failure who refused endotracheal intubation. Crit Care Med 22(10): 1584–1590
3. Meduri GU, Turner RE, bou-Shala N, Wunderink R, Tolley E (1996) Noninvasive positive pressure ventilation via face mask. First-line intervention in patients with acute hypercapnic and hypoxemic respiratory failure. Chest 109(1): 179–193
4. Levy M, Tanios MA, Nelson D et al (2004) Outcomes of patients with do-not-intubate orders treated with noninvasive ventilation. Crit Care Med 32(10):2002–2007
5. Chu CM, Chan VL, Wong IW, Leung WS, Lin AW, Cheung KF (2004) Noninvasive ventilation in patients with acute hypercapnic exacerbation of chronic obstructive pulmonary disease who refused endotracheal intubation. Crit Care Med 32(2):372–377
6. Scarpazza P, Incorvaia C, Di FG et al (2008) Effect of noninvasive mechanical ventilation in elderly patients with hypercapnic acute-on-chronic respiratory failure and a do-not-intubate order. Int J Chron Obstruct Pulmon Dis 3(4): 797–801
7. Fernandez R, Baigorri F, Artigas A (2007) Noninvasive ventilation in patients with "do-not-intubate" orders: medium-term efficacy depends critically on patient selection. Intensive Care Med 33(2):350–354
8. Schettino G, Altobelli N, Kacmarek RM (2005) Noninvasive positive pressure ventilation reverses acute respiratory failure in select "do-not-intubate" patients. Crit Care Med 33(9):1976–1982

9. Meert AP, Berghmans T, Hardy M, Markiewicz E, Sculier JP (2006) Non-invasive ventilation for cancer patients with life-support techniques limitation. Support Care Cancer 14(2):167–171
10. Cuomo A, Delmastro M, Ceriana P et al (2004) Noninvasive mechanical ventilation as a palliative treatment of acute respiratory failure in patients with end-stage solid cancer. Palliat Med 18(7):602–610
11. Sculier JP, Paesmans M, Markiewicz E, Berghmans T (2000) Scoring systems in cancer patients admitted for an acute complication in a medical intensive care unit. Crit Care Med 28(8):2786–2792
12. Sculier JP, Berghmans T, Meert AP (2007) Indications and results of intensive care in patients with lung cancer. Rev Mal Respir 24(8 Pt 2):6S114–6S119
13. Vallot F, Paesmans M, Berghmans T, Sculier JP (2003) Leucopenia is an independent predictor in cancer patients requiring invasive mechanical ventilation: a prognostic factor analysis in a series of 168 patients. Support Care Cancer 11(4):236–241
14. Meert AP, Sotiriou M, Berghmans T et al (2006) Non-invasive ventilation in cancer patients: a historically matched controlled study. Hosp Chron 1(2):93–98
15. Berghmans T, Meert AP, Markiewicz E, Sculier JP (2004) Continuous venovenous haemofiltration in cancer patients with renal failure: a single-centre experience. Support Care Cancer 12(5):306–311
16. Bach JR (2007) Palliative care becomes ‘uninformed euthanasia’ when patients are not offered noninvasive life preserving options. J Palliat Care 23(3):181–184
17. Farha S, Ghamra ZW, Hoisington ER, Butler RS, Stoller JK (2006) Use of noninvasive positive-pressure ventilation on the regular hospital ward: experience and correlates of success. Respir Care 51(11):1237–1243

Acute Kidney Injury in Cancer Patients

51

Michael Darmon, Laurent Camous, Camille Devanlay, Emmanuel Canet, Benoit Schlemmer, and Fabrice Zeni

Contents

M. Darmon (✉)
Medical Intensive Care Unit, Saint-Louis University Hospital, Paris, France and
Medical Intensive Care Unit, Saint-Etienne University Hospital, Avenue Albert Raymond, 42270 Saint-Priest-en-Jarez, Saint-Etienne, France
e-mail: michael.darmon@chu-st-etienne.fr

L. Camous, E. Canet, and B. Schlemmer
Medical Intensive Care Unit, Saint-Louis University Hospital, Paris, France and
University of Paris VII, Paris, France

C. Devanlay and F. Zeni
Medical Intensive Care Unit, Saint-Etienne University Hospital, Avenue Albert Raymond, 42270 Saint-Priest-en-Jarez, Saint-Etienne, France

51.1 Introduction

Acute kidney injury (AKI) is a serious complication during malignancies that causes substantial morbidity and mortality. Among critically ill cancer patients (CICPs), the prevalence of AKI may be as high as 49%, and up to one third (32%) of CICPs will require renal replacement therapy (RRT) during their ICU stay [1–7]. The risk of AKI seems higher in CICPs than in other critically ill patients [5,8]. The hospital mortality rate may be as high as 80% in studies of CICPs requiring RRT [3,6]. Moreover, AKI may preclude optimal cancer treatment by requiring a decrease in chemotherapy dosage or by contraindicating potentially curative treatment (e.g., high-dose methotrexate in patients with recently diagnosed Burkitt lymphoma).

Unresolved issues in this setting are similar to those in the overall population of patients with AKI, namely, the definition of AKI, the possible benefits from early RRT, and the optimal dialysis dose. Multiple causes are often present in combination, such as contrast nephropathy, toxicity of cancer chemotherapy, infiltration by cancer cells, and sepsis. These causes are listed in Table 51.1. We will discuss factors associated with specific aspects of renal disease in CICPs, and we will provide a comprehensive overview of the specific causes of AKI in this population, including acute tumor lysis syndrome (TLS), treatment toxicity, sinusoidal obstruction syndrome, and thrombotic microangiopathy syndrome.

É. Azoulay (ed.), *Pulmonary Involvement in Patients with Hematological Malignancies*,
DOI: 10.1007/978-3-642-15742-4_51,

Table 51.1 Causes of acute renal failure in cancer patients (ACE inhibitors: angiotensin-converting enzyme inhibitors; NSAIDs: nonsteroidal anti-inflammatory drugs

Prerenal failure
• Sepsis
• Extracellular dehydration (diarrhea, mucitis, vomiting)
• Sinusoidal obstruction syndrome (formerly called hepatic veno-occlusive disease)
• Drugs (calcineurin inhibitors, ACE inhibitors, NSAIDs, etc.)
• Capillary-leak syndrome (IL2)
Intrinsic failure
• Acute tubular necrosis
– *Ischemia (shock, severe sepsis)*
– *Nephrotoxic agents (contrast agents, aminoglycosides, amphotericin, ifosfamide, cisplatin)*
– *Disseminated intravascular coagulation*
– *Intravascular hemolysis*
• Acute interstitial nephritis
– *Immuno-allergic nephritis*
– *Pyelonephritis*
– *Cancer infiltration (lymphoma, metastasis, etc.)*
– *Nephrocalcinosis*
• Vascular nephritis
– *Thrombotic microangiopathy*
– *Vascular obstruction*
• Glomerulonephritis
– *Amyloidosis (AL: myeloma; AA: renal carcinoma or Hodgkin's disease)*
– *Immunotactoid glomerulopathy*
– *Membranous glomerulonephritis (pulmonary, breast, or gastric carcinoma))*
– *IgA glomerulonephritis, focal glomerulosclerosis*
Postrenal failure
• Intra-renal obstruction (urate crystals, light chain, acyclovir, methotrexate, etc.)
• Extrarenal obstruction (retroperitonal fibrosis, ureteral or bladder outlet obstruction)

51.2 Consequences of Acute Renal Failure

51.2.1 Prognostic Impact of AKI

Despite improvements in RRT technology and advances in supportive care, the morbidity and mortality associated with AKI have remained unchanged over the last decades [9,10]. Whether this poor prognosis in patients with AKI is a reflection of the severity of the underlying disease or should be attributed to the uremic state has long been debated. Several recent studies have suggested that AKI in itself, independently of underlying disease or its severity, and apart from the metabolic consequences of the uremic state, may influence patient prognosis. Indeed, several studies have demonstrated a consistently high relative risk of death associated with AKI despite adjustment for comorbid conditions and severity of illness [9,11,12]. In addition, several studies have underlined the impact of a prognosis of modest AKI [11,13–15]. A recent study demonstrated modest rises in serum creatinine (>26 μmol/L) to be associated with a 6.5 odds increase in the risk of hospital death (95% CI 5.0–8.5) [11]. In fact, the kidney is no longer considered a witness of multiple organ failure, but as an actor that may participate in organ dysfunction [16].

51.2.2 Kidney Lung Crosstalk

An increasing body of evidence suggests that detrimental interactions may develop between the kidney and lung. This lung-kindey crosstalk may help us to understand the natural history of multiple organ failure and underline the central role of AKI in this syndrome.

51.2.2.1 Kidney–Lung Interaction

Beside hydrostatic pulmonary edema that occurs as a consequence of volume overload in the setting of

AKI [17], experimental evidence suggests that pulmonary injury occurs during AKI [18]. Experimental models have demonstrated that ischemic/reperfusion kidney injury in rodents leads to an increase in pulmonary vascular permeability, a lesional pulmonary edema, and an increase in bronchoalveolar lavage protein concentration [19–21]. In addition, ischemic/reperfusion kidney injury leads to downregulation of the epithelial salt and water transporters, ENaC, Na+-K+-ATPase and aquaporin, in rodent lung [21]. These changes seems to be due to activation of proinflammatory and proapoptotic pathways specific to the ischemic/reperfusion injury rather than due to uremic syndrome [21].

Cytokines seem to play a major role in the initiation and progression of this response [22]. In mice, AKI or bilateral nephrectomy is associated with an increase in IL-6, IL-1β, and macrophage inflammatory protein 2 [23]. The critical role of IL-6 in distant organ dysfunction related to AKI has been further demonstrated by experimental studies [24].

51.2.2.2 Lung–Kidney Interaction

Beside changes in respiratory function occurring after AKI, acute lung injury (ALI) may influence renal function. The role of hemodynamic changes has been well established during mechanical ventilation. Indeed, mechanical ventilation may reduce cardiac output and modify renal blood flow (RBF) [25–27]. Positive pressure ventilation may modify cardiac preload and cardiac afterload, and has been associated with changes in glomerular filtration rate, RBF, and free water clearance [25–27]. In addition, positive pressure ventilation may activate sympathetic and renin-angiotensin systems, and suppress atrial natriuretic peptide release [28].

Beside modifications induced by positive pressure ventilation in itself, hypoxemia and hypercapnia can modify renal vascular resistances [29–31] and diuresis [32–34]. This effect, well demonstrated in healthy subjects, is retrieved in patients with ALI [35]. The mechanism of this effect remains controversial [32,34–36], and its long-term impact on mechanical ventilation remains to be evaluated.

Last, emerging data support the idea that biotrauma induced by mechanical ventilation affects not only the lung, but also leads to further systemic inflammation through the release of inflammatory cytokines [37,38]. In a recent study evaluating protective ventilation, higher tidal volumes were associated not only with a higher level of TNF-α, IL-1b, IL-6, and IL-8, but also with a higher rate of AKI [37–40].

51.2.3 AKI in Patients with ALI/ARDS and in Critically Ill Cancer Patients

The association of ALI or ARDS with AKI is particularly common. A recent study evaluated factors predictive of AKI occurrence in the first three studies of the ARDS network (876 patients evaluated) [39]. Of these patients, 209 (24%) developed an AKI according to the RIFLE definition [39]. When ALI and AKI are combined, mortality has been described to be as high as 80% [41].

In CICPs, up to 66% of the cancer patients requiring mechanical ventilation had an AKI accordingly to the RIFLE criteria [42]. In this population of patients, oliguria was associated with a longer duration of mechanical ventilation (odds ratio 2.51; 95% CI 1.24–5.08) after adjustment for confounding factors and was strongly predictive of hospital mortality (odds ratio 31; 95% CI 8–127) [42].

Beside the impact on prognosis of AKI in CICPs, the development of an AKI may preclude optimal cancer treatment and therefore chances for the patient to experience complete remission [43]. As a consequence, if AKI has been demonstrated to be independently associated with a poor prognosis in patients with acute myeloid leukemia, this effect is mainly due to frequent failure of the induction treatment [43].

51.3 Specific Causes of Acute Renal Failure in Onco-hematological Patient

51.3.1 Acute Tumor Lysis Syndrome

TLS is a potentially life-threatening complication of cancer treatment in patients with extensive, rapidly growing, chemosensitive malignancies. TLS results from the rapid destruction of malignant cells, which abruptly release intracellular ions, proteins, and metabolites into the extra-cellular space [44,45]. Potassium, calcium, phosphates, and uric acid are present in high concentrations within malignant cells. The result is a constellation of metabolic disturbances that can cause AKI of which the most common mechanism is uric-acid crystal formation in the renal tubules. Another cause of AKI is calcium-phosphate deposition related to hyperphosphatemia. AKI may, in itself, cause substantial morbidity and mortality [9]. In addition, AKI leads to further increases in the above-listed metabolites, most notably potassium and phosphate, which may lead to cardiac arrhythmia or sudden death [44,46].

51.3.1.1 Definition and Risk Factors

Until very recently, there was no diagnostic criterion for TLS. The first diagnostic classification was developed by Hande and Garrow in 1993, then modified by Cairo and Bishop (Table 51.2) [44]. According to this classification, a constellation of metabolic disturbances (hyperkalemia, hyperphosphatemia, hyperuricemia, and hyperkalemia) defines laboratory TLS in high-risk patients, whereas clinical manifestations (cardiac, renal, or neurological manifestations of TLS) in a patient with laboratory TLS defines clinical TLS. Guidelines developed in 2008 rest on this classification [45].

Table 51.2 Definition of acute tumor lysis syndrome

Laboratory TLS: at least two of the following in serum	
Nonionized calcium	<1.75 mmol/L or −25% from baseline
Potassium	>6 mmol/L or +25% from baseline
Uric acid	>476 μmol/L or +25% from baseline
Phosphate	>1.45 mmol/L or +25% from baseline
Clinical TLS: laboratory TLS (above) plus one of the following	
Renal involvement	Acute kidney injury
Cardiovascular involvement	Cardiac arrhythmia or sudden death
Neurological involvement	Seizure

TLS tumor lysis syndrome

Early recognition of high-risk patients may allow a risk-based strategy for preventing both TLS and AKI. TLS typically occurs in patients with high-grade hematological malignancies (acute leukemia, Burkitt's lymphoma, or other high-grade non-Hodgkin's lymphoma) [47–52]. Despite routine urate oxidase therapy, TLS develops in 10–50% of patients with these high-grade malignancies [53–56] and AKI in up to one third [54–56]. In addition to the type of tumor and to its sensitivity to chemotherapeutic agents, features related to the tumor burden (large tumor burden, lactate dehydrogenase >1,500 IU, and extensive bone marrow involvement) influence the risk of TLS [48]. Last, patient characteristics may affect the TLS risk. For example, preexisting renal failure is associated with an increased risk of laboratory and clinical TLS.

51.3.1.2 Treatment

Three steps must be distinguished: (1) prevention of TLS, (2) prevention of clinical manifestations in patients with laboratory TLS, and (3) prevention of further organ dysfunction in clinical TLS. The goal of these measures is to prevent AKI, which severely exacerbates the laboratory and clinical manifestations of TLS. In addition, this strategy may help to avoid not only excess mortality, but also residual organ dysfunction.

Therefore, hyperuricemia control and nephrocalcinosis prevention are key treatment goals. Although this strategy is not supported by interventional study, we believe that RRT should be started if the metabolic disorders are not controlled within 6 h of treatment initiation. If AKI develops despite prevention, extra-renal therapy should be initiated quickly to clear the excess of phosphates, thus limiting further kidney impairment [57]. Patients with highly aggressive tumors may have hypophosphatemia and hypokalemia before cancer chemotherapy initiation. These abnormalities indicate a high risk of TLS; therefore, they should not be corrected. Preventive and curative measures are summarized in Table 51.3.

Although no scientific proof exists to support this statement, ICU admission should be discussed routinely for high-risk patients and patients with overt TLS, especially spontaneous TLS. In addition, close metabolic monitoring should be performed, including measurement of serum potassium, calcium, phosphate, urea, creatinine, and uric acid at least every 8 h.

Table 51.3 Definitions of laboratory and clinical tumor lysis syndrome in adults, according to Cairo and Bishop [44]

General measures
Avoid correcting of hypokalemia or hypophosphatemia before induction
Avoid urine alkalinization
Avoid correcting hypocalcemia, unless symptomatic
Prevention of TLS
Volume expansion
Urate oxidase if high risk for TLS, allopurinol otherwise
No phosphate, potassium, or calcium in the intravenous fluids
Prevention of clinical TLS
Volume expansion
Urate oxidase
No phosphate, potassium, or calcium in the intravenous fluids
Initiate RRT if phosphatemia remains high after 6 h of management
Treatment of clinical TLS
Volume expansion
Urate oxidase
No phosphate, potassium, or calcium in the intravenous fluids
Initiate RRT:
After 6 h in patients with persistent hyperphosphatemia or renal function impairment
Immediately in patients with cardiac or neurological manifestations

TLS tumor lysis syndrome, *RRT* renal replacement therapy

Fluid Expansion

The mainstay for TLS prophylaxis or treatment is aggressive hydration with saline solution to maintain a high urinary output capable of flushing out uric acid and phosphate [44,57,58]. In patients whose urinary output decreases despite adequate fluid intake, diuretic therapy with or without mannitol has been suggested [44,45]. In our experience, the effectiveness of diuretics is limited. In addition, the development of oliguria usually indicates AKI, which requires RRT as opposed to diuretics, especially when oliguria develops despite adequate prevention. As a general rule, caution is required when using diuretics in critically ill patients [59].

Urine Alkalinization

Urine alkalinization has long been used to promote the elimination of uric acid. However, the introduction of fast-acting urate oxidase has considerably reduced the risk of urate nephropathy [52,60]. In addition, urine alkalinization may promote calcium-phosphate deposition [61,62]. Furthermore, the efficacy of urine alkalinization remains unclear. High tubular fluid flow is the key to protecting against acute uric-acid nephropathy, and urine alkalinization may play only a minor preventive role, at least in animal models of hyperuricemia [58]. Given the limited effectiveness and potential adverse effects of urine alkalinization, this method is no longer recommended routinely when urate oxidase is available (level of evidence V; grade D recommendation) [45]. However, the role for urine alkalinization in patients treated with allopurinol remains unclear [45].

Hypouricemic Agents

Several agents are available for decreasing uric acid levels. Recombinant urate oxidase converts uric acid to allantoin, which is five to ten times more soluble in urine [44]. Recombinant urate oxydase (rasburicase) decreases the median uric acid concentration from 577 to 60 μmol/L within 4 h [51]. Moreover, recombinant urate oxidase significantly decreases the uric-acid exposure time compared to allopurinol in children at high risk for TLS [52]. Recombinant urate oxidase ensures the control of plasma uric acid within 4 h [51,60,63]. Last, urate oxidase has long been known to decrease the risk of AKI during TLS [64]. Although very effective, recombinant urate oxidase is costly. In 2003, the cost of rasburicase treatment for a 70-kg adult for 4 days was estimated at 2,200 € in Europe [64,65]. Whereas rasburicase treatment of established TLS in adults was highly cost-effective, the cost-effectiveness of TLS prevention with rasburicase varied widely, being extremely sensitive to TLS risk [64,65]. Therefore, rasburicase should be restricted to the prevention of TLS in high-risk patients, the treatment of established TLS, and the prevention of TLS in low- or intermediate-risk patients who have preexisting hyperuricemia or who develop hyperuricemia despite allopurinol [45,65]. Rasburicase is contraindicated in patients with glucose-6-phosphate dehydrogenase (G6PD) deficiency, as uric acid breakdown leads to excessive hydrogen peroxide production with a risk of hemolysis [66].

In patients at low or intermediate risk for TLS, allopurinol can be used as a hypouricemic agent. Allopurinol is a xanthine analog that decreases the conversion of xanthine to uric acid [63]. However, although allopurinol may decrease the risk of uric acid nephropathy in some patients, it also increases serum xanthine and hypoxanthine concentrations. Both compounds are less soluble in water than uric acid, so that xanthine nephropathy may develop [62]. This complication is uncommon, however, and allopurinol is still recommended provided the treatment is started 24–48 h before cancer chemotherapy and continued for 3–7 days after the cancer chemotherapy initiation (level of evidence: II; grade B recommendation) [45]. In addition, since allopurinol prevents the formation of uric acid but does not decrease the amount of uric acid present before treatment initiation, rasburicase should be preferred in patients with baseline hyperuricemia (>450 μmol/L) (level of evidence: II; grade B recommendation) [45].

Prevention of Nephrocalcinosis

Nephrocalcinosis prevention requires the correction of hyperphosphatemia. Calcium should not be administered. Apart from hydration, few methods are available for preventing or treating hyperphosphatemia. The persistence of hyperphosphatemia 4–6 h after the initiation of a saline infusion should lead to RRT. Although hyperphosphatemia remains a good marker for the response to hydration, the occurrence of hypocalcemia with persistent hyperphosphatemia usually indicates calcium-phosphate crystal deposition.

Indication and Timing of Renal Replacement Therapy

Although the indications of RRT in TLS have not been the focus of specific studies, emergency RRT is probably appropriate when hydration fails to promptly improve the metabolic disturbances or when AKI develops. AKI carries a poor prognosis in patients with TLS [55]. RRT may prove effective in controlling the metabolic disturbances and preventing AKI. A few case reports and case series suggest that phosphate clearance may be higher with sequential dialysis than with hemofiltration. However, phosphate rebound is common 30–60 min after the end of hemodialysis [46]. Extended daily dialysis or isolated sequential dialysis followed by continuous hemofiltration may therefore be helpful in patients with TLS requiring RRT.

Management of Cancer Chemotherapy in Patients with Tumor Lysis Syndrome

In patients at high risk for TLS or with spontaneous TLS, the appropriateness of delaying cancer chemotherapy until preventive measures are initiated should be discussed based on patient status and on the nature of the underlying malignancy (level of evidence: II; grade A recommendation) [45]. In addition, increasing the time over which cancer chemotherapy is administered may deserve consideration, especially in patients with overt TLS. However, in our experience, the full chemotherapy dose can be given to most patients. Dose reduction should be avoided whenever possible in order to minimize the risk of failed induction treatment.

51.3.2 AKI and Myeloma

51.3.2.1 Epidemiology

Up to 50% of patients with newly diagnosed multiple myeloma have renal failure and up to 10% require dialysis [67]. The two major causes of AKI in patients with myeloma are urinary light chain excretion and hypercalcemia. However, several factors may contribute to AKI in these patients, including dehydration, infection, nonsteroidal anti-inflammatory agents, nephrotoxic agents, and contrast media [68,69]. Renal failure is reversible in half of these patients (most of them having cast nephropathy), usually within the first 3 months [70–72].

Cast nephropathy is the most common cause of renal failure in myeloma patients. The clinical presentation usually combines AKI and Bence-Jones proteinuria. When renal biopsy is performed, numerous casts are present in the renal tubules. Casts are formed when light chains bind to a specific peptide domain on the Tamm-Horsfall protein [67]. Hypovolemia, sepsis, urinary pH<7.00, or hypercalciuria can promote cast formation.

51.3.2.2 Prevention and Treatment

Recent guidelines have evaluated preventive and curative measures in patients with multiple myeloma [73]. Grade of recommendation as well as more recent data from the literature will be mentioned whenever possible.

The prevention of renal failure rests on fluid infusion (saline; grade D recommendation [73]), elimination of nephrotoxic compounds, and correction of hypercalcemia or hyperuricemia (grade D recommendation [73]).

In patients with AKI, fluid infusion (saline) should be proposed (grade B recommendation [73]) with the aim of maintaining diuresis >3 L/day. Despite its potential interest for limiting cast formation, authors of the recent published guidelines considered that the evidence was not sufficient to support the use of urine alkalinization in these patients [73].

Since it may transiently remove light chains, plasma exchange has been supposed to be beneficial and recommended (grade B recommendation [73]). However, a recent large randomized study published after the guidelines found no conclusive evidence that five to seven plasma exchanges substantially reduce the death rate or dialysis dependence at 6 month [74]. Although further research in this field may be required, we therefore believe that plasma exchange should not be recommended anymore as routine therapy, except in patients with a hyperviscosity syndrome.

Although renal failure has been considered to indicate a poor prognosis, several studies have demonstrated that long-term survival can be achieved. Therefore, prompt evaluation of these patients for autologous stem cell transplantation should be performed, and dependency on dialysis is no longer considered a contraindication to autologous bone marrow transplantation [75,76] (Fig. 51.1).

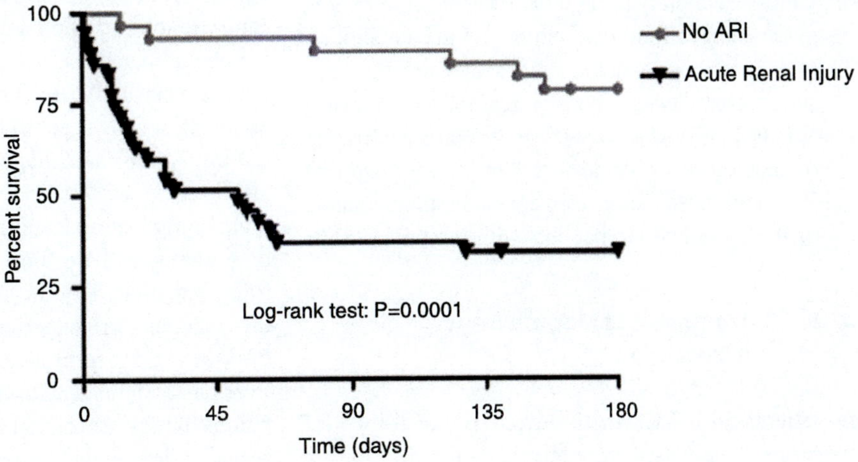

Fig. 51.1 Cumulative survival in patients with an acute renal injury at ICU admission (ARI; $n=35$) and patients without ARI (no ARI; $n=28$). Log rank test: $P=0.0001$ (From Darmon et al. [99])

51.3.3 Methotrexate Intoxication

51.3.3.1 Toxicity of Methotrexate

Methotrexate is widely used to treat cancer. High-dose methotrexate (>1 g/m^2) is part of the treatment of acute lymphoid leukemia, high-grade lymphoma, and sarcoma. These high doses are associated with a 2–4% prevalence of AKI due to precipitation of methotrexate or its metabolite 7-OH-methotrexate within the renal tubules [77]. When AKI occurs, the resulting decrease in methotrexate clearance leads to extrarenal toxicity (neutropenia, hepatitis, orointestinal mucositis, and/or neurological impairment). Thus, methotrexate toxicity may manifest as multiple organ failure [24].

51.3.3.2 Prevention Measures

Prevention of nephrotoxicity, together with methotrexate level monitoring, is crucial to prevent extrarenal methotrexate toxicity:

1. During methotrexate infusion and elimination, fluids should be given to maintain a high urinary output.
2. Urinary alkalization to keep the urinary pH above 7.5 should be given.
3. Rescue with folinic acid (25 mg×4/day) should be started 24 h after each high-dose methotrexate infusion.
4. Serum methotrexate concentrations should be measured every day. Patients are considered at high risk for methotrexate toxicity when serum levels are greater than 15 μM/L at 24 h, 1.5 μM/L at 48 h, or 0.5 μM/L at 72 h.
5. Unless absolutely necessary, patients should not be given medications that inhibit folate metabolism (e.g., trimethoprim-sulfamethoxazole), exhibit intrinsic renal toxicity (e.g., nonsteroidal anti-inflammatory agents and contrast agents) or decrease the fraction of methotrexate bound to albumin (e.g., aspirin). When all these measures were taken, the incidence of AKI was 1.8% in patients with sarcoma [78].

51.3.3.3 Treatment of Methotrexate Intoxication

In patients with AKI, methotrexate removal by RRT (peritoneal dialysis, hemodialysis, hemofiltration, or hemoperfusion) has been used, with disappointing results. Although hemodialysis may achieve a 52% reduction in plasma methotrexate concentrations, post-dialysis rebound has been described [78]. Carboxypeptidase-G2 (CPDG2) is a bacterial enzyme that converts methotrexate into an inactive metabolite (2,4-diamino-*N*10-methylpteroic acid), thus providing an alternative route of elimination. Its use lowered plasma methotrexate concentrations to nontoxic levels (by 98% in 15 min), although rebounds (with an increase no greater than 10% in plasma methotrexate concentrations) occurred in 60% of patients [79]. CPDG2 and high-dose leucovorin have been tested in patients with methotrexate intoxication and AKI, with similar results [79,80]. Therefore, RRT cannot be recommended in patients with methotrexate intoxication. High dose leucovirine (100 mg×4 to 8) should be started on an emergency basis [80]. Although highly effective biologically, clinical interest of CPDG2 remains to be evaluated.

51.3.4 Veno-occlusive Disease/Sinusoidal Obstruction Syndrome

Liver damage is a common complication of cytoreductive therapy and develops in 20–40% of alloBMT recipients [81]. The main site of liver damage in this setting is the hepatic sinusoid, and the resulting clinical syndrome is called veno-occlusive disease/sinusoidal obstruction syndrome (VOD/SOS). Numerous risk factors for VOD/SOS have been identified, including alloBMT, prior exposure to gemtuzumab ozogamicin and mTOR-inhibitor (Sirolimus) (Table 51.4) [82,83]. Injury to the endothelial cells and hepatocytes by cancer chemotherapy seems to be the primary event in the pathogenesis of VOD/SOS [84]. Although sinusoidal endothelial cells seem to be the pivotal site of the initial injury, the exact diagnostic and prognostic criteria are listed in Table 51.5. VOD/SOS after BMT is the main complication leading to AKI [85,86]. Up to 14% of patients will develop VOD/SOS after stem cell transplantation [87]. In addition, as many as half of these patients will experience AKI [85,86]. Most cases of VOD/SOS are clinically obvious, with jaundice, liver pain, edema, and ascites. These clinical manifestations may be associated with AKI mimicking hepatorenal syndrome, with normal kidney histology [88].

Table 51.4 Factors associated with veno-occlusive disease/sinusoidal obstruction syndrome

Patient characteristics
• Age
• Preexisting liver disease
• Hormonal treatment
Conditioning regimen and GVHD prevention
• *Cyclophosphamide*
• *Total body irradiation*
• *Busulfan*
• *BCNU*
• Carboplatin
• Thiotepa
• Melphalan
• *Gemtuzumab ozogamicin*
• *Sirolimus*
Transplant source
• HLA-identical non-related donor
• HLA mismatch donor
Infection or antibiotics
• Cytomegalovirus reactivation
• Amphotericin during conditioning
• Acyclovir during conditioning
• Vancomycin during conditioning

GVHD graft-versus-host disease

Table 51.5 Diagnostic and severity criteria for veno-occlusive disease/sinusoidal obstruction syndrome

Diagnostic criteria
• Hepatomegaly
• Sudden weight gain (+2% of body weight)
• Jaundice (total bilirubin >34 μmol/L)
• Right upper quadrant pain
• No other cause:
– Budd-Chiari syndrome
– Sepsis
– Heart failure
– Graft versus host disease
Other symptoms
• Cytolysis
• Gall bladder wall thickening
• Portal hypertension
• Multiple organ failure
• Thrombocytopenia
Severe sinusoidal obstruction syndrome
• Multiple organ failure
• Thrombocytopenia
• Cytolysis with ASAT or ALAT >750 IU/L
• Confusion or disorientation
• Maximum total bilirubin or severity of weight gain

VOD/SOS can be classified as mild (clinically obvious, requires no treatment, and resolves completely), moderate (signs and symptoms require treatment but resolve completely), or severe (requires treatment but does not resolve before death or day 100). Severe VOD/SOS carries a bleak prognosis, with 98% mortality in a cohort study [81]. AKI, similar to any other organ failure, influences the prognosis of VOD/SOS. In patients with moderate VOD/SOS, diuretic therapy and/or analgesics are usually sufficient. In patients with severe VOD/SOS, the treatment rests on supportive care. No satisfactory specific treatments are available. Defibrotide (a polydeoxyribonucleotide with anti-ischemic, anti-thrombotic, and thrombolytic properties) produced promising results in an open-label study [89]. Results of a more recent dose-finding phase II study involving 150 patients with VOD/SOS have been recently released, suggesting that the complete remission rate was 46% and the day-100 survival of 41% when defibrotide was used [90]. Efficacy of defibrotide remains however to be demonstrated, and a pivotal phase III study is ongoing [91]. Thrombolytic therapy has been tested with disappointing efficacy and a high rate of severe bleeding [92]. Its routine use should therefore not be recommended [92].

51.3.5 Thrombotic Microangiopathy

The association between TMA and cancer was first described in 1973 and is now well established. TMA may be associated with the cancer itself, with cancer chemotherapy, or with allogeneic BMT [93].

Thrombocytopenia with microangiopathic hemolytic anemia (peripheral non-autoimmune anemia with schizocytes) and no alternative diagnosis is considered sufficient to establish a presumptive diagnosis of TMA. In this setting, disseminated intravascular coagulopathy must be ruled out. The incidence of TMA associated with cancer is difficult to estimate because of possible confusion with disseminated intravascular coagulopathy. It may be as high as 5% [94]. Most of the cases occur in patients with solid tumors, the most common type being adenocarcinoma (stomach, breast, and lung) [94]. However, TMA has been reported in patients with other solid tumors or hematological malignancies [93]. The pathophysiology of the TMA-malignancy association remains controversial, although many studies suggest an insult to the vascular endothelium. Nevertheless, studies have demonstrated that disseminated cancer was associated with decreased ADAMTS13 activity, without anti-ADAMTS13 antibody [95].

The link between TMA and cancer chemotherapy was first described with mitomycin C. Subsequently, TMA was reported with many anticancer agents including gemcitabine, bleomycin, cisplatin, CCNU, cytosine arabinoside, daunorubicin, deoxycoformycin, 5-FU, azathioprine, and interferon [93].

Last, the association between TMA and bone marrow transplantation has been known since 1980. Although the prognosis has been described as poor, the clinical presentation is heterogeneous, with some patients having renal failure as the only manifestation and others experiencing remissions [96]. Typically, TMA starts 2–12 months after BMT and is unresponsive to plasma therapy [97]. Total body irradiation and graft-versus-host disease are the main factors associated with TMA in BMT recipients. Therefore, radiation nephritis may be a contributor, although cases of TMA related to CMV infection have been reported [85,96].

The optimal treatment of this highly specific subtype of TMA is unknown. Plasma exchanges are known to be rarely effective in this setting [98]. The recent guidelines of the British Society of Haematology did not recommend plasmatherapy in cancer-related TMA or in TMA after bone marrow transplantation [98]. Effective treatment for this group of patients is, however, lacking. Protein-A column immunoadsorption has been proposed as a possible treatment, without strong evidence of its effectiveness (British Society of Haematology grade of recommendation: C) [98]. Causative factors should be looked for and antihypertensive treatment given. Last, in the absence of a guideline, we believe that plasma exchange should be proposed in patients with severe cancer-treatment associated TMA.

51.4 Conclusion

AKI is a common and severe complication in CICPs. It results from various causes, including metabolic disturbances secondary to the tumor burden, renal infiltration by malignant cells, sepsis, and drug-induced toxicity. Prognosis of AKI in this particular setting remains poor, especially when AKI occurs in association with acute respiratory failure. In addition, lung-kidney crosstalk may lead to further organ deterioration. In regard to the poor prognosis associated with AKI in this setting, prevention of AKI remains crucial in this population of patients.

Fluid expansion and uricolytic treatment in patients with a high risk of acute TLS, prevention of contrast nephropathy, elimination of nephrotoxic drugs in high-risk patients, and monitoring of serum methotrexate concentrations are among the main measures that may reduce the risk of AKI, limit further AKI, or reduce residual long-term organ dysfunction.

Acknowledgment We thank A. Wolfe, M.D., for helping with this manuscript.

References

1. Azoulay E, Moreau D, Alberti C, Leleu G, Adrie C, Barboteu M, Cottu P, Levy V, Le Gall JR, Schlemmer B (2000) Predictors of short-term mortality in critically ill patients with solid malignancies. Intensive Care Med 26:1817–1823
2. Azoulay E, Recher C, Alberti C, Soufir L, Leleu G, Le Gall JR, Fermand JP, Schlemmer B (1999) Changing use of intensive care for hematological patients: the example of multiple myeloma. Intensive Care Med 25:1395–1401
3. Benoit DD, Hoste EA, Depuydt PO, Offner FC, Lameire NH, Vandewoude KH, Dhondt AW, Noens LA, Decruyenaere JM (2005) Outcome in critically ill medical patients treated with renal replacement therapy for acute renal failure: comparison between patients with and those without haematological malignancies. Nephrol Dial Transplant 20:552–558

4. Darmon M, Thiery G, Ciroldi M, de Miranda S, Galicier L, Raffoux E, Le Gall JR, Schlemmer B, Azoulay E (2005) Intensive care in patients with newly diagnosed malignancies and a need for cancer chemotherapy. Crit Care Med 33:2488–2493
5. Darmon M, Thiery G, Ciroldi M, de Miranda S, Ksibi H, Adda M, Coquet I, Schlemmer B, Azoulay E (2006) Prognosis of acute kidney injury in a cohort of non-allotransplanted critically-ill cancer patients. Intensive Care Med 32:S10
6. Lanore JJ, Brunet F, Pochard F, Bellivier F, Dhainaut JF, Vaxelaire JF, Giraud T, Dreyfus F, Dreyfuss D, Chiche JD et al (1991) Hemodialysis for acute renal failure in patients with hematologic malignancies. Crit Care Med 19:346–351
7. Soares M, Salluh JI, Carvalho MS, Darmon M, Rocco JR, Spector N (2006) Prognosis of critically ill patients with cancer and acute renal dysfunction. J Clin Oncol 24: 4003–4010
8. Bagshaw SM, Laupland KB, Doig CJ, Mortis G, Fick GH, Mucenski M, Godinez-Luna T, Svenson LW, Rosenal T (2005) Prognosis for long-term survival and renal recovery in critically ill patients with severe acute renal failure: a population-based study. Crit Care 9:R700–R709
9. Metnitz PG, Krenn CG, Steltzer H, Lang T, Ploder J, Lenz K, Le Gall JR, Druml W (2002) Effect of acute renal failure requiring renal replacement therapy on outcome in critically ill patients. Crit Care Med 30:2051–2058
10. Palevsky PM, Zhang JH, O'Connor TZ, Chertow GM, Crowley ST, Choudhury D, Finkel K, Kellum JA, Paganini E, Schein RM, Smith MW, Swanson KM, Thompson BT, Vijayan A, Watnick S, Star RA, Peduzzi P (2008) Intensity of renal support in critically ill patients with acute kidney injury. N Engl J Med 359:7–20
11. Chertow GM, Burdick E, Honour M, Bonventre JV, Bates DW (2005) Acute kidney injury, mortality, length of stay, and costs in hospitalized patients. J Am Soc Nephrol 16: 3365–3370
12. Levy EM, Viscoli CM, Horwitz RI (1996) The effect of acute renal failure on mortality. A cohort analysis. JAMA 275:1489–1494
13. Bates DW, Su L, Yu DT, Chertow GM, Seger DL, Gomes DR, Dasbach EJ, Platt R (2001) Mortality and costs of acute renal failure associated with amphotericin B therapy. Clin Infect Dis 32:686–693
14. Lassnigg A, Schmidlin D, Mouhieddine M, Bachmann LM, Druml W, Bauer P, Hiesmayr M (2004) Minimal changes of serum creatinine predict prognosis in patients after cardiothoracic surgery: a prospective cohort study. J Am Soc Nephrol 15:1597–1605
15. Loef BG, Epema AH, Smilde TD, Henning RH, Ebels T, Navis G, Stegeman CA (2005) Immediate postoperative renal function deterioration in cardiac surgical patients predicts in-hospital mortality and long-term survival. J Am Soc Nephrol 16:195–200
16. Li X, Hassoun HT, Santora R, Rabb H (2009) Organ crosstalk: the role of the kidney. Curr Opin Crit Care 15: 481–487
17. Wiedemann HP, Wheeler AP, Bernard GR, Thompson BT, Hayden D, deBoisblanc B, Connors AF Jr, Hite RD, Harabin AL (2006) Comparison of two fluid-management strategies in acute lung injury. N Engl J Med 354:2564–2575
18. Rabb H, Wang Z, Nemoto T, Hotchkiss J, Yokota N, Soleimani M (2003) Acute renal failure leads to dysregulation of lung salt and water channels. Kidney Int 63: 600–606
19. Deng J, Hu X, Yuen PS, Star RA (2004) Alpha-melanocyte-stimulating hormone inhibits lung injury after renal ischemia/reperfusion. Am J Respir Crit Care Med 169:749–756
20. Hassoun HT, Grigoryev DN, Lie ML, Liu M, Cheadle C, Tuder RM, Rabb H (2007) Ischemic acute kidney injury induces a distant organ functional and genomic response distinguishable from bilateral nephrectomy. Am J Physiol Renal Physiol 293:F30–F40
21. Kramer AA, Postler G, Salhab KF, Mendez C, Carey LC, Rabb H (1999) Renal ischemia/reperfusion leads to macrophage-mediated increase in pulmonary vascular permeability. Kidney Int 55:2362–2367
22. Feltes CM, Van Eyk J, Rabb H (2008) Distant-organ changes after acute kidney injury. Nephron Physiol 109:p80–p84
23. Hoke TS, Douglas IS, Klein CL, He Z, Fang W, Thurman JM, Tao Y, Dursun B, Voelkel NF, Edelstein CL, Faubel S (2007) Acute renal failure after bilateral nephrectomy is associated with cytokine-mediated pulmonary injury. J Am Soc Nephrol 18:155–164
24. Klein CL, Hoke TS, Fang WF, Altmann CJ, Douglas IS, Faubel S (2008) Interleukin-6 mediates lung injury following ischemic acute kidney injury or bilateral nephrectomy. Kidney Int 74:901–909
25. Hall SV, Johnson EE, Hedley-Whyte J (1974) Renal hemodynamics and function with continuous positive-pressure ventilation in dogs. Anesthesiology 41:452–461
26. Kuiper JW, Groeneveld AB, Slutsky AS, Plotz FB (2005) Mechanical ventilation and acute renal failure. Crit Care Med 33:1408–1415
27. Murdaugh HV Jr, Sieker HO, Manfredi F (1959) Effect of altered intrathoracic pressure on renal hemodynamics, electrolyte excretion and water clearance. J Clin Invest 38: 834–842
28. Annat G, Viale JP, Bui Xuan B, Hadj Aissa O, Benzoni D, Vincent M, Gharib C, Motin J (1983) Effect of PEEP ventilation on renal function, plasma renin, aldosterone, neurophysins and urinary ADH, and prostaglandins. Anesthesiology 58:136–141
29. Baudouin SV, Bott J, Ward A, Deane C, Moxham J (1992) Short term effect of oxygen on renal haemodynamics in patients with hypoxaemic chronic obstructive airways disease. Thorax 47:550–554
30. Sharkey RA, Mulloy EM, O'Neill SJ (1998) Acute effects of hypoxaemia, hyperoxaemia and hypercapnia on renal blood flow in normal and renal transplant subjects. Eur Respir J 12: 653–657
31. Sharkey RA, Mulloy EM, O'Neill SJ (1999) The acute effects of oxygen and carbon dioxide on renal vascular resistance in patients with an acute exacerbation of COPD. Chest 115:1588–1592
32. Hildebrandt W, Ottenbacher A, Schuster M, Swenson ER, Bartsch P (2000) Diuretic effect of hypoxia, hypocapnia, and hyperpnea in humans: relation to hormones and O(2) chemosensitivity. J Appl Physiol 88:599–610
33. Hohne C, Boemke W, Schleyer N, Francis RC, Krebs MO, Kaczmarczyk G (2002) Low sodium intake does not impair renal compensation of hypoxia-induced respiratory alkalosis. J Appl Physiol 92:2097–2104

34. Hohne C, Krebs MO, Boemke W, Arntz E, Kaczmarczyk G (2001) Evidence that the renin decrease during hypoxia is adenosine mediated in conscious dogs. J Appl Physiol 90: 1842–1848
35. Darmon M, Schortgen F, Leon R, Moutereau S, Mayaux J, Di Marco F, Devaquet J, Brun-Buisson C, Brochard L (2009) Impact of mild hypoxemia on renal function and renal resistive index during mechanical ventilation. Intensive Care Med 35:1031–1038
36. Olsen NV (1995) Effect of hypoxaemia on water and sodium homeostatic hormones and renal function. Acta Anaesthesiol Scand Suppl 107:165–170
37. The Acute Respiratory Distress Syndrome Network (2000) Ventilation with lower tidal volumes as compared with traditional tidal volumes for acute lung injury and the acute respiratory distress syndrome. N Engl J Med 342: 1301–1308
38. Ranieri VM, Suter PM, Tortorella C, De Tullio R, Dayer JM, Brienza A, Bruno F, Slutsky AS (1999) Effect of mechanical ventilation on inflammatory mediators in patients with acute respiratory distress syndrome: a randomized controlled trial. JAMA 282:54–61
39. Liu KD, Glidden DV, Eisner MD, Parsons PE, Ware LB, Wheeler A, Korpak A, Thompson BT, Chertow GM, Matthay MA (2007) Predictive and pathogenetic value of plasma biomarkers for acute kidney injury in patients with acute lung injury. Crit Care Med 35:2755–2761
40. Ranieri VM, Giunta F, Suter PM, Slutsky AS (2000) Mechanical ventilation as a mediator of multisystem organ failure in acute respiratory distress syndrome. JAMA 284: 43–44
41. Mehta RL, Pascual MT, Gruta CG, Zhuang S, Chertow GM (2002) Refining predictive models in critically ill patients with acute renal failure. J Am Soc Nephrol 13: 1350–1357
42. Vieira JM Jr, Castro I, Curvello-Neto A, Demarzo S, Caruso P, Pastore L Jr, Imanishe MH, Abdulkader RC, Deheinzelin D (2007) Effect of acute kidney injury on weaning from mechanical ventilation in critically ill patients. Crit Care Med 35:184–191
43. Munker R, Hill U, Jehn U, Kolb HJ, Schalhorn A (1998) Renal complications in acute leukemias. Haematologica 83: 416–421
44. Cairo MS, Bishop M (2004) Tumour lysis syndrome: new therapeutic strategies and classification. Br J Haematol 127: 3–11
45. Coiffier B, Altman A, Pui CH, Younes A, Cairo MS (2008) Guidelines for the management of pediatric and adult tumor lysis syndrome: an evidence-based review. J Clin Oncol 26: 2767–2778
46. Davidson MB, Thakkar S, Hix JK, Bhandarkar ND, Wong A, Schreiber MJ (2004) Pathophysiology, clinical consequences, and treatment of tumor lysis syndrome. Am J Med 116:546–554
47. Jeha S (2001) Tumor lysis syndrome. Semin Hematol 38: 4–8
48. Cohen LF, Balow JE, Magrath IT, Poplack DG, Ziegler JL (1980) Acute tumor lysis syndrome. A review of 37 patients with Burkitt's lymphoma. Am J Med 68:486–491
49. Altman A (2001) Acute tumor lysis syndrome. Semin Oncol 28:3–8
50. Flombaum CD (2000) Metabolic emergencies in the cancer patient. Semin Oncol 27:322–334
51. Pui CH (2001) Urate oxidase in the prophylaxis or treatment of hyperuricemia: the United States experience. Semin Hematol 38:13–21
52. Goldman SC, Holcenberg JS, Finklestein JZ, Hutchinson R, Kreissman S, Johnson FL, Tou C, Harvey E, Morris E, Cairo MS (2001) A randomized comparison between rasburicase and allopurinol in children with lymphoma or leukemia at high risk for tumor lysis. Blood 97:2998–3003
53. Annemans L, Moeremans K, Lamotte M, Garcia Conde J, van den Berg H, Myint H, Pieters R, Uyttebroeck A (2003) Incidence, medical resource utilisation and costs of hyperuricemia and tumour lysis syndrome in patients with acute leukaemia and non-Hodgkin's lymphoma in four European countries. Leuk Lymphoma 44:77–83
54. Mato AR, Riccio BE, Qin L, Heitjan DF, Carroll M, Loren A, Porter DL, Perl A, Stadtmauer E, Tsai D, Gewirtz A, Luger SM (2006) A predictive model for the detection of tumor lysis syndrome during AML induction therapy. Leuk Lymphoma 47:877–883
55. Montesinos P, Lorenzo I, Martin G, Sanz J, Perez-Sirvent ML, Martinez D, Orti G, Algarra L, Martinez J, Moscardo F, de la Rubia J, Jarque I, Sanz G, Sanz MA (2008) Tumor lysis syndrome in patients with acute myeloid leukemia: identification of risk factors and development of a predictive model. Haematologica 93:67–74
56. Razis E, Arlin ZA, Ahmed T, Feldman EJ, Puccio C, Cook P, Chun HG, Helson L, Mittelman A (1994) Incidence and treatment of tumor lysis syndrome in patients with acute leukemia. Acta Haematol 91:171–174
57. Humphreys BD, Soiffer RJ, Magee CC (2005) Renal failure associated with cancer and its treatment: an update. J Am Soc Nephrol 16:151–161
58. Conger JD, Falk SA (1977) Intrarenal dynamics in the pathogenesis and prevention of acute urate nephropathy. J Clin Invest 59:786–793
59. Mehta RL, Pascual MT, Soroko S, Chertow GM (2002) Diuretics, mortality, and nonrecovery of renal function in acute renal failure. JAMA 288:2547–2553
60. Coiffier B, Mounier N, Bologna S, Ferme C, Tilly H, Sonet A, Christian B, Casasnovas O, Jourdan E, Belhadj K, Herbrecht R (2003) Efficacy and safety of rasburicase (recombinant urate oxidase) for the prevention and treatment of hyperuricemia during induction chemotherapy of aggressive non-Hodgkin's lymphoma: results of the GRAAL1 (Groupe d'Etude des Lymphomes de l'Adulte Trial on Rasburicase Activity in Adult Lymphoma) study. J Clin Oncol 21:4402–4406
61. Baeksgaard L, Sorensen JB (2003) Acute tumor lysis syndrome in solid tumors – a case report and review of the literature. Cancer Chemother Pharmacol 51:187–192
62. Haas M, Ohler L, Watzke H, Bohmig G, Prokesch R, Druml W (1999) The spectrum of acute renal failure in tumour lysis syndrome. Nephrol Dial Transplant 14: 776–779
63. Goldman SC (2003) Rasburicase: potential role in managing tumor lysis in patients with hematological malignancies. Expert Rev Anticancer Ther 3:429–433
64. Patte C, Sakiroglu C, Ansoborlo S, Baruchel A, Plouvier E, Pacquement H, Babin-Boilletot A (2002) Urate-oxidase in

the prevention and treatment of metabolic complications in patients with B-cell lymphoma and leukemia, treated in the Societe Francaise d'Oncologie pediatrique LMB89 protocol. Ann Oncol 13:789–795

65. Annemans L, Moeremans K, Lamotte M, Garcia Conde J, van den Berg H, Myint H, Pieters R, Uyttebroeck A (2003) Pan-European multicentre economic evaluation of recombinant urate oxidase (rasburicase) in prevention and treatment of hyperuricaemia and tumour lysis syndrome in haematological cancer patients. Support Care Cancer 11: 249–257
66. Browning LA, Kruse JA (2005) Hemolysis and methemoglobinemia secondary to rasburicase administration. Ann Pharmacother 39:1932–1935
67. Winearls CG (1995) Acute myeloma kidney. Kidney Int 48:1347–1361
68. McCarthy CS, Becker JA (1992) Multiple myeloma and contrast media. Radiology 183:519–521
69. Sakhuja V, Jha V, Varma S, Joshi K, Gupta KL, Sud K, Kohli HS (2000) Renal involvement in multiple myeloma: a 10-year study. Ren Fail 22:465–477
70. Alexanian R, Barlogie B, Dixon D (1990) Renal failure in multiple myeloma. Pathogenesis and prognostic implications. Arch Intern Med 150:1693–1695
71. Knudsen LM, Hjorth M, Hippe E, Nordic Myeloma Study Group (2000) Renal failure in multiple myeloma: reversibility and impact on the prognosis. Eur J Haematol 65: 175–181
72. Rota S, Mougenot B, Baudouin B, De Meyer-Brasseur M, Lemaitre V, Michel C, Mignon F, Rondeau E, Vanhille P, Verroust P et al (1987) Multiple myeloma and severe renal failure: a clinicopathologic study of outcome and prognosis in 34 patients. Medicine (Baltimore) 66: 126–137
73. Barosi G, Boccadoro M, Cavo M, Corradini P, Marchetti M, Massaia M, Merlini G, Tosi P, Tura S (2004) Management of multiple myeloma and related-disorders: guidelines from the Italian Society of Hematology (SIE), Italian Society of Experimental Hematology (SIES) and Italian Group for Bone Marrow Transplantation (GITMO). Haematologica 89:717–741
74. Clark WF, Stewart AK, Rock GA, Sternbach M, Sutton DM, Barrett BJ, Heidenheim AP, Garg AX, Churchill DN (2005) Plasma exchange when myeloma presents as acute renal failure: a randomized, controlled trial. Ann Intern Med 143: 777–784
75. Attal M, Harousseau JL, Stoppa AM, Sotto JJ, Fuzibet JG, Rossi JF, Casassus P, Maisonneuve H, Facon T, Ifrah N, Payen C, Bataille R (1996) A prospective, randomized trial of autologous bone marrow transplantation and chemotherapy in multiple myeloma. Intergroupe Francais du Myelome. N Engl J Med 335:91–97
76. Lee CK, Zangari M, Barlogie B, Fassas A, van Rhee F, Thertulien R, Talamo G, Muwalla F, Anaissie E, Hollmig K, Tricot G (2004) Dialysis-dependent renal failure in patients with myeloma can be reversed by high-dose myeloablative therapy and autotransplant. Bone Marrow Transplant 33:823–828
77. Widemann BC, Adamson PC (2006) Understanding and managing methotrexate nephrotoxicity. Oncologist 11: 694–703
78. Widemann BC, Balis FM, Kempf-Bielack B, Bielack S, Pratt CB, Ferrari S, Bacci G, Craft AW, Adamson PC (2004) High-dose methotrexate-induced nephrotoxicity in patients with osteosarcoma. Cancer 100:2222–2232
79. Buchen S, Ngampolo D, Melton RG, Hasan C, Zoubek A, Henze G, Bode U, Fleischhack G (2005) Carboxypeptidase G2 rescue in patients with methotrexate intoxication and renal failure. Br J Cancer 92:480–487
80. Flombaum CD, Meyers PA (1999) High-dose leucovorin as sole therapy for methotrexate toxicity. J Clin Oncol 17: 1589–1594
81. McDonald GB, Hinds MS, Fisher LD, Schoch HG, Wolford JL, Banaji M, Hardin BJ, Shulman HM, Clift RA (1993) Veno-occlusive disease of the liver and multiorgan failure after bone marrow transplantation: a cohort study of 355 patients. Ann Intern Med 118:255–267
82. Cutler C, Stevenson K, Kim HT, Richardson P, Ho VT, Linden E, Revta C, Ebert R, Warren D, Choi S, Koreth J, Armand P, Alyea E, Carter S, Horowitz M, Antin JH, Soiffer R (2008) Sirolimus is associated with veno-occlusive disease of the liver after myeloablative allogeneic stem cell transplantation. Blood 112:4425–4431
83. McKoy JM, Angelotta C, Bennett CL, Tallman MS, Wadleigh M, Evens AM, Kuzel TM, Trifilio SM, Raisch DW, Kell J, DeAngelo DJ, Giles FJ (2007) Gemtuzumab ozogamicin-associated sinusoidal obstructive syndrome (SOS): an overview from the research on adverse drug events and reports (RADAR) project. Leuk Res 31:599–604
84. DeLeve LD (1996) Cellular target of cyclophosphamide toxicity in the murine liver: role of glutathione and site of metabolic activation. Hepatology 24:830–837
85. Noel C, Hazzan M, Noel-Walter MP, Jouet JP (1998) Renal failure and bone marrow transplantation. Nephrol Dial Transplant 13:2464–2466
86. Zager RA (1994) Acute renal failure in the setting of bone marrow transplantation. Kidney Int 46:1443–1458
87. Coppell JA, Richardson PG, Soiffer R, Martin PL, Kernan NA, Chen A, Guinan E, Vogelsang G, Krishnan A, Giralt S, Revta C, Carreau NA, Iacobelli M, Carreras E, Ruutu T, Barbui T, Antin JH, Niederwieser D (2009) Hepatic veno-occlusive disease following stem cell transplantation: incidence, clinical course and outcome. Biol Blood Marrow Transplant 16(2):157–168
88. Zager RA, O'Quigley J, Zager BK, Alpers CE, Shulman HM, Gamelin LM, Stewart P, Thomas ED (1989) Acute renal failure following bone marrow transplantation: a retrospective study of 272 patients. Am J Kidney Dis 13: 210–216
89. Richardson PG, Murakami C, Jin Z, Warren D, Momtaz P, Hoppensteadt D, Elias AD, Antin JH, Soiffer R, Spitzer T, Avigan D, Bearman SI, Martin PL, Kurtzberg J, Vredenburgh J, Chen AR, Arai S, Vogelsang G, McDonald GB, Guinan EC (2002) Multi-institutional use of defibrotide in 88 patients after stem cell transplantation with severe veno-occlusive disease and multisystem organ failure: response without significant toxicity in a high-risk population and factors predictive of outcome. Blood 100:4337–4343
90. Richardson P, Soiffer R, Antin JH, Jin Z, Kurtzberg J, Martin PL, Steinbach G, Murray KF, Vogelsang GB, Chen A, Krishnan A, Kernan NA, Avigan D, Spitzer TR, Warren D, Revta C, Wei LJ, Iacobelli M, McDonald GB, Guinan EC

(2006) Defibrotide (DF) for the treatment of severe veno-occlusive disease (sVOD) and multi-organ failure (MOF) post SCT: final results of a multi-center, randomized, dose-finding trial. Blood 108:Abstract 43
91. http://clinicaltrials.gov/ct2/show/NCT00358501?term=defibrotide&rank=5
92. Bearman SI, Lee JL, Baron AE, McDonald GB (1997) Treatment of hepatic veno-occlusive disease with recombinant human tissue plasminogen activator and heparin in 42 marrow transplant patients. Blood 89:1501–1506
93. Kwaan HC, Gordon LI (2001) Thrombotic microangiopathy in the cancer patient. Acta Haematol 106:52–56
94. Gordon LI, Kwaan HC (1997) Cancer- and drug-associated thrombotic thrombocytopenic purpura and hemolytic uremic syndrome. Semin Hematol 34:140–147
95. Oleksowicz L, Bhagwati N, DeLeon-Fernandez M (1999) Deficient activity of von Willebrand's factor-cleaving protease in patients with disseminated malignancies. Cancer Res 59:2244–2250
96. Chappell ME, Keeling DM, Prentice HG, Sweny P (1988) Haemolytic uraemic syndrome after bone marrow transplantation: an adverse effect of total body irradiation? Bone Marrow Transplant 3:339–347
97. Sarode R, McFarland JG, Flomenberg N, Casper JT, Cohen EP, Drobyski WR, Ash RC, Horowitz MM, Camitta B, Lawton C et al (1995) Therapeutic plasma exchange does not appear to be effective in the management of thrombotic thrombocytopenic purpura/hemolytic uremic syndrome following bone marrow transplantation. Bone Marrow Transplant 16:271–275
98. Allford SL, Hunt BJ, Rose P, Machin SJ (2003) Guidelines on the diagnosis and management of the thrombotic microangiopathic haemolytic anaemias. Br J Haematol 120: 556–573
99. Darmon M, Guichard I, Vincent F, Schlemmer B, Azoulay E (2010) Prognostic significance of acute renal injury in acute tumor lysis syndrome. Leuk Lymphoma 51:221–227

52 Septic Shock

David Grimaldi and Frédéric Pène

Contents

D. Grimaldi and F. Pène (✉)
Medical Intensive Care Unit, Cochin Hospital, AP-HP and University Paris Descartes 27 rue du Faubourg Saint-Jacques, 75014, Paris, France
e-mail: frederic.pene@cch.aphp.fr

52.1 Introduction

Severe infections account for the majority of complications that warrant ICU admission in the course of hematological malignancies. Sepsis represents the physiological inflammatory response induced by infections, and can result in tissue hypoperfusion and organ failures that define the entities of severe sepsis and septic shock. Septic shock is characterized by acute circulatory failure requiring vasopressive drugs and carries the highest mortality rate. Regardless of underlying comorbidities and of the mode of acquisition (community-acquired or nosocomial), the lung represents the primary site of infection responsible for septic shock. Whereas the overall prognosis of severe sepsis and septic shock has been moderately improved over the last 2 decades, it is noteworthy that the most impressive improvements in outcome have been achieved in specific populations of vulnerable patients, including those with malignancies. Since studies in the field often mix patients with hematological malignancies and solid tumors, most of the issues discussed here will refer to cancer patients in general, irrespective of the type of malignancy, with emphasis on patients with hematological malignancies when available.

52.2 Epidemiology of Septic Shock in Patients with Malignancies

52.2.1 Incidence

Sepsis is a frequent disorder whose overall incidence is steadily increasing. A nationally representative study of 750 millions acute care hospitalizations in the United

É. Azoulay (ed.), *Pulmonary Involvement in Patients with Hematological Malignancies*,
DOI: 10.1007/978-3-642-15742-4_52, © Springer-Verlag Berlin Heidelberg 2011

States reported a 8.7% annual increase in the sepsis incidence during the 1979–2000 period, from 0.8 per 1,000 in 1979 to 2.4 per 1,000 in 2000 [1]. At the same time, the prevalence of severe presentations with organ failures (severe sepsis and septic shock) also increased. Accordingly, the rate of hospitalization for severe sepsis more than doubled between 1993 (0.6 per 1,000) and 2003 (1.3 per 1,000) [2]. Likewise, a large French study reported an increase from 7% to 9.7% in the prevalence of septic shock among ICU admissions within the period 1993–2000 [3]. This trend has been mainly ascribed to the population aging and to the growing frequency of underlying comorbidities (immunosuppression, cancer, diabetes, chronic organ failures). Cancer is associated with a considerable increased risk of sepsis, especially in patients with hematological malignancies. Cancer patients have been estimated to have a 9.8-fold increased risk for sepsis (annual incidence rate 14.6 per 1,000 vs 1.5 per 1,000 in the noncancer population) [4]. In 1999, national US projections estimated a similar incidence of severe sepsis of 16.4 cases per 1,000 cancer patients per year [5]. When compared to the noncancer population (annual incidence rate 4.2 per 1,000), the risk of severe sepsis moderately increased in patients with solid tumors (annual incidence rate 7.6 per 1,000 patients, relative risk 1.81 [1.79–1.82]), but dramatically increased in patients with hematological malignancies (annual incidence rate 66.4 per 1,000 patients, relative risk 15.71 [15.55–15.88]), the higher risk being carried by acute myeloid leukemia (66.15 [63.95–66.36]) and multiple myeloma (33.61 [32.87–34.38]). As a result, cancer patients now represent a considerable proportion of septic patients in unselected cohorts, 17% of medical admissions associated with severe sepsis in the United States [6] and 15.4% of septic shock patients in a French ICU cohort [3].

52.2.2 Site of Infection and Type of Pathogens

52.2.2.1 Infections in Patients with Hematological Malignancies

Most of our knowledge about the type of pathogens causing severe infections and septic shock in cancer patients stems from epidemiological surveys of bloodstream infections in neutropenic or non-neutropenic cancer patients. Before the mid-1980s, gram-negative organisms were the most commonly encountered pathogens. Since then, gram-positive bacteria became the predominant pathogens [7]. Several reasons accounted for this change: increasing use of long-term indwelling central venous catheters, gut decontamination with antibiotics and intensive chemotherapy resulting in severe mucosal damage such as high-dose cytarabine [8]. Nonetheless, a significant proportion of bacteremia is related to coagulase-negative staphylococci whose pathogenic role remains questionable in this setting. Severe infections due to *Streptococcus pneumoniae* predominantly affect patients with impaired humoral immunity or functional hyposplenism, such as those with multiple myeloma or hematopoietic stem cell transplantation (HSCT) recipients. However, bloodstream infections do not recapitulate the complete picture of infections among neutropenic patients. Other common sites of infections include the respiratory tract, the urinary tract and the gastrointestinal tract where gram-negative organisms predominate. Furthermore, polymicrobial infections represent a significant proportion of documented infections among patients with neutropenia and are associated with greater morbidity and mortality than monomicrobial infections [9]. In addition, invasive fungal infections such as candidiasis with or without candidemia frequently occur in cancer patients, and remain associated with higher mortality rates than bacterial infections [10, 11]. Of note, non-albicans *Candida* species now account for more than half of fungal isolates as a result of the extensive use of fluconazole prophylaxis [12]. Invasive aspergillosis preferentially occurs during prolonged neutropenia, in corticosteroid-treated patients and in allogeneic hematopoietic stem cell transplant recipients [13].

Of increasing concern is the development of antibiotic resistance in many hospitals. Likewise, increasing rates of drug resistance among gram-positive and gram-negative pathogens are being documented in patients with hematological malignancies [14–18]. In the same way, the highly resistant gram-negative bacteria *Stenotrophomonas maltophilia* emerged as a cause of serious infection in cancer patients [19]. The development of drug resistance in these patients can be ascribed to the frequent and prolonged courses of broad-spectrum antibiotics. Therefore, cancer patients hospitalized in the ICU are at increased risk of acquisition of multidrug-resistant bacteria, including extended spectrum β-lactamase enterobacteriaceae, methicillin-resistant *Staphylococcus aureus*, imipenem-resistant *Pseudomonas aeruginosa*, *Acinetobacter baumanii* and *Stenotrophomonas maltophilia* [20].

52.2.2.2 Particularities of Septic Shock in Cancer Patients

Among unselected patients, the epidemiology of severe sepsis and septic shock is characterized by a grossly balanced proportion of gram-negative and gram-positive bacteria and by the increasing number of cases caused by fungal organisms [1, 3, 21–23]. Interestingly, recent studies consistently reported that gram-negative bacteria still account for the vast majority of documented episodes of septic shock in cancer patients [24–27]. Indeed, gram-negative organisms are more likely to cause severe organ infections, such as pneumonia or enterocolitis in the setting of neutropenia or other immune defects, while gram-positive bacteremic episodes more likely result from mucosal damage. Some specific virulence factors or a higher bacterial load might also account for the susceptibility towards gram-negative infections in immunocompromised patients. In addition, a large proportion of severe sepsis among patients with hematological malignancies and bone marrow transplantation recipients are related to hospital- or ICU-acquired infections inherent to the impaired immune system and to prolonged periods of hospitalization imposed by intensive treatments [23].

52.2.3 Risk Factors of Septic Shock in Patients with Hematological Malignancies

52.2.3.1 Acquired Immune Disorders

Depending on the nature of malignancy, its status and its treatments, various mechanisms, such as impaired phagocytosis or defective cellular or humoral immune responses, account for the increased incidence and the poor outcome of sepsis in cancer patients [28]. Neutropenia is a frequent and unavoidable side effect of chemotherapy. Especially when profound and prolonged, neutropenia represents a major risk factor for severe bacterial and fungal infections. T and B cells are also directly impaired by corticosteroids, cytotoxic drugs such as methotrexate or nucleosides analogs, and anti-lymphocyte monoclonal antibodies, with increased risk of opportunistic infections. In addition, indwelling catheters and chemotherapy- and radiotherapy-induced mucosal damage contribute to the increased risk of severe infections in these patients. Allogeneic HSCT recipients combine several immune defects that result in a complex and sustained immunodeficiency. The engraftment period is characterized by prolonged and profound neutropenia and mucosal damage, very similar to that observed after high-dose chemotherapy for induction of acute leukemia. The use of peripheral stem cell and nonmyeloablative conditioning regimens can significantly reduce the duration of neutropenia. After hematological recovery, immunosuppressive drugs, graft-versus-host disease, cytomegalovirus reactivation and radiation-induced functional asplenia result in delayed T and B immune reconstitution.

52.2.3.2 Genetic Predisposition

Besides environmental and acquired factors, several epidemiological studies have highlighted the individual variability in the susceptibility towards severe infections. Recently, numerous studies have highlighted the role of genetic variants that are likely to affect interactions between hosts and pathogens. These genetic variants, named polymorphisms when present in more than 1% of the population, involve genes implicated in the recognition of pathogens, in the inflammatory response or in the coagulation system. Recognition of invading pathogens is an essential phase of anti-infective host defense and triggers a potent inflammatory response that is required in order to clear the pathogen, but that can contribute to tissue damage and organ failures. Functional genetic variants of membrane and soluble receptors for pathogen-associated molecular patterns have been involved in the severity of various infections. Thus, polymorphisms of Toll-like receptors (TLR) involved in recognition of bacteria (TLR1, TLR2, TLR4, TLR5) have been associated with increased susceptibility towards bacterial infections and severe sepsis [29–32]. In the same way, polymorphisms of the TLR4-associated co-receptor CD14 and of the downstream kinase protein IRAK-1 have also been associated with increased severity of severe sepsis [33, 34]. A polymorphism responsible for decreased concentrations of mannose-binding lectin has been associated with susceptibility and poor outcome towards septic shock [35]. While the inflammatory response results from the controlled and coordinated production of pro- and anti-inflammatory cytokines, some genetic polymorphisms can disrupt this balance, leading to increased severity of septic shock [36]. Some genetic variants that contribute to a sepsis-induced hypercoagulable state through increased generation of fibrin (Leiden factor) or inhibition of fibrinolysis (PAI-1) have also been associated with a worse outcome in this setting [37].

Some recent data suggest that inherited genetic variants are also associated with increased susceptibility to severe infections in patients with hematological malignancies. Thus, mannose-binding lectin deficiency has been associated with an increased risk of severe bacterial infections and invasive aspergillosis in patients with hematological malignancies, including allogeneic HSCT recipients [38–41]. In the same way, Bochud and colleagues reported that common polymorphisms of TLR4 in donors were independently associated with an increased risk of invasive aspergillosis in allogeneic HSCT recipients [42]. Although acquired comorbid conditions remain the major predisposing factors underlying the increased susceptibility to severe infections, these data suggest that inherited genetic variants might contribute to the pathophysiology and to the prognosis of septic shock in patients with hematological malignancies.

52.3 Outcomes of Septic Shock in Patients with Malignancies

With respect to advances in antimicrobial treatments and advanced life supports, large epidemiological studies reported a modest but noticeable decrease in the overall mortality rate of severe sepsis and septic shock over the last 2 decades. Thus, the mortality rate of severe sepsis decreased from 45% to 37.7% between 1993 and 2003 [2]. A similar trend was observed in septic shock whose mortality rate decreased from 62.1% to 55.9% between 1993 and 2001 [3]. Recently, management of severe sepsis and septic shock has been improved by protocolized procedures including rapid and appropriate initiation of antimicrobial treatments and therapeutic interventions, and the emergence of adjuvant therapies (mechanical ventilation with low tidal volumes, activated protein C, intensive insulin therapy, corticosteroid supplementation) that have been retained in international recommendations [43]. Implementation of these guidelines has been associated with improved survival in unselected cohorts of patients in before-after studies.

Cancer patients with severe sepsis and septic shock represent a high-risk subgroup affected with a particularly high mortality rate (Table 52.1). Although the

Table 52.1 Characteristics of cancer patients with severe sepsis and septic shock

Study	Period	Number of patients	Type of malignancy: hematological/solid tumor	Sepsis stage: septic shock/severe sepsis	Short-term mortality (%)
[86]	1994–1999	73	31/42	73/0	53.4[a]
[24]	1995–1997	34	79/9	34/0	79.4[b]
	1998–2000	54		54/0	55.5[b]
[5]	1999	34,684	10,405/24,279	na	37.8[c]
[25]	1998–2001	90	47/43	90/0	78.9[c]
	2002–2005	148	85/63	148/0	63.5[c]
[27]	2002	230	63/167	80/150	44.6[a,e]
[54]	2002–2004	80	na[d]	80/0	78[c]
[26]	2000–2006	186	186/0	109/77	52.2[c]
[88]	2001–2006	50	50/0	50/0	60[a]
[87]	1995–2007	4,177	4,177/0	na	66.6[c]

[a]Mortality in ICU

[b]28-day mortality

[c]Hospital mortality

[d]The overall study population included 132 patients with hematological malignancies and 56 patients with solid tumors. na = non-available

[e]Personal unpublished data from F. Taccone, reproduced with permission

case fatality rate of severe sepsis remains considerably higher in cancer patients than in noncancer patients, it is noteworthy that relatively impressive improvements in outcome have been achieved in this vulnerable subgroup. Thus, the crude mortality rate of cancer patients with sepsis dropped from 44.7% to 23.8% over the 1979–2001 period [4]. Accordingly, favorable trends in outcome were reported among cancer patients with septic shock within recent periods. In a center particularly experienced in the management of critically ill cancer patients, the overall 30-day mortality of cancer patients with septic shock decreased from 79.4% in 1995–1997 to 55.5% in 1998–2000 [24]. In the same way, a recent study assessed the trend in outcomes of cancer patients with septic shock between two consecutive 4-year periods in 1998–2001 and 2002–2005. The 28-day and hospital mortality rates were 52.7% and 63.5%, respectively, during 2002–2005, as compared to 72.2% and 78.9%, respectively, during 1998–2001. Although the latter period was characterized with implementation of new therapeutic interventions for sepsis, factors that accounted for improvement in survival remained unclear and also potentially involved an early and judicious selection of patients more likely to benefit from intensive care [25].

52.4 Prognostic Factors of Septic Shock: The Critical Role of Organ Failures

Prognostic factors for critically ill cancer patients have been extensively assessed by multiple studies, but relatively few specifically focused on patients with septic shock. However, these studies defined the general principles that actually influence the decision-making process of ICU admission and "do not resuscitate" orders in this subgroup of patients. While the prognostic influence of age is attenuated in critically ill cancer patients, the performance status prior to acute illness appears to be a more relevant prognostic factor [44]. Of note, characteristics of malignancy (grade, stage and response to treatment) have little or no impact on short-term outcome and rather determine the long-term outcome after ICU and hospital discharge [45]. In contrast, allogeneic HSCT represents a notable condition associated with a desperately worse in-ICU outcome when invasive mechanical ventilation is required, especially when associated with extra-pulmonary organ failures such as shock or liver failure [46]. Accordingly, a reliable and thorough assessment of the underlying disease status remains central to the triage decision.

Despite its dreaded reputation, neutropenia by itself does not seem to confer an increased risk of death in cancer patients [47]. For instance, the outcome of patients that developed severe sepsis and septic shock following recent intravenous chemotherapy was relatively good despite the high frequency of neutropenia, and was even better than that of patients without neutropenia [26]. Furthermore, bacterial infections that commonly arise during neutropenia have been associated with a more favorable outcome than nonbacterial complications in critically ill patients with hematological malignancies, including those requiring vasoactive drugs and mechanical ventilation [48]. The relatively fast and efficient identification of bacterial infections combined with the widespread policy of early broad-spectrum empirical antibiotic treatment for neutropenic fever probably accounted in part for these paradoxical observations. Indeed, inadequacy of antimicrobial treatment has been clearly associated with worse outcomes in patients with septic shock. Kumar and coworkers thus identified the time to initiation of effective antimicrobial therapy as the strongest predictor of outcome in septic shock. Survival in severe sepsis decreased linearly if antimicrobial treatment was initiated more than 1 h after the onset of hypotension (mean decrease of 7.6% per hour of delay) [49]. In the same way, inadequacy of empirical antimicrobial treatment has been associated with increased mortality in ventilator-associated pneumonia or ICU-acquired bacteremia [50, 51]. Likewise, time to antibiotic administration >2 h was an independent poor prognostic factor in cancer patients with septic shock, thereby highlighting the critical role of rapidly effective antimicrobial treatment in immunocompromised patients [24].

Finally, the number and extent of organ failures are the main prognostic factors in critically ill cancer patients with or without septic shock [52]. However, requirements of invasive mechanical ventilation, vasopressive drugs or renal replacement therapy (RRT) imperfectly predict outcomes at the time of ICU admission. Accordingly, single measurements of severity scores on ICU admission, such as the logistic organ dysfunction (LOD) or sequential organ failure assessment (SOFA) scores that comprise variables related to organ failures, perform poorly for the prediction of outcome. In contrast, a more reliable assessment of the prognosis through repetition of these scores is made possible after a few days of stay in the ICU [53]. In the same way, delayed initiation of life supports such as vasopressive drugs, invasive mechanical ventilation or RRT after 72 h of ICU admission is associated with almost constant mortality [54].

52.5 Intended Management of Septic Shock in Patients with Hematological Malignancies

Routine management of severe sepsis and septic shock was recently modified by the emergence of therapeutic strategies that demonstrated an improvement in survival in septic shock patients. Most of the measures described below originated from randomized control trials (RCT) and were retained in the Surviving Sepsis Campaign Guidelines [43]. However, the actual benefits of some of these strategies were challenged in subsequent studies and remain controversial. Nonetheless, implementation of these guidelines has been associated with improvement in survival of severe sepsis and septic shock in unselected cohorts of patients. Of note, none of these therapeutic measures have been specifically assessed in cancer patients who were either excluded or underrepresented in the aforementioned studies. The impact of these guidelines in cancer patients with septic shock was assessed in a single center study. As compared to the 1998–2001 period, the mortality rate dropped between 2002 and 2005 when new therapeutic strategies were commonly applied, suggesting that cancer patients also benefited from improvement in care of septic shock [25]. Therefore, most of these treatments are applicable to patients with hematological malignancies. We will discuss the current management of patients with septic shock and the relevance or applicability for patients with hematological malignancies.

52.5.1 Antimicrobial Treatment and Source of Infection Control

Outcome of severe sepsis and septic shock is highly dependent on time to efficient antimicrobial treatment, especially in immunocompromised patients with phagocytosis defects such as neutropenia, whose immune system is less likely to prevent the spread of infection. Depending on the focus of infection, removal of infected devices or surgical excision of infected tissues might also be required. In patients with hematological malignancies, many factors are likely to influence the choice of antimicrobial drugs: type and extent of immune defects, previously received and ongoing antibiotics at the onset of shock, known colonization by resistant pathogens, focus of infection and risk factors for infection by specific pathogens.

A potent antibiotic combination including a broad-spectrum antipseudomonal beta-lactam and an aminoglycoside forms the basis of antimicrobial treatment. The synergistic effect of this combination on bacterial killing is supported by numerous experimental data, and several clinical studies reported that neutropenic patients with gram-negative bacterial infections were likely to benefit from a combination of beta-lactam and aminoglycoside [55, 56]. Since then, a number of studies comparing monotherapy with beta-lactams and combination therapy with beta-lactams plus aminoglycosides failed to show any differences in response rates of febrile neutropenic patients, including those with gram-negative infections. However, the fast bactericidal activity of aminoglycosides and their synergistic effect with beta-lactams justify an aminoglycoside-containing regimen in most patients with severe infections, especially in immunocompromised patients for whom efficient containment of infection is critical. Risk factors for infections due to potentially resistant gram-positive bacteria (neutropenia, intravascular devices, extensive mucosal damage, systemic or digestive prophylaxis with antibiotics, skin and soft tissue involvement) are almost constantly present in septic shock patients with hematological malignancies. Therefore, glycopeptides (or other antibiotics targeted against potentially resistant gram-positive cocci) should be included in the initial treatment regimen. Finally, given the high frequency and the poor prognosis of invasive fungal infections in this setting, it seems wise to include antifungal drugs in the first-line antimicrobial regimen, especially when risk factors for candidiasis or aspergillosis are present. Hence, the multiplicity of potential etiologies of septic shock in immunocompromised patients often imposes a broad-spectrum empirical antimicrobial regimen. However, the respective indications of antimicrobial agents should be subsequently reassessed on the basis of the results of microbiological investigations.

Clinical conditions, such as sepsis and neutropenia, may influence the pharmacokinetics of antibiotics through enhanced renal clearance and enhanced distribution volume related to parenteral nutrition, hypoprotidemia and fluid overload, thereby resulting in insufficient dosing of antibiotics [57]. This risk is particularly relevant to concentration-dependent antibiotics such as aminoglycosides or fluoroquinolones. Since the ratio of serum concentration peak/bacterial minimal inhibitory concentration determines the aminoglycoside efficacy, such antibiotics should be preferentially administered through a high-dose, single daily infusion in order to achieve an efficient concentration peak. Residual concentrations should be monitored for further administrations in order to minimize renal and cochlear toxicities.

52.5.2 Hemodynamic Support

Besides antimicrobial treatment, management of the circulatory status is the cornerstone of septic shock treatment. The importance of early and aggressive restoration of hemodynamics was highlighted by a randomized controlled study in which a protocolized resuscitation strategy aimed to achieve therapeutic goals (central venous pressure 8–12 mmHg, mean arterial pressure >65 mmHg, urine output >0.5 mL/kg/h and central venous saturation >70%) within 6 h after recognition of tissue hypoperfusion was associated with improved survival in patients with severe sepsis [58]. Therefore, patients with severe sepsis or septic shock with malignancies should be referred as early as possible to the ICU where optimal management of hemodynamics is feasible. Since colloids have been associated with adverse side effects, cristalloids are preferentially used for fluid resuscitation. The choice of catecholamine regimen depends on the presence of preexisting or sepsis-induced myocardial dysfunction. Mokart and colleagues reported an incidence of cardiac dysfunction (left ventricle ejection fraction <45%) of 75% in a cohort of cancer patients with septic shock. In this study, the level of NT-proBNP as a marker of myocardial dysfunction was independently associated with increased mortality, although it was not adjusted to renal function [59]. Associated cardiac dysfunction indicates a combination of vasopressor and inotropic drugs (either epinephrine or a combination of norepinephrine and dobutamine) [60].

52.5.3 Ventilatory Support

Most patients with septic shock require endotracheal intubation and mechanical ventilation. Although non-invasive ventilation (NIV) has been shown to decrease the rate of intubation and finally the ICU mortality in immunocompromised patients with early acute respiratory failure, this study excluded patients with associated extrapulmonary failures [61]. The need for vasopressors is clearly a risk factor for failure of NIV, and avoiding invasive mechanical ventilation at any cost may lead to applying NIV beyond its indications and may contribute to unreasonably delaying endotracheal intubation, to preventing adequate diagnostic procedures and thus to interfering with optimal management of septic shock [62]. Therefore, NIV should be cautiously used in the setting of septic shock. Following intubation, protective ventilatory settings should then apply as this strategy has been associated with improved survival in patients with acute respiratory distress syndrome (low tidal volume of 6 mg/kg of predicted body weight with a plateau pressure <30 cmH_2O) [63].

52.5.4 Renal Replacement Therapy

Acute renal failure remains a major prognostic factor of septic shock. Accordingly, a study reported that recent improvement in survival of cancer patients with septic shock was mostly restricted to those who did not require RRT [25]. Several studies compared continuous RRT and intermittent hemodialysis in nonseptic and septic patients and concluded the equivalence of the two procedures without any differences in survival or renal function recovery [64]. Regardless of the choice of the procedure, the prognosis rather seems to be dependent on the intensity of RRT (dialysis dose or volume of filtration). Although continuous therapies may allow better tolerance and thereby may facilitate the management of fluid balance in hemodynamically unstable patients, they require continuous efficient anticoagulation and induce platelet consumption. Since thrombocytopenia is frequently present in septic shock patients with malignancies, it seems logical to favor intermittent hemodialysis, or alternatively to use continuous methods with regional citrate anticoagulation in patients with high bleeding risk [65].

52.5.5 Steroid Supplementation

Adrenal insufficiency as assessed by the short corticotropin test occurs in more than half of patients with septic shock. In a multicenter RCT, a substitutive treatment combining low-dose hydrocortisone (200 mg per day) and fludrocortisone was shown to improve survival in patients with septic shock when administered within the first 8 h of shock [66]. However, these results were not confirmed by the recently published CORTICUS study in which hydrocortisone at the same dose was administered within the first 48 h of shock in less severe cases [67]. In contrast, treatment with hydrocortisone was associated with an increase in the incidence of secondary infections. Altogether, these studies suggest that most patients with septic shock may not benefit from corticosteroid substitution, which is potentially associated with adverse side effects. Hence, the more recent guidelines restricted the use of hydrocortisone to patients with blood pressure poorly responsive to vasopressor therapy [43]. Nonetheless, it should be remembered that patients with hematological malignancies are frequently treated with corticosteroids and may exhibit functional adrenal insufficiency at the time of life-threatening complications, thereby indicating corticosteroid supplementation.

52.5.6 Blood Glucose Control

Hyperglycemia is almost constantly encountered in critically ill patients with septic shock and is related to stress hormone release and insulin resistance. Two randomized controlled studies concluded that tight glycemic control aimed to maintain glucose levels <1.1 g/L was associated with improved survival rates as compared to a permissive glycemic control (<2 g/L) in surgical ICU patients, and in medical ICU patients with a length of ICU stay >3 days [68, 69]. Since then, several multicenter RCTs evaluated tight glycemic control by intensive insulin therapy in critically ill patients with or without sepsis, but failed to demonstrate any improvement in outcome [70–72]. In contrast, some of these studies reported unacceptable rates of hypoglycemia in the intensive insulin arm. Of note, control groups from these recent trials were assigned to lower glycemic targets, which may explain in part the absence of an additive effect of intensive insulin therapy. Interestingly, hyperglycemia has also been associated with an increased risk of posttransplant complications in allogeneic HSCT [73], and a retrospective study suggested intensive glucose control might decrease the rate of infections during engraftment period [74]. Altogether, these data suggest that hyperglycemia should be controlled by intensive insulin therapy in septic shock patients with hematological malignancies, the optimal glycemia target remaining to be established.

52.5.7 Recombinant Activated Protein C

Recombinant Activated Protein C (rhAPC) is an anticoagulant protein aimed at antagonizing the sepsis-induced procoagulant state, but that also carries some anti-inflammatory and hemodynamic properties. In the PROWESS randomized controlled trial, a 96-h treatment with rhAPC was associated with a 6.1% absolute decrease of the 28-day mortality rate and a relative risk reduction of 19.4% (CI 6.6–30.5%) [75]. A post-hoc subgroup analysis revealed that the benefit was restricted to the most severe patients with an APACHE II score >25 and at least two organ failures. This was confirmed by a second RCT that did not observe any difference in outcome between rhAPC- and placebo-treated patients with severe sepsis and a low risk of death [76]. Since then, some observational studies also suggested an improvement in survival of severe sepsis patients treated with rhAPC [77]. However, there remain considerable controversies about the real efficacy of the drug, and whether rhAPC may also improve survival of immunocompromised patients with septic shock has not been established. Furthermore, the increased risk of serious bleeding of rhAPC limits its widespread use in patients with hematological malignancies in whom underlying coagulation disorders such as thrombocytopenia and other clotting disorders are frequently encountered. Therefore, it is difficult to provide any firm recommendation about the use of rhAPC in this setting, but whenever indicated, we strongly recommend maintaining a safe platelet count in rhAPC-treated patients.

52.5.8 Blood Product Administration

Medullar insufficiency caused by the malignancy itself or imposed by cytostatic treatments is frequently encountered in critically ill patients with hematological malignancies. With respect to the shortage and the cost of blood products on one hand, and to the number of potential adverse effects on the other hand, red blood cell and platelet transfusions became major issues in this setting. In order to decrease transfusion-related reactions, subsequent alloimmunization and transmission of intracellular viruses, leukodepletion of blood products became a standard practice in Europe and in North American countries, especially for high-risk recipients that are likely to receive multiple transfusions, such as hematological patients. In addition, irradiation of blood products aimed at preventing transfusion-related graft-versus-host disease may be required in some severely immunocompromised patients, such as hematopoietic stem cell transplant recipients or those treated with anti-lymphocyte drugs such as monoclonal antibodies (Campath anti-CD52) or nucleoside analogs (2CDA, pentostatine, fludarabine).

Red blood cell transfusions have potential side effects ranging from fluid overload, TRALI, severe mismatch-related reactions or immunization that may affect the efficiency of further transfusions. In addition, red blood cell transfusions may carry adverse immunomodulatory properties that seem to favor the development of ICU-acquired infections. A restrictive strategy aiming to maintain hemoglobin levels between 7 and 9 g/dL in critically ill patients allowed a significant sparing of red blood cell units, and was possibly associated with improved survival as compared to a standard strategy to maintain hemoglobin levels between 10 and 12 g/dL [78]. However, achievement of $ScVO_2$ objectives during the early resuscitation period may require temporarily increasing the transfusion threshold towards a hematocrit level of 30% [58].

There is actually no reliable evaluation of platelet transfusion thresholds in critically ill patients. Hence, triggers for platelet transfusions largely derive from randomized trials where patients with acute leukemia were prophylactically transfused at thresholds of either 10,000 or 20,000 platelets/mm^3. There was no difference in terms of incidence of severe and fatal hemorrhage, but the lower threshold was associated with a significant decrease in platelet transfusion. Some data suggest that the risk of bleeding in critically ill patients not only depends on platelet count, but also on the presence of associated conditions such as high urea serum levels, making it difficult to recommend any definitive transfusion threshold [79, 80].

52.5.9 Immune Defense Restoration

Besides standard treatment of septic shock combining antimicrobial treatment and extensive life support, restoration of immune defense in an attractive alternative strategy aimed at improving the clearance of the pathogen. The hematopoietic growth factor G-CSF is a regulatory cytokine capable of stimulating the production of neutrophils from bone marrow progenitors, and thus may accelerate neutropenia recovery. In addition, G-CSF enhances and primes many neutrophil functions, including antimicrobial activity. In neutropenic patients with fever, G-CSF is able to shorten the time to neutrophil recovery, and might possibly slightly reduce infection-related mortality [81]. A few studies evaluated the role of G-CSF in neutropenic patients with severe infections in the ICU and reported deceiving results without any improvement in survival or any reduction in time to neutrophil recovery [47]. In the same way, enhancement of neutrophil functions by administration of G-CSF did not improve the outcome of septic shock in non-neutropenic patients [82]. On the other hand, G-CSF has been associated with deterioration of respiratory status through lung infiltration by activated neutrophils at the time of neutropenia recovery [83–85]. Apart from G-CSF, transfusion of leukocytes collected by leukapheresis from G-CSF-stimulated healthy donors has been proposed as a supportive treatment in case of uncontrolled infections in neutropenic patients, especially when impaired pathogen clearance accounts for the severity of infection (necrotic extensive cellulitis, invasive fungal infections, etc.). However, the procedure is frequently associated with potential side effects, such as transfusion-associated lung injury and anti-HLA immunization. To date, uncertainties about the real efficacy and the potential adverse side effects of both G-CSF and leukocyte transfusion argue against the routine application of these immunomodulatory treatments in septic shock.

52.6 Conclusion

Regardless of underlying immune status, we now have numerous reliable data that highlight the critical impact of the "golden hours" of severe sepsis and septic shock, thereby supporting early and aggressive management of organ failures. Although no study reliably assessed the influence of early ICU admission on outcome in septic shock patients with hematological malignancies, we assume that the prognosis is in part dependent on early recognition of organ failures. Early identification of patients who are likely to benefit from intensive care in this setting requires close collaboration between hematologists and intensive care physicians. Besides patients with favorable hematological prognosis, such a policy of early ICU admission might also be relevant to patients with progressive malignancy for whom unlimited life support would not be justified, but for whom early management of severe sepsis might prevent the dreaded evolution towards septic shock and multiple organ failures.

References

1. Martin GS, Mannino DM, Eaton S, Moss M (2003) The epidemiology of sepsis in the United States from 1979 through 2000. N Engl J Med 348(16):1546–1554
2. Dombrovskiy VY, Martin AA, Sunderram J, Paz HL (2007) Rapid increase in hospitalization and mortality rates for severe sepsis in the United States: a trend analysis from 1993 to 2003. Crit Care Med 35(5):1244–1250
3. Annane D, Aegerter P, Jars-Guincestre MC, Guidet B (2003) Current epidemiology of septic shock: the CUB-Rea Network. Am J Respir Crit Care Med 168(2):165–172
4. Danai PA, Moss M, Mannino DM, Martin GS (2006) The epidemiology of sepsis in patients with malignancy. Chest 129(6):1432–1440
5. Williams MD, Braun LA, Cooper LM, Johnston J, Weiss RV, Qualy RL, Linde-Zwirble W (2004) Hospitalized cancer patients with severe sepsis: analysis of incidence, mortality, and associated costs of care. Crit Care 8(5):R291–R298
6. Angus DC, Linde-Zwirble WT, Lidicker J, Clermont G, Carcillo J, Pinsky MR (2001) Epidemiology of severe sepsis in the United States: analysis of incidence, outcome, and associated costs of care. Crit Care Med 29(7):1303–1310
7. Elting LS, Rubenstein EB, Rolston KV, Bodey GP (1997) Outcomes of bacteremia in patients with cancer and neutropenia: observations from two decades of epidemiological and clinical trials. Clin Infect Dis 25(2): 247–259
8. Cordonnier C, Buzyn A, Leverger G, Herbrecht R, Hunault M, Leclercq R, Bastuji-Garin S (2003) Epidemiology and risk factors for gram-positive coccal infections in neutropenia: toward a more targeted antibiotic strategy. Clin Infect Dis 36(2):149–158
9. Yadegarynia D, Tarrand J, Raad I, Rolston K (2003) Current spectrum of bacterial infections in patients with cancer. Clin Infect Dis 37(8):1144–1145
10. Wisplinghoff H, Seifert H, Wenzel RP, Edmond MB (2003) Current trends in the epidemiology of nosocomial bloodstream infections in patients with hematological malignancies and solid neoplasms in hospitals in the United States. Clin Infect Dis 36(9):1103–1110
11. Tortorano AM, Peman J, Bernhardt H, Klingspor L, Kibbler CC, Faure O, Biraghi E, Canton E, Zimmermann K, Seaton S, Grillot R (2004) Epidemiology of candidaemia in Europe: results of 28-month European Confederation of Medical Mycology (ECMM) hospital-based surveillance study. Eur J Clin Microbiol Infect Dis 23(4):317–322
12. Hachem R, Hanna H, Kontoyiannis D, Jiang Y, Raad I (2008) The changing epidemiology of invasive candidiasis: Candida glabrata and Candida krusei as the leading causes of candidemia in hematologic malignancy. Cancer 112(11): 2493–2499
13. Neofytos D, Horn D, Anaissie E, Steinbach W, Olyaei A, Fishman J, Pfaller M, Chang C, Webster K, Marr K (2009) Epidemiology and outcome of invasive fungal infection in adult hematopoietic stem cell transplant recipients: analysis of Multicenter Prospective Antifungal Therapy (PATH) Alliance registry. Clin Infect Dis 48(3):265–273
14. Cattaneo C, Quaresmini G, Casari S, Capucci MA, Micheletti M, Borlenghi E, Signorini L, Re A, Carosi G, Rossi G (2008) Recent changes in bacterial epidemiology and the emergence of fluoroquinolone-resistant *Escherichia coli* among patients with haematological malignancies: results of a prospective study on 823 patients at a single institution. J Antimicrob Chemother 61(3):721–728
15. Chen CY, Tsay W, Tang JL, Tien HF, Chen YC, Chang SC, Hsueh PR (2010) Epidemiology of bloodstream infections in patients with haematological malignancies with and without neutropenia. Epidemiol Infect 138(7)): 1044–1051
16. Morris PG, Hassan T, McNamara M, Hassan A, Wiig R, Grogan L, Breathnach OS, Smyth E, Humphreys H (2008) Emergence of MRSA in positive blood cultures from patients with febrile neutropenia – a cause for concern. Support Care Cancer 16(9):1085–1088
17. Trecarichi EM, Tumbarello M, Spanu T, Caira M, Fianchi L, Chiusolo P, Fadda G, Leone G, Cauda R, Pagano L (2009) Incidence and clinical impact of extended-spectrum-beta-lactamase (ESBL) production and fluoroquinolone resistance in bloodstream infections caused by *Escherichia coli* in patients with hematological malignancies. J Infect 58(4): 299–307
18. Tumbarello M, Spanu T, Caira M, Trecarichi EM, Laurenti L, Montuori E, Fianchi L, Leone F, Fadda G, Cauda R, Pagano L (2009) Factors associated with mortality in bacteremic patients with hematologic malignancies. Diagn Microbiol Infect Dis 64(3):320–326
19. Safdar A, Rolston KV (2007) Stenotrophomonas maltophilia: changing spectrum of a serious bacterial pathogen in patients with cancer. Clin Infect Dis 45(12):1602–1609
20. Nseir S, Di Pompeo C, Diarra M, Brisson H, Tissier S, Boulo M, Durocher A (2007) Relationship between immunosuppres-

sion and intensive care unit-acquired multidrug-resistant bacteria: a case-control study. Crit Care Med 35(5):1318–1323

21. Brun-Buisson C, Meshaka P, Pinton P, Vallet B (2004) EPISEPSIS: a reappraisal of the epidemiology and outcome of severe sepsis in French intensive care units. Intensive Care Med 30(4):580–588
22. Vincent JL, Sakr Y, Sprung CL, Ranieri VM, Reinhart K, Gerlach H, Moreno R, Carlet J, Le Gall JR, Payen D (2006) Sepsis in European intensive care units: results of the SOAP study. Crit Care Med 34(2):344–353
23. Alberti C, Brun-Buisson C, Burchardi H, Martin C, Goodman S, Artigas A, Sicignano A, Palazzo M, Moreno R, Boulme R, Lepage E, Le Gall R (2002) Epidemiology of sepsis and infection in ICU patients from an international multicentre cohort study. Intensive Care Med 28(2):108–121
24. Larche J, Azoulay E, Fieux F, Mesnard L, Moreau D, Thiery G, Darmon M, Le Gall JR, Schlemmer B (2003) Improved survival of critically ill cancer patients with septic shock. Intensive Care Med 29(10):1688–1695
25. Pene F, Percheron S, Lemiale V, Viallon V, Claessens YE, Marque S, Charpentier J, Angus DC, Cariou A, Chiche JD, Mira JP (2008) Temporal changes in management and outcome of septic shock in patients with malignancies in the intensive care unit. Crit Care Med 36(3):690–696
26. Vandijck DM, Benoit DD, Depuydt PO, Offner FC, Blot SI, Van Tilborgh AK, Nollet J, Steel E, Noens LA, Decruyenaere JM (2008) Impact of recent intravenous chemotherapy on outcome in severe sepsis and septic shock patients with hematological malignancies. Intensive Care Med 34(5):847–855
27. Taccone FS, Artigas AA, Sprung CL, Moreno R, Sakr Y, Vincent JL (2009) Characteristics and outcomes of cancer patients in European ICUs. Crit Care 13(1):R15
28. Dhainaut JF, Claessens YE, Janes J, Nelson DR (2005) Underlying disorders and their impact on the host response to infection. Clin Infect Dis 41(Suppl 7):S481–S489
29. Lorenz E, Mira JP, Cornish KL, Arbour NC, Schwartz DA (2000) A novel polymorphism in the toll-like receptor 2 gene and its potential association with staphylococcal infection. Infect Immun 68(11):6398–6401
30. Lorenz E, Mira JP, Frees KL, Schwartz DA (2002) Relevance of mutations in the TLR4 receptor in patients with gram-negative septic shock. Arch Intern Med 162(9):1028–1032
31. Texereau J, Chiche JD, Taylor W, Choukroun G, Comba B, Mira JP (2005) The importance of Toll-like receptor 2 polymorphisms in severe infections. Clin Infect Dis 41(Suppl 7): S408–S415
32. Wurfel MM, Gordon AC, Holden TD, Radella F, Strout J, Kajikawa O, Ruzinski JT, Rona G, Black RA, Stratton S, Jarvik GP, Hajjar AM, Nickerson DA, Rieder M, Sevransky J, Maloney JP, Moss M, Martin G, Shanholtz C, Garcia JG, Gao L, Brower R, Barnes KC, Walley KR, Russell JA, Martin TR (2008) Toll-like receptor 1 polymorphisms affect innate immune responses and outcomes in sepsis. Am J Respir Crit Care Med 178(7):710–720
33. Gibot S, Cariou A, Drouet L, Rossignol M, Ripoll L (2002) Association between a genomic polymorphism within the CD14 locus and septic shock susceptibility and mortality rate. Crit Care Med 30(5):969–973
34. Arcaroli J, Silva E, Maloney JP, He Q, Svetkauskaite D, Murphy JR, Abraham E (2006) Variant IRAK-1 haplotype is associated with increased nuclear factor-kappaB activation and worse outcomes in sepsis. Am J Respir Crit Care Med 173(12):1335–1341
35. Garred P, Strom J, Quist L, Taaning E, Madsen HO (2003) Association of mannose-binding lectin polymorphisms with sepsis and fatal outcome, in patients with systemic inflammatory response syndrome. J Infect Dis 188(9): 1394–1403
36. Mira JP, Cariou A, Grall F, Delclaux C, Losser MR, Heshmati F, Cheval C, Monchi M, Teboul JL, Riche F, Leleu G, Arbibe L, Mignon A, Delpech M, Dhainaut JF (1999) Association of TNF2, a TNF-alpha promoter polymorphism, with septic shock susceptibility and mortality: a multicenter study. JAMA 282(6):561–568
37. Texereau J, Pene F, Chiche JD, Rousseau C, Mira JP (2004) Importance of hemostatic gene polymorphisms for susceptibility to and outcome of severe sepsis. Crit Care Med 32(5 Suppl):S313–S319
38. Vekemans M, Robinson J, Georgala A, Heymans C, Muanza F, Paesmans M, Klastersky J, Barette M, Meuleman N, Huet F, Calandra T, Costantini S, Ferrant A, Mathissen F, Axelsen M, Marchetti O, Aoun M (2007) Low mannose-binding lectin concentration is associated with severe infection in patients with hematological cancer who are undergoing chemotherapy. Clin Infect Dis 44(12):1593–1601
39. Mullighan CG, Heatley S, Doherty K, Szabo F, Grigg A, Hughes TP, Schwarer AP, Szer J, Tait BD, Bik To L, Bardy PG (2002) Mannose-binding lectin gene polymorphisms are associated with major infection following allogeneic hemopoietic stem cell transplantation. Blood 99(10): 3524–3529
40. Mullighan CG, Heatley SL, Danner S, Dean MM, Doherty K, Hahn U, Bradstock KF, Minchinton R, Schwarer AP, Szer J, Bardy PG (2008) Mannose-binding lectin status is associated with risk of major infection following myeloablative sibling allogeneic hematopoietic stem cell transplantation. Blood 112(5):2120–2128
41. Lambourne J, Agranoff D, Herbrecht R, Troke PF, Buchbinder A, Willis F, Letscher-Bru V, Agrawal S, Doffman S, Johnson E, White PL, Barnes RA, Griffin G, Lindsay JA, Harrison TS (2009) Association of mannose-binding lectin deficiency with acute invasive aspergillosis in immunocompromised patients. Clin Infect Dis 49(10):1486–1491
42. Bochud PY, Chien JW, Marr KA, Leisenring WM, Upton A, Janer M, Rodrigues SD, Li S, Hansen JA, Zhao LP, Aderem A, Boeckh M (2008) Toll-like receptor 4 polymorphisms and aspergillosis in stem-cell transplantation. N Engl J Med 359(17):1766–1777
43. Dellinger RP, Levy MM, Carlet JM, Bion J, Parker MM, Jaeschke R, Reinhart K, Angus DC, Brun-Buisson C, Beale R, Calandra T, Dhainaut JF, Gerlach H, Harvey M, Marini JJ, Marshall J, Ranieri M, Ramsay G, Sevransky J, Thompson BT, Townsend S, Vender JS, Zimmerman JL, Vincent JL (2008) Surviving sepsis campaign: international guidelines for management of severe sepsis and septic shock: 2008. Intensive Care Med 34(1):17–60
44. Soares M, Salluh JI, Spector N, Rocco JR (2005) Characteristics and outcomes of cancer patients requiring mechanical ventilatory support for >24 hrs. Crit Care Med 33(3):520–526
45. Massion PB, Dive AM, Doyen C, Bulpa P, Jamart J, Bosly A, Installe E (2002) Prognosis of hematologic malignancies

does not predict intensive care unit mortality. Crit Care Med 30(10):2260–2270
46. Pene F, Aubron C, Azoulay E, Blot F, Thiery G, Raynard B, Schlemmer B, Nitenberg G, Buzyn A, Arnaud P, Socie G, Mira JP (2006) Outcome of critically ill allogeneic hematopoietic stem-cell transplantation recipients: a reappraisal of indications for organ failure supports. J Clin Oncol 24(4):643–649
47. Darmon M, Azoulay E, Alberti C, Fieux F, Moreau D, Le Gall JR, Schlemmer B (2002) Impact of neutropenia duration on short-term mortality in neutropenic critically ill cancer patients. Intensive Care Med 28(12): 1775–1780
48. Benoit DD, Vandewoude KH, Decruyenaere JM, Hoste EA, Colardyn FA (2003) Outcome and early prognostic indicators in patients with a hematologic malignancy admitted to the intensive care unit for a life-threatening complication. Crit Care Med 31(1):104–112
49. Kumar A, Roberts D, Wood KE, Light B, Parrillo JE, Sharma S, Suppes R, Feinstein D, Zanotti S, Taiberg L, Gurka D, Cheang M (2006) Duration of hypotension before initiation of effective antimicrobial therapy is the critical determinant of survival in human septic shock. Crit Care Med 34(6): 1589–1596
50. Ibrahim EH, Sherman G, Ward S, Fraser VJ, Kollef MH (2000) The influence of inadequate antimicrobial treatment of bloodstream infections on patient outcomes in the ICU setting. Chest 118(1):146–155
51. Iregui M, Ward S, Sherman G, Fraser VJ, Kollef MH (2002) Clinical importance of delays in the initiation of appropriate antibiotic treatment for ventilator-associated pneumonia. Chest 122(1):262–268
52. Blot F, Guiguet M, Nitenberg G, Leclercq B, Gachot B, Escudier B (1997) Prognostic factors for neutropenic patients in an intensive care unit: respective roles of underlying malignancies and acute organ failures. Eur J Cancer 33(7): 1031–1037
53. Lamia B, Hellot MF, Girault C, Tamion F, Dachraoui F, Lenain P, Bonmarchand G (2006) Changes in severity and organ failure scores as prognostic factors in onco-hematological malignancy patients admitted to the ICU. Intensive Care Med 32(10):1560–1568
54. Lecuyer L, Chevret S, Thiery G, Darmon M, Schlemmer B, Azoulay E (2007) The ICU trial: a new admission policy for cancer patients requiring mechanical ventilation. Crit Care Med 35(3):808–814
55. De Jongh CA, Joshi JH, Newman KA, Moody MR, Wharton R, Standiford HC, Schimpff SC (1986) Antibiotic synergism and response in gram-negative bacteremia in granulocytopenic cancer patients. Am J Med 80(5C):96–100
56. The EORTC International Antimicrobial Therapy Cooperative Group (1987) Ceftazidime combined with a short or long course of amikacin for empirical therapy of gram-negative bacteremia in cancer patients with granulocytopenia. N Engl J Med 317(27):1692–1698
57. Lortholary O, Lefort A, Tod M, Chomat AM, Darras-Joly C, Cordonnier C (2008) Pharmacodynamics and pharmacokinetics of antibacterial drugs in the management of febrile neutropenia. Lancet Infect Dis 8(10):612–620
58. Rivers E, Nguyen B, Havstad S, Ressler J, Muzzin A, Knoblich B, Peterson E, Tomlanovich M (2001) Early goal-directed therapy in the treatment of severe sepsis and septic shock. N Engl J Med 345(19):1368–1377
59. Mokart D, Sannini A, Brun JP, Faucher M, Blaise D, Blache JL, Faucher C (2007) N-terminal pro-brain natriuretic peptide as an early prognostic factor in cancer patients developing septic shock. Crit Care 11(2):R37
60. Annane D, Vignon P, Renault A, Bollaert PE, Charpentier C, Martin C, Troche G, Ricard JD, Nitenberg G, Papazian L, Azoulay E, Bellissant E (2007) Norepinephrine plus dobutamine versus epinephrine alone for management of septic shock: a randomised trial. Lancet 370(9588):676–684
61. Hilbert G, Gruson D, Vargas F, Valentino R, Gbikpi-Benissan G, Dupon M, Reiffers J, Cardinaud JP (2001) Noninvasive ventilation in immunosuppressed patients with pulmonary infiltrates, fever, and acute respiratory failure. N Engl J Med 344(7):481–487
62. Adda M, Coquet I, Darmon M, Thiery G, Schlemmer B, Azoulay E (2008) Predictors of noninvasive ventilation failure in patients with hematologic malignancy and acute respiratory failure. Crit Care Med 36(10):2766–2772
63. The Acute Respiratory Distress Syndrome Network. (2000) Ventilation with lower tidal volumes as compared with traditional tidal volumes for acute lung injury and the acute respiratory distress syndrome. N Engl J Med 342(18): 1301–1308
64. Vinsonneau C, Camus C, Combes A, Costa de Beauregard MA, Klouche K, Boulain T, Pallot JL, Chiche JD, Taupin P, Landais P, Dhainaut JF (2006) Continuous venovenous haemodiafiltration versus intermittent haemodialysis for acute renal failure in patients with multiple-organ dysfunction syndrome: a multicentre randomised trial. Lancet 368(9533): 379–385
65. Monchi M, Berghmans D, Ledoux D, Canivet JL, Dubois B, Damas P (2004) Citrate vs. heparin for anticoagulation in continuous venovenous hemofiltration: a prospective randomized study. Intensive Care Med 30(2):260–265
66. Annane D, Sebille V, Charpentier C, Bollaert PE, Francois B, Korach JM, Capellier G, Cohen Y, Azoulay E, Troche G, Chaumet-Riffaut P, Bellissant E (2002) Effect of treatment with low doses of hydrocortisone and fludrocortisone on mortality in patients with septic shock. JAMA 288(7):862–871
67. Sprung CL, Annane D, Keh D, Moreno R, Singer M, Freivogel K, Weiss YG, Benbenishty J, Kalenka A, Forst H, Laterre PF, Reinhart K, Cuthbertson BH, Payen D, Briegel J (2008) Hydrocortisone therapy for patients with septic shock. N Engl J Med 358(2):111–124
68. van den Berghe G, Wouters P, Weekers F, Verwaest C, Bruyninckx F, Schetz M, Vlasselaers D, Ferdinande P, Lauwers P, Bouillon R (2001) Intensive insulin therapy in the critically ill patients. N Engl J Med 345(19):1359–1367
69. Van den Berghe G, Wilmer A, Hermans G, Meersseman W, Wouters PJ, Milants I, Van Wijngaerden E, Bobbaers H, Bouillon R (2006) Intensive insulin therapy in the medical ICU. N Engl J Med 354(5):449–461
70. Brunkhorst FM, Engel C, Bloos F, Meier-Hellmann A, Ragaller M, Weiler N, Moerer O, Gruendling M, Oppert M, Grond S, Olthoff D, Jaschinski U, John S, Rossaint R, Welte T, Schaefer M, Kern P, Kuhnt E, Kiehntopf M, Hartog C, Natanson C, Loeffler M, Reinhart K (2008) Intensive insulin therapy and pentastarch resuscitation in severe sepsis. N Engl J Med 358(2):125–139

71. Finfer S, Chittock DR, Su SY, Blair D, Foster D, Dhingra V, Bellomo R, Cook D, Dodek P, Henderson WR, Hebert PC, Heritier S, Heyland DK, McArthur C, McDonald E, Mitchell I, Myburgh JA, Norton R, Potter J, Robinson BG, Ronco JJ (2009) Intensive versus conventional glucose control in critically ill patients. N Engl J Med 360(13):1283–1297
72. Preiser JC, Devos P, Ruiz-Santana S, Melot C, Annane D, Groeneveld J, Iapichino G, Leverve X, Nitenberg G, Singer P, Wernerman J, Joannidis M, Stecher A, Chiolero R (2009) A prospective randomised multi-centre controlled trial on tight glucose control by intensive insulin therapy in adult intensive care units: the Glucontrol study. Intensive Care Med 35(10):1738–1748
73. Fuji S, Kim SW, Mori S, Fukuda T, Kamiya S, Yamasaki S, Morita-Hoshi Y, Ohara-Waki F, Honda O, Kuwahara S, Tanosaki R, Heike Y, Tobinai K, Takaue Y (2007) Hyperglycemia during the neutropenic period is associated with a poor outcome in patients undergoing myeloablative allogeneic hematopoietic stem cell transplantation. Transplantation 84(7):814–820
74. Fuji S, Kim SW, Mori S, Kamiya S, Yoshimura K, Yokoyama H, Kurosawa S, Saito B, Takahashi T, Kuwahara S, Heike Y, Tanosaki R, Takaue Y, Fukuda T (2009) Intensive glucose control after allogeneic hematopoietic stem cell transplantation: a retrospective matched-cohort study. Bone Marrow Transplant 44(2):105–111
75. Bernard GR, Vincent JL, Laterre PF, LaRosa SP, Dhainaut JF, Lopez-Rodriguez A, Steingrub JS, Garber GE, Helterbrand JD, Ely EW, Fisher CJ Jr (2001) Efficacy and safety of recombinant human activated protein C for severe sepsis. N Engl J Med 344(10):699–709
76. Abraham E, Laterre PF, Garg R, Levy H, Talwar D, Trzaskoma BL, Francois B, Guy JS, Bruckmann M, Rea-Neto A, Rossaint R, Perrotin D, Sablotzki A, Arkins N, Utterback BG, Macias WL (2005) Drotrecogin alfa (activated) for adults with severe sepsis and a low risk of death. N Engl J Med 353(13):1332–1341
77. Ferrer R, Artigas A, Suarez D, Palencia E, Levy MM, Arenzana A, Perez XL, Sirvent JM (2009) Effectiveness of treatments for severe sepsis: a prospective, multicenter, observational study. Am J Respir Crit Care Med 180(9): 861–866
78. Hebert PC, Wells G, Blajchman MA, Marshall J, Martin C, Pagliarello G, Tweeddale M, Schweitzer I, Yetisir E, Transfusion Requirements in Critical Care Investigators, Canadian Critical Care Trials Group (1999) A multicenter, randomized, controlled clinical trial of transfusion requirements in critical care. N Engl J Med 340(6): 409–417
79. Vanderschueren S, De Weerdt A, Malbrain M, Vankersschaever D, Frans E, Wilmer A, Bobbaers H (2000) Thrombocytopenia and prognosis in intensive care. Crit Care Med 28(6):1871–1876
80. Strauss R, Wehler M, Mehler K, Kreutzer D, Koebnick C, Hahn EG (2002) Thrombocytopenia in patients in the medical intensive care unit: bleeding prevalence, transfusion requirements, and outcome. Crit Care Med 30(8):1765–1771
81. Clark OA, Lyman GH, Castro AA, Clark LG, Djulbegovic B (2005) Colony-stimulating factors for chemotherapy-induced febrile neutropenia: a meta-analysis of randomized controlled trials. J Clin Oncol 23(18):4198–4214
82. Stephens DP, Thomas JH, Higgins A, Bailey M, Anstey NM, Currie BJ, Cheng AC (2008) Randomized, double-blind, placebo-controlled trial of granulocyte colony-stimulating factor in patients with septic shock. Crit Care Med 36(2):448–454
83. Gruson D, Hilbert G, Vargas F, Valentino R, Chene G, Boiron JM, Reiffers J, Gbikpi-Benissan G, Cardinaud JP (2000) Impact of colony-stimulating factor therapy on clinical outcome and frequency rate of nosocomial infections in intensive care unit neutropenic patients. Crit Care Med 28(9):3155–3160
84. Bouchama A, Khan B, Djazmati W, Shukri K (1999) Hematopoietic colony-stimulating factors for neutropenic patients in the ICU. Intensive Care Med 25(9): 1003–1005
85. Karlin L, Darmon M, Thiery G, Ciroldi M, de Miranda S, Lefebvre A, Schlemmer B, Azoulay E (2005) Respiratory status deterioration during G-CSF-induced neutropenia recovery. Bone Marrow Transplant 36(3):245–250
86. Regazzoni CJ, Irrazabal C, Luna CM, Poderoso JJ (2004) Cancer patients with septic shock: mortality predictors and neutropenia. Support Care Cancer 12(12):833–839
87. Hampshire PA, Welch CA, McCrossan LA, Francis K, Harrison DA (2009) Admission factors associated with hospital mortality in patients with haematological malignancy admitted to UK adult, general critical care units: a secondary analysis of the ICNARC Case Mix Programme Database. Crit Care 13(4):R137
88. Park HY, Suh GY, Jeon K, Koh WJ, Chung MP, Kim H, Kwon OJ, Kim K, Jang JH, Jung CW, Kang E, and Kim MJ (2008) Outcome and prognostic factors of patients with acute leukemia admitted to the intensive care unit for septic shock. Leuk Lymphoma 49(10):1929–34

Prognostic Factors for Mortality in the Critically Ill Cancer Patient

53

Kathleen N.S. Cathcart and Jeffrey S. Groeger

Contents

K.N.S. Cathcart (✉) and J.S. Groeger
Urgent Care Service, Department of Medicine, Memorial Sloan-Kettering Cancer Center, 1275 York Avenue, New York, NY 10065, USA
e-mail: cathcark@mskcc.org; groegerj@mskcc.org

53.1 Introduction

As more people in industrialized societies are living longer, more people are also being diagnosed with cancer. It has been estimated that one in eight deaths worldwide is due to cancer, with malignancy as cause of death second to heart disease in developed countries, and tertiary to heart disease and diarrheal illnesses in developing countries. [2]. Many patients with hematologic and solid tumors are considered to have curable illness, or may live with their disease as a chronic process for a number of years while receiving chemotherapy, radiation, or surgical management. During their treatment courses, it can be expected that some patients will become critically ill and that there will be consideration for intensive care unit (ICU) management.

Historical outcomes for the critically ill cancer patient admitted to the ICU were dismal in the 1980s, leading to recommendations for discouragement of ICU admission [4, 13, 14, 41].

Cohorts of ICU patients with cancer fared poorly compared to other patients in comparative outcome studies [10, 15, 53]. In general, patients with incurable, progressive, or relapsed solid tumors or hematologic malignancies who require mechanical ventilation have a dismal prognosis, with hospital mortality rates approaching 70–90% [21]. Those admitted to the ICU for postoperative care have a lower mortality rate relative to those individuals admitted for a medical emergency. Subgroups of patients admitted for medical emergencies tend to fare better: metabolic problems (i.e., hypercalcemia, tumor lysis syndrome), cardiac arrhythmias, or those being monitored during drug administration have a mortality rate similar to that of nonventilated patients without cancer. With the

É. Azoulay (ed.), *Pulmonary Involvement in Patients with Hematological Malignancies*,
DOI: 10.1007/978-3-642-15742-4_53, © Springer-Verlag Berlin Heidelberg 2011

Table 53.1 Identified poor prognostic indicators and hospital mortality in critically ill patients with malignancy as reported in selected reports between 1999 and 2009

Author, year	Study type	*N*	Patient characteristics	Identified poor prognostic feature	Hospital mortality
Taccone et al. 2009 [49]	Cohort multicenter observational	473	85% ST, 15% heme	>3 organ failures	75%
Adda et al. 2008 [1]	Retrospective single center	99	Heme malignancy failing to NIV	Need for MV	79% (41% in patients not requiring MV)
Mendoza et al. 2008 [33]	Retrospective single center	147	ST malignancy	Metastatic disease, vasopressors needed	46%
Soares et al. 2008 [45]	Cohort single center	163	ICU LOS ≥21 days	No. of organ failures, poor PS	50%
Ferrà et al. 2007 [17]	Retrospective single center	100	Heme malignancy	Hemodynamic instability, need for MV	58% ICU mortality
Lecuyer et al. 2007 [27]	Prospective single center	188	30% ST, 70% heme	Survival to day 5	60% surviving to day 5
Massion et al. 2002 [32]	Prospective observational single center	84	Heme malignancy	Respiratory failure, fungal infection	61%
Groeger et al. 1999 [21]	Prospective observational multicenter	782	MV required	Progressive cancer, alloSCT, leukopenia, arrhythmia, DIC	76%

ST solid tumor, *MV* mechanical ventilation, *LOS* length of stay, *PS* performance status, *SCT* stem cell transplant, *DIC* disseminated intravascular coagulation

development of respiratory failure, however, prognosis declines. As in all critically ill patients, multiorgan system failure heralds increased mortality, with the overall death rate increasing with the number of organ systems affected [21, 30, 34, 43]. Table 53.1 presents identified poor prognostic indicators and hospital mortality in critically ill patients with malignancy as reported in selected reports between 1999 and 2009.

53.2 Reasons for ICU Admission

Acute respiratory failure (ARF) is the leading reason cancer patients are admitted to the ICU [5, 26]. Recent studies have described improved outcomes for critically ill patients with both hematologic and solid tumor malignancies [6–8, 26, 31, 46, 50]. Moreover, the characteristics of the underlying malignancy are not associated with ICU survival [6, 12, 32]. Critically ill cancer patients have shown comparable mortality rates compared to non-cancer-bearing, severity-of-illness-scored matched cohorts [48]. Additionally, a recent report found that 54% of solid tumor patients admitted to the ICU, of whom about half had metastatic disease, survived to hospital discharge [33]. Also, a multicenter study that included data from all adult patients admitted with sepsis to 1 of 198 participating European ICUs found the outcome of all cancer patients comparable to that of the non-cancer population, with a 27% mortality rate [49]. While this information cannot help evaluate individual patients as candidates for ICU admission, it does suggest that aggressive critical care intervention be considered for the cancer patient population [18].

Adding to the complexity of decision-making regarding who would best be served in receiving ICU care is the broad range in cancer mortality rates, which is reflective of the fact that cancer is a heterogeneous group of diseases. What is clear is that the coexistence of HIV infection and cancer or the modality of allogeneic stem cell transplant has a marked negative survival impact on those patients requiring mechanical ventilation [9, 22, 24, 37, 39, 51]. Indeed, many studies regarding outcomes of critically ill cancer patients have excluded these two patient groups.

Patients requiring mechanical ventilation after autologous or allogeneic hematopoietic stem cell transplant have a baseline probability of death of 82–96%. In the setting of combined hepatic and renal dysfunction, the probability of death rises to 98–100%. For patients who recover from respiratory failure, the proportion surviving 6 months or longer ranges from 27% to 88%, which argues for aggressive management of critically ill transplant recipients, as withholding ICU management might negatively impact the chance of survival for a sizable proportion of these patients [9].

As shown elsewhere, treatment of organ failure more that 30 days after allogeneic transplantation in patients on immunosuppressive agents was associated with a particularly poor outcome, in contrast to the survival of patients receiving mechanical ventilation during the first 30 days post-transplant [36]. Short-term prognosis in recipients of autologous stem cell transplants is similar to other critically ill patients with cancer, and is dependent on the number and type of organ failures [23, 35, 40, 52].

Primary pulmonary malignancies are the most common fatal cancers in adults, and these patients also have a lower ICU prognosis overall compared to patients with other solid tumor malignancies. Although the 5-year survival low is generally reported to be less than 20% [3], patients with lung cancer are often admitted to the medical ICU. The most common presenting organ dysfunction was pulmonary, and patients requiring mechanical ventilation or with advanced stage have worsened ICU survival, with mortality rates of 74% and 68%, respectively [38]. In this patient group, airway infiltration or obstruction by cancer, number of organ failures, cancer recurrence or progression, and severity of comorbidities were associated with increased mortality [44].

53.3 Withholding Admission

The general tenet regarding ICU admission is that those who will not benefit from critical care, because too well or too sick, should not be offered ICU care. Ideally, patients who might benefit from ICU care should receive it [11]. In many hospitals, cancer patients are considered to have a particularly poor prognosis and are frequently not admitted to the ICU [42]. Indeed, an editorial commenting on mechanically ventilated patients undergoing bone marrow transplant suggested that an appropriate response to request for ICU care might be to "just say no" [14].

Utilization of expensive resources means that ICU care should be offered to patients with reversible medical conditions who can reasonably be expected to recover [47]. Triaging patients as too well or too sick to benefit from critical care management may be difficult based solely on diagnosis.

Decision-making difficulty arises when it is unclear which patients are appropriate ICU candidates. This difficulty in accurately predicting consequences for critically ill cancer patients was demonstrated in a report on outcome of cancer patients considered for ICU admission. In that investigation, the 30-day survival of patients considered "too sick" for ICU admission was 26%, and more surprisingly, the survival of those patients considered to be "too well" was 78.7% at 30 days [50].

53.4 Predictors of Outcomes

Models such as the Acute Physiology and Chronic Health Evaluation II (APACHE), Mortality Probability Model II (MPMII), and Simplified Acute Physiology Score II (SAPS) have been shown to underestimate the mortality of cancer patients admitted to ICUs [25, 28, 29]. In addition, these measures are intended to study patient populations and therefore have limited value in the prediction of outcome in individual patients. Another cancer-specific model has been developed to predict hospital mortality in critically ill cancer patients on the basis of variables readily obtained on admission [19, 20]. Once more, although such a model may not accurately assess an individual patient's risk for death, models such as this may be of use in discussions regarding goals of care for an individual patient.

53.5 The ICU Trial

A strategy to improve the chances for survival in critically ill patients with cancer who had a reasonable performance status and who could receive potentially life-extending cancer treatment assuming the survival of the acute illness prompting ICU consideration has been developed [27]. Admission was not offered for bedridden patients or those for whom no lifespan-extending therapy is obtainable. The utility of full treatment was reappraised on day 5 of ICU care. There was no reported significant difference in cancer characteristics between surviving and deceased patients during the first 4 ICU days. However, no patient requiring the initiation of mechanical ventilation, vasopressors, or dialysis after 3 days in the ICU survived. Overall survival in ventilated patients surviving to day 5 was 40%, and overall survival was 21.8%, leading to the recommendation that ICU care in appropriate critically ill cancer patients be offered, with reappraisal of management strategies on day 6. Of note, HIV-positive cancer patients and recipients of allogeneic hematopoietic transplant were not included in the study population. In a recent review, the authors reiterate the assertion that critically ill cancer patients for whom ICU care offers potential benefit should receive a trial of full ICU management, with reassessment of goals of care after at least 3 days [16].

53.6 Conclusion

As people are living longer, more individuals can be expected to develop cancer. With increasing therapeutic options available, more of these patients can be expected to be living with their diseases as chronic processes. Over time, patients may develop complications of their treatment or their disease that necessitates consideration of critical care management. Although historical data reveal that cancer patients had a poor outcome with ICU care in the past, more current observations conclude that these patients have outcomes that approach that of nonmalignant-associated critically ill patient populations. Allogeneic stem cell transplant recipients and patients with advanced or progressed lung cancer continue to have poor prognoses should more serious illness develop. While further study regarding long-term survival after critical care admission and quality of life when ICU care yields positive outcomes is necessary, it may be prudent to offer selected patients a trial of full-support management.

References

1. Adda M, Coquet I, Darmon M, Thiery G, Schlemmer B, Azoulay E (2008) Predictors of noninvasive ventilation failure in patients with hematologic malignancy and acute respiratory failure. Crit Care Med 36(10):2766–2772
2. American Cancer Society (2007) Global cancer facts and figures
3. American Cancer Society (2009) Cancer facts and figures
4. Anonymous (1999) Guidelines for intensive care unit admission, discharge, and triage. Task Force of the American College of Critical Care Medicine, Society of Critical Care Medicine. Crit Care Med 27:633–638
5. Azoulay E, Alberti C, Bornstain C, Leleu G, Moreau D, Recher C, Chevret S, LeGall JR, Brochard L, Schlemmer B (2001) Improved survival in cancer patients requiring mechanical ventilatory support: impact of noninvasive mechanical ventilatory support. Crit Care Med 29:519–525
6. Azoulay E, Moreau D, Alberti C, Leleu G, Adrie C, Barboteu M, Cottu P, Levy V, LeGall JR, Schlemmer B (2000) Predictors of short-term mortality in critically ill patients with solid malignancies. Intensive Care Med 26(12):1817–23
7. Azoulay E, Recher C, Alberti C, Soufir L, Leleu G, Le Gall JR, Fermand JP, Schlemmer B (1999) Changing use of intensive care for hematological patients: the example of multiple myeloma. Intensive Care Med 25:1395–1401
8. Azoulay E, Thiery G, Chevret S, Moreau D, Darmon M, Bergeron A, Yang K, Meignin V, Ciroldi M, LeGall J-R, Tazi A, Schlemmer B (2004) The prognosis of acute respiratory failure in critically ill cancer patients. Medicine 83:360–370
9. Bach PB, Schrag D, Nierman DM, Horak D, White P Jr, Young JW, Groeger JS (2001) Identification of poor prognostic features among patients requiring mechanical ventilation after hematopoietic stem cell transplantation. Blood 98:3234–3240
10. Bellamy PE, Oye RK (1984) Adult respiratory distress syndrome: Hospital charges and outcome according to underlying disease. Crit Care Med 12:622–625
11. Bone RC, McElwee NE, Eubanks DH, Gluck EH (1993) Analysis of indications for intensive care admission. Clinical efficacy project: American College of Physicians. Chest 104:1806–1811
12. Boussat S, El'rini T, Dubiez A, Depierre A, Barale F, Capellier G (2000) Predictive factors of death in primary lung cancer patients on admission to the intensive care unit. Intensive Care Med 26:1811–1816
13. Carlon GC (1988) Admitting cancer patients to the intensive care unit. Crit Care Clin 4:183–191
14. Carlon GC (1989) Just say no. Crit Care Med 17(1): 106–107
15. Cox SC, Norwood SH, Duncan CA (1985) Acute respiratory failure: Mortality associated with underlying disease. Crit Care Med 13:1005–1008
16. Darmon M, Azoulay E (2009) Critical care management of cancer patients: cause for optimism and need for objectivity. Curr Opin Oncol 21:318–326
17. Ferra C, Marcos P, Misis M, Morgades M, Bordeje ML, Oriol A, Lloveras N, Sancho JM, Xicoy B, Battle M, Klamburg J, Feliu E, Ribera JM (2007 Apr) Outcome and

prognostic factors in patients with hematologic malignancies admitted to the intensive care unit: a single center experience. Int J Hematol 85(3):195–202
18. Groeger JS, Bach PB (2003) Consider saying yes. Crit Care Med 31(1):320–321
19. Groeger JS, Glassman J, Nierman DM, Wallace SK, Price K, Horak D, Landsberg D (2003) Probability of mortality of critically ill cancer patients at 72 h of intensive care unit (ICU) management. Support Care Cancer 11:686–695
20. Groeger JS, Lemeshow S, Price K, Nierman DM, White P Jr, Klar J, Granovsky S, Horak D, Kish SK (1998) Multicenter outcome study of cancer patients admitted to the intensive care unit: a probability of mortality model. J Clin Oncol 16:761–770
21. Groeger JS, White P Jr, Nierman DM, Glassman J, Shi W, Horak D, Price K (1999) Outcome for cancer patients requiring mechanical ventilation. J Clin Oncol 17:991–997
22. Huaringa AJ, Levya FJ, Giralt SA, Blanco J, Signes-Costa J, Velarde H, Champlin RE (2000) Outcome of bone marrow transplantation patients requiring mechanical ventilation. Crit Care Med 28:1014–1017
23. Khassawaneh BY, White P Jr, Anaissie EJ, Barlogie B, Hiller FC (2002) Outcome from mechanical ventilation after autologous peripheral blood stem cell transplantation. Chest 121:185–188
24. Khouli H, Afrasiabi A, Shibli M, Hajal R, Barrett CR, Homel P (2005) Outcome of critically ill human immunodeficiency virus-infected patients in the era of highly active antiretroviral therapy. J Intensive Care Med 20:327–333
25. Knaus WA, Draper EA, Wagner DP, Zimmerman JE (1985) Apache II: a severity of disease classification system. Crit Care Med 13:818–829
26. Kress JP, Christenson J, Pohlman AS, Linkin DR, Hall JB (1999) Outcomes of critically ill patients in a university hospital setting. Am J Respir Crit Care Med 160:1957–1961
27. Lecuyer L, Chevret S, Thiery G, Darmon M, Schlemmer B, Azoulay E (2007) The ICU Trial: A new admission policy for cancer patients requiring mechanical ventilation. Crit Care Med 35:808–814
28. LeGall J-R, Lemeshow S, Sauinier F (1993) A new Simplified Acute Physiology Score (SAPS II) based on a European/North American Multicenter Study. JAMA 270:2957–2963
29. Lemeshow S, Teres D, Klar J, Avrinin JS, Gehlbach SH, Rapoport J (1993) Mortality Probability Models (MPM II) based on an international cohort of intensive care unit patients. JAMA 270:2478–2486
30. Lloyd-Thomas AR, Wright I, Lister TA, Hinds CJ (1988) Prognosis of patients receiving intensive care for life threatening medical complications of haematological malignancy. BMJ 296:1025–1029
31. Maschmeyer G, Bertshat FL, Moesta KT, Häusler E, Held TK, Nolte M, Osterziel KJ, Papstein V, Peters M, Reich G, Schmutzler M, Sezer O, Stula M, Wauer H, Wörtz T, Wischnewsky M, Hohenberger P (2003) Outcome analysis of 189 consecutive cancer patients referred to the intensive care unit as emergencies during a 2-year period. Eur J Cancer 39:783–792
32. Massion PB, Dive AM, Doyen C, Bulpa P, Jamart J, Bosly A, Istalle E (2002 Oct) Prognosis of hematologic malignancies does not predict intensive care unit mortality. Crit Care Med 30(10):2260–70
33. Mendoza V, Lee A, Marik PE (2008) The hospital-survival and prognostic factors of patients with solid tumors admitted to an ICU. Am J Hosp Palliat Care 25(3):240–243
34. Paz HL, Crilley P, Weinar M, Brodsky I (1993) Outcome of patients requiring medical ICU admission following bone marrow transplantation. Chest 104:527–531
35. Peigne V, Rusinova K, Karlin L, Darmon M, Fermand JP, Schlemmer B, Azoulay E (2009) Continued survival gains in recent years among critically ill myeloma patients. Intensive Care Med 35:512–518
36. Pene F, Aubron C, Azoulay E, Blot F, Thiéry G, Raynard B, Schlemmer B, Nitenberg G, Buzyn A, Arnaud P, Socié G, Mira JP (2006) Outcome of critically ill allogeneic stem-cell transplantation recipients: a reappraisal of indications for organ failure supports. J Clin Oncol 24:643–649
37. Price KJ, Thall PF, Kish SK, Shannon VR, Andersson BS (1998) Prognostic indicators for blood and bone marrow transplant patients admitted to an intensive care unit. Am J Respir Crit Care Med 158:876–884
38. Reichner CA, Thompson JA, O'Brien S, Kuru T, Anderson ED (2006) Outcome and code status of lung cancer patients admitted to the medical ICU. Chest 130:719–723
39. Rubenfeld GD, Crawford SW (1996) Withdrawing life support from mechanically ventilated recipients of bone marrow transplants: A case for evidence-based guidelines. Ann Intern Med 125:625–633
40. Scales DC, Thiruchelvam D, Kiss A, Sibbald WJ, Redelmeier DA (2008) Intensive care outcomes in bone marrow transplant recipients: a population-based cohort analysis. Crit Care 12:R77
41. Schuster DP (1992) Everything that should be done-not everything that can be done. Am Rev Respir Dis 145: 508–509
42. Sculier JP, Markiewicz E (1995) Intensive care in anticancer centres: an international inquiry. Support Care Cancer 3:130–134
43. Snow RM, Miller WC, Rice DL, Ali MK (1979) Respiratory failure in cancer patients. JAMA 241:2039–2042
44. Soares M, Darmon M, Salluh JIF, Ferreira CG, Thiery G, Schlemmer B, Spector N, Azoulay E (2007) Prognosis of lung cancer patients with life-threatening complications. Chest 131:840–846
45. Soares M, Salluh JI, Torres VB, Leal JV, Spector N (2008) Short- and long-term outcomes of critically ill patients with cancer and prolonged ICU length of stay. Chest 134(3): 520–526
46. Soubani AO, Kseibi E, Bander JJ, Klein JL, Khanchandani G, Ahmed HP, Guzman JA (2004) Outcome and prognostic factors of hematopoietic stem cell transplantation recipients admitted to a medical ICU. Chest 126:1604–1611
47. Sprung CL, Geber D, Eidelman LA, Baras M, Pizov R, Nimrod A, Oppenheim A, Epstein L, Cotev S (1999) Evaluation of triage decisions for intensive care admission. Crit Care Med 27:1073–1079
48. Staudinger T, Stoiser B, Mullner M, Locker GJ, Laczika K, Knapp S, Burgmann H, Wilfing A, Kofler J, Thalhammer F, Frass M (2000) Outcome and prognostic factors in critically ill cancer patients admitted to the intensive care unit. Crit Care Med 28:1322–1328
49. Taccone FS, Artigas AA, Sprung CL, Moreno R, Sakr Y, Vincent JL (2009 Feb 6) Characteristics and outcomes of cancer patients in European ICUs. Crit Care 13(1):R15

50. Thiery G, Azoulay E, Darmon M, Ciroldi M, De Miranda S, Lévy V, Fieux F, Moreau D, Le Gall JR, Schlemmer B (2005) Outcome of cancer patients considered for intensive care unit admission: a hospital-wide prospective study. J Clin Oncol 23:4406–4413
51. Torrecilla C, Cortes JL, Chamorro C, Rubio JJ, Galdos P, Dominguez de Villota E (1988) Prognostic assessment of the acute complications of bone marrow transplantation requiring intensive therapy. Intensive Care Med 14:393–398
52. Trinkaus MA, Lapinsky SE, Crump M, Keating A, Reece DE, Chen C, Hallett DC, Franke N, Winter A, Mikhael JR (2009) Predictors of mortality in patients undergoing autologous hematopoietic cell transplantation admitted to the intensive care unit. Bone Marrow Transplant 43:411–415
53. Van Keen A, Karstens A, van der Hoek AC, Tibboel D, Hahlen K, van der Voort E (1996) The prognosis of oncologic patients in the pediatric intensive care unit. Intensive Care Med 22:237–241

Managing Critically Ill Cancer Patients: Another Medical Success Story

54

Élie Azoulay, Marcio Soares, Michael Darmon, Dominique Benoit, Stephen Pastores, and Bekele Afessa

Contents

É. Azoulay (✉)
Service de Réanimation Médicale, Hôpital Saint-Louis, 1 avenue Claude Vellefaux, 75010, Paris, France and Medical Intensive Care Units, Saint-Louis Hospital, Paris 7 University, Paris, France
e-mail: elie.azoulay@sls.aphp.fr

M. Soares
Intensive Care Unit and Postgraduate Program, Instituto Nacional de Câncer, Rio de Janeiro, Brazil

M. Darmon
AP-HP, Hôpital Saint-Louis, Medical ICU, 1 avenue Claude Vellefaux, 75010 Paris, France, and Medical ICU, Saint-Etienne University Hospital, 42000, Saint-Etienne, France

D. Benoit
Department of Intensive Care Medicine, Medical Unit, 12K12IB, Ghent University Hospital, De Pintelaan 185, 9000 Gent, Belgium

S. Pastores
Memorial Sloan-Kettering Cancer Center Critical Care Medicine Service, Department of Anesthesiology and Critical Care Medicine, 1275 York Avenue C-1179, New York, NY 10065

B. Afessa
Division of Pulmonary and Critical Care Medicine, Department of Internal Medicine, Mayo Clinic College of Medicine, Rochester, MN 55905, USA

54.1 Introduction

The number of patients living with cancer has been rising [1, 2]. The aging population, improved diagnostic tools, and decrease in cancer-related mortality have contributed to this rise. The age-adjusted invasive cancer incidence rate in the USA is 533.8 per 100,000 population [3]. Over 1.4 million people were projected to be

Supported by a grant from the Assistance-Publique Hôpitaux de Paris (AOM 04139) and the French Society for Intensive Care Medicine. Dr. Soares is supported in part by an individual research grant from CNPq.

É. Azoulay (ed.), *Pulmonary Involvement in Patients with Hematological Malignancies*,
DOI: 10.1007/978-3-642-15742-4_54, © Springer-Verlag Berlin Heidelberg 2011

diagnosed with cancer in the US in 2009 [2]. In Europe, there were an estimated 3,191,600 cancer cases diagnosed and 1,703,000 deaths from cancer in 2006 [4]. In 2005, over 100,000 cases of hematological malignancies were diagnosed in the USA and approximately 230,000 in Europe [3, 5]. Intensive chemotherapy regimens [6] and the use of new and more targeted therapeutic drugs have resulted in high cancer cure rates. However, the treatment often leads to drug-related organ toxicities and increased susceptibility to infection. As a consequence, intensivists are increasingly managing cancer patients admitted to the intensive care unit (ICU) for organ dysfunction [7]. Timely recognition and early ICU admission offer opportunities to prevent and manage cancer-related life-threatening complications, such as tumor lysis syndrome [8], leukostasis [9], and macrophage activation syndrome [10]. Managing organ dysfunction in critically ill cancer patients requires close collaboration between the intensivist and oncologist.

The mortality rates of critically ill cancer patients are not higher compared to critically ill patients with other comorbidities [11]. Recent studies have shown a survival improvement in ICU patients with cancer [12–14]. Health-care providers and patients often discuss the worthiness of life-sustaining treatments in patients with cancer [15]. More recently, the lack of survival benefit in cancer patients admitted to the ICU with multiple organ failure [13, 16] has raised concerns about the timing of ICU admission [7].

In this review, we will appraise the most recent literature on ICU management of cancer patients. We will highlight the following issues: (1) the low survival rate of a subgroup of critically ill cancer patients, despite overall improvement; (2) the need for the development and implementation of broader ICU admission policies; (3) The need to document patients' preferences for resuscitation and end-of-life issues at the time of ICU admission [17].

54.2 Prognosis of Cancer Patients Requiring ICU Support: The Ten Truths

54.2.1 *Short-Term Survival After a Critical Care Illness Has Improved*

Several studies of cancer patients have reported improvement in hospital survival over the last decade [7, 16, 18–21] (Fig. 54.1). Acceptable survival rates have been reported in patients requiring mechanical ventilation [18, 22–24], renal replacement therapy [25–27], and vasopressors [19, 20]. Most of these studies are retrospective and single-centered. Only two prospective multiple center studies have been published [24, 28]. Other limitations of these studies include heterogeneity in patient case mix and ICU admission and discharge criteria as well as the settings and timing for the implementation of end-of-life decisions, making it difficult to compare the results [29] (Tables 54.1 and 54.2).

Four hypotheses have been proposed to explain the decreased mortality rate in critically ill cancer patients [15]: (1) an overall improved survival with the use of a more intense therapeutic regimen and the development of more potent and targeted therapies [30]; (2) improved ICU management with the development of noninvasive diagnostic [28] and therapeutic strategies [18, 31, 32]; (3) ability to make the specific etiological diagnosis in patients with acute respiratory failure [28, 33, 34] and bacterial infection [35]; (4) improved performance status in cancer patients managed using watch and wait policies, or immunotherapy that may be associated with less organ-related toxicity and epithelial and endothelial dysfunction with its increased propensity for cardiovascular, renal, and lung dysfunctions [36].

54.2.2 *Classic Predictors of Mortality Are No Longer Relevant*

Prognostic factors in critically ill cancer patients are often unreliable and are derived from inconsistent results. A British multicenter study of patients with hematologic malignancy admitted to the ICU showed that BMT was a risk factor for increased hospital death [37]. However, among patients with cancer admitted to the ICU, those who underwent autologous BMT had the same prognosis as those who did not [15]. Benoit and colleagues reported neutropenia to be an independent risk factor for increased mortality in ICU patients with hematologic malignancy [12]. However, this finding has been refuted by others [24, 38]. The prognostic importance of other classic mortality predictors, such as age or characteristics of the malignancy, vary among studies and may mainly depend on ICU admission criteria [14, 29]. We recommend not denying ICU admission to elderly patients based on age alone.

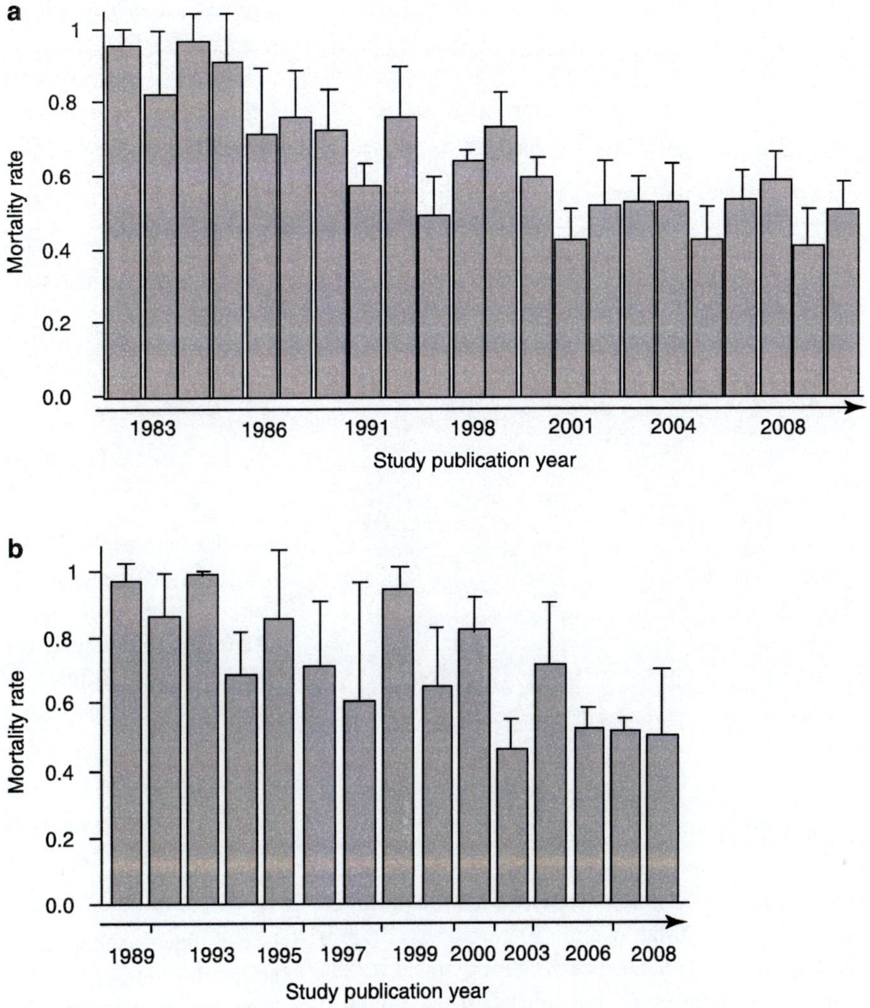

Fig. 54.1 Trends of mortality in critically ill cancer patients over the last 2 decades. (**a**) Unadjusted hospital mortality rates in critically ill cancer patients by year of study publication. (**b**) Unadjusted ICU mortality rates in bone marrow transplant recipients by year of study publication (Adapted from [52]. Permission obtained from Current Opinion in Oncology)

54.2.3 Improved Understanding of Organ Dysfunction

Close collaboration between hematologists/oncologists and intensivists has resulted in an improved understanding of organ dysfunction and probably survival [39]. Clinical experience in managing cancer patients has led to better understanding of acute tumor lysis syndrome [8, 40–42], macrophage activation syndrome [10], and acute respiratory failure [43]. Although the cause-effect relationship cannot be proven, we believe that the improved understanding has translated into better survival (Table 54.2).

54.2.4 Some Groups of Patients Have High and Unchanged Mortality

In addition to bedridden patients and those with no lifespan-expanding therapy (see point 5 below), there are three groups of patients in whom survival rates remain low. These include allogeneic BMT recipients with severe, unresponsive graft-versus-host disease (GVHD) [20], patients with multiple organ failure related to delayed ICU admission [16], and solid tumor patients with pulmonary carcinomatous lymphangitis with acute respiratory failure, carcinomatous meningitis with coma, or bone involvement.

Table 54.1 Prognosis in cancer patients needing intensive care support: the ten truths

1. Short-term survival after critical care illness has improved.
2. Classic predictors of mortality are no longer relevant.
3. Clinicians' understanding of organ dysfunction has improved.
4. Some subgroups of patients continue to have high and unchanged mortality.
5. The usually used triage criteria for ICU admission are ineffective.
6. Three days of ICU management are warranted before making a final decision (ICU trial).
7. Attempt should be made to find a balance between non-invasive treatments and avoiding delays in optimal therapies.
8. Close relationship and collaboration need to be developed between intensivists and hematologist/oncologists to increase skills of all sides in the global management of cancer patients.
9. Early admission to the ICU for cancer patients is recommended.
10. Doing everything that can be done, even cancer chemotherapy, may improve outcome.

Table 54.2 Recent ICU advances in the management of critically ill cancer patients

1. Less restrictive admission policies [13]
2. Noninvasive mechanical ventilation [18, 31, 32]
3. Acute respiratory failure [28, 33, 43, 63]
4. Tumor lysis syndrome [8, 41, 42]
5. Acute kidney injury [25–27]
6. Antifungal agents [64]
7. Transfusion policies [65]
8. Drug-related organ toxicities [66, 67]
9. Macrophage activation syndrome [10]
10. Neurological involvement [21]

Several studies have assessed the outcomes of allogeneic BMT recipients admitted to the ICU over the last 3 decades [44]. Despite careful selection for ICU admission and advances in critical care, the prognosis remains grim, with an overall 1-year survival rate of less than 10% in patients receiving mechanical ventilation [44]. Outcomes are not related to the source of stem cells (bone marrow vs peripheral blood vs cord blood donors), the underlying malignancy for which BMT was performed, or patient-related characteristics such as age or comorbidities. Ten factors have been associated with mortality after a critical care illness, most of them being surrogate markers of GVHD. These are (1) BMT from unrelated donor; (2) GVHD with toxic and infectious complications from immunosuppression; (3) the need for mechanical ventilation; (4) acute respiratory failure and the need for mechanical ventilation 4–6 weeks after BMT (GVHD period, 10% survival); (5) the association of severe sepsis and resistant GVHD; (6) thrombotic microangiopathy by endothelial activation triggered by GVHD, total body irradiation, immunosuppressive regimen and infectious diseases; (7) multiple organ failure in the setting of severe veno-occlusive disease; (8) acute respiratory failure from pulmonary aspergillosis; (9) late non-infectious pulmonary complications including diffuse alveolar hemorrhage [45] and bronchiolitis obliterans [46]; and (10) relapse of the underlying malignancy. Patients developing multiple organ failure are at higher risk for death if their ICU admission is delayed [16]. In patients with multiple myeloma, delayed ICU admission was associated with increased mortality [7].

54.2.5 Triage Criteria That Are Usually Used Are Ineffective

In bedridden patients and in patients with no lifespan-prolonging anti-cancer therapy, care should transition from cure to comfort. However, triage criteria for ICU admission remain ineffective. In a prospective study evaluating the outcomes of patients proposed for ICU admission, 20% of the patients who were not admitted because they were considered "too well" died before hospital discharge (mainly after a delayed ICU admission), and 25% of the patients who were not admitted because they were too sick survived [47]. A striking finding of this study was that it highlighted the inadequacy of the triage criteria and the need for the development and implementation of new ICU admission policies.

54.2.6 At Least 3 Days of ICU Management Before Making End-of-Life Decisions (ICU Trial)

The use of life-sustaining therapies in most cancer patients is no longer futile. However, recent data suggest that the duration of mechanical ventilation, vasopressor administration, and dialysis are strong predictors of death. Identifying patients with no improvement (or with worsening condition) after 3 days of full ICU support may be more effective to appraise outcomes [13, 15]. During the "golden hours" of resuscitation, which are associated with improved outcome, everything should be done. After these golden hours, the continuation or introduction of life-sustaining therapies in patients whose conditions are worsening may not be beneficial.

54.2.7 Finding a Balance Between Non-invasive Treatments and Avoiding Delays in Optimal Therapies

Early ICU admission offers the opportunity to use non-invasive diagnostic tests and non-invasive mechanical ventilation [31, 32]. Although bronchoscopy and BAL can be avoided in a large proportion of patients, those who may benefit should be identified early after admission to the ICU.

54.2.8 Close Relationship and Collaboration Need to Be Developed Between Hematologists and Oncologists to Increase the Skills of Both Sides in the Overall Management of Cancer Patients

Part of the improvement in the outcome of critically ill cancer patients can be attributed to exchange of ideas between intensivists and hemato-oncologists. The hemato-oncologists are able to appraise outcomes and to update the intensivists about therapeutic options and potentials for cure of the underlying malignancies. Intensivists may be more knowledgeable and experienced in setting goals of life-sustaining therapies based on the reversibility of single organ dysfunction. ICU admission decisions as well as decisions to withhold or withdraw life-sustaining therapies should be undertaken by both parties based on the acute medical disease, as well as the underlying disease prognosis and patients' preferences and values.

54.2.9 Early Admission to the ICU for Cancer Patients

We are not aware of any study designed to assess the impact of early ICU admission. Existing data suggest that early admission may improve outcome. Over the past decade, decreased mortality was observed along with earlier ICU admission [7]. There is a linear relationship between the number of organ dysfunctions and patients' mortality, suggesting that patients should best be admitted as early as possible rather than at a time of multiple organ failure.

54.2.10 Doing Everything That Can Be Done, Including Cancer Chemotherapy

When ICU admission is warranted, patients should be treated with a full code status or according to an ICU trial. In both situations, patients receive everything they need during the first few ICU days and then have their situation reappraised after 3–5 days. This full code status includes the administration of cancer chemotherapy along with life-sustaining therapies. Patients with tumor lysis syndrome, pulmonary or renal infiltration by the malignancy, sepsis related to obstructive pneumonia or ureteral compression may require life-sustaining therapies until the cancer chemotherapy becomes effective. Studies have shown the feasibility of administering chemotherapy in the ICU with acceptable short- and long-term outcomes [48, 49]. They have also demonstrated that when patients present with severe sepsis or septic shock after recent chemotherapy, outcomes may be better than in those who did not receive recent cancer chemotherapy [49, 50].

54.3 Broadening ICU Admission Policies and Clarifying the Patient's Code Status at the Time of Admission

Most critically ill cancer patients are admitted to the ICU during the early management period of aggressive malignancies. Some patients with low-grade hematological malignancies may be admitted at any time of their disease course, mainly for infectious or

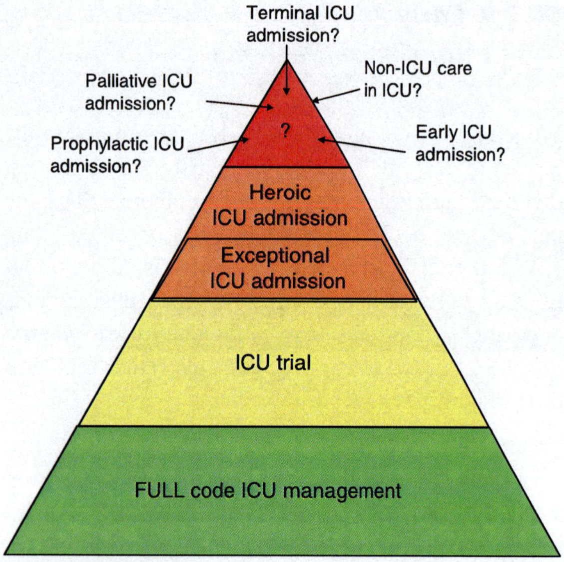

Fig. 54.2 Alternative to ICU refusal in cancer patients proposed for ICU admission

toxic life-threatening complications. Patients with partial remission (myeloma) or high-risk solid tumors (metastatic breast or ovarian cancer) can be admitted at a later course of their disease, even after several courses of chemotherapy, providing significant and sustained response with improved long-term survival [51]. All these patients are admitted to the ICU with a full code status. The decision-making process is similar to that of other ICU patients without malignancy (Fig. 54.2, Table 54.3). We also recommend unrestricted ICU support of allogeneic BMT recipients at the earliest phase of transplantation (before GVHD develops), after 1 year of transplant if they have no or controlled GVHD, and those requiring mechanical ventilation for status epilepticus related to posterior reversible encephalopathy syndrome. It seems reasonable to discourage ICU admission and mechanical ventilation in patients with severe sepsis or acute respiratory failure and uncontrolled GVHD.

Table 54.3 Different ICU admission policies

Type of ICU admission	Code status	Clinical situation
1. Full code ICU management	Full code	Newly diagnosed malignancies; malignancies in complete remission
2. ICU trial	Unlimited for a limited time period that should last at least 3–5 days	Clinical response to therapy not available or undetermined
3. Exceptional ICU admission	Same as ICU trial	Newly available effective therapy that should be tested in a patient who becomes critically ill
4. Heroic ICU admission	ICU management until conflict resolution	Both hematologists/oncologists and intensivists agree that ICU admission is not appropriate, but patients or relatives disagree about the appropriate level of care
5. Other admission modalities that are performed but not yet formally evaluated		
(a) Prophylactic ICU admission	Full code. Intensive clinical and biological monitoring. Invasive procedures under safer conditions	Earliest phase of high-risk malignancies. Admission to the ICU is warranted to avoid development of organ dysfunction (acute respiratory failure, tumor lysis syndrome, etc.)
(b) Early ICU admission	Full code. Intensive clinical and biological monitoring. Invasive procedures under safe conditions	Admission to the ICU in patients with no organ dysfunction but physiological disturbances. ICU is warranted to avoid late ICU admission (a condition associated with higher mortality)
(c) Palliative ICU admission	No life-sustaining therapies. Noninvasive strategies only	Admission to the ICU for the purpose of undergoing noninvasive mechanical ventilation as the ceiling of therapy
(d) In-ICU non ICU care	No life-sustaining therapies	Short ICU admission to help for optimal and prompt management (catheter withdrawal, early antibiotics, etc.)
(e) Terminal ICU admission	No life-sustaining therapies	ICU admission is required to best provide palliative care and symptom control. Controversial issue

In some patients with cancer, the usual ICU admission triage criteria may be ineffective. Nevertheless, establishing the goals of therapy at the time of ICU admission is crucial to optimize their management. The ICU trial is an alternative to ICU refusal in cancer patients [13]. It consists of unlimited ICU support for a limited time, for at least 3–5 days [15]. In a study performed at Saint-Louis Hospital in Paris, France, clinicians made clear to patients and families that the ICU trial was an alternative to ICU refusal and that as soon as the situation was considered irreversible with no hope for survival, the level of care was transitioned from cure to comfort. The major result from this ICU trial was that none of the variables available at ICU admission was significantly different between ICU survivors and non-survivors. Only after day 3, non-survivors had significantly more organ dysfunction than ICU survivors. We advocate the use of the ICU trial in patients with newly diagnosed malignancies, but with a life expectancy of less than 1 year [52]. In the evaluation of the ICU trial [13], survival was 20% overall, but 40% in patients who were alive and in the ICU after day 3.

We suggest three other ICU admission statuses that need to be evaluated (Fig. 54.2, Table 54.3). The first status is the "*exceptional ICU.*" We propose this status of admission for patients in whom severe limitation of the performance status is attributable to the malignancy itself and may improve in response to chemotherapy. Another place for this status is when evidence emerges from new trials that a new effective therapy is available for a patient without lifespan-prolonging therapy. Formal discussions between hemato-oncologists and intensivists must address the statuses of ICU management and the time with which a response to therapy can be expected. As for the ICU trial, patients and relatives must agree with ICU admission and fully grasp its objectives. The second new status of ICU admission that we sometimes adopt is the "*Heroic ICU.*" This is used to resolve conflicts between ICU clinicians and hemato-oncologists, or between clinicians and patients/relatives about the actual prognosis and the appropriate level of care. The philosophy of this type of ICU admission is that 1 or 2 days of ICU management will make the prognosis more evident to create mutual trust. We must bear in mind that if this status of ICU admission is used more than two to three times a year, conflict resolution strategies or attempts to increase the understanding and knowledge about the actual prognoses of malignancies and organ dysfunctions are in order.

The common characteristic of all the previous ICU admission statuses is that patients receive full code management for an unlimited or a limited time. Other admission policies need to be evaluated before specific recommendations are made. Such policies include early ICU admission, prophylactic ICU admission, palliative ICU admission, ICU admission for non-ICU care, and terminal ICU admission (Fig. 54.2, Table 54.3). The terminal admission policy is based on a controversial assumption that the ICU is the best place to die in the hospital and ICU clinicians are skilled at performing adequate palliative care for dying patients. Details on code status are reported in Table 54.3 and Fig. 54.3.

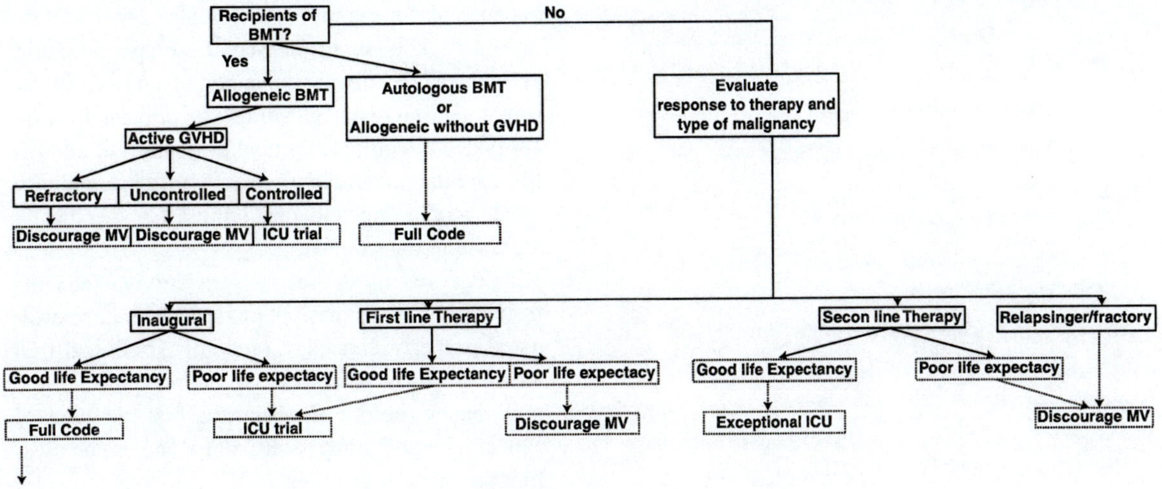

Fig. 54.3 Code status in cancer patients receiving mechanical ventilation

54.4 Unanswered Questions and Research Agenda

Many unanswered questions deserve future observational and interventional studies (Table 54.4). As experts in the management of critically ill cancer patients, we recommend a research agenda to address the following issues:

1. The first issue is the lack of studies on long-term outcomes in cancer patients who survive their ICU stay. The ICU benefits in the overall long-term and disease-free survival are unknown. We do not know whether the improved survival reflects a prolongation of the dying process or an actual increase in survival with good quality of life. Very few studies have addressed ICU survivors' quality of life. Cancer treatment decisions are influenced by the clinical condition of the patient. In critically ill cancer patients, poor performance status may prevent the use of optimally aggressive treatment regimens thereby shortening long-term survival. We need studies evaluating outcomes up to 2 years after critical illness, to investigate survival, treatments that have been implemented, and remission from the malignancy.
2. In addition to physical outcomes, mental health and quality of life outcomes must be assessed in ICU survivors. At this time, no study has specifically evaluated health-related quality of life and post-ICU burden in cancer patients who survived the ICU. Nelson et al. investigated self-reported symptom experience of cancer patients at the time they were receiving intensive care support [53]. Most patients reported experiencing pain, discomfort, anxiety, sleep disturbance, or unsatisfied hunger or thirst. About one third reported depression and dyspnea. Significant pain and discomfort were associated with common ICU procedures. Inability to communicate, sleep disruption, and limitations on visiting were particularly stressful among ICU conditions studied. However, no study has assessed the prevalence of these symptoms 6 months or 1 year after ICU discharge.
3. Studies in relatives of critically ill cancer patients should be performed to seek for specific needs and communication strategies. Determinants of ICU and post-ICU burden on relatives of ICU survivors should be evaluated because relatives of critically ill patients may become actual caregivers.
4. Existing ICU admission criteria need to be described and appraised. New modalities of ICU admission should be evaluated. Controversial issues such as palliative or terminal ICU admission must be discussed at a global level, including patient and family participation. We recognize broadening ICU admission criteria may be obviously associated with increased mortality [54], clinician burnout, demoralization, and further exhausting the limited available resources.
5. One of the most difficult issues in the ICU trial is determining the appropriate time for making end-of-life decisions [17]. Transition from curative to palliative care is complex in cancer patients because of their young age, complex medical conditions, doubts about the actual therapeutic plans, and pressures from consultants and relatives. Implementing new ICU admission policies for cancer patients requires a critical evaluation of end-of-life care that occurs in up to 80% of these patients. Quality of dying and death must be specifically assessed in this context.
6. Although recent studies suggest survival benefits from early ICU admission, this has never been evaluated properly. Indeed, a randomized clinical trial aimed at cancer patients at the earliest phase of the malignancy (before or within the first few days of cancer chemotherapy) with only one organ dysfunction may be in order.

Table 54.4 Unanswered questions and research agenda

1.	Establishing long-term outcomes in oncology and hematology patients who survive their ICU stay. Do we prolong the dying process or do we actually increase survival?
2.	Addressing qualitative outcomes.
3.	Searching for specific family needs and communication strategies.
4.	Evaluating new admission policies.
5.	Improving transition from curative to palliative care.
6.	Evaluating the impact of the ICU on an overall long-term and disease-free survival.
7.	Defining the appropriate timing for ICU admission (avoiding delays).
8.	Appraising prognostic factors of mortality.
9.	Evaluating outcomes in patients receiving intensive care (NIV, vasopressor, etc.) in the wards.
10.	Performing qualitative studies before any recommendation on the use of NIV as the ceiling of therapy.

7. An appraisal of classic prognostic factors is timely. There are data suggesting that neutropenia and autologous BMT may no longer have prognostic importance [24]. New determinants of outcome have emerged from recent studies. These new determinants include our ability to make the actual etiological diagnosis rather than treating empirically [28, 31, 33, 34], delayed ICU admission [7], cytogenetic data in patients with aggressive malignancies [55], and the extent of organ dysfunctions [13, 19]. Future multicenter cohort studies are needed to identify predictors of death in cancer patients admitted to the ICU controlling for the ASSESS criteria that we have recently proposed (Table 54.5) [14].
8. There is emerging interest in adding noninvasive mechanical ventilation (NIV) to routine supportive care provided in hematology/oncology wards. This is partly due to the shortage of ICU beds and ICU physicians' reluctance to admit cancer patients with acute respiratory failure, as well as the unconfirmed assumption that ICU admission may hamper patients' chances of receiving good hematology/oncology care and appropriate infection prevention. We advise caution when implementing NIV in hypoxemic patients with cancer [56]. Unless NIV is the ceiling of therapy [57], we believe NIV should be initiated only in an ICU or high-dependency unit (HDU) setting, where endotracheal intubation and invasive mechanical ventilation can be performed safely and in a timely manner if NIV fails [58].
9. Mortality in patients receiving palliative NIV has been reported in various subgroups of patients [59– 61]. Cancer patients remain poor candidates for palliative NIV, even if some of them may derive some benefit [62]. However, these studies report no qualitative outcomes, including quality of life, ICU burden and quality of dying for the majority of patients who die after NIV. We believe that qualitative studies are mandatory before establishing any recommendation on the use of NIV as the ceiling of therapy in cancer patients.

Table 54.5 The ASSESS approach: a five-step framework for a comprehensive evaluation in studies of ICU patients with cancer (Adapted from [14])

Domain	Description
Triage for ICU *admission*	Triage criteria for ICU admission used by onco-hematologists and intensivists. Detailed evaluation of ICU admission process, including data on the effects of early ICU admission, and also information about non-ICU cancer patients with various levels of organ dysfunction on the wards
Code *status*	Code status to be implemented at ICU admission: full code, ICU trial for a short period (3–5 days with full-code status then re-evaluation), or early provision of palliative care
ICU *support* and patient's *evolution*	Data on ICU management, including reappraisal of the intensity, duration, and nature of life-supporting treatments provided in the ICU. Evaluation of incidence, nature, outcome, and post-ICU residual organ dysfunctions
Survival	Go beyond short- and medium-term survival, by evaluating long-term outcomes (up to 1 year)
Picture of *survivors*	Detailed description of ICU survivors, including qualitative evaluation of the ability to undergo anticancer treatments, disease-free survival, functional status, health-related quality of life, and post-ICU burden (stress-related disorders, anxiety, and depression)

54.5 Conclusions

In cancer patients requiring ICU admission, the survival rate has improved. Besides refinements in the selection criteria of patients for ICU admission, advances in hematology/oncology and ICU management have contributed to this improved survival. In this changing context, clinicians' beliefs regarding the results of ICU management of cancer patients must be appraised. Also, admission policies must be broadened and closely evaluated to avoid depriving patients who may benefit from life-sustaining therapies.

References

1. Coleman MP, Quaresma M, Berrino F, Lutz JM, De Angelis R, Capocaccia R, Baili P, Rachet B, Gatta G, Hakulinen T, Micheli A, Sant M, Weir HK, Elwood JM, Tsukuma H, Koifman S, GA ES, Francisci S, Santaquilani M, Verdecchia A, Storm HH, Young JL (2008) Cancer survival in five continents: a worldwide population-based study (CONCORD). Lancet Oncol 9(8):730–756, Epub 2008 July 17

2. Jemal A, Siegel R, Ward E, Hao Y, Xu J, Murray T, Thun MJ (2008) Cancer statistics, 2008. CA Cancer J Clin 58(2): 71–96, Epub 2008 Feb 20
3. Atlanta: US Department of Health and Human Services CfDCaPaNCI (2010) US Cancer Statistics Working Group. United States Cancer Statistics: 1999–2005 Incidence and Mortality Web-based Report Aug 1. www.cdc.gov/uscs2009
4. Ferlay J, Autier P, Boniol M, Heanue M, Colombet M, Boyle P (2007) Estimates of the cancer incidence and mortality in Europe in 2006. Ann Oncol 18(3):581–592
5. Rodriguez-Abreu D, Bordoni A, Zucca E (2007) Epidemiology of hematological malignancies. Ann Oncol 18(Suppl 1):i3–i8
6. Linker C, Damon L, Ries C, Navarro W (2002) Intensified and shortened cyclical chemotherapy for adult acute lymphoblastic leukemia. J Clin Oncol 20(10):2464–2471
7. Peigne V, Rusinova K, Karlin L, Darmon M, Fermand JP, Schlemmer B, Azoulay E (2009) Continued survival gains in recent years among critically ill myeloma patients. Intensive Care Med 35(3):512–518
8. Darmon M, Guichard I, Vincent F, Schlemmer B, Azoulay E (2010) Prognostic significance of acute renal injury in acute tumor lysis syndrome. Leuk Lymphoma 51(2):221–227
9. Azoulay E, Fieux F, Moreau D, Thiery G, Rousselot P, Parrot A, Le Gall JR, Dombret H, Schlemmer B (2003) Acute monocytic leukemia presenting as acute respiratory failure. Am J Respir Crit Care Med 167(10):1329–1333
10. Creput C, Galicier L, Buyse S, Azoulay E (2008) Understanding organ dysfunction in hemophagocytic lymphohistiocytosis. Intensive Care Med 34(7):1177–1187
11. Tanvetyanon T, Leighton JC (2003) Life-sustaining treatments in patients who died of chronic congestive heart failure compared with metastatic cancer. Crit Care Med 31(1):60–64
12. Benoit DD, Vandewoude KH, Decruyenaere JM, Hoste EA, Colardyn FA (2003) Outcome and early prognostic indicators in patients with a hematologic malignancy admitted to the intensive care unit for a life-threatening complication. Crit Care Med 31(1):104–112
13. Lecuyer L, Chevret S, Thiery G, Darmon M, Schlemmer B, Azoulay E (2007) The ICU trial: a new admission policy for cancer patients requiring mechanical ventilation. Crit Care Med 35(3):808–814
14. Soares M, Azoulay E (2009) Critical care management of lung cancer patients to prolong life without prolonging dying. Intensive Care Med 35(12):2012–2014
15. Azoulay E, Afessa B (2006) The intensive care support of patients with malignancy: do everything that can be done. Intensive Care Med 32(1):3–5, Epub 2005 Nov 25
16. Khassawneh BY, White P Jr, Anaissie EJ, Barlogie B, Hiller FC (2002) Outcome from mechanical ventilation after autologous peripheral blood stem cell transplantation. Chest 121(1):185–188
17. Gaeta S, Price KJ (2010) End-of-life issues in critically ill cancer patients. Crit Care Clin 26(1):219–227
18. Azoulay E, Alberti C, Bornstain C, Leleu G, Moreau D, Recher C, Chevret S, Le Gall JR, Brochard L, Schlemmer B (2001) Improved survival in cancer patients requiring mechanical ventilatory support: impact of noninvasive mechanical ventilatory support. Crit Care Med 29(3): 519–525
19. Larche J, Azoulay E, Fieux F, Mesnard L, Moreau D, Thiery G, Darmon M, Le Gall JR, Schlemmer B (2003) Improved survival of critically ill cancer patients with septic shock. Intensive Care Med 29(10):1688–1695, Epub 2003 Sep 12
20. Pene F, Aubron C, Azoulay E, Blot F, Thiery G, Raynard B, Schlemmer B, Nitenberg G, Buzyn A, Arnaud P, Socie G, Mira JP (2006) Outcome of critically ill allogeneic hematopoietic stem-cell transplantation recipients: a reappraisal of indications for organ failure supports. J Clin Oncol 24(4):643–649, Epub 2005 Dec 27
21. Legriel S, Marijon H, Darmon M, Lemiale V, Bedos JP, Schlemmer B, Azoulay E (2010) Central neurological complications in critically ill patients with malignancies. Intensive Care Med 36(2):232–240
22. Soares M, Salluh JI, Spector N, Rocco JR (2005) Characteristics and outcomes of cancer patients requiring mechanical ventilatory support for >24 h. Crit Care Med 33(3):520–526
23. Depuydt PO, Benoit DD, Vandewoude KH, Decruyenaere JM, Colardyn FA (2004) Outcome in noninvasively and invasively ventilated hematologic patients with acute respiratory failure. Chest 126(4):1299–1306
24. Soares M, Caruso P, Silva E, Teles JM, Lobo SM, Friedman G, Dal Pizzol F, Mello PV, Bozza FA, Silva UV, Torelly AP, Knibel MF, Rezende E, Netto JJ, Piras C, Castro A, Ferreira BS, Rea-Neto A, Olmedo PB, Salluh JI (2010) Characteristics and outcomes of patients with cancer requiring admission to intensive care units: a prospective multicenter study. Crit Care Med 38(1):9–15
25. Benoit DD, Hoste EA, Depuydt PO, Offner FC, Lameire NH, Vandewoude KH, Dhondt AW, Noens LA, Decruyenaere JM (2005) Outcome in critically ill medical patients treated with renal replacement therapy for acute renal failure: comparison between patients with and those without haematological malignancies. Nephrol Dial Transplant 20(3): 552–558, Epub 2005 Jan 25
26. Darmon M, Thiery G, Ciroldi M, Porcher R, Schlemmer B, Azoulay E (2007) Should dialysis be offered to cancer patients with acute kidney injury? Intensive Care Med 33(5): 765–772
27. Soares M, Salluh JI, Carvalho MS, Darmon M, Rocco JR, Spector N (2006) Prognosis of critically ill patients with cancer and acute renal dysfunction. J Clin Oncol 24(24): 4003–4010
28. Azoulay E, Mokart D, Rabbat A, Pene F, Kouatchet A, Bruneel F, Vincent F, Hamidfar R, Moreau D, Mohammedi I, Epinette G, Beduneau G, Castelain V, de Lassence A, Gruson D, Lemiale V, Renard B, Chevret S, Schlemmer B (2008) Diagnostic bronchoscopy in hematology and oncology patients with acute respiratory failure: prospective multicenter data. Crit Care Med 36(1):100–107
29. Massion PB, Dive AM, Doyen C, Bulpa P, Jamart J, Bosly A, Installe E (2002) Prognosis of hematologic malignancies does not predict intensive care unit mortality. Crit Care Med 30(10):2260–2270
30. Brenner H, Gondos A, Arndt V (2007) Recent major progress in long-term cancer patient survival disclosed by modeled period analysis. J Clin Oncol 25(22):3274–3280
31. Hilbert G, Gruson D, Vargas F, Valentino R, Chene G, Boiron JM, Pigneux A, Reiffers J, Gbikpi-Benissan G, Cardinaud JP (2000) Noninvasive continuous positive airway

pressure in neutropenic patients with acute respiratory failure requiring intensive care unit admission. Crit Care Med 28(9):3185–3190
32. Hilbert G, Gruson D, Vargas F, Valentino R, Gbikpi-Benissan G, Dupon M, Reiffers J, Cardinaud JP (2001) Noninvasive ventilation in immunosuppressed patients with pulmonary infiltrates, fever, and acute respiratory failure. N Engl J Med 344(7):481–487
33. Azoulay E, Thiery G, Chevret S, Moreau D, Darmon M, Bergeron A, Yang K, Meignin V, Ciroldi M, Le Gall JR, Tazi A, Schlemmer B (2004) The prognosis of acute respiratory failure in critically ill cancer patients. Medicine (Baltimore) 83(6):360–370
34. Hilbert G, Gruson D, Vargas F, Valentino R, Favier JC, Portel L, Gbikpi-Benissan G, Cardinaud JP (2001) Bronchoscopy with bronchoalveolar lavage via the laryngeal mask airway in high-risk hypoxemic immunosuppressed patients. Crit Care Med 29(2):249–255
35. Benoit DD, Depuydt PO, Peleman RA, Offner FC, Vandewoude KH, Vogelaers DP, Blot SI, Noens LA, Colardyn FA, Decruyenaere JM (2005) Documented and clinically suspected bacterial infection precipitating intensive care unit admission in patients with hematological malignancies: impact on outcome. Intensive Care Med 31(7):934–942
36. Ardeshna KM, Smith P, Norton A, Hancock BW, Hoskin PJ, MacLennan KA, Marcus RE, Jelliffe A, Vaughan G, Hudson, Linch DC (2003) Long-term effect of a watch and wait policy versus immediate systemic treatment for asymptomatic advanced-stage non-Hodgkin lymphoma: a randomised controlled trial. Lancet 362(9383):516–522
37. Hampshire PA, Welch CA, McCrossan LA, Francis K, Harrison DA (2009) Admission factors associated with hospital mortality in patients with haematological malignancy admitted to UK adult, general critical care units: a secondary analysis of the ICNARC Case Mix Programme Database. Crit Care 13(4):R137
38. Meyer S, Gortner L, Gottschling S (2008) Comment on "impact of recent intravenous chemotherapy on outcome in severe sepsis and septic shock patients with haematological malignancies" by Vandijck et al. Intensive Care Med 34(10):1929; author reply 1930–1931
39. Azoulay E, Recher C, Alberti C, Soufir L, Leleu G, Le Gall JR, Fermand JP, Schlemmer B (1999) Changing use of intensive care for hematological patients: the example of multiple myeloma. Intensive Care Med 25(12):1395–1401
40. Wossmann W, Schrappe M, Meyer U, Zimmermann M, Reiter A (2003) Incidence of tumor lysis syndrome in children with advanced stage Burkitt's lymphoma/leukemia before and after introduction of prophylactic use of urate oxidase. Ann Hematol 82(3):160–165
41. Coiffier B, Altman A, Pui CH, Younes A, Cairo MS (2008) Guidelines for the management of pediatric and adult tumor lysis syndrome: an evidence-based review. J Clin Oncol 26(16):2767–2778
42. Tosi P, Barosi G, Lazzaro C, Liso V, Marchetti M, Morra E, Pession A, Rosti G, Santoro A, Zinzani PL, Tura S (2008) Consensus conference on the management of tumor lysis syndrome. Haematologica 93(12):1877–1885
43. Azoulay E, Schlemmer B (2006) Diagnostic strategy in cancer patients with acute respiratory failure. Intensive Care Med 32(6):808–822, Epub 2006 Apr 29
44. Afessa B, Azoulay E (2010) Critical care of the hematopoietic stem cell transplant recipient. Crit Care Clin 26(1):133–150
45. Afessa B, Tefferi A, Litzow MR, Peters SG (2002) Outcome of diffuse alveolar hemorrhage in hematopoietic stem cell transplant recipients. Am J Respir Crit Care Med 166(10):1364–1368
46. Afessa B, Litzow MR, Tefferi A (2001) Bronchiolitis obliterans and other late onset non-infectious pulmonary complications in hematopoietic stem cell transplantation. Bone Marrow Transplant 28(5):425–434
47. Thiery G, Azoulay E, Darmon M, Ciroldi M, De Miranda S, Levy V, Fieux F, Moreau D, Le Gall JR, Schlemmer B (2005) Outcome of cancer patients considered for intensive care unit admission: a hospital-wide prospective study. J Clin Oncol 23(19):4406–4413
48. Darmon M, Thiery G, Ciroldi M, de Miranda S, Galicier L, Raffoux E, Le Gall JR, Schlemmer B, Azoulay E (2005) Intensive care in patients with newly diagnosed malignancies and a need for cancer chemotherapy. Crit Care Med 33(11):2488–2493
49. Benoit DD, Depuydt PO, Vandewoude KH, Offner FC, Boterberg T, De Cock CA, Noens LA, Janssens AM, Decruyenaere JM (2006) Outcome in severely ill patients with hematological malignancies who received intravenous chemotherapy in the intensive care unit. Intensive Care Med 32(1):93–99
50. Vandijck DM, Benoit DD, Depuydt PO, Offner FC, Blot SI, Van Tilborgh AK, Nollet J, Steel E, Noens LA, Decruyenaere JM (2008) Impact of recent intravenous chemotherapy on outcome in severe sepsis and septic shock patients with hematological malignancies. Intensive Care Med 34(5): 847–855
51. Kinsey T, Jemal A, Liff J, Ward E, Thun M (2008) Secular trends in mortality from common cancers in the United States by educational attainment, 1993-2001. J Natl Cancer Inst 100(14):1003–1012, Epub 2008 July 8
52. Darmon M, Azoulay E (2009) Critical care management of cancer patients: cause for optimism and need for objectivity. Curr Opin Oncol 21(4):318–326
53. Nelson JE, Meier DE, Oei EJ, Nierman DM, Senzel RS, Manfredi PL, Davis SM, Morrison RS (2001) Self-reported symptom experience of critically ill cancer patients receiving intensive care. Crit Care Med 29(2):277–282
54. Azoulay E, Timsit JF, Sprung CL, Soares M, Rusinova K, Lafabrie A, Abizanda R, Svantesson M, Rubulotta F, Ricou B, Benoit D, Heyland D, Joynt G, Francais A, Azeivedo-Maia P, Owczuk R, Benbenishty J, de Vita M, Valentin A, Ksomos A, Cohen S, Kompan L, Ho K, Abroug F, Kaarlola A, Gerlach H, Kyprianou T, Michalsen A, Chevret S, Schlemmer B (2009) Prevalence and factors of intensive care unit conflicts: the conflicus study. Am J Respir Crit Care Med 180(9):853–860
55. Prebet T, Boissel N, Reutenauer S, Thomas X, Delaunay J, Cahn JY, Pigneux A, Quesnel B, Witz F, Thepot S, Ugo V, Terre C, Recher C, Tavernier E, Hunault M, Esterni B, Castaigne S, Guilhot F, Dombret H, Vey N (2009) Acute myeloid leukemia with translocation (8;21) or inversion (16) in elderly patients treated with conventional chemotherapy: a collaborative study of the French CBF-AML intergroup. J Clin Oncol 27(28):4747–4753

56. Truwit JD, Bernard GR (2004) Noninvasive ventilation–don't push too hard. N Engl J Med 350(24):2512–2515
57. Tanvetyanon T (2004) Which patient with a do-not-intubate order is a candidate for noninvasive ventilation? Crit Care Med 32(10):2148–2150
58. Adda M, Coquet I, Darmon M, Thiery G, Schlemmer B, Azoulay E (2008) Predictors of noninvasive ventilation failure in patients with hematologic malignancy and acute respiratory failure. Crit Care Med 36(10):2766–2772
59. Cuomo A, Delmastro M, Ceriana P, Nava S, Conti G, Antonelli M, Iacobone E (2004) Noninvasive mechanical ventilation as a palliative treatment of acute respiratory failure in patients with end-stage solid cancer. Palliat Med 18(7):602–610
60. Curtis JR, Cook DJ, Sinuff T, White DB, Hill N, Keenan SP, Benditt JO, Kacmarek R, Kirchhoff KT, Levy MM (2007) Noninvasive positive pressure ventilation in critical and palliative care settings: understanding the goals of therapy. Crit Care Med 35(3):932–939
61. Levy M, Tanios MA, Nelson D, Short K, Senechia A, Vespia J, Hill NS (2004) Outcomes of patients with do-not-intubate orders treated with noninvasive ventilation. Crit Care Med 32(10):2002–2007
62. Meert AP, Berghmans T, Hardy M, Markiewicz E, Sculier JP (2006) Non-invasive ventilation for cancer patients with life-support techniques limitation. Support Care Cancer 14(2):167–171, Epub 2005 Jun 10
63. Rano A, Agusti C, Jimenez P, Angrill J, Benito N, Danes C, Gonzalez J, Rovira M, Pumarola T, Moreno A, Torres A (2001) Pulmonary infiltrates in non-HIV immunocompromised patients: a diagnostic approach using non-invasive and bronchoscopic procedures. Thorax 56(5):379–387
64. Herbrecht R, Denning DW, Patterson TF, Bennett JE, Greene RE, Oestmann JW, Kern WV, Marr KA, Ribaud P, Lortholary O, Sylvester R, Rubin RH, Wingard JR, Stark P, Durand C, Caillot D, Thiel E, Chandrasekar PH, Hodges MR, Schlamm HT, Troke PF, de Pauw B (2002) Voriconazole versus amphotericin B for primary therapy of invasive aspergillosis. N Engl J Med 347(6):408–415
65. Hebert PC, Wells G, Blajchman MA, Marshall J, Martin C, Pagliarello G, Tweeddale M, Schweitzer I, Yetisir E (1999) A multicenter, randomized, controlled clinical trial of transfusion requirements in critical care. Transfusion Requirements in Critical Care Investigators, Canadian Critical Care Trials Group. N Engl J Med 340(6):409–417
66. Chagnon K, Boissel N, Raffoux E, Dombret H, Tazi A, Bergeron A (2009) A new pattern of cytosine-arabinoside-induced lung toxicity. Br J Haematol 147(5):771–774
67. Bergeron A, Rea D, Levy V, Picard C, Meignin V, Tamburini J, Bruzzoni-Giovanelli H, Calvo F, Tazi A, Rousselot P (2007) Lung abnormalities after dasatinib treatment for chronic myeloid leukemia: a case series. Am J Respir Crit Care Med 176(8):814–818

Palliative Care and Dyspnea Management in Patients with Hematological Malignancies and Acute Respiratory Failure

55

Amy P. Abernethy, Jane L. Wheeler, and David C. Currow

Contents

A.P. Abernethy (✉)
Division of Medical Oncology, Department of Medicine, Duke University Medicine Center, Durham, NC 27710, USA and
Department of Palliative and Supportive Services, Division of Medicine, Flinders University, Bedford Park, South Australia, Australia
e-mail: amy.abernethy@duke.edu

J.L. Wheeler
Division of Medical Oncology, Department of Medicine, Duke University Medicine Center, Durham, NC 27710, USA
e-mail: jane.wheeler@duke.edu

D.C. Currow
Department of Palliative and Supportive Services, Division of Medicine, Flinders University, Adelaide, South Australia, Australia
e-mail: david.currow@health.sa.gov.au

55.1 Introduction

Among patients with hematological malignancies, acute respiratory failure (ARF) exacts a huge toll. The incidence of ARF in patients with acute leukemia or lymphoma ranges from 10% to 20%; this proportion increases to approximately 50% in patients with neutropenia or bone marrow transplantation [1, 2]. ARF is the most common reason for admitting hematological patients to the intensive care setting [3–5], and prognosis at this point is poor [6], with an overall mortality rate of more than 50%. Higher mortality rates (75–85%) occur among patients who have undergone allogeneic bone marrow transplantation or who require mechanical ventilation [6–9].

Although life-saving medical intervention is appropriate for a small percentage of selected patients with hematological malignancies and ARF [6, 9], in the majority of cases the clinical emphasis shifts toward palliation. In the palliative care phase, the goals of care shift from cure of disease to improvement of the patient's experience of living and of dying, and optimization of the patient's quality of life (QOL). Among the multiple symptoms that require careful management in the context of palliative care, dyspnea (breathlessness), which frequently accompanies respiratory failure, is particularly prevalent and distressing for cancer patients entering the last stages of life. Patients whose dyspnea cannot be alleviated through further treatment of their illness are said to have "intractable" or "refractory" dyspnea [10]. At this point, palliative care focuses on relief of breathlessness and improvement in function, rather than extension of survival.

É. Azoulay (ed.), *Pulmonary Involvement in Patients with Hematological Malignancies*,
DOI: 10.1007/978-3-642-15742-4_55, © Springer-Verlag Berlin Heidelberg 2011

55.2 Dyspnea

A consensus panel of the American Thoracic Society has described dyspnea as follows: "a subjective experience of breathing discomfort that consists of qualitatively distinct sensations that vary in intensity. The experience derives from interactions among multiple physiological, psychological, social, and environmental factors, and may induce secondary physiological and behavioral responses" [11]. Building on earlier efforts to develop a working definition of dyspnea, Harver et al. identified three dimensions of breathlessness: depth and frequency of breathing, perceived urge of need to breathe, and difficulty breathing and phase of respiration [12]. The experience of dyspnea arises from activation of neural pathways, inflected by the patient-specific perception [11]. The physical mechanisms and parameters of dyspnea have proven difficult to define; the phenomenon contains a significant subjective component; and factors such as underlying disease, racial/ethnic background, previous experience, and emotional state further influence the individual patient's experience of this distressing symptom.

55.2.1 Assessment

The subjective intensity of dyspnea can be assessed with single-item scales such as a visual analogue scale (VAS), numerical rating scale (NRS), or modified Borg scale. These scales are useful in the clinical setting, enabling longitudinal within-patient monitoring of dyspnea, its course, and therapeutic response. The functional impact of breathlessness can be gauged by physical measurements, such as a 6-min walking test or shuttle test, or through categorical functional scales (e.g., the Medical Research Council Dyspnea Scale). The Cancer Dyspnea Scale (CDS) was recently developed by Tanaka et al. to define dyspnea from the patient's perspective, including effort, anxiety, and discomfort; it can be easily deployed in real-world clinical settings [13]. The CDS was originally developed and validated in Japanese; an English-language validation study has recently been completed.

55.2.2 Mechanisms

While the pathophysiological mechanisms involved in its development remain unclear, dyspnea is currently understood to result from a mismatch of respiratory motor activity and incoming afferent activity, including information from chemo-, vagal, mechano-, pulmonary stretch, and muscle receptors [11]. The mechanistic interactions among these factors have yet to be mapped, and certain puzzling scenarios imply the involvement of additional factors. For example, dyspnea is associated with an increase in $PaCO_2$ and a decrease in the detection of PaO_2 and/or pH by peripheral chemoreceptors; however, many patients with abnormal blood gas levels do not experience dyspnea, and many dyspneic patients have normal blood gas levels [14–16].

55.3 Palliative Care for Intractable Dyspnea

In palliative care, minimization of symptom burden and enhancement of quality of life (QOL) replace cure and extension of survival as the primary treatment goals. For dyspneic patients, palliative interventions specifically aim to alleviate the patient's sensation of breathlessness and/or to improve his or her functional status. From this perspective, the fact that patients often complain of dyspnea that seems out of proportion to their objective physical disability or functional impairment is irrelevant. In determining what symptoms are to be treated in the palliative care setting, the clinician prioritizes *the patient's report* of his/her experience, then chooses the palliative approaches that best address these self-reported symptoms and, correspondingly, improve the patient's QOL.

55.4 Pharmacological Interventions

Approaches to management of refractory dyspnea have focused on several primary options: opioids, psychotropic drugs, inhaled frusemide, and Heliox 28 [17]. Current evidence supports the use of opioids (oral, parenteral), but the data remain insufficient with regard to nebulized opioids, anxiolytics, selective serotonin reuptake inhibitors (SSRIs), inhaled frusemide (also known as furosemide), or Heliox28. The data do not support use of phenothiazines.

55.4.1 Oral and Parenteral Opioids

Although opioids have long been used to alleviate intractable dyspnea, this practice remains controversial, safety being the primary concern, due to risk of respiratory depression [18, 19]. The mechanism of action of opioids in alleviating dyspnea is poorly understood; they may act centrally, peripherally, or by reducing anxiety [20].

Opioids diminish ventilatory response to carbon dioxide [21], hypoxia [22, 23], inspiratory flow-resistive loading [24], and exercise. Morphine has been shown to reduce oxygen consumption in healthy individuals both at rest and during exercise [25]. According to a systematic review and meta-analysis, oral and parenteral opioids produce a statistically significant effect on the sensation of breathlessness (overall pooled effect size –0.31, 95% confidence interval [CI] –0.50 to –0.13, $p=0.0008$), although the clinical effect was relatively small (approximately 8 mm on a 100 mm VAS with baseline levels of dyspnea of 50 mm) [26]. The authors proposed several reasons for this minimal effect: opioid doses were often low, doses were not titrated, dosing intervals were long, and single-dose studies would fail to achieve steady state. In their analyses, the use of opioids was not associated with changes in arterial blood gas measurements or oxygen saturation.

A subsequent trial assessed oral morphine's effect on intractable dyspnea among opioid-naïve adults [10]. Forty-eight outpatients with refractory dyspnea were enrolled in an 8-day, randomized, double-blind, crossover study of 20 mg once-daily sustained-release oral morphine sulfate or placebo. The primary outcome was the sensation of breathlessness measured on a 100 mm VAS. Participants were elderly (mean age 76, standard deviation [SD] 5); 71% were receiving oxygen therapy; the mean baseline morning dyspnea score was 43 (SD 26). Patients receiving morphine experienced a significant decrease in dyspnea, with mean improvements in dyspnea intensity of 6.6 mm in the morning ($p=0.011$) and 9.5 mm in the evening ($p=0.006$), a relative improvement over baseline dyspnea of 15–22%. Morphine did not depress the respiratory rate (RR; mean RR for morphine vs placebo = 20 [SD 5] vs 21 [SD 4], $p=0.143$). No episodes of severe sedation or obtundation were recorded. The primary side effect was constipation (9 vs 1, $p=0.021$), but neither treatment caused more vomiting, confusion, sedation, or appetite suppression. Patients who received morphine described better sleep at night ($p=0.039$).

In practice, for opioid-naïve patients with refractory dyspnea, clinicians initiate treatment with a 20-mg, once daily, sustained-release, oral morphine preparation (provided the patient has no contraindication to morphine). Alternatively, if this preparation is unavailable, clinicians can substitute a 15-mg, twice daily, long-acting morphine product, initially administered once per day; after 5–7 days, the treatment can be increased to twice daily if the medication is well-tolerated and the patient is experiencing residual breathlessness. For patients who have a contraindication to morphine, clinicians prescribe long-acting oxycodone, starting at 10 mg once a day and, after 5–7 days, increasing to twice a day as tolerated and needed. As an alternative, hydromorphone can be used in analgesic doses equal to 20–30 mg of morphine around the clock. The 25-µg fentanyl transdermal patch provides over 80 morphine equivalents per day, so it is not advisable to begin with this approach. For opioid-tolerant patients already receiving regular doses of morphine or opioids, clinicians can sequentially increase the opioid dose by 20% of the total daily dose every 3–5 days until the breathlessness is relieved or side effects occur [27].

55.4.2 Psychotropic Drugs

In the treatment of refractory dyspnea, the use of psychotropic agents is based on two assumptions: that dyspnea involves a significant psychological component and that anxiety contributes substantially to the functional impairment associated with dyspnea [28]. The principal psychotropic agents used in the management of dyspnea are anxiolytics, phenothiazines, and selective serotonin reuptake inhibitors (SSRIs).

55.4.2.1 Benzodiazepines

Benzodiazepine studies in the context of dyspnea have been small scale and somewhat inconclusive. While an exploratory study found diazepam to have beneficial effects in four patients [29], two subsequent studies failed to replicate these results [30, 31]. Several other studies investigated the efficacy of alprazolam, a shorter acting and potentially less-sedating medication than diazepam; one controlled study found no improvement in breathlessness [32], whereas a case report did document benefit [33]. In a randomized controlled trial of terminally ill cancer patients given morphine 2.5 mg every 4 h, midazolam 5.0 mg every 4 h, or the combination, the combined intervention was the most effective in alleviating breathlessness [34]. Side effects, especially sedation, were most problematic in the morphine-only arm, which may have been due to the bolus rescue doses provided in accordance with the study protocol. These patients were quite near the end of life, and the results may not be applicable earlier in the palliative care period.

When anxiety obviously and substantially aggravates dyspnea, the clinician can prescribe benzodiazepines. Midazolam carries risk and may be disallowed in some clinical areas, so alprazolam is generally preferable as a short-acting product, and clonazepam is acceptable for longer-acting control.

55.4.2.2 Other Anxiolytics

The serotonergic anxiolytic agent buspirone has been shown in animal studies to be a respiratory stimulant [35, 36]. Two small studies evaluated the effects of buspirone on breathlessness, exercise tolerance, and anxiety in human patients with severe COPD [37, 38]. Although these studies included slightly different patient populations (only one of the studies required baseline anxiety among its eligibility criteria) and yielded conflicting results (one finding improvement in all three domains, the other finding no difference), the data nevertheless suggest that anxiolytic agents may have a possible role in selected patients with refractory dyspnea.

In clinical practice, it is advisable to conduct an "n of 1" trial for patients who are potential candidates for anxiolytics, as well as other interventions for refractory dyspnea, carefully monitoring each patient for benefit (relief of breathlessness, improvement in function) without undue adverse effects. When an identical-looking placebo is unavailable, the best option may be a single-sided "n of 1" trial, with outcomes documented thoroughly for clinician review in concert with the patient and caregivers.

55.4.2.3 Selective Serotonin Reuptake Inhibitors (SSRIs)

SSRIs first attracted attention in the 1990s for their potential to alleviate breathlessness. A pilot study found that 6 weeks of sertraline resulted in symptom improvement in six patients (three of whom had psychiatric disorders) [39]. In a series of case studies, seven patients with obstructive lung disease, three of whom met criteria for panic disorder, were treated with sertraline; while no formal measures were performed, all patients reported a decrease in breathlessness, and several additionally reported improved exercise tolerance [40].

SSRIs may improve dyspnea and exercise tolerance by direct influence on respiration, by relieving anxiety symptoms, or both. Many patients whose dyspnea seems disproportionate to their measurable pulmonary compromise also experience depression and/or anxiety; data suggest that dyspnea responds to treatment of these symptoms [41]. According to data from animal research, serotonin may act at the level of the brainstem respiratory center, which could in turn affect the sensation of breathlessness [42]. However, current evidence is insufficient to indicate SSRIs for relief of dyspnea in the absence of an underlying psychiatric diagnosis.

55.4.2.4 Inhaled Frusemide

Due to its low chloride content, frusemide inhibits the cough response [43], and it exerts a preventive effect on bronchoconstriction in patients with asthma [44–46]. Inhaled frusemide may also act indirectly on the vagally mediated sensory nerve ending in the airway epithelium [47]. Inhaled frusemide has been studied in healthy individuals [48] and in COPD patients [49]. In healthy individuals, inhaled frusemide increases breath-holding time and the period of no respiratory sensation, slowing as well the onset of discomfort during loaded breathing [48]. Examining 42 articles published between 1988 and 2004, one systematic review reported that, while nebulized frusemide appeared to have a positive effect on the symptom of dyspnea and its physiological measurements, such data have thus far been generated only by small-scale clinical trials or observation trials [50]. While frusemide appears promising as an intervention for dyspnea, more evidence is required to sufficiently establish its benefit.

55.4.2.5 Heliox28

Heliox28 is a mixed gas comprising 72% helium and 28% oxygen. A Phase II crossover trial involving 12 lung cancer patients with intractable dyspnea evaluated breathlessness during a 6-min walk test while the participants breathed either Heliox28, 28% oxygen, or medical air [51]. These patients rated their breathlessness significantly lower on a VAS when breathing Heliox28 compared to medical air (40.2% [SD 4.8] vs 59.3% [SD 5.3], $p<0.05$); the same patients reported no significant difference (VAS, Borg) in breathlessness when they breathed Heliox28 vs oxygen (47.0% [SD 5.6]) or oxygen vs medical air. Patients walked farther when breathing Heliox28 (214.2 m [SD 9.6]) than they did when breathing either oxygen (174.6 m [SD 11.2], $p<0.05$) or medical air (128.8 m [SD 10.3], $p<0.0001$). While these results suggest that Heliox28 may have some role in managing refractory dyspnea, the evidence remains limited.

55.5 Oxygen Therapy

Long-term oxygen therapy is indicated for patients with severe hypoxemia (resting $PaO_2 \leq 55$ mmHg); in this setting, it improves survival, dyspnea, and functional status [52–54]. For patients approaching the end of life, palliative oxygen is often prescribed to manage breathlessness regardless of PaO_2 levels [55, 56]. More than 70% of physicians caring for palliative care patients with dyspnea report prescribing oxygen, usually for refractory symptoms (65%) or at patient request (30%); [57] in one study, over 40% of patients who were administered long-term oxygen therapy failed to meet current therapeutic guidelines [53].

Belief in the effectiveness of palliative oxygen for the alleviation of breathlessness is widespread. Of 214 respondents to an e-mail survey of palliative care specialists and respiratory physicians in Australia and New Zealand, 58% reported a belief that palliative oxygen is beneficial (69% of palliative medicine clinicians and 48% of respiratory physicians surveyed); 65% cited intractable dyspnea as the most common reason for prescription [57]. Similar convictions were reported among Canadian clinicians [58].

An international double-blind randomized controlled trial assessed the effectiveness of palliative oxygen vs medical (room) air, delivered by concentrator, for relief of breathlessness in patients with end-stage illness, refractory dyspnea, and PaO_2 >55 mmHg (manuscript submitted [68]). Patients were recruited from outpatient pulmonary, palliative care, oncology, and primary care clinics at nine sites in Australia, the United States, and England; of the 239 participants, 64% had COPD. Neither medical gas proved superior. Over the 7-day intervention period, mean morning and evening dyspnea scores on a 0–10 numerical rating scale (NRS) decreased by –0.81 (SD 2.6) and –0.40 (SD 2.1), respectively ($p<0.001$), regardless of intervention, reflecting 18% and 9% relative improvement with either medical gas. QOL showed parallel improvement ($p<0.001$). Most improvement in dyspnea occurred within the first 3 days; for example, 55% of improvement in evening dyspnea took place in the first 24 h, 88% in the first 72 h. Baseline dyspnea predicted improvement; participants with moderate (4–6 NRS) and severe (7–10 NRS) baseline dyspnea experienced average decreases in morning dyspnea of 1.0 and 1.3, respectively. The results of this study suggest that a medical gas may help some patients, particularly those who present with more severe baseline breathlessness, and that a 3–4 day therapeutic trial should effectively identify patients who may benefit.

Current standard practice is to first establish the goals of therapy (e.g., alleviation of breathlessness, improvement in function, improvement in QOL), then to determine the optimal course of therapy for the individual patient, guided by best available evidence. Ideally, a blinded "n of 1" trial will help to determine effectiveness of the selected treatment option for patients who are candidates for pharmacologic agents; in these cases, the clinician should carefully monitor for benefit, burden, and adverse effects. When placebos are not available, clinicians should consider a single-sided n of 1 trial in which they carefully document outcomes in concert with the patient and caregiver(s).

An n of 1trial, applied to palliative oxygen therapy, might proceed as follows: The patient is randomly assigned to receive either oxygen or medical air from a concentrator, via nasal cannulae. The patient's assignment is not revealed to the clinician, patient, or caregiver. A respiratory therapist or nurse administers the appropriate gas for 15 min, then allows the patient to undergo a 5-min washout period before delivering the other gas. When medical air is unavailable, the test can be conducted using a fan as the comparator (at which point the trial is no longer blinded). The patient scores his/her dyspnea on a VAS or NRS. When function is a primary concern, assessment should include a baseline exertional test that is consistent with the patient's best functional status (i.e., shuttle test [59], 3-min walking test, reading a paragraph aloud), with the same functional test being repeated after the patient has received 10 min of each gas. Unblinded results are reported to the clinician and patient. For patients who experience superior results on oxygen, the attending clinician prescribes palliative oxygen after an informative discussion about cost. A fan is prescribed if air produces superior results. When both treatments are equally helpful, the decision is left to the patient. Patients receiving oxygen are asked to evaluate QOL improvements and therapy-related limitations over the course of 1 week, which helps guide the decision as to whether to continue the intervention. Clinicians should bear in mind that oxygen therapy is not without burden; patients may have an uncomfortable sense of being tied to a machine, feel anxiety about the power supply, and experience limitations on their ability to take excursions outside the house.

55.6 Non-pharmacological Interventions

Several alternative, non-pharmacological treatments have been investigated for their role in assisting patients with the symptoms or burden of dyspnea. The most promising strategies are psychosocial support and breathing techniques.

55.6.1 Psychosocial Support

Although essential in the treatment of all chronically ill patients, psychosocial support becomes more important as patients approach the end of life and their functional limitations increase. At this stage, patients often need help coming to terms with their illness and the life changes that occur as a result. Relatives and family members, too, may require guidance to navigate the shifting relationships and family roles that accompany disease progression and escalating symptom burden.

Several qualitative studies have examined the support needs of caregivers for dyspneic individuals. In one study, the investigators interviewed ten COPD patients and their caregivers; many caregivers reported that taking care of a breathless person was "preoccupying, restricting, and a major cause of anxiety." The investigators concluded that clinicians must not forget about the needs of their patients' families and that patients with disabling symptoms are often best managed using a multidisciplinary approach that includes psychosocial care [60]. A similar study, also describing the experiences of ten patients with COPD and their caregivers, found that caregivers experienced losses similar to those of the patients, felt burdened by multiple roles, and felt an unfairness that strained the patient/caregiver relationship [61].

Existing guidelines do not stipulate protocols for psychosocial care of patients with dyspnea or their caregivers. Clinicians caring for dyspneic patients must evaluate and attend to needs for increased psychosocial support, and respond to patient/family concerns when they arise with appropriate intervention and/or referral.

55.6.1.1 Breathing Techniques

Controlled breathing techniques, especially postural positioning and pursed lip breathing (PLB), are useful for managing dyspnea. In the "forward-leaning position," the posture most frequently used to alleviate breathlessness, patients lean forward (e.g., onto a table) and support their weight with their arms and upper body. This posture increases abdominal pressure and may enhance respiratory muscle function; [11] it has also been found to increase the strength of inspiratory muscle [62], improve diaphragmatic function [63], reduce the use of accessory muscles, and decrease abdominal breathing [63–65].

In PLB, the patient inhales through the nose and then exhales slowly, usually for 4–6 seconds, through pursed lips. By stenting the airways and preventing dynamic airway collapse, PLB decreases air trapping [66]. Moreover, it can help the patient manage or prevent the panic attacks that accompany severe breathlessness [67]. While studies have demonstrated the benefit of these techniques for relieving dyspnea in controlled research settings, results in actual clinical practice vary [11].

Given the potential benefit of breathing techniques, clinicians are advised to provide dyspneic patients with instruction in positioning and PLB and to review patients' skill with these techniques as well as their perceptions of benefit during subsequent clinic visits.

55.7 Conclusions

Intractable or refractory dyspnea contributes substantially to the suffering of patients with hematological malignancies and ARF. Palliative therapies, which aim to reduce symptom burden and to improve both functional status and QOL, have the potential to minimize this suffering. At this time, several treatment options are available to treat dyspnea in the palliative phase of care, with evidence most strongly supporting the use of oral or parenteral opioids, particularly morphine, for relief of breathlessness. Some patients, especially those with severe breathlessness, may benefit from palliative oxygen delivered via concentrator or from medical air delivered either through concentrator or by use of a fan. Insufficient and sometimes conflicting data limit the use of anxiolytics and SSRIs, which should be employed cautiously until further research provides more solid information. Evidence for Heliox28 is currently inconclusive, and feasibility issues may limit its utility regardless of any benefit that may be demonstrated in the future. Therapy with inhaled frusemide requires further evidence before it can be recommended. Finally, positioning and pursed-lip breathing constitute simple, cost-free interventions that have the potential to be very effective for certain patients.

References

1. Azoulay E, de Miranda S, Bele N, Schlemmer B (2008) Diagnostic strategy for acute respiratory failure in patients with haematological malignancy. Rev Mal Respir 25: 433–449
2. Azoulay E, Thiery G, Chevret S et al (2004) The prognosis of acute respiratory failure in critically ill cancer patients. Medicine 83:360–370
3. Kress JP, Christenson J, Pohlman AS, Linkin DR, Hall JB (1999) Outcomes of critically ill cancer patients in a university hospital setting. Am J Respir Crit Care Med 160: 1957–1961
4. Lecuyer L, Chevret S, Thiery G et al (2007) The ICU trial: a new admission policy for cancer patients requiring mechanical ventilation. Crit Care Med 35:808–814
5. Soares M, Salluh JI, Spector N et al (2005) Characteristics and outcomes of cancer patients requiring mechanical ventilatory support for >24 hrs. Crit Care Med 33: 520–526
6. Benoit DD, Vandewoude KH, Decruyenaere JM et al (2003) Outcome and early prognostic indicators in patients with a hematologic malignancy admitted to the intensive care unit for a life-threatening complication. Crit Care Med 31: 104–112
7. Azoulay E, Schlemmer B, Azoulay E, Schlemmer B (2006) Diagnostic strategy in cancer patients with acute respiratory failure. Intensive Care Med 32:808–822
8. Lecuyer L, Chevret S, Guidet B et al (2008) Case volume and mortality in haematological patients with acute respiratory failure. Eur Respir J 32:748–754
9. Pastores SMP, Voigt LP (2010) Acute respiratory failure in the patient with cancer: Diagnostic and management strategies. Crit Care Clin 26:21–40
10. Abernethy AP, Currow DC, Frith P et al (2003) Randomised, double blind, placebo controlled crossover trial of sustained release morphine for the management of refractory dyspnea. BMJ 327:523–528
11. ATS. Dyspnea (1999) Mechanisms, assessment, and management: a consensus statement. American Thoracic Society. Am J Respir Crit Care Med 159:321–340
12. Harver A, Mahler DA, Schwartzstein RM, Baird JC (2000) Descriptors of breathlessness in healthy individuals: distinct and separable constructs. Chest 118:679–690
13. Tanaka K, Akechi T, Okuyama T, Nishiwaki Y, Uchitomi Y (2000) Development and validation of the Cancer Dyspnea Scale: a multidimensional, brief, self-rating scale. Br J Cancer 82:800–805
14. Kikuchi Y, Okabe S, Tamura G et al (1994) Chemosensitivity and perception of dyspnea in patients with a history of near-fatal asthma. N Engl J Med 330:1329–1334
15. Mountain R, Zwillich C, Weil J (1978) Hypoventilation in obstructive lung disease. The role of familial factors. N Engl J Med 298:521–525
16. Stulbarg MS, Winn WR, Kellett LE (1989) Bilateral carotid body resection for the relief of dyspnea in severe chronic obstructive pulmonary disease. Physiologic and clinical observations in three patients [Erratum appears in Chest 1989 Sep;96(3):706]. Chest 95:1123–1128
17. Burdon JG, Pain MC, Rubinfeld AR, Nana A (1994) Chronic lung diseases and the perception of breathlessness: a clinical perspective. Eur Respir J 7:1342–1349

18. Currow D, Abernethy AP, Frith P (2003) Morphine for management of refractory dyspnea: authors' reply. BMJ 327:1288–1289
19. Pauwels RA, Buist AS, Calverley PM, Jenkins CR, Hurd SS, Committee GS (2001) Global strategy for the diagnosis, management, and prevention of chronic obstructive pulmonary disease. NHLBI/WHO Global Initiative for Chronic Obstructive Lung Disease (GOLD) Workshop summary. Am J Respir Crit Care Med 163:1256–1276
20. Leach RM (2005) Palliative medicine and non-malignant, end-stage respiratory disease. In: Doyle D (ed) Oxford textbook of palliative medicine, 3dth edn. Oxford University Press, Oxford
21. Eckenhoff JE, Oech SR (1960) The effects of narcotics and antagonists upon respiration and circulation in man. A review. Clin Pharmacol Ther 1:483–524
22. Santiago TV, Pugliese AC, Edelman NH (1977) Control of breathing during methadone addiction. Am J Med 62: 347–354
23. Weil JV, McCullough RE, Kline JS, Sodal IE (1975) Diminished ventilatory response to hypoxia and hypercapnia after morphine in normal man. N Engl J Med 292: 1103–1106
24. Kryger MH, Yacoub O, Dosman J, Macklem PT, Anthonisen NR (1976) Effect of meperidine on occlusion pressure responses to hypercapnia and hypoxia with and without external inspiratory resistance. Am Rev Respir Dis 114: 333–340
25. Santiago TV, Johnson J, Riley DJ, Edelman NH (1979) Effects of morphine on ventilatory response to exercise. J Appl Physiol Respir Environ Exerc Physiol 47: 112–118
26. Jennings AL, Davies AN, Higgins JP et al (2002) A systematic review of the use of opioids in the management of dyspnea. Thorax 57:939–944
27. Bruera E, MacEachern T, Ripamonti C, Hanson J (1993) Subcutaneous morphine for dyspnea in cancer patients. Ann Intern Med 119:906–907
28. Kim HF, Kunik ME, Molinari VA et al (2000) Functional impairment in COPD patients: the impact of anxiety and depression. Psychosomatics 41:465–471
29. Mitchell-Heggs P, Murphy K, Minty K et al (1980) Diazepam in the treatment of dyspnea in the 'Pink Puffer' syndrome. Q J Med 49:9–20
30. Sen D, Jones G, Leggat PO (1983) The response of the breathless patient treated with diazepam. Br J Clin Pract 37:232–233
31. Woodcock AA, Gross ER, Geddes DM (1981) Drug treatment of breathlessness: contrasting effects of diazepam and promethazine in pink puffers. Br Med J Clin Res Ed 283: 343–346
32. Man GC, Hsu K, Sproule BJ (1986) Effect of alprazolam on exercise and dyspnea in patients with chronic obstructive pulmonary disease. Chest 90:832–836
33. Greene JG, Pucino F, Carlson JD, Storsved M, Strommen GL (1989) Effects of alprazolam on respiratory drive, anxiety, and dyspnea in chronic airflow obstruction: a case study. Pharmacotherapy 9:34–38
34. Navigante AH, Cerchietti LC, Castro MA et al (2006) Midazolam as adjunct therapy to morphine in the alleviation of severe dyspnea perception in patients with advanced cancer. J Pain Symptom Manage 31:38–47
35. Garner SJ, Eldridge FL, Wagner PG, Dowell RT (1989) Buspirone, an anxiolytic drug that stimulates respiration. Am Rev Respir Dis 139:946–950
36. Mendelson WB, Martin JV, Rapoport DM (1990) Effects of buspirone on sleep and respiration. Am Rev Respir Dis 141: 1527–1530
37. Argyropoulou P, Patakas D, Koukou A, Vasiliadis P, Georgopoulos D (1993) Buspirone effect on breathlessness and exercise performance in patients with chronic obstructive pulmonary disease. Respiration 60:216–220
38. Singh NP, Despars JA, Stansbury DW, Avalos K, Light RW (1993) Effects of buspirone on anxiety levels and exercise tolerance in patients with chronic airflow obstruction and mild anxiety. Chest 103:800–804
39. Papp LA, Weiss JR, Greenberg HE et al (1995) Sertraline for chronic obstructive pulmonary disease and comorbid anxiety and mood disorders. Am J Psychiatry 152:1531
40. Smoller JW, Pollack MH, Systrom D, Kradin RL (1998) Sertraline effects on dyspnea in patients with obstructive airways disease. Psychosomatics 39:24–29
41. Burns BH, Howell JB (1969) Disproportionately severe breathlessness in chronic bronchitis. Q J Med 38:277–294
42. Mueller RA, Lundberg DB, Breese GR, Hedner J, Hedner T, Jonason J (1982) The neuropharmacology of respiratory control. Pharmacol Rev 34:255–285
43. Ventresca PG, Nichol GM, Barnes PJ, Chung KF (1990) Inhaled furosemide inhibits cough induced by low chloride content solutions but not by capsaicin. Am Rev Respir Dis 142:143–146
44. Bianco S, Pieroni MG, Refini RM, Rottoli L, Sestini P (1989) Protective effect of inhaled furosemide on allergen-induced early and late asthmatic reactions. N Engl J Med 321:1069–1073
45. Bianco S, Vaghi A, Robuschi M, Pasargiklian M (1988) Prevention of exercise-induced bronchoconstriction by inhaled frusemide. Lancet 2:252–255
46. Robuschi M, Gambaro G, Spagnotto S, Vaghi A, Bianco S (1989) Inhaled frusemide is highly effective in preventing ultrasonically nebulised water bronchoconstriction. Pulm Pharmacol 1:187–191
47. Chung KF, Barnes PJ (1992) Loop diuretics and asthma. Pulm Pharmacol 5:1–7
48. Nishino T, Ide T, Sudo T, Sato J (2000) Inhaled furosemide greatly alleviates the sensation of experimentally induced dyspnea. Am J Respir Crit Care Med 161:1963–1967
49. Ong KC, Kor AC, Chong WF et al (2004) Effects of inhaled furosemide on exertional dyspnea in chronic obstructive pulmonary disease. Am J Respir Crit Care Med 169: 1028–1033
50. Newton PJ, Davidson PM, Macdonald P et al (2008) Nebulized furosemide for the management of dyspnea: does the evidence support its use? J Pain Symptom Manage 36: 424–441
51. Ahmedzai SH, Laude E, Robertson A, Troy G, Vora V (2004) A double-blind, randomised, controlled Phase II trial of Heliox28 gas mixture in lung cancer patients with dyspnea on exertion. Br J Cancer 90:366–371
52. Cranston JM, Crockett A, Currow D, Cranston JM, Crockett A, Currow D (2008) Oxygen therapy for dyspnea in adults. Cochrane Database of Systematic Reviews 2008:CD004769
53. Guyatt GH, McKim DA, Austin P et al (2000) Appropriateness of domiciliary oxygen delivery. Chest 118:1303–1308

54. O'Donohue WJ Jr, Plummer AL (1995) Magnitude of usage and cost of home oxygen therapy in the United States. Chest 107:301–302
55. Booth S, Wade R, Johnson M et al (2004) The use of oxygen in the palliation of breathlessness. A report of the expert working group of the Scientific Committee of the Association of Palliative Medicine. Respir Med 98:66–77
56. Luce JM, Luce JA (2001) Perspectives on care at the close of life. Management of dyspnea in patients with far-advanced lung disease: "once I lose it, it's kind of hard to catch it...". JAMA 285:1331–1337
57. Abernethy AP, Currow DC, Frith P et al (2005) Prescribing palliative oxygen: a clinician survey of expected benefit and patterns of use. Palliat Med 19:168–170
58. Stringer E, McParland C, Hernandez P, Stringer E, McParland C, Hernandez P (2004) Physician practices for prescribing supplemental oxygen in the palliative care setting. J Palliat Care 20:303–307
59. Booth S, Adams L (2001) The shuttle walking test: a reproducible method for evaluating the impact of shortness of breath on functional capacity in patients with advanced cancer. Thorax 56:146–150
60. Booth S, Silvester S, Todd C, Booth S, Silvester S, Todd C (2003) Breathlessness in cancer and chronic obstructive pulmonary disease: using a qualitative approach to describe the experience of patients and carers. Palliat Support Care 1: 337–344
61. Seamark DA, Blake SD, Seamark CJ, Halpin DM (2004) Living with severe chronic obstructive pulmonary disease (COPD): perceptions of patients and their carers. An interpretative phenomenological analysis. Palliat Med 18:v 619–625
62. O'Neill S, McCarthy DS (1983) Postural relief of dyspnea in severe chronic airflow limitation: relationship to respiratory muscle strength. Thorax 38:595–600
63. Sharp JT, Drutz WS, Moisan T, Foster J, Machnach W (1980) Postural relief of dyspnea in severe chronic obstructive pulmonary disease. Am Rev Respir Dis 122: 201–211
64. Barach AL (1974) Chronic obstructive lung disease: postural relief of dyspnea. Arch Phys Med Rehabil 55: 494–504
65. Barach AL, Beck GJ (1954) The ventilatory effects of the head-down position in pulmonary emphysema. Am J Med 16:55–60
66. Tiep BL, Burns M, Kao D, Madison R, Herrera J (1986) Pursed lips breathing training using ear oximetry. Chest 90:218–221
67. Madge S, Esmond G (2001) End-stage management of respiratory disease. In: Esmond G (ed) Respiratory nursing. Bailliere Tindall, London, pp 229–240
68. Abernethy AP, McDonald CF, Frith PA, Clark K, Herndon JE, Marcello J, Young IH, Bull J, Wilcock A, Booth S, Wheeler JL, Tulsky JA, Crockett AJ, Currow DC. Effect of palliative oxygen versus medical (room) air in relieving breathlessness in patients with refractory dyspnoea: a double-blind randomised controlled trial (NCT00327873). Lancet; 2010; 376:784–93

End-of-Life Decisions in Cancer Patients

56

Lieve Van den Block, Agnes Van der Heide, and Luc Deliens

Contents

L. Van den Block (✉)
End-of-Life Care Research Group, Ghent University & Vrije Universiteit Brussel, Brussels, Belgium and
Department of General Practice, Vrije Universiteit Brussel, Laarbeeklaan 103, 1090 Brussels, Belgium
e-mail: lvdblock@vub.ac.be

A. Van der Heide
Department of Public Health, Erasmus University, Rotterdam, The Netherlands
e-mail: a.vanderheide@erasmusmc.nl

L. Deliens
End-of-Life Care Research Group, Ghent University & Vrije Universiteit Brussel, Brussels, Belgium and
Department of Public and Occupational Health, EMGO Institute for Health and Care Research, VU University Medical Centre, Amsterdam, The Netherlands
e-mail: luc.deliens@vub.ac.be

56.1 Introduction

Curing disease and prolonging life have traditionally been the main goals of medical care. Progress in diagnostic and therapeutic options has decreased deaths from acute diseases and considerably increased life expectancy. However, as the population ages, more and more people are dying from serious chronic conditions, which raises a wide range of physical, psychosocial, and spiritual problems [1, 2]. Currently, one-third of all deaths in most European countries occur suddenly and totally unexpectedly [3, 4]; the remaining two-thirds are non-sudden and thus eligible for some type of end-of-life care. This number is expected to increase in the near future [5, 6]; hence, delivery of optimal end-of-life care has become another important goal of medicine. Meanwhile, palliative care – an approach that improves the quality of life of patients and their families facing the problems associated with life-threatening illness, through the prevention and relief of suffering by means of early identification and painstaking assessment and treatment of pain and other physical, psychosocial, and spiritual problems – was recently identified by the World Health Organization as a priority public health issue for all countries [1, 2]. These aspects of care are extensively described in Chap. 55 about dyspnea.

Additionally, it is increasingly recognized that prolonging life might not always benefit the patient. End-of-life care and decision-making are best guided by the patient's quality of life and aimed at relieving suffering. In some cases, shortening of life may therefore be an

Financial Support: This study was supported by a grant from the Fifth Framework Program of the European Commission (contract QLRT-1999-30859) and the Fund for Scientific Research, Flanders, Belgium.

É. Azoulay (ed.), *Pulmonary Involvement in Patients with Hematological Malignancies*,
DOI: 10.1007/978-3-642-15742-4_56, © Springer-Verlag Berlin Heidelberg 2011

accepted, and for some people a desired, result [3, 4, 7]. Making decisions that can shorten a patient's life entails complex decision-making processes, which have received increasing attention in public, professional, and political debates, especially when they involve euthanasia or physician-assisted suicide [8, 9]. Belgium, Luxemburg, and the Netherlands are the only countries in the world with laws regulating the practice of euthanasia [10, 11]. Switzerland and the state of Oregon in the US permit or do not prosecute physician-assisted suicide under certain conditions, but do not allow euthanasia [12, 13].

Cancer stands out as a particular type of chronic illness. Cancer is the cause of approximately one in four deaths overall and one in three non-sudden deaths [3]. Previous research has also identified a distinct dying trajectory for cancer patients compared with those dying from other chronic diseases [1, 2, 14, 15]. While people with heart failure or chronic obstructive respiratory disease, for example, often have intermittent episodes of illness and often die with little warning after a rapid deterioration, cancer patients have a relatively predictable course with a fairly short period of evident decline just before death [16]. Hence, the incidence and characteristics of end-of-life decision-making may differ substantially between cancer patients and patients with other illnesses.

Previous studies have shown that cancer was the cause of death in over 70% of legal physician-assisted suicide cases in 1999 in Oregon [8], and in 82.5% and 88% of legal euthanasia and physician-assisted suicide cases in Belgium and the Netherlands, respectively, in 2002–2003 [9, 10]. Studies showing that oncologists receive more requests for, and have performed more euthanasia and physician-assisted suicides, than other physicians further support the epidemiological data [11–13].

In this report we will analyze data from the European Study on End-of-Life Decisions (EURELD) and focus on end-of-life decisions among cancer patients. The study was performed in 2001 and provides incidence estimates of end-of-life decisions among all deaths in six European countries: Belgium (Flanders), Denmark, Italy (four areas), Sweden, Switzerland (German-speaking part), and the Netherlands [3].

Firstly, we will provide a full description of the conceptual framework used in the EURELD study (Sect. 56. 2) and outline the methodology (Sect. 56.3). Secondly, incidence figures of end-of-life decisions among cancer patients in these six European countries will be compared (Sect. 56.4). Finally, cancer and non-cancer patients will be compared (Sect. 56.5), and we will end with some concluding remarks (Sect. 56.6).

56.2 Conceptual Framework of End-of-Life Decisions

Medical end-of-life decisions can be defined as medical decisions that probably or certainly hasten the death of a patient [3, 4, 17–19]. They are usually classified into the following categories: euthanasia, physician-assisted suicide, administration of life-ending drugs not explicitly requested by the patient, intensification of treatments to alleviate pain or other symptoms, and treatment limitation decisions with a possible or certain life-shortening intention.

The defining elements in categorizing a decision are whether the physician committed or omitted an act, the intention of the physician, and the request of the patient. The first dimension, the medico-technical dimension, involves "what the physician actually does." Two kinds of actions can be distinguished: the withholding or withdrawing of potentially life-prolonging treatment, and the use of potentially life-shortening drugs. The physician's intention and the patient's involvement in the decision-making process belong to the second, medico-ethical dimension. The physician can make a decision with the knowledge that it may hasten death but without the intention of hastening death, with the co-intention of hastening death, or with the explicit intention of hastening death. The patient may explicitly request the physician to make, or not to make, a specific type of decision. On the basis of the possible combinations of these dimensions, end-of-life decisions can be classified as shown in Box 56.1.

Another important practice at the end of life, which has been differentiated from medical end-of-life decisions, is the practice of *continuous deep sedation until death*, i.e., the administration of drugs to keep the patient continuously in deep sedation or coma until death, with or without giving artificial nutrition or hydration (when nutrition and hydration are not given, this practice is often called "terminal sedation") [17, 20]. The status of continuous deep sedation with respect to possibly life-shortening end-of-life decisions is unclear and much debated. An important issue is whether or not sedation can hasten death in some cases [21, 22]. Regarding terminal sedation, research has shown that, in most cases, death is expected, but not explicitly intended [17, 20]. There are also indications that terminal sedation is sometimes used as an alternative to euthanasia [20].

This conceptual framework has been carefully and extensively tested and has repeatedly been proven valid and robust in international and nationwide studies [3, 4, 18, 23–27].

Box 56.1 Conceptual framework for medical end-of-life decisions with a possible or certain life-shortening effect [3, 4, 17–19]

Euthanasia or physician-assisted suicide	The prescription, supply, or administration of drugs with the explicit intention of ending life at the explicit request of the patient or of enabling the patient to end his/her own life
Administration of life-ending drugs without explicit request by the patient	The administration of drugs with the explicit intention of ending life without an explicit request from the patient
Intensification of the alleviation of pain or other symptoms	The use of drugs to alleviate pain or other symptoms, taking into account the possible life-shortening side effects, or with a co-intention of hastening death
Treatment limitation decisions	The withholding or withdrawal of treatment, taking into account the possible life-shortening effect, or with the explicit intention of hastening death

56.3 Methodology of the European Study on End-of-Life Decisions (EURELD) Study 2001

In 2001, the EURELD study was conducted in six European countries (Belgium, Denmark, Italy, Sweden, German-speaking Switzerland, and the Netherlands) to investigate the incidence and background characteristics of end-of-life decisions. The EURELD study is a death-certificate study that used a quantitative mortality follow-back design, looking backward from death. In each participating country, a random sample of death certificates for people aged 1 year or older (18 years or older for Italy) was obtained from the death registries to which all deaths were reported in each country. Deaths occurred between June 2001 and February 2002. In all countries except Switzerland, the sample taken was stratified for the likelihood of an end-of-life decision with a possible life-shortening effect, i.e., larger samples of deaths were taken for strata in which the cause of death made an end-of-life decision more likely. Standardized questionnaires were mailed to the physicians who signed the death certificates. A complex mailing procedure ensured the anonymity of the physician and patient. The study protocol was approved by an ethics committee in each country.

Response rates varied between 44% (Italy) and 75% (The Netherlands) [3].

56.3.1 Questionnaire

To identify the cases in which an end-of-life decision was not possible, the physician was asked if the patient died "suddenly and totally unexpectedly." If the answer was "no," the following questions were asked to investigate the incidence of end-of-life decisions:

(a) Did you withhold or withdraw medical treatment while taking into account the possibility or certainty that this would hasten the patient's death or with the explicit intention of hastening the patient's death?
(b) Did you intensify the alleviation of pain and suffering while taking into account the possibility or certainty that this would hasten the patient's death, or partly with the intention of hastening the patient's death?
(c) Was death the result of the administration, supply, or prescription of drugs with the explicit intention of hastening the patient's death?

The second part of the questionnaire surveyed the decision-making process leading to the end-of-life decision, if there had been one. The physician was asked if the patient was competent to make decisions (incompetence was defined as "not or not entirely able to judge his or her situation and to make adequate decisions accordingly"), whether he or she had made an explicit request, whether the decision was discussed with the patient without him or her making an explicit request, and whether the decision was discussed with the patients' relatives and other professional caregivers.

The case was classified as a treatment limitation decision when at least one of the questions under (a) was answered "yes." When at least one of the questions under (b) was answered "yes," the case was classified as intensification of pain and symptom alleviation with a possible life-shortening effect. When question (c) was answered "yes," the case was classified as euthanasia if the drug was given by the physician at the patient's explicit request, as physician-assisted suicide if the patient had taken the drug himself or herself, and as a life-ending act without the patient's explicit request if the drug was administered without the patient's explicit request. To classify cases in which more than one end-of-life decision was reported, the decision with the most explicit intention was considered. When the same life-shortening intentions were reported, explicit life-shortening acts prevailed over symptom alleviation with a possible life-shortening effect, which prevailed over treatment limitation decisions.

The final question dealing with continuous deep sedation was as follows: Did the patient receive drugs, such as barbiturates or benzodiazepines, to keep him/her continuously in deep sedation or coma until death? Answer options were "yes, and artificial nutrition and hydration were not given;" "yes, and artificial nutrition or hydration were given;" and "no." This question was asked for all non-sudden deaths, except in the Netherlands, where, due to a routing difference, the question was asked only if an end-of-life decision preceded death.

The underlying cause of death on the death certificates (ICD10 codes) was anonymously linked to the questionnaires completed by the physicians. Data were corrected for stratification and weighted for sex, age, place of death, and cause of death according to all deaths during the study period. Results for euthanasia and physician-assisted suicide were combined because the physician-assisted suicide occurred for only 12 cancer patients in all countries.

Further details on the methodology, stratification, and weighting procedure can be found in previous publications [3, 17, 28].

56.4 Epidemiology of End-of-Life Decisions Among Cancer Patients: European Study on End-of-Life Decisions (EURELD) 2001

The EURELD study showed that the percentage of all deaths of persons aged 1 year and older (18 years and older in Italy) preceded by any end-of-life decision varied between 23% (Italy) and 51% (Switzerland). The administration of drugs with explicit life-shortening intention, with or without an explicit request from the patient, occurred in all countries, ranging from less than 1% of all deaths in Denmark to 3.4% in the Netherlands. In all countries, intensified symptom alleviation while taking into account or co-intending the hastening of death occurred much more frequently than the use of lethal drugs, ranging from 19% (Italy) to 26% (Denmark). Treatment-limitation decisions were also more common than the use of lethal drugs in most countries, but these decisions showed greater variability across countries, ranging from 4% (Italy) to 28% (Switzerland) [3]. Prevalence figures for continuous deep sedation while food or fluid were given ranged from 0.9 (Denmark) to 5.5 (Italy), and sedation while forgoing food and fluid ranged from 1.6 (Denmark) to 3.7 (The Netherlands) [17].

These previously reported incidence figures are estimates for all deaths due to cancer and other illnesses. Incidence figures for cancer patients only have not been published so far.

Table 56.1 displays the incidence rates of end-of-life decisions among cancer deaths per country. At least one possibly life-shortening end-of-life decision was made for more than half of all cancer deaths in Belgium, Denmark, Switzerland, and the Netherlands. For Italy and Sweden, the proportions fell between 40% and 50%. End-of-life decisions were most common in Switzerland (69%) and least common in Italy (41%).

Euthanasia or physician-assisted suicide, described as the prescription, supply, or administration of drugs with the explicit intention of ending life at the explicit request of the patient, was most prevalent in the Netherlands (7.5% of cancer deaths) and occurred in 1% or fewer deaths in the other countries. The high percentage in the Netherlands can probably be explained by the historical context of the law on euthanasia. Although the law was passed in 2002, it was the outcome of a 2-decade long societal process, whereas in Belgium the legislation was finalized rather quickly in 2002 [29].

Life-ending acts without an explicit request from the patient were most common among cancer deaths in Belgium (2.8%), but occurred in all other countries in 1% or fewer cases and mainly involved patients who were judged incompetent at the end of life (data not shown).

Table 56.1 Frequencies of end-of-life decisions among 5,664 cancer deaths

	Country					
	Belgium	Denmark	Italy	Sweden	Switzerland	The Netherlands
Number of cancer deaths studied	783	793	863	879	822	1,524
At least one end-of-life decision	499 (63.7%)	457 (57.6%)	351 (40.7%)	392 (44.6%)	570 (69.3%)	884 (58.0%)
Euthanasia/ physician-assisted suicide	9 (1.1%)	4 (.5%)	1 (.1%)	0 (.0%)	6 (.7%)	115 (7.5%)
Life-ending without explicit patient request	22 (2.8%)	10 (1.3%)	2 (0.2%)	3 (0.3%)	5 (.6%)	14 (0.9%)
Intensified alleviation of pain and symptoms	354 (45.2%)	342 (43.1%)	306 (35.5%)	274 (31.2%)	320 (38.9%)	509 (33.4%)
Treatment limitation decisions	113 (14.4%)	102 (12.9%)	43 (5.0%)	115 (13.1%)	239 (29.1%)	246 (16.1%)

Data are weighted percentages

The frequency of intensified alleviation of pain or other symptoms with possible life-shortening effect ranged from 31% (Sweden) to 45% (Belgium). The frequency of treatment limitation decisions varied more substantially across countries, from 5% in Italy to 29% in Switzerland.

Overall across Europe, end-of-life decisions that may possibly, or are explicitly intended to, shorten a patient's life seem to be made very often among patients dying from cancer. Also, the country-specific patterns found for all deaths are reflected in the figures for cancer deaths. In particular, the use of lethal drugs and the decision to withhold or withdraw possibly life-prolonging treatments at the end of life seem to differ across countries. These are decisions that are highly constrained by legal and cultural-ethical factors. Decisions aimed at ending patient suffering, e.g., intensified symptom alleviation, varied less substantially. This is also reflected in the results for continuous deep sedation.

Regarding the results for continuous deep sedation until death, a striking finding was the high rate of use of this technique at the end of life in cancer patients in Europe (Table 56.2). Sedating an individual continuously until death without administering food or fluid occurred most often in Italy (10.5%) and least often in Denmark (1.1%). Continuous deep sedation while administering food and/or fluid was reported most often in the Netherlands (11.5%) and least often in Sweden (3.7%). Variations across countries appear to be highest for the use of continuous deep sedation while deciding to stop or not to initiate artificial feeding or hydration. In this form of terminal sedation, life-shortening effects are more likely than if food and/or fluid are continued.

56.5 A Comparison of End-of-Life Decisions Between Cancer and Non-cancer Patients in Belgium

In a secondary analysis of the EURELD data for Belgium, the prevalence of end-of-life decisions among cancer patients who died non-suddenly was compared with the prevalence among non-cancer patients who died non-suddenly [28]. Sudden and totally unexpected deaths, which preclude end-of-life decision-making, were excluded from this analysis to allow meaningful comparisons [28].

The results showed that end-of-life decisions in general occurred more frequently among non-sudden cancer deaths (74%) than among non-sudden non-cancer deaths (50%), particularly decisions involving intensified symptom alleviation (53% vs 23%, respectively) (Table 56.3). This difference probably stems from the different dying trajectories between the two groups and the associated recognition of differences in patient needs [1, 2, 14, 16, 30, 31]. Because of the less predictable

Table 56.2 Frequencies of continuous deep sedation among 5,664 cancer deaths

	Country					
	Belgium	Denmark	Italy	Sweden	Switzerland	The Netherlands[a]
Number of cancer deaths studied	783	793	863	879	822	1,524
Continuous deep sedation with food and fluid	49 (7.5%)	25 (3.9%)	60 (7.9%)	27 (3.7%)	49 (7.0%)	85 (11.5%)
Continuous deep sedation without food or fluid	28 (4.3%)	7 (1.1%)	80 (10.5%)	17 (2.4%)	25 (3.6%)	17 (2.3%)

Data are weighted percentages

[a]Due to a technical problem in the questionnaire, data from the Netherlands refer only to deep sedation until death combined with another end-of-life decision

Table 56.3 End-of-life decisions among non-sudden cancer versus noncancer deaths in Flanders, Belgium $n = 2{,}128$ [28]

	Cancer, $n = 1{,}140$	No cancer, $n = 988$
At least one end-of-life decision	844 (74.1%)	501 (50.1%)
Euthanasia or physician-assisted suicide	16 (1.2%)	0 (0%)
Life-ending acts without the patient's explicit request	39 (3.4%)	19 (1.8%)
Intensification of pain and/or symptom alleviation with a possible life-shortening effect	606 (53.1%)	234 (23.2%)
Treatment limitation decisions	183 (16.4%)	248 (25.1%)

Data are weighted percentages

dying course of non-cancer patients, a palliative care approach might be adopted less frequently and also later in the dying process [32]. Additionally, symptoms might more often go unreported and untreated among non-cancer patients, since these patients are often elderly people displaying increasing dependency and cognitive impairment at the end of life.

The study also shows that treatment limitation decisions were more prevalent among non-cancer patients (25%) than among cancer patients (16%), a difference that can also be ascribed to the differences in the dying process. In the case of chronic diseases with intermittent serious episodes of illness (e.g., heart failure or chronic obstructive respiratory disease), there may be a period of rapid deterioration at the very end of life, when explicit decisions about continuing or beginning possibly futile treatments will have to be made. In the case of elderly persons with several co-morbid conditions and increasing dependency and cognitive impairment at the end of life, similar questions about whether life-prolonging therapies will improve quality of life will come to the fore.

Regarding euthanasia or physician-assisted suicide, cancer patients were more likely to die after euthanasia or physician-assisted suicide (1.2% vs 0%, respectively), but this point could not be statistically evaluated because no occurrences were reported in the non-cancer group. This finding may be explained by the fact that cancer patients are generally younger and thus probably more assertive, while their prognosis is more certain, making them more aware of the terminal nature of their illness.

Finally, there was a higher prevalence of the use of life-ending drugs without explicit patient request among cancer patients (3.4% vs 1.8%, respectively). However, in a multivariate analysis correcting for differences in demographic characteristics between cancer and non-cancer deaths, the difference in prevalence was no longer significant.

56.6 Conclusion

End-of-life decisions are common in medical practice today. While curing illness and prolonging life have traditionally been the main goals of medical care, physicians sometimes need to make decisions that can, or are explicitly intended to, shorten a patient's life. The findings shown in this report indicate that these end-of-life decisions are particularly prevalent among patients dying from cancer. In most countries, decisions that possibly shorten life are made in more than half of all patients dying of cancer. This proportion is higher for non-sudden cancer deaths only, reaching three out of four patients, as data from Belgium have shown. Oncologists and other health-care workers dealing with cancer patients are relatively often confronted with complex medico-ethical decision-making at the end of life. This necessitates the integration of end-of-life care and medical decision-making into the basic curriculum for physicians worldwide.

References

1. World Health Organization (2004) Palliative care: the solid facts. WHO, Copenhagen, Denmark
2. World Health Organization (2004) Better palliative care for older people. WHO, Copenhagen, Denmark
3. van der Heide A, Deliens L, Faisst K, Nilstun T, Norup M, Paci E et al (2003 Aug 2) End-of-life decision-making in six European countries: descriptive study. Lancet 362(9381): 345–50
4. Deliens L, Mortier F, Bilsen J, Cosyns M, Vander Stichele R, Vanoverloop J et al (2000 Nov 25) End-of-life decisions in medical practice in Flanders, Belgium: a nationwide survey. Lancet 356(9244):1806–11
5. Abramowska A, Gourbin C, Wunsch G (2005) Projections of the dependent elderly population by age, sex, and household composition. Scenarios for Belgium. Archives of Public Health 63(5):243–57
6. van der Velden LFJ, Francke AL, Hingstman L, Willems DL (2007) Sterfte aan kanker en andere chronische aandoeningen: kenmerken in 2006 en trends vanaf 1996 [Death from cancer and other chronic conditions: characteristics in 2006 and trends since 1996]. NIVEL, Utrecht, The Netherlands
7. Emanuel EJ (2002 Jan 28) Euthanasia and physician-assisted suicide: a review of the empirical data from the United States. Arch Intern Med 162(2):142–52
8. van der Heide A, Onwuteaka-Philipsen BD, Emanuel EJ, van der Maas PJ, van der Wal G (2001) Clinical and epidemiological aspects of end-of-life decision-making. Royal Netherlands Academy of Arts and Sciences, Amsterdam, The Netherlands
9. Spreeuwenberg C, Bakker DJ, Dillmann RJM, Blijkham GH, Teunissen S, Zylicz Z (2002) Reference book palliative care [Handboek palliatieve zorg]. Elsevier Gezondheidszorg, Maarssen, The Netherlands
10. Wet betreffende euthanasie 28 mei 2002 [Law concerning euthanasia May 28, 2002] (in Dutch), Number Bill 2002009590, Brussels, Belgium, Belgisch Staatsblad 22 juni 2002 [Belgian official collection of the laws June 22, 2002] (2002)
11. Nys H (2002) Euthanasia in the Low Countries: a comparative analysis of the law regarding euthanasia in Belgium and The Netherlands. Ethical Perspect 9(2–3):73–85
12. Ganzini L, Nelson HD, Schmidt TA, Kraemer DF, Delorit MA, Lee MA (2000 Feb 24) Physicians' experiences with the Oregon Death with Dignity Act. N Engl J Med 342(8): 557–63
13. Bosshard G, Fischer S, Bar W (2002 Oct 12) Open regulation and practice in assisted dying. Swiss Med Wkly 132(37–38):527–34
14. Murray SA, Kendall M, Boyd K, Sheikh A (2005 Apr 30) Illness trajectories and palliative care. BMJ 330(7498): 1007–11
15. National Institute of Health (2004) State-of-the-science conference statement on improving end-of-life care, Bethesda, MD, USA
16. Lynn J, Adamson D (2003) Living well at the end of life: adapting health care to serious chronic illness in old age. RAND, Santa Monica, CA
17. Miccinesi G, Rietjens JA, Deliens L, Paci E, Bosshard G, Nilstun T et al (2006 Feb) Continuous deep sedation: physicians' experiences in six European countries. J Pain Symptom Manage 31(2):122–9
18. Seale C (2006 Jan) National survey of end-of-life decisions made by UK medical practitioners. Palliat Med 20(1): 3–10
19. Mitchell K, Owens RG (2003 July 26) National survey of medical decisions at end of life made by New Zealand general practitioners. BMJ 327(7408):202–3
20. Rietjens JA, van Delden JJ, van der Heide A, Vrakking AM, Onwuteaka-Philipsen BD, van der Maas PJ et al (2006 Apr 10) Terminal sedation and euthanasia: a comparison of clinical practices. Arch Intern Med 166(7):749–53
21. Rietjens J (2006) Medical decision-making at the end of life: experiences and attitudes of physicians and the general public. Erasmus Universiteit, Rotterdam
22. Van den Block L (2008) End-of-life care and medical decision-making in the last phase of life, Ph.D. Thesis. Vrije Universiteit Brussel
23. van der Maas PJ, van der Wal G, Haverkate I, de Graaff CL, Kester JG, Onwuteaka-Philipsen BD et al (1996 Nov 28) Euthanasia, physician-assisted suicide, and other medical practices involving the end of life in The Netherlands, 1990-1995. N Engl J Med 335(22):1699–705
24. Kuhse H, Singer P, Baume P, Clark M, Rickard M (1997 Feb 17) End-of-life decisions in Australian medical practice. Med J Aust 166(4):191–6
25. Meier DE, Emmons CA, Wallenstein S, Quill T, Morrison RS, Cassel CK (1998 Apr 23) A national survey of physician-assisted suicide and euthanasia in the United States. N Engl J Med 338(17):1193–201

26. Van den Block L, Deschepper R, Bilsen J, Bossuyt N, Van Casteren V, Deliens L (2009) Euthanasia and other end-of-life decisions: a mortality follow-back study in Belgium. BMC Public Health 9:79
27. Van den Block L, Deschepper R, Bilsen J, Bossuyt N, Van Casteren Viviane (2009) Deliens L. Euthanasia and other end of life decisions and care provided in final 3 months of life: nationwide retrospective study in Belgium. BMJ 339:b2772
28. Van den Block L, Bilsen J, Deschepper R, Van Der Kelen G, Bernheim JL, Deliens L (2006 June 20) End-of-life decisions among cancer patients compared with noncancer patients in Flanders, Belgium. J Clin Oncol 24(18):2842–8
29. Bilsen J, Vander Stichele R, Broeckaert B, Mortier F, Deliens L (2007 May 7) Changes in medical end-of-life practices during the legalization process of euthanasia in Belgium. Soc Sci Med 65:803–808
30. Murray SA, Boyd K, Kendall M, Worth A, Benton TF, Clausen H (2002 Oct 26) Dying of lung cancer or cardiac failure: prospective qualitative interview study of patients and their careers in the community. BMJ 325(7370):929
31. Murtagh FE, Preston M, Higginson I (2004 Jan) Patterns of dying: palliative care for non-malignant disease. Clin Med 4(1):39–44
32. Van den Block L, Deschepper R, Bossuyt N, Drieskens K, Bauwens S, Van Casteren V et al (2008 Sep 8) Care for patients in the last months of life: the Belgian Sentinel Network Monitoring End-of-Life Care study. Arch Intern Med 168(16):1747–54

Part VII

Pearls That You Should be Aware Of

An Unexpected Diagnosis of Pulmonary Tuberculosis

57

Virginie Lemiale, A. Seguin, and Élie Azoulay

Contents

V. Lemiale (✉), A. Seguin, and É. Azoulay
Medical ICU, Saint Louis Hospital, 1 av. Claude Vellefaux, 75010 Paris, France
e-mail: virginie.lemiale@sls.aphp.fr

57.1 Case Report

This 68-year-old man was admitted to our medical ICU for acute respiratory failure. He was from Tunisia and had been working in France for 40 years. He had a history of myocardial infarction 6 years earlier with persistent cardiomyopathy and an ejection fraction of 66%. His treatment consisted of a beta-blocker, aspirin, and pravastatin. He had been admitted 6 months earlier to the infectious diseases department for evaluation of a fever with weight loss. Investigations were negative for infection with the HIV, hepatitis B and C viruses, cytomegalovirus, *Mycobacterium tuberculosis*, *Cryptococcus neoformans*, and leishmaniasis. Osteomedullar biopsies showed Hodgkin's lymphoma. He had hepatomegaly and numerous enlarged lymph nodes in the mediastinum and mesentery, indicating dacarbazine stage 4 disease.

Over the next 6 months, he received chemotherapy including adriamycin, vinblastine, bleomycin, and dacarabazine. During the first episode of aplasia, he had sepsis of unknown origin with blood cultures positive for *Escherichia coli*. Computed tomography (CT) of the chest showed a response to chemotherapy with no other parenchymatous lesions (Fig. 57.1). When he was seen just before the seventh chemotherapy cycle, he reported a 15-day history of dyspnea, chills, and a cough. Oxygen saturation was 88% with 10 L/min oxygen. He had no evidence of shock, but his body temperature was 39.5°C. The chest X-ray disclosed alveolar lesions throughout the lung parenchyma (Fig. 57.2). He was admitted to the ICU and intubated within the first few hours. His PaO_2/FiO_2 ratio was 150, indicating acute respiratory distress syndrome (ARDS). He required vasopressors and developed acute renal failure requiring continuous venovenous hemodiafiltration on day 1.

É. Azoulay (ed.), *Pulmonary Involvement in Patients with Hematological Malignancies*,
DOI: 10.1007/978-3-642-15742-4_57, © Springer-Verlag Berlin Heidelberg 2011

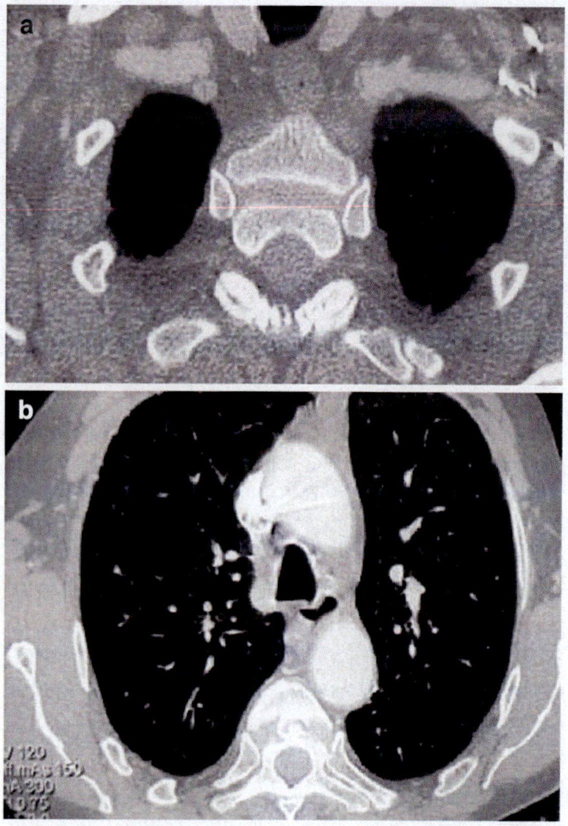

Fig. 57.1 Computed tomography of the chest 60 days before ICU admission. The patient had emphysema, but no other parenchymal lesions. (**a**) Upper lobes; (**b**) lower lobes

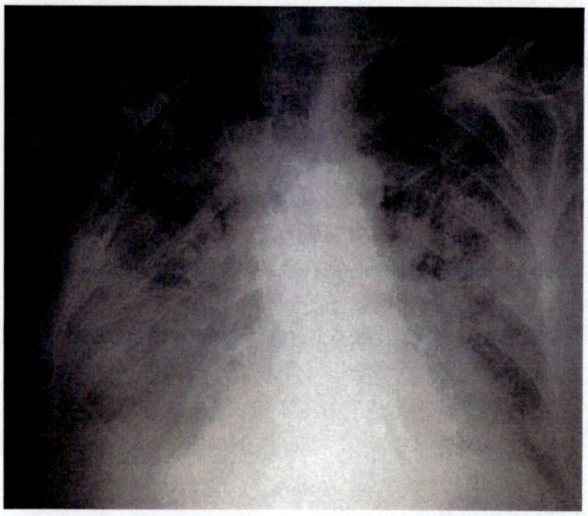

Fig. 57.2 Chest X-ray at ICU admission

57.2 Diagnoses Suspected at ICU Admission

57.2.1 Lung Infection

Bacterial pneumonia: he was immunocompromised and had a fever and chills. Infection is the leading complication during chemotherapy [1].

Pneumocystis jiroveci pneumonia: He received no prophylactic treatment, and Hodgkin's disease causes cellular immune deficiency. The 15-day symptom duration seemed long for this diagnosis, but the chest X-ray was compatible [2].

Invasive pulmonary aspergillosis: He had immunosuppression with a cellular immune deficiency and several episodes of neutropenia over the last few months. He reported no hemoptysis or chest pain, but this diagnosis remained consistent with the presence of Hodgkin's disease.

Pulmonary tuberculosis: He was from Tunisia, where tuberculosis is endemic. Nevertheless, CT of the chest done before chemotherapy showed no lesions of the lung parenchyma. Sputum cultures were negative for *M. tuberculosis* during the evaluation in the infectious diseases department. The rapid progression and severity of the pulmonary involvement were not typical for tuberculosis. Serial cultures were negative for *M. tuberculosis*.

Catheter-related bloodstream infection with acute lung injury: He had the same catheter for 6 months, but reported no symptoms during any of the chemotherapy infusions. Nevertheless, this diagnosis remained possible.

Viral pneumonia: Cytomegalovirus or herpes simplex virus pneumonia was considered, although there were no suggestive clinical findings. The patient was admitted during the influenza season, but reported no flu-like symptoms before the onset of respiratory failure.

57.2.2 Noninfectious Diseases

Heart failure: He had received Adriamycin and had ischemic cardiomyopathy before treatment onset. The symptoms and chest X-ray findings were compatible with cardiogenic edema.

Treatment toxicity: He received bleomycin during the first six chemotherapy cycles. This drug is associated with interstitial pneumonia and pulmonary fibrosis, particularly in smokers and in patients given granulocyte/macrophage colony-stimulating factor [3].

ARDS related to another condition: He reported no extrapulmonary symptoms before the onset of respiratory failure. Nevertheless, he was evaluated for the main causes of secondary ARDS (pancreatitis and extrapulmonary infections).

57.3 Outcome

During the first few days, he received cephalosporin, erythromycin, sulfamethoxazole-trimethoprim, and furosemide. Bronchoalveolar lavage (BAL) was performed on day 2 to look for infectious agents, such as *Pneumocystis*, and for arguments supporting bleomycin-related pulmonary toxicity. The BAL fluid exhibited a normal cytological pattern with no evidence of *Pneumocystis* by microscopic examination or PCR and no viruses. Bacteriological studies of the BAL fluid showed 2×10^4 *E. coli*/mm^3 with resistance to cephalosporin. He was then given imipenem and amikacin. His condition deteriorated, and he had multiorgan failure with fever. Abdominal pain prompted an ultrasound scan of the abdomen, which showed two abscesses in the spleen. Transesophageal echocardiography visualized a small vegetation on an aortic valve with no valve destruction, suggesting bacterial endocarditis. The patient died on the same day.

A postmortem lung biopsy was done and showed granulomas (Fig. 57.3). Tracheal aspirate cultures, done at admission, became positive for *M. tuberculosis* 4 weeks later.

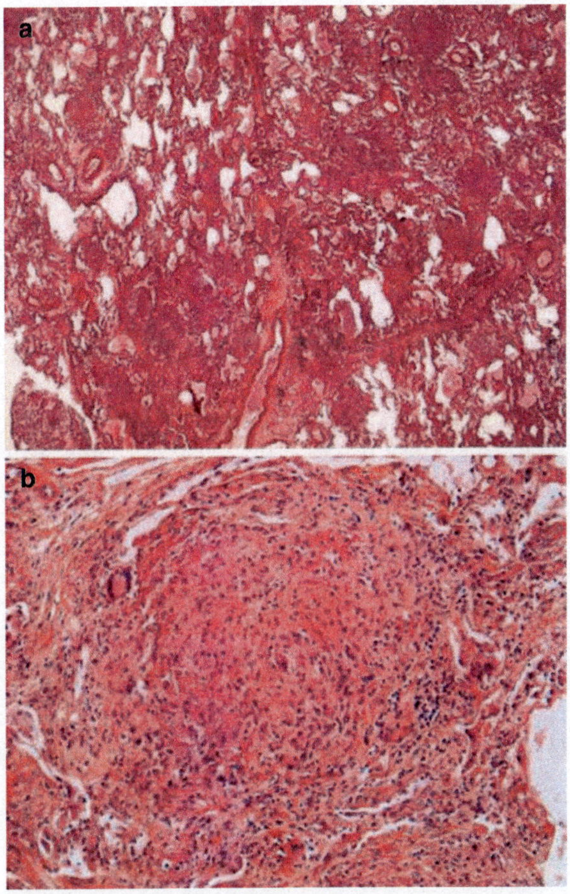

Fig. 57.3 Lung biopsy. (**a**) Inflammatory parenchyma with multiple nodular lesions (×10). (**b**) Granuloma composed of lymphocytes, multinucleate giant cells, and epithelioid macrophages (×40)

57.4 Discussion

Tuberculosis in ICU patients is still a severe disease associated with a high mortality rate. Few studies of pulmonary tuberculosis in patients requiring ICU admission are available. Our patient was no doubt exposed to *M. tuberculosis* during his childhood in Tunisia. Moreover, he had immunosuppression with altered cellular immunity because of Hodgkin's disease and chemotherapy [1]. Cellular immune deficiency increases the risk of tuberculosis. Nevertheless, infections with other bacteria are far more common [1].

Pulmonary tuberculosis is often fatal in critically ill patients. A 2006 retrospective study in 58 patients reported a 25% ICU mortality rate [4]. In that study, 45% of patients had respiratory symptoms for more than 2 weeks, 81% were admitted for respiratory distress, and 79% had respiratory specimens positive for *M. tuberculosis*. By multivariate analysis, factors associated with higher mortality were associated organ dysfunction ($P = 0.002$), sepsis ($P = 0.001$), nosocomial pneumonia ($P = 0.002$), and ARDS ($P = 0.008$). Our patient had three of these four risk factors.

A 2005 retrospective study in two French ICUs [5] enrolled 99 patients with pulmonary tuberculosis, including 22 with malignancies. Among them, 30% had tuberculosis diagnosed during the ICU stay. Symptom duration before the diagnosis was longer than 1 month in 34% of patients. Mortality was 26%

and was related to the number of organ failures (OR per additional failing organ, 3.11), the nutritional status (albumin <20 g/L had an OR of 3.73), and a time from symptom onset to treatment longer than 1 month (OR, 3.73).

More than 20 different causes may lead to acute respiratory failure in patients with hematological malignancies who are admitted to the ICU. The diagnosis relies on a systematic assessment of these possible causes using the DIRECT approach (Chap. 2 in the diagnosis strategy). In our patient, the time from symptom onset to admission was 15 days, and the alteration in cellular immune deficiency associated with Hodgkin's disease suggested infection with intracellular bacteria. Radiographic findings before ICU admission were normal. Our patient had a history of ischemic cardiomyopathy, and cardiogenic edema was therefore a possibility. He received bleomycin and was a smoker. Based on these features, the most likely diagnoses were infection (bacterial, viral, or parasitic), cardiogenic edema, and pulmonary toxicity [1]. Bleomycin toxicity has been evaluated in a study of patients with Hodgkin's disease [3]. Of 141 patients, 18% experienced bleomycin toxicity. The ABVD chemotherapy regimen, granulocyte/macrophage colony-stimulating factor, radiation therapy, and age older than 40 years were associated with bleomycin toxicity. Overall 5-year survival was 63% in the patients with bleomycin toxicity and 90% in the other patients ($P = 0.001$) [1].

M. tuberculosis could have been suspected in our patient based on his childhood spent in Tunisia [3]. Nevertheless, CT of the chest obtained 60 days before ICU admission showed no parenchymal lesions, nodules, or sequelae of tuberculosis. The rate of symptom progression was unusually fast for a patient with tuberculosis.

The cause of acute respiratory failure in ICU patients remains unknown despite extensive investigations in 10–20% of cases [1, 6]. A study has shown that postmortem examination supplied a previously unrecognized diagnosis in 4% of patients overall and in a higher proportion of immunocompromised patients [6, 7]. Also, a recent comprehensive review on rapid growing mycobacteria concluded that the approach to antimycobacterial drugs may be different for various patients with cancer [8]. We believe that similar data are needed in cancer patients with mycobacteria to recognize clinical vignettes highly suggestive of mycobacteria infections allowing early antimycobacterial therapy initiation in patients likely to receive a post-mortem diagnosis.

References

1. Azoulay É, Schlemmer B (2006) Diagnostic strategy in cancer patients with acute respiratory failure. ICM 32:808–822
2. Bollee G, Sarfati C, Thiery G, Bergeron A, de Miranda S, Menotti J, de Castro N, Taz A, Schlemmer B, Elie Azoulay (2007) Clinical picture of pneumocystis jirovecipneumonia in cancer patients. Chest 132:1305–1310
3. Martin WG, Ristow KM, Habermann TM, Colgan JP, Witzig TE, Ansell SM (2005 Oct 20) Bleomycin pulmonary toxicity has a negative impact on the outcome of patients with Hodgkin's lymphoma. J Clin Oncol 23(30):7614–20
4. Erbes R, Oettel K, Raffenberg M, Mauch H, Schmidt-Ioanas M, Lode H (2006 June) Characteristics and outcome of patients with active pulmonary tuberculosis requiring intensive care. Eur Respir J 27(6):1223–8
5. Zahar JR, Azoulay E, Klement E, De Lassence A, Lucet JC, Regnier B, Schlemmer B, Bedos JP (2001 Mar) Delayed treatment contributes to mortality in ICU patients with severe active pulmonary tuberculosis and acute respiratory failure. Intensive Care Med 27(3):513–20
6. Nadrous HF, Afessa B, Pfeifer EA, Peters SG (2003 Aug) The role of autopsy in the intensive care unit. Mayo Clin Proc 78(8):947–50
7. Sharma S, Nadrous HF, Peters SG, Tefferi A, Litzow MR, Aubry MC, Afessa B (2005 Sep) Pulmonary complications in adult blood and marrow transplant recipients: autopsy findings. Chest 128(3):1385–92
8. Redelman-Sidi G, Sepkowitz KA (2010) Rapidly growing mycobacteria infection in patients with cancer. Clin Infect Dis 51(4):422–434

Respiratory Symptoms Occurring 4 Months After Allogeneic Hematopoietic Stem Cell Transplantation

58

Anne Bergeron, Séverine Feuillet, Véronique Meignin, Patricia Ribaud, and Abdellatif Tazi

Contents

A. Bergeron (✉), S. Feuillet, and A. Tazi
Université Paris 7, UFR Denis Diderot; Assistance Publique-Hôpitaux de Paris, Service de Pneumologie, Hôpital Saint-Louis, 1, Avenue Claude Vellefaux, 75475, Paris Cedex 10, France
e-mail: anne.bergeron-lafaurie@sls.aphp.fr

V. Meignin
Université Paris 7, UFR Denis Diderot; Assistance Publique-Hôpitaux de Paris, Service de Pathologie, Hôpital Saint-Louis, Paris, France

P. Ribaud
Université Paris 7, UFR Denis Diderot; Assistance Publique-Hôpitaux de Paris, Service d'Hématologie-Greffe, Hôpital Saint-Louis, Paris, France

58.1 Case Study

A 46-year-old woman underwent a genoidentical bone marrow transplant for chronic myeloid leukemia with myeloablative conditioning that included busulfan and cyclophosphamide in January 1999. Her early course after transplantation was not complicated by infection or acute graft-versus-host disease (GVHD). She had no history of pulmonary disease and had stopped smoking at the time of the transplantation (30 packs/year).

In May 1999, while she was taking cyclosporine for GVHD prophylaxis, she presented with biological liver abnormalities that were attributed to chronic liver GVHD. At this time, she reported recent cough and insidious dyspnea on exertion. No further exploration of the lung was initially performed. Steroids were then introduced (1.2 mg/kg/day prednisone). Anti-infectious prophylaxis consisted in amoxicillin, valacyclovir, and trimethoprim/sulfamethoxazole. Despite steroids, both dyspnea and cough increased during the 2 following months; the liver biology remained stable. Subsequent workup revealed no abnormalities on lung high-resolution computed tomography (HRCT) both on inspiratory and expiratory cuts; pulmonary function testing (PFT) was within the normal range (Fig. 58.1a, b; Table 58.1). Bronchoalveolar lavage (BAL) recovered 180,000 cells/mL with 76% macrophages, 9% lymphocytes, 15% neutrophils, and scattered atypical epithelial cells resembling tumoral cells. An extensive search for infectious agents and for cancer was negative. Inhaled steroids were initiated with transient improvement of the respiratory symptoms.

Five months later, her liver biology had remained unchanged, but she presented with recurrent severe acute respiratory distress, similar to asthma exacerbations, that dramatically responded to β2 agonists. At this time, she was taking 0.5 mg/kg/day prednisone and 150 mg

É. Azoulay (ed.), *Pulmonary Involvement in Patients with Hematological Malignancies*, DOI: 10.1007/978-3-642-15742-4_58, © Springer-Verlag Berlin Heidelberg 2011

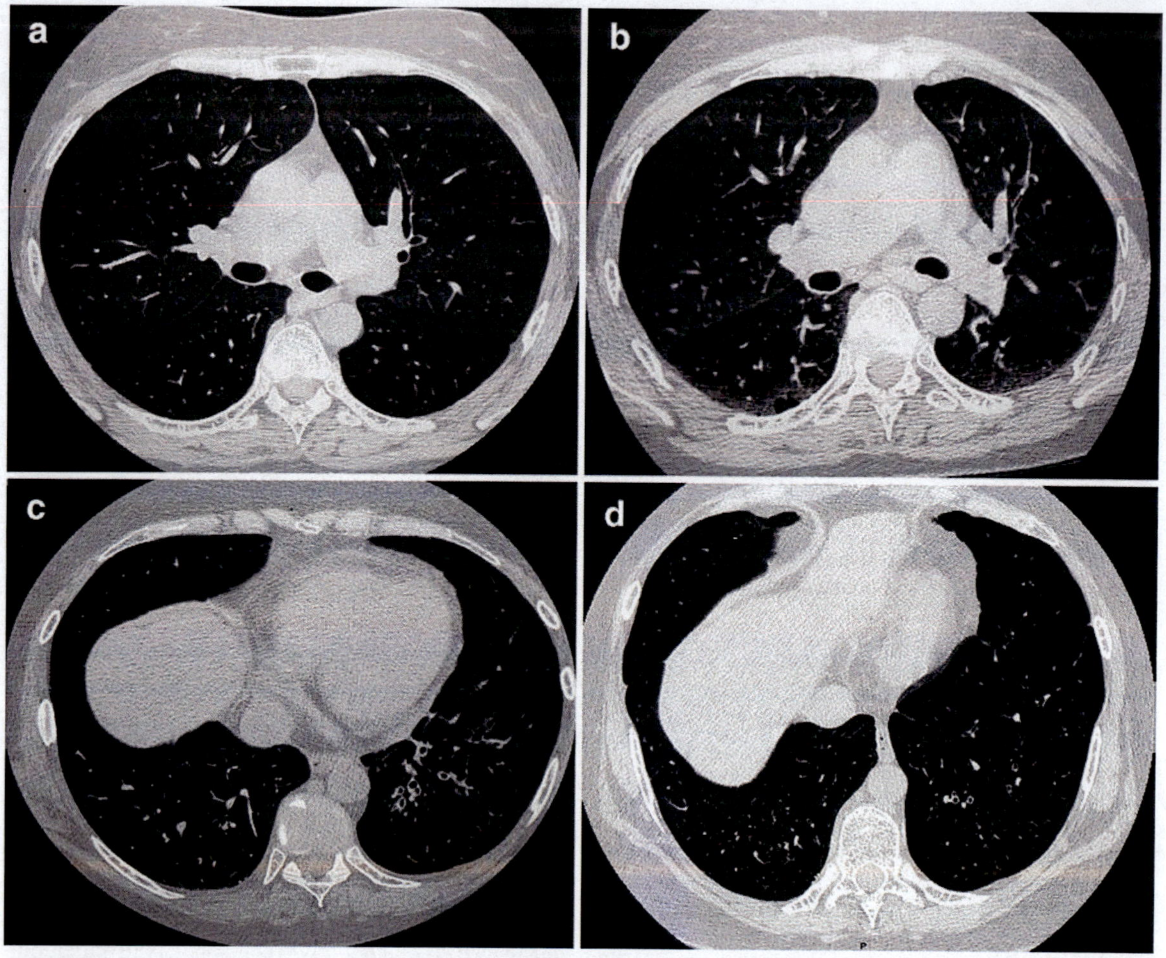

Fig. 58.1 Evolution of lung high-resolution computed tomography (HRCT). In April 1999, HRCT revealed no parenchymal abnormalities or air trapping on inspiratory (**a**) and expiratory cuts (**b**). Bronchiectasis further appeared in the lower regions of the lungs in December 2001 (**c**) and further regressed (**d**)

cyclosporine. PFT revealed new evidence of significant improvements of forced expiratory volume in 1 s (FEV1) and maximal expiratory flows at low lung volumes (FEF) after inhalation of bronchodilators, although these parameters remained within the normal ranges at baseline. Both the patient and her sibling donor had no history of asthma or allergy.

Because of the atypical clinical picture in the context of allogenic hematopoietic stem cell transplantation (AHSCT), a lung surgical biopsy was performed. Biopsy of the lung revealed changes consistent with the diagnosis of bronchiolitis obliterans (BO) (Fig. 58.2). As the pulmonary condition did not improve while she was taking steroids and she developed Cushing syndrome, steroids were progressively tapered. In parallel, after the lung biopsy, mycophenolate mofetil was introduced as well as inhaled corticosteroids and long-acting β2-adrenergic agonist combination therapy.

Her pulmonary clinical condition remained unchanged with stable dyspnea on exertion and several "asthma-like" exacerbations. Two years after the beginning of the respiratory symptoms, the frequency of the asthma-like exacerbations progressively decreased, but recurrent pulmonary infections occurred, including several presentations of bronchitis and pneumonia due to *Streptococcus pneumoniae* and *Pseudomonas aeruginosa*. At this time, steroids were stopped, and the serum γ immunoglobulin level was found to be 5 g/L. Exogenous immunoglobulin administration had been stopped 8 months prior. PFT showed a new mild obstructive ventilatory defect (Table 58.1); lung HRCT revealed new bronchiectasis in the lower lobes (Fig. 58.1c). Both inhaled therapy and mycophenolate mofetil were pursued, and tacrolimus was added to the regimen. During the following year, chronic cough, sputum, and dyspnea remained unchanged, and PFT

Table 58.1 Pulmonary functional testing during follow-up

	12/1998	07/1999	02/2000	02/2001	11/2001	12/2003	03/2004	09/2004	06/2005	03/2006	05/2007	06/2008
RV (mL)	1,730	2,277	1,480	2,900	2,030	2,870	2,330	3,240	2,690	3,010	3,060	2,020
% of predicted value	106	138	90	179	124	167	136	187	155	172	172	113
FVC (mL)	3,320	2,960	2,720	2,790	2,840	2,680	2,710	2,590	2,320	2,650	2,910	2,570
% of predicted value	111	99	91	97	101	93	94	91	82	95	105	87
FEV1 (mL)	2,640	2,170	2,280	1,920	2,100	1,780	1,890	1,900	1,610	1,730	1,830	1,850
% of predicted value	103	85	89	79	88	73	77	79	67	72	78	77
FEV1 after bronchodilators (mL)			2,550	2,040	2,550	1,880	2,180	2,220	1,870	2,040	2,110	2,020
FEV1/FVC	0.8	0.73	0.84	0.69	0.74	0.66	0.69	0.73	0.69	0.65	0.63	0.72
FEF 50% (mL)	3,690	1,560	2,910	1,460	1,860	1,310	1,490	1,460	1,200	1,230	1,120	1,460
% of predicted value	94	41	74	38	49	35	39	39	32	33	30	45%

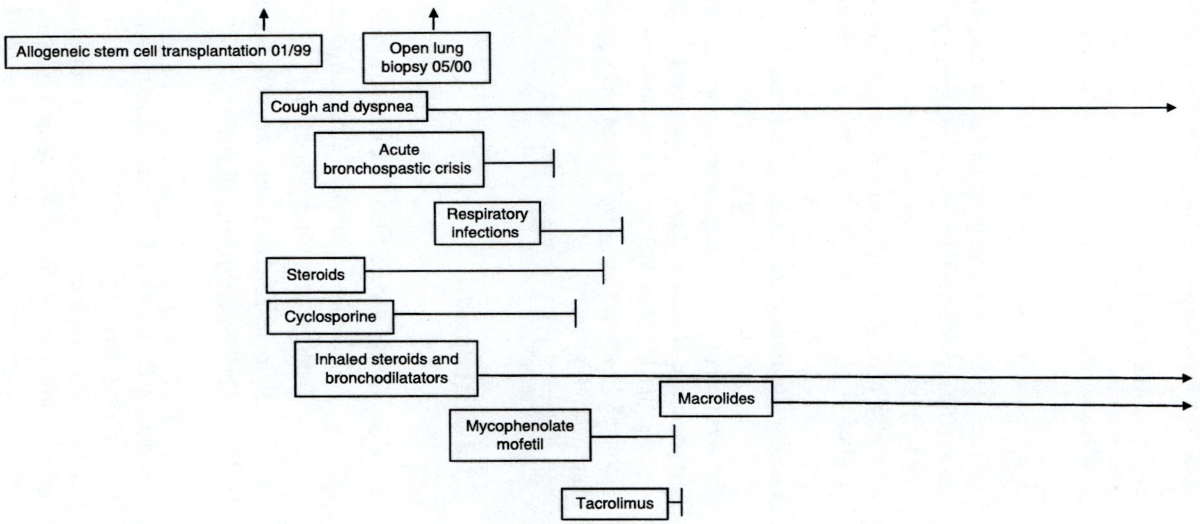

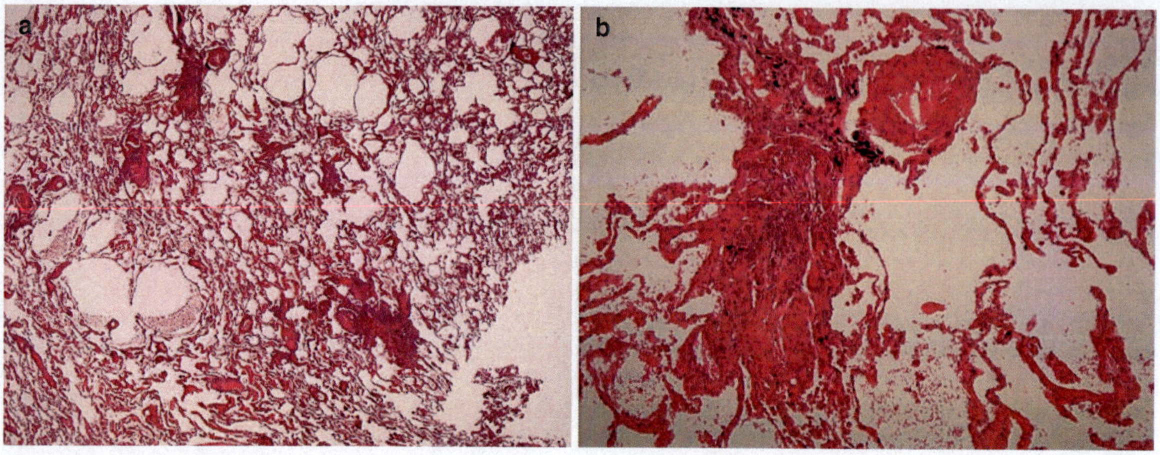

Fig. 58.2 Histopathological examination of surgical lung biopsy. (**a**) Fibrous scars are scattered in an otherwise normal lung parenchyma (H&E ×40). (**b**) The fibrous scar is adjacent to a pulmonary arterial section and corresponds to an entirely obliterated bronchiole (H&S ×100)

stabilized (Table 58.1).

Because of the numerous infectious events and the poor efficacy of systemic immunosuppressive treatment on both respiratory symptoms and PFT, tacrolimus and mycophenolate mofetil were progressively stopped 4 years after the beginning of respiratory symptoms. Combined inhaled treatment was pursued, and low-dose macrolides were introduced.

At the last follow-up, 10 years after the AHSCT, she was free of chronic respiratory symptoms, she had not presented at the emergency department for the last 4 years, her PFT had stabilized with no severe defect (Table 58.1), and her lung HRCT scan had significantly improved (Fig. 58.1d).

58.2 Discussion

58.2.1 *Was Our Patient's Clinical Picture Typical of Cases of Bronchiolitis Obliterans Complicating Allogeneic Hematopoietic Stem Cell transplantation?*

The clinical diagnosis of BO, which is the most frequent picture of pulmonary GVHD, is usually difficult to establish [1]. Dyspnea on exertion and cough are the most common symptoms [1]. However, within the many other complications related to the procedure of AHSCT, these symptoms may not be initially predominant for these patients. Furthermore, these symptoms may have several explanations in the context of recent AHSCT. First, infectious diseases must be ruled out. Next, in this context, shortness of breath may be associated with other causes, such as muscle impairment or anemia.

Our patient initially complained of usual cough and dyspnea on exertion. However, she subsequently presented with a more surprising clinical picture resembling acute asthma despite steroid therapy. Indeed, she presented several times at the emergency department for severe bronchospasms that responded dramatically to bronchodilators. Neither she nor her related donor had a history of asthma or allergy, in contrast to reported patients who developed asthma after AHSCT from an atopic donor [13]. Although wheezing may be part of the lung physical examination of patients with BO, sudden asthma-like exacerbations are unusual.

The occurrence of any respiratory symptoms in our patient should have led to the consideration of BO. In fact, our patient's pulmonary symptoms began 4 months after AHSCT, while most BOs usually occur within 18 months after AHSCT and rarely before the third month [1]. Furthermore, our patient had probable chronic liver GVHD at the time that she developed respiratory symptoms. Many risk factors have been proposed for the development of BO post-AHSCT based on retrospective studies. The only consistent one is an association with extra-thoracic chronic GVHD, leading to the recognition of BO as a chronic lung GVHD [8]. Interestingly, in this case, liver GVHD resolved after the administration of steroids, while BO continued to develop. The busulfan-based conditioning regimen received by our patient has also been proposed as a risk factor for BO [19]. Community viruses and respiratory tract infections have also been associated with airflow decline after AHSCT [7]. Of note, only a few nasal swabs in search of some viruses (respiratory syncytial virus, parainfluenza virus types 1–3, influenza virus A and B, adenovirus) were performed during the follow-up of our patient. Neither these samples nor the BAL recovered any of these viruses. Importantly, only conventional microbiological techniques were available at this time in our center (not molecular biology techniques); thus, we cannot formally conclude the absence of a respiratory virus at any moment.

58.2.2 Was Pulmonary Function Testing Consistent with the Diagnosis of BO?

Although histological examination remains the standard diagnostic criterion for BO, lung biopsy is rarely performed. In fact, the diagnosis of BO syndrome is routinely made following the development of an obstructive lung ventilatory defect on PFT after AHSCT [8]. Therefore, the recent NIH consensus definition of BO syndrome relies on the following lung functional pattern: (1) decreased FEV1 (<75% of predicted normal), (2) evidence of airway obstruction with a ratio of FEV1 to forced vital capacity (FVC) of less than 0.7, and (3) elevated residual volume (RV) of air (>120% of predicted normal), reflecting lung hyperinflation. Nevertheless, these criteria may be insufficient for diagnosing BO. It is important to note that, in the case of the collapse of small airways, which characterizes BO, air trapping may result in concomitant decreases of FEV1 and FVC. Thus, the FEV1/FVC ratio may be normal, whereas RV is ordinarily increased [16]. Measurement of slow vital capacity (VC) may then give a more correct estimate of the FEV1/VC ratio [16]. A decline in FEV1 of 10% to 15% of predicted normal and a decline in the predicted forced midexpiratory flow rate (FEF 25–75%) to less than 70%, which is nonspecific, have also been proposed to identify patients with BO syndrome [23]. Finally, it has been shown that, in a few cases, BO can be diagnosed in patients with normal PFT [1].

The PFT performed before AHSCT in our patient was within normal limits; in particular, FEV1 was 103%, of predicted. At the time she developed the first respiratory symptoms, the pulmonary functional NIH definition of BO could not be applied [8] because FEV1 was still within normal range, i.e., 90% of predicted value. Even if, interestingly, FEV1 had decreased by 10% of the predicted normal value, RV was 94% of the predicted normal value, and, unfortunately, $FEF_{25-75\%}$ was not available. When she began developing sudden bronchospasms, her PFT showed normal FEV1 at baseline, but revealed the appearance of a positive bronchodilator response with values of FEV1 >12% and 200 mL compared with baseline [16]. Reversibility of FEV1 after bronchodilator inhalation is unusual in patients with BO post-AHSCT. In one of the studies that first described this entity, less than 10% of the patients had this functional characteristic [5]. In some subsequent studies, some authors have included the restriction that FEV1 must remain unchanged after bronchodilator testing in their functional definition of BO [17].

Three years after the beginning of respiratory symptoms, the FEV1/FVC ratio declined to 65%, the RV increased until reaching 170%, and the $FEF_{25-75\%}$ was <50%, whereas FEV1 remained 75% of the predicted normal value. Interestingly, the pulmonary functional defect has remained stable, with a current follow-up of 10 years.

58.2.3 Was the Lung Computed Tomography Scan Informative for Diagnosing BO?

In regard to the difficulty in diagnosing small airway diseases, lung HRCT has been widely evaluated in different contexts, including lung transplantation, where BO is also a major problem [9]. Following these studies, air trapping, small airway thickening, and bronchiectasis on lung HRCT (with inspiratory and expiratory cuts) are part of the NIH definition of BO post-AHSCT [8]. Importantly, few studies have focused on BO post-AHSCT [20], and all of these studies have reported a high sensitivity of these abnormalities for the diagnosis of BO, especially air trapping. Several questions arise from this assertion. First, evaluation of air trapping is limited to subjective interpretation. Second, specificity of these signs has not been evaluated. Last, whether these lung HRCT abnormalities permit the diagnosis of BO before PFT is modified remains questionable. A recent study showed that the ranking of air trapping correlated with the severity of obstructive ventilatory defect and lung hyperinflation, suggesting a close correlation between PFT and air trapping [12].

At the time that our patient presented with cough, dyspnea, and normal PFT, the lung HRCT scan did not show significant abnormalities, such as air trapping, small airway thickening, or bronchiectasis. Subsequently, her successive lung HRCT scans revealed the development of bronchiectasis, while the PFT was only slightly altered. Unexpectedly, at the last follow-up, when the patient was free of respiratory symptoms, the bronchiectasis had decreased (Fig. 58.1).

58.2.4 What About the Cell Profile of Bronchoalveolar Lavage for Our patient?

In the context of AHSCT, the BAL is performed as an extensive search for a pulmonary infectious disease. Once an infection has been ruled out, very little is known about the diagnostic value of cellular analysis of BAL. Twenty years ago, St. John et al. reported two distinct BAL cell profiles in AHSCT recipients with obstructive lung ventilatory defects. In that study, some of the patients had neutrophil predominance, whereas others had lymphocyte predominance, with no correlation with the clinical outcome [21]. Consistent with these data, our patient had a slight increase in the neutrophil differential count of her BAL. Notably, we observed atypical cells in her BAL fluid. Immunohistochemical analysis revealed that these cells were of epithelial origin and resembled malignant cells. The hypothesis of neoplasm malignant cells was ruled out after an extensive search for a neoplasm failed to detect any such malignancy. Furthermore, no malignant disease was diagnosed in the following 10 years.

Marked cellular atypia may be seen in BAL fluid from patients with pulmonary infections, especially among those with viral or acute respiratory distress symptoms. In these settings, these cells correspond to bronchial cell hyperplasia and hyperplastic type II pneumocytes [11]. Our patient had no respiratory distress, and no pathogen was found in the BAL fluid. As reported for epidermal and gastrointestinal epithelial cells, the conditioning regimen for AHSCT may also be the cause of atypical cells in BAL fluids [11]. However, atypical bronchial cells after chemotherapy are usually seen within the first few weeks following chemotherapy, whereas our patient had undergone AHSCT 4 months prior. More interestingly, GVHD may be the source of atypical cells. Yousem noticed prominent alveolar pneumocyte atypia in all specimens obtained from patients with BO when he first described the spectrum of pulmonary GVHD [24]. In a recent study, Rochat et al. found that the presence of epithelial cell atypia in BAL fluid recovered from children who had undergone AHSCT, concomitant with respiratory symptoms and GVHD in other organs, may suggest the diagnosis of pulmonary GVHD [18]. Whether the cytology of BAL fluid may be a useful tool for diagnosing BO post-AHSCT needs further examination.

58.2.5 Was the Lung Biopsy Necessary for Our Patient?

Definitive diagnosis of BO post-AHSCT relies on histological examination of a lung biopsy, demonstrating more or less complete obliteration of the lumens of small airways with dense fibrous scar tissue together with damage of the epithelium and peribronchiolar mononuclear infiltrate.

The lung biopsy also permits the ruling out of a differential diagnosis, especially pulmonary infections. However, a lung biopsy may result in severe complications in AHSCT recipients, and thus noninvasive diagnostic tools are usually preferred, such as PFT or lung HRCT [22].

In our patient, a lung biopsy was performed 1 year after the beginning of respiratory symptoms. At that time, she had no fever, and the diagnosis of an infectious disease was unlikely. However, we indicated the lung biopsy for several reasons: (1) the clinical picture was unusual, with an uncertainty of whether the symptoms could be related to the AHSCT; (2) we did not have decisive results from other diagnostic tools, such as PFT or lung HRCT; (3) in regard to the usual poor prognosis of BO post-AHSCT, it was important to make a definitive diagnosis in an attempt to better adapt the treatment.

Diagnosing BO is not always straightforward, even with a lung biopsy. At first look, histological examination of our patient's lung biopsy seemed to be normal. This observation underlines the necessity of carefully analyzing lung parenchyma in these patients. Indeed, in some cases of BO, the lumens of airways are entirely obliterated by dense fibrous scar tissue, and the atretic airways are identified only by their location adjacent to arterioles, which was the case for our patient (Fig. 58.1a) [24].

58.2.6 What A Posteriori Analysis Can Be Made for the Therapeutic Management of Our patient?

Our patient's pulmonary condition worsened despite immunosuppressive treatments. Interestingly, her respiratory symptoms were serious, whereas her PFT was only slightly altered. Surprisingly, she developed bronchospasms while taking steroids. Bronchodilator nebulization permitted the dramatic resolution of each asthma-like exacerbation. Our patient was taking inhaled steroids and bronchodilators throughout her follow-up. Low-dose macrolides were added when she developed recurrent pulmonary infections, which then became less frequent. As time went on, systemic immunosuppressive treatment was decreased and then stopped, and her respiratory symptoms progressively regressed.

Data from the evaluation of BO post-AHSCT treatment are presented only in small retrospective studies. In these studies, an increase of systemic immunosuppressive therapy is usual, similar to the treatment of extra-thoracic GVHD. Most of the patients do not respond to this treatment, and their prognosis is poor, with deaths due to both respiratory insufficiency and severe infections [4,6,17]. As illustrated by our case study, immunosuppressive treatment was probably associated with the development of infections.

By considering that immunosuppressive treatment is associated with an increased occurrence of infections and that its efficacy for the treatment of BO post-ASCHT is uncertain, this treatment must be carefully prescribed in the absence of progressive extra-thoracic GVHD. In this context, close evaluation of the effect of immunosuppressants on pulmonary condition must be performed to adapt their use.

We previously reported the efficacy of a combination of an inhaled long-acting bronchodilator and steroids in a group of patients with BO post-AHSCT [3]. Another study confirmed the potential utility of inhaled steroids in this context [2]. There are a few reports on the use of low-dose macrolides, which have anti-inflammatory as well as anti-infectious properties, to treat BO both after lung transplantation and after AHSCT [10,14,15].

Large prospective studies are necessary to confirm these preliminary data and to evaluate other treatments to determine the optimal line of treatment. In this context, the objective of these treatments should be determined: resolution of the pulmonary condition or stabilization. The main limitation of such an evaluation will be the lack of knowledge concerning BO post-AHSCT pathogenesis and its natural history.

58.3 Conclusion

The presented case illustrates that the diagnosis and treatment of BO post-AHSCT remain challenging. It also shows that, although BO is known to have a poor prognosis, the evolution can be positive, even if there is no evident correlation between the evolution of the disease and the treatments. It also illustrates the association between BO and pulmonary infections, raising the question of interactions between infections and BO in the pathogenesis of BO. New insights into the understanding of BO post-AHSCT are necessary, with respect to its pathogenesis and its clinical management.

References

1. Afessa B, Peters SG (2005) Chronic lung disease after hematopoietic stem cell transplantation. Clin Chest Med 26: 571–586, vi
2. Bashoura L, Gupta S, Jain A et al (2008) Inhaled corticosteroids stabilize constrictive bronchiolitis after hematopoietic stem cell transplantation. Bone Marrow Transplant 41: 63–67
3. Bergeron A, Belle A, Chevret S et al (2007) Combined inhaled steroids and bronchodilatators in obstructive airway disease after allogeneic stem cell transplantation. Bone Marrow Transplant 39:547–553
4. Chan CK, Hyland RH, Hutcheon MA et al (1987) Small-airways disease in recipients of allogeneic bone marrow transplants. An analysis of 11 cases and a review of the literature. Medicine (Baltimore) 66:327–340
5. Clark JG, Crawford SW, Madtes DK et al (1989) Obstructive lung disease after allogeneic marrow transplantation. Clinical presentation and course. Ann Intern Med 111: 368–376

6. Dudek AZ, Mahaseth H, DeFor TE et al (2003) Bronchiolitis obliterans in chronic graft-versus-host disease: analysis of risk factors and treatment outcomes. Biol Blood Marrow Transplant 9:657–666
7. Erard V, Chien JW, Kim HW et al (2006) Airflow decline after myeloablative allogeneic hematopoietic cell transplantation: the role of community respiratory viruses. J Infect Dis 193:1619–1625
8. Filipovich AH, Weisdorf D, Pavletic S et al (2005) National Institutes of Health consensus development project on criteria for clinical trials in chronic graft-versus-host disease: I. Diagnosis and staging working group report. Biol Blood Marrow Transplant 11:945–956
9. Franquet T, Muller NL (2003) Disorders of the small airways: high-resolution computed tomographic features. Semin Respir Crit Care Med 24:437–444
10. Gerhardt SG, McDyer JF, Girgis RE et al (2003) Maintenance azithromycin therapy for bronchiolitis obliterans syndrome: results of a pilot study. Am J Respir Crit Care Med 168: 121–125
11. Gulbahce HE, Baker KS, Kumar P et al (2003) Atypical cells in bronchoalveolar lavage specimens from bone marrow transplant recipients. A potential pitfall. Am J Clin Pathol 120:101–106
12. Gunn ML, Godwin JD, Kanne JP et al (2008) High-resolution CT findings of bronchiolitis obliterans syndrome after hematopoietic stem cell transplantation. J Thorac Imaging 23:244–250
13. Hallstrand TS, Sprenger JD, Agosti JM et al (2004) Long-term acquisition of allergen-specific IgE and asthma following allogeneic bone marrow transplantation from allergic donors. Blood 104:3086–3090
14. Khalid M, Al Saghir A, Saleemi S et al (2005) Azithromycin in bronchiolitis obliterans complicating bone marrow transplantation: a preliminary study. Eur Respir J 25:490–493
15. Maimon N, Lipton JH, Chan CK et al (2009) Macrolides in the treatment of bronchiolitis obliterans in allograft recipients. Bone Marrow Transplant 44:69–73
16. Pellegrino R, Viegi G, Brusasco V et al (2005) Interpretative strategies for lung function tests. Eur Respir J 26:948–968
17. Philit F, Wiesendanger T, Archimbaud E et al (1995) Post-transplant obstructive lung disease ("bronchiolitis obliterans"): a clinical comparative study of bone marrow and lung transplant patients. Eur Respir J 8:551–558
18. Rochat I, Posfay-Barbe KM, Kumar N et al (2008) Bronchoalveolar cytology for diagnosing pulmonary GVHD after bone marrow transplant in children. Pediatr Pulmonol 43:697–702
19. Santo Tomas LH, Loberiza FR Jr, Klein JP et al (2005) Risk factors for bronchiolitis obliterans in allogeneic hematopoietic stem-cell transplantation for leukemia. Chest 128: 153–161
20. Sargent MA, Cairns RA, Murdoch MJ et al (1995) Obstructive lung disease in children after allogeneic bone marrow transplantation: evaluation with high-resolution CT. AJR Am J Roentgenol 164:693–696
21. St John RC, Gadek JE, Tutschka PJ et al (1990) Analysis of airflow obstruction by bronchoalveolar lavage following bone marrow transplantation. Implications for pathogenesis and treatment. Chest 98:600–607
22. White DA, Wong PW, Downey R (2000) The utility of open lung biopsy in patients with hematologic malignancies. Am J Respir Crit Care Med 161:723–729
23. Williams KM, Chien JW, Gladwin MT et al (2009) Bronchiolitis obliterans after allogeneic hematopoietic stem cell transplantation. JAMA 302:306–314
24. Yousem SA (1995) The histological spectrum of pulmonary graft-versus-host disease in bone marrow transplant recipients. Hum Pathol 26:668–675

Pulmonary Complications of Chronic Lymphocytic Leukemia

59

Melhem Solh and Punit Wadhwa

Contents

M. Solh
Division of Hematology, Oncology and Transplantation, University of Minnesota, One Veterans Drive, 111E, Minneapolis, MN 55417, USA

P. Wadhwa (✉)
Division of Hematology, Oncology and Transplantation, University of Minnesota, One Veterans Drive, 111E, Minneapolis, MN 55417, USA and
Minneapolis VA Medical Center, One Veterans Drive, 111E, Minneapolis, MN 55417, USA
e-mail: punit.wadhwa@med.va.gov

59.1 Introduction

Chronic lymphocytic leukemia (CLL) remains the most common type of leukemia in the western world, accounting for almost 30% of leukemias [31]. CLL accounts for 15,000 new cases and 4,400 deaths in the United States annually [31]. The actual incidence of CLL is thought to be underestimated as most CLL patients are asymptomatic and discovered incidentally on the basis of abnormalities detected on a routine blood count [53]. CLL was considered to be a disease of older age (median age at diagnosis of 55 years), but it is not unusual to diagnose CLL in patients as young as 35 years of age [27].

CLL is a disorder of malignant B lymphocytes characterized by expression of the B cell antigens CD19 and CD20, and expression of the T cell antigen CD5. The majority of patients present with lymphocytosis without any other disease manifestations. As the disease progresses, patients develop lymphadenopathy, hepatosplenomegaly and cytopenias. As the disease often runs an indolent course, the majority of patients are observed and followed clinically, and treatment is generally deferred in the absence of bulky adenopathy, B symptoms (fevers, night sweats or weight loss), debilitating fatigue or significant cytopenias.

Over the last two decades, there has been a dramatic increase in the number of neoplastic agents available to treat CLL, ranging from the purine analogues such as fludarabine, pentostatin and cladribine to monoclonal antibodies rituximab and alemtuzumab [67]. These agents bring about impressive complete remission rates when used to treat newly diagnosed CLL patients [32, 38]. These advances in achieving durable remissions, coupled with the chronic nature of this disease, have led to an increased frequency of complications in

É. Azoulay (ed.), *Pulmonary Involvement in Patients with Hematological Malignancies*,
DOI: 10.1007/978-3-642-15742-4_59, © Springer-Verlag Berlin Heidelberg 2011

survivors, of which pulmonary complications are an important cause of acute and long-term sequelae.

59.2 Pulmonary Complications of CLL

Pulmonary complications are a common cause of morbidity and mortality in CLL patients. The respiratory tract illnesses manifest a wide array of abnormalities radiographically and clinically. Pulmonary infiltrates remain the most common radiographic presentation and are usually secondary to infectious complications [7, 47]. Other underlying etiologies for the radiographic presentation of pulmonary infiltrates include parenchymal involvement by leukemia, alveolar hemorrhage, drug-related toxicity, arterial thrombosis with pulmonary embolism, pulmonary leukostasis and secondary malignancies [26, 28, 51]. Airway obstruction by hilar and mediastinal lymphadenopathy, pleural effusions and atelectasis are among other complications seen in CLL (Table 59.1).

In a study by Ahmed et al. [1], pulmonary complications accounted for 22.3% of hospital admissions in CLL patients between 1993 and 2001. The common presenting symptoms were dyspnea (61%), cough (58%), fever (56%), chest pain (12%), altered mental status (10%), decreased oral intake (6%), and stridor or hoarseness (3%). Pulmonary infiltrates were the most common radiographic abnormality (65% of patients) with multilobar involvement in 24% of the cases. Other radiographic findings included pleural effusions (24%), lung nodules, lymphadenopathy and lung abscesses. The median duration of hospital stay was 11 days. Thirty-five percent of patients developed respiratory failure, and 40% of the patients died during the same hospital stay. Mortality was associated with absolute neutrophil count $ANC \leq 0.5 \times 10^9/L$ ($p < 0.001$), $BUN \geq 20$ mg/dL ($p < 0.003$), secondary malignancy ($p < 0.005$) and CLL ≥ stage III ($p < 0.05$). The array of common diagnoses included pneumonias (75%), malignant pleural effusion and/or lung infiltrate due to CLL (9%), pulmonary leukostasis (4%), Richter transformation or nonsmall cell lung carcinoma (3%), and upper airway obstruction (2%).

Table 59.1 Pulmonary complications in CLL

Infectious complications	• Bacterial infections: encapsulated organisms, gram negative • Opportunistic infections: listeria, nocardia, PCP, mycobacteria • Fungal infections: candida, aspergillus • Viral infections: CMV (mainly with alemtuzumab)
Noninfectious complications	• Pulmonary leukostasis • Pleural effusion • Leukemic infiltrates • Drug-related pneumonitis • Bronchiolitis obliterans • Airway obstruction (intrinsic or extrinsic) • Lung cancer

59.3 Infectious Pulmonary Complications

Infections are the most common pulmonary complication, accounting for 75% of respiratory illnesses among hospitalized CLL patients [1]. The pathogenesis of infections in patients with CLL is complex and multifactorial.

CLL patients have inherent defects in multiple arms of the immune system, including qualitative and quantitative defects in B and T lymphocytes, complement defects and hypogammaglobulinemia. These defects are compounded by the immunosuppressive effects of chemotherapy and monoclonal antibodies, such as purine analogs and alemtuzumab, as well as neutropenia secondary to alkylating agents and purine analogs [64].

Bacterial infections are the most common type of infection in CLL patients treated with either alkylator agents or purine analogues. These infections have a tendency to occur at mucosal sites, mainly the respiratory tract. The most common encountered bacterial organisms are those that require opsonization for killing (*Streptococcus pneumoniae*, *Staphylococcus* spp. and *Haemophilus influenza*) [11]; however, posttherapy and hospitalizations, there is an increased risk of gram-negative infections, including *Pseudomonas* spp., *Klebsiella* spp., *Serratia* spp. *and Enterobacter* spp. [1]. The incidence of pneumonia differs among different series and is related to the therapeutic agent used. In earlier studies patients treated with alkylators (such as chlorambucil) and steroids were mostly susceptible to develop pneumonia with bacterial organisms, such as *Staphylococcus aureus*, *Streptococcus pneumoniae*, *Haemophilus influenza*, *Klebsiella pneumonia*, *Pseudomonas and Escherichia coli* [64]. Lung infections caused by opportunistic infection such as nocardia, PCP and mycobacteria are uncommon among patients treated with alkylator therapy alone. Respiratory fungal infections with candida and aspergillus could be seen in the context of prolonged cytotoxic therapy related to an extended period of neutropenia.

Purine analogues induce qualitative and quantitative T-cell abnormalities with a significant drop in CD4 count [36]. This explains why patients treated with fludarabine are at higher risk of such opportunistic lung infections as listeria, nocardia, mycobacteria, candida, aspergillous, Cryptococcus and pneumocystis. In an early report by Keating [34], among 68 patients who were treated with fludarabine, 25 patients developed pneumonia during the course of their therapy. The same group described one case of nocardia pneumonia among 33 patients treated with fludarabine [35]. Anaissie and colleagues studied 402 patients at a single center who received fludarabine therapy alone or with steroids. They identified an increased incidence of opportunistic infections with pneumocytosis, as well as fungal infections with candida and aspergillus. The risk of developing these infections was higher in the context of advanced stage disease (stage III, IV), a history of previous chemotherapy and elevated serum creatinine [3]. The incidence of PCP infection was less than 1% among 544 previously untreated CLL patients who received either fludarabine and/or chlorambucil on the CALGB 9011 study (despite no prophylaxis). No cases of aspergillus infections and only two mycobacterial infections were identified. The risk of lung infections and other severe infections was significantly higher when steroids were part of the therapy in conjunction with purine analogues (cladribine or fludarabine), and the incidence has been as high as 31% with cladribine therapy [66].

Although the addition of rituximab (a monoclonal antibody against CD20) to purine analogues worsens immunosuppression by depleting B cells, the incidence of pulmonary infections with combinations of rituximab and purine analogs does not seem to be higher than that of patients treated with fludarabine alone. In a study of 224 CLL patients who received rituximab plus purine analogues, only three patients developed PCP pneumonia, two developed aspergillosis and one developed a CMV infection [38].

Alemtuzumab is a monoclonal antibody directed against the phosphatidylinositolglycan (PIG)-anchored CD52 glycoprotein, which is expressed in high density on most of normal and malignant B and T-lymphocytes, NK cells, neutrophils and monocytes, hence leading to neutropenia, a profound deficit in cellular immunity and a decrease in all of the mentioned cell lines [24]. Immune dysfunction associated with alemtuzumab begins shortly after initiation of therapy and can last as long as 9 months posttreatment [43]. In earlier studies where alemtuzumab was used in patients who had failed fludarabine therapy, 27% of the 93 patients sustained grade 3/4 infectious complications, including cases of aspergillosis, zygomycosis, candidiasis, *Listeria* meningitis, *Pneumocystis* pneumonia and CMV reactivation despite prohpylaxis with trimethoprim/sulfamethoxazole and famciclovir or the equivalent [37]. In another study, PCP pneumonia was seen in 7%, while bacterial pneumonia was seen in 14% among 29 patients treated with alemtuzumab without antimicrobial prophylaxis [50].

The diagnosis and treatment of lung infections in CLL patients does not differ significantly from similar infections in other patients; however there are a few unique modalities in the context of CLL worth emphasizing. The benefit of prophylactic intravenous immunoglobulin (IVIG) therapy at a dose of 400 mg/kg every 3 weeks, as well as other dose schedules, was evaluated [14,46]. Patients treated with IVIG had fewer minor or moderate bacterial infections, but this did not translate into a reduction in major infections or mortality. It was found that the benefit related to IVIG administration did not improve quality or length of life and was not cost effective. There are no clear guidelines to direct the use of IVIG as there is no clear mortality benefit with this intervention.

Prophylactic antibiotics, antiviral and antifungal agents have not been studied in randomized trials in the setting of CLL. The common practice guidelines are derived from several CLL treatment trials and anecdotal reports. It has been recommended that elderly patients treated with fludarabine receive routine antimicrobial prophylaxis due to the increased risk of severe infections in these patients [57]. Antiviral and *Pneumocystis* prophylaxis is recommended for therapy with fludarabine plus cyclophosphamide (FC) as well as with FC plus rituximab. As the immune defects rendered by purine analog therapy as well as alemtuzumab may persist for several months to a year or two after discontinuation of therapy, prophylaxis in this setting should be continued for some months after treatment is stopped [48]. With alemtuzumab therapy, weekly PCR screening for CMV antigen has been advocated, with prompt institution of ganciclovir therapy for PCR positive cases.

59.4 Noninfectious Lung Complications

59.4.1 Pulmonary Leukostasis

Pulmonary leukostasis is a potentially serious problem for patients with hematologic malignancies whose blast count exceeds 50,000/mm^3 [69]. An entire chapter of this book from Dr. Vincent is dedicated to pulmonary leukostasis. These patients usually present with pulmonary infiltrates, which can mimic an acute pneumonia. The lung and the central nervous system are the most commonly affected sites, and symptoms can be attributed to microvascular obstruction and sludging by leukemic cells. Respiratory failure can also be related to pulmonary hemorrhage or to direct damage to the pulmonary endothelium by the lysed leukemic cells [58]. Patients usually present with new onset shortness of breath or worsening dyspnea. On physical exam, patients are tachypneic, and lung exam reveals diffuse rales. If severe, patients with leukostasis can develop hypoxia, fever and progressive respiratory acidosis, all of which indicate a worse prognosis [21].

Although leukostasis is more common in acute leukemias where the blast count is elevated, it can still be seen in patients with CLL with extremely elevated white cell counts. In a report by Ahmed et al. [1], 5 (3.5%) of 142 hospitalized CLL patients developed leukostasis. Four patients had an extremely elevated white count of >500,000/mm^3, and one patients had a count of 300,000/mm^3 [1]. Other reports of leukostasis in CLL patients are similar to the previous one and are mostly seen in cases where the white count exceeded 300,000/mm^3 [5]. Diagnosis of leukostasis is based on a high degree of suspicion in a patient with elevated white count, combined with the presenting symptomatology and clinical signs. Timely diagnosis is essential to prevent respiratory failure. The treatment is directed at immediate lowering of the white count, correcting any underlying coagulopathy and avoiding measures that might increase blood viscosity, such as blood transfusions. Leukopheresis could be considered when the white count exceeds 500,000/mm^3 or when symptoms develop even at lower counts [40]. Cytotoxic chemotherapy should be administered simultaneously because the effect of leukopheresis is short lived. Five CLL patients with leukostasis were successfully treated with leukapheresis and chemotherapy or chemotherapy alone [1].

59.4.2 Pleural Effusion

Malignant pleural effusions are not uncommon in patients with CLL and have been reported in 7% of hospitalized CLL patients with advanced stage disease [1]. CLL effusions are difficult to diagnose since the malignant lymphocytes in the pleural fluid are similar morphologically to reactive lymphocytes [65]. The diagnosis of CLL pleural effusion is confirmed by immunophenotyping [65]. Malignant pleural effusions are usually related to direct pleural involvement by CLL. The treatment of CLL effusion is directed at treatment of the underlying leukemia [4].

Chylothorax and hemorrhagic pleural effusions have also been reported in rare instances with CLL as complications or as presenting symptoms [63]. CLL should also be included in the differential diagnosis of patients with atraumatic chylous effusions. Chylous effusions in the setting of CLL have been successfully treated with irradiation to the mediastinum [2], with surgical ligation of the thoracic duct [20] or with talc pleurodesis [70].

As patients with CLL are at a higher risk of developing other malignancies, including lung cancer [52], synchronous malignancies can present as a pleural effusion in CLL and should always be considered during the course of the workup [42, 59].

59.4.3 Leukemic Infiltrates

Autopsy studies showed that 30–40% of CLL patients have leukemia infiltrates in the lungs [6, 7, 51]. Nine percent of hospitalized CLL patients had direct lung or pleural involvement with CLL [1]. As reported in the chapter from Dr. Bouros in this book, in most patients, leukemic infiltrates are asymptomatic, and overall these account for <20% of radiographic infiltrates noted in patients with CLL [18]. Diagnosis of leukemic CLL infiltrates requires tissue confirmation and exclusion of infectious etiology. Lymphoid pulmonary involvement can be either nodular (in a perilymphatic distribution) or diffuse [12, 62]. Diffuse involvement also shows a predilection for lymphatic routes, and hence involvement of the bronchovascular bundles is common. Bronchiolocentric involvement has also been described with CLL [51]. CLL patients with leukemic infiltrates can present with cough, chest pain, hemoptysis or pleural effusions. Wheezing has also been described as a presenting symptom in patients with bronchiolocentric involvement [51]. Pulmonary involvement was also reported in the setting of nonprogressive, therapy-responsive CLL and in one case was the sole site of recurrence. Berkman et al. reported three cases of lung involvement with low peripheral counts and responsive disease that were diagnosed by transbronchial biopsy and bronchoalveolar lavage [7]. The treatment of leukemic pulmonary involvement with CLL is directed towards systemic treatment of the leukemia [1]. Patients usually have a good response to chemotherapy with or without steroids, with radiologic evidence of clearance of the infiltrates [54].

59.4.4 Airway Obstruction

Airway obstruction is a rare complication seen among patients with CLL. It is more likely to occur in patients with bulky adenopathy, but tracheal obstruction was also reported as a presenting symptom in one patient [17, 68]. Airway obstruction could be related to extrinsic compression as in the previously reported cases or could be related to direct involvement of the airway. In 5,319 patients with malignant lymphomas seen at the Mayo Clinic, Desanto found only nine with primary laryngeal involvement [19]. Firestone reported a case of a CLL patient presenting with airway obstruction secondary to subglottic involvement [22]. Management of airway obstruction in the setting of CLL should consist initially of securing the airway and then directing attention towards treatment of the leukemia with chemotherapy with or without radiation.

59.4.5 Constrictive Bronchiolitis

Constrictive brochiolitis is defined as the presence of new respiratory symptoms, irreversible airflow obstruction on pulmonary function testing and presence of patchy or diffuse air trapping on CT scan with no other identifiable cause for these findings [44]. It is an obstructive lung disease observed in different contexts, such as connective tissue diseases, solid organ transplant, hematopoietic cell transplant, viral infections and drug-induced lung injury [56]. It can also be a rare manifestation of paraneoplastic pemphigus or paraneoplastic autoimmune multi-organ syndrome (PAMS), which is a paraneoplastic syndrome with a tendency to involve the skin, lungs, muscles and kidneys [8]. In a study of 17 patients with PAMS, two thirds were secondary to either non-Hodgkin's lymphoma or CLL. One patient developed bronchiolitis obliterans 2 years after the onset of CLL and was alive at 16 months of follow-up [44]. Management of bronchiolitis obliterans includes effective treatment of the underlying neoplasm with immunosuppressive or immunomodulatory agents, but this has not been effective in controlling the disease [29]. Further studies to understand the pathogenesis of this disorder may improve the morbidity and mortality associated with it.

59.4.6 Drug-Related Pulmonary Toxicity

Another etiology of pulmonary complications in CLL patients relates to the agents used in the treatment of this leukemia. Identifying drug-induced lung toxicity in cancer patients is always challenging due to the confounding factors of pulmonary malignancy, infection, hemorrhage and radiation toxicity. Alkylating agents have been known to cause pulmonary toxicity [55]. Cyclophosphamide has been well documented to cause pneumonitis in several reports [45]. Clinical features of cyclophosphamide toxicity include dyspnea, fever, cough, parenchymal infiltrates, gas exchange abnormalities on pulmonary function tests and pleural thickening on chest roentgenogram. Over a 20-year period, six patients at the Mayo Clinic were identified with cyclophosphamide-induced pneumonitis. Two patterns were described, early and late onset, with late onset pneumonitis having a less favorable response to drug discontinuation and steroids. Late onset pneumonitis was more likely to be associated with pleural thickening and to progress into pulmonary fibrosis [45].

Chlorambucil has also been reported to induce pneumonitis [13, 16, 23]. The clinical presentation is nonspecific including cough, dyspnea, fever and anorexia. Bibasilar crackles are common on physical exam, and chest imaging reveals a diffuse reticulonodular bibasilar pattern. Diagnosis of alkylator toxicity is based on a histopathologic pattern including hyperplasia of the alveolar lining with mononuclear cell infiltrate and focal interstitial fibrosis [13]. There is no correlation between the cumulative total dose and the development of lung toxicity since toxicity has been reported across a wide range of cumulative doses, ranging from 540 to 8,340 mg [39]. Fludarabine has also been associated with pulmonary toxicity [10, 26, 30, 33, 41]. Helman et al. reported a series of 105 patients treated with fludarabine between 1989 and 2000. Of these patients, 8.6% developed fludarabine-related lung toxicity defined as new onset fever, hypoxia, dyspnea and pulmonary infiltrates, for which there was no alternative explanation. There was no increased risk based on gender, age, history of underlying lung disease, previous chemotherapy and fludarabine regimen (fludarabine alone or in combination with other agents). Patients who received fludarabine for CLL treatment had a 13.3-fold higher risk of developing lung toxicity compared to those who received fludarabine for another indication. The most common radiographic finding was diffuse interstitial infiltrates or diffuse interstitial-alveolar infiltrates. The onset of symptoms after fludarabine treatment ranged from 3 days after the first cycle to 6 days after the seventh cycle. Patients had a good subjective and objective response to steroid therapy with either oral prednisone or intravenous methylprednisolone with a median time to response of 4 days [26].

Alemtuzumab has been described in one case report as a cause of fatal pulmonary pneumonitis [15]. The patient developed acute respiratory failure 3 weeks after the administration of alemtuzumab. The workup was suggestive of interstitial pneumonitis, and the patient died of progressive respiratory failure 2 months after hospitalization.

59.4.7 CLL and Lung Cancer

Patients with CLL are at increased risk of second primary malignancies, including lung cancer [25, 52, 61]. A report from the National Cancer Institute end result program showed an excess risk for the development of a second malignancy among 9,456 patients with CLL when compared to the general population. The common tumors were melanoma, lung carcinoma and brain cancers. There was a significant excess for the development of lung cancer with an observed over expected (O/E) ratio of 1.90 [60]. Another report from M.D. Anderson Cancer Center showed an 11% incidence of cancer among 2,028 CLL patients followed from 1985 to 2005. Lung cancer accounted for 6% of the tumors with an O/E ratio of 1.12. The reason for the increased risk of malignancies and in particular lung cancer in patients with CLL is not well understood. Independent factors predicting development of secondary cancers among the CLL population were older age, male sex and elevated levels of β_2-microglobulin, lactate dehydrogenase and creatinine [61]. One study reports an association of CLL with smoking and hence the increased risk of lung cancer, but immunologic impairment with CLL could contribute to the overall risk [9].

Parekh and colleagues studied the clinical course of lung cancer in CLL patients. During a 22-year follow-up period between 1977 and 1998, 1,329 CLL patients were evaluated at Memorial Sloan Kettering Cancer Center, and 26 patients (1.9%) developed lung cancer. Twenty-two out of the twenty-six secondary lung cancer patients (85%) were either current or former smokers. The median age for diagnosis of CLL was 61 years, and the median age for diagnosis of lung cancer was 68 years. Histologically, the 26 lung carcinomas included six squamous cell carcinomas, 16 adenocarcinomas, three large cell carcinomas and one small cell carcinoma. Ten patients had a third primary tumor. Thirteen patients were treated surgically, but not all patients with early stage lung cancer were able to undergo surgery. Three out of the nine patients diagnosed with stage I lung cancer were not able to undergo resection because of their poor performance status secondary to the underlying CLL. Those with advanced stage disease who required chemotherapy tolerated it poorly, despite treatment with less toxic chemotherapy (mitomycin and vinblastine) to accommodate for the overall performance status [52]. Among nonsurgical patients, the median survival was 6 months, whereas the median survival of the surgical group was 25 months. The 6-month survival of nonsurgical CLL patients was substantially worse compared to advanced lung cancer patients without CLL [49].

59.5 Conclusions

1. Pulmonary complications are an important cause of morbidity and mortality in CLL patients, and account for more than 20% of hospitalizations.
2. The symptoms of pulmonary involvement (fevers, cough, dyspnea and pulmonary infiltrates) are nonspecific, and hence accurate identification of the correct etiology is critical to ensure an optimal patient outcome.
3. An understanding of the immunosuppressive nature of the disease itself, as well as awareness of the immunosuppression and toxicity associated with its therapy, is required to ensure timely diagnosis and treatment.
4. Infections remain the most common cause of pulmonary complications and should be considered to be causative till proven otherwise. While bacterial infections with encapsulated organisms are common in untreated CLL or CLL treated with alkylating agents, opportunistic infections are common in patients treated with purine analogs and alemtuzumab, and the period of susceptibility often lasts for several months after the cessation of treatment.
5. Noninfectious complications are less frequent and, with some exceptions, usually need to be confirmed with a tissue diagnosis.
6. Overall, the outcome of CLL patients hospitalized for pulmonary complication remains poor, and urgent attention should be directed towards these patients.

References

1. Ahmed S, Siddiqui AK et al (2003) Pulmonary complications in chronic lymphocytic leukemia. Cancer 98(9): 1912–1917
2. Ampil FL, Burton GV et al (1993) Chylous effusion complicating chronic lymphocytic leukemia. Leuk Lymphoma 10(6):507–510
3. Anaissie EJ, Kontoyiannis DP et al (1998) Infections in patients with chronic lymphocytic leukemia treated with fludarabine. Ann Intern Med 129(7):559–566
4. Andrieu V, Encaoua R et al (1998) Leukemic pleural effusion in B-cell prolymphocytic leukemia. Hematol Cell Ther 40(6):275–278
5. Baer MR, Stein RS et al (1985) Chronic lymphocytic leukemia with hyperleukocytosis. The hyperviscosity syndrome. Cancer 56(12):2865–2869
6. Barcos M, Lane W et al (1987) An autopsy study of 1206 acute and chronic leukemias (1958 to 1982). Cancer 60(4): 827–837
7. Berkman N, Polliack A et al (1992) Pulmonary involvement as the major manifestation of chronic lymphocytic leukemia. Leuk Lymphoma 8(6):495–499
8. Billet SE, Grando SA et al (2006) Paraneoplastic autoimmune multiorgan syndrome: review of the literature and support for a cytotoxic role in pathogenesis. Autoimmunity 39(7):617–630
9. Brown LM, Gibson R et al. (1992) Smoking and risk of leukemai 135(7): 763–768
10. Cervantes F, Salgado C et al (1990) Fludarabine for prolymphocytic leukaemia and risk of interstitial pneumonitis. Lancet 336(8723):1130
11. Cheson BD (1995) Infectious and immunosuppressive complications of purine analog therapy. J Clin Oncol 13(9): 2431–2448
12. Colby TV, Carrington CB (1983) Pulmonary lymphomas: current concepts. Hum Pathol 14(10):884–887
13. Cole SR, Myers TJ et al (1978) Pulmonary disease with chlorambucil therapy. Cancer 41(2):455–459
14. Cooperative Group for the Study of Immunoglobulin in Chronic Lymphocytic Leukemia (1988) Intravenous immunoglobulin for the prevention of infection in chronic lymphocytic leukemia. A randomized, controlled clinical trial. N Engl J Med 319(14):902–907
15. Creelan B, Ferber A (2008) A fatal case of alemtuzumab-associated interstitial pneumonitis. Am J Ther 15(1): 82–84
16. Crestani B, Jaccard A et al (1994) Chlorambucil-associated pneumonitis. Chest 105(2):634–636
17. Dean MG, Cunningham I et al (1996) Chronic lymphocytic leukaemia with upper airway obstruction. Leuk Lymphoma 20(5–6):505–507
18. Dear A, Goldstein D et al (1995) Pulmonary chronic lymphocytic leukemia: difficulty in establishing a tissue diagnosis. Eur J Haematol 54(2):130–133
19. DeSanto LW, Weiland LH (1970) Malignant lymphoma of the larynx. Laryngoscope 80(6):966–978
20. Doerr CH, Staats BA et al (2002) Chylothorax in chronic lymphocytic leukemia patient. Am J Hematol 70(3): 237–240

21. Dombret H, Hunault M et al (1992) Acute lysis pneumopathy after chemotherapy for acute myelomonocytic leukemia with abnormal marrow eosinophils. Cancer 69(6): 1356–1361
22. Firestone FN, Robinson MJ (1972) Upper airway obstruction: a rare presentation of chronic lymphocytic leukemia. Chest 61(5):505–507
23. Giles FJ, Smith MP et al (1990) Chlorambucil lung toxicity. Acta Haematol 83(3):156–158
24. Gilleece MH, Dexter TM (1993) Effect of Campath-1 H antibody on human hematopoietic progenitors in vitro. Blood 82(3):807–812
25. Greene MH, Hoover RN et al (1978) Subsequent cancer in patients with chronic lymphocytic leukemia – a possible immunologic mechanism. J Natl Cancer Inst 61(2): 337–340
26. Helman DL Jr, Byrd JC et al (2002) Fludarabine-related pulmonary toxicity: a distinct clinical entity in chronic lymphoproliferative syndromes. Chest 122(3):785–790
27. Hernandez JA, Land KJ et al (1995) Leukemias, myeloma, and other lymphoreticular neoplasms. Cancer 75(1 Suppl): 381–394
28. Hisada M, Biggar RJ et al (2001) Solid tumors after chronic lymphocytic leukemia. Blood 98(6):1979–1981
29. Hoffman MA, Qiao X et al (2003) CD8+ T lymphocytes in bronchiolitis obliterans, paraneoplastic pemphigus, and solitary Castleman's disease. N Engl J Med 349(4):407–408
30. Hurst PG, Habib MP et al (1987) Pulmonary toxicity associated with fludarabine monophosphate. Invest New Drugs 5(2):207–210
31. Jemal A, Murray T et al (2003) Cancer statistics, 2003. CA Cancer J Clin 53(1):5–26
32. Johnson S, Smith AG, The French Cooperative Group on CLL et al (1996) Multicentre prospective randomised trial of fludarabine versus cyclophosphamide, doxorubicin, and prednisone (CAP) for treatment of advanced-stage chronic lymphocytic leukaemia. Lancet 347(9013):1432–1438
33. Kane GC, McMichael AJ et al (1992) Pulmonary toxicity and acute respiratory failure associated with fludarabine monophosphate. Respir Med 86(3):261–263
34. Keating MJ, Kantarjian H et al (1989) Fludarabine: a new agent with major activity against chronic lymphocytic leukemia. Blood 74(1):19–25
35. Keating MJ, Kantarjian H et al (1991) Fludarabine: a new agent with marked cytoreductive activity in untreated chronic lymphocytic leukemia. J Clin Oncol 9(1):44–49
36. Keating MJ, O'Brien S et al (1998) Long-term follow-up of patients with chronic lymphocytic leukemia (CLL) receiving fludarabine regimens as initial therapy. Blood 92(4): 1165–1171
37. Keating MJ, Flinn I et al (2002) Therapeutic role of alemtuzumab (Campath-1 H) in patients who have failed fludarabine: results of a large international study. Blood 99(10): 3554–3561
38. Keating MJ, O'Brien S et al (2005) Early results of a chemoimmunotherapy regimen of fludarabine, cyclophosphamide, and rituximab as initial therapy for chronic lymphocytic leukemia. J Clin Oncol 23(18):4079–4088
39. Khong HT, McCarthy J (1998) Chlorambucil-induced pulmonary disease: a case report and review of the literature. Ann Hematol 77(1–2):85–87
40. Lester TJ, Johnson JW et al (1985) Pulmonary leukostasis as the single worst prognostic factor in patients with acute myelocytic leukemia and hyperleukocytosis. Am J Med 79(1):43–48
41. Levin M, Aziz M et al (1997) Steroid-responsive interstitial pneumonitis after fludarabine therapy. Chest 111(5): 1472–1473
42. Lucivero G, Pierucci G et al (1986) B cell chronic lymphocytic leukemia and lung carcinoma with T-lymphocyte-rich pleural effusion in a single patient. Acta Haematol 75(2): 110–112
43. Lundin J, Osterborg A (2004) Advances in the use of monoclonal antibodies in the therapy of chronic lymphocytic leukemia. Semin Hematol 41(3):234–245
44. Maldonado F, Pittelkow MR et al (2009) Constrictive bronchiolitis associated with paraneoplastic autoimmune multiorgan syndrome. Respirology 14(1):129–133
45. Malik SW, Myers JL et al (1996) Lung toxicity associated with cyclophosphamide use. Two distinct patterns. Am J Respir Crit Care Med 154(6 Pt 1):1851–1856
46. Molica S, Musto P et al (1996) Prophylaxis against infections with low-dose intravenous immunoglobulins (IVIG) in chronic lymphocytic leukemia. Results of a crossover study. Haematologica 81(2):121–126
47. Morrison VA (1998) The infectious complications of chronic lymphocytic leukemia. Semin Oncol 25(1):98–106
48. Morrison VA (2007) Management of infectious complications in patients with chronic lymphocytic leukemia. Hematology Am Soc Hematol Educ Program 2007: 332–338
49. Mountain CF (1986) A new international staging system for lung cancer. Chest 89(4 Suppl):225S–233S
50. Osterborg A, Dyer MJ, European Study Group of CAMPATH-1H Treatment in Chronic Lymphocytic Leukemia et al (1997) Phase II multicenter study of human CD52 antibody in previously treated chronic lymphocytic leukemia. J Clin Oncol 15(4):1567–1574
51. Palosaari DE, Colby TV (1986) Bronchiolocentric chronic lymphocytic leukemia. Cancer 58(8):1695–1698
52. Parekh K, Rusch V et al (1999) The clinical course of lung carcinoma in patients with chronic lymphocytic leukemia. Cancer 86(9):1720–1723
53. Rawstron AC, Green MJ et al (2002) Monoclonal B lymphocytes with the characteristics of "indolent" chronic lymphocytic leukemia are present in 3.5% of adults with normal blood counts. Blood 100(2):635–639
54. Rollins SD, Colby TV (1988) Lung biopsy in chronic lymphocytic leukemia. Arch Pathol Lab Med 112(6): 607–611
55. Rubio FA Jr (1972) Possible pulmonary effects of alkylating agents. N Engl J Med 287(22):1150–1151
56. Ryu JH, Myers JL et al (2003) Bronchiolar disorders. Am J Respir Crit Care Med 168(11):1277–1292
57. Shvidel L, Shtalrid M et al (2003) Conventional dose fludarabine-based regimens are effective but have excessive toxicity in elderly patients with refractory chronic lymphocytic leukemia. Leuk Lymphoma 44(11):1947–1950
58. Stucki A, Rivier AS et al (2001) Endothelial cell activation by myeloblasts: molecular mechanisms of leukostasis and leukemic cell dissemination. Blood 97(7):2121–2129

59. Sur N, Silverman JF (1998) Synchronous malignancies detected by effusion cytology. Diagn Cytopathol 18(3): 184–187
60. Travis LB, Curtis RE et al (1992) Second cancers in patients with chronic lymphocytic leukemia. J Natl Cancer Inst 84(18):1422–1427
61. Tsimberidou AM, Wen S et al (2009) Other malignancies in chronic lymphocytic leukemia/small lymphocytic lymphoma. J Clin Oncol 27(6):904–910
62. Turner RR, Colby TV et al (1984) Well-differentiated lymphocytic lymphoma. A study of 47 patients with primary manifestation in the lung. Cancer 54(10):2088–2096
63. van den Berge M, Tinga CJ et al (2001) A 73-year-old man with chronic lymphocytic leukaemia and a haemorrhagic pleural effusion. Ann Hematol 80(3):183–186
64. Wadhwa PD, Morrison VA (2006) Infectious complications of chronic lymphocytic leukemia. Semin Oncol 33(2): 240–249
65. Walts AE, Marchevsky AM (1989) Computerized interactive morphometry. An expert system for the diagnosis of lymphoid-rich effusions. Am J Clin Pathol 92(6): 765–772
66. Robak T, Błoński JZ et al (2000) Cladribine with prednisone versus chlorambucil with prednisone as first-line therapy in chronic lymphocytic leukemia: report of a prospective, randomized, multicenter trial 96(8):2723–2729
67. Wierda W, O'Brien S et al (2005) Chemoimmunotherapy with fludarabine, cyclophosphamide, and rituximab for relapsed and refractory chronic lymphocytic leukemia. J Clin Oncol 23(18):4070–4078
68. Winkler CF, Corpus R (1980) Tracheal obstruction in chronic lymphocytic leukemia. Chest 77(2):244–245
69. Wurthner JU, Kohler G et al (1999) Leukostasis followed by hemorrhage complicating the initiation of chemotherapy in patients with acute myeloid leukemia and hyperleukocytosis: a clinicopathologic report of four cases. Cancer 85(2): 368–374
70. Zimhony O, Davidovitch Y et al (1994) Chronic lymphocytic leukaemia complicated by chylothorax. J Intern Med 235(4):375–377

Clinical Pearls: Pulmonary Veno-occlusive Disease

60

Jonathan Gutman

Contents

Herein, we describe a case of pulmonary veno-occlusive disease (PVOD) following reduced-intensity cord blood transplantation (CBT). A 51-year-old woman was hospitalized for progressive dyspnea on exertion and hypoxia 80 days following a second reduced-intensity double unit CBT. Five months before, the patient underwent the first reduced-intensity double unit CBT for high-risk AML in first CR. Conditioning was 200 mg/m^2 fludarabine, 50 mg/kg CY, 2 Gy TBI and 90 mg/kg antithymocyte globulin. GVHD prophylaxis was cyclosporine (CSP) and mycophenolate mofetil (MMF). Although the patient engrafted neutrophils on day 6, she subsequently developed graft failure with marginal autologous hematopoietic recovery by day 50. Three months after her initial CBT, the patient underwent salvage, second reduced-intensity CBT following conditioning with 200 mg/m^2 fludarabine, 50 mg/kg CY and 4 Gy total body irradiation (TBI). GVHD prophylaxis was CSP and MMF. The patient engrafted neutrophils on day 25 and developed 100% single donor chimerism by day 28. Computed tomography (CT) of the chest before the second CBT demonstrated only sub-5-mm pulmonary nodules, stable compared to prior imaging, and echocardiogram revealed normal left and right ventricular function without evidence of pulmonary hypertension (estimated pulmonary artery [PA] systolic pressure 19.4 mmHg). Her post-transplantation course was notable only for intermittently positive reactivation of CMV by PCR treated with foscarnet

J. Gutman
Fred Hutchinson Cancer Research Center, Seattle, WA, USA
e-mail: jgutman@fhcrc.org

Portions of the following case have been previously published as cited belowGutman JA, Allen CT, Madtes DK, Schramm J, Delaney C (2008) Pulmonary veno-occlusive disease following reduced-intensity cord blood transplantation. Bone Marrow Transplant 42(8):559–561

É. Azoulay (ed.), *Pulmonary Involvement in Patients with Hematological Malignancies*,
DOI: 10.1007/978-3-642-15742-4_60, © Springer-Verlag Berlin Heidelberg 2011

and ganciclovir, and spontaneously resolved cystitis associated with BK virus viruria.

Two months after her second CBT, the patient was admitted with cough, wheezing, dyspnea and room air arterial oxygen saturation of 88%. The chest CT showed septal thickening, small bilateral pleural effusions, scattered multifocal ground-glass opacities and patchy left lower lobe airspace opacities (Fig. 60.1). Bronchoscopy was negative for infections. In spite of improvement in the airspace disease on levofloxacin and furosemide, dyspnea and hypoxia persisted and the pleural effusions enlarged. The patient was readmitted 80 days following the second CBT, at which time CT angiography revealed no evidence of pulmonary embolus, and inferior vena cava and bilateral lower extremity Doppler imaging revealed no evidence of deep venous thrombosis. Echocardiogram revealed moderate PA hypertension (estimated PA systolic pressure 56.2 mmHg) with normal left ventricular size and function. Pulmonary function tests demonstrated forced vital capacity (FVC) 1.61 L (42% predicted), forced expiratory volume (FEV1) 1.4 L (46% predicted) and corrected diffusing capacity of the lung for carbon monoxide (DLCO) 5.2 mL/mmHg/min (18% predicted; baseline pre-transplantation values FVC 3.45 l [91% predicted], FEV1 2.85 l [94% predicted], corrected DLCO 20.3 mL/mmHg/min [71% predicted]). Right heart catheterization demonstrated moderate PA hypertension (PA systolic pressure 48 mmHg, PA diastolic pressure 15 mmHg, mean PA pressure 29 mmHg) with normal pulmonary capillary wedge pressure (4 mmHg).

Lung biopsy by thoracoscopic wedge resection showed PVOD affecting small venules and tiny parenchymal vessels primarily as well as mild hemosiderin deposition in intra-alveolar septa (Fig. 60.2). Autoimmune and vasculitis testing, including antinuclear antibody (ANA), anti-SCL 70, C and P anti-neutrophil cytoplasmic antibody (ANCAs), were negative.

The patient was placed on therapeutic unfractionated heparin followed by warfarin and prednisone at 1 mg/kg orally per day. Prednisone was continued at 1 mg/kg for 6 weeks followed by tapering over 6 weeks. Warfarin was discontinued upon echocardiographic resolution of pulmonary hypertension. Eight months after the diagnosis of PVOD, the patient's pulmonary symptoms had largely resolved. The chest CT demonstrated resolution of pleural effusions and septal thickening. FVC had improved to 3.74 L (66% predicted), FEV1 had improved to 2.84 L (77% predicted), and DLCO remained stable. Echocardiogram revealed normal right ventricular function without evidence of PA hypertension. Two years post transplant, the patient remains well without recurrence of pulmonary symptoms.

Though PVOD is a rare reported complication of myeloablative SCT, it has been presumed to be a regimen-related toxicity [1–7]. Our patient had undergone two CBTs, but both were of reduced intensity. Infection has also been suggested as a possible cause of PVOD, and though our patient did not exhibit an obvious infection, CBT patients are particularly immunocompromised following transplantation. The possibility of occult viral infection contributing to the condition must be considered. Finally, autoimmunity has also

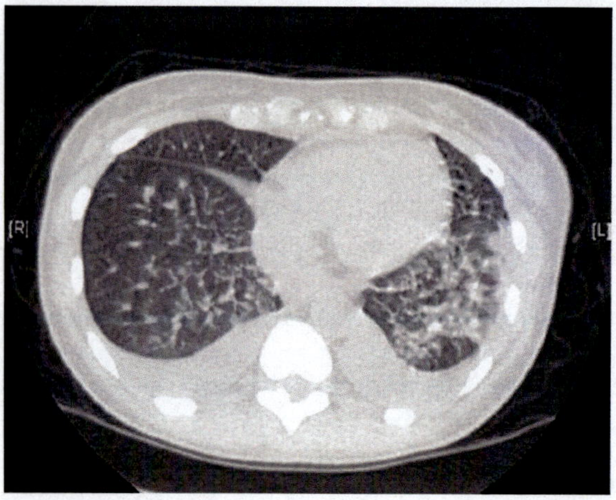

Fig. 60.1 Chest CT showing septal thickening, small bilateral pleural effusions, scattered multifocal ground-glass opacities and patchy left lower lobe airspace opacities

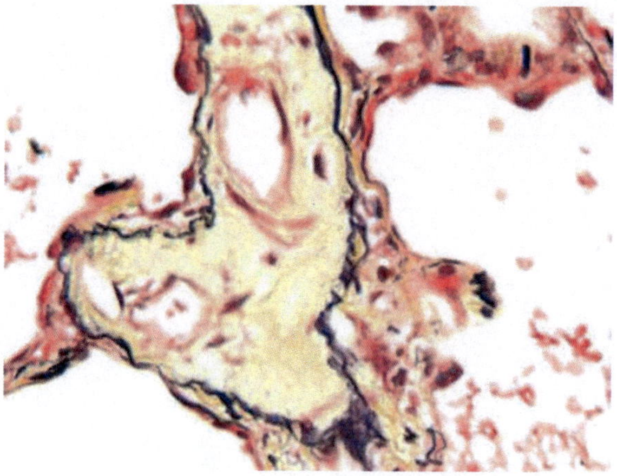

Fig. 60.2 Lung biopsy by thoracoscopic wedge resection showing PVOD affecting small venules and tiny parenchymal vessels primarily as well as mild hemosiderin deposition in intra-alveolar septa

been suggested as a contributing factor associated with PVOD, and although our patient experienced no significant GVHD, the possibility exists of donor/host interactions contributing to the condition [8, 9].

The diagnosis of PVOD requires a high index of suspicion. Patients typically present with dyspnea on exertion and fatigue. CT scans may reveal smooth septal thickening, diffuse or mosaic ground-glass opacities, pleural effusions or areas of alveolar consolidation. Cardiac catheterization reveals normal or decreased PA wedge pressure with elevated pulmonary capillary pressures. Surgical lung biopsy provides definitive diagnosis [9].

Treatment recommendations for PVOD are anecdotal. Owing to the rarity of the condition, its natural history is not well defined, and milder and nonfatal forms with spontaneous resolution of pulmonary venular obstruction may be an under-recognized course of the disease. Our patient did demonstrate evidence of some recanalization of pulmonary vasculature on biopsy, and this finding may portend a more favorable prognosis. Steroids and heparin have been reported to possibly improve outcomes [3], and our patient appears to have had stabilization and improvement of disease on these agents. Defibrotide and N-acetylcysteine hold appeal as potential therapeutic agents, but no data have been reported regarding their efficacy. The role of PA dilators in treating PVOD is controversial. Although sildenafil, prostacyclins and calcium channel blockers have been reported to improve the symptoms in isolated case reports, use of these agents warrants significant caution given the fixed venular obstruction in PVOD. Dilation of the PA tree in this setting may lead to profound pulmonary edema [9].

PVOD should be included in the differential diagnosis of dyspnea and hypoxia following reduced-intensity transplantation and CBT. Additional case reports describing the condition may yield further insights into its etiology.

References

1. Bunte MC, Patnaik MM, Pritzker MR, Burns LJ (2008) Pulmonary veno-occlusive disease following hematopoietic stem cell transplantation: a rare model of endothelial dysfunction. Bone Marrow Transplant 41:677–686
2. Troussard X, Bernaudin JF, Cordonnier C, Fleury J, Payen D, Briere J et al (1984) Pulmonary veno-occlusive disease after bone marrow transplantation. Thorax 39:956–957
3. Hackman RC, Madtes DK, Petersen FB, Clark JG (1989) Pulmonary veno-occlusive disease following bone marrow transplantation. Transplantation 47:989–992
4. Williams LM, Fussell S, Vieth RW, Nelson S, Mason CM (1996) Pulmonary veno-occlusive disease in an adult following bone marrow transplantation. Case report and review of the literature. Chest 109:1388–1391
5. Trobaugh-Lotrario AD, Greffe B, Detering R, Deutsch G, Quinones R (2003) Pulmonary veno-occlusive disease after autologous bone marrow transplant in a child with stage IV neuroblastoma: case report and literature review. J Pediatr Hematol Oncol 25:405–409
6. Mukai M, Kondo M, Bohgaki T, Notoya A, Kohno M (2003) Pulmonary veno-occlusive disease following allogeneicperipheral blood stem cell transplantation for chronic myeloid leukaemia. Br J Haematol 123:1
7. Doll DC, Yarbro JW (1992) Vascular toxicity associated with antineoplastic agents. Semin Oncol 19:580–596
8. Johnson SR, Patsios D, Hwang DM, Granton JT (2006) Pulmonary veno-occlusive disease and scleroderma associated hypertension. J Rheumatol 33:2347–2350
9. Mandel J, Mark EJ, Hales CA (2000) Pulmonary veno-occlusive disease. Am J Respir Crit Care Med 162: 1964–1973

Cytarabine-Induced Pulmonary Toxicity in Leukemic Patients

61

Fabio Forghieri, Leonardo Potenza, Monica Morselli, Monica Maccaferri, Giuseppe Torelli, and Mario Luppi

Contents

A 66-year-old male patient successfully treated with remission induction and consolidation chemotherapeutic regimens for acute myeloid leukemia (AML) with myelodysplasia-related changes according to the WHO classification [1] relapsed 5 months after autologous bone marrow transplantation. The patient, receiving prophylaxis with isoniazide for a latent tuberculosis infection documented by a Quantiferon-TB serological test, was admitted to our department in order to undergo a salvage chemotherapeutic regimen (FLAG) consisting of cytarabine (2 g/m^2 on days +1 to +5), fludarabine (30 mg/m^2 on days +1 to +3) and granulocyte-colony stimulating factor (G-CSF, 5 mcg/kg/day from day −1 to day +5). At admission the patient was asymptomatic, and his physical examination was unremarkable. Moreover, the chest X-ray performed before starting chemotherapy was negative. On day +1 the patient showed mild dyspnea and bilateral inspiratory crackles on chest auscultation, despite normal pO_2 on blood gas analysis. On day +2 after the administration of high-dose cytarabine had been started, he became febrile (temperature 38.4°C) (Fig. 61.1) and continued to show mild dyspnea in the absence of chest pain or cough. Blood tests were consistent with self-limiting disseminated intravascular coagulation in the absence of bleeding, probably due to leukemic cell lysis. Blood gas analysis on room air documented moderate hypoxemia (pO_2 62 mmHg), and chest X-ray showed an area of consolidation in the left lower lobe and bilateral pleural effusions, especially on the left side (Fig. 61.2a). Chest high-resolution computerized tomography (HRCT) was performed on day +3 (Fig. 61.2b), confirming the presence of

F. Forghieri, L. Potenza, M. Morselli, M. Maccaferri, G. Torelli, and M. Luppi (✉)
Department of Oncology, Hematology and Respiratory Diseases, Section of Hematology, University of Modena and Reggio Emilia, Azienda Ospedaliera-Universitaria Policlinico, Via del Pozzo 71, 41100 Modena, Italy
e-mail: mario.luppi@unimore.it

Authors' disclosures of potential conflict of interest: The authors indicated no potential conflict of interest.

É. Azoulay (ed.), *Pulmonary Involvement in Patients with Hematological Malignancies*, DOI: 10.1007/978-3-642-15742-4_61, © Springer-Verlag Berlin Heidelberg 2011

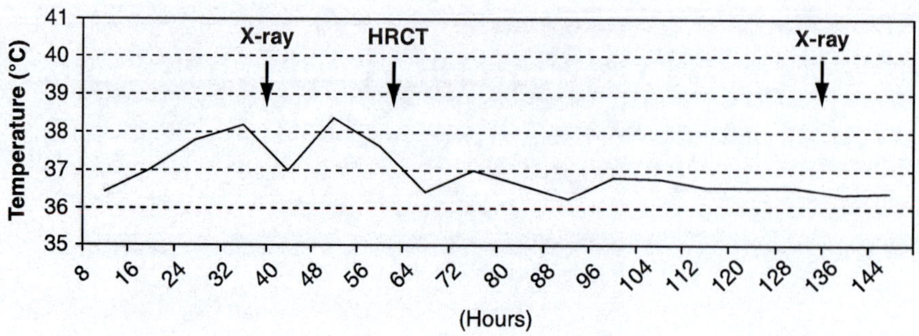

Fig. 61.1 Fever chart of the leukemic patient treated with high-dose cytarabine. Graph shows onset and subsequent resolution of fever and the timing of radiological examinations (chest X-ray and HRCT) indicated by *arrows*. "O hours" indicates the start of administration of chemotherapy

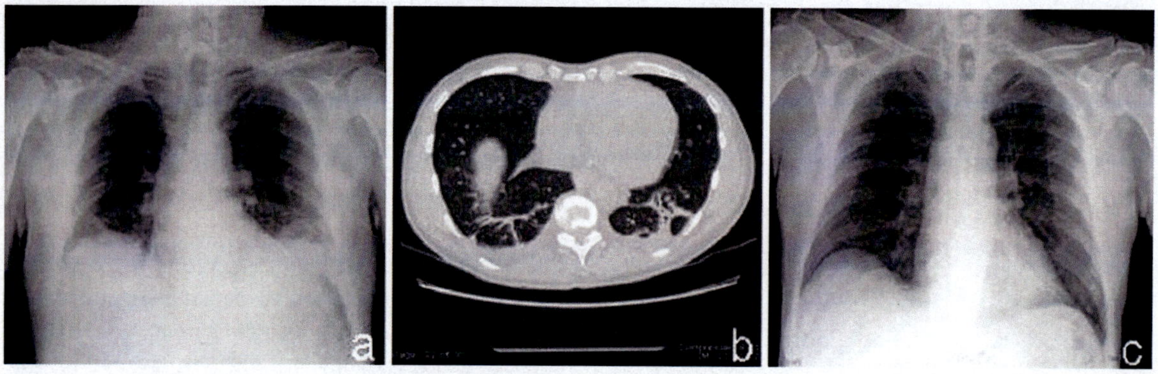

Fig. 61.2 Radiological examinations in the leukemic patient receiving high-dose cytarabine. Early lung infiltrates (bilateral patchy consolidations in lower lobes and bilateral pleural effusions) characterized by chest X-ray and HRCT (**a**, **b**); complete and spontaneous resolution in 72 h documented on chest X-ray (**c**)

bilateral pleural effusions and showing bilateral patchy consolidations in the lower lobes. The occurrence of respiratory symptoms in leukemic patients accompanied by lung infiltrates documented on either chest X-ray or HRCT may be attributed to either infectious or noninfectious causes [2–4]. The radiological findings disclosed in our patient are not pathognomonic for a specific process, so that an early and appropriate differential diagnosis is essential for clinical management. Patchy consolidations, with or without areas of ground-glass opacities, and pleural effusions, may be caused by several infectious agents [4], including bacteria, fungi, *Pneumocystis jiroveci* and, although rarely, viruses [4, 5]. An empirical antibiotic therapy with piperacillin-tazobactam and azithromycin was started in our patient, who was febrile and considered at high risk for systemic infections because of leukemia relapse, even though he was not neutropenic, with neutrophils being 4.6×10^9/L at that time point under treatment with G-CSF. Serological, cultural and molecular examinations (SCME) of biologic fluids (namely blood, urine, feces cultures, CMV and Galactomannan antigenemia, and urinary Legionella antigen) did not disclose any infectious agent. Furthermore, the patient underwent bronchoscopy with bronchoalveolar lavage (BAL). BAL samples were not hemorrhagic, and their extensive microbiologic analyses showed negative results for the most common bacterial, fungal and viral pathogens. When an infectious agent is not detected, several other noninfectious causes of lung infiltrates should be considered and investigated in leukemic patients, such as pulmonary edema due to heart failure [4], metabolic dysfunctions (namely renal failure, hypoalbuminemia and pancreatitis) [6], pulmonary leukostasis or leukemic infiltrates, even in the absence of leukocytosis or peripheral blastosis [7], alveolar hemorrhage and transfusion-related acute lung injury [4]. The above-mentioned causes of lung infiltrates were excluded in our patient (Table 61.1). From day +3 he became apyretic (Fig. 61.1), asymptomatic and blood gas analysis normalized, without stopping the administration of chemotherapy. A chest X-ray, performed 72 h later, showed complete resolution of the radiological features described above (Fig. 61.2c).

Table 61.1 Clinical evaluation of possible causes of lung infiltrates (cardiac or metabolic dysfunctions, infectious agents) other than cytarabine in our leukemic patient

Patient age/diagnosis	SCME on biological fluids	Echocardiogram before starting chemotherapy (EF%)	ECG at presentation of symptoms	Renal function at presentation of symptoms, creatinine (mg/dL)	Albuminemia on the day before starting chemotherapy (g/dL)	Pancreatic enzymes (U/L)
66 years/ AML	Negative	Normal (55%)	Normal	Normal (0.80)	Normal (3.9)	Amylase 16 lipase NA

Normal values in our laboratory: creatinine 0.6–1.4 mg/dL for male, 0.6–1.2 mg/dL for female; albumin 3.5–5 g/dL; amylase 1–100 U/L; lipase 1–60 U/L

SCME indicates serological, cultural and molecular examination of biologic fluids (blood, urine, feces, BAL cultures, CMV and Galactomannan antigenemia, urinary Legionella antigen), *AML* acute myeloid leukemia. *EF%* ejection fraction, *ECG* electrocardiogram, *NA* not available

The prompt resolution of the febrile condition, in the absence of disclosure of infectious agents by biologic fluid SCME, as well as the very early and complete disappearance of clinical symptoms and of radiological findings, as documented by subsequent chest X-ray, cannot be ascribed to the few days of empirical antibiotic therapy and argue against an infectious etiology. Having excluded other noninfectious causes, the pulmonary symptoms and radiological features demonstrated by our patient 24 h after starting chemotherapy were most likely induced by the administration of high-dose cytarabine.

Cytarabine, a pyrimidine nucleoside analogue introduced into clinical regimens for cancer therapy in 1964, is still one of the most effective drugs for the treatment of adult acute leukemia. The toxicity of cytarabine can be represented either by minor side effects like exanthema, fever and elevation of hepatic enzymes, which are relatively frequent although rarely represent a therapeutic problem, or by major adverse effects, including myelosuppression, oral and gastrointestinal mucosal damage, keratoconjunctivitis and neurotoxicity, which can determine serious clinical problems, sometimes requiring the definitive interruption of treatment [8, 9].

Several cancer therapeutic drugs are known to induce pulmonary toxicity, which may result in a broad spectrum of clinico-pathologic syndromes with minor to severe consequences for the patient. Potentially fatal pulmonary toxicity has been described in leukemia patients treated with cytarabine, especially at intermediate to high doses. This clinical entity, occurring in about 12–20% of patients a median of 1–2 weeks (range 1–21 days) after chemotherapy, has been defined as noncardiogenic pulmonary edema (NCPE) or acute lung injury [6, 10–19]. It typically presents as a subacute syndrome characterized by severe dyspnea, cough, tachypnea, low grade fever, severe hypoxemia, crackles on chest auscultation and confluent alveolar consolidation on standard chest X-ray. NCPE is usually characterized by abrupt onset of severe symptoms, which, if not fatal, can be reversed only with discontinuation of the administration of cytarabine and immediate start of intensive support treatment, including high-dose systemic steroids, mechanical ventilation and pressure support [6, 10–19]. Anecdotally, the association between administration of cytarabine and the onset of organizing pneumonia (COP) has been reported in the literature [20, 21]. COP is an uncommon fibrotic diffuse lung disorder, histopathologically defined as granulation tissue plugging into the lumens of small airways, extending, in a continuous fashion into alveolar ducts and alveoli. It is generally characterized by the subacute onset of respiratory symptoms resolving in the majority of cases (65–80%) with the administration of steroids. The response to corticosteroids is impressive, because clinical manifestations improve within 48 h, but complete resolution of radiographic pulmonary infiltrates takes several weeks. However, spontaneous, slow improvement only occasionally occurs, whereas in other cases, symptoms may persist with chronic and disabling cough and dyspnea and may be life threatening, especially in the case of recurrence [22–25].

We have recently widened the spectrum of clinical features of cytarabine-related pulmonary toxicity, reporting on three leukemic patients who developed fever, mild dyspnea, moderate hypoxemia on blood gas analysis and lung infiltrates documented by either chest X-ray or HRCT 24 h after the administration of high-dose cytarabine [26]. The disappearance of symptoms and the complete resolution of radiological signs were obtained in 48–72 h. While the radiological signs resemble those typically detected in both NCPE and COP, which can be characterized by signs of alveolar or interstitial opacification, surrounded sometimes by ground-glass areas, and pleural effusions, our cases showed a more indolent behavior and a benign clinical outcome compared to cases previously reported in the literature. Of note, our patients developed a sudden onset of symptoms after starting to receive the drug, but, despite the severity of radiological findings, the symptoms rapidly improved and were self-limiting, with only mild dyspnea and moderate hypoxemia on blood gas analysis [26].

Cytarabine-induced pulmonary toxicity is probably related to a cytokine-mediated mechanism involving tumor necrosis factor-alpha and platelet-activating factor, which determine inflammatory response with alveolar damage and increased vascular permeability [27]. Most of the reported patients were affected with relapsed leukemia (Table 61.2), so it cannot be

Table 61.2 Revision of the clinical data available from cases of cytarabine-related lung toxicity reported in the literature

Reference	Patients presenting lung toxicity (*N*)	Median age (years) of patients (range)	Status of hematologic disease (*N*)	Cytarabine dosage	Median time (days) of onset of symptoms from start of chemotherapy (range)	Clinical outcome (*N*)
Haupt et al. [10]	10 early; 18 late occurrence	39 (1–85)	28 REL	Intermediate (7.5–30 mg/kg/day)	0–3; 4–30	28 Deaths (autoptic data)
Andersson et al. [11]	16	35 (16–68)	16 REL	High (3 g/m^2 every 12 h for 4–12 doses)	16 (2–21)	15 Recoveries, 1 death[a]
Tham et al. [15]	15	29 (15–57)	15 first-line therapy	Intermediate (1 g/m^2 every 12 h for 6 days); high (3 g/m^2 every 12 h for 4 days)	16 (8–20)	13 Recoveries, 2 deaths[a]
Jehn et al. [16]	7	40 (17–64)	7 REL/REF	Intermediate (1 g/m^2 every 12 h for 6 days); high (3 g/m^2 every 12 h for 4 days)	NA (1–14)	3 Recoveries, 4 deaths
Andersson et al. [12]	14	39 (22–66)	14 REL	High (3 g/m^2 every 6–12 h for 6–12 doses OR 3 g/m^2 every 12 h for 2 doses, followed by 1.5 g/m^2 over 24 h for 3–4 days)	8 (1–29)	4 Recoveries, 10 deaths
Shearer et al. [17]	5	NA (4–12)	5 REL	Intermediate/high (1.0–1.5 g/m^2 over 24 h for 5 days)	8 (3–38)[b]	2 Recoveries, 3 deaths
Salvucci et al. [14]	2	14, 31	1 PR 1 REL	High (4 g/day for 5 days)	1, 7	2 Recoveries[a]
Larouche et al. [18]	1	72	1 First-line therapy	Standard (200 mg/m^2 over 24 h for 7 days)	3	1 Recovery[a]
Forghieri et al. [26]	3	53, 51, 66	2 First-line therapy 1 REL	High (3 g/m^2 every 12 h on day 1, 3, 5, 7 OR 2 g/m^2 for 5 days)	1	3 Recoveries[a]
Yegln et al. [19]	1	17	First-line therapy	High (3 g/m^2 every 12 h on days 2, 3)	4	1 Recovery[a]

Patients affected with BOOP secondary to cytarabine administration were not included in this table

N number of cases, *PR* partial remission, *REL* relapsed, *REF* refractory, *NA* not available

[a]Indicates that some patients of the series received corticosteroids

[b]Indicates that one patient presented respiratory symptoms 38 days after the first course of cytarabine, but a second course had been already administered just before the onset of symptoms

excluded that heavily pretreated patients could be more exposed to a possibly more severe pulmonary toxicity. From the review of the literature [6, 10–19, 26], cytarabine-related pulmonary toxicity occurs more frequently in patients with relapsed leukemia (72 out of 92 reported cases) than in patients with "de novo" leukemia (20 out of 92 patients). In the former group, a more severe course, often fatal (46 out of 72), is observed; in the latter group, only 2 out of 20 patients died from lung toxicity. Of note, most of the reported patients underwent standard chest X-ray examinations, whereas the performance of HRCT at a very early phase would probably allow better characterization of severe radiological findings in the absence of a corresponding severity of the clinical symptoms. Thus, the incidence of cytarabine-related lung infiltrates may be underestimated so that the early performance of HRCT in leukemic patients treated with intermediate to high-dose cytarabine at onset of respiratory symptoms, even if of mild entity, should be recommended. Recently, mild dyspnea in a febrile context has been reported as an early complication of Ara C therapy, with diffuse bilateral centrilobular micronodules with upper lobe predominance [28].

Because the diagnosis of cytarabine-induced pulmonary toxicity in the setting of leukemic patients is an exercise of exclusion of several other causes of lung infiltrates, an aggressive diagnostic approach, including invasive procedures such as bronchoscopy with BAL and transbronchial biopsy sampling, unless contraindicated, should be performed [4, 6]. Of note, the subsequent complete resolution of radiological findings should be promptly documented by either chest X-ray or HRCT as soon as the fever and the respiratory symptoms disappear.

As far as the therapeutic approach to patients with cytarabine-related pulmonary toxicity is concerned, it is not possible to define a formal management guideline simply based on the scanty data reported from the literature. Decisions about temporary or definitive discontinuation of cytarabine or about the introduction of systemic steroid therapy, which could lead to dramatic improvement and favorable outcomes, also in the most critical patients [6, 18, 19], should be based upon a careful evaluation of the clinical status (respiratory symptoms, fever, blood gas analysis and state of hematologic disease). The role of corticosteroids or any other therapeutic support in this clinical setting should be evaluated in clinical trials. However, the reported high incidence of cytarabine-related lung toxicity in relapsed leukemia patients may suggest introducing pre-medication with low-dose dexamethasone in this patient subgroup. In conclusion, cytarabine-related toxicity should be considered among the possible causes of lung infiltrates in patients with hematologic malignancies.

References

1. Vardiman JW, Thiele J, Arber DA, Brunning RD, Borowitz MJ, Porwit A et al (2009) The 2008 revision the World Health Organization (WHO) classification of myeloid neoplasms and acute leukemia: rationale and important changes. Blood 114:937–951
2. Heussel CP, Kauczor HU, Heussel GE, Fisher B, Begrich M, Mildenberger P et al (1999) Pneumonia in febrile neutropenic patients and in bone marrow and blood stem-cell transplant recipients: use of high-resolution computed tomography. J Clin Oncol 17:796–805
3. Maschmeyer G, Beinert T, Buchheidt D et al (2009) Diagnosis and antimicrobial therapy of lung infiltrates in febrile neutropenic patients: guidelines of the infectious diseases working party of the German Society of Haematology and Oncology. Eur J Cancer. doi:10.1016/j.ejca.2009.05.001
4. Vento S, Cainelli F, Temesgen Z (2008) Lung infections after cancer chemotherapy. Lancet Oncol 9:982–992
5. Ferrari A, Luppi M, Potenza L, Riva G, Morselli M, Imovilli A et al (2005) Herpes simplex virus pneumonia during standard induction chemotherapy for acute leukemia: case report and review of literature. Leukemia 19:2019–2021
6. Briasoulis E, Pavlidis N (2001) Noncardiogenic pulmonary edema: an unusual and serious complication of anticancer therapy. Oncologist 6:153–161
7. Potenza L, Luppi M, Morselli M, Tonelli S, D'Apollo N, Facchini L et al (2003) Leukaemic pulmonary infiltrates in adult acute myeloid leukaemia: a high-resolution computerized tomography study. Br J Haematol 120:1058–1061
8. Barrios NJ, Tebby CK, Freeman AI, Brecher ML (1987) Toxicity of high dose Ara-C in children and adolescents. Cancer 60:165–169
9. Stentoft J (1990) The toxicity of cytarabine. Drug Saf 5:7–27
10. Haupt HM, Hutchins GM, Moore GW (1981) Ara-C lung: non-cardiogenic pulmonary edema complicating cytosine arabinoside therapy of leukemia. Am J Med 70:256–261
11. Andersson BS, Cogan BM, Keating MJ, Estey EH, McCredie KB, Freireich EJ (1985) Subacute pulmonary failure complicating therapy with high-dose Ara-C in acute leukemia. Cancer 56:2181–2184
12. Andersson BS, Luna MA, Yee C, Hui KK, Keating MJ, McCredie KB (1990) Fatal pulmonary failure complicating high-dose cytosine arabinoside therapy in acute leukemia. Cancer 65:1079–1084

13. Kopterides P, Lignos M, Mentzelopoulos S, Armaganidis A, Pappa V (2005) Cytarabine-induced lung injury: case report. Anticancer Drugs 16:743–745
14. Salvucci M, Zanchini R, Molinari AL, Zuffa E, Poletti V, Poletti G et al (2000) Lung toxicity following fludarabine, cytosine arabinoside and mitoxantrone (FLAN) treatment for acute leukemia. Haematologica 85:769–770
15. Tham RT, Peters WG, de Bruine FT, Willemze R (1987) Pulmonary complications of cytosine-arabinoside therapy: radiographic findings. Am J Roentgenol 149:23–27
16. Jehn U, Goldel N, Rienmuller R, Wilmanns W (1988) Non-cardiogenic pulmonary edema complicating intermediate and high-dose Ara C treatment for relapsed acute leukemia. Med Oncol Tumor Pharmacother 5:41–47
17. Shearer P, Katz J, Bozeman P, Jenkins J, Laver J, Krance R et al (1994) Pulmonary insufficiency complicating therapy with high dose cytosine arabinoside in five pediatric patients with relapsed acute myelogenous leukemia. Cancer 74: 1953–1958
18. Larouche G, Denault A, Prenovault J (2000) Corticosteroids and serious cytarabine-induced pulmonary edema. Pharma_ cotherapy 20:1396–1399
19. Yegln ZA, Aki S, Sucak G, Yagci M (2007) Cytarabine induced noncardiogenic pulmonary edema in a case of acute lymphoblastic leukemia. Int J Lab Hematol 29:482–483
20. Patel M, Ezzat W, Pauw KL, Lowsky R (2001) Bronchiolitis obliterans organizing pneumonia in a patient with chronic myelogenous leukemia developing after initiation of interferon and cytosine arabinoside. Eur J Haematol 67: 318–321
21. Battistini E, Dini G, Savioli C, Morando A, Gandolfo A, Kotitsa Z et al (1997) Bronchiolitis obliterans organizing pneumonia in three children with acute leukaemias treated with cytosine arabinoside and anthracyclines. Eur Respir J 10:1187–1190
22. Cordier JF (2005) Organizing pneumonia. Thorax 55: 318–328
23. Epler GR, Colby TV, McLoud TC, Carrington CB, Gaensler EA (1985) Bronchiolitis obliterans organizing pneumonia. N Engl J Med 312:152–158
24. King TE (2005) Clinical advances in the diagnosis and therapy of the interstital lung disease. Am J Respir Crit Care Med 172:268–279
25. Daniels CE, Myers JL, Utz JP, Markovic SN, Ryu JH (2007) Organizing pneumonia in patients with hematologic malignancies: a steroid-responsive lesion. Respir Med 101: 162–168
26. Forghieri F, Luppi M, Morselli M, Potenza L, Volzone F, Riva G et al (2007) Cytarabine-related lung infiltrates on high resolution computerized tomography: a possible complication with benign outcome in leukemic patients. Haematologica 92:e85–e90
27. Chiche D, Pico JL, Bernaudin JF, Chouaib S, Wollman E, Arnoux A et al (1993) Pulmonary edema and shock after high-dose aracytine-C for lymphoma; possible role of TNF-alpha and PAF. Eur Cytokine Netw 4:147–151
28. Chagnon K, Boissel N, Raffoux E, Dombret H, Tazi A, Bergeron A (2009) A new pattern of cytosine-arabinoside-induced lung toxicity. Br J Haematol 147(5):771–774

Histoplasmosis in a Patient with Chronic Myelogenous Leukemia

62

Vincent Peigne, Benoît Schlemmer, and Olivier Lortholary

Contents

V. Peigne (✉)
Medical Intensive Care Unit, Saint-Louis Hospital,
Paris, France and National Reference Center for Mycoses and Antifungals, Institut Pasteur,
Paris, France
e-mail: vincent.peigne@sls.aphp.fr

B. Schlemmer
Medical Intensive Care Unit, Saint-Louis Hospital,
Paris, France

O. Lortholary
National Reference Center for Mycoses and Antifungals,
Institut Pasteur, Paris, France and Université Paris Descartes,
Centre d'Infectiologie Necker-Pasteur, Service des Maladies Infectieuses et Tropicales, Hôpital Necker-Enfants malades,
Paris, France

62.1 Case Presentation

A 66-year-old woman was admitted to the ICU because of acute respiratory failure with a fever. She was from French Guyana, where she had last traveled 20 years earlier, and she had been living in Europe for 50 years. Chronic myelogenous leukemia had been diagnosed 10 years earlier and treated with hydroxyurea and mercaptopurine. Transition to the accelerated phase had occurred 8 months before admission (8% blast cells in bone marrow). She had a history of retinal vasculitis 4 years earlier with a good outcome after 2 years of corticosteroid therapy.

She had been in her usual state of health until 3 months before admission, when she started experiencing a fever and arthritis of the right knee. She was treated first with antibiotics and nonsteroidal antiinflammatory drugs. The knee aspirate contained abundant protein (42 g/L) and polymorphonuclear cells (50,000/mm^3) without crystals or pathogens. Prednisone (0.5 mg/kg/day) failed to improve the symptoms, and she was admitted to an infectious diseases ward. Her body temperature was 40°C. The right knee was swollen and painful, and she had several oral ulcers. The lung and heart sounds were normal. She had hepatomegaly without lymphadenopathy or splenomegaly. Routine laboratory values were unremarkable except for high C-reactive protein (143 mg/L) and tenfold increases in alkaline phosphatase and gamma-glutamyltransferase. Serological tests for *Yersinia*, *Brucella*, and HIV were negative. Examination of a surgical synovial biopsy from the right knee revealed a polymorphonuclear cell infiltrate without pathogens. The hepatic biopsy was considered normal. Antituberculosis therapy was begun. The fever persisted, and the patient was referred to a hematology ward. Fever related to the hematological malignancy was considered, and chemotherapy with

É. Azoulay (ed.), *Pulmonary Involvement in Patients with Hematological Malignancies*,
DOI: 10.1007/978-3-642-15742-4_62, © Springer-Verlag Berlin Heidelberg 2011

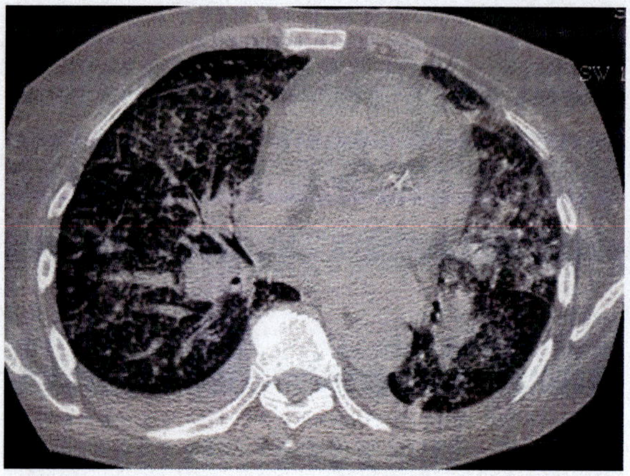

Fig. 62.1 CT scan aspect of histoplasmosis in a patient at the accelerated phase of chronic myelogenous leukemia

thiotepa and etoposide was administered. The following day, her respiratory status deteriorated with polypnea, hypoxemia, bilateral crackles, and diffuse infiltrates on the chest X-ray. She was admitted to the ICU.

Empirical antibiotic therapy with cefepime, vancomycin, and gentamicin was initiated. Histoplasmosis was suspected because of the combination of oral ulcers, fever, and pneumonia in a patient from an endemic area. Amphotericin B deoxycholate (1 mg/kg/day) was begun. CT of the chest showed micronodules and ground-glass opacities with peribronchovascular thickening (Fig. 62.1). Fiberoptic bronchoscopy with bronchoalveolar lavage and knee aspiration were performed. The diagnosis of *Histoplasma capsulatum* var. *capsulatum* histoplasmosis was confirmed by visualization of small budding yeasts in the bronchoalveolar fluid and knee aspirate. Similar yeasts were identified in the liver when the hepatic biopsy was reexamined. Two days later, her respiratory status worsened, requiring mechanical ventilation. Blood and tracheal aspirate cultures were negative. Multiorgan failure developed, and the patient died 1 week later.

62.2 Comment

This case report emphasizes the diagnostic challenges raised by histoplasmosis [1], particularly outside endemic areas.

Histoplasma capsulatum var. *capsulatum* is a dimorphic fungus. Histoplasmosis is endemic in certain areas of North, Central, and South America, Africa, and Southeast Asia [2, 3]. A few native cases have been reported in northern Italy. Contamination occurs via the inhalation of aerosols containing the mycelial phase of *H. capsulatum*. Activities at risk for exposure include caving, cleaning chicken coops, and building demolition [4]. Outbreaks have been related to public works and air-conditioning-system contamination. Laboratory staff can be contaminated by inhalation or percutaneous inoculation. Transmission of histoplasmosis by organ transplantation has also been reported [5]. Except in this last situation, inter-human transmission never occurs, and histoplasmosis develops only in patients who are living or have lived in endemic areas after acute exogenous exposure or reactivation of a latent infection.

Pulmonary and disseminated histoplasmosis may occur in immunocompromised hosts including, in rare cases, patients with hematological malignancies [2, 3]. Cases have been reported in patients with Hodgkin's or non-Hodgkin's lymphoma, acute leukemia, chronic leukemia, and hairy cell leukemia [6]. Histoplasmosis may be the first manifestation of the hematological malignancy or may appear as an opportunistic infection following immunosuppressive therapy [7]. Few epidemiological data are available, but histoplasmosis seems uncommon in patients with hematological malignancies, even in endemic areas. Only 1% of pediatric patients treated for hematological malignancies at an oncology center in an endemic area had histoplasmosis [7]. No patients were diagnosed with histoplasmosis in a review of 137 allogeneic bone marrow transplant recipients from a hyperendemic area [8]. Hematological malignancy was the risk factor for histoplasmosis in 10% of patients with disseminated histoplasmosis managed at a medical center in a nonendemic area [9].

Acute pulmonary histoplasmosis usually follows airborne contamination (incubation, 1–3 weeks). Symptoms include fatigue, a fever, and a dry cough. The chest X-ray and CT scan show diffuse reticulonodular infiltrates and, in some cases, lymphadenopathy (Fig. 62.2). Severe disease with acute respiratory distress may occur in the event of massive inoculation or in immunocompromised hosts. Other complications consist of arthritis, pericarditis, and mediastinal syndromes (mediastinal granuloma, mediastinal fibrosis, broncholithiasis).

Fever, night sweats, weight loss, and fatigue are the most frequent symptoms of disseminated histoplasmosis.

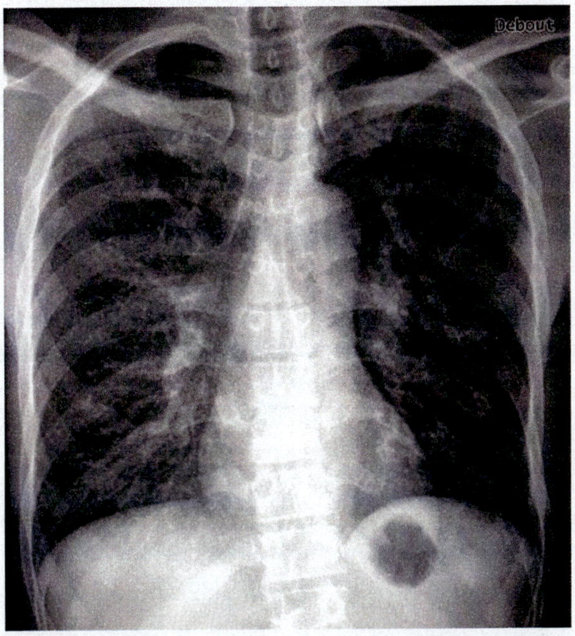

Fig. 62.2 Chest X-ray of a 46-year-old man with disseminated histoplasmosis showing diffuse reticulo-nodular infiltrate

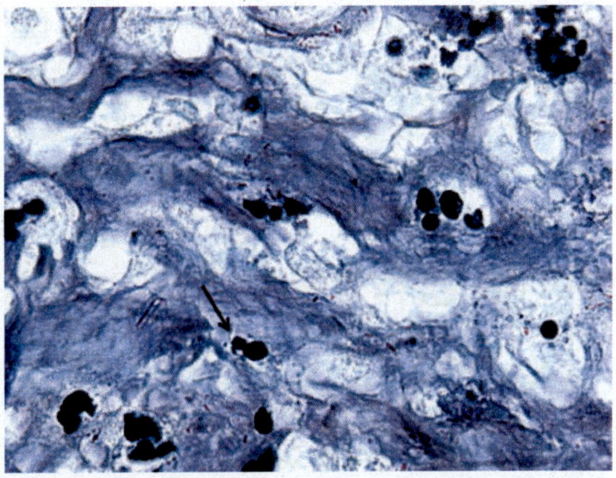

Fig. 62.3 Yeast form of *Histoplasma capsulatum* var. *capsulatum.* Skin biopsy of a patient with disseminated histoplasmosis. Grocott staining, magnification × 100. The *arrow* indicates a small budding yeast typical of *Histoplasma capsulatum* var. *capsulatum*

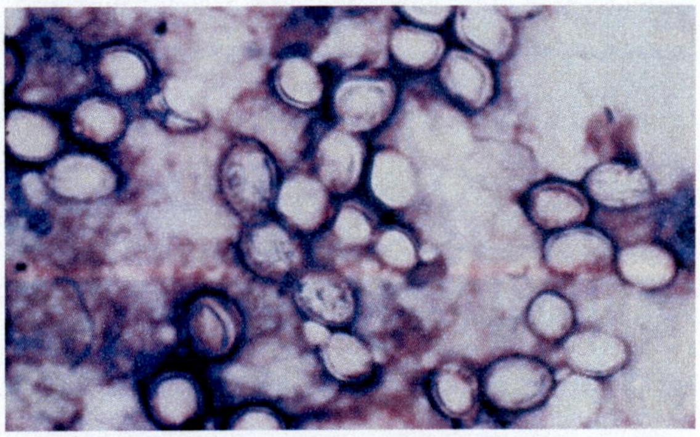

Fig. 62.4 Yeast form of *Histoplasma capsulatum* var. *duboisii.* Skin biopsy of a patient with disseminated histoplasmosis. Grocott staining, magnification × 100

The presentation is usually subacute (1–3 months), but acute illness is not rare. Adenomegaly and hepatosplenomegaly are commonly noted. Mucocutaneous lesions including oral ulcers, papules, maculopapules, and ulcerated plaques are highly evocative [10, 11]. Gastrointestinal signs are frequent but nonspecific (diarrhea, abdominal pain) [12]. Central nervous system involvement, including lymphocytic meningitis, focal brain or spinal lesions, and seizures, is severe but rare [13]. Hemophagocytic syndrome has been associated with disseminated histoplasmosis [14].

The diagnosis relies on culturing, histopathology, and antigen and antibody tests [15]. Culturing is the definitive test for establishing the diagnosis of histoplasmosis, but *H. capsulatum* grows slowly (up to several weeks) and should be manipulated in P3 laboratories as the mycelial phase can cause human contamination. Cultures can be performed on samples of blood, bone marrow, or any affected site. Blood culture sensitivity is enhanced by using the lysis-centrifugation system. Histopathology and direct examination provide faster results. *H. capsulatum* var. *capsulatum* appears as characteristic intracellular yeasts within tissue macrophages. The Gomori-Grocott stain is positive (Fig. 62.3). *Histoplasma capsulatum* var. *capsulatum* yeasts are small (2–5 μm), ovoid, budding yeasts (Fig. 62.3), whereas *Histoplasma capsulatum* var. *duboisii* yeasts are larger (8–15 μm) and oval (Fig. 62.4). Yeasts may be visible in a peripheral blood smear phagocyte in patients with T-lymphocyte impairment, resulting in a high fungal burden. Detection of the *Histoplasma* antigen is available only in the USA and can be performed in blood, urine, cerebrospinal fluid, and bronchoalveolar lavage fluid. This test is highly sensitive and specific [16]. *Histoplasma* antigen level monitoring may be useful to detect relapses early [17]. The galactomannan test may be positive in patients with disseminated histoplasmosis [18, 19]. This cross-reactivity must be known to avoid diagnostic delays [20] and may be useful for physicians outside the USA [18]. The β-glucan test may be positive, but its specificity is too low (0.68) to provide the diagnosis, and its sensitivity is not high enough (0.87) for screening [21]. In immunocompromised patients, antibody detection performs less well than in normal hosts and therefore should not be used. Immunodiffusion assays and complement fixation assays are available, the latter being less specific and more sensitive [15]. A positive test indicates that the patient is at risk for histoplasmosis. A negative test does not rule out histoplasmosis.

Diagnostic criteria for histoplasmosis have been proposed by the Mycoses Study Group of the European Organization for Research and Treatment of Cancer (EORTC/MSG) [22] and are summarized in Table 62.1.

Prognostic factors have been investigated in AIDS patients [23–26]. Renal failure, dyspnea, requirement for mechanical ventilation, albumin level <3.5 g/dL, hemoglobin level <8 g/dL, platelet count <100 g/L, and lactate dehydrogenase level more than twice the upper limit of normal have been associated with severe disease or death [23–26].

Amphotericin B and itraconazole are the best evaluated drugs for the treatment of histoplasmosis and should be used as first-line therapy. Voriconazole [27] and posaconazole [28, 29] have been used successfully. Fluconazole should not be used because of the risk of failure related to the emergence of resistant strains [30]. Similar recommendations have been issued for voriconazole [31, 32]. No data support the use of combination antifungal therapy. Maintenance therapy is required because of the high relapse rate in immunocompromised patients as long as the immune deficiency persists. Guidelines for the management of patients with histoplasmosis were recently endorsed by the Infectious Diseases Society of America [32]. Data about immunocompromised patients are mainly extrapolated from studies of AIDS patients with disseminated histoplasmosis. The initial treatment should be guided by the severity of the disease in both pulmonary and disseminated histoplasmosis. Liposomal amphotericin B (3 mg/kg/day) proved superior to the deoxycholate formulation of amphotericin B in AIDS patients with disseminated histoplasmosis (significant decreases in mortality and renal failure) [33] and should be used in patients with severe disease [32]. Patients who have moderately severe disease and who are at low risk for nephrotoxicity may receive amphotericin B deoxycholate (0.7–1 mg/kg/day), whereas patients with mild disease may receive oral itraconazole (200 mg twice daily). The duration of initial amphotericin B treatment can be reduced to 1–2 weeks, after which itraconazole is given. The total treatment duration should be at least 12 months in case of disseminated disease, and probably of pulmonary disease in an immunocompromised host. Lifelong therapy with itraconazole (200 mg/day) may be required if the immunosuppression persists. Monitoring of the itraconazole blood concentration is recommended [32].

Table 62.1 EORTC/MSG criteria for the diagnosis of histoplasmosis [22]

Proven histoplasmosis
Illness consistent with histoplasmosis
And one of the following
Recovery of *Histoplasma capsulatum* in culture from an affected site or from blood
Presence of characteristic intracellular yeasts in a phagocyte in a peripheral blood smear or in tissue macrophages
Probable histoplasmosis
Host factors including prolonged use of corticosteroids at a mean minimum dose of 0.3 mg/kg/day of prednisone equivalent for >3 weeks, treatment with recognized T-cell immunosuppressants, such as cyclosporine, TNF-blockers, inherited severe immunodeficiency
And illness consistent with histoplasmosis
And mycological evidence such as a positive *Histoplasma* antigen test result from urine, blood or cerebrospinal fluid

Prophylaxis may be discussed in patients scheduled to receive immunosuppressive therapy [32]. No criteria for identifying patients at high risk for histoplasmosis are available. However, patients with a recent history of histoplasmosis are probably at higher risk for a new episode and may benefit from itraconazole prophylaxis.

Histoplasmosis is a rare but severe opportunistic infection in patients with hematological malignancies. Awareness of this disease among clinicians is crucial to avoid diagnostic delays. Patients should be asked routinely about previous places of residence and travel in order to identify individuals at risk for histoplasmosis.

References

1. Gulati M, Saint S, Tierney LM Jr (2000) Clinical problem-solving. Impatient inpatient care. N Engl J Med 342(1):37–40, 6 Jan 2000
2. Cano MV, Hajjeh RA (2001) The epidemiology of histoplasmosis: a review. Semin Respir Infect 16(2):109–118
3. Kauffman CA (2007) Histoplasmosis: a clinical and laboratory update. Clin Microbiol Rev 20(1):115–132
4. Wheat LJ, Kauffman CA (2003) Histoplasmosis. Infect Dis Clin North Am 17(1):1–19, vii
5. Limaye AP, Connolly PA, Sagar M et al (2000) Transmission of *Histoplasma capsulatum* by organ transplantation. N Engl J Med 343(16):1163–1166, 19 Oct 2000
6. Kauffman C, Israel K, Smith J, White A, Schwarz J, Brooks G (1978) Histoplasmosis in immunosuppressed patients. Am J Med 64(6):923–932
7. Adderson EE (2004) Histoplasmosis in a pediatric oncology center. J Pediatr 144(1):100–106
8. Vail GM, Young RS, Wheat LJ, Filo RS, Cornetta K, Goldman M (2002) Incidence of histoplasmosis following allogeneic bone marrow transplant or solid organ transplant in a hyperendemic area. Transpl Infect Dis 4(3):148–151
9. Assi MA, Sandid MS, Baddour LM, Roberts GD, Walker RC (2007) Systemic histoplasmosis: a 15-year retrospective institutional review of 111 patients. Medicine (Baltimore) 86(3):162–169
10. Couppie P, Clyti E, Nacher M et al (2002) Acquired immunodeficiency syndrome-related oral and/or cutaneous histoplasmosis: a descriptive and comparative study of 21 cases in French Guiana. Int J Dermatol 41(9):571–576
11. Ramdial PK, Mosam A, Dlova NC, Satar NB, Aboobaker J, Singh SM (2002) Disseminated cutaneous histoplasmosis in patients infected with human immunodeficiency virus. J Cutan Pathol 29(4):215–225
12. Kahi CJ, Wheat LJ, Allen SD, Sarosi GA (2005) Gastrointestinal histoplasmosis. Am J Gastroenterol 100(1): 220–231
13. Wheat LJ, Musial CE, Jenny-Avital E (2005) Diagnosis and management of central nervous system histoplasmosis. Clin Infect Dis 40(6):844–852, 15 Mar 2005
14. Rouphael NG, Talati NJ, Vaughan C, Cunningham K, Moreira R, Gould C (2007) Infections associated with haemophagocytic syndrome. Lancet Infect Dis 7(12):814–822
15. Kauffman CA (2008) Diagnosis of histoplasmosis in immunosuppressed patients. Curr Opin Infect Dis 21(4):421–425
16. Wheat LJ, Witt J 3rd, Durkin M, Connolly P (2007) Reduction in false antigenemia in the second generation Histoplasma antigen assay. Med Mycol 45(2):169–171
17. Wheat LJ, Connolly-Stringfield P, Blair R, Connolly K, Garringer T, Katz BP (1991) Histoplasmosis relapse in patients with AIDS: detection using *Histoplasma capsulatum* variety capsulatum antigen levels. Ann Intern Med 115(12):936–941, 15 Dec 1991
18. Ranque S, Pelletier R, Michel-Nguyen A, Dromer F (2007) *Platelia Aspergillus* assay for diagnosis of disseminated histoplasmosis. Eur J Clin Microbiol Infect Dis 26(12): 941–943
19. Wheat LJ, Hackett E, Durkin M et al (2007) Histoplasmosis-associated cross-reactivity in the BioRad Platelia Aspergillus enzyme immunoassay. Clin Vaccine Immunol 14(5): 638–640
20. Jones O, Cleveland K, Gelfand M (2009) A case of disseminated histoplasmosis following autologous stem cell transplantation for Hodgkin's lymphoma: an initial misdiagnosis with a false-positive serum galactomannan assay. Transpl Infect Dis 11(3):281–283
21. Egan L, Connolly P, Wheat LJ et al (2008) Histoplasmosis as a cause for a positive Fungitell (1–>3)-beta-D-glucan test. Med Mycol 46(1):93–95
22. De Pauw B, Walsh TJ, Donnelly JP et al (2008) Revised definitions of invasive fungal disease from the European Organization for Research and Treatment of Cancer/Invasive Fungal Infections Cooperative Group and the National Institute of Allergy and Infectious Diseases Mycoses Study Group (EORTC/MSG) Consensus Group. Clin Infect Dis 46(12):1813–1821, 15 Jun 2008
23. Couppie P, Sobesky M, Aznar C et al (2004) Histoplasmosis and acquired immunodeficiency syndrome: a study of prognostic factors. Clin Infect Dis 38(1):134–138, 1 Jan 2004
24. de Francesco Daher E, de Sousa Barros FA, da Silva Junior GB et al (2006) Risk factors for death in acquired immunodeficiency syndrome-associated disseminated histoplasmosis. Am J Trop Med Hyg 74(4):600–603
25. Hajjeh RA, Pappas PG, Henderson H et al (2001) Multicenter case-control study of risk factors for histoplasmosis in human immunodeficiency virus-infected persons. Clin Infect Dis 32(8):1215–1220, 15 Apr 2001
26. Wheat LJ, Chetchotisakd P, Williams B, Connolly P, Shutt K, Hajjeh R (2000) Factors associated with severe manifestations of histoplasmosis in AIDS. Clin Infect Dis 30(6): 877–881
27. Srinivasan J, Ooi WW (2008) Successful treatment of histoplasmosis brain abscess with voriconazole. Arch Neurol 65(5):666–667
28. Clark B, Foster R, Tunbridge A, Green S (2005) A case of disseminated histoplasmosis successfully treated with the investigational drug posaconazole. J Infect 51(3): e177–e180
29. Restrepo A, Tobon A, Clark B et al (2007) Salvage treatment of histoplasmosis with posaconazole. J Infect 54(4): 319–327
30. Wheat LJ, Connolly P, Smedema M, Brizendine E, Hafner R (2001) Emergence of resistance to fluconazole as a cause of failure during treatment of histoplasmosis in patients with acquired immunodeficiency disease syndrome. Clin Infect Dis 33(11):1910–1913, 1 Dec 2001
31. Wheat LJ, Connolly P, Smedema M et al (2006) Activity of newer triazoles against *Histoplasma capsulatum* from patients with AIDS who failed fluconazole. J Antimicrob Chemother 57(6):1235–1239
32. Wheat LJ, Freifeld AG, Kleiman MB et al (2007) Clinical practice guidelines for the management of patients with histoplasmosis: 2007 update by the Infectious Diseases Society of America. Clin Infect Dis 45(7):807–825, 1 Oct 2007
33. Johnson PC, Wheat LJ, Cloud GA et al (2002) Safety and efficacy of liposomal amphotericin B compared with conventional amphotericin B for induction therapy of histoplasmosis in patients with AIDS. Ann Intern Med 137(2):105–109, 16 July 2002

Pulmonary Toxicity of Imatinib and Other BCR-ABL Tyrosine Kinase Inhibitors

63

François Vincent

Contents

F. Vincent
Medico-surgical Intensive Care Unit, Avicenne Teaching Hospital, 125 rue de Stalingrad, 93009 Bobigny Cedex, France
e-mail: francois.vincent@avc.aphp.fr

63.1 Case Report

This 77-year-old man had a history of hypertension well controlled by hydrochlorothiazide and ranipril and of prostate cancer treated with hormonotherapy. A routine blood count showed 52 × 10^9/L leukocytes with an increase in intermediate myeloid cells, indicating chronic myelogenous leukemia. A bone marrow examination revealed mye-loid hyperplasia and presence of the Philadelphia chromosome. He was started on imatinib at a dosage of 400 mg/day. Over the next 3 weeks, the leukocyte count dropped to 2.2 × 10^9/L.

Four weeks after starting imatinib therapy, he developed dyspnea on exertion that worsened to the point where he was unable to perform the activities of daily living. He was comfortable at rest and denied cough, orthopnea, or paroxysmal nocturnal dyspnea. He was seen at the emergency department, where he was afebrile with a respiratory rate of 26/min, 85% oxygen saturation on room air, and scattered rhonchi by lung auscultation. The chest radiograph visualized bilateral patchy interstitial infiltrates and a focal infiltrate in the lower right lung (Fig. 63.1). He was admitted to the medical intensive care unit (ICU) for respiratory support and a diagnostic workup after undergoing high-resolution computed tomography (HRCT) of the lungs, which ruled out pulmonary embolism and showed bilateral interstitial infiltrates with ground-glass opacities and pleural thickening (Fig. 63.2). He was started on oxygen therapy and noninvasive mechanical ventilation (NIV). Imatinib was discontinued. Furosemide was started despite normal findings from echocardiography and a brain natriuretic peptide (BNP) assay. Cefotaxime and azythromycin were started. His leukocyte count was 5.7 × 10^9/L, his hemoglobin level was 10.8 g/dL, and his platelet count was 503 × 10^9/L. Findings were

É. Azoulay (ed.), *Pulmonary Involvement in Patients with Hematological Malignancies*,
DOI: 10.1007/978-3-642-15742-4_63, © Springer-Verlag Berlin Heidelberg 2011

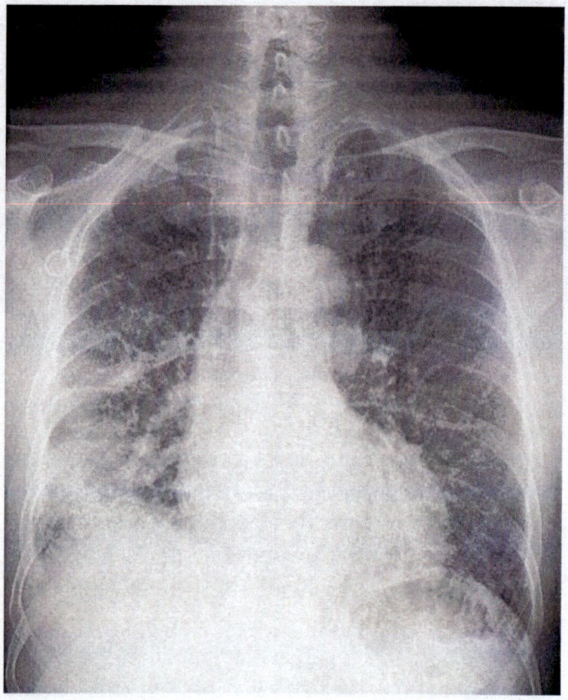

Fig. 63.1 The chest radiograph visualized bilateral patchy interstitial infiltrates and a focal infiltrate in the lower right lung

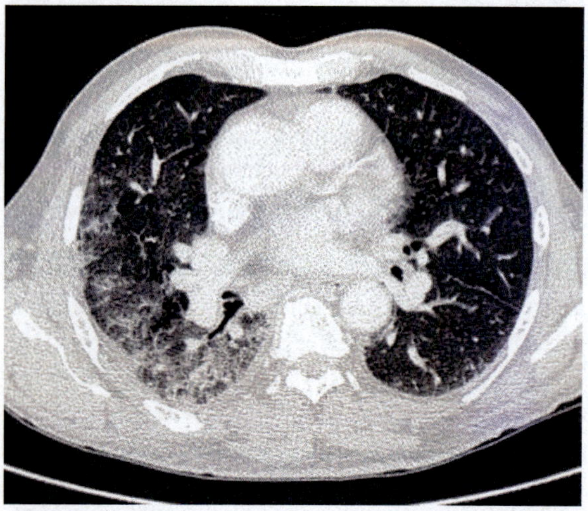

Fig. 63.2 High-resolution computed tomography (HRCT) of the lungs, which ruled out pulmonary embolism and showed bilateral interstitial infiltrates with ground-glass opacities and pleural thickening

negative from blood cultures and tests for urinary antigens of *Legionella pneumophila* and *Streptococcus pneumonia*. Bronchoscopy with bronchoalveolar lavage (BAL) was performed on day 2 after ICU admission. No macroscopic abnormalities were seen. The BAL fluid was clear and contained 360 × 10^9/L with 70% macrophages, 15% eosinophils, 10% lymphocytes (CD4/CD8 ratio, 0.9), 5% neutrophils, no hemosiderin-laden macrophages, and no proteinaceous material. Bacterial BAL cultures showed no growth. Stains and cultures were negative for *Pneumocystis jiroveci* and other fungi, *Toxoplasma gondii*, viruses (adenovirus, respiratory syncytial virus, influenza virus, parainfluenzae virus, herpes virus, and cytomegalovirus). Bronchial biopsies showed no specific lesions. No malignant cells were identified. Clinically, volume depletion developed, and the dyspnea and hypoxemia remained unchanged. Hypersensitivity pneumonitis related to imatinib was suspected, and prednisone was introduced at a dosage of 1 mg/kg/day. Over the next 4 days, the dyspnea began to improve, allowing NIV discontinuation and discharge from the ICU on day 7. A chest radiograph and HRCT done about 2 weeks later showed fading of the pulmonary infiltrates. The dyspnea and oxygen requirement diminished over the next month. Imatinib was reintroduced and prednisone tapered to 0.2 mg/kg/day without recurrent pulmonary symptoms.

Imatinib mesylate is a targeted therapy that is highly active in patients with CML or GIST. Some CML are characterized by constitutive activation of a tyrosine kinase (Abelson murine leukemia viral oncogene homolog or ABL) in a fusion oncoprotein (BCR-ABL) produced by the Philadelphia chromosome; Some GIST are characterized by a c-transmembrane receptor tyrosine kinase known as C-KIT. Imatinib inhibits both BCR-ABL and C-KIT, as well as the tyrosine kinase of the platelet-derived growth factor (PDGF) receptor and its associated pathways. Commonly reported side effects include nausea, diarrhea, fluid retention, fatigue, skin rash and, in 5% of cases, gastrointestinal or intraabdominal hemorrhage [1]. The mechanisms underlying TKI toxicity are unclear. Nausea and vomiting may be related to local irritation by the compound and the other side effects to pharmacological effects of tyrosine kinase inhibition. For example, diarrhea may be ascribable to inhibition of C-KIT, which is highly expressed by the intestinal pacemaker cells. Inhibition of C-KIT, which is also expressed on skin basal cells, melanocytes, and mast cells, has been implicated in the occurrence of imatinib-associated skin rash [2, 3]. Furthermore, prolonged PDGF inhibition by imatinib has also been implicated in imatinib-related skin toxicity [4]. Fluid retention may be related to inhibition of the PDGF receptor, whose pathways regulate interstitial fluid homeostasis by modulating the tension between cells and extracellular matrix structures [5].

63.2 Incidence of Lung Manifestations During the Course of Treatment with Imatinib

Most of the lung complications reported during imatinib therapy are related to pulmonary edema, a rare manifestation of the fluid retention syndrome associated with this medication. Pulmonary edema occurred in 2.3% of patients in the phase II study of chronic-phase Ph+CML that had failed to respond to interferon therapy [6]. Dyspnea and cough ascribed to pulmonary edema have been reported in 7–10% and 10–14% of patients receiving imatinib, respectively [7]. Severe fluid retention (grade 3/4) resulting in pleural or pericardial effusions, pulmonary edema, ascites, or severe superficial edema are rare in Chronic-phase Ph+ CML (<1%), but more common at the advanced phases (up to 3%), probably as a result of higher drug dosages and greater severity of concomitant conditions [8]. ILD occurs more rarely during the course of imatinib therapy. As of October 2003, approximately 5,000 patients with CML and 500 patients with GIST had been estimated to have received imatinib since its approval in Japan (November 2001 for CML and July 2003 for GIST) [9]. Of 3,023 adverse events reported spontaneously, 39 (1.29%) were cases of ILD. The median time to ILD development was 49 days (range, 10–282 days), and the median daily imatinib dosage was 400 mg (range, 200–600 mg) at the time ILD was diagnosed. There was no clear correlation between ILD development and either the dose or the duration of imatinib therapy. Only anecdotal case reports have been reported in Europe and North America. This distribution of cases suggests that imatinib-related ILD might be more common in Asians than in other ethnic groups.

63.3 Clinical and Radiological Findings

Fluid retention is a very common side effect of imatinib. Most patients (54–65%) given imatinib have some degree of superficial edema, which is usually mild (grade 1/2), dose-dependent, and limited to the periorbital regions and lower legs [10]. Pleural or pericardial effusions are revealed by dyspnea and chest pain. Although the symptoms suggest congestive heart failure, imatininib-related fluid retention is not due to impaired ventricular function but is instead a specific side effect [11]. IPD produces symptoms similar to those seen in fluid retention syndrome. Consequently, the development of nonspecific respiratory symptoms in a patient taking imatinib should prompt a chest radiograph. ILD produces ground-glass infiltrates and a decrease in carbon-dioxyde capacity [9]. In one study of 27 patients with ILD, 11 (41%) had preexisting lung disease [9].

63.4 Histopathological Findings

Imatinib-related ILD was first described in a 64-year-old man with CML. Increasing dyspnea developed on day 78 of imatinib therapy 400 mg/day. A transbronchial lung biopsy (TBLB) showed destruction of the alveolar septa and mixed intraalveolar and interstitial fibrosis with eosinophilic infiltration [12]. The prominent eosinophil infiltrate suggested an immunoallergic mechanism. Subsequently, a histopathological pattern without eosinophils was documented by TBLB [13]. In the largest Japanese series, TBLB was performed in 5/27 (18.5%) patients [9] and showed interstitial inflammation; intraluminal-organizing fibrosis; destruction of alveolar septa; mixed intraalveolar and interstitial fibrosis with eosinophil infiltrates; and alveolitis with lymphocytes, plasma cells, mild type II pneumocyte hyperplasia and organization. Video-assisted thoracoscopic surgery was performed in a patient whose chest CT showed a nodular pattern. Histopathology showed focal lymphocyte infiltrates and mixed intraalveolar and interstitial fibrosis. TBLB confirmed the clinical suspicion of interstitial pneumonitis, showing alveolar wall thickening by moderately dense fibrous tissue and mild patchy lymphocytic infiltrates [13]. Lymphomatoid granulomatosis with lung involvement was described in a 39-year-old man with a history of recurrent GIST of the small bowel treated with imatinib (400 mg once daily). He presented with a 2-week history of shortness of breath, fluctuating fever, pancytopenia, and bilateral airspace opacities. He was treated for pneumonia, but his condition deteriorated, and he died 6 weeks after admission Autopsy revealed bilateral pleural effusions and partially or well-defined pale gray/tan nodules of variable size showing central necrosis and focal cavitation in all lobes of the two lungs. Large areas of necrosis were found. Viable tissue showed large CD20+ atypical lymphoid cells and CD3+ small lymphocytes around the blood vessels. The atypical cells contained the Epstein-Barr virus [14]. A similar picture was reported in an 89-year-old woman with liver metastases from GIST in whom cutaneous and pulmonary lesions consistent with lymphomatoid granulomatosis occurred after 9 months on imatinib 400 mg/day [15].

63.5 Management

In patients with respiratory manifestations (cough, chest pain, dyspnea, or other), imatinib should be discontinued and a chest X-ray performed. When a pleural effusion without parenchymal involvement is found, echocardiography and a BNP or NT-proBNP assay are useful to rule out cardiotoxicity [16, 17], although congestive heart failure may be rare with imatinib therapy, particularly in patients treated for GIST [18].

After ILD resolution, several patients were successfully re-treated with imatinib, often in combination with corticosteroids [13, 19–21]. However, reintroduction of the drug has also been shown to induce ILD progression and should therefore be avoided [9, 22]. In the largest Japanese series of patients with imatinib-related ILD, the drug was reintroduced in a lower dosage in 11 patients, among whom 4 experienced recurrent ILD [9].

63.6 Pulmonary Manifestations Associated with the Other BCR-ABL Tyrosine Kinase Inhibitors

Dasatinib is a multitargeted kinase inhibitor against BCR-ABL and SRC that was recently approved for the treatment of CML and Ph+ALL with resistance or intolerance to prior imatinib therapy [23]. Dasatinib is being investigated in clinical trials for patients with solid tumors. Pleural effusions and other manifestations of fluid retention syndromes were shown in phase II/III studies to be typical and frequent side effects of dasatinib [11]. The incidence of grade 3–4 pleural effusions in patients with chronic-phase Ph+CML included in the clinical studies ($n=1{,}150$) was 4% [24]. The incidence rate of grade 3–4 pleural effusion was 5% in acute-phase CML, 10% in myeloid chronic-phase Ph+CML, and 6% in lymphoid chronic-phase Ph+CML or Ph+ALL [24]. Phase III dose optimization studies showed that diminishing the dosage from 70 mg twice daily to 100 mg/day reduced the incidence of pleural effusion from 16% to 7% ($P=0.024$) [25]. However, pleural effusion has been reported in up to 35% of patients with Ph+CML, usually at the accelerated or blast phase [26]. In a cohort of Ph+CML patients treated with dasatinib, the only variables associated with fluid retention were a history of autoimmune disease (relative risk, 1.3; 95% confidence interval, 1.6–103) and the dasatinib dosage (7.4; 1.2–44.3) [27]. Guidelines for managing pleural effusions during dasatinib treatment have been developed (Fig. 63.1) [24, 28]. Parenchymal lung disease associated with dasatinib is rare. The first case was described in a 60-year-old man with chronic-phase Ph+CML who had taken dasatinib 70 mg bid for 27 days [29]. He presented with a fever, acute episodes of bronchospasm, arthritis of the interphalangeal joints, and roundish papules over the legs. Gas exchange was impaired, and chest X-rays revealed bilateral pleural effusions. Specimens recovered by thoracocentesis were negative for pathogens. Neither BAL nor biopsies were performed. Dasatinib was discontinued, and broad-spectrum antimicrobials with corticosteroids were given. He improved rapidly after the introduction of corticosteroid therapy, suggesting an immunoallergic mechanism. Of 40 patients who received dasatinib (70 mg bid) for Ph+CML with imatinib resistance or intolerance, 9 (22.5%) developed dyspnea, cough, and chest pain [30]. Of these nine patients, six had pleural effusions (all were exudates), and seven had lung parenchyma abnormalities consisting of ground-glass or alveolar opacities or septal thickening (four patients had both). High lymphocyte counts were found in pleural and BAL fluids from eight patients; the remaining patient had neutrophilic alveolitis. Pleural biopsies revealed lymphocytic infiltration in one patient and myeloid infiltration in another. After dasatinib interruption, the lung manifestations resolved in all patients and did not recur in three of the four patients who were re-treated with dasatinib at a lower dosage (40 mg twice daily). The available data on pleural effusions during dasatinib treatment are reported in Tables 63.1–63.3. No respiratory adverse effects or lung involvement was described in preliminary studies of nilotinib [31–33]. Pleural effusion was reported in only 1% of patients with chronic-phase Ph+CML given nilotinib after imatinib resistance and intolerance [34]. In a phase I study of dasatinib plus nilotinib in 34 patients with advanced non-small-cell lung cancer, 18 patients had pleural effusions, which were grade 2–4 [35]. None had ILD. Pulmonary and upper respiratory side effects, which were not described in any detail, were reported in 17.9% of patients in a phase I study of INNO-406, a dual kinase inhibitor (against ABL and the yes-1 Yamaguchi sarcoma viral-related oncogene homolog Lyn) used for Ph+CML after imatinib resistance or intolerance [36].

63.7 Conclusion

Imatinib-related ILD varies in severity but responds well to corticosteroid treatment. Pre-existing pulmonary disease may be a risk factor. Therefore, the chest radiographs should be evaluated carefully before initiating imatinib treatment. Physicians should pay careful attention to clinical symptoms such as unexplained fever, cough, and dyspnea during the first few months after starting imatinib therapy. These symptoms warrant imatinib discontinuation and investigations for toxicity including ILD. When ILD is found, concomitant infection must be ruled out, and corticosteroid therapy is in order after an in-depth evaluation.

Table 63.1 Reported cases of interstitial lung diseases associated with imatinib

Authors	Reference	Country	*n*	Incidence	Previous respiratory disorders	Indication	Imatinib dosage (mg/day)	Length of treatment
Bergeron et al. (2002)	[37]	Africa*	1	–	No	CML	600	9 months
Rosado et al. (2003)	[38]	USA	1	–	No	CML	400	5 months
Ma et al. (2003)	[19]	USA	1	–	No	CML	400	2 weeks
Yokoyama et al. (2004)	[12]	Japan	1	–	No	CML	400	78 days
Isshiki et al. (2004)	[39]	Japan	1	–	No	CML	400	1 month
Grimison et al. (2005)	[13]	Australia	1	–	No	GIST	400	4 months
Rajda et al. (2005)	[40]	USA	1	–	No	CML	400	4 weeks
Ohnishi et al. (2006)	[9]	Japan	27	27/5 500 (0.5%)	11/27 (41%)	23 CML 4 GIST	400 (200–600)	49 days (10–282)
Lin et al. (2006)	[41]	Taiwan	1	–	No	CML	100	3 days
Seki et al. (2007)	[22]	Japan	1	–	No	CML	–	–
Yamasawa et al. (2008)	[20]	Japan	1	–	IPF	CML	400	28 days
Loong et al. (2008)	[42]	China	1	–	No	GIST	400	1 month
Izumiyama et al. (2009)	[21]	Japan	2	–	No	GIST	–	2 months

* Reported in France, patient borned in Africa

IPF idiopathic pulmonary fibrosis, *CML* chronic myelogenous leukemia, *GIST* gastrointestinal stromal tumors

Table 63.2 Reported cases of interstitial lung disease associated with imatinib (continued) including follow-up

Authors	Reference	Imatinib discontinuation	Adjunctive corticosteroids	Reintroduction of imatinib	Imatinib dosage at reintroduction	Adjunctive corticosteroids	ILD recurrence	Follow-up duration
Bergeron et al. (2002)	[37]	Yes	No	No	–	–	–	–
Rosado et al. (2003)	[38]	Yes	Yes, prednisone 1 mg/kg/day	No	–	–	–	–
Ma et al. (2003)	[19]	Yes	Yes, prednisone 100 mg/day	Yes	–	Yes, prednisone 20 mg/day tapered to 9 mg/day	No	7 months
Yokoyama et al. (2004)	[12]	Yes	No	No	–	–	–	–
Isshiki et al. (2004)	[39]	Yes	Yes dosage?	No	–	–	–	–
Grimison et al. (2005)	[13]	Yes	Yes, prednisone 50 mg/day	Yes	400 mg/day	Prednisone 50 mg/day tapered to dexamethasone 1 mg/day	No	–
Rajda et al. (2005)	[40]	Yes	Yes, prednisone 30 mg/day	No	–	–	–	–
Ohnishi et al. (2006)	[9]		Yes, dosage?	Yes, 11/27	Reduced (not specified)	No	Yes, 5/11	–
Lin et al. (2006)	[41]	Yes	No	No	–	–	–	–
Seki et al. (2007)	[22]	Yes	–	Yes	–	–	–	4 years
Yamasawa et al. (2008)	[20]	Yes	Methylprednisolone (1 g/day i.v. for 3 days), followed by prednisone 60 mg/day	No	–	–	–	–
Loong et al. (2008)	[42]	Yes	Yes Dosage?	No	–	–	–	–
Izumiyama et al. (2009)	[21]	Yes	No (dosage?)	Yes	Half the previous dosage	Yes (dosage?)	No	–

Table 63.3 Reported cases of pleural effusions associated with dasatinib

Author	Reference	Patients	Incidence pleural effusion, *n* (%)	Male (%)	Initial drug dosage	Side	Most common associated symptoms
Talpaz et al. (2006)	[23]	84	30 (36%)	47	15–240 mg/day, 5 days on, 2 off	–	Cytopenia, GI[b] symptoms, edema, dyspnea, rash, headache
Radaelli et al. (2006)	[29]	1	1 (100%)	100	70 mg bid[a]	1/1 bilateral	Fever, lung infiltrates, dyspnea, rash, arthritis
Guilhot et al. (2007)	[43]	107	25 (23%)	51	70 mg bid[a]	–	Cytopenia, GI[b] symptoms, headache, fatigue, fever, rash
Kantarjian et al. (2007)	[44]	101	17 (17%)	53	70 mg bid[a]	–	Cytopenia, GI[b] symptoms, fatigue, headache, dyspnea
Bergeron et al. (2007)	[30]	40	6 (15%)	–	70 mg bid[a]	2/6 bilateral	–
Quintas-Cardarama et al. (2007)	[26]	138	48 (35%)	–	Varying doses	39/48 bilateral	–
Ottman et al. (2007)	[45]	36	7 (19%)	23	70 mg bid[a]	–	Cytopenia, GI[b] symptoms, asthenia, fever
Hochhaus et al. (2008)	[46]	387	106 (27%)	–	Median: 101–104 mg/day	–	Cytopenia, diarrhea, headaches, fatigue, dyspnea, rash
De Lavallade et al. (2008)	[47]	62	17 (27%)	–	100–140 mg/day	2/17 bilateral	2/17 pericardial effusions
Shah et al. (2008)	[25]	335	31 (9%)	50	100 mg qd[a]	–	Cytopenia, headaches, GI[b] symptoms, fatigue, rash
Cortes et al. (2008)	[48]	109	39 (36%)	58	70 mg bid[a]	–	Cytopenia, GI[b] symptoms, fever, fatigue, edema
Goldblatt et al. (2009)	[49]	2	2 (100%)	50	70 mg bid[a]	1/2 bilateral	Cytopenia, GI[b] toxicity

[a]*bid* twice daily, *qd* once daily
[b]Gastrointestinal

References

1. Demetri GD, von Mehren M, Blanke CD, Van den Abbeele AD, Eisenberg B, Roberts PJ, Heinrich MC, Tuveson DA, Singer S, Janicek M et al (2002) Efficacy and safety of imatinib mesylate in advanced gastrointestinal stromal tumors. N Engl J Med 347(7):472–480
2. Deininger MW, O'Brien SG, Ford JM, Druker BJ (2003) Practical management of patients with chronic myeloid leukemia receiving imatinib. J Clin Oncol 21(8):1637–1647
3. Valeyrie L, Bastuji-Garin S, Revuz J, Bachot N, Wechsler J, Berthaud P, Tulliez M, Giraudier S (2003) Adverse cutaneous reactions to imatinib (STI571) in Philadelphia chromosome-positive leukemias: a prospective study of 54 patients. J Am Acad Dermatol 48(2):201–206
4. Schaich M, Schakel K, Illmer T, Ehninger G, Bornhauser M (2003) Severe epidermal necrolysis after treatment with imatinib and consecutive allogeneic hematopoietic stem cell transplantation. Ann Hematol 82(5):303–304
5. Heuchel R, Berg A, Tallquist M, Ahlen K, Reed RK, Rubin K, Claesson-Welsh L, Heldin CH, Soriano P (1999) Platelet-derived growth factor beta receptor regulates interstitial fluid homeostasis through phosphatidylinositol-3' kinase signaling. Proc Natl Acad Sci USA 96(20):11410–11415
6. Kantarjian H, Sawyers C, Hochhaus A, Guilhot F, Schiffer C, Gambacorti-Passerini C, Niederwieser D, Resta D, Capdeville R, Zoellner U et al (2002) Hematologic and cytogenetic responses to imatinib mesylate in chronic myelogenous leukemia. N Engl J Med 346(9):645–652
7. O'Brien SG, Guilhot F, Larson RA, Gathmann I, Baccarani M, Cervantes F, Cornelissen JJ, Fischer T, Hochhaus A, Hughes T et al (2003) Imatinib compared with interferon and low-dose cytarabine for newly diagnosed chronic-phase chronic myeloid leukemia. N Engl J Med 348(11):994–1004
8. Silver RT, Cortes J, Waltzman R, Mone M, Kantarjian H (2009) Sustained durability of responses and improved progression-free and overall survival with imatinib treatment for accelerated phase and blast crisis chronic myeloid leukemia: long-term follow-up of the STI571 0102 and 0109 trials. Haematologica 94(5):743–744
9. Ohnishi K, Sakai F, Kudoh S, Ohno R (2006) Twenty-seven cases of drug-induced interstitial lung disease associated with imatinib mesylate. Leukemia 20(6):1162–1164
10. Druker BJ, Guilhot F, O'Brien SG, Gathmann I, Kantarjian H, Gattermann N, Deininger MW, Silver RT, Goldman JM, Stone RM et al (2006) Five-year follow-up of patients receiving imatinib for chronic myeloid leukemia. N Engl J Med 355(23):2408–2417
11. Mauro MJ, Deininger MW (2009) Management of drug toxicities in chronic myeloid leukaemia. Best Pract Res Clin Haematol 22(3):409–429
12. Yokoyama T, Miyazawa K, Kurakawa E, Nagate A, Shimamoto T, Iwaya K, Akata S, Aoshima M, Serizawa H, Ohyashiki K (2004) Interstitial pneumonia induced by imatinib mesylate: pathologic study demonstrates alveolar destruction and fibrosis with eosinophilic infiltration. Leukemia 18(3):645–646
13. Grimison P, Goldstein D, Schneeweiss J, Murray N (2005) Corticosteroid-responsive interstitial pneumonitis related to imantinib mesylate with successful rechallenge, and potential causative mechanisms. Intern Med J 35(2): 136–137
14. Salmons N, Gregg RJ, Pallalau A, Woolhouse I, Geh I, Taniere P (2007) Lymphomatoid granulomatosis in a patient previously diagnosed with a gastrointestinal stromal tumour and treated with imatinib. J Clin Pathol 60(2): 199–201
15. Yazdi AS, Metzler G, Weyrauch S, Berneburg M, Bitzer M, Muller-Hermelink HK, Rocken M (2007) Lymphomatoid granulomatosis induced by imatinib-treatment. Arch Dermatol 143(9):1222–1223
16. Kerkela R, Grazette L, Yacobi R, Iliescu C, Patten R, Beahm C, Walters B, Shevtsov S, Pesant S, Clubb FJ et al (2006) Cardiotoxicity of the cancer therapeutic agent imatinib mesylate. Nat Med 12(8):908–916
17. Orphanos GS, Ioannidis GN, Ardavanis AG (2009) Cardiotoxicity induced by tyrosine kinase inhibitors. Acta Oncol 48(7):964–970
18. Trent JC, Patel SS, Zhang J, Araujo DM, Plana JC, Lenihan DJ, Fan D, Patel SR, Benjamin RS, Khakoo AY (2010) Rare incidence of congestive heart failure in gastrointestinal stromal tumor and other sarcoma patients receiving imatinib mesylate. Cancer 116(1):184–192
19. Ma CX, Hobday TJ, Jett JR (2003) Imatinib mesylate-induced interstitial pneumonitis. Mayo Clin Proc 78(12): 1578–1579
20. Yamasawa H, Sugiyama Y, Bando M, Ohno S (2008) Drug-induced pneumonitis associated with imatinib mesylate in a patient with idiopathic pulmonary fibrosis. Respiration 75(3):350–354
21. Izumiyama N, Noguchi K, Takahashi H, Shishikura Y, Saitou W, Nishimaki K, Kikuchi T, Sasamori K, Miki H, Tezuka F et al (2009) Successful reintroduction of mesylate imatinib after pneumonitis in two patients with gastrointestinal stromal tumor (GIST). Nihon Kokyuki Gakkai Zasshi 47(10):918–923
22. Seki N, Ito A, Watanabe K, Shibakuki R, Seto T, Uematsu K, Mine T, Eguchi K (2007) Irreversible imatinib-induced pneumonitis following long-term imatinib administration. Intern Med 46(23):1941–1942
23. Talpaz M, Shah NP, Kantarjian H, Donato N, Nicoll J, Paquette R, Cortes J, O'Brien S, Nicaise C, Bleickardt E et al (2006) Dasatinib in imatinib-resistant Philadelphia chromosome-positive leukemias. N Engl J Med 354(24): 2531–2541
24. Masiello D, Gorospe G 3rd, Yang AS (2009) The occurrence and management of fluid retention associated with TKI therapy in CML, with a focus on dasatinib. J Hematol Oncol 2:46
25. Shah NP, Kantarjian HM, Kim DW, Rea D, Dorlhiac-Llacer PE, Milone JH, Vela-Ojeda J, Silver RT, Khoury HJ, Charbonnier A et al (2008) Intermittent target inhibition with dasatinib 100 mg once daily preserves efficacy and improves tolerability in imatinib-resistant and -intolerant chronic-phase chronic myeloid leukemia. J Clin Oncol 26(19):3204–3212
26. Quintas-Cardama A, Kantarjian H, O'Brien S, Borthakur G, Bruzzi J, Munden R, Cortes J (2007) Pleural effusion in patients with chronic myelogenous leukemia treated with dasatinib after imatinib failure. J Clin Oncol 25(25): 3908–3914

27. de Lavallade H, Punnialingam S, Milojkovic D, Bua M, Khorashad JS, Gabriel IH, Chaidos A, Olavarria E, Goldman JM, Apperley JF et al (2008) Pleural effusions in patients with chronic myeloid leukaemia treated with dasatinib may have an immune-mediated pathogenesis. Br J Haematol 141(5): 745–747
28. Cony-Makhoul P, Bergeron A, Corm S, Dubruille V, Rea D, Rigal-Huguet F, Nicolini FE (2008) Guidelines for the management of dasatinib (Sprycel)-induced side effects in chronic myelogenous leukemia and Philadelphia positive acute lymphoblastic leukemias. Bull Cancer 95(9): 805–811
29. Radaelli F, Bramanti S, Fantini NN, Fabio G, Greco I, Lambertenghi-Deliliers G (2006) Dasatinib-related alveolar pneumonia responsive to corticosteroids. Leuk Lymphoma 47(6):1180–1181
30. Bergeron A, Rea D, Levy V, Picard C, Meignin V, Tamburini J, Bruzzoni-Giovanelli H, Calvo F, Tazi A, Rousselot P (2007) Lung abnormalities after dasatinib treatment for chronic myeloid leukemia: a case series. Am J Respir Crit Care Med 176(8):814–818
31. Cortes JE, Jones D, O'Brien S, Jabbour E, Konopleva M, Ferrajoli A, Kadia T, Borthakur G, Stigliano D, Shan J et al (2010) Nilotinib as front-line treatment for patients with chronic myeloid leukemia in early chronic phase. J Clin Oncol 28(3):392–397
32. Kantarjian H, Giles F, Wunderle L, Bhalla K, O'Brien S, Wassmann B, Tanaka C, Manley P, Rae P, Mietlowski W et al (2006) Nilotinib in imatinib-resistant CML and Philadelphia chromosome-positive ALL. N Engl J Med 354(24): 2542–2551
33. Rosti G, Palandri F, Castagnetti F, Breccia M, Levato L, Gugliotta G, Capucci A, Cedrone M, Fava C, Intermesoli T et al (2009) Nilotinib for the frontline treatment of Ph + chronic myeloid leukemia. Blood 114(24): 4933–4938
34. Kantarjian HM, Giles F, Gattermann N, Bhalla K, Alimena G, Palandri F, Ossenkoppele GJ, Nicolini FE, O'Brien SG, Litzow M et al (2007) Nilotinib (formerly AMN107), a highly selective BCR-ABL tyrosine kinase inhibitor, is effective in patients with Philadelphia chromosome-positive chronic myelogenous leukemia in chronic phase following imatinib resistance and intolerance. Blood 110(10): 3540–3546
35. Haura EB, Tanvetyanon T, Chiappori A, Williams C, Simon G, Antonia S, Gray J, Litschauer S, Tetteh L, Neuger A et al (2010) Phase I/II study of the Src inhibitor dasatinib in combination with erlotinib in advanced non-small-cell lung cancer. J Clin Oncol 28(8):1387–1394
36. Kantarjian H, Coutre PL, Cortes J, Pinilla-Ibarz J, Nagler A, Hochhaus A, Kimura S, Ottmann O (2010) Phase 1 study of INNO-406, a dual Abl/Lyn kinase inhibitor, in Philadelphia chromosome-positive leukemias after imatinib resistance or intolerance. Cancer 116(11):2665–2672
37. Bergeron A, Bergot E, Vilela G, Ades L, Devergie A, Esperou H, Socie G, Calvo F, Gluckman E, Ribaud P et al (2002) Hypersensitivity pneumonitis related to imatinib mesylate. J Clin Oncol 20(20):4271–4272
38. Rosado MF, Donna E, Ahn YS (2003) Challenging problems in advanced malignancy: case 3 Imatinib mesylate-induced interstitial pneumonitis. J Clin Oncol 21(16): 3171–3173
39. Isshiki I, Yamaguchi K, Okamoto S (2004) Interstitial pneumonitis during imatinib therapy. Br J Haematol 125(4): 420
40. Rajda J, Phatak PD (2005) Reversible drug-induced interstitial pneumonitis following imatinib mesylate therapy. Am J Hematol 79(1):80–81
41. Lin JT, Yeh KT, Fang HY, Chang CS (2006) Fulminant, but reversible interstitial pneumonitis associated with imatinib mesylate. Leuk Lymphoma 47(8):1693–1695
42. Loong HH, Yeo W (2008) Imatinib-induced interstitial lung disease and sunitinib-associated intra-tumour haemorrhage. Hong Kong Med J 14(6):495–498
43. Guilhot F, Apperley J, Kim DW, Bullorsky EO, Baccarani M, Roboz GJ, Amadori S, de Souza CA, Lipton JH, Hochhaus A et al (2007) Dasatinib induces significant hematologic and cytogenetic responses in patients with imatinib-resistant or -intolerant chronic myeloid leukemia in accelerated phase. Blood 109(10):4143–4150
44. Kantarjian H, Pasquini R, Hamerschlak N, Rousselot P, Holowiecki J, Jootar S, Robak T, Khoroshko N, Masszi T, Skotnicki A et al (2007) Dasatinib or high-dose imatinib for chronic-phase chronic myeloid leukemia after failure of first-line imatinib: a randomized phase 2 trial. Blood 109(12):5143–5150
45. Ottmann O, Dombret H, Martinelli G, Simonsson B, Guilhot F, Larson RA, Rege-Cambrin G, Radich J, Hochhaus A, Apanovitch AM et al (2007) Dasatinib induces rapid hematologic and cytogenetic responses in adult patients with Philadelphia chromosome positive acute lymphoblastic leukemia with resistance or intolerance to imatinib: interim results of a phase 2 study. Blood 110(7):2309–2315
46. Hochhaus A, Baccarani M, Deininger M, Apperley JF, Lipton JH, Goldberg SL, Corm S, Shah NP, Cervantes F, Silver RT et al (2008) Dasatinib induces durable cytogenetic responses in patients with chronic myelogenous leukemia in chronic phase with resistance or intolerance to imatinib. Leukemia 22(6):1200–1206
47. de Lavallade H, Apperley JF, Khorashad JS, Milojkovic D, Reid AG, Bua M, Szydlo R, Olavarria E, Kaeda J, Goldman JM et al (2008) Imatinib for newly diagnosed patients with chronic myeloid leukemia: incidence of sustained responses in an intention-to-treat analysis. J Clin Oncol 26(20):3358–3363
48. Cortes JE, Jones D, O'Brien S, Jabbour E, Ravandi F, Koller C, Borthakur G, Walker B, Zhao W, Shan J et al (2010) Results of dasatinib therapy in patients with early chronic-phase chronic myeloid leukemia. J Clin Oncol 28(3):398–404
49. Goldblatt M, Huggins JT, Doelken P, Gurung P, Sahn SA (2009) Dasatinib-induced pleural effusions: a lymphatic network disorder? Am J Med Sci 338(5):414–417

Rituximab-Related Pulmonary Toxicity

64

Yair Herishanu, Chava Perry, and Aaron Polliack

Contents

Y. Herishanu (✉) and C. Perry
Department of Hematology, Tel Aviv Sourasky Medical Center, 6 Weizmann Street, Tel Aviv 64239, Israel
e-mail: herishanu@yahoo.com

A. Polliack
Department of Hematology, Tel Aviv Sourasky Medical Center, 6 Weizmann Street, Tel Aviv 64239, Israel and
Department of Hematology, Hadassah University Hospital, Jerusalem, Israel

64.1 The Case

An 80-year-old man was generally healthy until 2004, when he noticed progressive enlargement of a growing right sub-mandibular mass. On physical examination and in computerized tomography (CT) scan, the patient was found to have generalized lymphadenopathy on both sides of the diaphragm. A lymph node biopsy from the right sub-mandibular mass revealed a follicular grade 3B non-Hodgkin's lymphoma (NHL) that was in clinical stage 3A with an international prognostic index (IPI) of 2. The patient was treated with cycles of combination immunochemotherapy with rituximab (375 mg/m^2)-CHOP (cyclophosphamide, doxorubicin, vincristine and prednisone) every 21 days. After three uneventful cycles of therapy, he had a good clinical response, and an interim mid-treatment positron emission tomography-computed tomography (PET-CT) was performed, which showed disappearance of all the previous imaging findings, and no uptake of ^{18}F-deoxyfluoroglucose (^{18}F-FDG) was detected in these sites. However, on the same PET-CT scan, new abnormal sites of ^{18}F-FDG uptake were detected as opacities in the sub-pleural areas of the lung, mostly on the right side (Fig. 64.1).

At the same time, the patient complained of mild dyspnea on effort, and bilateral basilar crackles were present on physical examination. Pulse oximetry and chest X-ray were performed, which were within normal limits. Treatment with rituximab-CHOP was continued as scheduled, but 2 days after starting the fifth cycle of therapy, the patient was admitted to the hospital because of a dry cough and worsening dyspnea. On examination, the patient had a normal body temperature, but was tachypneic, and hypoxemic and bilateral basal inspiratory crackles were present. Chest X-ray showed reticulo-nodular infiltrates (Fig. 64.2), and

É. Azoulay (ed.), *Pulmonary Involvement in Patients with Hematological Malignancies*,
DOI: 10.1007/978-3-642-15742-4_64, © Springer-Verlag Berlin Heidelberg 2011

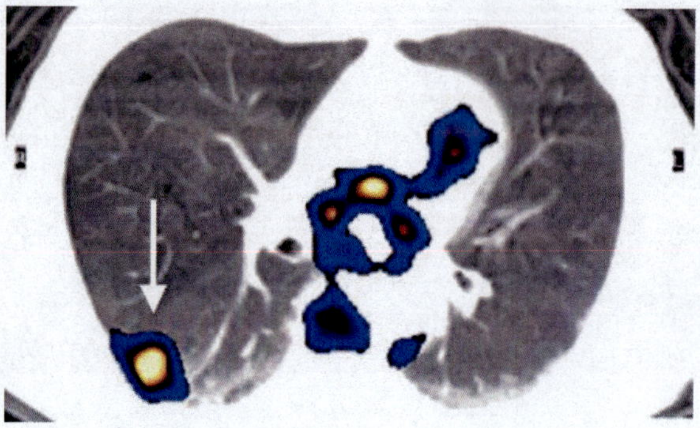

Fig. 64.1 Early radiological findings of rituximab-related pulmonary toxicity as detected in mid-treatment PET-CT. Abnormal uptake of ^{18}F-FDG is evident in sub-pleural lung opacities, mostly on the right side

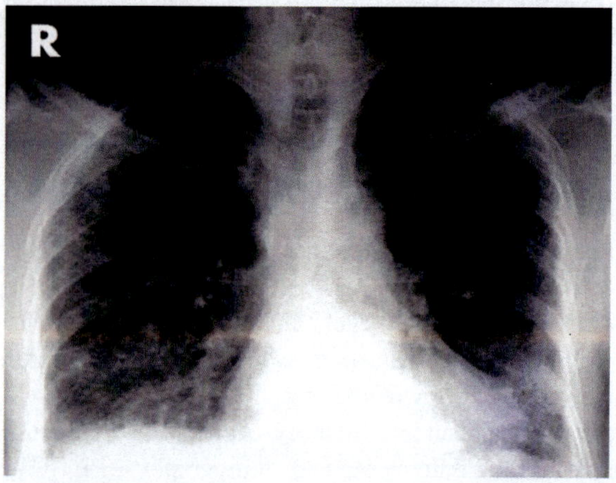

Fig. 64.2 Chest X-ray. Showing bilateral reticulo-nodular infiltrates

a contrast-enhanced chest CT scan revealed further progression of the sub-pleural air-space consolidation. "Ground-glass" opacities, small pulmonary cysts and thickening of the interlobular septa were also evident (Fig. 64.3).

Bronchoscopy was performed and was within normal limits, and the bronchoalveolar lavage revealed no evidence of bacteria; acid-fast bacilli, *Pneumocystis jirovecii* (*P. jirovecii*) and cytomegalovirus (CMV) were also negative. Trans-bronchial biopsy was performed and revealed interstitial inflammation of the lung parenchyma, as well as swelling and hyperplasia of atypical type II alveolar cells, which showed increased nuclear size and hyperchromasia, and an accumulation of foamy histiocytes with cytoplasmic vacuoles was evident within the alveoli (Fig. 64.4). Treatment with intravenous methylprednisolone (1 mg/kg) was started, but the patient developed rapidly progressive respiratory insufficiency requiring mechanical ventilation and unfortunately died 10 days after admission.

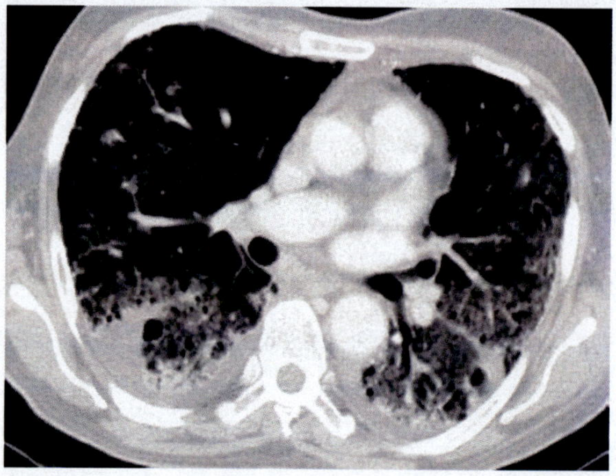

Fig. 64.3 Contrast-enhanced chest CT scan. Progression of the sub-pleural areas of intraalveolar consolidation, "ground-glass" opacities, small pulmonary cysts and thickening of the interlobular septa

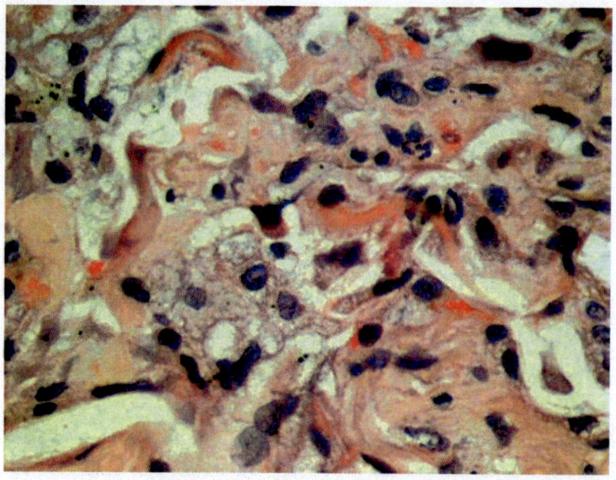

Fig. 64.4 Transbronchial biopsy. Showing interstitial inflammation as well as swelling and hyperplasia of atypical type II alveolar cells. Accumulation of foamy histiocytes with cytoplasmic vacuoles is seen in alveoli

64.1.1 Rituximab-Related Pulmonary Toxicity

Rituximab is a genetically engineered, chimeric murine/human monoclonal IgG_1 antibody that binds specifically to the CD20 antigen, which is expressed on normal B-cells and on the vast majority of malignant cells in B-cell lymphoproliferative disorders [1]. The binding of rituximab to the CD20 ligand causes cell lysis through a variety of mechanisms, including complement-mediated cytotoxicty, antibody-dependent cell (e.g., NK cells)-mediated cytoxicity and direct induction of cell apoptosis [1]. Rituximab has been extensively studied and used to treat CD20 positive, B-cell lymphoproliferative disorders, either as a single agent or more commonly in combination with chemotherapy; in recent years it has also been used for the treatment of autoimmune disorders. It has currently been approved by the Food and Drug Administration (FDA) and/or by the European Medicines Agency (EMEA) for the treatment of: (1) low-grade/follicular non-Hodgkin's lymphoma (NHL) as first-line treatment as well as for relapsed or refractory disease and for maintenance therapy in this disorder; (2) diffuse large B-cell NHL as first-line treatment in combination with anthracycline-based chemotherapy regimens; (3) chronic lymphocytic leukemia (CLL) in previously untreated patients, in combination with chemotherapy; (4) rheumatoid arthritis, in combination with methotrexate, for patients with an inadequate response to one or more of the TNF antagonist therapies [1]. In addition to rheumatoid arthritis, rituximab has been shown to be effective in the treatment of a variety of other autoimmune disorders, including autoimmune cytopenias, such as immune thrombocytopenic purpura (ITP) and autoimmune hemolytic anemia (AIHA), as well as in systemic lupus erythematosus (SLE), Sjorgen's syndrome, vasculitides, and autoimmune neurologic and dermatologic disorders [2].

Rituximab is generally well tolerated and safe to use. Its major adverse effects appear to be infusion-related reactions [1]. During the first infusion, patients may develop fever, chills and dyspnea, and occasionally hypotension; however, it rarely causes anaphylactic shock or acute respiratory distress syndrome (ARDS). Patients with high numbers of circulating neoplastic lymphoid cells may develop cytokine-release syndrome [3] and/or tumor lysis syndrome [4]. Other infrequent adverse affects include delayed neutropenia [5], hepatitis B virus reactivation [6], Stevens Johnson syndrome [7] and serum sickness [8].

With regard to pulmonary toxicity, more than 40 cases, most probably related to therapy with rituximab, have been reported until now [9–26]. Rituximab-associated lung toxicity has been described more commonly in elderly patients (mean age 65 years, range, 43–80 years), with a slight male predominance (male:female ratio of 2:1) [9]. These patients had either received rituximab as a single agent [11, 14, 16] or in combination with different chemotherapy regimens (COP, CHOP, CEOP, ACVBP, VNCOP, fludarabine, cladribine) [9–12, 15, 16, 22] with or without the addition of growth factors for NHL, CLL, ITP, rheumatoid arthritis and SLE [10–12, 14–16, 23, 24]. In most cases the patients developed acute or subacute symptoms after one or more cycles of therapy [10–12, 14–16].

64.1.2 Acute Pulmonary Reactions

Rituximab-associated acute adverse pulmonary reactions were reported during or shortly after the first infusion of the agent and included bronchospasm, hypoxia, pulmonary infiltrates as well as ARDS [27– 29]. The latter syndrome has been reported in several patients within a few hours after initiating rituximab infusion. All these patients required mechanical ventilation, and although all were treated with corticosteroids, this complication was associated with a high mortality rate of around 40% [27–29]. In one patient, in whom a lung biopsy was performed, diffuse alveolar damage and hemorrhages were also seen [29].

64.1.3 Subacute Pulmonary Reactions

The majority of cases of rituximab-associated pulmonary toxicity occurred within days and up to 3 weeks after the first infusion of the antibody or following subsequent cycles with rituximab treatment. It appeared to occur most commonly after the fourth cycle of therapy and within a mean of 12 weeks after the initial rituximab infusion [9]. Patients usually presented with dyspnea, dry cough, signs of hypoxemia and occasional fever [10–16]. Crackles are present on physical examination in approximately a third of the patients [9]. Chest radiographs may reveal patchy or diffuse mixed interstitial and alveolar infiltrates [8, 18, 23, 24, 26, 30], while CT scan typically shows multiple focal alveolar infiltrates and areas of "ground-glass" shadowing [11, 15, 17, 23, 24, 26]. Pulmonary function tests are mostly compatible with restrictive abnormalities associated with a reduced diffusion capacity [11, 14, 30]. In some cases, a PET scan, performed for the evaluation of lymphoma response to treatment, showed some form of uptake, thereby detecting early pulmonary changes [8, 31, 32] while patients were still basically asymptomatic. In other cases, a PET-CT scan revealed late-onset pulmonary infiltrates, occurring between 1 and 3 months after the treatment of rituximab was discontinued, appearing as linear subpleural FDG uptake, which sometimes persisted for several months [33]. Bronchoaleveolar lavage (BAL) fluid was negative for infectious disease, and cytology was negative for malignant cells, whereas normal CD4+ T-lymphocytes predominated [15, 18, 25]. Transbronchial or lung biopsies most commonly showed histological findings compatible with organizing pneumonia and interstitial pneumonitis [9, 19–21, 23, 30, 34]; diffuse alveolar hemorrhage and acute pulmonary fibrosis were less commonly observed [15, 16, 18].

64.1.4 Mechanism of Toxicity

Acute lung toxicity, mostly ARDS, is considered to be the result of a cytokine release syndrome with tumor necrosis factor-α (TNF- α), interferon-γ (INF-γ), interleukin-6 (IL-6) or interleukin-8 (IL-8)] [3, 9] released in high concentrations. This clinical picture occurs shortly after the first infusion of rituximab, at a time when the patient still has a large tumor burden [9]. The more insidious onset reactions described appear to be due to hypersensitivity reactions, and continuing treatment with rituximab results in recurrence of the same symptoms, but of increasing severity [9, 15, 26]. This type of rituximab-associated pulmonary toxicity seems to respond favorably to corticosteroid therapy [9]. It has also been suggested that the mechanism of toxicity seen in the latter reaction may also be linked to the release of inflammatory cytokines, including TNF- α, INF-γ, IL-6 and IL-8 [11, 35], complement activation [15] or indirect cytotoxic T lymphocyte activation [15], all of which are known to occur during therapy with rituximab [36, 37]. Along this line, results of an experimental in vitro model have suggested that apoptotic lymphoma cells undergo phagocytosis by dendritic cells (DC). This leads to DC maturation and thereafter promotes induction of a cytotoxic T-cell response against these lymphoma cell-associated antigens [37, 38].

64.1.5 Differential Diagnosis

The appearance of pulmonary infiltrates in lymphoma patients receiving rituximab is a challenging situation. Several diagnoses can be considered, namely cardiogenic pulmonary edema, infection, progressive lymphoma, exacerbation of underlying chronic lung disease and drug-related pulmonary toxicity. Rituximab-related pulmonary toxicity is basically a diagnosis of exclusion. In immunocompromised patients, infectious causes, such as bacterial pneumonia, mycobacterial infections, viral pneumonits including CMV, *P. jirovecii* pneumonia (PCP) and fungal infection, should all be considered in the differential diagnosis. In this respect, the development of PCP has been reported during rituximab therapy, particularly in patients with NHL co-treated with the antibody and combination chemotherapy [39–44]. A few cases of cytomegalovirus (CMV) reactivation have also been recorded in the rituximab-treated patients [45–47]. After excluding the above-mentioned infectious causes, special consideration should be given to the possibility of drug-related pulmonary toxicity. Many cytotoxic agents are known to cause lung injury. In this respect, cyclophosphamide in particular, one of the most common agents used in combination with rituximab for the treatment of NHL and CLL, should be considered as one of the possible agents causing this clinical and radiological picture. As in the case of rituximab, the incidence of cyclophosphamide induced-pulmonary toxicity is low [48, 49], and the interval between exposure to cyclophosphamide and the appearance of the pulmonary insult varies from weeks to several years [48]. Early onset toxicity usually appears about 1–6 months after exposure to cyclophosphamide, and typically patients present with 1–2 weeks of dyspnea on effort and a dry cough [48, 49]. Bilateral basal reticular or reticulo-nodular infiltrates are seen on chest X-ray [49], "ground-glass" shadowing is evident on CT scan [49], and pulmonary function tests show restrictive abnormalities with reduced diffusion capacity [49]. Late-onset toxicity generally appears in patients who had received relatively low doses of cyclophosphamide given over a prolonged period of time [49], and these may occur years after discontinuation of the drug [49]. While the prognosis of early onset toxicity is generally good and corticosteroids are beneficial, late-onset toxicity has a poorer outcome and often progresses despite therapy with steroids [48, 49]. The histopathological spectrum of cyclophosphamide-induced lung injury includes: nonspecific interstitial pneumonia, organizing pneumonia, diffuse alveolar damage and diffuse alveolar hemorrhage [49]. In this regard, the endogenous production of reactive oxygen radicals was suggested as the most probable underlying mechanism for this pulmonary toxicity [48]. G-CSF is a growth factor commonly used in cancer patients to shorten the period of neutropenia following chemotherapy and is also utilized to mobilize hematopoietic progenitor cells for stem cell transplantation. Common adverse effects of G-CSF include fever, bone pain and fatigue. Pulmonary toxicities attributed to G-CSF include cough, dyspnea, interstitial pneumonitis and ARDS [50]. When used as a single agent, among 1,801 published cases of healthy stem cell donors given G-CSF for stem cell mobilization, lung toxicity was reported in 1 case only [50]. G-CSF-related pulmonary toxicity is more frequently reported in patients receiving this growth factor in combination with chemotherapeutic agents, and in these cases G-CSF may actually exacerbate chemotherapy-related pulmonary toxicity, particularly when cyclophosphamide, bleomycin or methotrexate is the chemotherapeutic agent involved [50]. G-CSF related-pulmonary toxicity can be fatal, with a relatively high mortality rate (24.6%) [50]. Because neutropenic patients treated with G-CSF frequently develop their pulmonary symptoms during or after recovery from the neutropenia, it was suggested that neutrophils play a central role in mediating this toxicity [50]. Treatment with G-CSF not only increases the number of neutrophils, but also enhances their functions [51, 52], thereby promoting neutrophil entrapment in the pulmonary vascular capillaries, and release of their oxygen radicals and proteolytic enzymes, which may cause subsequent endothelial and pulmonary damage [53–57]. G-CSF is commonly given for patients who have been treated with rituximab-containing regimens, and these combinations of drugs may potentially increase the risk of pulmonary toxicity [19, 30].

64.1.6 Clinical Investigations

Non-invasive studies such as arterial blood gas analysis, sputum examination, chest X-ray, pulmonary function tests, echocardiogram and chest CT scans are all helpful in determining the pattern of the pulmonary insult. However, bronchoscopy with BAL and biopsy of the lung tissue are eventually required to establish a more definitive diagnosis to be sure to rule out any infection before deciding for drug-related pulmonary toxicity. Sputum as well as the BAL fluid should be evaluated by direct smear and cultures for bacterial infections, including mycobacterium, and for possible opportunistic pathogens, such as fungi (Pneumocystis, Aspergillus, Candida). In addition, nasopharyngeal aspirates should also be evaluated for viral antigens, such as respiratory syncytial virus, adenovirus, influenza and parainfluenza viruses. The peripheral blood should also be sent for cultures and evaluated for CMV antigenemia or CMV-DNA PCR titer, β-D-glucan (antigens for Candida and Aspergillus), serology test for viruses, *Mycoplasma pneumonia* and *Chlamydophila pneumoniae*, while the urine should be tested for Legionella antigen.

An early lung biopsy either by open or a thoracoscopic approaches may be helpful to define the lung pathology more precisely as well as to exclude other alternative diagnoses, such as opportunistic infection or lymphoma. Trans-bronchial biopsy can be an alternative to lung biopsy; however, it has the disadvantage of ending up more frequently without an adequate sample for diagnosis.

64.1.7 Clinical Course and Treatment

In all the reported cases of pulmonary toxicity, rituximab was discontinued after the appearance of toxicity, and the majority of patients gradually recovered within a few days. Nevertheless, this complication is known to be fatal in 20% of the patients [9], and although some of these patients developed lung toxicity while receiving corticosteroids [10, 14], most appeared to respond favorably to early corticosteroid treatment [9]. Re-treatment with rituximab was uneventful in a proportion of these cases [12], whereas in others, re-treatment with rituximab, as a single agent or in combination with chemotherapeutic drugs, did cause pulmonary deterioration [10, 15], which was fatal in some cases [8, 15]. Accordingly, it is recommended that in patients suspected of having rituximab-related pulmonary toxicity, any possible agent known to cause pulmonary toxicity should be stopped. Furthermore, in addition to any empirical anti-infectious therapy given, corticosteroid therapy should also be initiated early on. After pulmonary recovery, rituximab re-challenge is best avoided.

References

1. Rastetter W, Molina A, White CA (2004) Rituximab: expanding role in therapy for lymphomas and autoimmune diseases. Annu Rev Med 55:477–503
2. Dorner T, Radbruch A, Burmester GR (2009) B-cell-directed therapies for autoimmune disease. Nat Rev Rheumatol 5(8):433–441
3. Winkler U et al (1999) Cytokine-release syndrome in patients with B-cell chronic lymphocytic leukemia and high lymphocyte counts after treatment with an anti-CD20 monoclonal antibody (rituximab, IDEC-C2B8). Blood 94(7): 2217–2224
4. Byrd JC et al (1999) Rituximab therapy in hematologic malignancy patients with circulating blood tumor cells: association with increased infusion-related side effects and rapid blood tumor clearance. J Clin Oncol 17(3):791–795
5. Voog E, Morschhauser F, Solal-Celigny P (2003) Neutropenia in patients treated with rituximab. N Engl J Med 348(26): 2691–2694, discussion 2691-4
6. Westhoff TH et al (2003) Fatal hepatitis B virus reactivation by an escape mutant following rituximab therapy. Blood 102(5):1930
7. Lowndes S et al (2002) Stevens-Johnson syndrome after treatment with rituximab. Ann Oncol 13(12):1948–1950
8. Herishanu Y (2002) Rituximab-induced serum sickness. Am J Hematol 70(4):329
9. Liote H et al (2010) Rituximab-induced lung disease: a systematic literature review. Eur Respir J 35(3):681–687
10. Kanelli S et al (2001) Rituximab toxicity in patients with peripheral blood malignant B-cell lymphocytosis. Leuk Lymphoma 42(6):1329–1337
11. Burton C, Kaczmarski R, Jan-Mohamed R (2003) Interstitial pneumonitis related to rituximab therapy. N Engl J Med 348(26):2690–2691, discussion 2690-1
12. Byrd JC et al (2003) Randomized phase 2 study of fludarabine with concurrent versus sequential treatment with rituximab in symptomatic, untreated patients with B-cell chronic lymphocytic leukemia: results from Cancer and Leukemia Group B 9712 (CALGB 9712). Blood 101(1):6–14
13. Hainsworth JD et al (2003) First-line treatment with brief-duration chemotherapy plus rituximab in elderly patients with intermediate-grade non-Hodgkin's lymphoma: phase II trial. Clin Lymphoma 4(1):36–42
14. Swords R et al (2004) Interstitial pneumonitis following rituximab therapy for immune thrombocytopenic purpura (ITP). Am J Hematol 77(1):103–104
15. Alexandrescu DT et al (2004) Fatal intra-alveolar hemorrhage after rituximab in a patient with non-Hodgkin lymphoma. Leuk Lymphoma 45(11):2321–2325
16. Leon RJ et al (2004) Rituximab-induced acute pulmonary fibrosis. Mayo Clin Proc 79(7):949–953
17. Heresi GA, Farver CF, Stoller JK (2008) Interstitial pneumonitis and alveolar hemorrhage complicating use of rituximab: case report and review of the literature. Respiration 76(4):449–453
18. Hiraga J et al (2005) A case of interstitial pneumonia induced by rituximab therapy. Int J Hematol 81(2):169–170
19. Mian M et al (2006) Extensive organizing pneumonia during chemo-immunotherapy containing rituximab and G-CSF in a patient with diffuse large B-cell lymphoma: case report and review of the literature. Leuk Lymphoma 47(8): 1683–1685
20. Biehn SE et al (2006) Bronchiolitis obliterans with organizing pneumonia after rituximab therapy for non-Hodgkin's lymphoma. Hematol Oncol 24(4):234–237
21. Maeng CH et al (2007) A case of organizing pneumonia associated with rituximab. Cancer Res Treat 39(2):88–91
22. Ghesquieres H (2005) Severe interstitial pneumonitis following rituximab and bleomycin-containing combination chemotherapy. Ann Oncol 16(8):1399
23. Soubrier M et al (2008) Organizing pneumonia after rituximab therapy: Two cases. Joint Bone Spine 75(3):362–365
24. Kishi J et al (2009) A case of rituximab-induced interstitial pneumonitis observed in systemic lupus erythematosus. Rheumatology (Oxford) 48(4):447–448
25. Lee Y et al (2006) Two cases of interstitial pneumonitis caused by rituximab therapy. Korean J Intern Med 21(3): 1836
26. Tonelli AR et al (2009) Rituximab-induced hypersensitivity pneumonitis. Respiration 78(2):225–229
27. Saito B et al (2004) Acute respiratory distress syndrome during the third infusion of rituximab in a patient with follicular lymphoma. Int J Hematol 80(2):164–167
28. Montero AJ et al (2005) Acute respiratory distress syndrome after rituximab infusion. Int J Hematol 82(4):324–326
29. Wu SJ et al (2007) Severe pulmonary complications after initial treatment with Rituximab for the Asian-variant of intravascular lymphoma. Haematologica 92(1):141–142
30. Macartney C et al (2005) Bronchiolitis obliterans organizing pneumonia in a patient with non-Hodgkin's lymphoma following R-CHOP and pegylated filgrastim. Leuk Lymphoma 46(10):1523–1526
31. Nieuwenhuizen L et al (2008) A possible role of 18F-FDG positron-emission tomography scanning in the early detection of rituximab-induced pneumonitis in patients with non-Hodgkin's lymphoma. Haematologica 93(8):1267–1269
32. Yamane T et al (2008) Drug-induced pneumonitis detected earlier by 18F-FDG-PET than by high-resolution CT: a case report with non-Hodgkin's lymphoma. Ann Nucl Med 22(8):719–722
33. Kalkanis D et al (2009) [18F]-fluorodeoxyglucose positron emission tomography combined with computed tomography detection of asymptomatic late pulmonary toxicity in patients with non-Hodgkin lymphoma treated with rituximab-containing chemotherapy. Leuk Lymphoma 50(6):904–911

34. Liote H (2008) Organizing pneumonia associated with rituximab: Challenges raised by establishing causality. Joint Bone Spine 75(3):260–262
35. Bienvenu J et al (2001) Tumor necrosis factor alpha release is a major biological event associated with rituximab treatment. Hematol J 2(6):378–384
36. van der Kolk LE et al (2001) Complement activation plays a key role in the side-effects of rituximab treatment. Br J Haematol 115(4):807–811
37. Selenko N et al (2001) CD20 antibody (C2B8)-induced apoptosis of lymphoma cells promotes phagocytosis by dendritic cells and cross-priming of CD8+ cytotoxic T cells. Leukemia 15(10):1619–1626
38. Selenko N et al (2002) Cross-priming of cytotoxic T cells promoted by apoptosis-inducing tumor cell reactive antibodies? J Clin Immunol 22(3):124–130
39. Kolstad A et al (2007) Pneumocystis jirovecii pneumonia in B-cell lymphoma patients treated with the rituximab-CHOEP-14 regimen. Haematologica 92(1):139–140
40. Venhuizen AC et al (2008) Three cases of Pneumocystis jirovecii pneumonia (PCP) during first-line treatment with rituximab in combination with CHOP-14 for aggressive B-cell non-Hodgkin's lymphoma. Eur J Haematol 80(3): 275–276
41. Chang H et al (2008) Pneumocystis jiroveci pneumonia in patients with non-Hodgkin's lymphoma receiving chemotherapy containing rituximab. J Chin Med Assoc 71(11): 579–582
42. Teichmann LL et al (2008) Fatal Pneumocystis pneumonia following rituximab administration for rheumatoid arthritis. Rheumatology (Oxford) 47(8):1256–1257
43. Brusamolino E et al (2006) Dose-dense R-CHOP-14 supported by pegfilgrastim in patients with diffuse large B-cell lymphoma: a phase II study of feasibility and toxicity. Haematologica 91(4):496–502
44. Ennishi D et al (2008) Increased incidence of interstitial pneumonia by CHOP combined with rituximab. Int J Hematol 87(4):393–397
45. Aksoy S et al (2007) Rituximab-related viral infections in lymphoma patients. Leuk Lymphoma 48(7):1307–1312
46. Lee MY et al (2008) Rituximab therapy increased post-transplant cytomegalovirus complications in Non-Hodgkin's lymphoma patients receiving autologous hematopoietic stem cell transplantation. Ann Hematol 87(4):285–289
47. Sharma M et al (2009) Fatal CMV pneumonitis in a lymphoma patient treated with rituximab. Am J Hematol 84(9):614–616
48. Cooper JA Jr, White DA, Matthay RA (1986) Drug-induced pulmonary disease. Part 1: Cytotoxic drugs. Am Rev Respir Dis 133(2):321–340
49. Malik SW et al (1996) Lung toxicity associated with cyclophosphamide use. Two distinct patterns. Am J Respir Crit Care Med 154(6 Pt 1):1851–1856
50. Azoulay E et al (2001) Granulocyte colony-stimulating factor or neutrophil-induced pulmonary toxicity: myth or reality? Systematic review of clinical case reports and experimental data. Chest 120(5):1695–1701
51. Kerst JM et al (1993) Recombinant granulocyte colony-stimulating factor administration to healthy volunteers: induction of immunophenotypically and functionally altered neutrophils via an effect on myeloid progenitor cells. Blood 82(11):3265–3272
52. de Haas M et al (1994) Granulocyte colony-stimulating factor administration to healthy volunteers: analysis of the immediate activating effects on circulating neutrophils. Blood 84(11):3885–3894
53. Balazovich KJ, Almeida HI, Boxer LA (1991) Recombinant human G-CSF and GM-CSF prime human neutrophils for superoxide production through different signal transduction mechanisms. J Lab Clin Med 118(6):576–584
54. Pajkrt D et al (1997) Modulation of cytokine release and neutrophil function by granulocyte colony-stimulating factor during endotoxemia in humans. Blood 90(4): 1415–1424
55. Terashima T et al (1994) Granulocyte colony-stimulating factor exacerbates acute lung injury induced by intratracheal endotoxin in guinea pigs. Am J Respir Crit Care Med 149(5):1295–1303
56. Azoulay E et al (2002) Exacerbation by granulocyte colony-stimulating factor of prior acute lung injury: implication of neutrophils. Crit Care Med 30(9):2115–2122
57. Azoulay E et al (2003) Effect of granulocyte colony-stimulating factor on bleomycin-induced acute lung injury and pulmonary fibrosis. Crit Care Med 31(5):1442–1448

Cardiogenic Causes of Respiratory Failure in Patients with Hematological Malignancies

65

Julien Maizel, Berengere Gruson, Jean-Pierre Marolleau, and Michel Slama

Contents

J. Maizel (✉) and M. Slama
Medical Intensive Care Unit, Department of Nephrology, University Hospital of Amiens, France and INSERM, ERI 12, Amiens University, France
e-mail: maizel.julien@chu-amiens.fr

B. Gruson and J.-P. Marolleau
Department of Clinical Hematology, University Hospital of Amiens, 1 pl Victor Pauchet, 80000 Amiens, France

65.1 Case Report

A 54-year-old woman was admitted for dyspnea. She had a history of hypertension treated with propranolol; breast cancer treated 2 years earlier by surgery, chemotherapy (including anthracyclines), and radiotherapy, then by chronic tamoxifen; and acute myeloid leukemia. Blood cell counts at admission showed 100,000/mm^3 leukocytes with 90% monoblasts, anemia (7.9 g/dL), thrombocytopenia (12,000/mm^3), acute kidney injury (serum creatinine, 200 μmol/L and urea, 8 mmol/L), and hyperuricemia (1,064 μmol/L). Pulmonary leukemic infiltration or leukostasis was suspected, and 50 mg of daunorubicin was therefore given at admission combined with large amounts of intravenous saline to prevent tumor lysis syndrome. The next day, she had worsening dyspnea with polypnea, jugular vein distension, bibasilar rales, tachycardia, and oliguria. Her body temperature was normal. The chest X-ray revealed bibasilar interstitial infiltrates and a subnormal cardiothoracic ratio (Fig. 65.1). The leukocyte count had decreased to 81,000/mm^3, the hemoglobin level was stable at 7.1 g/dL, and the platelet count was 11,000/mm^3. Serum brain natriuretic peptide (BNP) was 222 ng/L, troponin Ic was 0.1 μg/L, and C-reactive protein was 76 mg/L.

Initial diagnostic hypotheses were acute cardiogenic pulmonary edema (requiring diuretic therapy) and pulmonary leukemic infiltration or leukostasis (requiring chemotherapy and corticosteroids). This case illustrates the importance of rapidly determining the etiology of acute respiratory failure to ensure appropriate treatment. Furthermore, acute cardiogenic pulmonary edema can coexist with leukemic infiltration or leukostasis.

É. Azoulay (ed.), *Pulmonary Involvement in Patients with Hematological Malignancies*,
DOI: 10.1007/978-3-642-15742-4_65, © Springer-Verlag Berlin Heidelberg 2011

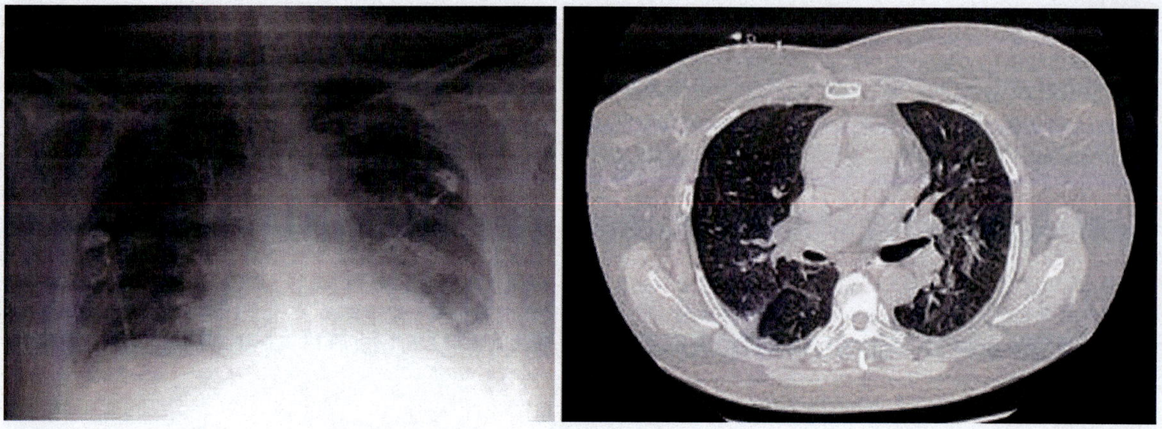

Fig. 65.1 The chest X-ray revealed bibasilar interstitial infiltrates and a subnormal cardiothoracic ratio. CT disclosed ground-glass opacities, septal lines, and bilateral pleural effusion

65.2 Introduction

Severe dyspnea indicating acute respiratory failure (ARF) is common in patients with hematological malignancies. Determining the cause of ARF, although often difficult, is crucial to ensure appropriate treatment. Because patients with hematological malignancies are at risk for cardiogenic dyspnea, the first step is to determine whether the cause of ARF is cardiogenic or noncardiogenic. Risk factors for cardiogenic ARF include the use of cardiotoxic chemotherapeutic agents, hyperhydration during chemotherapy, and specific clinical situations (e.g., acute tumor lysis syndrome or bone marrow transplantation). The role of comorbidities should also be considered. Early identification of the cause followed by appropriate treatment improves the outcomes of patients with ARF [1]. Several conditions may cause cardiogenic ARF in patients with hematological malignancies. The main cause is acute or chronic congestive heart failure (CHF). Acute CHF may be related to acute coronary syndrome, arrhythmia, or hyperhydratation. Chronic CHF is usually due to the use of cardiotoxic chemotherapeutic agents, radiotherapy, or cardiovascular complications of the hematological malignancy (amyloidosis). Other cardiogenic causes of ARF include tamponade and pulmonary embolism, which are associated with specific chemotherapeutic agents.

In this chapter, we will describe the cardiogenic causes of ARF and discuss the best diagnostic strategies for identifying them in patients with hematological malignancies.

65.3 Acute Heart Failure

Cardiogenic pulmonary edema results from a rapid hydrostatic pressure increase in the pulmonary capillaries, which is usually due to elevations in left ventricular diastolic pressure and left atrial pressure. Left atrial pressure elevation above 18 mmHg can cause interstitial edema and flood the alveoli [2]. Left atrial pressure elevation can be the result of systolic or diastolic dysfunction.

Similar to patients with other clinical conditions, individuals with hematological malignancies may experience pulmonary edema due to myocardial ischemia, arrhythmia, exacerbation of chronic systolic or diastolic heart failure, valvular dysfunction, or volume overload. In addition, pulmonary edema due to left ventricular systolic dysfunction in patients with hematological malignancies may result from preexisting cardiomyopathy and/or cardiomyopathy induced by a cardiotoxic chemotherapeutic agent and/or radiation therapy.

65.3.1 Acute Coronary Syndromes

Acute coronary syndromes can cause dyspnea due to acute ischemic heart failure. Patients with ARF should be routinely asked about chest pains, and an electrocardiogram and troponin assay should be obtained. Although myocardial ischemia may occur in any

Table 65.1 Chemotherapeutic agents associated with cardiac toxicity

Drug/therapy	Cardiac event	Comments
Anthracyclines *Doxorubicin* *Daunorubicin* *Epirubicin* *Idarubicin*	CHF	Prevention based on minimizing the cumulative dose, administration by continuous infusion, and dexrazoxane
Cyclophosphamide	CHF Pericarditis Myocarditis	Risk factors are high cumulative dose, chest radiation, and prior anthracycline therapy
Busulfan	Pericardial effusion Endomyocardial fibrosis	
Cisplatin	CHF CAD	Risk factors are older age, chest radiation, and prior anthracycline therapy
All-transretinoic acids	CHF Pericardial effusion	All-transretinoic acid syndrome
Tyrosine kinase inhibitors *Imatinib* *Dasatinib* *Nilotinib*	CHF Pericardial effusion	
Thalidomide	DVT	
Arsenic trioxide	Arrhythmias	QT prolongation
Radiation	CHF CAD Arrhythmias Pericardial effusion	Time since exposure ranging from 2 to 145 months

CHF chronic heart failure, *CAD* coronary artery disease, *DVT* deep vein thrombosis

patient, those having received the chemotherapeutic agents listed in Table 65.1 are at increased risk. Radiation therapy promotes the development of coronary artery disease, and cases of sudden death due to diffuse intimal hyperplasia of all the coronary arteries have been reported [3]. Cisplatin can induce acute coronary syndromes ranging from angina to acute myocardial infarction. The mechanism leading to ischemia is unclear, as some patients have no coronary artery lesions by coronary angiography [4]. The treatment consists of cisplatin withdrawal and introduction of antiischemic treatment.

65.3.2 Arrhythmias

Rituximab is a drug used in various lymphoproliferative disorders, including non-Hodgkin's lymphoma. Infusion-related side effects are common within the first few hours, especially after the first administration. Hypotension, hypoxia, distributive shock, bronchospasm, angioedema, and arrhythmias have been reported. Ventricular tachycardia and severe atrioventricular blockade may occur [5, 6]. Interruption of rituximab treatment combined with supportive care is usually effective.

Arsenic trioxide is used for refractory or relapsed acute promyelocytic leukemia. Arsenic prolongs the QT interval, leading to an increased risk of ventricular tachycardia and torsades de pointes [7]. Complete heart block and sudden death have been reported several hours after arsenic trioxide infusions, highlighting the need for continued cardiac monitoring after each infusion [8]. To prevent severe arrhythmia, electrolyte levels must be kept within the normal range, and any QT-prolonging medications must be stopped.

65.3.3 Fluid Overload

Patients with hematological malignancies may experience pulmonary edema due to fluid overload. Large amounts of fluids are given to prevent tumor lysis syndrome or chemotherapy-related renal toxicity. Patients with pre-existing systolic and/or diastolic dysfunction are at increased risk, as they have high baseline left ventricular diastolic pressures and a steep left ventricular pressure–volume relationship. Thus, the infusion of small amounts of fluid may increase the left ventricular diastolic pressure, thereby precipitating acute pulmonary edema. Diastolic dysfunction is common in elderly patients with hypertension and/or coronary artery disease [9]. Moreover, several chemotherapeutic agents can alter left ventricular relaxation (see below). The fluid balance should be carefully monitored in the patients who have a history of systolic or diastolic heart failure or risk factors for altered left ventricular relaxation.

65.4 Chronic Heart Failure

We will focus on specific situations seen in patients with hematological malignancies. However, comorbidities may also cause heart disease in these patients.

65.4.1 Chemotherapy-Related Cardiotoxicity

Several chemotherapeutic agents can alter left ventricular contractility. In this book, Dr. Khakoo provides an in-depth review of cardiac disorders related to anticancer drugs. Table 65.1 lists drugs associated with cardiotoxicity and Table 65.2 risk factors for chemotherapy-induced cardiotoxicity. Cardiotoxicity depends on both the pharmacological properties of the drug and factors related to the individual patient. The time from chemotherapy (or radiotherapy) to manifestations of cardiotoxicity varies widely and can reach several months to several years.

Anthracyclines are the most extensively studied drugs associated with acute and late cardiotoxicity with left ventricular dilatation and a decline in the left ventricular ejection fraction (LVEF) [10]. The pathogenesis of anthracycline-induced cardiotoxicity is highly controversial. Myocardial production of reactive oxygen species is the most widely accepted hypothesis. Anthracyclines induce the production of reactive oxygen species via redox cycling of aglycones and anthracycline-iron complexes [11]. The prevention of anthracycline-induced cardiotoxicity relies on restricting the cumulative dose (doxorubicin equivalent, 550 mg/m^2) and administering the drug as a continuous infusion [12]. Cardiac function monitoring is crucial in anthracycline-treated patients. Echocardiography or radionuclide ventriculography should be obtained regularly, starting before anthracycline initiation and continuing beyond the end of the treatment [13]. For patients given more than 300 mg/m^2 of doxorubicin-based therapy, dexrazoxane has been recommended to reduce the amount of free iron in myocytes, thereby protecting against anthracycline-induced cardiotoxicity [14]. However, this recommendation remains controversial. The development of left ventricular systolic dysfunction during anthracycline therapy requires treatment discontinuation, administration of appropriate

Table 65.2 Risk factors for cardiovascular complications due to chemotherapy

Patient-related factors
Age
Previous cardiovascular disease
Previous or concomitant radiation therapy
Metabolic abnormalities
Drug-related factors
Dose of the drug during each session
Cumulative dose
Route of administration

medications for left ventricular dysfunction, caution with fluid loading, and close fluid balance monitoring.

In addition to systolic dysfunction, chemotherapy may induce diastolic dysfunction. Echocardiography studies have established that diastolic dysfunction (sometimes followed by systolic dysfunction) can develop during cardiotoxic chemotherapy or after stem cell transplantation. Tissue Doppler imaging findings and the mitral inflow pattern are important parameters that can undergo gradual alteration during chemotherapy or many years later [15–17]. Risk factors for diastolic dysfunction seem to be the same as those for systolic dysfunction. As with systolic dysfunction, the presence of any such risk factors and/or a history of diastolic heart failure require great caution during fluid loading and close monitoring of the fluid balance. No accurate data are available about chemotherapy dosage adjustment in patients with isolated relaxation abnormalities without clinical pulmonary edema.

Allogeneic or autologous hematopoietic stem cell transplantation is associated with cardiac complications, including arrhythmia and heart failure. The use of high-dose cyclophosphamide in the myeloablative conditioning regimen has been convincingly shown to increase the risk for cardiovascular events [18, 19]. The strongest risk factors are anthracycline therapy and/or a LVEF lower than 45% before stem cell transplantation.

Imatinib has revolutionized the treatment of chronic myeloid leukemia, Philadelphia-positive acute lymphoblastic leukemia, FIP1L1-PDGFRα transcript-positive hypereosinophilic syndrome, and gastrointestinal stromal tumors. A preclinical animal study indicated that chronic heart failure was a potential complication of imatinib treatment [20]. However, a retrospective study in humans found no increase in the incidence of chronic heart failure among imatinib-treated patients compared to the general population [21]. Thus, the cardiotoxic potential of imatinib remains unclear.

65.4.2 Radiation

Cardiogenic pulmonary edema may develop several months or years after radiotherapy to the chest. Radiation can induce systolic or diastolic dysfunction, coronary artery disease, valvular damage, or a pericardial effusion. Concomitant doxorubicin administration increases the risk of radiation-induced cardiotoxicity. Coronary ischemia and/or myocardial fibrosis may be involved early on or after many years.

65.4.3 Cardiac Manifestations of Amyloidosis

Systemic AL amyloidosis can lead to myocardial infiltration with chronic heart failure. Amyloidosis is associated with cardiac involvement in up to 90% of cases and with clinical diastolic heart failure in 50% of cases [22]. Symptoms of cardiac amyloidosis may consist of dizziness, syncope, postural hypotension, and heart failure. Half the patients with cardiac amyloidosis die from heart failure or arrhythmia. The diagnosis of cardiac amyloidosis is difficult and relies on a combination of findings from the clinical examination, echocardiography, electrocardiography, and cardiovascular magnetic resonance imaging (CMR). Echocardiographic findings of concentric left ventricular wall thickening with a granular appearance, thickened mitral valve leaflets, biventricular dilatation, and pericardial effusion are suggestive in a patient with clinically compatible manifestations. The electrocardiogram may show atrial fibrillation or flutter, low voltage, and a pseudo-infarct pattern (in an anterior, inferior, or lateral distribution). CMR is useful for distinguishing among various cardiomyopathies. In patients with histologically proven cardiac amyloidosis, CMR shows late gadolinium enhancement of the myocardium, which may be diffuse or focal, and transmural or confined to the subendocardium [23]. However, none of the echocardiographic, electrocardiographic, or CMR findings in cardiac amyloidosis is highly specific. Therefore, the diagnosis relies on a combination of findings from these various sources. Troponin I and BNP levels are elevated in cardiac amyloidosis, and their levels at diagnosis and during treatment provide important prognostic information. The treatment consists of diminishing the deposition of amyloid fibrils and supporting the failing organs. Heart failure requires high-dose diuretic therapy in patients with concomitant nephrotic syndrome. The risk of bradycardia and hypotension limits the use of beta-blockers, angiotensin-converting enzyme, and angiotensin II inhibitors. Digoxin and some of the calcium-channel blockers can bind to amyloid fibrils, leading to an increased risk of digoxin toxicity and to declining cardiac function with calcium-channel blockers [24, 25].

65.5 Other Causes of Cardiogenic Acute Respiratory Failure

65.5.1 Tamponade

Tamponade presents as cardiogenic shock with hypotension, dyspnea, tachycardia, diminished heart sounds, jugular vein distension, a pericardial rub, and pulsus paradoxus. Since most of these manifestations are nonspecific, tamponade should be considered in many clinical situations, including ARF. The chest X-ray may show cardiomegaly, usually without lung opacities. Tamponade usually complicates a pericardial effusion. As illustrated by our case report, the pericardium may be involved in patients with acute leukemia [26]. The best means of preventing life-threatening tamponade is routine echocardiography to detect pericardial effusion, followed by close monitoring should such an effusion be found. Among hematological malignancies, Hodgkin's and non-Hodgkin's lymphomas are often associated with pericardial involvement or chemotherapy/radiation-induced pericardial effusion (Table 65.1).

Tyrosine kinase inhibitors (dasatinib, imatinib, and nilotinib) are associated with an increased risk of pericardial effusion [27]. All-transretinoic acid (ATRA), which is used to treat acute promyelocytic leukemia, can induce ATRA syndrome, characterized by a fever, dyspnea, hypotension, and pericardial or pleural effusion [28]. The treatment rests on corticosteroids. Cardiogenic shock and tamponade have been reported in patients with ATRA syndrome [29].

Lethal tamponade has been reported in patients with thalassemia after busulfan administration during conditioning for allogeneic stem cell transplantation. Cases of tamponade occurred between conditioning initiation and 30 days after stem cell transplantation [30].

Radiation therapy carries a high risk of pericardial effusion or pericarditis, with a time to onset ranging from 2 to 145 months. Pericardial constriction may develop over time [31].

Pericardial effusion and the associated risk of tamponade constitute a major challenge given the unpredictability of this complication, substantial variability in time to onset, and frequent need for invasive therapeutic procedures. In a patient with a pericardial effusion, whether the chemotherapeutic regimen is involved and should be stopped may be difficult to determine. Close echocardiographic monitoring to detect and monitor this complication is the only means of preventing life-threatening tamponade. Tamponade requires immediate needle aspiration of the pericardial fluid. Surgical drainage may be necessary in patients with clotted hemopericardium, thoracic abnormalities contraindicating needle aspiration, or abundant and recurrent pericardial effusion [32].

65.5.2 Pulmonary Embolism

Similar to patients with solid malignancies, those with hematological malignancies are at increased risk for pulmonary embolism. Thrombocytopenia has not been reported as a significant protective factor [33].

Patients with suspected pulmonary embolism should be investigated for deep vein thrombosis and central venous catheter thrombosis [34]. Chemotherapeutic agents may promote venous thrombosis by altering coagulation factors and anticoagulant proteins, and by damaging the endothelium [35–37]. Moreover, several non-cytotoxic medications such as thalidomide are associated with a high rate of deep vein thrombosis, warranting routine prevention with warfarin, heparin, or aspirin [38]. In our patient, the clinical presentation and the lung opacities by chest X-ray were not suggestive of pulmonary embolism.

Anticoagulant therapy for pulmonary embolism carries a high risk of severe bleeding in patients with marked thrombocytopenia. Despite the absence of specific data in the literature, a reasonable strategy may be to confirm the presence of thromboembolism (Doppler and/or computed tomography) before starting anticoagulant therapy.

65.6 Clinical, Laboratory, and Imaging Findings

We will first briefly discuss the diagnostic value of clinical, laboratory, and imaging findings before making the case that echocardiography is at present the best tool for ruling in or out a cardiogenic cause of ARF.

65.6.1 Clinical, Laboratory, and X-Ray Findings

In theory, clinical findings indicating hypervolemia suggest hydrostatic pulmonary edema. However, several studies have established that the clinical examination has limited diagnostic accuracy for volemic status assessment in patients with severe dyspnea [39, 40]. An S3 gallop has 90–97% specificity for cardiogenic pulmonary edema, but only 9–51% sensitivity [2]. Edema, rales, and jugular turgescence have insufficient sensitivity and specificity. In addition, several factors in patients with hematological malignancies can alter the blood volume distribution, causing concomitant accumulation of blood in the venous compartment and intraarterial hypovolemia, a situation known as relative hypovolemia. Factors associated with relative hypovolemia include hypoalbuminemia, hepatic failure, acute (or chronic) cor pulmonale, sepsis, and capillary leak syndrome.

Hypoalbuminemia and anemia have limited value for diagnosing hemodilution in patients with hematological malignancies. BNP is a marker for left ventricular end-diastolic pressure (LVEDP) elevation. In an unselected population of emergency room patients with severe dyspnea, BNP was highly effective in distinguishing cardiogenic and noncardiogenic causes [41]. However, several limitations in interpreting BNP or N-terminal prohormone BNP (NT-proBNP) concentrations have been reported. More specifically, these concentrations may be affected by renal failure, inflammation, isolated right heart failure (i.e., related to pulmonary embolism), atrial fibrillation, and body mass index. Moreover, in critically ill cancer patients, NT proBNP failed to reliably identify cardiac dysfunction [42]. Nevertheless, NT-proBNP concentrations lower than 500 pg/mL in a critically ill cancer patient with ARF is a strong argument against a cardiogenic cause [42]. The troponin concentration and ECG may suggest myocardial ischemia or infarction. However, both tests are normal in patients with nonischemic cardiogenic pulmonary edema.

Although chest X-ray findings may provide diagnostic orientation, none is specific of hydrostatic pulmonary edema. The main difficulty in a patient with bilateral interstitial infiltrates is differentiating hydrostatic from lesional pulmonary edema. Acute respiratory distress syndrome (ARDS) may be caused by intersititial pneumonitis; drug-induced lung injury; or graft-versus-host disease presenting as idiopathic pneumonia after allogeneic stem cell transplantation, nonspecific interstitial pneumonitis, organized pneumonia, or bronchiolitis. The X-ray findings in patients with ARDS may be indistinguishable from those produced by hydrostatic pulmonary edema.

When seeking to distinguish cardiogenic from noncardiogenic ARF, a crucial step is the evaluation of heart function and, more specifically, of LVEDP. As discussed above, clinical, laboratory, and X-ray findings are not satisfactory diagnostic tools. Heart function in patients with ARF is best assessed using echocardiography.

65.6.2 Echocardiography

Pulmonary edema may be cardiogenic (i.e., hydrostatic or hemodynamic) or noncardiogenic (i.e., related to acute lung injury/ARDS with increased blood-vessel permeability). LVEDP is elevated in hydrostatic pulmonary edema, but not in noncardiogenic pulmonary edema. Direct measurement of LVEDP requires pulmonary artery catheterization to measure the pulmonary arterial occlusion pressure (PAOP), which is not recommended as a routine investigation, given the risk of adverse events [43].

Since the 1980s, the role for echocardiography in the management of patients with hemodynamic or respiratory failure has increased considerably [44]. Echocardiography provides real-time information about systolic function, diastolic function, and left ventricular pressure. Several studies have validated echocardiography versus pulmonary artery catheterization for estimating cardiac output and PAOP in patients with a variety of conditions, including ICU patients. Contrary to pulmonary artery catheterization, echocardiography is noninvasive and can be used easily in many clinical situations. The LVEF is not sufficient to distinguish cardiogenic from noncardiogenic dyspnea, as it may be normal or elevated in patients with cardiologic pulmonary edema and, conversely, diminished in patients with ARDS or septic shock. Parameters that specifically reflect LVEDP must be used instead.

Several echocardiography parameters are available for estimating LVEDP (i.e., PAOP) from Doppler echocardiography measurements during ventricular loading. Values suggesting a PAOP greater than 18 mmHg strongly suggest hydrostatic pulmonary edema. Several indices of ventricular preload have been evaluated comparatively to PAOP in ICU patients. However, some of these parameters require considerable time and experience to obtain reliable values [45, 46]. Furthermore, the correlation with PAOP depends on various factors, such as whether the LVEF is altered [47]. We recently looked for an echocardiographic parameter that was easy to determine accurately and both sensitive and specific for distinguishing cardiogenic from noncardiogenic dyspnea in ICU patients with ARF [48]. We found that the best parameters were the ratio of early mitral inflow peak velocity (*E*) over early diastolic velocity of the lateral mitral annulus (Ea) recorded by Doppler tissue imaging (*E*/Ea) and the ratio of *E* over the *E* wave deceleration time (*E*/EDT) (Fig. 65.2) [48]. For predicting cardiogenic ARF, an *E*/Ea ratio greater than 8 was 88% sensitive and 80% specific, and an E/EDT ratio greater than 5 was 92% sensitive and 87% specific.

Echocardiography is also the noninvasive method that is most widely used to detect and monitor myocardial toxicity induced by anthracyclines or other chemotherapeutic agents. The LVEF is the most commonly used parameter. However, studies have demonstrated the importance of detecting diastolic dysfunction, which precedes systolic dysfunction in patients with anthracycline cardiotoxicity [49].

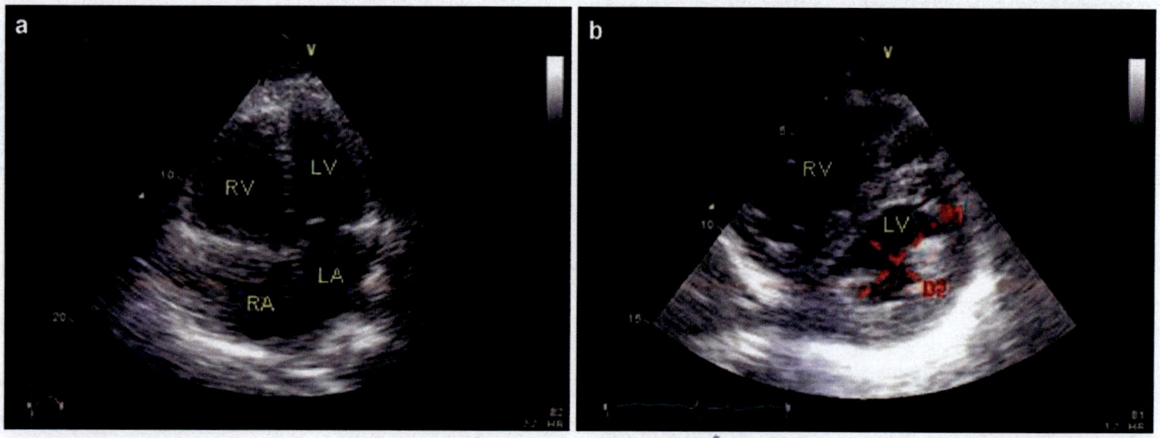

Fig. 65.2 Acute cor pulmonale in a patient admitted for acute pulmonary embolism. (**a**) Apical four-chamber view showing severe right ventricular dilatation (right/left ventricle diameter >1). (**b**) Parasternal short-axis view showing an eccentricity index (*EI*) >1 (EI = D1/D2). *RV* right ventricle, *LV* left ventricle, *RA* right atrium, *LA* left atrium

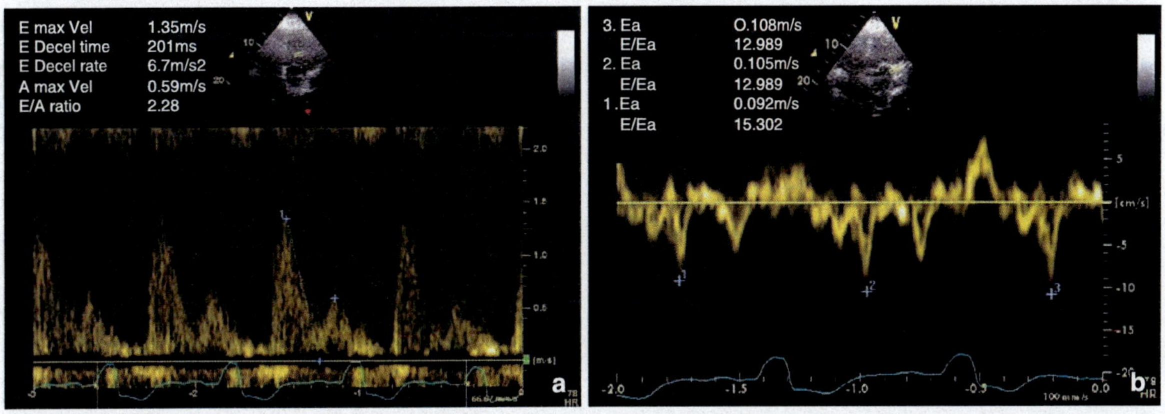

Fig. 65.3 Mitral inflow pattern recorded using pulsed Doppler (**a**) and early diastolic velocity of the lateral mitral annulus recorded using tissue Doppler imaging (**b**) in a patient with elevated left ventricular end-diastolic pressure

Detection of pericardial effusion was among the first indications for echocardiography, which is still considered the best noninvasive tool for diagnosing tamponade. Echocardiography cannot establish the diagnosis of pulmonary embolism (except in the rare cases where a thrombus is visible in the proximal pulmonary artery), but can detect the consequences of pulmonary embolism on the right ventricle. Features that are useful for the diagnosis and treatment of pulmonary embolism include right ventricular dilatation, paradoxical septal movement, and pulmonary hypertension with normal (or low) LVEDP (Fig. 65.3). However, none of these findings is specific for pulmonary embolism, and all can occur in ARDS.

65.7 Conclusion

ARF is a common event in patients with hematological malignancies. The first step in the diagnostic strategy is to determine whether the cause is cardiogenic edema, of which the main causes are acute and chronic heart failure, pericardial effusion, and pulmonary embolism. Based on the data in this chapter, we have developed a diagnostic algorithm (Fig. 65.4). Clinical, laboratory, and X-ray findings are helpful but not sufficient. Echocardiography is at present the best noninvasive tool for easily and rapidly providing reliable information on the cause of ARF.

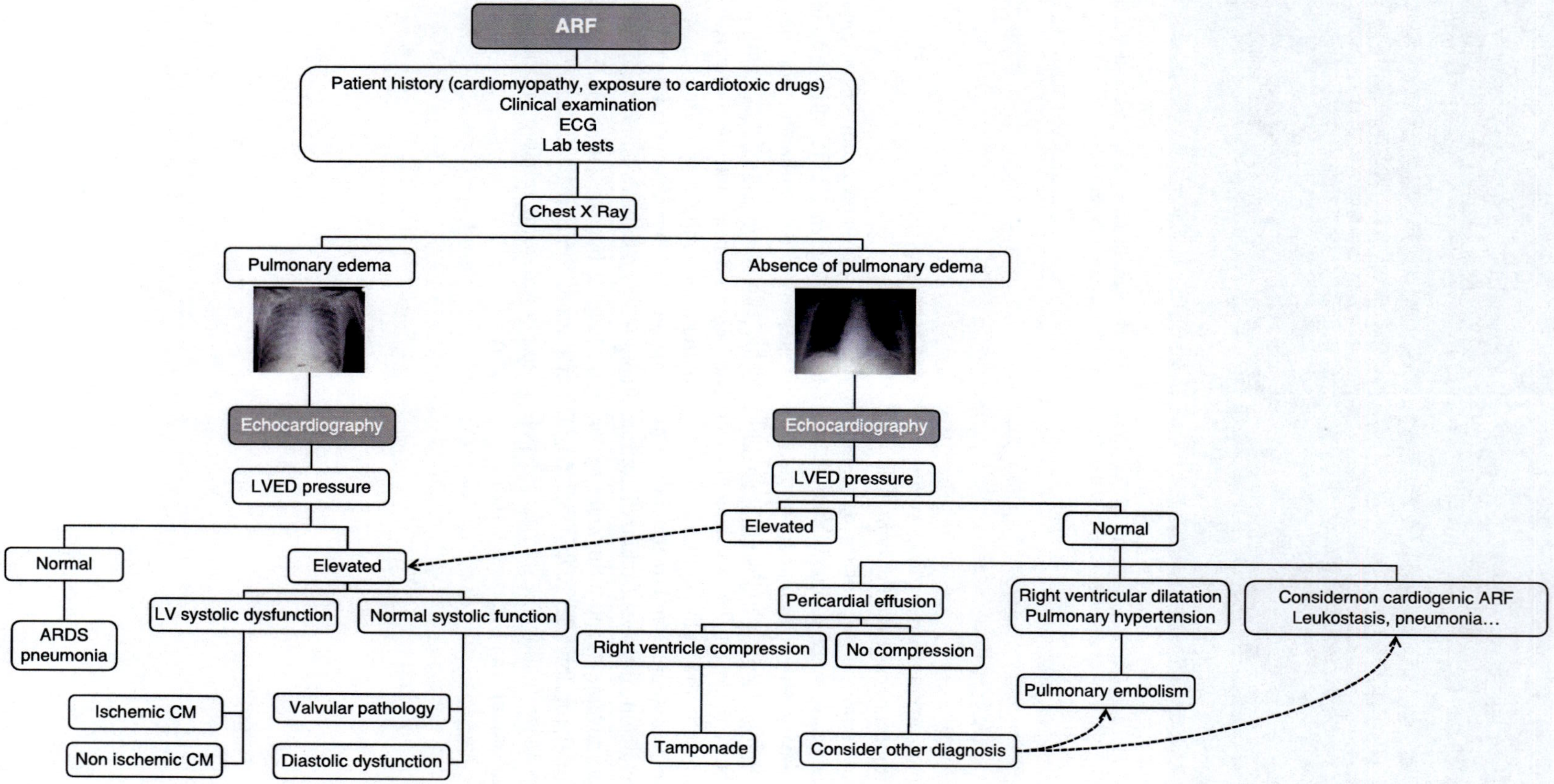

Fig. 65.4 An integrated approach to the evaluation of patients with acute severe dyspnea using echocardiography. *ARF* acute respiratory failure, LVED left ventricular end diastolic

References

1. Bales AC, Sorrentino MJ (1997) Causes of congestive heart failure. Prompt diagnosis may affect prognosis. Postgrad Med 101(44–9):54–56
2. Ware LB, Matthay MA (2005) Clinical practice. Acute pulmonary edema. N Engl J Med 353:2788–2796
3. Orzan F, Brusca A, Conte MR, Presbitero P, Figliomeni MC (1993) Severe coronary artery disease after radiation therapy of the chest and mediastinum: clinical presentation and treatment. Br Heart J 69:496–500
4. Berliner S, Rahima M, Sidi Y, Teplitsky Y, Zohar Y, Nussbaum B, Pinkhas J (1990) Acute coronary events following cisplatin-based chemotherapy. Cancer Invest 8:583–586
5. Cervera Grau JM, Esquerdo Galiana G, Belso Candela A, Llorca Ferrándiz C, Juárez Marroquí A, Maciá Escalante S (2008) Complete atrioventricular block induced by rituximab in monotherapy in an aged patient with non-Hodgkin's diffuse large B-cell lymphoma. Clin Transl Oncol 10: 298–299
6. Arai Y, Tadokoro J, Mitani K (2005) Ventricular tachycardia associated with infusion of rituximab in mantle cell lymphoma. Am J Hematol 78:317–318
7. Ohnishi K, Yoshida H, Shigeno K, Nakamura S, Fujisawa S, Naito K et al (2000) Prolongation of the QT interval and ventricular tachycardia in patients treated with arsenic trioxide for acute promyelocytic leukemia. Ann Intern Med 133:881–885
8. Westervelt P, Brown RA, Adkins DR, Khoury H, Curtin P, Hurd D et al (2001) Sudden death among patients with acute promyelocytic leukemia treated with arsenic trioxide. Blood 98:266–271
9. Redfield MM, Jacobsen SJ, Burnett JC, Mahoney DW, Bailey KR, Rodeheffer RJ (2003) Burden of systolic and diastolic ventricular dysfunction in the community: appreciating the scope of the heart failure epidemic. JAMA 289: 194–202
10. Hayek ER, Speakman E, Rehmus E (2005) Acute doxorubicin cardiotoxicity. N Engl J Med 352:2456–2457
11. Simnek T, Stérba M, Popelová O, Adamcová M, Hrdina R, Gersl V (2009) Anthracycline-induced cardiotoxicity: overview of studies examining the roles of oxidative stress and free cellular iron. Pharmacol Rep 61:154–171
12. Ewer MS, Ali MK, Mackay B, Wallace S, Valdivieso M, Legha SS et al (1984) A comparison of cardiac biopsy grades and ejection fraction estimations in patients receiving Adriamycin. J Clin Oncol 2:112–117
13. Yeh ETH, Tong AT, Lenihan DJ, Yusuf SW, Swafford J, Champion C et al (2004) Cardiovascular complications of cancer therapy: diagnosis, pathogenesis, and management. Circulation 109:3122–3131
14. Hensley ML, Hagerty KL, Kewalramani T, Green DM, Meropol NJ, Wasserman TH et al (2009) American Society of Clinical Oncology 2008 clinical practice guideline update: use of chemotherapy and radiation therapy protectants. J Clin Oncol 27:127–145
15. Pudil R, Horacek JM, Strasova A, Jebavy L, Vojacek J (2008) Monitoring of the very early changes of left ventricular diastolic function in patients with acute leukemia treated with anthracyclines. Exp Oncol 30:160–162
16. Radulescu D, Pripon S, Radulescu LI, Duncea C (2008) Left ventricular diastolic performance in breast cancer survivors treated with anthracyclines. Acta Cardiol 63:27–32
17. Tassan-Mangina S, Codorean D, Metivier M, Costa B, Himberlin C, Jouannaud C et al (2006) Tissue Doppler imaging and conventional echocardiography after anthracycline treatment in adults: early and late alterations of left ventricular function during a prospective study. Eur J Echocardiogr 7:141–146
18. Gottdiener JS, Appelbaum FR, Ferrans VJ, Deisseroth A, Ziegler J (1981) Cardiotoxicity associated with high-dose cyclophosphamide therapy. Arch Intern Med 141:758–763
19. Schrama JG, Holtkamp MJ, Baars JW, Schornagel JH, Rodenhuis S (2003) Toxicity of the high-dose chemotherapy CTC regimen (cyclophosphamide, thiotepa, carboplatin): The Netherlands Cancer Institute experience. Br J Cancer 88:1831–1838
20. Kerkelä R, Grazette L, Yacobi R, Iliescu C, Patten R, Beahm C et al (2006) Cardiotoxicity of the cancer therapeutic agent imatinib mesylate. Nat Med 12:908–916
21. Atallah E, Durand JB, Kantarjian H, Cortes J (2007) Congestive heart failure is a rare event in patients receiving imatinib therapy. Blood 110:1233–1237
22. Selvanayagam JB, Hawkins PN, Paul B, Myerson SG, Neubauer S (2007) Evaluation and management of the cardiac amyloidosis. J Am Coll Cardiol 50:2101–2110
23. Perugini E, Rapezzi C, Piva T, Leone O, Bacchi-Reggiani L, Riva L et al (2006) Non-invasive evaluation of the myocardial substrate of cardiac amyloidosis by gadolinium cardiac magnetic resonance. Heart 92:343–349
24. Rubinow A, Skinner M, Cohen AS (1981) Digoxin sensitivity in amyloid cardiomyopathy. Circulation 63:1285–1288
25. Gertz MA, Skinner M, Connors LH, Falk RH, Cohen AS, Kyle RA (1985) Selective binding of nifedipine to amyloid fibrils. Am J Cardiol 55:1646
26. Chaves FP, Quillen K, Xu D (2004) Pericardial effusion: a rare presentation of adult T-cell leukemia/lymphoma. Am J Hematol 77:381–383
27. Kelly K, Swords R, Mahalingam D, Padmanabhan S, Giles FJ (2009) Serosal inflammation (pleural and pericardial effusions) related to tyrosine kinase inhibitors. Target Oncol 4:99–105
28. Tallman MS, Andersen JW, Schiffer CA, Appelbaum FR, Feusner JH, Ogden A et al (2000) Clinical description of 44 patients with acute promyelocytic leukemia who developed the retinoic acid syndrome. Blood 95:90–95
29. Larrea L, de la Rubia J, Jiménez C, Martín G, Sanz MA (1997) Cardiac tamponade and cardiogenic shock as a manifestation of all-trans retinoic acid syndrome: an association not previously reported. Haematologica 82:463–464
30. Angelucci E, Mariotti E, Lucarelli G, Baronciani D, Cesaroni P, Durazzi SM et al (1992) Sudden cardiac tamponade after chemotherapy for marrow transplantation in thalassaemia. Lancet 339:287–289
31. Veinot JP, Edwards WD (1996) Pathology of radiation-induced heart disease: a surgical and autopsy study of 27 cases. Hum Pathol 27:766–773
32. Mercé J, Sagristà-Sauleda J, Permanyer-Miralda G, Soler-Soler J (1998) Should pericardial drainage be performed routinely in patients who have a large pericardial effusion without tamponade?. Am J Med 105:106–109

33. Needleman SW, Stein MN, Hoak JC (1981) Pulmonary embolism in patients with acute leukemia and severe thrombocytopenia. West J Med 135:9–13
34. Cortelezzi A, Moia M, Falanga A, Pogliani EM, Agnelli G, Bonizzoni E et al (2005) Incidence of thrombotic complications in patients with haematological malignancies with central venous catheters: a prospective multicentre study. Br J Haematol 129:811–817
35. Lee AY, Levine MN (1999) The thrombophilic state induced by therapeutic agents in the cancer patient. Semin Thromb Hemost 25:137–145
36. Rogers JS, Murgo AJ, Fontana JA, Raich PC (1988) Chemotherapy for breast cancer decreases plasma protein C and protein S. J Clin Oncol 6:276–281
37. Kuzel T, Esparaz B, Green D, Kies M (1990) Thrombogenicity of intravenous 5-fluorouracil alone or in combination with cisplatin. Cancer 65:885–889
38. Zangari M, Fink LM, Elice F, Zhan F, Adcock DM, Tricot GJ (2009) Thrombotic events in patients with cancer receiving antiangiogenesis agents. J Clin Oncol 27:4865–4873
39. Stevenson LW, Perloff JK (1989) The limited reliability of physical signs for estimating hemodynamics in chronic heart failure. JAMA 261:884–888
40. Chakko S, Woska D, Martinez H, de Marchena E, Futterman L, Kessler KM, Myerberg RJ (1991) Clinical, radiographic, and hemodynamic correlations in chronic congestive heart failure: conflicting results may lead to inappropriate care. Am J Med 90:353–359
41. Morrison LK, Harrison A, Krishnaswamy P, Kazanegra R, Clopton P, Maisel A (2002) Utility of a rapid B-natriuretic peptide assay in differentiating congestive heart failure from lung disease in patients presenting with dyspnea. J Am Coll Cardiol 39:202–209
42. Lefebvre A, Kural-Menasché S, Darmon M, Thiéry G, Feugeas JP, Schlemmer B, Azoulay E (2008) Use of N-terminal pro-brain natriuretic peptide to detect cardiac origin in critically ill cancer patients with acute respiratory failure. Intensive Care Med 34:833–839
43. Rubenfeld GD, McNamara-Aslin E, Rubinson L (2007) The pulmonary artery catheter, 1967-2007: rest in peace? JAMA 298:458–461
44. Vieillard-Baron A, Slama M, Cholley B, Janvier G, Vignon P (2008) Echocardiography in the intensive care unit: from evolution to revolution? Intensive Care Med 34:243–249
45. Bouhemad B, Nicolas-Robin A, Benois A, Lemaire S, Goarin JP, Rouby JJ (2003) Echocardiographic Doppler assessment of pulmonary capillary wedge pressure in surgical patients with postoperative circulatory shock and acute lung injury. Anesthesiology 98:1091–1100
46. Khan S, Bess RL, Rosman HS, Nordstrom CK, Cohen GI, Gardin JM (2004) Which echocardiographic Doppler left ventricular diastolic function measurements are most feasible in the clinical echocardiographic laboratory? Am J Cardiol 94:1099–1101
47. Appleton CP, Galloway JM, Gonzalez MS, Gaballa M, Basnight MA (1993) Estimation of left ventricular filling pressures using two-dimensional and Doppler echocardiography in adult patients with cardiac disease. Additional value of analyzing left atrial size, left atrial ejection fraction and the difference in duration of pulmonary venous and mitral flow velocity at atrial contraction. J Am Coll Cardiol 22: 1972–1982
48. Feissel M, Maizel J, Robles G, Badie J, Faller JP, Slama M (2009) Clinical relevance of echocardiography in acute severe dyspnea. J Am Soc Echocardiogr 22:1159–1164
49. Marchandise B, Schroeder E, Bosly A, Doyen C, Weynants P, Kremer R, Pouleur H (1989) Early detection of doxorubicin cardiotoxicity: interest of Doppler echocardiographic analysis of left ventricular filling dynamics. Am Heart J 118:92–98

Pulmonary Alveolar Proteinosis

66

François Vincent, H. Tandjaoui, and P.Y. Brillet

Contents

F. Vincent (✉)
Medico-surgical Intensive Care Unit, Avicenne Teaching Hospital, 125, rue de Stalingrad, 93009 Bobigny Cedex, France
e-mail: francois.vincent@avc.aphp.fr

H. Tandjaoui
Department of Pulmonary Diseases, Avicenne Teaching Hospital, 125, rue de Stalingrad, 93009 Bobigny Cedex, France

P.Y. Brillet
Department of Radiology, Avicenne Teaching Hospital, 125, rue de Stalingrad, 93009 Bobigny Cedex, France

66.1 Introduction

Pulmonary alveolar proteinosis (PAP), also known as alveolar proteinosis, alveolar lipoproteinosis, or pulmonary alveolar phospholipoproteinosis, is a rare lung disorder characterized by the abnormal accumulation of lipid-rich granular eosinophilic material (surfactant-like) within the alveoli. This material is made up of surfactant lipids and proteins, tubular myelin, membranous vesicles, and structures resembling lamellar bodies [1]. Three forms of PAP have been recognized: acquired (idiopathic) PAP, secondary PAP, and congenital PAP. Acquired PAP is the most common form, accounting for 90% of cases, and presents as a pulmonary disorder without any associated disease. The acquired form was first described in 1958 [2]. Secondary PAP (5–10%) occurs in association with immunodeficiency syndromes (including AIDS and various malignancies, especially hematological) or complicates exposure to environmental antigens: inhalation of mineral dusts (e.g., silica, titanium oxide, and aluminum) or insecticides, or exposure to various medications (Table 66.1). An association with cigarette smoking has also been suggested [3]. Congenital PAP is rare (2%). Affected neonates suffer from very rare gene mutations encoding for surfactant B or C proteins, receptors α or β of granulocyte macrophage-colony stimulating factor (GM-CSF), or ATP-binding cassette transporter A3 [4–6]. The prevalence of acquired PAP has been estimated to be 0.002–0.37 per 100,000 persons [7, 8].

66.2 Case Report

A 39-year-old woman was admitted to the intensive care unit (ICU) for acute respiratory insufficiency. She had smoked one pack of cigarettes daily since the age

É. Azoulay (ed.), *Pulmonary Involvement in Patients with Hematological Malignancies*,
DOI: 10.1007/978-3-642-15742-4_66, © Springer-Verlag Berlin Heidelberg 2011

Table 66.1 Secondary causes of PAP

Immune deficiency syndromes/chronic inflammation	Malignancies	Infectious diseases	Exposures
Acquired immunodeficiency syndrome	Acute lymphocytic leukemia	*Nocardia asteroides*	Agricultural dust
Amyloidosis	Acute myeloid leukemia	*Mycobacterium tuberculosis*	Aluminum dust
Subacute combined immunodeficiency disease	Chronic lymphocytic leukemia	*Mycobacterium avium-intracellulare*	Bakery flour dust
Fanconi's syndrome	Non-Hodgkin's lymphoma	*Streptococcus pneumoniae*	Cement dust
Hypogammaglobulinemia	Multiple myeloma	*Aspergillus* sp.	Chlorine
Idiopathic thrombocytopenic purpura	Waldenström's macroglobulinemia	*Pneumocystis jiroveci*	Cleaning products
Juvenile dermatomyositis	Myelodysplatic syndromes	*Candida* sp.	Fertilizer dust
Renal tubular acidosis	Adenocarcinoma	*Cryptococcus neoformans*	Gasoline fumes
Congenital lymphoplasia	Glioblastoma	*Histoplasma capsulatum*	Nitrogen dioxide
Aplastic anemia	Melanoma	*Cytomegalovirus*	Paint Petroleum Sawdust Silica Synthetic plastic fumes Titanium Varnish

Adapted from Ref. [19]

of 20. She had no previous disease. She had been admitted 17 days earlier because of the diagnosis of acute myeloid leukemia (unclassified). Chemotherapy with idarubicine and cytosine arabinoside was immediately instituted, and treatment with granulocyte-stimulating factor (G-CSF) was started on day 10. Echocardiography performed before treatment was unremarkable. Because of fever without microbiological documentation, a broad-spectrum anti-infectious treatment was initiated at ICU admission: ceftazidime, amikacin, vancomycin, and amphotericine B deoxycholate. One day before ICU admission, signs of respiratory failure developed, and high-resolution computed tomography (HRCT) was performed (Fig. 66.1). It revealed diffuse ground-glass opacities and bilateral pleural effusion. On ICU admission, the respiratory rate was 30 breaths/min, temperature 36.3°C, blood pressure 97/60 mmHg, and pulse 115/min. Chest auscultation revealed diffuse crackles. There were no heart murmurs, lymphadenopathy, or enlargements of the spleen and the liver. No skin rash or wounds were detected. Neurological examination was normal. Arterial blood gas analysis when breathing 100% oxygen via a non-rebreathing mask showed: pH 7.54, PaO_2 92.8 mmHg, $PaCO_2$ 23.4 mmHg, HCO_3^- 20.6 mmol/L, and lactate 0.6 mmol/L. The white blood cells count was 0.1 Giga/L, platelet count 41 Giga/L, hemoglobin 9.1 g/dL, and hematocrit 24.6%. Renal

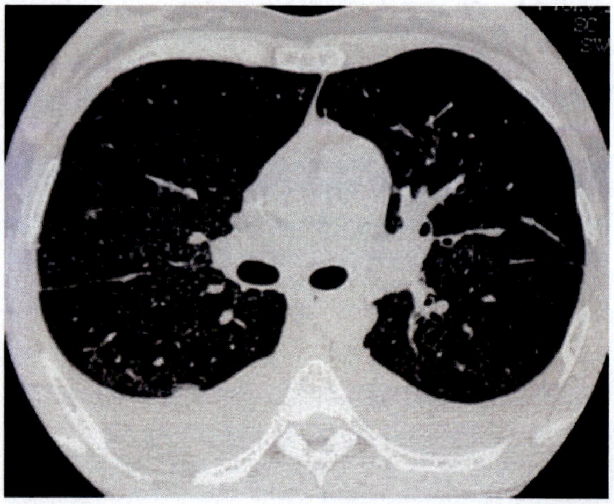

Fig. 66.1 High-resolution computed tomography (HRCT) revealing diffuse ground-glass opacities and bilateral pleural effusion

and hepatic functions were normal. Chest X-ray showed bilateral mid and lower lung field opacities with blunting of the lateral costophrenic angles (Figs. 66.2 and 66.3). The evolution was rapidly unfavorable despite noninvasive ventilation and orotracheal intubation and mechanical ventilation was needed on day 2 after ICU admission. A fiberoptic bronchoscopy with bronchoalveolar lavage (BAL) was performed in the right inferior lobe. There was no macroscopic abnormality. The BAL fluid was noted to be hemorrhagic. Microbiological analysis (bacteriology, virology, and mycology) remained negative, except for a positive *Pneumocystis jiroveci* polymerase chain reaction. Cytological study revealed 500,000 cells/mL (macrophages: 82%, lymphocytes: 17%, mastocytes 1%). There were no siderophages. Coloration with periodic acid-Schiff (PAS) was positive and revealed granular material compatible with PAP. Treatment with sulfametoxazole trimethoprime and steroids was initiated. The evolution was rapidly unfavorable, and acute respiratory distress syndrome developed. On day 10, because of a positive *Aspergillus* antigenemia test and the occurrence of a generalized seizure, high-resolution cerebral CT was performed revealing bilateral focal lesions compatible with *Aspergillus* infection. Treatment with voriconazole was added. Despite this, the patient died on day 14 of multiple organ failure. She was still profoundly neutropenic. No autopsy was performed.

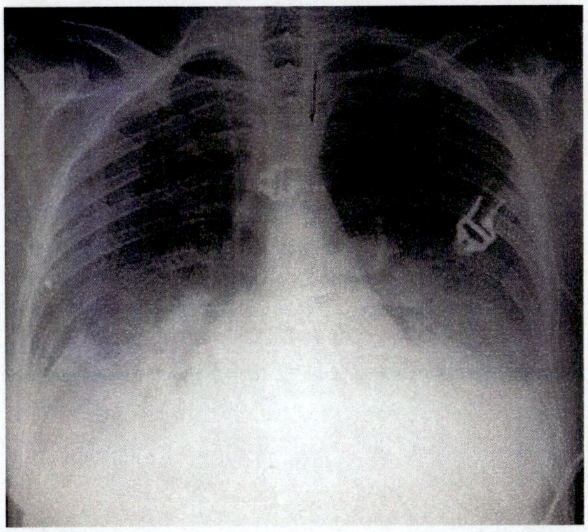

Fig. 66.2 Chest X-ray showing bilateral mid and lower lung field opacities with blunting of the lateral costophrenic angles

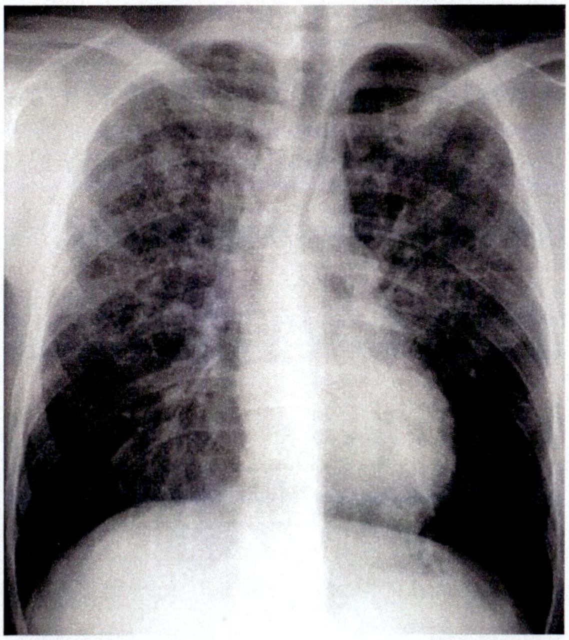

Fig. 66.3 Idiopathic PAP; X-ray shows bilateral mid- and lower-lung field opacities in a butterfly distribution with normal hila

This observation emphasizes many points about PAP:

- Its association with hematological malignancies, especially myeloid ones
- The existence of atypical radiological features in secondary forms
- The association of PAP with opportunistic agents, such as *P. jiroveci* or *Aspergillus fumigatus*
- The existence of neurological complications of PAP, first in relation to opportunistic infections with potential cerebral localizations, such as *Aspergillus* sp. *Cryptococcus neoformans* or *N. asteroides*

66.3 Clinical Presentation of PAP

The clinical presentation is variable and nonspecific, often leading to months or years of misdiagnosis in primary cases of PAP. A recent study from Japan disclosed important clinical features of primary PAP: a male-to-female ratio of 2.1:1, median age at diagnosis of 51 years, and a 56% history of cigarette smoking [9]. Symptoms are frequently milder than expected

Table 66.2 Symptoms and signs of pulmonary alveolar proteinosis

Symptoms and signs	% of patients ($n=167$)
Dyspnea	64
Cough	41
Crackles	28
Hemoptysis	21
Weight loss	18
Fever	16
Clubbing	15
Chest pain	14
Cyanosis	14

Adapted from Ref. [7]

from the radiographic findings, with up to 30% of patients having no symptoms. Others, however, present with acute symptoms suggestive of pneumonia or subacute to chronic symptoms with nonresolving radiographic infiltrates. Dyspnea and cough are the most common presenting symptoms (Table 66.2) [3, 7, 9]. The lung examination is frequently normal despite grossly abnormal chest radiographs, although crackles, clubbing, and cyanosis may be detected. Uncommon but reported features include pneumothorax and cor pulmonale.

66.4 Radiological Features

Many patterns of abnormalities on chest radiography can be seen. The classical description is a bilateral asymmetric alveolar filling pattern with perihilar infiltrates extending to the periphery (lower more than upper), sparing the costophrenic angles and yielding a "butterfly" distribution. The absence of pleural effusion, cardiomegaly, and adenopathy may suggest PAP. HRCT shows patchy, ground-glass opacifications with superimposed interlobular septal and intralobular thickening, a pattern commonly referred as "crazy paving" (Figs. 66.4a–c, 66.5, 66.6). This pattern is not

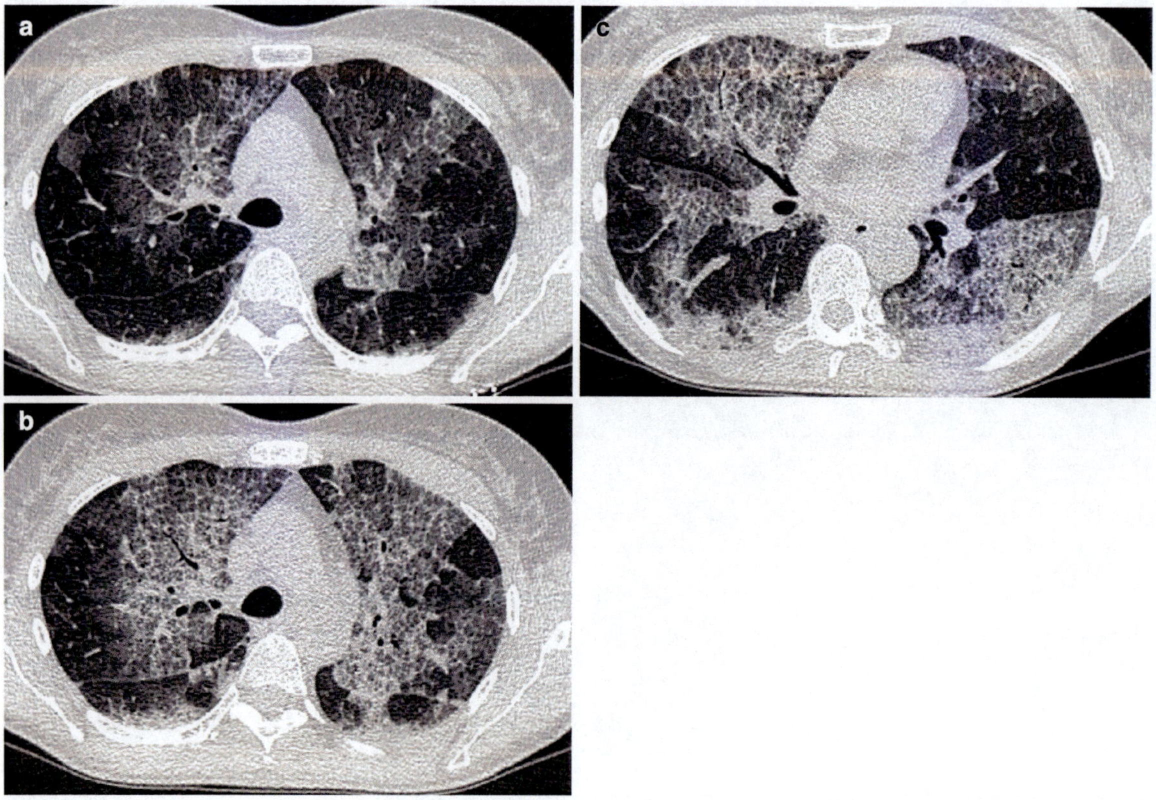

Fig. 66.4 (**a–c**) High-resolution computed tomography (HRCT) in a 59-year-old woman with progressive primitive alveolar proteinosis despite therapeutic whole lung lavage. Initial HRCT (**a**) typically shows diffuse ground-glass attenuation with superimposed intra- and interlobular septal thickening and a patchy geographic distribution (i.e., "crazy paving" pattern). After whole lung lavage, an extension of images was observed (**b**) leading to subpleural consolidations (**c**)

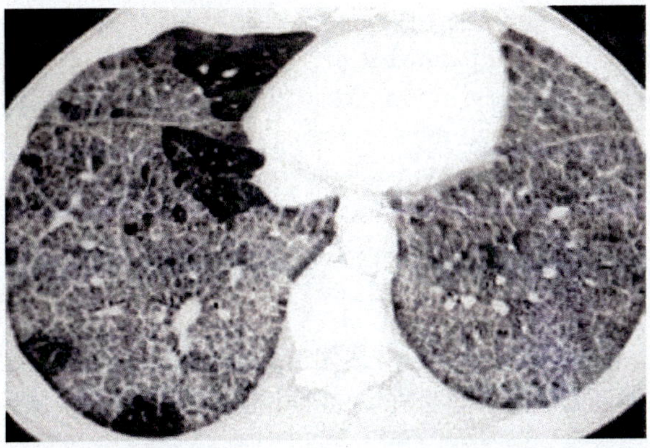

Fig. 66.5 High-resolution computed tomography scan in 65-year-old man hospitalized for acute respiratory distress. It was related to secondary PAP related to silica exposure. This image demonstrates "crazy paving," which refers to bilateral ground-glass opacity that is associated with marked interlobular septal thickening and a sharp nonanatomic demarcation between normal and abnormal lung

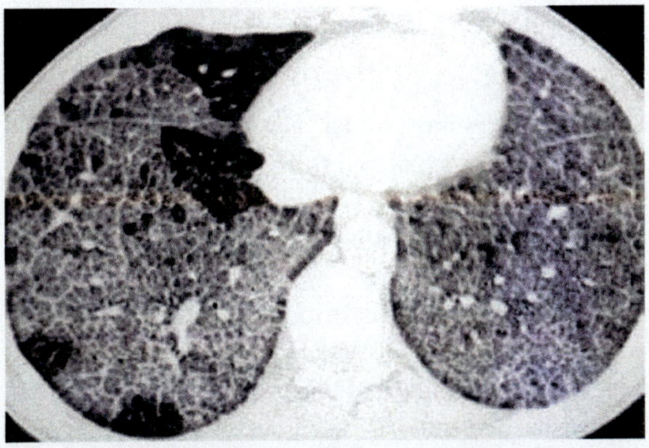

Fig. 66.6 High-resolution computed tomography scan in 65-year-old man hospitalized for acute respiratory distress. It was related to secondary PAP related to silica exposure. This image demonstrates "crazy paving," which refers to bilateral ground-glass opacity that is associated with marked interlobular septal thickening and a sharp nonanatomic demarcation between normal and abnormal lung

specific of PAP. Different diseases have been identified in association with "crazy paving" (Table 66.3) [10, 11]. Recent data also suggest that such a finding is frequent in autoimmune PAP (ground glass and "crazy paving": 71% each), but rather infrequent in patients with secondary PAP (ground-glass 14% and crazy paving 33%) [12].

Table 66.3 Differential diagnosis of "crazy-paving" pattern on high-resolution computed tomography (HRCT)

Mechanism	Causes
Infectious	*Pneumocystis jiroveci* pneumonia
Neoplasm	Mucinous bronchioloalveolar carcinoma
Idiopathic	Pulmonary alveolar proteinosis
	Sarcoidosis
	Nonspecific interstitial pneumonia
	Cryptogenic organizing pneumonia
Inhalation	Exogenous lipoid pneumonia
"Systemic"	Acute respiratory distress syndrome
	Pulmonary hemorrhage syndromes
	Wegener granulomatosis
	Goodpasture's syndrome
	Collagen-vascular diseases
	Coagulopathy
	Malignancies
	Bone marrow transplantation

66.5 Pulmonary Function

The most common disorders of PAP are mild restriction with a disproportionate reduction in diffusing capacity. Patients are often mildly hypoxemic with an elevated alveolar-arterial oxygen gradient and compensated respiratory alkalosis (Table 66.4) [7]. The

Table 66.4 Physiological measures in pulmonary alveolar proteinosis

Measure	Mean value ($n=140$)
Forced vital capacity	78% of predicted
Total lung capacity	77% of predicted
FEV_1/FVC	0.85
DLCO	57% of predicted
PaO_2	67 mmHg
$PaCO_2$	34 mmHg

Adapted from Ref. [7]

FEV_1/FVC forced expiratory volume in 1 s divided by forced vital capacity, *DLCO* diffusing capacity for lung carbon monoxide

shunt fraction is often elevated compared with patients with other diffuse lung diseases.

66.6 Diagnosis

Clinical and radiographic findings often suggest the diagnosis of PAP [12]. Laboratory data are of little utility in diagnosis. Serum lactate dehydrogenase, carcinoembryonic antigen, cytokeratin 19, surfactant proteins A, B, or D, and mucin KL-6 may be elevated [13]. These findings are usually not helpful in making the diagnosis, and their value in predicting the severity of PAP or monitoring disease activity is actually unknown. In about 75% of suspected cases, findings on examination of BAL can establish the diagnosis. The fluid is usually opaque and milky in appearance, and spontaneously separates into a pale yellow, almost translucent supernatant and thick sediment. A cytospin preparation demonstrates the presence of amorphous, granular, and eosinophilic material that stains with PAS. The alveolar macrophages are large and foamy [13]. Open lung biopsy, traditionally considered to be the gold standard, is now largely unnecessary. When BAL is not sufficient for diagnosis, transbronchial biopsy specimens are usually sufficient. Biopsy specimens reveal multiple nodular areas of consolidation, with PAS-positive acellular material filling the alveoli and terminal bronchioles. Importantly, the underlying architecture of the lung is usually preserved, with fibrotic changes leading to architectural distortion occurring only in advanced cases.

66.7 Complications

Secondary infections are the main complication of PAP, accounting for 18% of attributable mortality. No specific pathogen has been identified [3]. Although there is likely to be some degree of publication bias favoring the reporting of "unusual" organisms, opportunistic pathogens are over-represented among patients with PAP (*Mycobacterium tuberculosis, M. avium-intracellulare complex, Streptomyces* sp., *C. Neoformans, N. asteroides, Mucorales, Histoplasma* sp., *Coccidioidies immitis, Aspergillus* sp., *Blastomyces demartidis*, and *Acinetobacter* sp.). No disease- *or* patient-related factors (especially duration of symptoms, treatment with corticosteroids, or smoking) could be identified as associated with the occurrence of infections to these unusual organisms [3]. Notably, a number of infections were disseminated, particularly those involving the central nervous system. Cerebral involvement has been reported in a few cases of PAP [14, 15]. There appear to be three main ways in which this can occur: cerebral infarction due to hypoxia (diffusion limitation in the lungs), vessel blockage with mucomycin protein, and having a predisposition to unusual pulmonary infections (mainly *N. asteroides* and *Aspergillus* sp.), which spread to form cerebral abscesses. Neurological signs are often seen, specific to the vascular territory in which the event occurred. Development of pulmonary fibrosis has been reported in isolated cases. Other complications include the development of pneumothorax or emphysematous bullas [16].

66.8 Treatment

Whole-lung lavage (WLL), allowing the removal of lipoproteinaceous material from the lungs, has boosted survival rates of patients with idiopathic PAP from 70% to 100% [3, 17]. It has been proposed since the early 1960s, when segmental lavage was reported, and remains the standard of care today [12, 18, 19]. Because no prospective study of WLL is available, it is difficult to determine the effects of this procedure on prognosis. A retrospective analysis of 231 cases revealed significant improvement in blood gases, physiological and radiological data, and survival [3]. WLL is associated with improvement in macrophage functions and a decreased incidence of opportunistic infections [16]. The median duration of freedom from recurrent symptoms, such as exertional dyspnea, appears to be approximately 15 months, but is highly variable, with many patients needing only a single lavage [3]. A small number of patients do not respond to WLL, with younger age appearing to be the major predictor of poor response [3]. Moreover, it is difficult to determine exactly when WLL must be performed. In practice, reasonable indications seem to be dyspnea affecting the patient's daily activities, a $PaO_2 < 60$ mmHg on room air, or a shunt fraction greater than 12% [19]. WLL is performed under general anesthesia with a double-lumen endotracheal tube. One lung is lavaged with warm (36–37°C) neutral sterile saline (0.9% saline with 0.6 mmol sodium bicarbonate/l) while the other is being ventilated. Serial aliquots of saline are infused until the effluent is almost totally clear. This requires 20–40 L of saline. The second lung undergoes the same procedure either the same day or 3–7 days later [16]. Complications of WLL are overspill of lavage fluid in the ventilated lung related to a misplacement of the endotracheal tube, hypoxemia, barotraumas, pleural collections, hydropneumothorax, and emphysema. The lavage may also be done with fiberoptic bronchoscopy [20]. Treatment for secondary PAP involves treatment of the underlying condition or removal from exposure to the suspected environmental agent [21]. In the congenital forms, lung transplantation seems to be the only therapeutic option, with possible recurrence. Gene therapy is being researched [22].

66.9 Idiopathic PAP and GM-CSF

The first indication that GM-CSF may be central to idiopathic PAP pathogenesis derived from observations of GM-CSF knockout mices (GM-/GM-), who have normal life spans and normal circulating numbers of red and white blood cells, but were found at 3 weeks of age to have lung alveolar spaces filled with material like in PAP in humans [23, 24]. The role of GM-CSF in lung tissue was further confirmed when PAP developed, also without abnormal hematopoiesis, in genetically modified mice lacking one chain of the GM-CSF receptor (GM $R_{\beta c}$) [25]. The GM-CSF receptor is expressed on type II pneumocytes and alveolar macrophages. Pulmonary epithelial cells are a source of GM-CSF. Local intrapulmonary delivery of exogenous GM-CSF or alveolar overexpression of GM-CSF can correct the pulmonary pathology observed in GM-/GM- mices. Notably, such mices also have other abnormalities, including a predisposition to infections and impaired macrophage functions [13]. Analysis of blood and BAL in patients with PAP revealed normal levels of GM-CSF and no detectable defects in gene-encoding GM-CSF [13]. Advances in understanding the condition in humans were made in 1999 when the presence of circulating antibodies in both the serum and BAL of patients with idiopathic PAP was found [26]. These antibodies were IgG and neutralizing, binding to GM-CSF with a high affinity and specificity. A large cohort study showed that 90% of patients with idiopathic PAP have such antibodies [9]. However, the presence of anti-GM-CSF antibodies is not 100% specific of idiopathic PAP, with very low rates having been reported in healthy subjects [27]. The precise mechanisms by which the lack of GM-CSF, either due to its complete absence in GM-/GM- mices or to its binding by antibodies (in idiopathic PAP), leads to surfactant accumulation is not yet known. It has been demonstrated that alveolar macrophages from GM-/GM- mices exhibit decreased expression of PU.1, a transcription factor required for maturation of these cells [28]. These cells were unable to metabolize surfactant; however, when provided with GM-CSF in vitro, they expressed PU.1 and cell surface markers characteristic of mature macrophages, and acquired the ability to metabolize surfactant. Use of the anti-GM-CSF assay seems to be very interesting in patients with idiopathic PAP, with a sensitivity of 100% and specificity greater than 91% [29]. Furthermore, the anti-GM-CSF antibody titer correlates with PAP activity and may predict the response to therapy with GM-CSF replacement. Comprehensive reviews of the role of GM-SF in idiopathic PAP are available in Refs. [3, 27, 30–32]. The discovery of anti-GM-CSF neutralizing antibodies led to multiple trials evaluating the usefulness of GM-CSF, using subcutaneous or nebulized administration, eventually in association with WLL [13, 19]. Another approach to this "autoimmune" disease is to try to eliminate antibodies using plasma exchange or to limit the overproduction using rituximab (http://www.clinicaltrials.gov/).

66.10 PAP and Hematological Malignancies

The association of PAP and hematological disorders is well established, and these forms are considered secondary PAP. The incidence of PAP in patients with respiratory symptoms was estimated to be 5.3% among all patients with hematological malignancies and to be 10% in patients with myeloid disorders [33]. Such incidences have never been reported since this publication. In a review of 3,500 children treated between 1962 and 2007 at one pediatric oncological institution, only five patients were diagnosed with secondary PAP [34]. Four of them had acute leukemia (three myeloid, one lymphoid) and one chronic myeloid leukemia (CML). In a review of 241 cases of PAP in China from 1965 to 2006, only three were associated with hematological malignancies (two chronic and one acute leukemia) [35]. PAP is most commonly encountered in acute myeloid leukemia (AML), CML, myelodysplastic syndrome (MDS), and lymphoblastic leukemia [33, 36–38]. The frequency of each hematological malignancy is difficult to determine specifically. In a recent radiological study concerning 21 patients with secondary PAP, 12 were related to MDS, 1 to CML, 1 to acute lymphoid leukemia, and 1 to aplastic anemia [12]. This secondary form is not well characterized. Pulmonary alveolar macrophages are largely bone marrow derived. One cause of PAP in leukemia patients is alveolar infiltration by leukemic blast cells that lack functional GM-CSF signaling [38]. In pediatric patients who developed PAP at the onset of AML, the common β and/or α chain of the GM-CSF receptor was found to be deficient on leukemic blast cells obtained from bone marrow and BAL fluid [39, 40]. The second cause is a profound depression in the development of alveolar macrophages. Third, the role of cytarabine and total body irradiation has been advocated as a precipitating factor. Fourth, high titers of anti GM-CSF antibodies of multiple isotypes are often found in patients with active myeloid leukemia without PAP [41]. They are usually non-neutralizing and probably independent of the development of PAP. Especially in these patients PAP may be misinterpreted as infection, particularly by *P. jiroveci* and viral pneumonia, given its nonspecific radiographic findings [42]. PAP associated with hematological malignancies is potentially reversible without undergoing WLL. The prognosis of such secondary forms appears to be related to the prognosis of underlying hematological malignancy and the curability of associated infections (Fig. 66.7). Resolution of PAP can occur after recovery of neutropenia or successful bone marrow transplantation (BMT) [32, 33, 43]. WLL may be used with success, but always in association with the treatment of the underlying disease [44]. There is no report of GM-CSF therapy for hematological malignancies associated with PAP, although PAP symptoms resolved in one patient who received G-CSF [45].

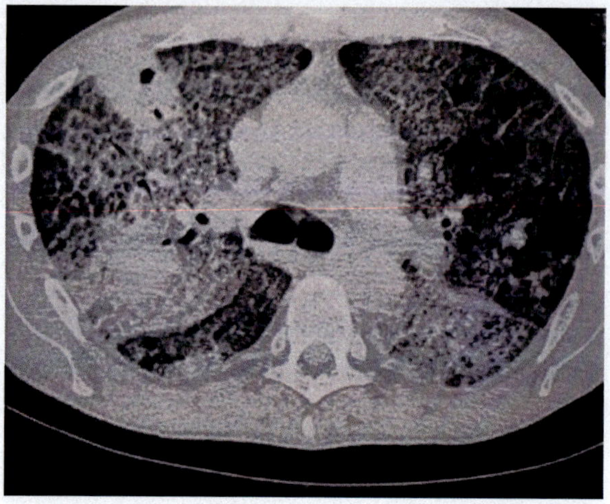

Fig. 66.7 High-resolution computed tomography (HRCT) in a 34-year-old man with idiopathic pulmonary alveolar proteinosis diagnosed 1 month ago. The patient was hospitalized in intensive care unit for respiratory distress. HRCT demonstrated extensive lesions with multiple consolidation and cavitated nodules consistent with the presence of *Aspergillus fumigatus* on bronchoalveolar lavage

66.11 Conclusion

PAP is a rare disease. Because of a lack of specificity in clinical and radiological presentation in the forms secondary to hematological malignancies, especially myeloid, it should be systematically considered in the diagnosis of acute respiratory failure in patients treated for such diseases. The prognosis seems to be related to the prognosis of the underlying malignancy, recovery of neutropenia and the curability of any associated infection.

References

1. Mazzone PJ, Jane Thomassen M, Kavuru MS (2002) Pulmonary alveolar proteinosis: recent advances. Semin Respir Crit Care Med 23(2):115–26
2. Rosen SH, Castleman B, Liebow AA (1958) Pulmonary alveolar proteinosis. N Engl J Med 258(23):1123–42
3. Seymour JF, Presneill JJ (2002) Pulmonary alveolar proteinosis: progress in the first 44 years. Am J Respir Crit Care Med 166(2):215–35, Review
4. Martinez-Moczygemba M, Doan ML, Elidemir O, Fan LL, Cheung SW, Lei JT, Moore JP, Tavana G, Lewis LR, Zhu Y, Muzny DM, Gibbs RA, Huston DP (2008) Pulmonary alveolar proteinosis caused by deletion of the GM-CSFR alpha gene in the X chromosome pseudoautosomal region 1. J Exp Med 205(12):2711–6

5. Suzuki T, Sakagami T, Rubin BK, Nogee LM, Wood RE, Zimmerman SL, Smolarek T, Dishop MK, Wert SE, Whitsett JA, Grabowski G, Carey BC, Stevens C, van der Loo JC, Trapnell BC (2008) Familial pulmonary alveolar proteinosis caused by mutations in CSF2RA. J Exp Med 205(12): 2703–10
6. Yokota T, Matsumura Y, Ban N, Matsubayashi T, Inagaki N (2008) Heterozygous ABCA3 mutation associated with non-fatal evolution of respiratory distress. Eur J Pediatr 167(6): 691–3
7. Mazzone P, Thomassen MJ, Kavuru M (2001) Our new understanding of pulmonary alveolar proteinosis: what an internist needs to know. Cleve Clin J Med 68(12):977–8, 981–2, 984–5, Review
8. Ben-Dov I, Kishinevski Y, Roznman J, Soliman A, Bishara H, Zelligson E, Grief J, Mazar A, Perelman M, Vishnizer R, Weiler-Ravel D (1999) Pulmonary alveolar proteinosis in Israel: ethnic clustering. Isr Med Assoc J 1(2):75–8
9. Inoue Y, Trapnell BC, Tazawa R, Arai T, Takada T, Hizawa N, Kasahara Y, Tatsumi K, Hojo M, Ichiwata T, Tanaka N, Yamaguchi E, Eda R, Oishi K, Tsuchihashi Y, Kaneko C, Nukiwa T, Sakatani M, Krischer JP, Nakata K, Japanese Center of the Rare Lung Diseases Consortium (2008) Characteristics of a large cohort of patients with autoimmune pulmonary alveolar proteinosis in Japan. Am J Respir Crit Care Med 177(7): 752–62
10. Johkoh T, Itoh H, Müller NL, Ichikado K, Nakamura H, Ikezoe J, Akira M, Nagareda T (1999) Radiology. Crazy-paving appearance at thin-section CT: spectrum of disease and pathologic findings. Radiology 211(1):155–60
11. Rossi SE, Erasmus JJ, Volpacchio M, Franquet T, Castiglioni T, McAdams HP (2003) "Crazy-paving" pattern at thin-section CT of the lungs: radiologic-pathologic overview. Radiographics 23(6):1509–19, Review
12. Ishii H, Trapnell BC, Tazawa R, Inoue Y, Akira M, Kogure Y, Tomii K, Takada T, Hojo M, Ichiwata T, Goto H, Nakata K (2009) Japanese Center of the Rare Lung Disease Consortium. Comparative study of high-resolution CT findings between autoimmune and secondary pulmonary alveolar proteinosis. Chest 136(5):1348–55
13. Trapnell BC, Whitsett JA, Nakata K (2003) Pulmonary alveolar proteinosis. N Engl J Med 349(26):2527–39
14. Wolman L (1961) The cerebral complications of pulmonary alveolar proteinosis. Lancet 2(7205):733–5
15. McDermott H, Aitchison F, Nathan N, Bhatnager A. A case report of pulmonary alveolar proteinosis (2009). BMJ Case Reports. doi:10.1136/bcr.04.2009.1796
16. Shah PL, Hansell D, Lawson PR, Reid KB, Morgan C (2000) Pulmonary alveolar proteinosis: clinical aspects and current concepts on pathogenesis. Thorax 55(1):67–77
17. Ioachimescu OC, Kavuru MS (2006) Pulmonary alveolar proteinosis. Chron Respir Dis 3(3):149–59
18. Ramirez J, Schultz RB, Dutton RE (1963) Alveolar proteinosis: a new technique and rationale for treatment. Arch Intern Med 112:419–31
19. Huizar I, Kavuru MS (2009) Alveolar proteinosis syndrome: pathogenesis, diagnosis, and management. Curr Opin Pulm Med 15(5):491–8
20. Cheng SL, Chang HT, Lau HP, Lee LN, Yang PC (2002) Pulmonary alveolar proteinosis: treatment by bronchofiberscopic lobar lavage. Chest 122(4):1480–5
21. Ladeb S, Fleury-Feith J, Escudier E, Tran Van Nhieu J, Bernaudin JF, Cordonnier C (1996) Secondary alveolar proteinosis in cancer patients. Support Care Cancer 4(6):420–6, Review
22. Kleff V, Sorg UR, Bury C, Suzuki T, Rattmann I, Jerabek-Willemsen M, Poremba C, Flasshove M, Opalka B, Trapnell B, Dirksen U, Moritz T (2008) Gene therapy of beta(c)-deficient pulmonary alveolar proteinosis (beta(c)-PAP): studies in a murine in vivo model. Mol Ther 16(4):757–64
23. Dranoff G, Crawford AD, Sadelain M, Ream B, Rashid A, Bronson RT, Dickersin GR, Bachurski CJ, Mark EL, Whitsett JA et al (1994) Involvement of granulocyte-macrophage colony-stimulating factor in pulmonary homeostasis. Science 264(5159):713–6
24. Stanley E, Lieschke GJ, Grail D, Metcalf D, Hodgson G, Gall JA, Maher DW, Cebon J, Sinickas V, Dunn AR (1994) Granulocyte/macrophage colony-stimulating factor-deficient mice show no major perturbation of hematopoiesis but develop a characteristic pulmonary pathology. Proc Natl Acad Sci USA 91(12):5592–6
25. Nishinakamura R, Nakayama N, Hirabayashi Y, Inoue T, Aud D, McNeil T, Azuma S, Yoshida S, Toyoda Y, Arai K et al (1995) Mice deficient for the IL-3/GM-CSF/IL-5 beta c receptor exhibit lung pathology and impaired immune response, while beta IL3 receptor-deficient mice are normal. Immunity 2(3):211–22
26. Kitamura T, Tanaka N, Watanabe J, Uchida, Kanegasaki S, Yamada Y, Nakata K (1999) Idiopathic pulmonary alveolar proteinosis as an autoimmune disease with neutralizing antibody against granulocyte/macrophage colony-stimulating factor. J Exp Med 190(6):875–80
27. Greenhill SR, Kotton DN (2009) Pulmonary alveolar proteinosis: a bench-to-bedside story of granulocyte-macrophage colony-stimulating factor dysfunction. Chest 136(2):571–7
28. Shibata Y, Berclaz PY, Chroneos ZC, Yoshida M, Whitsett JA, Trapnell BC (2001) GM-CSF regulates alveolar macrophage differentiation and innate immunity in the lung through PU.1. Immunity 15(4):557–67
29. Bonfield TL, Russell D, Burgess S, Malur A, Kavuru MS, Thomassen MJ (2002) Autoantibodies against granulocyte macrophage colony-stimulating factor are diagnostic for pulmonary alveolar proteinosis. Am J Respir Cell Mol Biol 27(4):481–6
30. Uchida K, Beck DC, Yamamoto T, Berclaz PY, Abe S, Staudt MK, Carey BC, Filippi MD, Wert SE, Denson LA, Puchalski JT, Hauck DM, Trapnell BC (2007) GM-CSF autoantibodies and neutrophil dysfunction in pulmonary alveolar proteinosis. N Engl J Med 356(6):567–79
31. Greenhill SR, Kotton DN (2009) Pulmonary alveolar proteinosis: a bench-to-bedside story of granulocyte-macrophage colony-stimulating factor dysfunction. Chest 136(2):571–7
32. Trapnell BC, Carey BC, Uchida K, Suzuki T (2009) Pulmonary alveolar proteinosis, a primary immunodeficiency of impaired GM-CSF stimulation of macrophages. Curr Opin Immunol 21(5):514–21
33. Cordonnier C, Fleury-Feith J, Escudier E, Atassi K, Bernaudin JF (1994) Secondary alveolar proteinosis is a reversible cause of respiratory failure in leukemic patients. Am J Respir Crit Care Med 149(3 Pt 1):788–94

34. Inaba H, Jenkins JJ, McCarville MB, Morrison RR, Howard SC, Pui CH, Ribeiro RC (2008) Pulmonary alveolar proteinosis in pediatric leukemia. Pediatr Blood Cancer 51(1): 66–70
35. Xu Z, Jing J, Wang H, Xu F, Wang J (2009) Pulmonary alveolar proteinosis in China: a systematic review of 241 cases. Respirology 14(5):761–6
36. Gacouin A, Le Tulzo Y, Suprin E, Briens E, Bernard M, Camus C, Thomas R (1998) Acute respiratory failure caused by secondary alveolar proteinosis in a patient with acute myeloid leukemia: a case report. Intensive Care Med 24(3):265–7
37. Ohnishi T, Yamada G, Shijubo N, Takagi-Takahashi Y, Itoh T, Takahashi H, Satoh M, Koba H, Nakata K, Abe S (2003) Secondary pulmonary alveolar proteinosis associated with myelodysplastic syndrome. Intern Med 42(2):187–90
38. Pamuk GE, Turgut B, Vural O, Demir M, Hatipoğlu O, Unlü E, Altaner S, Gerenli M, Cakir B (2003) Pulmonary alveolar proteinosis in a patient with acute lymphoid leukemia regression after G-CSF therapy. Leuk Lymphoma 44(5):871–4
39. Dirksen U, Hattenhorst U, Schneider P, Schroten H, Göbel U, Böcking A, Müller KM, Murray R, Burdach S (1998) Defective expression of granulocyte-macrophage colony-stimulating factor/interleukin-3/interleukin-5 receptor common beta chain in children with acute myeloid leukemia associated with respiratory failure. Blood 92(4):1097–103
40. Seymour JF, Begley CG, Dirksen U, Presneill JJ, Nicola NA, Moore PE, Schoch OD, van Asperen P, Roth B, Burdach S, Dunn AR (1998) Attenuated hematopoietic response to granulocyte-macrophage colony-stimulating factor in patients with acquired pulmonary alveolar proteinosis. Blood 92(8):2657–67
41. Sergeeva A, Ono Y, Rios R, Molldrem JJ (2008) High titer autoantibodies to GM-CSF in patients with AML, CML and MDS are associated with active disease. Leukemia 22(4):783–90
42. Chung JH, Pipavath SJ, Myerson DH, Godwin D (2009) Secondary pulmonary alveolar proteinosis: a confusing and potentially serious complication of hematologic malignancy. J Thorac Imaging 24(2):115–8
43. Tabata S, Shimoji S, Murase K, Takiuchi Y, Inoue D, Kimura T, Nagai Y, Mori M, Togami K, Kurata M, Ito K, Hashimoto H, Matushita A, Nagai K, Takahashi T (2009) Successful allogeneic bone marrow transplantation for myelodysplastic syndrome complicated by severe pulmonary alveolar proteinosis. Int J Hematol Oct;90(3):407–12
44. Numata A, Matsuishi E, Koyanagi K, Saito S, Miyamoto Y, Irie K, Gondo H, Harada M (2006) Successful therapy with whole-lung lavage and autologous peripheral blood stem cell transplantation for pulmonary alveolar proteinosis complicating acute myelogenous leukemia. Am J Hematol 81(2): 107–9
45. Pamuk GE, Turgut B, Vural O, Demir M, Hatipoğlu O, Unlü E, Altaner S, Gerenli M, Cakir B (2003) Pulmonary alveolar proteinosis in a patient with acute lymphoid leukemia regression after G-CSF therapy. Leuk Lymphoma 44(5): 871–4

Pneumocystis jiroveci Pneumonia in a Patient with Diffuse Large B-Cell Lymphoma

67

Hung Chang and Lee-Yung Shih

Contents

67.1 Case Presentation

A 70-year-old male was diagnosed with stage I_A diffuse large B-cell lymphoma. The tumor cells were CD3−, CD20+, CD10−, BCL−6+, CD5−, and cyclin D1−. He received rituximab 375 mg/m^2 and combination chemotherapy with cyclophosphamide 750 mg/m^2, epirubicin 50 mg/m^2, vincristine 2 mg, and prednisolone 100 mg/day for 5 days (R-CEOP). The cycle was repeated every 3 weeks. He developed fever and dry cough 14 days after the second cycle. Blood cultures, the chest radiograph (Fig. 67.1), and urine analysis failed to

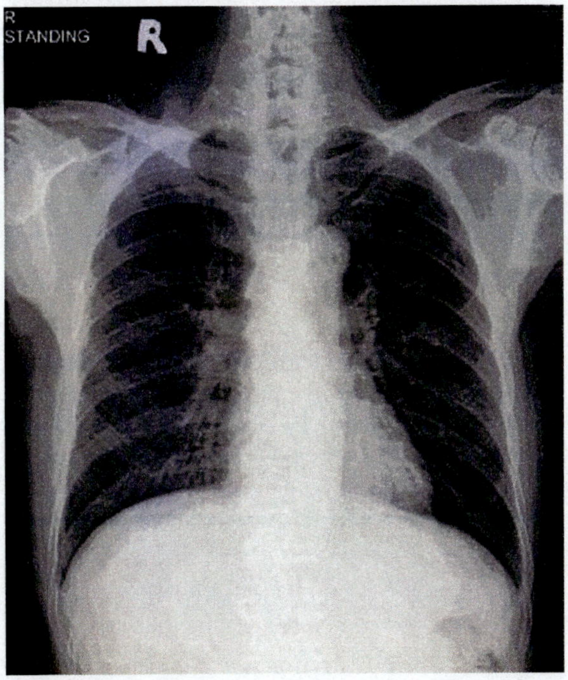

Fig. 67.1 A chest radiograph showed unremarkable findings. No lung infiltrates, nodules, or tumors were visible

H. Chang and L.-Y. Shih (✉)
Division of Hematology-Oncology, Department of Internal Medicine, Chang Gung Memorial Hospital, and College of Medicine, Chang Gung University, 5 Fu-Shing Street, Kweishan, Taoyuan 333, Taiwan
e-mail: sly7012@adm.cgmh.org.tw

É. Azoulay (ed.), *Pulmonary Involvement in Patients with Hematological Malignancies*, DOI: 10.1007/978-3-642-15742-4_67, © Springer-Verlag Berlin Heidelberg 2011

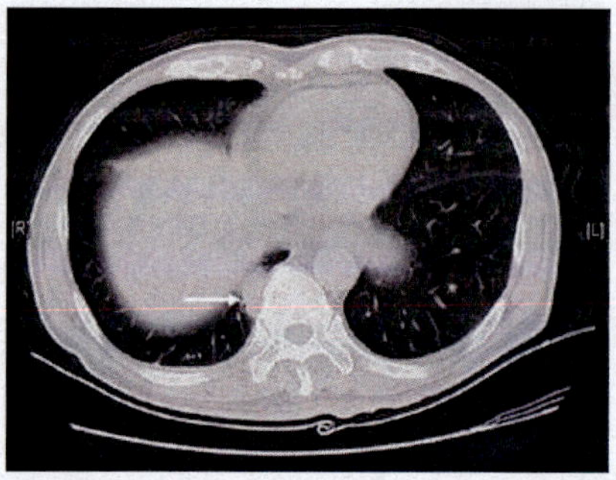

Fig. 67.2 Computed tomography showed sub-segmental consolidation (*arrow*) in the posterior basal segment of the right lower lobe with homogeneous enhancement

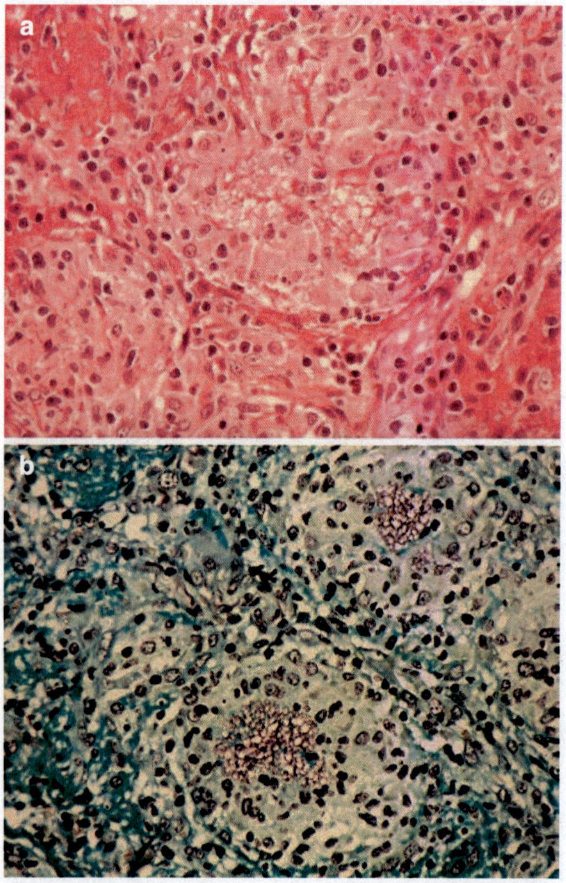

Fig. 67.3 Histology of the wedge resection specimen. (**a**) Frothy exudate in the center of a granuloma (hematoxylin and eosin stain, ×400). (**b**) *Pneumocystis jiroveci* cysts in the exudate (Gomori's methenamine-silver nitrate stain, ×400)

identify the cause. Despite empirical antibiotic therapy (ceftriaxone 1 g every 12 h), the fever persisted for 5 days. A whole-body computed tomography (CT) scan revealed a solitary pulmonary nodule measuring 2.3 × 1.0 cm in the right lower lung (Fig. 67.2). At that time, the CD4 lymphocyte count was 187/mm^3, serum immunoglobulin G level was 507 mg/dL, and screening for HIV was negative. Video-assisted thoracic wedge resection of the nodule was performed. Microscopic examination of the nodule showed non-necrotizing granulomatous inflammation with eosinophilic frothy exudates in the centers of the granulomas (Fig. 67.3a). *Pneumocystis jiroveci* cysts were demonstrated by Gomori's methenamine-silver nitrate stain (Fig. 67.3b). A diagnosis of granulomatous *P. jiroveci* pneumonia (PJP) was given. The fever subsided after surgery. Trimethoprim–sulfamethoxazole was given for 21 days. In all, six R-CEOP cycles were given, and no further infections developed after the additional cycles.

67.2 Discussion

Hematological malignancies raise challenges in pulmonary care. The patients often have immunosuppression related both to the disease and to the treatment. Although bacterial and fungal infections predominate, opportunistic infections such as PJP may occur [1], as illustrated by our case report.

Patients with PJP typically have diffuse interstitial pulmonary infiltrates. However, atypical features such as cavitary or granulomatous lesions have been reported [2, 3]. Granulomatous PJP occurs in patients with acquired immunodeficiency syndrome (AIDS) and, less frequently, in patients with lymphoma or leukemia. In a retrospective report, granulomatous PJP was found in 5% of lung biopsy specimens from AIDS patients with PJP [3]. The incidence among patients with hematological malignancies is unclear. Even in its granulomatous form, PJP usually manifests as diffuse multiple infiltrates. A solitary pulmonary nodule as the only radiological finding is unusual [4].

Granulomatous PJP has been reported in patients with various hematological malignancies, including chronic lymphocytic leukemia (CLL), small lymphocytic lymphoma (SLL), prolymphocytic leukemia (PLL) [2, 5, 6], non-Hodgkin lymphoma [4, 7], Hodgkin's lymphoma [5], multiple myeloma [8], and acute and chronic myeloid leukemias [8, 9]. In the English-language literature, 14 cases of granulomatous PJP in patients with hematological malignancies have been reported. The clinical features in these patients are summarized in Table 67.1. It is noteworthy

Table 67.1 Clinical features of patients with hematological malignancies and granulomatous *Pneumocystis jiroveci* pneumonia

Age/sex	Hematological malignancy	Chemotherapy or immunosuppressive therapy	BAL	CD4 count (/mm^3)	IgG (mg/dL)	Treatment for PJP	Outcome	Radiological findings	Reference
Stem cell transplant recipients									
40/M	AML	ASCT	Non-diagnostic	NA	NA	TMX-SMX	Improved[a]	Diffuse nodules	[9]
39/M	CML	ASCT	Non-diagnostic	NA	NA	TMX-SMX	Improved	Infiltrate	[8]
39/F	AML	ASCT	Non-diagnostic	NA	NA	TMX-SMX	Improved	Nodule consolidation	[8]
55/M	MM	ABCT	Non-diagnostic	NA	NA	TMX-SMX	Improved	Diffuse infiltrate	[8]
Nontransplanted patients									
57/F	Lymphoma	COP	ND	NA	NA	Resection	Improved	Solitary nodule	[4]
62/M	Lymphoma	None	Non-diagnostic	NA	NA	TMP-SMX	Improved	Diffuse infiltrate	[7]
74/M	CLL/PLL	COP	Non-diagnostic	NA	NA	TMP-SMX →Dapsone/ TMP →atovaquone	Improved	Nodules	[14]
57/M	SLL	Fludarabine, steroid CHOP	Non-diagnostic	0	NA	TMP-SMX→ dapsone/TMP	Improved	Diffuse infiltrate	[14]
52/F	CLL	Cyclophosphamide steroid	Positive	1700	52	TMX-SMX	Improved[a]	Bilateral nodules	[6]
17/NA	HL	Combination CT steroid	Non-diagnostic	NA	NA	TMX-SMX	Improved	Reticulonodular infiltrate	[5]
42/NA	CLL	Fludarabine, steroid	Non-diagnostic	NA	NA	TMX-SMX	Improved	Reticulonodular infiltrate	[5]
NA/NA	CLL	NA	Non-diagnostic	NA	NA	NA	Died[b]	NA	[13]
75/F	CLL	Alemtuzumab				TMX-SMX	Improved	Bilateral infiltrate	[2]
70/M	DLBL	R-CEOP	ND	187	507	Resection →TMX-SMX	Improved	Solitary nodule	[20]

AML acute myeloid leukemia, *CLL* chronic lymphocytic leukemia, *SLL* small lymphocytic lymphoma, *PLL* prolymphocytic leukemia, MM multiple myeloma, *CML* chronic myeloid leukemia, *HL* Hodgkin's lymphoma, *DLBL* diffuse large B-cell lymphoma, *C(H)OP* cyclophosphamide/(adriamycin)/vincristine/prednisolone, *ASCT* allogeneic stem cell transplantation, *ABCT* autologous blood stem cell transplantation, *R-CEOP* rituximab/cyclophosphamide/epirubicin/vincristine/prednisolone, *NA* not available, *ND* not done, *TMP/SMX* trimethoprim–sulfamethoxazole

[a]With residual pulmonary lesion

[b]Only abstract available in English

that bronchoscopy with bronchoalveolar lavage, which is frequently performed in an attempt to isolate the offending microorganism in patients with pulmonary infections, was positive in only 1 of the 11 patients who had this procedure. Thus, a biopsy is often needed to establish the diagnosis. The patients fall into two main groups depending on whether they received stem cell transplantation ($n = 4$) or chemotherapy or target therapies without transplantation ($n = 10$). It is well recognized that autologous or allogeneic stem-cell transplantation is associated with profound immunosuppression. Opportunistic infections, including PJP, are of considerable concern in stem cell transplant recipients, in whom routine prophylaxis is therefore recommended [10–12]. Granulomatous PJP in these patients may be more closely related to stem cell transplantation than to the underlying disease (Table 67.1). However, in nontransplanted patients, both the underlying disease and the cytotoxic chemotherapy or immunotherapy contribute substantially to suppressing the immune system. As shown in Table 67.1, no patient in this group had acute myeloid leukemia, myelodysplastic syndrome, or chronic myeloid leukemia. All patients in this group had lymphocytic leukemia or lymphoma. Because prolymphocytic leukemia (PLL) and small lymphocytic lymphoma (SLL) represent different phases of chronic lymphocytic leukemia (CLL), similar or identical treatments are used in these three diseases. The CLL/PLL/SLL constellation accounted for six of the ten nontransplanted patients (4 CLLs, 1 SLLs, and 1 CLL with PLL progression) [2, 5, 6, 13, 14]. Thus, CLL/SLL/PLL may be associated with greater susceptibility to granulomatous PJP infection. Such susceptibility may be related to several factors. CLL is associated with impaired T-cell and B-cell functions [15]. In addition, CLL patients are often older, and many of them receive corticosteroids at some point of their treatment.

Rituximab is a monoclonal antibody against CD20, a marker expressed by nearly all B-cells and B-lineage lymphoid neoplasms. The use of rituximab in addition to chemotherapy increases the risk of viral reactivation (e.g., cytomegalovirus and hepatitis B virus) [16] and of opportunistic infections, including PJP. Because rituximab significantly increases the efficacy of chemotherapy for diffuse large B-cell lymphoma, adding rituximab to treatment protocols is becoming standard practice [17, 18]. Currently, routine PJP prophylaxis has not been suggested for patients receiving rituximab-based treatment, except selected patients on highly intensive regimens [19]. There are increasing reports of PJP following rituximab and chemotherapy [1, 19–22]. It is likely that PJP will become a potentially serious threat in such patients. Clinicians must be aware that PJP does not always manifest as typical diffuse interstitial infiltrates, as illustrated by our case report.

The mechanism of granuloma formation in PJP is unclear. In a study by Totet et al., granuloma formation was not related to any specific *P. jiroveci* genotype [23]. Therefore, it was suggested that granuloma formation may be mediated by host factors [23]. This possibility remains to be investigated, however.

In conclusion, our experience illustrates the difficulty of diagnosing PJP in patients with atypical radiological features. Invasive diagnostic procedures are often required to establish the definitive diagnosis. Clinicians should be aware that PJP can manifest as a solitary pulmonary nodule.

Acknowledgment We acknowledge S. Karger AG, Basel, for permission to use the content from Acta Haematologica.

References

1. Chang H, Yeh HC, Su YC, Lee MH (2008) Pneumocystis jiroveci pneumonia in patients with non-Hodgkin's lymphoma receiving chemotherapy containing rituximab. J Chin Med Assoc 71:579–582
2. Otahbachi M, Nugent K, Buscemi D (2007) Granulomatous Pneumocystis jiroveci Pneumonia in a patient with chronic lymphocytic leukemia: a literature review and hypothesis on pathogenesis. Am J Med Sci 333:131–135
3. Travis WD, Pittaluga S, Lipschik GY et al (1990) Atypical pathologic manifestations of Pneumocystis carinii pneumonia in the acquired immune deficiency syndrome. Review of 123 lung biopsies from 76 patients with emphasis on cysts, vascular invasion, vasculitis, and granulomas. Am J Surg Pathol 14:615–625
4. Hartz JW, Geisinger KR, Scharyj M, Muss HB (1985) Granulomatous pneumocystosis presenting as a solitary pulmonary nodule. Arch Pathol Lab Med 109:466–469
5. Bondoc AY, White DA (2002) Granulomatous Pneumocystis carinii pneumonia in patients with malignancy. Thorax 57:435–437
6. Oki Y, Kami M, Kishi Y et al (2001) Pneumocystis carinii pneumonia with an atypical granulomatous response in a patient with chronic lymphocytic leukemia. Leuk Lymphoma 41:435–438
7. Cupples JB, Blackie SP, Road JD (1989) Granulomatous Pneumocystis carinii pneumonia mimicking tuberculosis. Arch Pathol Lab Med 113:1281–1284

8. Gal AA, Plummer AL, Langston AA, Mansour KA (2002) Granulomatous Pneumocystis carinii pneumonia complicating hematopoietic cell transplantation. Pathol Res Pract 198:553–558
9. Leroy X, Copin MC, Ramon P, Jouet JP, Gosselin B (2000) Nodular granulomatous Pneumocystis carinii pneumonia in a bone marrow transplant recipient. Case report. APMIS 108:363–366
10. Fishman JA (2001) Prevention of infection caused by Pneumocystis carinii in transplant recipients. Clin Infect Dis 33:1397–1405
11. Momin F, Chandrasekar PH (1995) Antimicrobial prophylaxis in bone marrow transplantation. Ann Intern Med 123: 205–215
12. Winston DJ, Ho WG, Gale RP, Champlin RE (1988) Prophylaxis of infection in bone marrow transplants. Eur J Cancer Clin Oncol 24(Suppl 1):S15–S23
13. Pontier S, Busato F, Daste G et al (2004) Granulomatous pneumocystis pneumonia. Rev Mal Respir 21:989–992
14. Kester KE, Byrd JC, Rearden TP et al (1996) Granulomatous Pneumocystis carinii pneumonia in patients with low-grade lymphoid malignancies: a diagnostic dilemma. Clin Infect Dis 22:1111–1112
15. Ramsay AG, Johnson AJ, Lee AM et al (2008) Chronic lymphocytic leukemia T cells show impaired immunological synapse formation that can be reversed with an immunomodulating drug. J Clin Invest 118:2427–2437
16. Aksoy S, Harputluoglu H, Kilickap S et al (2007) Rituximab-related viral infections in lymphoma patients. Leuk Lymphoma 48:1307–1312
17. Coiffier B, Lepage E, Briere J et al (2002) CHOP chemotherapy plus rituximab compared with CHOP alone in elderly patients with diffuse large-B-cell lymphoma. N Engl J Med 346:235–242
18. Pfreundschuh M, Trumper L, Osterborg A et al (2006) CHOP-like chemotherapy plus rituximab versus CHOP-like chemotherapy alone in young patients with good-prognosis diffuse large-B-cell lymphoma: a randomised controlled trial by the MabThera International Trial (MInT) Group. Lancet Oncol 7:379–391
19. Kolstad A, Holte H, Fossa A et al (2007) Pneumocystis jirovecii pneumonia in B-cell lymphoma patients treated with the rituximab-CHOEP-14 regimen. Haematologica 92:139–140
20. Chang H, Shih LY, Wang CW, Chuang WY, Chen CC (2010) Granulomatous Pneumocystis jiroveci pneumonia in a patient with diffuse large B-cell lymphoma: case report and review of the literature. Acta Haematol 123: 30–33
21. Venhuizen AC, Hustinx WN, van Houte AJ, Veth G, van der Griend R (2008) Three cases of Pneumocystis jirovecii pneumonia (PCP) during first-line treatment with rituximab in combination with CHOP-14 for aggressive B-cell non-Hodgkin's lymphoma. Eur J Haematol 80:275–276
22. Lim KH, Yoon HI, Kang YA et al (2010) Severe pulmonary adverse effects in lymphoma patients treated with cyclophosphamide, doxorubicin, vincristine, and prednisone (CHOP) regimen plus rituximab. Korean J Intern Med 25: 86–92
23. Totet A, Duwat H, Daste G et al (2006) Pneumocystis jirovecii genotypes and granulomatous pneumocystosis. Méd Mal Infect 36:229–231

Pulmonary Infiltration in Anaplastic T-Cell Lymphoma

68

Christophe Cracco, Julien Mayaux, Sylvain Choquet, Catherine Beigelman, and Frédéric Charlotte

Contents

C. Cracco (✉) and J. Mayaux
Unité de Réanimation, Service de Pneumologie, Groupe Hospitalier Pitié-Salpêtrière, 47–83 Boulevard de l'Hôpital, 75651 Paris Cedex 13, France
e-mail: christophe.cracco@psl.aphp.fr; julien.mayaux@psl.aphp.fr

S. Choquet
Service d'Hématologie clinique, Groupe Hospitalier Pitié-Salpêtrière, 47–83 Boulevard de l'Hôpital, 75651 Paris Cedex 13, France
e-mail: sylvain.choquet@psl.aphp.fr

C. Beigelman
Service de Radiologie générale, Groupe Hospitalier Pitié-Salpêtrière, 47–83 Boulevard de l'Hôpital, 75651 Paris Cedex 13, France
e-mail: catherine.beigelman@psl.aphp.fr

F. Charlotte
Service d'Anatomie et Cytologie Pathologique, Groupe Hospitalier Pitié-Salpêtrière, 47–83 Boulevard de l'Hôpital, 75651 Paris Cedex 13, France
e-mail: frederic.charlotte@psl.aphp.fr

68.1 Background

Pulmonary infiltrates are common during the course of hematological malignancies [1, 2]. Diagnosing the cause of these infiltrates can be difficult, given the large number of possibilities and the difficulties raised by invasive pulmonary investigations, most notably in patients with severe respiratory function impairment [3]. Bronchoalveolar lavage (BAL) performed during fiberoptic bronchoscopy (FOB) can provide information about the cells involved in the alveolar process. It can also identify pathogens. In most cases, however, BAL fails to indicate the specific type of reaction or inflammatory process [4]. Transbronchial or surgical lung biopsy is difficult to perform in this setting. Moreover, lung biopsy histology usually indicates the pattern of the disorder but not the cause. For instance, inflammation with predominant alveolar CD8+ T lymphocytes may be related to drug toxicity [5], a viral infection [6], lymphocyte activation associated with a B- or T-cell proliferation, or lymphomatous lung infiltration [7].

Lymphoproliferative disorders, most notably T-cell lymphoma and other T-cell lymphoproliferative disorders, may manifest as parenchymal lung infiltration [8–11]. Anaplastic large T-cell lymphoma (ALCL) belongs to the peripheral T-cell lymphoma group in the WHO classification [12] and accounts for about 2–8% of non-Hodgkin's lymphomas in adults and about 15% in children [13]. ALCL may be peripheral (cutaneous) or systemic. Immunohistochemistry shows a CD30+, CD 20−, EMA + pattern; highly chemosensitive ALCLs are also positive for anaplastic lymphoma kinase (ALK+). The clinical manifestations may include lymph node enlargement, hemophagocytosis, and lung infiltrates. Determining whether the lung infiltrates are due to the tumor cells or to an inflammatory T-cell response is difficult.

É. Azoulay (ed.), *Pulmonary Involvement in Patients with Hematological Malignancies*,
DOI: 10.1007/978-3-642-15742-4_68, © Springer-Verlag Berlin Heidelberg 2011

68.2 Case Description

We describe the case of a 60-year-old woman who was admitted to the intensive care unit (ICU) of our respiratory diseases department for respiratory distress with lung infiltrates on the chest roentgenogram. She had a smoking history of eight pack-years. In June 2006, panniculitis developed. She was found to have hemophagocytic lymphohistiocytosis syndrome and was diagnosed with anaplastic T-cell lymphoma with CD 30+ cells (ALCL) based on a skin lesion biopsy done in March 2007. She tested negative for HIV. First-line treatment was with six courses of CHOP chemotherapy (cyclophosphamide, adriamycin, vincristine, and prednisone). She achieved complete remission with normal findings by fluorine-18-fluorodeoxyglucose positron emission tomography (FDG-PET). In September 2007, she underwent autologous stem cell transplantation for consolidation.

A cutaneous relapse with hemophagocytic lymphohistiocytosis syndrome occurred in June 2008. She received second-line treatment with ESHAP chemotherapy (etoposide, methylprednisolone, cytarabine, and cisplatin). A new FDG-PET scan showed resolution of the skin lesions after three courses of ESHAP chemotherapy; however, soft tissue infiltration with increased lymph node uptake was noted in one leg.

The fourth ESHAP course scheduled for early October 2008 was not performed because she had a fever. Dyspnea developed rapidly, worsening over the next week. Computed tomography (CT) of the chest showed subtle ground-glass opacities predominating in the left upper lobe and sparing the subpleural area, with tiny superimposed micronodules (Fig. 68.1a). She

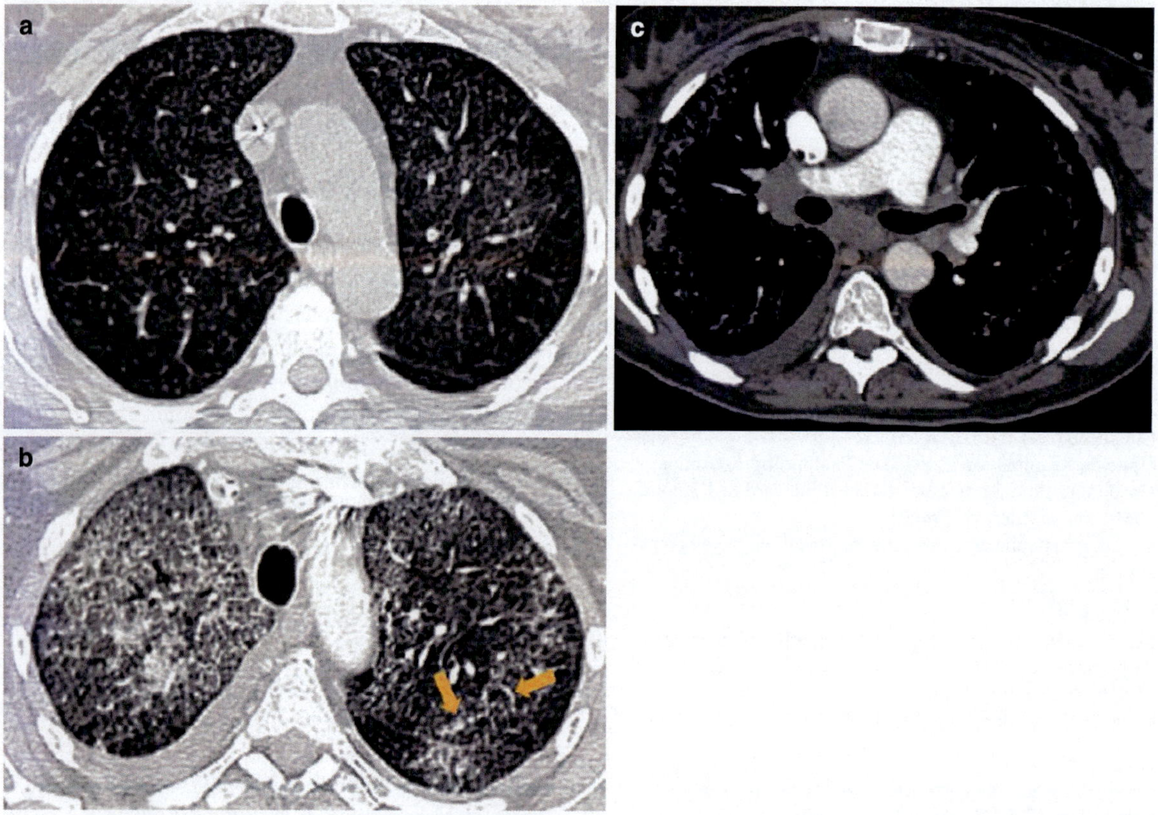

Fig. 68.1 Findings by computed tomography (CT) of the chest. (**a**) Initial CT scan, thin axial slice with lung window. Subtle ground-glass opacities predominating on the *left side* with tiny superimposed micronodules. Note the sparing of the subpleural area. (**b**) Follow-up CT scan, thin axial slice with lung window. Note the increased ground-glass opacities with some alveolar consolidation at the level of the apical segment of the right upper lobe. In addition, the micronodules are more numerous, and some of them have a perilymphatic distribution along the interlobular septa (*arrows*). Note the bilateral pleural effusion predominating on the *right side*. (**c**) Follow-up CT scan, axial slice with soft window after contrast medium administration. Subcarinal and bilateral hilar lymph nodes and bilateral pleural effusion predominating on the *right side*

was admitted to the ICU because of increasing oxygen requirements (partial arterial oxygen pressure [PaO_2], 61 mmHg on 15 L/min oxygen flow). FOB-BAL was performed. No pathogens were recovered from microbiological samples. BAL fluid cytology indicated lymphocytic alveolitis (380,000 cells/mL with 24% lymphocytes and a predominance of CD8+ cells). The initial diagnosis was drug-induced pneumonitis due either to cytarabine or to rosuvastatin, which she was taking for hypercholesterolemia. The rosuvastatin was stopped, and prednisone 1 mg/kg/day was started 7 days later. Her clinical condition improved. She did not require mechanical ventilatory support and was discharged from the ICU in late October 2008, although she still needed supplemental oxygen.

Two weeks later, gradually worsening respiratory distress developed. Increased ground-glass opacities with some alveolar consolidation were noted in the apical segment of the right upper lobe, as well as increased numbers of micronodules, some of which had a perilymphatic distribution. Moreover, mediastinal and hilar lymphadenopathy was visible on a follow-up CT scan, as well as a bilateral pleural effusion predominating on the right side (Fig. 68.1b and c). She was readmitted to the ICU with high-flow oxygen support. Magnetic resonance imaging of the legs visualized two soft tissue lesions on the right foot and bone marrow infiltration in both legs. A repeat FOB-BAL procedure again indicated lymphocytic alveolitis (45% of total cells, with a predominance of CD8+ cells). She had hemophagocytic lymphohistiocytosis syndrome. A bone marrow biopsy showed massive infiltration by the ALCL (Fig. 68.2). A treatment withholding decision was taken, and she died a few days later.

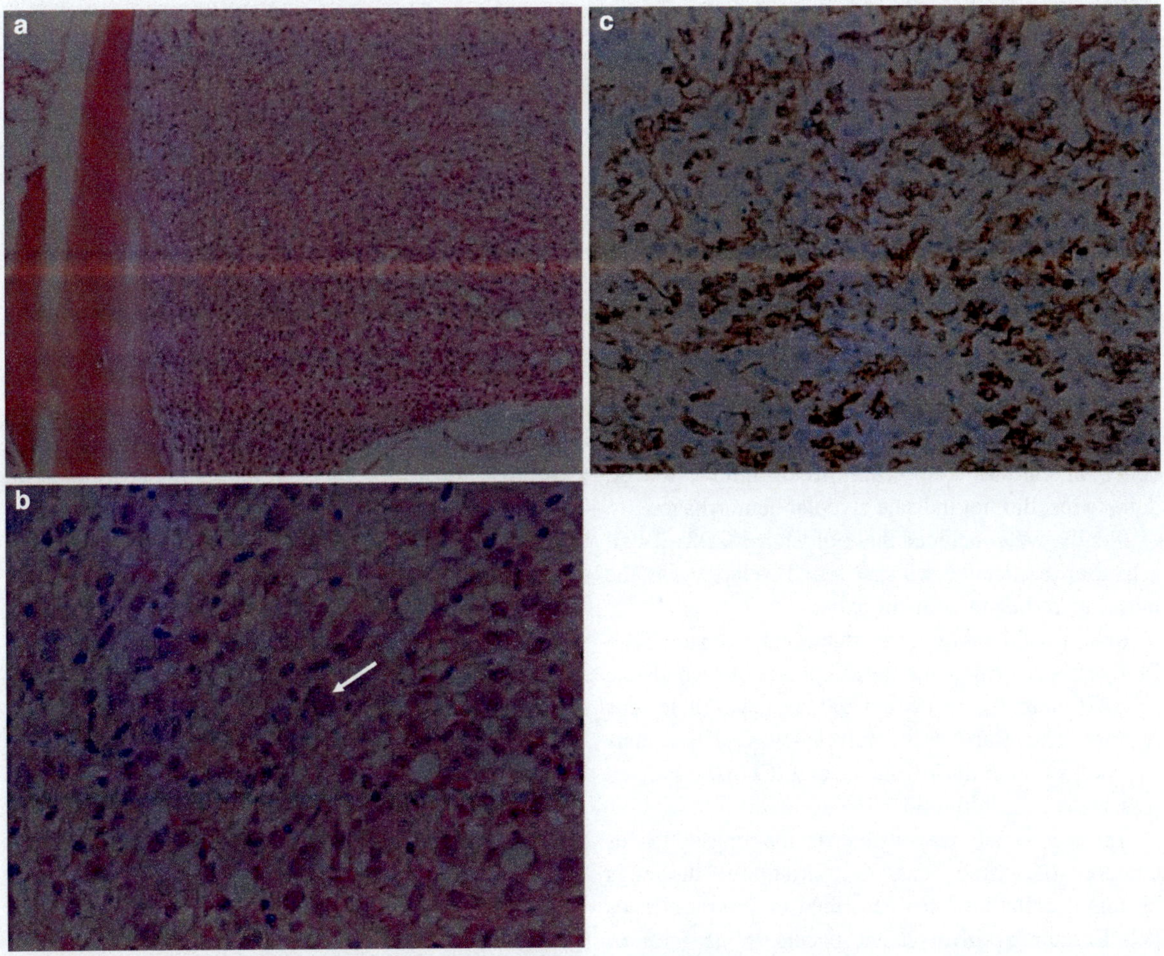

Fig. 68.2 Anaplastic large cell lymphoma, bone marrow involvement. (**a**) Massive infiltration of the marrow spaces by malignant cells (H&E, original magnification × 100). (**b**) The cells are large with nuclei containing prominent nucleoli. There is a hallmark cell (*arrow*) with a horseshoe-shaped nucleus (H&E, original magnification × 400). (**c**) The tumor cells express CD30 (immunoperoxidase technique, original magnification × 200)

68.3 Discussion

Respiratory distress with parenchymal lung involvement is a common complication during the course of hematological malignancies. A number of causes must be considered.

The main cause of respiratory symptoms in patients with hematological malignancies is infection with opportunistic or pyogenic bacteria [1, 3]. In our patient, the extensive search for infectious agents included blood cultures for bacteria and fungi; serum PCR tests for cytomegalovirus and *Toxoplasma gondii*; and tests on BAL fluid for bacteria, fungi, and viruses, performed on two occasions. Moreover, the presence of compromised T-cell functions and the limited ground-glass opacities on the first chest CT scan contrasting with severe hypoxia prompted testing for *Pneumocystis jirovecii* using silver stain, immunofluorescence, and PCR on BAL fluid samples. No pathogens were found.

Several drugs are known to cause respiratory distress with lung infiltrates [14], including cytarabine and rosuvastatin, both used by our patient. In addition, the timing of the manifestations relative to the drug exposures, the chest CT scan findings, and the BAL cytological pattern supported drug-induced pneumonitis. The symptoms improved initially with discontinuation of the two drugs and steroid therapy, but worsened 2 weeks later, although neither drug had been reintroduced and the steroid dose had remained unchanged. Thus, the course did not support drug toxicity as the cause of the respiratory symptoms.

Transthoracic echocardiography showed no evidence of cardiac dysfunction. BAL fluid cytology, done twice, did not indicate alveolar hemorrhage.

Finally, we concluded that polyclonal CD8+ T-cell activation associated with an ALCL relapse was the most likely diagnosis in our patient.

Relapse of the ALCL was suspected when an FDG-PET scan performed after three courses of second-line ESHAP chemotherapy visualized two new skin lesions on a leg. The relapse was confirmed when a bone marrow biopsy done during the second ICU stay showed massive ALCL infiltration.

The mechanism responsible for the lung infiltrates deserves discussion. Massive infiltration of the lungs by tumor cells has been described in several articles [9]. Extranodal involvement occurs in 25–65% of patients with ALCL [9]. Although the skin is selectively affected, lung involvement has been reported in up to 12% of patients [9]. Several patients with ALCL had lung involvement as the only manifestation, with masses and nodules because of infiltration by the tumor [11]. In our patient, ground-glass opacities were seen on the first chest CT, and consolidations were also present subsequently, but only micronodules (and no nodules) were visible. FDG-PET showed no lung uptake, despite the presence of respiratory symptoms. Finally, no ALCL cells were found in either of the BAL fluids. The CD8+ T cells found in both BAL fluids were polyclonal activated cells.

Although none of these findings definitively rules out massive lung parenchyma infiltration by the ALCL, a more likely explanation is polyclonal CD8+ T-cell activation associated with the ALCL relapse. Hemophagocytic lymphohistiocytosis syndrome is common in ALCL and was found in our patient initially and when the ALCL relapsed. T-cell-receptor activation of CD8+ cytotoxic T cells has been described during hemophagocytic lymphohistiocytosis syndrome. Thus, the lung involvement in our patient may have been one of the manifestations of hemophagocytic lymphohistiocytosis syndrome [15]. However, this entity is controversial [15]. Pulmonary infiltrates associated with hemophagocytic lymphohistiocytosis are considered manifestations of capillary leak syndrome. One possibility is that CD8+ T cells infiltrated the lungs of our patient as a result of ALCL-related upregulation of CD8+ cytotoxic T cells. BAL fluid cytology on both samples indicated lymphocytic alveolitis with a predominance of activated CD8+ T cells and no tumor cells. Furthermore, CD8+ T-cell activation has been described in peripheral T-cell lymphoma [16].

Regardless of the cause of the lung involvement in our patient, controlling or curing the underlying malignancy would have been the only effective treatment. However, the ALCL relapsed during second-line chemotherapy. The family, hematology department team, and ICU team decided together that withholding life-support while providing optimal comfort care was the best course of action.

References

1. Mayaud C, Cadranel J (2000) A persistent challenge: the diagnosis of respiratory disease in the non-AIDS immunocompromsed host. Thorax 55:511–517
2. Afessa B, Peters SG (2008) Noninfectious pneumonitis after blood and marrow transplant. Curr Opin Oncol 20: 227–233

3. Azoulay E, Schlemmer B (2006) Diagnostic strategy in cancer patients with acute respiratory failure. Intensive Care Med 32:808–822
4. Poletti V, Poletti G, Murer B, Saragoni L, Chilosi M (2007) Bronchoalveolar lavage in malignancy. Semin Respir Crit Care 28:534–545
5. Fuhrman C, Parrot A, Wislez M, Prigent H, Boussaud V, Bernaudin JF, Mayaud C, Cadranel J (2001) Spectrum of CD4 to CD8 T-cell ratios in lymphocytic alveolitis associated with methotrexate-induced pneumonitis. Am J Respir Crit Care Med 164:1186–1191
6. Bruder D, Srikiatkhachorn A, Enelow RI (2006) Cellular immunity and lung injury in respiratory virus infection. Viral Immunol 19:147–155
7. Berti E, Tomasini D, Vermeer MH, Meijer CJ, Alessi E, Willemze R (1999) Primary cutaneous CD8-positive epidermotropic cytotoxic T cell lymphomas. A distinct clinicopathological entity with an aggressive clinical behavior. Am J Pathol 155:483–492
8. Chott A, Kasere K, Augustin I, Vesely M, Heinz R, Oehlinger W, Hanak H, Radaszkiewicz T (1990) Ki-1 positive large cell lymphoma. A clinicopathologic study of 41 cases. Am J Surg Pathol 14:439–448
9. Greer JP, Kinney MC, Collins RD, Salhany KE, Wolff SN, Hainsworth JD, Flexner JM, Stein RS (1991) Clinical features of 31 patients with Ki-1 anaplastic large-cell lymphoma. J Clin Oncol 9:539–547
10. Chadburn A, Cesarman E, Jagirdar J, Subar M, Mir RM, Knowles DM (1993) CD30 (Ki-1) positive anaplastic large cell lymphoma in individuals infected with the human immunodeficiency virus. Cancer 72:3078–3090
11. Rush W, Andriko JAW, Taubenberger JK, Nelson AM, Abbondanzo SL, Travis WD, Koss MN (2000) Primary anaplastic large cell lymphoma of the lung: a clinicopathologic study of five patients. Mod Pathol 13:1285–1292
12. Fornari A, Piva R, Chiarle R, Novero D, Inghirami G (2009) Anaplastic large cell lymphoma: one or more entities among T-cell lymphoma? Hematol Oncol (www.interscience.wiley.com)
13. Sevilla D, Choi JK, Gong JZ (2007) Mediastinal adenopathy, lung infiltrates, and hemophagocytosis. Am J Clin Pathol 127:458–464
14. Vahid B, Marik PE (2008 Feb) Pulmonary complications of novel antineoplastic agents for solid tumors. Chest 133(2):528–538
15. Ohta H, Yumara-Yagi K, Sakata N, Inoue M, Kawa-Ha K (1994) Capillary leak syndrome in patients with hemophagocytic lymphohistiocytosis. Acta Paediatr 83:1113–1114
16. Costello R, Sanchez C, Le Treut T, Rihet P, Imbert J, Sébahoun G (2009) Peripheral T-cell lymphoma gene expression profiling and potential therapeutic exploitations. Br J Haematol Nov 12 [Epub ahead of print]

A Rapidly Reversible Cause of Pulmonary Embolism

69

Sophie Georgin-Lavialle, Élie Azoulay, Fabrice Zeni, and Michael Darmon

Contents

69.1 Introduction

Intravascular lymphoma (IVL) is an intravascular proliferation of clonal lymphocytes with minimal or absent parenchymal involvement. The clinical presentation is highly variable, ranging from little or no organ involvement to multiple organ failure. Therefore, the diagnosis is often difficult. Proliferation of lymphoma cells in the blood vessels of parenchymal organs results in vessel occlusion and ischaemia. We report the case of a patient who had intravascular lymphoma with predominant pulmonary involvement, presenting as acute respiratory failure and malignant pulmonary embolism.

69.2 Case Report

A 38-year-old man was admitted to the intensive care unit in May 2005 for acute respiratory failure and prolonged fever. He had had an unremarkable medical history until 5 months earlier, when he was evaluated for weight loss of 15 kg and a fever. Physical findings were normal at the time. Appropriate investigations failed to demonstrate any bacterial, viral, parasitic, or mycobacterial infection, including infection due to intra-cellular bacteria, HIV, hepatitis B virus, hepatitis C virus, tuberculosis, typhoid, syphilis, or brucellosis. Tests were negative for antinuclear antibodies, rheumatoid factors, and anti-neutrophil cytoplasmic antibodies. No monoclonal immunoglobulin was detected in the serum or urine. Thoracic and abdominal computed tomography (CT) was normal except for homogeneous splenomegaly. In April 2005, bone marrow

S. Georgin-Lavialle
AP-HP, Hôpital Saint-Louis, Medical ICU,
75010 Paris, France

É. Azoulay
Service de Réanimation Médicale, Hôpital Saint-Louis,
1 avenue Claude Vellefaux, 75010, Paris, France and
Medical Intensive Care Units, Saint-Louis Hospital,
Paris 7 University, Paris, France
e-mail: elie.azoulay@sls.aphp.fr

F. Zeni
Medical ICU, Saint-Etienne University Hospital,
42000 Saint-Etienne, France and
Saint-Etienne University, 42000 Saint-Etienne, France

M. Darmon (✉)
AP-HP, Hôpital Saint-Louis, Medical ICU,
75010 Paris, France and
Medical ICU, Saint-Etienne University Hospital,
42000 Saint-Etienne, France and
Medical Intensive Care Unit, Saint-Etienne University
Hospital, Avenue Albert Raymond, 42270
Saint-Priest-en-Jarez, France
e-mail: michael.darmon@chu-st-etienne.fr

Conflict of interest: None

É. Azoulay (ed.), *Pulmonary Involvement in Patients with Hematological Malignancies*,
DOI: 10.1007/978-3-642-15742-4_69, © Springer-Verlag Berlin Heidelberg 2011

aspiration demonstrated haemophagocytosis with no other abnormalities, and a lymphoproliferative disorder was therefore suspected. The bone marrow biopsy was normal and diagnostic splenectomy was performed, but the pathologic examination of the spleen was inconclusive. The high suspicion of histiocytic lymphohistiocytosis and lymphoproliferation prompted steroid therapy, which transiently improved the clinical condition.

In May 2005, he developed acute respiratory failure with profound hypoxemia (PaO_2 35 mmHg on room air) and a shunt effect that was only partly corrected by oxygen (PaO_2 51 mmHg and $PaCO_2$ 25 mmHg on 5 L/min O_2). He was referred to the ICU with a clinical diagnosis of highly probable pulmonary embolism with acute right heart failure.

In addition to persistent fever (39.3°C), the physical findings consisted of an exanthema and jugular vein distension, with no other signs of heart failure. The clinical examination was otherwise unremarkable. The clinical and radiological examination found no evidence of pneumonia or bronchiolitis. Ultrasonography of the deep leg veins was normal. The haemoglobin level was 10.6 g/dL (mean corpuscular volume, 94 fl; mean corpuscular haemoglobin 31.2 pg), and the platelet count was 117 g/L. The peripheral blood picture was unremarkable. The serum lactate dehydrogenase level was elevated (1,164 U/L).

Chest CT ruled out proximal or sub-segmental pulmonary embolism, but the ventilation/perfusion lung scan indicated a high probability of pulmonary embolism with multiple bilateral and distal perfusion defects and no evidence of a right-to-left shunt (Fig. 69.1, left panel). Cytological examination of skin biopsy smears showed several abnormal lymphocytes suggesting lymphoma. Skin biopsy histological studies identified large pleiomorphic cells expressing CD20 and located within the blood vessels, establishing the diagnosis of intravascular lymphoma (Fig. 69.2).

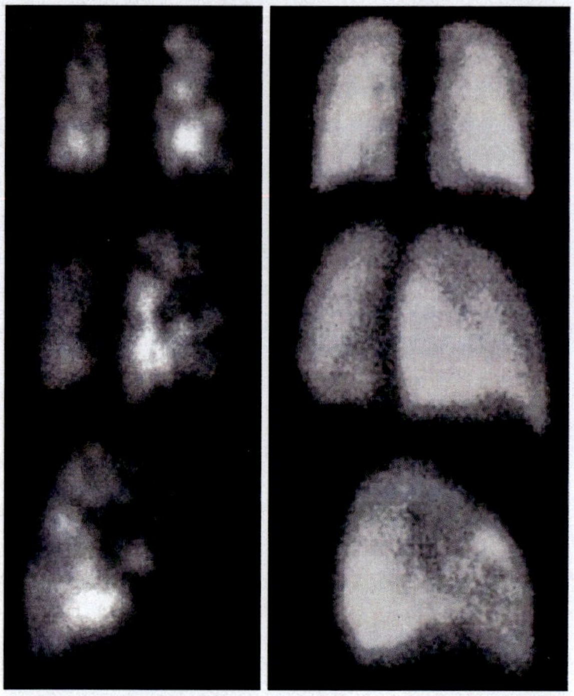

Fig. 69.1 Perfusion lung scan before (*left panel*) and after (*right panel*) cancer chemotherapy

69.3 Discussion

Intravascular large B-cell lymphoma is a rare disease characterised by exclusive or predominant growth of the neoplastic cells within the lumina of small blood vessels [1]. Lymphoma cell proliferation within the blood vessels of parenchymal organs results in vessel obstruction and ischaemia. The diagnosis is established antemortem in fewer than half the patients. Lung involvement seems common but is rarely at the forefront of the clinical picture [2,3]. To the best of our knowledge, only four cases with pulmonary hypertension or suspected pulmonary embolism have been described [2,4,5]. Anthracycline-based chemotherapy has been reported to produce a nearly 60% response rate and a 3-year overall survival rate higher than 30%. Therefore, CHOP and CHOP-like regimens are considered effective [6]. Fever of unknown origin is the presenting feature in 60% of patients with intravascular lymphoma and is frequently associated with haemophagocytic lymphohistiocytosis [6]. Although our patient did not meet all the usual criteria for this syndrome, the clinical presentation (bicytopenia, prolonged fever, and splenomegaly), together with the typical appearance of haemophagocytosis in the bone marrow aspirate, was highly suggestive of haemophagocytic lymphohistiocytosis and, therefore, of lymphoma [6,7]. Pulmonary involvement with haemophagocytic lymphohistiocytosis may occur in up to 30% of patients, but is usually associated with pulmonary infiltrates [8]. In our patient, the clinical course, negativity of

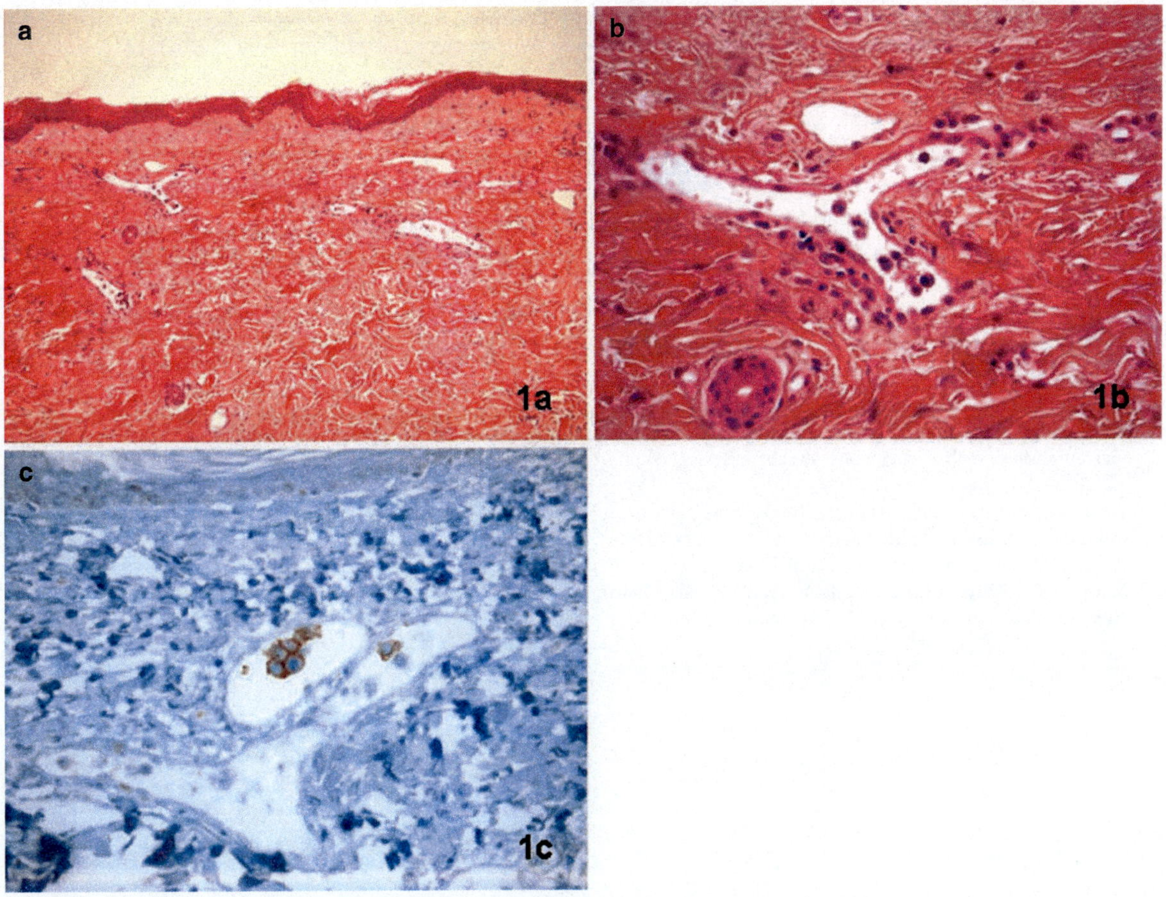

Fig. 69.2 Cutaneous punch biopsy showing an intra-vascular lymphocytic infiltrate (**a**) composed of large atypical cells (**b**) that were CD20 positive on an IHC stain (**c**).

extensive investigations for acute and chronic pulmonary infections, and absence of pneumonia or bronchiolitis allowed us to rule out an infectious disease. Non-thrombotic pulmonary embolism was diagnosed based on the high-probability ventilation/perfusion lung scan with normal CT findings, absence of deep vein thrombosis, and presence of abnormal lymphocytes.

Cancer chemotherapy (cyclophosphamide, adriamycine, VP16; and steroids [CHOP]) for malignant vascular pulmonary involvement was started immediately. The patient's clinical condition improved dramatically. Five days after ICU admission, he needed no oxygen, and a repeat perfusion lung scan was normal (Fig. 69.1, right panel). After six chemotherapy cycles (CHOP-methotrexate with rituximab), he was considered in complete remission. High-dose chemotherapy with autologous stem cell transplantation was carried out. He was alive and in complete remission at last follow-up 52 months after ICU admission.

69.4 Conclusion

In patients with malignancy-related organ failure and a high suspicion of active malignancy, emergent chemotherapy combined with appropriate supportive care is the only means of ensuring recovery. In a recent series of selected patients, we found that survival was 50% in cancer patients with malignancy-related organ failure treated with immediate cancer chemotherapy, mechanical ventilation, vasopressors, and dialysis [9]. The case reported here indicates that intravascular lymphoma can result in pre-capillary pulmonary arterial hypertension and can cause life-threatening manifestations requiring emergent chemotherapy. In the sickest patients with life-threatening complications, a high suspicion of malignancy together with the presence of abnormal cells should prompt appropriate cancer therapy before the definitive diagnosis is established in order to restore organ function and to increase the chances of survival.

References

1. Ferreri AJ, Campo E, Seymour JF et al (2004) Intravascular lymphoma: clinical presentation, natural history, management and prognostic factors in a series of 38 cases, with special emphasis on the "cutaneous variant". Br J Haematol 127:173–183
2. Aouba A, Diop S, Saadoun D et al (2005) Severe pulmonary arterial hypertension as initial manifestation of intravascular lymphoma: case report. Am J Hematol 79:46–49
3. Wick MR, Mills SE, Scheithauer BW et al (1986) Reassessment of malignant "angioendotheliomatosis." Evidence in favor of its reclassification as "intravascular lymphomatosis." Am J Surg Pathol 10:112–123
4. Owa M, Koyama J, Asakawa K et al (2000) Intravascular lymphomatosis presenting as reversible severe pulmonary hypertension. Int J Cardiol 75:283–284
5. Snyder LS, Harmon KR, Estensen RD (1989) Intravascular lymphomatosis (malignant angioendotheliomatosis) presenting as pulmonary hypertension. Chest 96: 1199–1200
6. Ponzoni M, Ferreri AJ, Campo E et al (2007) Definition, diagnosis, and management of intravascular large B-cell lymphoma: proposals and perspectives from an international consensus meeting. J Clin Oncol 25:3168–3173
7. Creput C, Galicier L, Buyse S et al (2008) Understanding organ dysfunction in hemophagocytic lymphohistiocytosis. Intensive Care Med 34:1177–1187
8. Ohta H, Yumara-Yagi K, Sakata N et al (1994) Capillary leak syndrome in patients with hemophagocytic lymphohistiocytosis. Acta Paediatr 83:1113–1114
9. Darmon M, Thiery G, Ciroldi M et al (2005) Intensive care in patients with newly diagnosed malignancies and a need for cancer chemotherapy. Crit Care Med 33: 2488–2493

Hairy Cell Leukemia with Pulmonary Infiltrates

70

Virginie Lemiale, Véronique Meignin, and Élie Azoulay

Contents

V. Lemiale (✉) and É. Azoulay
Medical ICU, Saint Louis Hospital, 1 av. Claude Vellefaux, 75010 Paris, France
e-mail: virginie.lemiale@sls.aphp.fr

V. Meignin
Anatomopathology Department, Saint Louis Hospital, 1 av. Claude Vellefaux, 75010 Paris, France

70.1 Case Report

A 44-year-old woman was admitted to the ICU with hypotension, respiratory failure, and abdominal pain. She had been diagnosed 1 month earlier with hairy cell leukemia and admitted to the hematology department, where she was given cladribine, with no short-term complications. Two days after returning home, she started having a fever and took amoxicillin and ciprofloxacin. Her fever persisted, and she was readmitted. She had a cough and a maculopapular rash on the arms, legs, and trunk. Findings were negative from all microbiologic samples, including sputum, nasopharyngeal aspirates, and blood and urine samples for antigen detection (*Legionella*) and PCRs (CMV, HSV, and HHV6). Computed tomography of the chest was normal. She was switched to piperacillin and tazobactam. Her fever and rash persisted, and 3 days later her treatment was changed to aztreonam, teicoplanin, and caspofungin. The rash faded, and 1 week later she became afebrile. At the time, she had neutropenia and received granulocyte colony-stimulating factor (G-CSF).

One week later, she again became febrile and had abdominal pain and jaundice. Hypotension and respiratory failure developed, prompting ICU admission. At admission, her breathing rate was 27/min, her blood pressure was 116/51 mmHg after fluid resuscitation, her heart rate was 139 bpm/min, and her body temperature was 38°C. The physical examination showed dyspnea with orthopnea and crackles in the lower right lung field, as well as jaundice and abdominal pain predominating in the left upper quadrant. She had no skin lesions, urinary symptoms, mucitis, or peritoneal effusion. She started having diarrhea on the day of ICU admission. The central venous catheter was unremarkable. She had normal serum levels of electrolytes,

É. Azoulay (ed.), *Pulmonary Involvement in Patients with Hematological Malignancies*,
DOI: 10.1007/978-3-642-15742-4_70, © Springer-Verlag Berlin Heidelberg 2011

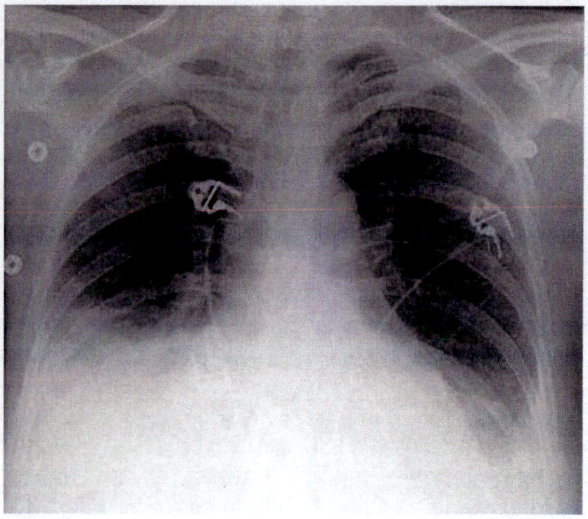

Fig. 70.1 Chest X-ray at ICU admission showing bilateral interstitial pneumonia and lower right lobar alveolar syndrome with atelectasis

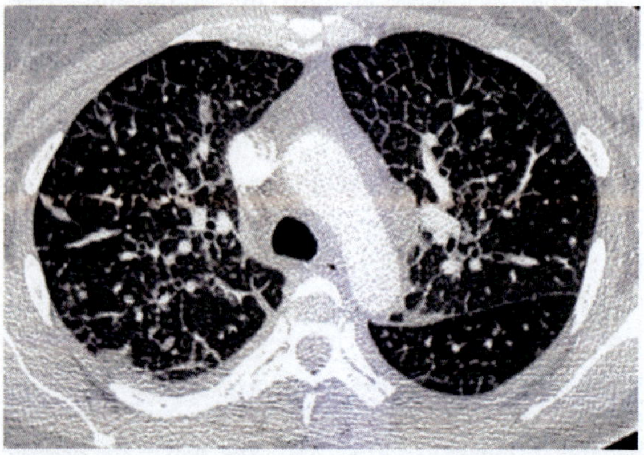

Fig. 70.2 Computed tomography at ICU admission showing interstitial pneumonia with reticulation and no pleural effusion

calcium, urea, and creatinine, and high serum levels of alkaline phosphatase, gamma-glutamyl transferase, and biluribin (twice the upper limit of normal). Blood cell counts showed 1,200 leukocytes/mm^3 with 800 eosinophils/mm^3. Bilateral interstitial disease with alveolar consolidation of the lower right lobe with pleural effusion was seen on chest X-ray (Fig. 70.1). Computed tomography (CT) of the chest visualized signs of interstitial pneumonia with visible interlobular septa and nodular lesions in the lower lobes, but no ground-glass opacities or pleural effusion (Fig. 70.2). Findings were normal on the CT of the abdomen, with no evidence of peritonitis or lesions in the liver, bladder, or pancreas. An ultrasound scan of the abdomen visualized multiple micronodules in the liver.

Over the first 12 h, her dyspnea worsened, and her oxygen requirements increased to 10 L/min. She also required norepinephrine at a dosage of up to 0.45 μg/kg/min. Her antibiotic treatment was a combination of aztreonam, teicoplanin, spiramycin, caspofungin, and gentamicin. G-CSF therapy was discontinued.

70.2 Suspected Diagnoses

At ICU admission, a number of diagnoses were suspected.

1. Infection

   (a) Pulmonary infection was the most likely diagnosis given the recent history in our patient. Hairy cell leukemia is associated with alterations in humoral immunity and monocyte function [1], which increase the risk of infections due to intracellular bacteria (i.e., *Legionella*, *Mycobacteria*, *Chlamydia*, *Listeria monocytogenes*, fungi, and tuberculosis). In addition, cladribine therapy is associated with leukopenia. The combination of pulmonary involvement and abdominal symptoms at admission was consistent with pulmonary legionellosis, but two urine tests for *Legionella* antigen were negative, and spiramycin therapy was consequently stopped on day 2. *Legionella* urine antigen detection is highly sensitive for *Legionella* type 1, the most common subtype found in patients with community-acquired legionellosis in France [2]. This patient did not have risk factors for hospital-acquired legionellosis.

   (b) Catheter-related infection or bloodstream infection-related acute lung injury. The catheter was removed and cultured, with negative results.

   (c) Gastrointestinal infection. Colitis and typhlitis occur during neutropenia. However, neutropenia in this patient was mild and brief. In addition, she had no abdominal symptoms during neutropenia. The abdominal pain and diarrhea developed during neutropenia recovery. The likelihood of neutropenia-related colitis was therefore low. Angiocholitis was considered because she had jaundice and small liver nodules. Septic shock due to abdominal infection can cause respiratory symptoms. However, this diagnosis was ruled out by the ultrasound findings and clinical follow-up. The laboratory tests showed no evidence of acute pancreatitis.

(d) Candidiasis. Hepatic cholestasis with nodular liver lesions and pulmonary involvement can be caused by deep-seated *Candida* infection. The patient was neutropenic and had a fever, abdominal symptoms, hepatic lesions, and abnormal liver function tests.

(e) Viral infection. The liver dysfunction and respiratory distress were consistent with a viral infection due, for instance, to the cytomegalovirus or to a herpes virus.

2. Noninfectious diseases

(a) Cardiogenic pulmonary edema. Acute respiratory failure with abnormal liver function tests can be related to heart failure. Fluid resuscitation was followed by increased dyspnea, and the patient had orthopnea. However, at admission her ECG and cardiac enzyme levels were normal.

(b) Hypersensitivity. The rash and increased eosinophil count suggested an allergic reaction. She received several antibiotics after cladribine therapy. The rash developed during penicillin treatment. The elevated eosinophil count after neutropenia recovery was highly suggestive of an allergy. The respiratory and hepatic symptoms were consistent with hypersensitivity to cladribine and/or antibiotics.

70.3 Results of Investigations and Outcome

The following investigations were performed to evaluate the above-listed diagnostic hypotheses.

- Bronchoalveolar lavage: The fluid contained 55,000 cells/mm^3, with 32% lymphocytes, 4% macrophages, 62% eosinophils, and 20% siderophages. No pathogens were found (Fig. 70.3).
- Transthoracic echocardiography showed a left ventricular ejection fraction of 45% with systolic and diastolic dysfunction, but no dilated cardiomyopathy.
- Blood PCR tests were negative for cytomegalovirus, herpes viruses, and parvovirus B19.
- A liver biopsy on day 3 was normal, with no infection, veno-occlusive disease, eosinophilic infiltrate, fibrosis, or inflammation.
- Bone marrow smears showed a low cell count with 10% of eosinophils, no pathogens, and a positive PCR test for HHV6 (5 log).

On day 2, her peripheral leukocyte count was less than 500/mm^3, but her clinical status was improved. She was given G-CSF until her leukocyte count returned to normal. On day 3, her liver tests were normal.

The diagnosis was respiratory failure related to cardiac pulmonary edema and cladribine pulmonary toxicity. Skin and liver symptoms were related to cladribine and penicillin hypersensitivity. The BAL fluid exhibited a high eosinophil count; however, it contained blood, and the peripheral blood eosinophil count was very high. Extensive investigations for viral and fungal

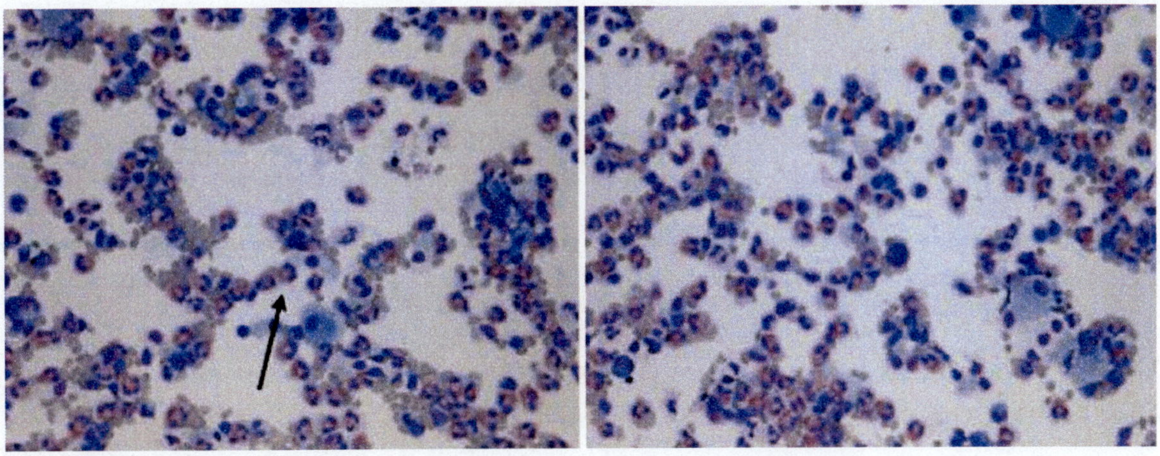

Fig. 70.3 Bronchoalveolar lavage fluid containing a high cell count with a high percentage of eosinophils (↑)

infections were negative. She chiefly responded to diuretic therapy and cladribine withdrawal, without steroid therapy.

70.4 Discussion

In our patient, both infections and noninfectious conditions were possible diagnoses. An original feature of this patient was that BAL and liver biopsy done to look for infections led to the diagnosis of two non-infectious conditions. The high eosinophil count may have been be related to cladribine therapy.

Cladribine is associated with numerous adverse events, among which the most common are fever, skin rash, and infection [3–5]. An allergic reaction and eosinophilia are less common. Although a skin rash and eosinophilia have been reported in patients receiving cladribine for hairy cell leukemia, only one patient had these two manifestations at the same time [4]. In our patient, eosinophilia was seen during recovery from bone marrow suppression and was probably exacerbated by G-CSF treatment. The respiratory failure and hepatic lesions were related to heart failure with pulmonary edema. Echocardiography showed left ventricular dysfunction. The high eosinophil count in BAL fluid was due to the presence of blood in this patient with peripheral eosinophilia. The liver biopsy ruled out candidiasis of the liver. The patient recovered a few days later and experienced no relapses.

References

1. Azoulay E, Schlemmer B (2007) Diagnostic strategy in cancer patients with respiratory failure. ICM 32:808–822
2. Campèse C, Jaraud S, Che D (2007) Legionnaire'disease: surveillance in France in 2005. Med Mal Inf Nov: 716–721
3. Rutella S, Sica S, Rumi C, Martucci R, Etuk B, De Stefano V, Testa U, Leone G, Peschle C (1996) Hypereosinophilia during 2-chlorodeoxyadenosine treatment for hairy cell leukemia. Br J Haematol 92:426–428
4. Rossini M, De Sousa E, Cintra M, Pagnano K, Chiari A, Lorant-Metzet I (2004) Cutaneous adverse reaction to 2-chlorodeoxyadenosine with histologic flame figures in patients with chronic lymphocytic leukaemia. JEDAV 18:538–542
5. Chubar Y, Bennett M (2003 Sept) Cutaneous reactions in hairy cell leukaemia treated with 2-chlorodeoxyadenosine and allopurinol. Br J Haematol 122(5):768–70

Trichosporon asahii Infection in a Neutropenic Patient

71

Djamel Mokart, Antoine Sannini, Jean-Paul Brun, Laurent Chow-chine, and Jean-Louis Blache

Contents

In immunocompromised patients, acute respiratory distress syndrome (ARDS) due to infectious causes remains associated with a high risk of death. Early diagnosis and adapted treatment may improve outcomes [1]. *Trichosporon* spp., a fungus usually found in soil and fresh water, is known to cause invasive infections in immunocompromised patients. Six different species are considered responsible for human disease [2]: *Trichosporon asahii*, *T. asteroides*, *T. cutaneum*, *T. inkin*, *T. mucoides*, and *T. ovoides*. Trichosporonosis has been recognized increasingly over the past decade. Both the clinical and the histopathological findings may mimic disseminated candidiasis [3]. *T. asahii* is the main cause of disseminated trichosporonosis and usually fails to respond to antifungal treatment [4]. Here, we describe the first reported case of disseminated *T. asahii* infection in a neutropenic patient with septic shock and ARDS who was successfully treated with amphotericin B, voriconazole, and splenectomy.

71.1 Case Report

A 17-year-old woman was admitted to the intensive care unit (ICU) because of septic shock and ARDS with severe neutropenia. She had a history of acute myeloid leukemia and had received induction chemotherapy with daunorubicin and cytarabin 35 days earlier. Ten days before ICU admission, she started having a fever, with no other abnormalities. Laboratory tests showed a total leukocyte count of 100/mm^3, a hemoglobin level of 7.2 g/dL, and a platelet count of 15,000/mm^3. She was given granulocyte colony-stimulating factor (400 μg/day), ceftazidime (4 g/day), nebcin (300 mg/day), and vancomycin (2 g/day). Persistence of the fever prompted the addition of amphotericin B

D. Mokart (✉), A. Sannini, J.-P. Brun, L. Chow-chine, and J.-L. Blache
Department of Anesthesiology and Intensive Care Unit, Paoli-Calmette Institute, 232 bd Sainte Marguerite, 13273 Marseille Cedex 9, France
e-mail: mokartd@marseille.fnclcc.fr

É. Azoulay (ed.), *Pulmonary Involvement in Patients with Hematological Malignancies*, DOI: 10.1007/978-3-642-15742-4_71, © Springer-Verlag Berlin Heidelberg 2011

48 h later. At ICU admission, she had ARDS (Fig. 71.1) and septic shock. She was started on endotracheal mechanical ventilation. The administration of low-dose norepinephrine increased her blood pressure to 125/70 mmHg. On day 1 after ICU admission, five blood cultures, BAL cultures, and a sternal puncture culture yielded *T. asahii*. Intravenous amphotericin B (1 mg/kg/day) was continued, and flucytosine was added. The central venous catheter was removed and was also found positive for *T. asahii*. After 2 weeks of treatment, she still had a fever, septic shock, and ARDS. Microbiological study results showed the following minimal inhibitory concentration values: fluconazole, 16 μg/mL; itraconazole, 1 μg/mL; voriconazole, 0.25 μg/mL; caspofungin, 8 μg/mL; flucytosine, 32 μg/mL; and amphotericin B, 1 μg/mL. Therefore, the flucytosine was replaced by intravenous voriconazole (600 mg on the first day then 400 mg/day), and the amphotericin B was continued. During the next 2 weeks, the number of neutrophils increased, and the septic shock and ARDS improved, but the fever persisted. Pulmonary and abdominal computed tomography scans showed ARDS resolution and numerous splenic abscesses (Figs. 71.2 and 71.3). On day 31, splenectomy was performed. Defervescence was obtained within 10 days. Voriconazole was given per os (400 mg/day) after 1 month of intravenous administration for 6 months (the patient stopped the treatment of her own accord). She has had no further febrile episodes, and her leukemia is in complete remission.

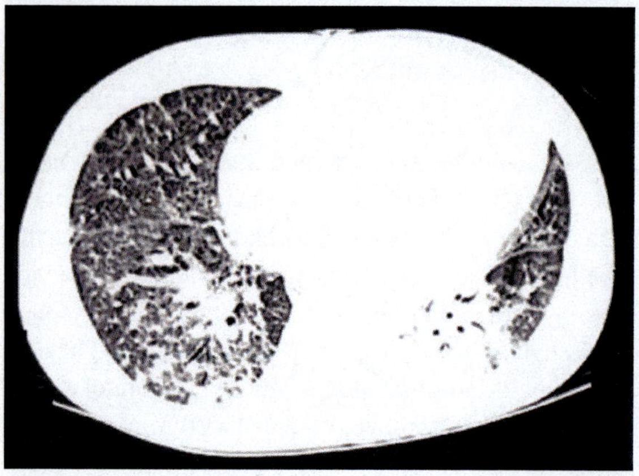

Fig. 71.1 Computed tomography of the chest showing bilateral lesions of ARDS with dense opacities in dependent parts of the lungs and ground-glass opacification of the non-dependent lung with interstitial thickening

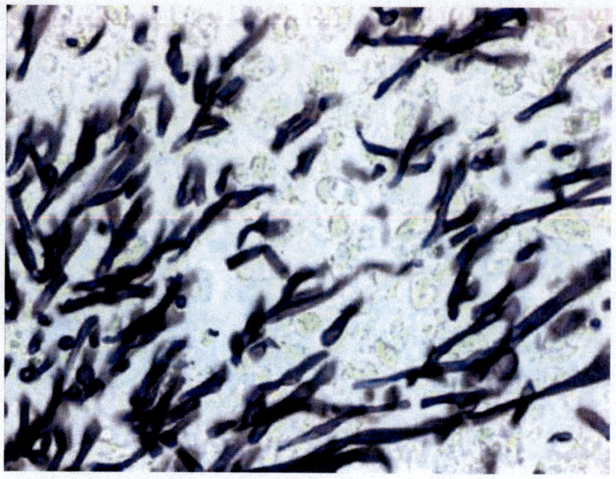

Fig. 71.2 Gomori methenamine silver stain ×40: numerous septate fungal hyphae and spores in an inflammatory splenic granuloma

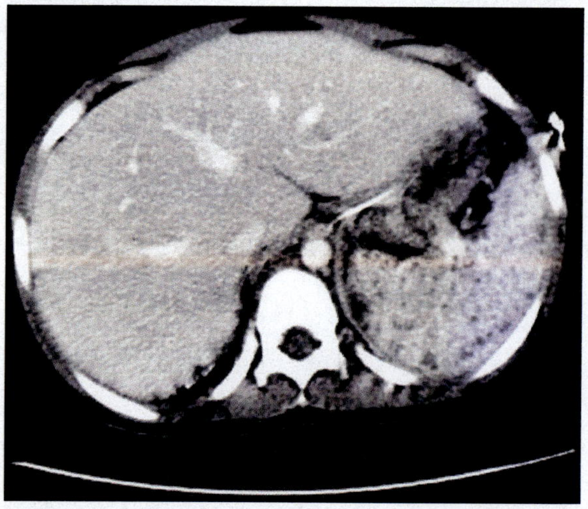

Fig. 71.3 Contrast-enhanced computed tomography of the abdomen showing numerous low-attenuation splenic abscesses

71.2 Discussion

Neutropenic patients with ARDS are profoundly immunocompromised [5] and are more susceptible to severe fungal infections than non-neutropenic patients [6]. *Trichosporon* sepsis in neutropenic patients was first described by Rivera and Cangir in 1974 [7]. When disseminated, this rare infection is life threatening. The predisposing factors for *Trichosporon* infection are cancer, leukemia, and neutropenia [8]. The mortality rate is very high in immunocompromised patients

(80%) [4, 9], and *Trichosporon* infection may also be life threatening in non-neutropenic patients [10]. A previous review described two neutropenic patients with splenic abscesses [11] or documented pulmonary lesions [9]. To our knowledge, our case is the first report of disseminated *T. asahii* infection with septic shock, ARDS, and multiple splenic lesions, as well as a response to amphotericin B and voriconazole. Despite the increasing frequency and severity of trichosporonosis, data on the susceptibility of *Trichosporon* spp. to antifungal agents are limited, and no recommendations are available [11]. In vitro, *Trichosporon* spp. seems sensitive to fluconazole, itraconazole, amphotericin B, and flucytosine [11–13]. In vitro, voriconazole may be superior to amphotericin B [11]. To date, no studies have compared amphotericin B to azoles or combinations of antifungal agents. In our patient, the course of septic shock and ARDS was clearly improved by combining amphotericin B and voriconazole. However, despite the clinical improvements and total neutrophil recovery, the patient still exhibited a persistent fever related to splenic abscesses. Splenic abscess is an infrequent complication in immunocompromised patients and requires splenectomy when systemic antifungal treatment alone fails [14].

References

1. Azoulay E, Mokart D, Rabbat A et al (2008) Diagnostic bronchoscopy in hematology and oncology patients with acute respiratory failure: prospective multicenter data. Crit Care Med 36:100–107
2. Gueho E, Improvisi L, de Hoog GS et al (1994) Trichosporon on humans: a practical account. Mycoses 37:3–10
3. Krcmery V, Krupova I, Denning DW (1999) Invasive yeast infections other than Candida spp. in acute leukaemia. J Hosp Infect 41:181–194
4. Hoy J, Hsu KC, Rolston K et al (1986) Trichosporon beigelii infection: a review. Rev Infect Dis 8:959–967
5. Mokart D, Guery BP, Bouabdallah R et al (2003) Deactivation of alveolar macrophages in septic neutropenic ARDS. Chest 124:644–652
6. Vento S, Cainelli F (2003) Infections in patients with cancer undergoing chemotherapy: aetiology, prevention, and treatment. Lancet Oncol 4:595–604
7. Rivera R, Cangir A (1975) Trichosporon sepsis and leukemia. Cancer 36:1106–1110
8. Krcmery V Jr, Mateicka F, Kunova A et al (1999) Hematogenous trichosporonosis in cancer patients: report of 12 cases including 5 during prophylaxis with itraconazol. Support Care Cancer 7:39–43
9. Fournier S, Pavageau W, Feuillhade M et al (2002) Use of voriconazole to successfully treat disseminated Trichosporon asahii infection in a patient with acute myeloid leukaemia. Eur J Clin Microbiol Infect Dis 21: 892–896
10. Ebright JR, Fairfax MR, Vazquez JA (2001) Trichosporon asahii, a non-Candida yeast that caused fatal septic shock in a patient without cancer or neutropenia. Clin Infect Dis 33:E28–E30
11. Paphitou NI, Ostrosky-Zeichner L, Paetznick VL et al (2002) In vitro antifungal susceptibilities of Trichosporon species. Antimicrob Agents Chemother 46:1144–1146
12. Walsh TJ, Melcher GP, Rinaldi MG et al (1990) Trichosporon beigelii, an emerging pathogen resistant to amphotericin B. J Clin Microbiol 28:1616–1622
13. Canales MA, Sevilla J, Ojeda GE et al (1998) Successful treatment of *Trichosporon beigelii* pneumonia with itraconazole. Clin Infect Dis 26:999–1000
14. Bhansali S, Karanes C, Palutke W et al (1986) Successful treatment of disseminated Trichosporon beigelii (cutaneum) infection with associated splenic involvement. Cancer 58:1630–1632

Part VIII
Post Face

Who Is This Book for? Reserved to Highly Specialized Teams?

72

Laurent Brochard

At first sight, a book dealing with pulmonary problems in patients with hematological malignancies would seem to be reserved to specialized teams working in specialized centers. Because this might reflect a misconception of the delivery of modern medicine, I would like to argue against this idea. Because I am an intensivist, I will mainly take the standpoint of the intensive care unit, but this concerns other disciplines.

There is little doubt that intensive care units admitting patients with hematological disorders for impending respiratory failure in large university centers managing patients with complex and resistant forms of hematological malignancies and providing bone-marrow transplant are highly concerned by the topics discussed in this book. The different chapters superbly illustrate the complexity of respiratory problems possibly encountered in these patients and also the need for organizing modern intensive care medicine from a multidisciplinary standpoint. Patients' respiratory problems must be approached from the respiratory angle, but also with knowledge of hematology, infectious diseases, cardiology, nephrology, and pharmacology, among other aspects of medicine. The fascinating complexity of situations described in this book implies that the intensivists managing these patients have potentially to deal with any one of these problems, and also that the ICU is probably the only place where all these problems can be observed.

L. Brochard
Medical Intensive Care Unit, AP-HP, Centre Hospitalier Henri Mondor, Créteil, France and
INSERM Unit 955, Créteil, France and
Université Paris-Est, Créteil, France
e-mail: laurent.brochard@hmn.aphp.fr

Hematological malignancies are, however, both frequent and frequently urgent to treat. Acute myeloid leukemia, whose incidence tends to increase with age, is rapidly fatal if left untreated. It must be considered a vital medical emergency requiring urgent medical management, and patients certainly cannot be put on a waiting list for admission to highly specialized centers. Also, the rising incidence of non-Hodgkin's lymphoma, especially in elderly patients, and the fact that its clinical presentation varies tremendously sometimes mean that the diagnosis of this cancer has to be made in the ICU where the patient has been admitted for potentially lethal organ dysfunction. In addition, chemotherapy-induced neutropenia in the course of solid cancer therapy is nowadays considered a frequent event in modern therapy and does not even require hospitalization in itself. As a consequence, the appropriate management of a patient presenting with febrile neutropenia and respiratory distress must be known and mastered by physicians in every location where this situation can be encountered, especially in the ICU. Having to face this problem happens in far more places than just the highly specialized centers described above.

Modern epidemiological studies have often come to the conclusion that the volume of cases treated has an important influence on the outcome of patients for a given disease or for a given specific therapy. This seems to be true for different forms of cancer, for some complex surgical procedures, for transplantation, and even for some medical therapies delivered specifically in intensive care units. It is based on relatively straightforward grounds, especially for complex procedures where skills and experience likely matter. Though interesting and important, these large studies are, however, difficult to conduct and to interpret. Multiple statistical adjustments are needed, trying to control for

É. Azoulay (ed.), *Pulmonary Involvement in Patients with Hematological Malignancies*,
DOI: 10.1007/978-3-642-15742-4_72, © Springer-Verlag Berlin Heidelberg 2011

bias referral and preselection of patients, misclassifications, and confounders. Last, statistical correlations do not imply a unique cause–effect relationship and can be difficult to extrapolate to individual centers. More importantly, because the theory looks like it is just common sense, it could easily lead to erroneous and potentially dangerous conclusions. The first one is to conclude that bigger is always better. For this to be true, one needs at least to ensure that a continuously growing activity in a specific area is associated with a continuous and homogeneous spreading of the specific knowledge required for this activity among all the personnel and also that this is not obtained at the expense of a less efficient management of other still present patients. The second mistake would be to naively think that the only solution relies in grouping the patients in specialized centers and to forget that an important part of the response to these findings is education. Sometimes necessitating important changes in hospital structures, referring patients to specialized centers may be a solution for specific activities but cannot be a universal solution. Therefore, spreading adequate knowledge into places where such difficult cases will be encountered and where a rapid and specific management is needed must be a major goal for academic physicians, especially those working in these highly specialized places.

This why such a book is important and why it might not be reserved only to already highly trained teams. Congratulations to Elie Azoulay, who has been working in this area for many years, for making it possible with this book.

73 Pulmonary Involvement in Patients with Hematological Malignancies: And Now?

Patricia Ribaud and Gérard Socié

Many of us remember the time when we had to warm up the blood gas analyzer, use polymyxin methylene sulfonic acid as the antibiotic of last resort, fear chicken pox like the plague, and wait for the autopsy results to diagnose most cases of cytomegalovirus or *Aspergillus* spp. pneumonia. We remember what it was like before computed tomography, magnetic resonance imaging, positron emission tomography, and molecular biology. Since then, 30 years have elapsed, although it feels more like a century. In those days, providing care to a hematology patient was not for the faint of heart. Failure enveloped us in a dreadful solitude that was bearable only because our occasional successes (complete remissions with hope for a cure) brought a profound sense of joy. We seem to recall feeling like the Lone Ranger, prepared to take on the enemy single-handed. The solitude, or rather the self-imposed isolation, was very real. We thought we were the only ones who "knew." We worked closely with the pathologists, cytologists, and geneticists, but we categorized our other colleagues (pulmonologists, gastroenterologists, nephrologists, radiologists, microbiologists, etc.) as mere service providers. We suspected the infectious disease specialists of not understanding our patients or, even worse, of not being interested in them, and we called in the intensivists only when all else had failed.

Those days are over, which is fortunate for everyone, primarily the patients. Lung involvement in patients with hematological malignancies is still a potentially serious event, but major strides have been made in the fields of pathophysiology, etiological diagnosis, and therapeutic management. Pulmonary aspergillosis is a good example, especially if we simplify things a bit. The diagnosis of pulmonary aspergillosis was made by autopsy (a frequently performed procedure at the time) or shortly before the patient died either from the *Aspergillus* infection or, more rarely, from the hematological malignancy after further chemotherapy courses were delayed or canceled. Now, recovery rates in patients with invasive aspergillosis range from 60% to more than 90% depending on the underlying disease, and a history of invasive aspergillosis is by no means a contraindication to hematopoietic stem cell transplantation. Has aspergillosis become a mere bump in the road? Almost. This achievement stemmed from improved knowledge of the clinical presentations and risk factors, the development of effective diagnostic tools, and the introduction of medications that were both potent and safe. In addition, aspergillosis prophylaxis is now fairly effective, and the incidence of the disease is on the decline. Nevertheless, much remains to be done, and emerging fungal and nonfungal infections are raising diagnostic and therapeutic challenges.

Although these beneficial changes can be ascribed in part to scientific advances achieved in the field of medicine, they are largely related to close cooperation among all those involved. This cooperation is wonderfully illustrated by this book, in which about 70 specialists working in a wide range of fields throughout the world dissect the currently available data on each of the many facets of lung disease in patients with hematological malignancies. The topic of this book is the hematology patient viewed holistically through the window provided by specific lung conditions. This commitment to meeting the full scope of patient needs

P. Ribaud (✉)
Service Hématologie-Greffe de Moelle, Hôpital Saint Louis, 1 av. Claude Vellefaux, 75475 Paris Cedex 10, France
e-mail: patricia.ribaud@paris7.jussieu.fr

G. Socié
Service Hématologie-Greffe de Moelle, Hôpital Saint Louis, 1 av. Claude Vellefaux, 75475 Paris Cedex 10, France

É. Azoulay (ed.), *Pulmonary Involvement in Patients with Hematological Malignancies*,
DOI: 10.1007/978-3-642-15742-4_73, © Springer-Verlag Berlin Heidelberg 2011

is also a form of progress. The book also offers a timely opportunity to think about a serene, evidence-based, rational, and multidisciplinary approach to the full range of debates surrounding the indications for life-supporting treatments (and even more crucially for their withdrawal), comfort care, and end-of-life care.

Where do we want to go now and how can we get there? We can hope that, in the future, screening for genetic and environmental risks will be performed well before disease develops. Cancer, viewed globally, together with other diseases (e.g., cardiovascular and neurological diseases), will be effectively prevented for the most part. Cancer chemotherapy, with its train of side effects, will fall into disuse. Targeted treatments will be increasingly accurate, and the risks of infection and organ toxicities will exist only in our memories. Then – in the twenty-first century perhaps – a cancer diagnosis will be a minor event. Until then, basic scientists must continue to move forward, and much more work will have to be done at the bedside and within collaborative clinician networks. This book, by bringing together a vast amount of data and experience, is a unique opportunity to enrich ourselves and thereby to contribute to the dissemination of much needed knowledge. We are grateful to Professor Élie Azoulay for this opportunity.

Index

É. Azoulay (ed.), *Pulmonary Involvement in Patients with Hematological Malignancies*,
DOI: 10.1007/978-3-642-15742-4, © Springer-Verlag Berlin Heidelberg 2011

I

R

S